DIAGNOSTIC PATHOLOGY

FAMILIAL CANCER SYNDROMES

AMIRSYS®

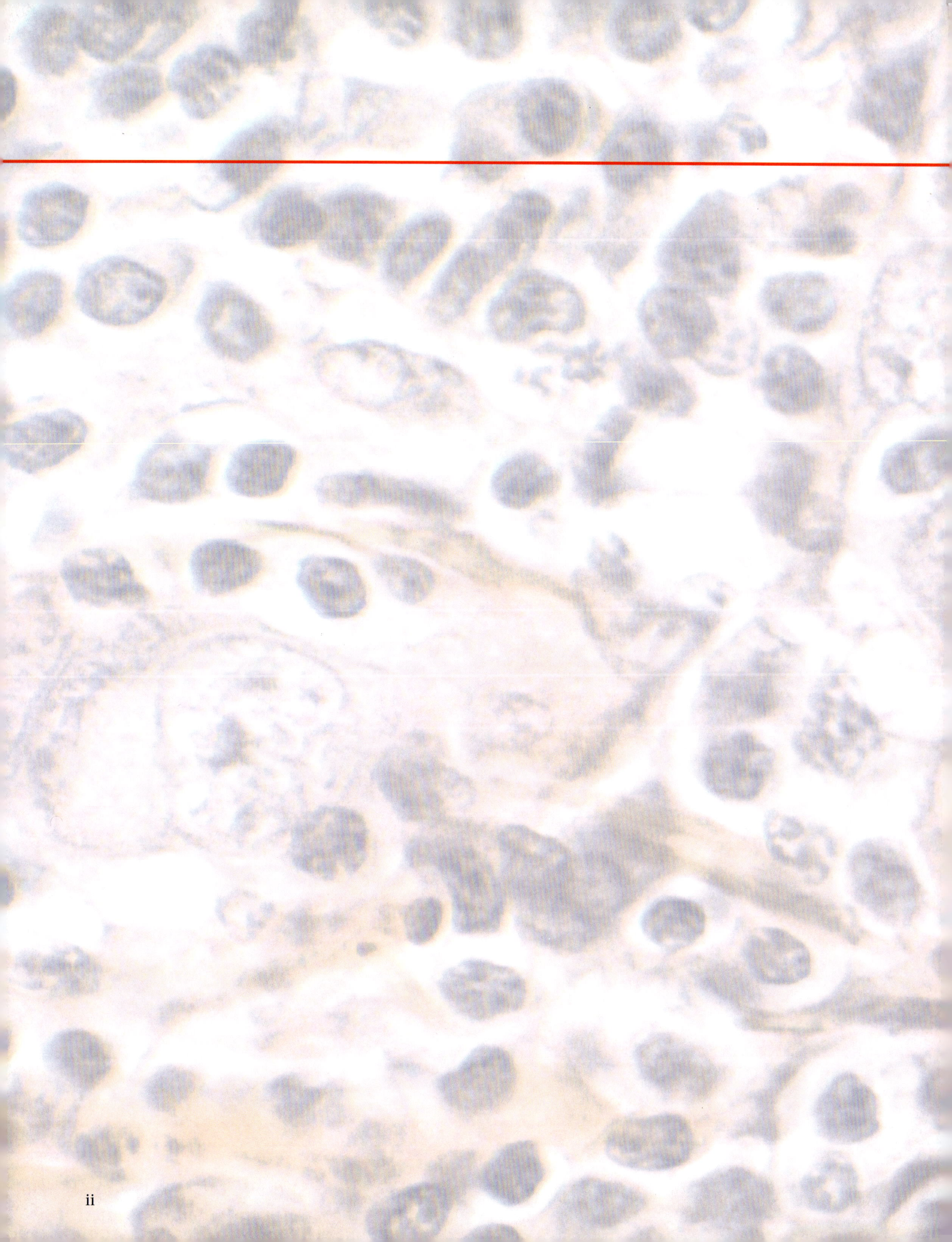

DIAGNOSTIC PATHOLOGY

FAMILIAL CANCER SYNDROMES

AMIRSYS®

Vania Nosé, MD, PhD
Director of Anatomic and Molecular Pathology
Associate Chief of Pathology
Massachusetts General Hospital
Professor of Pathology
Harvard Medical School
Boston, Massachusetts

Gladell P. Paner, MD
Assistant Professor
Departments of Pathology and Surgery
Section of Urology
University of Chicago Medical Center
Chicago, Illinois

Joel K. Greenson, MD
Professor of Pathology
Director of Gastrointestinal Pathology
Department of Pathology
University of Michigan Medical School
Ann Arbor, Michigan

Fausto J. Rodríguez, MD
Assistant Professor of Pathology and Oncology
Johns Hopkins University School of Medicine
Baltimore, Maryland

Christine J. Ko, MD
Associate Professor of Dermatology and Pathology
Yale University
New Haven, Connecticut

Elizabeth Morgan, MD
Instructor, Harvard Medical School
Department of Pathology
Brigham and Women's Hospital
Boston, Massachussetts

Matthew R. Lindberg, MD
Assistant Professor of Pathology
Department of Pathology
Directory of Immunohistochemistry
University of Arkansas for Medical Sciences
Little Rock, Arkansas

David G. Hicks, MD
Professor
Director, Surgical Pathology Unit
Department of Pathology and Laboratory Medicine
University of Rochester Medical Center
Rochester, New York

Susan C. Lester, MD, PhD
Chief, Breast Pathology Services
Brigham and Women's Hospital
Assistant Professor, Harvard Medical School
Staff Pathologist, Dana Farber Cancer Institute
Boston, Massachussetts

Fabiola Medeiros, MD
Assistant Professor of Pathology
University of Southern California
Los Angeles, California

AMIRSYS®
Names you know. Content you trust.®

First Edition

Printed in Canada by Friesens, Altona, Manitoba, Canada

ISBN: 978-1-931884-96-9

Notice and Disclaimer

Publisher Cataloging-in-Publication Data

Diagnostic pathology. Familial cancer syndromes / [edited by] Vania Nosé.
pages ; cm
Familial cancer syndromes
Includes bibliographical references and index.
ISBN 978-1-931884-96-9 (hardback)
1. Cancer--Genetic aspects. 2. Cancer--Diagnosis. 3. Cancer--Pathophysiology--Atlases. 4. Tumors--Diagnosis. 5. Familial diseases. I. Nosé, Vania. II. Title: Familial cancer syndromes.
[DNLM: 1. Neoplasms--genetics--Atlases. 2. Neoplasms--diagnosis--Atlases. 3. Neoplastic Syndromes, Hereditary--Atlases. QZ 202]
RC268.4.D515 2014
616.994/071--dc23

To my wonderful sons and best friends, Gustave, Erick, and Philip, for making my life complete.

To my dear parents, Dalva and Antonio, for their teaching, continuous support, and guidance.

To my brothers, Dalton and Walton, and their families, for their tremendous support and invaluable friendship.

I would like to thank my coauthors, Drs. Joel Greenson, Gladell Paner, Fausto Rodríguez, Christine Ko, Elizabeth Morgan, Matthew Lindberg, Susan Lester, David Hicks, and Fabiola Medeiros, for their contributions, wonderful work, and dedication in completing this project.

To Dr. J. Aidan Carney, for sharing his knowledge on familial cancer syndromes with us.

To Dr. A. John Iafrate, for his careful chapter review on the clinical and molecular aspects of familial cancer syndromes.

A special thank you to Dave Chance, Kellie Heap, and Laura Sesto from the Amirsys team for their patience and careful work in helping us make this book a reality.

VN

CONTRIBUTORS

Cesar A. Moran, MD
Professor and Deputy Chair
Chief, Thoracic Pathology
Department of Pathology
University of Texas MD Anderson Cancer Center
Houston, Texas

David S. Cassarino, MD, PhD
Consultant Dermatopathologist and Staff Pathologist
Southern California Permanente Medical Group
Los Angeles, California
Clinical Professor
Department of Dermatology
University of California at Irvine
Irvine, California

Lori A. Erickson, MD
Associate Professor of Pathology
Department of Laboratory Medicine and Pathology
Mayo Clinic
Rochester, Minnesota

Elizabeth A. Montgomery, MD
Professor of Pathology and Oncology and
Orthopedic Surgery
Johns Hopkins University Medical Institutions
Baltimore, Maryland

Mari Mino-Kenudson, MD
Associate Professor, Harvard Medical School
Department of Pathology
Massachusetts General Hospital
Boston, Massachusetts

Michiya Nishino, MD, PhD
Department of Pathology
Beth Israel Deaconess Medical Center
Instructor in Pathology, Harvard Medical School
Boston, Massachusetts

Arthur S. Tischler, MD
Professor of Pathology
Tufts University School of Medicine
Tufts Medical Center
Boston, MA

Carla S. Wilson, MD, PhD
Professor of Pathology
Department of Pathology
University of New Mexico Health Sciences Center
Albuquerque, NM

C. Cameron Yin, MD, PhD
Associate Professor
Department of Hematopathology
University of Texas MD Anderson Cancer Center
Houston, Texas

Qian-Yun Zhang, MD, PhD
Associate Professor of Pathology
Department of Pathology
University of New Mexico Health Sciences Center
Albuquerque, New Mexico

Carlos E. Bueso-Ramos, MD, PhD
Professor of Pathology
Department of Hematopathology
University of Texas MD Anderson Cancer Center
Houston, Texas

Jessica M. Comstock, MD
Assistant Professor
University of Utah Department of Pathology
Division of Pediatric Pathology
Primary Children's Hospital
Salt Lake City, Utah

Soheil Sam Dadras, MD, PhD
Associate Professor of Dermatology and
Genetics and Developmental Biology
UCONN Heath Center
Farmington, Connecticut

Cyril Fisher, MD, DSc, FRCPath
Consultant Histopathologist
Royal Marsden NHS Foundation Trust
Professor of Tumor Pathology
Institiue of Cancer Reasearch
University of London
London, United Kingdom

Aliya N. Husain, MD
Professor of Pathology
University of Chicago
Chicago, Illinois

Grace E. Kim, MD
Professor of Pathology
Department of Pathology
University of California San Francisco
San Francisco, California

Gregory Y. Lauwers, MD
Vice Chair of Pathology
Massachusetts General Hospital
Professor of Pathology
Harvard Medical School
Boston, Massachusetts

Ozgur Mete, MD
Assistant Professor
Consultant Endocrine Pathologist
Department of Laboratory Medicine & Patholobiology
University Health Network
University of Toronto
Toronto, Canada

Joseph Misdraji, MD
Associate Pathologist
Pathology Service
Massachusetts General Hospital
Boston, Massachusetts

Alexandros D. Polydorides, MD, PhD
Associate Professor
Department of Pathology
Icahn School of Medicine at Mount Sinai
New York, New York

Steven S. Shen, MD, PhD
Associate Director, Surgical Pathology
Houston Methodist Hospital
Professor of Pathology and Laboratory Medicine
Weill Medical College of Cornell University
Houston, Texas

Francisco Vega, MD, PhD
Professor (ranking pending)
Director of Hematopathology
Department of Pathology and Laboratory Medicine
University of Miami Hospital/Sylvester Cancer Center
Miami, Florida

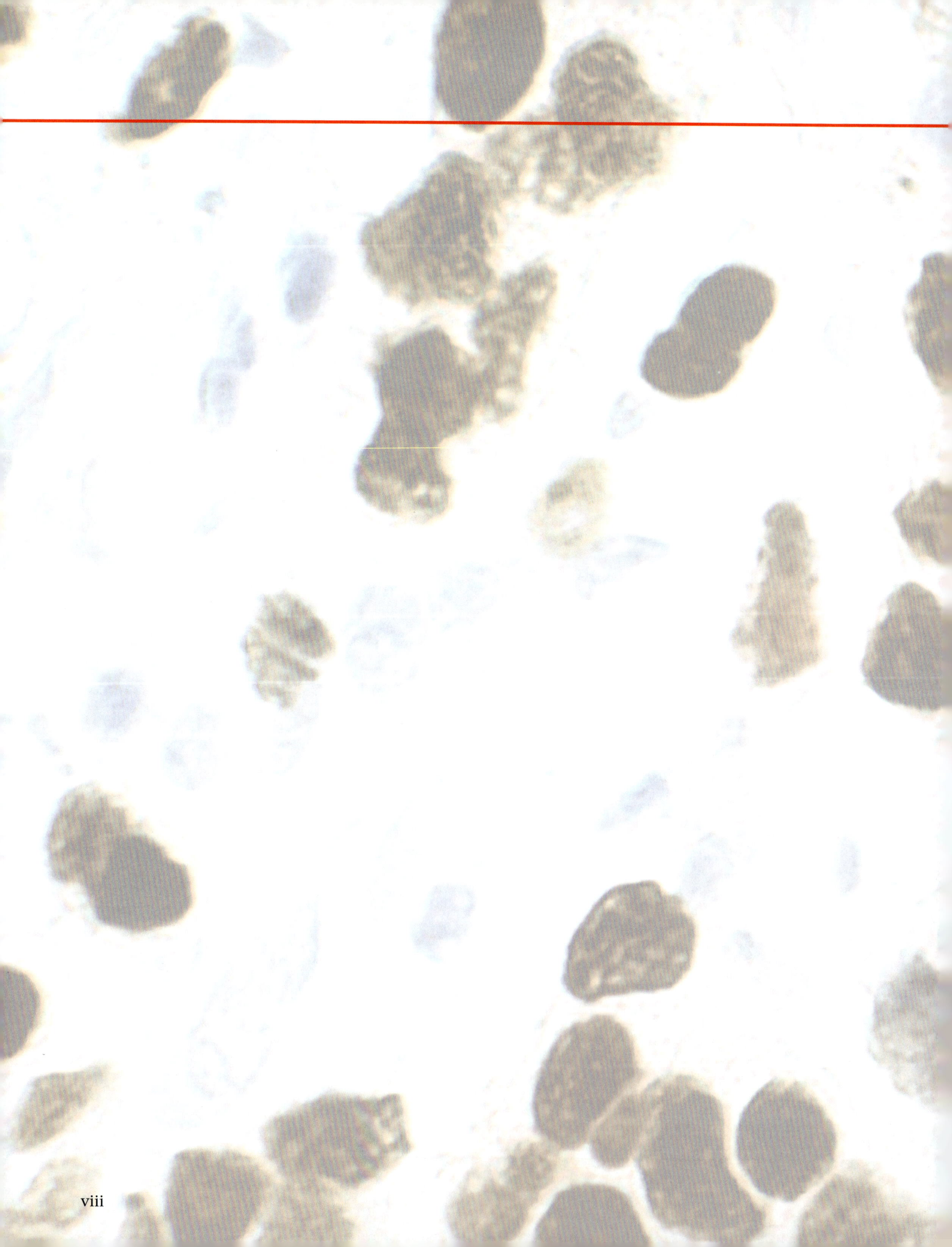

PREFACE

Welcome to *Diagnostic Pathology: Familial Cancer Syndromes*!

Diagnostic Pathology: Familial Cancer Syndromes features a comprehensive review of the top inherited tumor syndromes. It is becoming increasingly well recognized that a given familial tumor syndrome may be very heterogenous in clinical appearance and that unrecognized patients may present initially with an apparently isolated tumor. Therefore, it is crucial for surgical pathologists to be aware of the specific gross and microscopic findings that suggest a possible syndromic association.

Written by well-known experts in the field, this book with over 164 chapters will help surgical pathologists, clinicians, fellows, and residents understand the critical aspects of diagnosing familial tumors and differentiating these from their sporadic counterpart. It includes detailed gross and histologic features of syndromic-associated neoplasms with associated manifestations and clinical implications.

The book is organized in 3 parts:

The first part, "Overview of Syndromes," has the detailed description of the major syndromes within 56 chapters, genes involved, associated tumors, and diagnostic criteria. This part also contains tables that may be helpful in better classifying the diseases and the associated syndromes. Each syndrome discussed includes all benign and malignant tumors occurring in that specific syndrome as well as the differential diagnosis.

The second part, "Diagnoses Associated with Specific Syndromes," discusses in detail the diseases occurring within the syndromes described on part 1. The diagnoses are conveniently grouped according to the gland/organ/tissue involved. Distinct diseases are described, highlighting the characteristics of the tumors according to the different syndromes. The book points out some of the distinct characteristics of tumors found in inherited tumor syndrome that distinguishes these tumors from tumors in a sporadic setting.

The third part, "Syndromes by Organ Location," is also divided by organ/subspecialty and distributed in 26 chapters. This part has tables with "easy to find" possible syndromes by organ, including the differential diagnosis.

We hope that *Diagnostic Pathology: Familial Cancer Syndromes* will guide pathologists and clinicians to master diagnostic criteria when diagnosing tumors associated with inherited tumor syndromes.

Vania Nosé, MD, PhD
Director of Anatomic and Molecular Pathology
Associate Chief of Pathology
Massachusetts General Hospital
Professor of Pathology
Harvard Medical School
Boston, Massachusetts

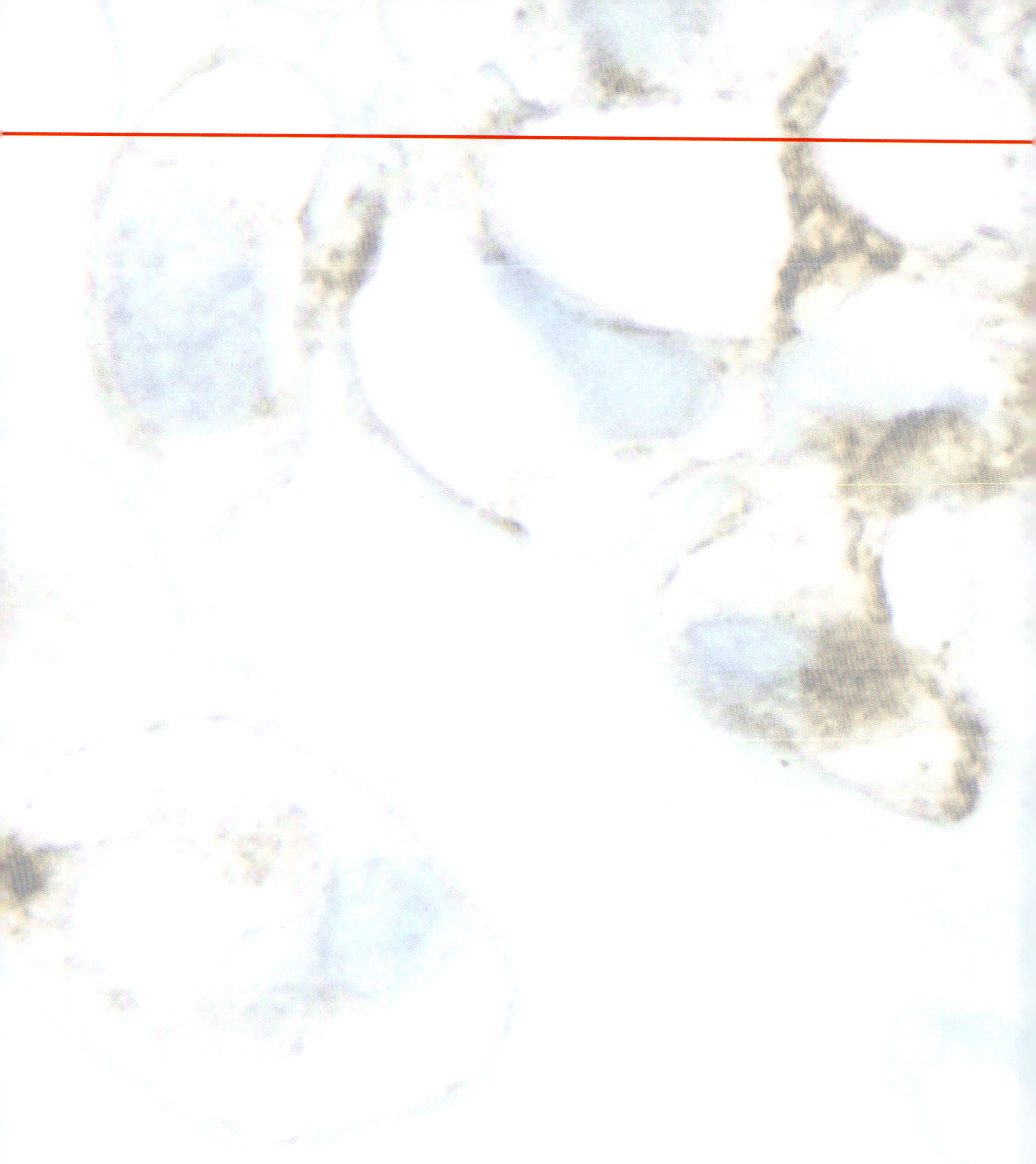

ACKNOWLEDGMENTS

Editors

Arthur G. Gelsinger, MA
Lorna Kennington, MS
Rebecca L. Hutchinson, BA
Angela M. Green Terry, BA
Kalina K. Lowery, MS
Sarah J. Connor, BA

Image Editors

Jeffrey J. Marmorstone, BS
Lisa A. M. Steadman, BS

Medical Editors

Michiya Nishino, MD, PhD

Illustrations

Laura C. Sesto, MA
Lane R. Bennion, MS
Richard Coombs, MS

Art Direction and Design

Laura C. Sesto, MA
Lisa A. M. Steadman, BS

Lead Editor

Dave L. Chance, MA, ELS

Publishing Lead

Katherine L. Riser, MA

AMIRSYS®
Names you know. Content you trust.®

SECTIONS

TABLE OF CONTENTS

PART I
Overview of Syndromes

SECTION 1
Introduction

SECTION 2
Syndromes

PART II
Diagnoses Associated With Specific Syndromes

SECTION 1
Breast

SECTION 2
Blood and Bone Marrow

Hepatobiliary and Pancreas

SECTION 7
Genitourinary

Collecting System

Genital Tract

Kidney

SECTION 8
Gynecology

SECTION 9
Nervous System

SECTION 10
Pulmonary

SECTION 10
Pulmonary

SECTION 11
Skin

PART IV
Reference

SECTION 1
Molecular Factors

DIAGNOSTIC PATHOLOGY

FAMILIAL CANCER SYNDROMES

AMIRSYS®

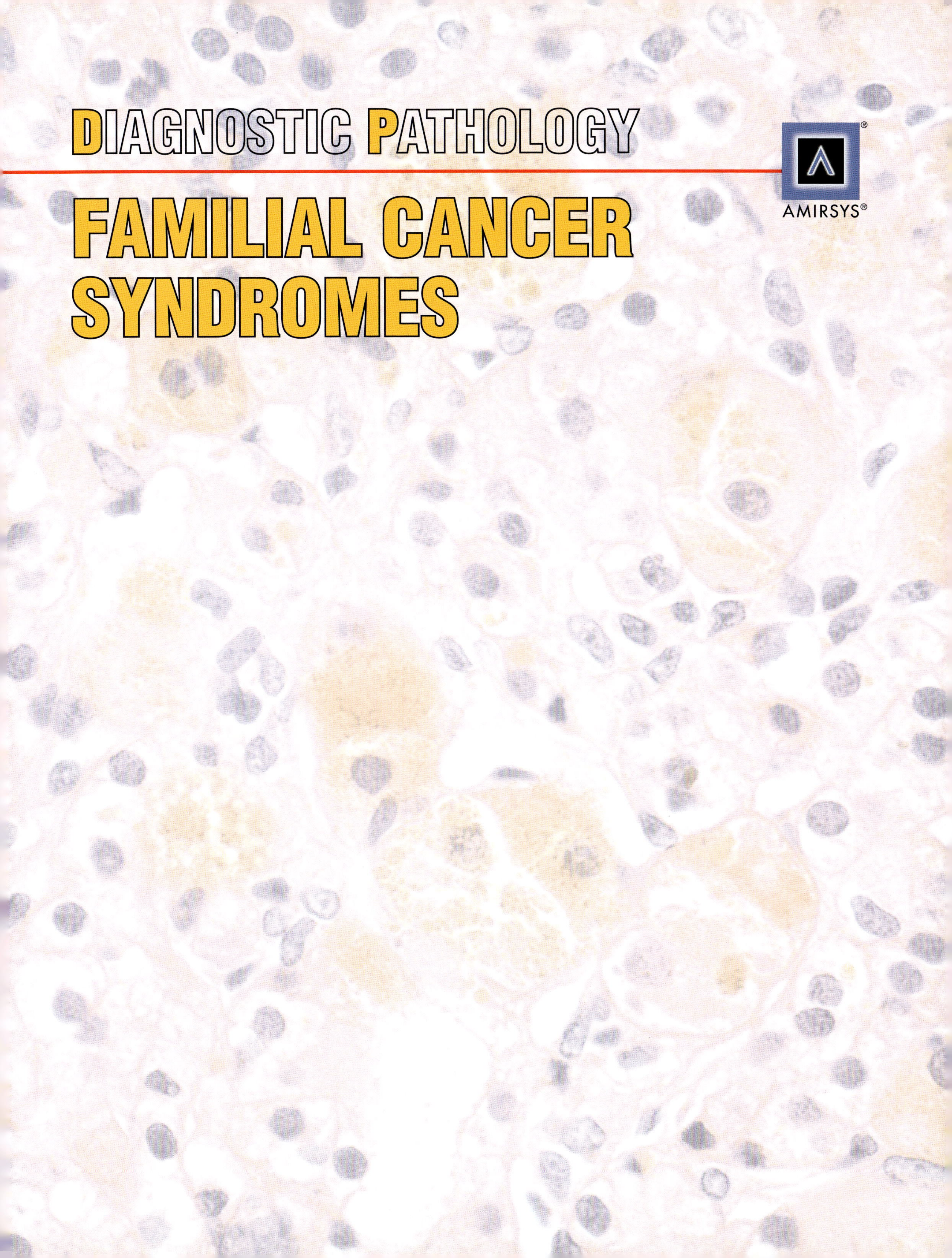

Introduction

PATHOLOGY OF FAMILIAL TUMOR SYNDROMES

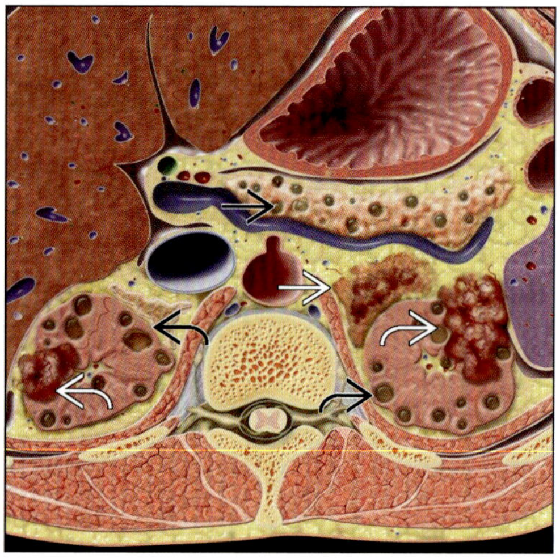

Graphic representation of abdominal lesions seen in patients with von Hippel-Lindau syndrome shows the bilateral and multiple renal cysts ➢, renal tumors ➢, pancreatic cysts ➔, and pheochromocytoma ➔.

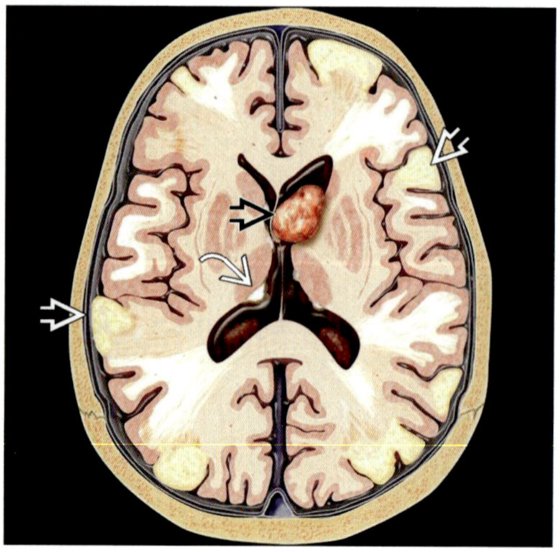

The characteristic lesions of tuberous sclerosis in the CNS include cortical tubers ➢, subependymal nodules identifiable in the walls of the lateral ventricles ➢, and a subependymal giant cell astrocytoma ➢.

INTRODUCTION

Hereditary Syndromes: Practical Guide to Pathological Recognition

- Diverse neoplasias are a common finding in patients with a genetic predisposition to cancer
- It is becoming increasingly well recognized that a given familial tumor syndrome may be very heterogeneous in clinical appearance
- Patients without overt clinical signs of their underlying syndrome may present initially for treatment of a tumor
- As molecular diagnostic testing for these familial diseases has become more readily available, the heterogeneous clinical appearance seen in many syndromes has become better recognized
- Awareness of important manifestations associated with each syndrome that might provide additional clues to a hereditary/familial neoplasia syndrome is also important
- Identification of hereditary cases and early diagnosis makes preventive surgery and adequate treatment possible
- Most of the patients with familial disease are asymptomatic and are discovered through genetic screening in predisposing families
- All patients identified as having familial tumors should then be screened for the familial disease's associated mutation
- Vast majority of tumors occurring in a familial setting are multiple, bilateral, and involve multiple organs
- Many surgical specimens are received from patients who have a known syndrome diagnosis at time of surgery
  - Pathologist may be 1st physician to suggest possibility of a syndromic association based on presence of unique pathologic findings in a tumor resection specimen
- Gross and histological features that are evaluated in routine tumor resection specimens might suggest each individual syndrome
- In their pathological examinations, it is important for surgical pathologists to be aware of specific gross and microscopic findings that suggest a possible syndromic association
- Some tumors frequently display characteristic clinical, biochemical, and histopathological features that, although not pathognomonic, can be helpful in suggesting an inherited disease as the underlying etiology and distinguishing these tumors from sporadic cases

Recognition of Morphological Characteristics That Indicate Familial Tumor Syndrome

- Awareness of pathologic features of neoplasms seen in a variety of hereditary/familial neoplasia syndromes is crucial for diagnosis
- Pathological findings suggestive of a familial or inherited tumor syndromes or findings specific for a syndrome are
  - Tumors occurring at a younger age than the sporadic counterpart
  - Multiple tumors
  - Bilateral tumors
  - Tumors involving multiple organs and systems
  - Tumors associated with multiple lesions
  - Tumors associated with multiple hamartomatous lesions
  - Specific location of a tumor
  - Unique morphological features of a tumor
  - Presence of precursor lesions
  - Presence of multiple benign lesions
- Characteristic and distinct pathology findings in some of these syndromes should alert the pathologist of a possible familial cancer syndrome

- Correct histologic interpretation may lead to further molecular genetic evaluation of patient and family members

Pathology Reporting

- If the constellation of pathology findings strongly suggests a potential syndromic association
  - Consult medical records for the diagnosis of a potential syndrome
  - Contact clinician to discuss possibility of a genetic syndrome
  - Pathologists should notify clinicians about this possibility, considering appropriate molecular testing
- For reporting purposes, diagnosis of a lesion or a neoplasm should use same criteria and terminology as for sporadic lesions and tumors
  - Comment suggesting a possible association with a genetic disease is recommended
    - To document possibility of specific genetic association
- Final diagnostic commentary to highlight differential diagnostic issues that frequently arise when these diagnoses are considered

HEREDITARY SYNDROMES KNOWN TO BE ASSOCIATED WITH NEOPLASIA

Hereditary Syndromes

- Some hereditary syndromes are known to be associated with neoplasia and have unique &/or characteristic pathological features
- Characteristic and distinct pathology findings in some of these syndromes should alert the pathologist of a possible familial cancer syndrome

ENDOCRINE SYSTEM

Hereditary Syndromes Known to be Associated With Thyroid Neoplasia

- Medullary thyroid carcinoma (MTC)
  - Multiple endocrine neoplasia 2A (MEN2A)
  - Multiple endocrine neoplasia 2B (MEN2B)
  - Familial medullary thyroid carcinoma (FMTC)
- Cribriform morular papillary thyroid carcinoma
  - Familial adenomatous polyposis (FAP) syndrome
    - Cribriform-morular variant of papillary thyroid carcinoma (CMV-PTC) was described originally as FAP-associated thyroid carcinoma
- Numerous adenomatous nodules, follicular adenomas, and follicular carcinoma
  - *PTEN*-hamartoma tumor syndrome (PHTS)/Cowden disease
    - Presence of numerous multiple adenomatous nodules (MANs) or follicular thyroid carcinoma (FC) in younger patients should raise suspicion for diagnosis of PHTS
  - Carney complex
- Oncocytic tumors
  - Li-Fraumeni syndrome
  - Familial oncocytic neoplasms
  - McCune-Albright syndrome
  - Tuberous sclerosis complex

Hereditary Syndromes Known to be Associated With Adrenal Neoplasia

- Adrenal cortical tumors
  - Beckwith-Wiedemann syndrome
  - Li-Fraumeni syndrome
  - Multiple endocrine neoplasia 1
  - Carney complex
  - Lynch syndrome
  - Congenital adrenal hyperplasia

Hereditary Syndromes Known to be Associated With Parathyroid Neoplasia

- Multiple endocrine neoplasia 1
- Hereditary hyperparathyroidism-jaw tumor syndrome
- Familial isolated hyperparathyroidism syndrome
- Multiple endocrine neoplasia 2A
- Neonatal severe primary hyperparathyroidism

Hereditary Syndromes Known to be Associated With Pituitary Neoplasia

- Multiple endocrine neoplasia 1
- Familial pituitary adenoma syndrome
- Familial isolated pituitary adenoma syndrome

Hereditary Syndromes Known to be Associated With Endocrine Pancreas Neoplasia

- Multiple endocrine neoplasia 1
- Familial adenomatous polyposis
- Tuberous sclerosis complex
- Von Hippel-Lindau syndrome

Hereditary Syndromes Known to be Associated With PGL/PCC

- Multiple endocrine neoplasia 2A
- Multiple endocrine neoplasia 2B
- von Hippel-Lindau syndrome
- Neurofibromatosis 1
- Familial paraganglioma type 1 (PGL1)
- Familial PGL2
- Familial PGL3
- Familial PGL4
- Carney-Stratakis syndrome
- Familial pheochromocytoma (PCC) 2q
- *MAX*-related
- *SDHA*-related

GENITOURINARY TRACT

Hereditary Syndromes Known to be Associated With Renal Neoplasia

- von Hippel-Lindau
- Hereditary papillary renal cell carcinoma (RCC)
- Hereditary leiomyomatosis RCC
- Birt-Hogg-Dubé

PATHOLOGY OF FAMILIAL TUMOR SYNDROMES

- Tuberous sclerosis complex
- Succinate dehydrogenase (*SDH*) germline mutation
- Lynch syndrome
- Heritable sickle cell hemoglobinopathy and medullary carcinoma of kidney
- Hyperparathyroidism-jaw tumor syndrome
- *PTEN*-hamartoma tumor syndrome
- Constitutional chromosome 3 translocation
- Wilms tumor syndrome

Hereditary Syndromes Known to be Associated With Testicle Neoplasia

- Carney complex
- Li-Fraumeni syndrome
- Peutz-Jeghers syndrome
- Renal cell carcinoma and leiomyomas
- Xeroderma pigmentosus

Hereditary Syndromes Known to be Associated With Bladder and Ureter Neoplasia

- Lynch syndrome

GASTROINTESTINAL TRACT

Hereditary Syndromes Known to be Associated With Esophagus, Stomach, and Intestinal Neoplasia

- Familial adenomatous polyposis
- Juvenile polyposis
- Familial gastrointestinal stromal tumor
- Hereditary diffuse gastric cancer
- *MYH*-associated polyposis
- Peutz-Jeghers syndrome
- Breast/ovarian *BRCA1* and *BRCA2*
- *PTEN*-hamartoma tumor syndrome
- Li-Fraumeni syndrome
- Bloom syndrome
- Dyskeratosis congenita
- Gastrointestinal stromal tumor syndrome
- Neurofibromatosis 1
- Multiple endocrine neoplasia 1

Hereditary Syndromes Known to be Associated With Pancreas Neoplasia

- von Hippel-Lindau syndrome
- Breast/ovarian *BRCA1* and *BRCA2*
- Li-Fraumeni syndrome
- Familial adenomatous polyposis
- Dyskeratosis congenita
- Juvenile polyposis
- Familial melanoma
- Multiple endocrine neoplasia 1
- Peutz-Jeghers syndrome
- Carney complex
- Tuberous sclerosis
- Hereditary pancreatic cancer syndrome

Hereditary Syndromes Known to be Associated With Liver Neoplasia

- Breast/ovarian *BRCA2*
- Familial adenomatous polyposis
- *PTEN*-hamartoma tumor syndrome
- Beckwith-Wiedemann syndrome
- von Hippel-Lindau syndrome
- Lynch syndrome

CENTRAL NERVOUS SYSTEM

Hereditary Syndromes Known to be Associated With CNS and PNS Neoplasia

- Ataxia-telangiectasia
- Familial uveal melanoma
- Hereditary retinoblastoma
- Neurofibromatosis type 1
- Neurofibromatosis type 2
- Rhabdoid predisposition syndrome
- Schwannomatosis
- Tuberous sclerosis complex
- von Hippel-Lindau syndrome
- Multiple meningoma syndrome
- Pleuropulmonary blastoma

SKIN

Hereditary Syndromes Known to be Associated With Skin Neoplasia

- Carney complex
- *PTEN*-hamartoma tumor syndrome
- Basal cell nevus syndrome
- Beckwith-Wiedemann syndrome
- Birt-Hogg-Dubé syndrome
- Dyskeratosis congenita
- Hereditary multiple melanoma
- Howell-Evans syndrome
- Melanoma pancreatic carcinoma syndrome
- Werner syndrome

BREAST

Hereditary Syndromes Known to be Associated With Breast Neoplasia

- *BRCA1* hereditary breast &/or ovarian cancer syndrome
- *BRCA2* hereditary breast &/or ovarian cancer syndrome
- Li-Fraumeni syndrome
- Familial gastric cancer and breast lobular cancer syndrome
- *PTEN*-hamartoma tumor syndrome
- Peutz-Jeghers syndrome
- Ataxia-telangiectasia syndrome

PATHOLOGY OF FAMILIAL TUMOR SYNDROMES

GYNECOLOGIC

Hereditary Syndromes Known to be Associated With Uterine Neoplasia

- *BRCA1* hereditary breast &/or ovarian cancer syndrome
- *BRCA2* hereditary breast &/or ovarian cancer syndrome
- Lynch syndrome
- *PTEN*-hamartoma tumor syndrome
- Peutz-Jeghers syndrome
- Hereditary leiomyomatosis and renal cell carcinoma
- von Hippel-Lindau syndrome

Hereditary Syndromes Known to be Associated With Ovarian Neoplasia

- *BRCA1* hereditary breast &/or ovarian cancer syndrome
- *BRCA2* hereditary breast &/or ovarian cancer syndrome
- von Hippel-Lindau syndrome
- Peutz-Jeghers syndrome
- Lynch syndrome

LUNG

Hereditary Syndromes Known to be Associated With Lung Neoplasia

- *BRCA2* hereditary breast &/or ovarian cancer syndrome
- Hereditary retinoblastoma syndrome
- Familial pleuropulmonary blastoma
- Tuberous sclerosis complex
- Carney triad
- Bloom syndrome
- Li-Fraumeni syndrome
- Xeroderma pigmentosum
- Peutz-Jeghers syndrome

HEAD AND NECK

Hereditary Syndromes Known to be Associated With Head and Neck Neoplasia

- Dyskeratosis congenita
- Fanconi anemia
- Xeroderma pigmentosum
- Bloom syndrome
- Hereditary retinoblastoma
- Neurofibromatosis 2
- Basal cell nevus syndrome/Gorlin syndrome
- Hyperparathyroidism-jaw tumor syndrome
- Familial adenomatous polyposis
- von Hippel-Lindau

Hereditary Syndromes Known to be Associated With Salivary Gland Neoplasia

- von Hippel-Lindau syndrome
- Ataxia-telangiectasia syndrome
- Hereditary retinoblastoma syndrome
- Brooke-Spiegler syndrome and familial cylindromatosis

CENTRAL NERVOUS SYSTEM

Hereditary Syndromes Known to be Associated With CNS Neoplasia

- Neurofibromatosis 1
- Neurofibromatosis 2
- von Hippel-Lindau syndrome
- Gorlin syndrome
- Lynch syndrome
- Familial adenomatous polyposis
- Tuberous sclerosis complex
- Li-Fraumeni syndrome
- Constitutional mismatch repair
- Melanoma astrocytoma syndrome
- Familial uveal melanoma
- Rhabdoid predisposition syndrome
- Hereditary retinoblastoma
- *PTEN*-hamartoma tumor syndrome
- Multiple meningoma syndrome
- Pleuropulmonary blastoma

BONE AND SOFT TISSUE

Hereditary Syndromes Known to be Associated With Bone Neoplasia

- Hereditary multiple exostosis
- Li-Fraumeni syndrome
- Hereditary retinoblastoma
- Familial chordoma syndrome
- Tuberous sclerosis complex
- Hyperparathyroidism-jaw tumor syndrome

Hereditary Syndromes Known to be Associated With Soft Tissue Neoplasia

- Basal cell nevus syndrome
- Li-Fraumeni syndrome
- Hereditary retinoblastoma
- Hereditary multiple exostosis
- Familial adenomatous polyposis
- Renal carcinoma with leiomyomas
- Neurofibromatosis 1
- Neurofibromatosis 2
- Carney complex
- Beckwith-Wiedemann syndrome

HEMATOLOGY

Hereditary Syndromes Known to be Associated With Blood and Bone Marrow Neoplasia

- Congenital amegakaryocytic thrombocytopenia
- Diamond-Blackfan anemia
- Dyskeratosis congenita
- Severe congenital neutropenia
- Shwachman-Diamond syndrome
- Fanconi anemia

Hereditary Syndromes Known to be Associated With Lymphoma/Leukemia

- Familial non-Hodgkin lymphoma
- Familial acute myeloid leukemia
- Familial chronic lymphocytic leukemia
- Familial Hodgkin lymphoma
- Fanconi anemia

SELECTED REFERENCES

1. Boedeker CC et al: Genetics of hereditary head and neck paragangliomas. Head Neck. Epub ahead of print, 2013
2. Burton-Chase AM et al: Changes in screening behaviors and attitudes toward screening from pre-test genetic counseling to post-disclosure in Lynch syndrome families. Clin Genet. 83(3):215-20, 2013
3. Busam KJ et al: Multiple epithelioid Spitz nevi or tumors with loss of BAP1 expression: a clue to a hereditary tumor syndrome. JAMA Dermatol. 149(3):335-9, 2013
4. Capatina C et al: The management of head-and-neck paragangliomas. Endocr Relat Cancer. 20(5):R291-305, 2013
5. Curtin K et al: Familial risk of childhood cancer and tumors in the li-fraumeni spectrum in the utah population database: Implications for genetic evaluation in pediatric practice. Int J Cancer. 133(10):2444-53, 2013
6. Daa T et al: PLAG1 and CYLD do not play a role in the tumorigenesis of adenoid cystic carcinoma. Mol Med Rep. 7(4):1086-90, 2013
7. Euhus DM et al: Genetic predisposition syndromes and their management. Surg Clin North Am. 93(2):341-62, 2013
8. Fang M et al: MEN1 is a melanoma tumor suppressor that preserves genomic integrity by stimulating transcription of genes that promote homologous recombination-directed DNA repair. Mol Cell Biol. 33(13):2635-47, 2013
9. Farley MN et al: A Novel Germline Mutation in BAP1 Predisposes to Familial Clear-Cell Renal Cell Carcinoma. Mol Cancer Res. 11(9):1061-71, 2013
10. Fendrich V et al: Familial pancreatic cancer-status quo. Int J Colorectal Dis. Epub ahead of print, 2013
11. Gaudineau A et al: Postnatal phenotype according to prenatal ultrasound features of Noonan syndrome: a retrospective study of 28 cases. Prenat Diagn. 33(3):238-41, 2013
12. Giusti F et al: Hereditary hyperparathyroidism syndromes. J Clin Densitom. 16(1):69-74, 2013
13. Greenup R et al: Prevalence of BRCA Mutations Among Women with Triple-Negative Breast Cancer (TNBC) in a Genetic Counseling Cohort. Ann Surg Oncol. 20(10):3254-8, 2013
14. Gupta A et al: Multifocal hepatic neoplasia in 3 children with APC gene mutation. Am J Surg Pathol. 37(7):1058-66, 2013
15. Gupta N et al: Pulmonary manifestations of Birt-Hogg-Dubé syndrome. Fam Cancer. Epub ahead of print, 2013
16. Höiom V et al: Hereditary uveal melanoma: a report of a germline mutation in BAP1. Genes Chromosomes Cancer. 52(4):378-84, 2013
17. Jones AV et al: Inherited predisposition to myeloproliferative neoplasms. Ther Adv Hematol. 4(4):237-53, 2013
18. Karamurzin Y et al: Histologic evaluation of prophylactic hysterectomy and oophorectomy in Lynch syndrome. Am J Surg Pathol. 37(4):579-85, 2013
19. Kessels K et al: Recording of family history is associated with colorectal cancer stage. Eur J Gastroenterol Hepatol. 25(4):482-7, 2013
20. Lucia-Casadonte C et al: An unusual case of pleuropulmonary blastoma in a child with jejunal hamartomas. Case Rep Pediatr. 2013:140508, 2013
21. Metcalfe K et al: Health care provider recommendations for reducing cancer risks among women with a BRCA1 or BRCA2 mutation. Clin Genet. Epub ahead of print, 2013
22. Mitchell G et al: High Frequency of Germline TP53 Mutations in a Prospective Adult-Onset Sarcoma Cohort. PLoS One. 8(7):e69026, 2013
23. Paparo L et al: Differential expression of PTEN gene correlates with phenotypic heterogeneity in three cases of patients showing clinical manifestations of PTEN hamartoma tumour syndrome. Hered Cancer Clin Pract. 11(1):8, 2013
24. Przybycin CG et al: Hereditary syndromes with associated renal neoplasia: a practical guide to histologic recognition in renal tumor resection specimens. Adv Anat Pathol. 20(4):245-63, 2013
25. Raizis AM et al: Trilateral retinoblastoma in a patient with Peutz-Jeghers syndrome. Am J Med Genet A. 161A(5):1096-100, 2013
26. Raymond VM et al: Elevated risk of prostate cancer among men with Lynch syndrome. J Clin Oncol. 31(14):1713-8, 2013
27. Sakurai N et al: Novel p53 splicing site mutation in Li-Fraumeni-like syndrome with osteosarcoma. Pediatr Int. 55(1):107-11, 2013
28. Stoffel EM et al: Familial CRC-Beyond the Lynch Syndrome. Clin Gastroenterol Hepatol. Epub ahead of print, 2013
29. Stojcev Z et al: Hamartomatous polyposis syndromes. Hered Cancer Clin Pract. 11(1):4, 2013
30. Sturgeon D et al: Increasing Lynch syndrome identification through establishment of a hereditary colorectal cancer registry. Dis Colon Rectum. 56(3):308-14, 2013
31. Win AK et al: Risks of colorectal and other cancers after endometrial cancer for women with Lynch syndrome. J Natl Cancer Inst. 105(4):274-9, 2013
32. Witkowski L et al: Familial rhabdoid tumour 'avant la lettre'-from pathology review to exome sequencing and back again. J Pathol. 231(1):35-43, 2013
33. Crispens MA: Endometrial and ovarian cancer in lynch syndrome. Clin Colon Rectal Surg. 25(2):97-102, 2012
34. Mishra N et al: Identification of patients at risk for hereditary colorectal cancer. Clin Colon Rectal Surg. 25(2):67-82, 2012
35. Son EJ et al: Familial follicular cell-derived thyroid carcinoma. Front Endocrinol (Lausanne). 3:61, 2012
36. Janeway KA et al: Defects in succinate dehydrogenase in gastrointestinal stromal tumors lacking KIT and PDGFRA mutations. Proc Natl Acad Sci U S A. 108(1):314-8, 2011
37. Laury AR et al: Thyroid pathology in PTEN-hamartoma tumor syndrome: characteristic findings of a distinct entity. Thyroid. 21(2):135-44, 2011
38. Nosé V: Familial thyroid cancer: a review. Mod Pathol. 24 Suppl 2:S19-33, 2011
39. Smith JR et al: Thyroid nodules and cancer in children with PTEN hamartoma tumor syndrome. J Clin Endocrinol Metab. 96(1):34-7, 2011
40. Zhang Y et al: Endocrine tumors as part of inherited tumor syndromes. Adv Anat Pathol. 18(3):206-18, 2011
41. Nosé V: Thyroid cancer of follicular cell origin in inherited tumor syndromes. Adv Anat Pathol. 17(6):428-36, 2010

Pathological Features in Familial Tumor Syndromes

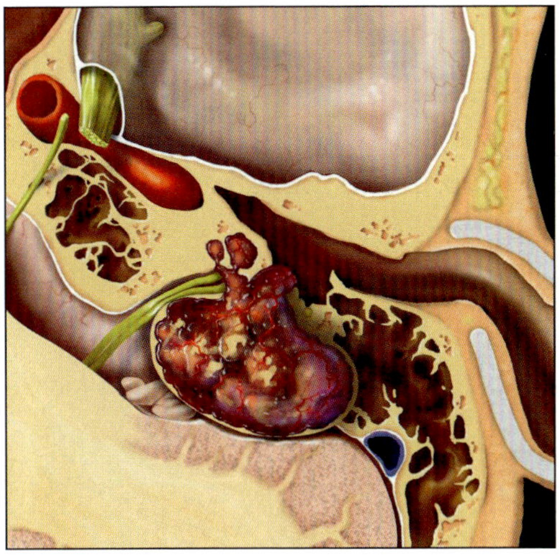

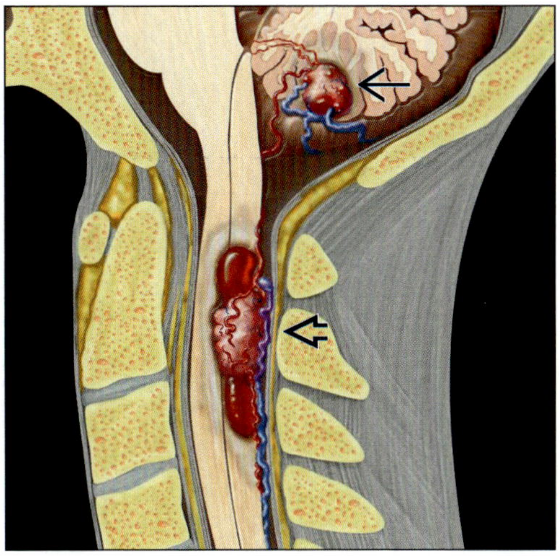

(Left) *The presence of unusual tumors is 1 of the characteristics of inherited tumor syndromes. Axial graphic of temporal bone shows the typical appearance of endolymphatic sac tumor seen in VHL patients. When diagnosing this tumor, VHL syndrome should be highly considered.* ***(Right)*** *Hemangioblastoma is the most frequently occurring tumor in VHL syndrome patients and is usually multiple. The main locations involved are the cerebellum → and spinal cord ⇨.*

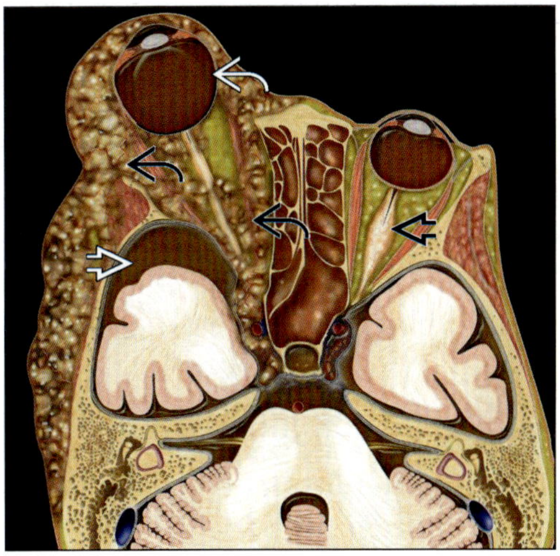

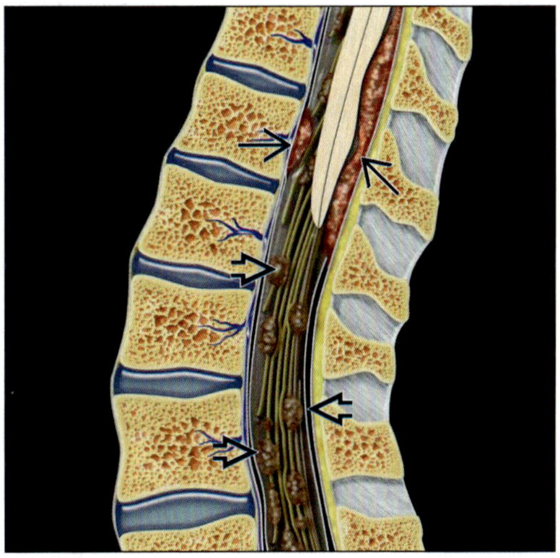

(Left) *The presence of multiple lesions, including multiple and bilateral tumors, is a characteristic feature of inherited tumor syndromes. Axial graphic depicts sphenoid dysplasia with arachnoid cyst ➡, optic nerve glioma ⇨, buphthalmos ➡, and multiple plexiform neurofibromas ↪, features associated with NF1.* ***(Right)*** *The combination of multiple meningiomas → and schwannomas ⇨ is characteristic of patients with NF2.*

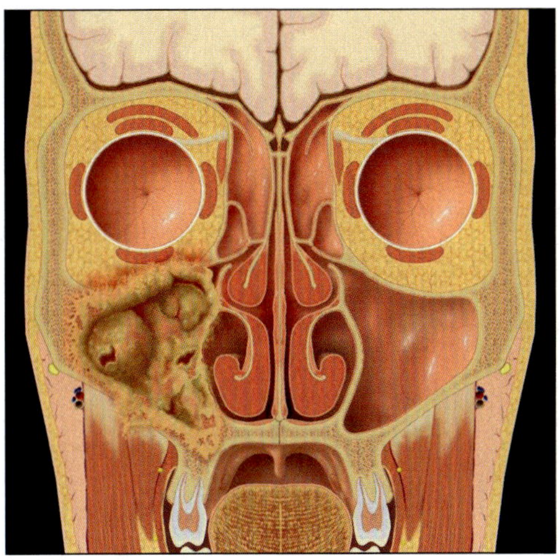

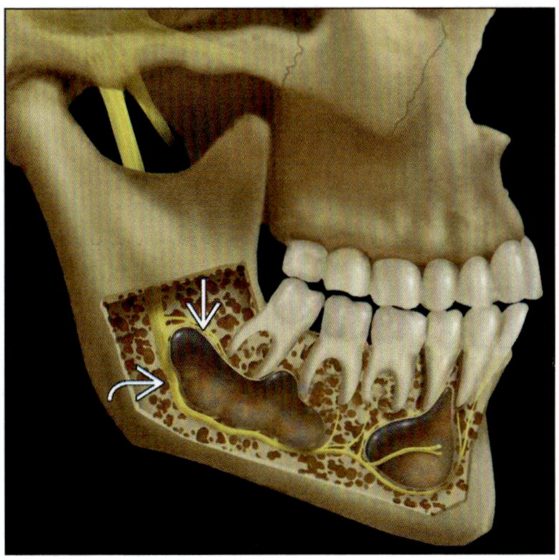

(Left) *This graphic depicts a squamous cell carcinoma of the maxillary sinus. These tumors may be present in patients with dyskeratosis congenita, Fanconi anemia, xeroderma pigmentosum, and Bloom syndrome, presenting at an earlier age than the sporadic tumors.* ***(Right)*** *Lateral graphic of the mandible illustrates features of a classic keratocystic odontogenic tumor (KOT) ➡, displacing the inferior alveolar nerve ➡. The diagnosis of KOT should prompt evaluation for Gorlin syndrome.*

Pathological Features in Familial Tumor Syndromes

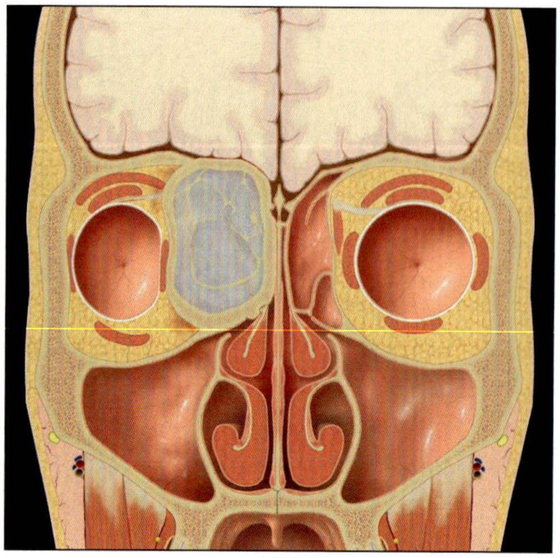

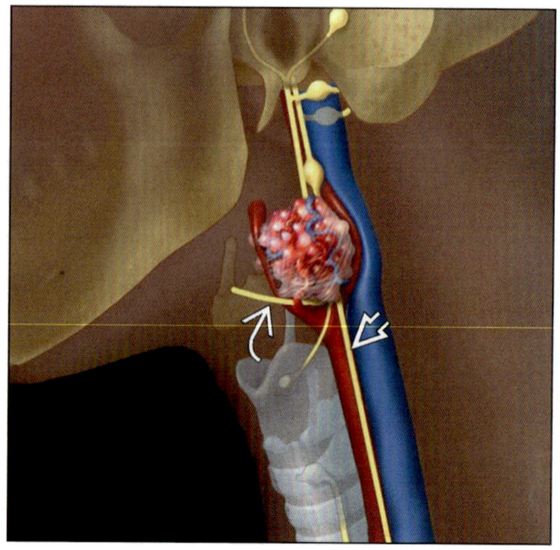

(Left) *Nonossifying fibroma shows a large, well-demarcated maxillary mass that obstructs 1 side of the nose and compresses the eye in a patient with hyperparathyroidism-jaw tumor syndrome. These patients present with hyperparathyroidism and also have distinct renal tumors.* ***(Right)*** *This lateral graphic depicts a carotid body paraganglioma at the carotid bifurcation. The main arterial feeder is the ascending pharyngeal artery. The vagus ⇨ and hypoglossal nerves ➚ are in close proximity.*

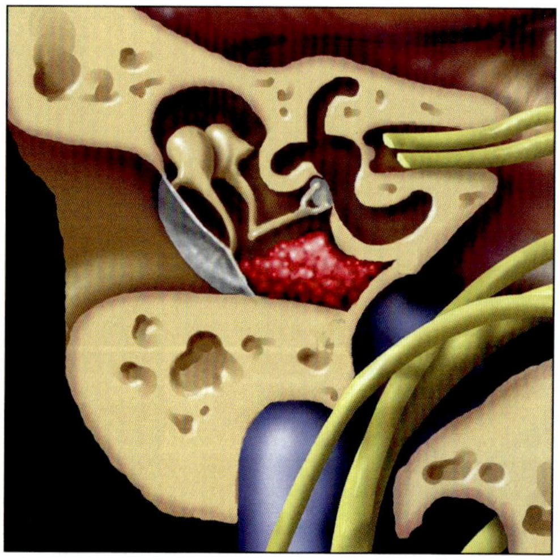

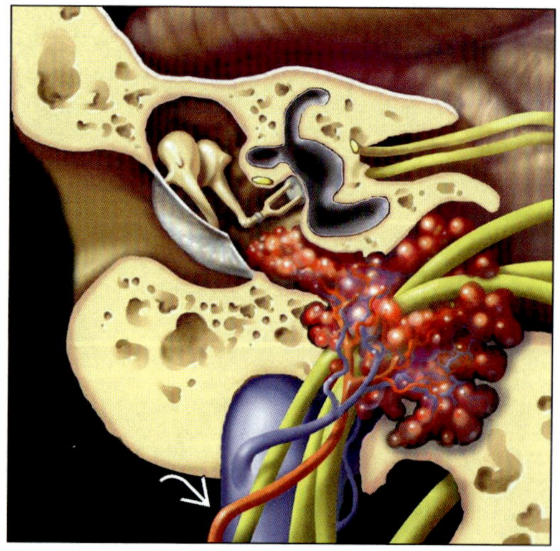

(Left) *This coronal graphic shows a highly vascular glomus tympanicum paraganglioma filling a portion of the middle ear cavity without involving adjacent structures and bone. The head and neck paragangliomas are mostly associated with succinate dehydrogenase (SDH) mutation.* ***(Right)*** *This coronal graphic shows a glomus jugulare paraganglioma centered in the jugular foramen with superolateral extension into the middle ear. The ascending parapharyngeal artery ➚ is feeding this vascular tumor.*

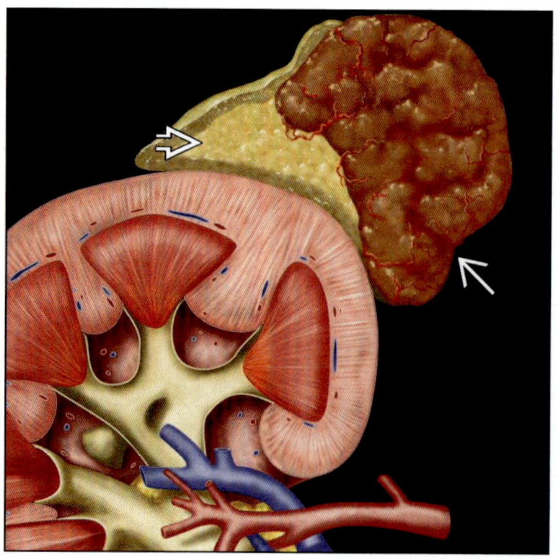

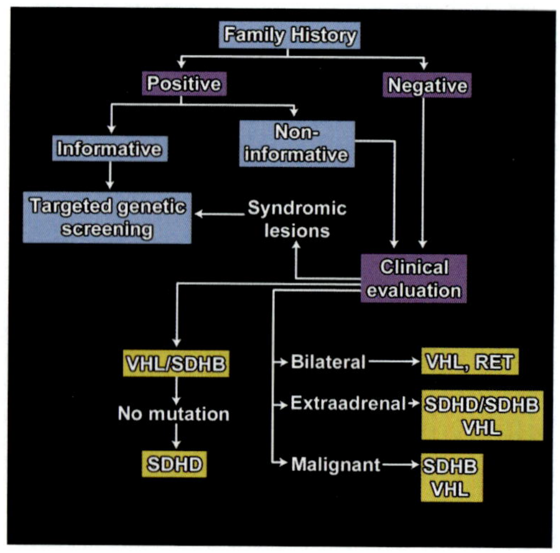

(Left) *This graphic shows both adrenal medullary hyperplasia ⇨ and MEN2 pheochromocytoma ➔. The presence of adrenal medullary hyperplasia should alert the pathologist for a MEN2-associated pheochromocytoma.* ***(Right)*** *Example shows an algorithmic approach for genetic testing in pheochromocytoma and paraganglioma for the evaluation and diagnosis of the most common and known pheochromocytoma/paraganglioma-associated syndromes.*

Pathological Features in Familial Tumor Syndromes

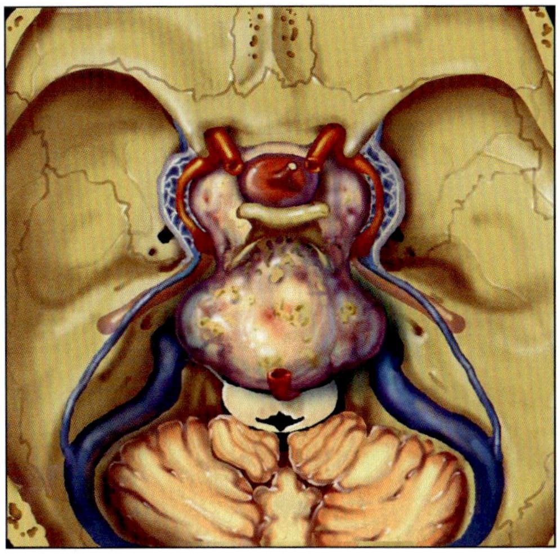

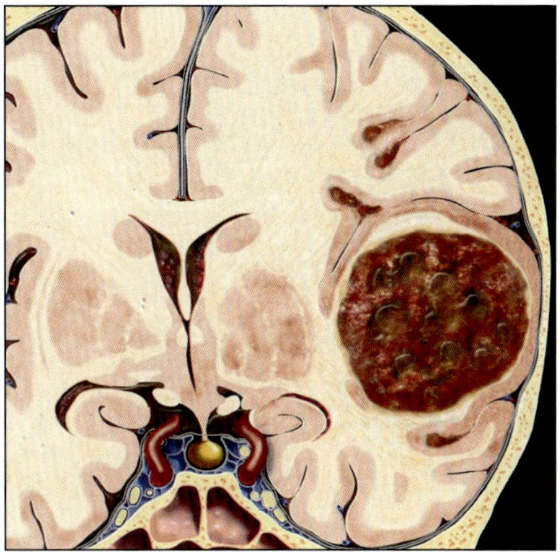

(Left) *Chordomas classically occur in the midline of the body, and 1 of the more common locations is at the base of the skull in the region of the clivus. In familial chordomas, there is an increased incidence of chordoma in patients with tuberous sclerosis.* ***(Right)*** *Atypical teratoid/rhabdoid tumors (AT/RT) form variably sized masses that may appear well circumscribed. Multiple foci of necrosis are common in these extremely aggressive pediatric tumors. They occur throughout the neural axis.*

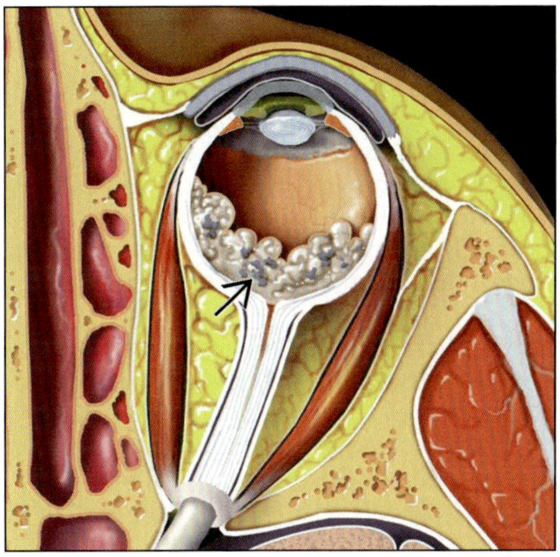

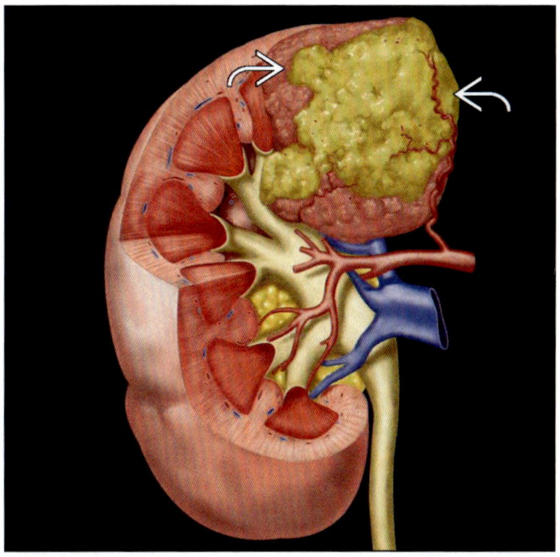

(Left) *Axial graphic shows retinoblastoma with lobulated tumor extending through the limiting membrane into the vitreous. Punctate calcifications ⇨ are characteristic. Hereditary retinoblastoma patients may develop carcinoma of the nasal cavity.* ***(Right)*** *Renal manifestations, including bilateral angiomyolipomas, are also typical of tuberous sclerosis complex. These are usually benign, but large tumors ➔ are associated with risk for life-threatening bleeding.*

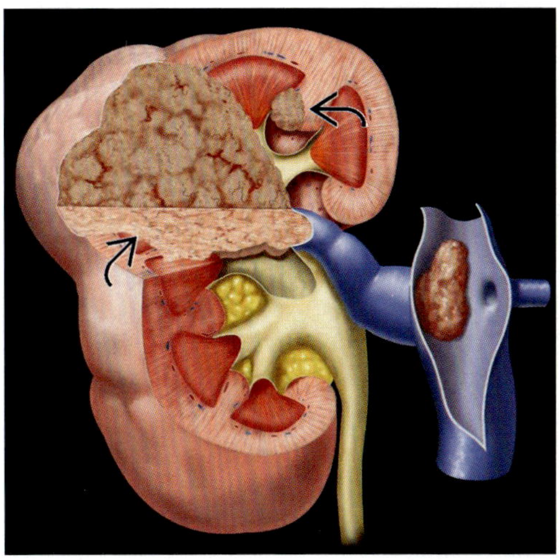

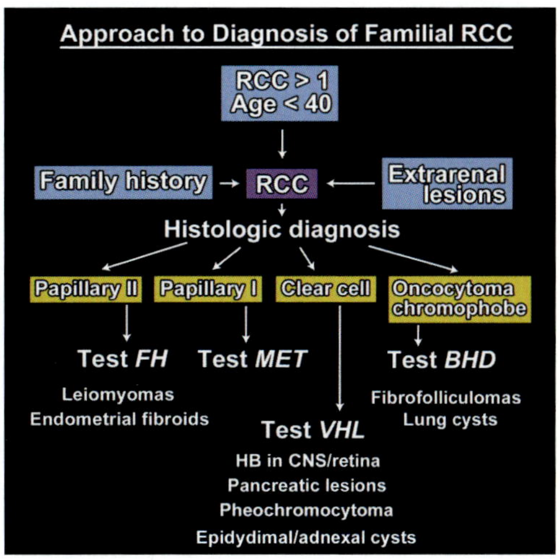

(Left) *The presence of renal cell carcinomas ⇨ in a young patient with specific histopathological features should alert the pathologist for the diagnosis of 1 of the familial renal tumor syndromes.* ***(Right)*** *Algorithmic approach for evaluation and genetic testing of patients with possible familial renal cell carcinoma by histopathological diagnosis is shown. The presence of extrarenal lesions and tumors help guide the proper testing and proper selection of candidate genes.*

CLINICAL DIAGNOSIS AND MANAGEMENT OF FAMILIAL/HEREDITARY TUMOR SYNDROMES

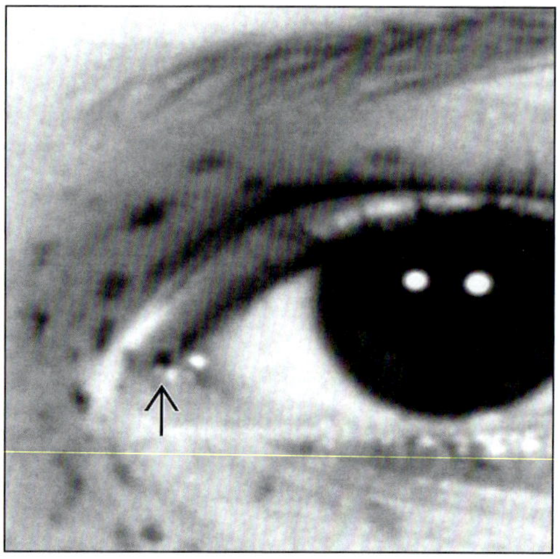

Mucocutaneous involvement in Carney complex is extensive and includes the characteristic pigmented skin lesions around the eye and in the inner canthus ➔. (Courtesy J. Carney, MD, PhD.)

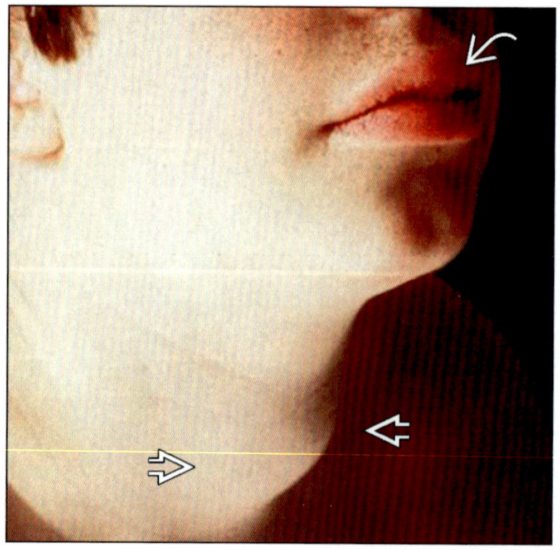

Patients with multiple endocrine neoplasia 2B (MEN2B) develop medullary thyroid carcinoma ➔, pheochromocytoma, and present with multiple neuromas of the tongue and lips ➔.

INTRODUCTION

Hereditary Cancer

- Characterized by mutations associated with a high probability of cancer development, vertical transmission through parents, and an association with other types of tumors
- Often have early age of onset
- Usually multiple and involve multiple organs
- Familial cancers may be associated with (or by combination of these)
  - Chance of clustering of sporadic cancer cases within a family
  - Genetic variation in lower penetrance genes
  - Shared environment
- Molecular genetics have identified a number of genes associated with inherited susceptibility to a specific cancer
  - Also provides a means of characterizing specific gene mutation or mutations present in certain individuals and families exhibiting an increased risk of cancer

Background

- ~ 10% of all cancers are attributable to a cancer predisposition gene
- Learning the clinical features that suggest possibility of an underlying genetic predisposition to cancer is another easily mastered diagnostic tool
  - It is crucial to raise awareness among oncologists and other health care providers about the importance of inherited cancer risk in the practice of oncology and cancer prevention
- Study of rare familial clusters became a remarkably productive scientific and clinical enterprise
  - These data have
    - Identified multiple new susceptibility genes
    - Informed understanding of pathogenesis of hereditary and nonhereditary cancers at individual, population, and laboratory levels
    - Defined clinical phenotypes of specific disorders more precisely
  - Much of the data that form basis of understanding of hereditary cancer syndromes are derived from evaluation of highly selected families
  - Single-gene hereditary syndromes account for only a small fraction of familial clustering on a population basis
  - Accuracy of reports from 1st-degree relatives is substantially better than for 2nd-degree relatives
- Diagnosis accuracy varies considerably, depending on
  - Age, gender, and cancer status of individual
  - Primary site of cancer origin
  - Degree of relatedness between individual and relative
  - Vital status of affected relative
  - Recentness of reported cancer diagnosis
- Need has never been greater for clinicians to be well grounded
  - In knowledge of biological and molecular bases of diseases they encounter
  - To become familiar with related new clinical issues, including predictive risk assessment, genetic counseling, and germline mutation testing for clinical decision making
  - To warn at-risk relatives vs. their high-risk patients' right to privacy and confidentiality, and the need for evidence-based, safe, and effective management recommendations for high-risk individuals

Identification of At-Risk Individuals

- Accurate identification of patients at increased risk for developing cancer is essential
- Assessment of an individual's risk of familial or hereditary cancer is based on a thorough evaluation of the family history

CLINICAL DIAGNOSIS AND MANAGEMENT OF FAMILIAL/HEREDITARY TUMOR SYNDROMES

- In the process of focusing on molecular biology of human cancer susceptibility, importance of taking a thoughtful family history cannot be emphasized sufficiently
  - Recording an appropriately focused family history must be performed in course of daily practice
- It is now increasingly routine to undertake a cancer genetics risk assessment, which includes the option of germline mutation testing for 1 or more relevant genes
- Identification of individuals at risk for cancer has become an integral part of medicine
  - Will allow health care providers to intervene with appropriate
    - Counseling and education
    - Increased cancer surveillance
    - Cancer prevention
- Genetic risk assessment in the context of childhood cancer represents a specific setting
  - Meticulous clinical evaluation often provides essential information upon which to base a syndromic diagnosis
- The National Comprehensive Cancer Network (NCCN) has established criteria for those individuals who need further genetic risk assessment
  - Multiple algorithmic approach for tumor syndromes are available at their website
    - http://www.nccn.org/professionals/physician_gls/pdf/genetics_screening

CANCER SUSCEPTIBILITY TESTING

American Society of Clinical Oncology (ASCO): Indications for Testing

- ASCO recommends that genetic testing be offered when
  - Individual has personal or family history features suggestive of a genetic cancer susceptibility condition
  - Test can be adequately interpreted, and
  - Results will aid in diagnosis or influence the medical or surgical management of the patient or family members at hereditary risk of cancer
- ASCO recommends that genetic testing only be done in setting of pre- and post-test counseling, which should include discussion of possible risks and benefits of early cancer detection and prevention modalities

ASCO: Policy Statement

- Advent of syndrome-specific germline mutation testing represents a major advance in the care of cancer-prone individuals
- ASCO reaffirms its commitment to integrating cancer risk assessment and management, including molecular analysis of cancer predisposition genes, into the practice of oncology and preventive medicine
  - Genetic testing for cancer susceptibility has become an accepted part of oncologic care
    - According to ASCO guidelines
    - Germline testing for inherited predisposition is well established as part of the care of individuals who may be at hereditary risk for cancers of the breast, ovary, colon, stomach, uterus, thyroid, and other primary sites
    - Germline genetic testing is distinct from somatic genetic profiling of cancer tissue to predict prognosis or treatment response
    - Germline testing involves analysis of DNA from blood or saliva for inherited mutations in specific genes that are associated with the type of cancer seen in the individual or family seeking assessment
    - When identified, such high-penetrance mutations usually result in a significant alteration in the function of the corresponding gene product and are associated with large increases in cancer risk
    - Other mutations result in less dramatic increases in risk (intermediate penetrance)
    - Identification of a high-penetrance mutation often justifies an adjustment of clinical care through the modification of surveillance or through preventive surgery
    - Germline testing for certain high-penetrance predispositions is now part of clinical guidelines and is reimbursed by most 3rd-party payers
    - Impact of intermediate penetrance mutations on clinical care is less clear

ASCO: Clinical Utility of Genetic Testing

- Genetic tests may benefit individuals by providing deeper self-knowledge and motivation to pursue healthy behaviors, even if the results do not inform clinical decision making
- Tests for high-penetrance mutations in appropriate populations have clinical utility, meaning that they inform clinical decision making and facilitate the prevention or amelioration of adverse health outcomes
- Genetic tests for intermediate-penetrance mutations and genomic profiles of SNPS linked to low-penetrance variants are of uncertain clinical utility

ASCO: Informed Consent

- Proposed elements of informed consent related to testing for inherited cancer susceptibility are set forth
- Basic elements of informed consent for cancer susceptibility testing
  - Information on specific genetic mutation(s) or genomic variant(s) being tested, including whether range of risk associated with variant will impact medical care
  - Implications of a positive and negative result
  - Possibility that test will not be informative
  - Options for risk estimation without genetic or genomic testing
  - Risk of passing a genetic variant to children
  - Technical accuracy of the test including, where required by law, licensure of the testing laboratory
  - Fees involved in testing and counseling and, for direct-to-consumer (DTC) testing, whether the counselor is employed by the testing company

- Psychological implications of test results (benefits and risks)
- Risks and protections against genetic discrimination by employers or insurers
- Confidentiality issues, including, for DTC testing companies, policies related to privacy and data security
- Possible use of DNA testing samples in future research
- Options and limitations of medical surveillance and strategies for prevention after genetic or genomic testing
- Importance of sharing genetic and genomic test results with at-risk relatives so that they may benefit from this information
- Plans for follow-up after testing

Special Issues Related to Genetic Testing Research

- Prospective clinical trials, large registries, and retrospective reviews are the most accurate methods for
  - Deriving relative risks of genetic variants
  - Measuring response to and effectiveness of clinical interventions based on genetic cancer risk assessment
- Tests with uncertain clinical utility become commercially available
  - It will be crucial to establish an evidence-based algorithm for clinically responsible use of these tests
    - For patient safety and effectiveness
- Wherever possible, genetic tests with uncertain clinical utility should be administered in the context of clinical trials
- Research should include basic studies of the functional significance of the genetic variants linked to disease risk
  - As well as prospective, randomized controlled trials of individual genomic markers
- At a translational level, it is important to establish criteria for technologic assessment of genetic and other diagnostic tests
- Research should focus on the extent to which personal benefits accrue to individuals who receive tests that have uncertain clinical utility
  - As well as the appropriate mechanism for measuring personal utility
- Establishing an evidence-based test for personal utility is particularly important for tests that would not be recommended based on clinical utility
- Research is also needed to demonstrate validity and reproducibility of some commercially available tests
- Because the algorithms used to convert genotypes into absolute risk estimates are empirically derived, prospective research is needed to confirm calibration of these estimates and to measure the effectiveness of interventions based on individual genomic profiling
- If genetic and genomic tests for cancer risk are going to be offered or justified on basis of personal utility, an effort should be made to establish evidence-based tests for these claims

Genetic Counseling

- Genetic testing should be conducted only in the setting of pre- and post-test counseling
  - **Pretest counseling**
    - Allows for advance consideration of medical options and the impact test results may have on family members
  - **Post-test counseling**
  - Provides a valuable opportunity for health care providers to interpret test results, recommend appropriate follow-up, and emphasize the importance of continuing regular prevention activities

DIAGNOSIS

Established Diagnostic Criteria

- Some examples of diagnostic criteria to characterize a syndrome present in individuals with multiple lesions and tumors
- **Diagnostic criteria for basal cell nevus syndrome**
- Diagnosis is established if 2 major or 1 major and 2 minor criteria are met
  - Multiple (> 2) basal cell carcinomas, or 1 basal cell carcinoma in patient < 30 years, or > 10 basal cell nevi
- Major criteria
  - Any odontogenic keratocyst (proven on histology) or polyostotic bone cyst
  - Palmar or plantar pits (≥ 3)
    - Ectopic calcification; lamellar or early (patient < 20 years) falx calcification
    - Family history of basal cell nevus syndrome (BCNS)
  - Minor criteria
    - Congenital skeletal anomaly: Bifid, fused, splayed, or missing rib; or bifid, wedged, or fused vertebrae
    - Head circumference > 97th percentile, with frontal bossing
    - Cardiac or ovarian fibroma
    - Medulloblastoma (primitive neuroectodermal tumor [PNET], most often of desmoplastic histology)
    - Lymphomesenteric or pleural cysts
    - Congenital malformation: Cleft lip &/or palate, polydactyly, eye anomaly (cataract, coloboma, microphthalmia)
- **Diagnostic criteria for von Hippel-Lindau (VHL) syndrome**
  - Diagnosis is established if there are
  - *VHL* mutation
  - ≥ 2 CNS or retinal hemangioblastomas or
  - Single CNS or retinal hemangioblastoma, plus 1 of the following
    - Multiple renal, pancreatic, or hepatic cysts
    - Pheochromocytoma (any location)
    - Renal cancer
    - Endolymphatic sac tumor of inner ear
    - Papillary cystadenoma of the epididymis or broad ligament

- Neuroendocrine tumor of the pancreas or
  - Definite family history of VHL plus 1 of the following
    - CNS or retinal hemangioblastoma
    - Multiple renal, pancreatic, or hepatic cysts
    - Pheochromocytoma
    - Renal cancer < age 60 years
    - Epididymal cystadenoma
  - Key diagnostic points
    - Multiple retinal and CNS hemangioblastomas
    - Multiple clear cell RCCs (bilateral), multiple renal cysts (bilateral) with clear cell lining, multiple pancreatic and hepatic cysts
    - May suspect possibility of syndrome based on constellation of pathologic findings
- **Diagnostic criteria for Carney complex**
  - *PRKAR1A* gene mutation
  - Patient must have at least 2 of the following
    - Spotty skin pigmentation with a typical distribution (often vermillion border of lips, conjunctiva and ocular canthi, vaginal or penile mucosa)
    - Myxoma (cutaneous: Often on the eyelid, external ear, nipple)
    - Cardiac myxoma
    - Breast myxomatosis or fat-suppressed MR findings suggestive of this diagnosis
    - Primary pigmented nodular adrenocortical disease or paradoxical positive response of urinary glucocorticosteroid to dexamethasone administration during Liddle diagnostic test for Cushing syndrome
    - Acromegaly due to GH-producing adenoma (somatotropinomas)
    - Large-cell calcifying Sertoli cell tumor of testis or characteristic calcification on testicular ultrasonography
    - Thyroid carcinoma or multiple hypoechoic nodules on thyroid ultrasonography in a young patient
    - Psammomatous melanotic schwannoma
    - Blue nevus, epithelioid blue nevus (multiple)
    - Breast ductal adenoma (multiple) (or mammary tumor with intraductal papilloma)
    - Osteochondromyxoma of bone (histological diagnosis)
  - Diagnostic criteria is also satisfied in a patient meeting any of these criteria and having either affected 1st-degree relative or inactivating mutation of *PRKAR1A* gene
- **Diagnostic criteria for neurofibromatosis type 1 (NF1)**
  - *NF1* mutation
  - Diagnosis requires 2 or more of the following
  - Café au lait macules
    - In children, ≥ 5 that are ≥ 0.5 cm in diameter
    - In adults, ≥ 6 that are ≥ 1.5 cm in diameter
  - ≥ 2 neurofibromas of any type or 1 plexiform neurofibroma
  - Multiple axillary or inguinal freckles
  - Sphenoid wing dysplasia or congenital bowing or thinning of long bone cortex (± pseudoarthrosis)
  - Bilateral optic nerve gliomas
  - ≥ 2 iris Lisch nodules (iris hamartomas)
  - 1st-degree relative with NF1 by these criteria
- **Diagnostic criteria for Li-Fraumeni syndrome (LFS)**
  - Population to be screened
    - When strict criteria are met, *TP53* mutations are found in 60-80%
    - If less strict criteria are used (Li-Fraumeni-like [LFL]), *TP53* mutations are found in up to 40%
  - Chompret criteria for screening
  - Individual (proband) must have 1 of the following tumors before age 46: Sarcoma, osteosarcoma, premenopausal breast cancer, brain tumor, adrenal cortical carcinoma, leukemia, or lung lepidic pattern carcinoma, and at least 1 of following 3 criteria
    - At least 1 first- or second-degree relative with an LFS tumor before age 56 or with multiple tumors
    - Breast cancer is not included if proband has breast cancer
    - Multiple tumors (not including breast cancers), 2 of which belong to LFS tumors and 1st of which occurred < age 46
    - Adrenal cortical carcinoma or choroid plexus tumor, irrespective of family history
  - 30% of individuals fulfilling these criteria have a germline *TP53* mutation
- **Diagnostic criteria for Lynch syndrome**
  - Mutations in genes coding for mismatch repair proteins (MLH1, PMS2, MSH2, MSH6)
  - Clinical features
    - Multiple epithelial cancers occur at average age of ~ 20 years younger than expected
  - Several guidelines have been proposed to help identify patients who should be tested for Lynch syndrome
    - **Amsterdam criteria II**
    - ≥ 3 relatives with a Lynch-associated cancer
    - ≥ 2 successive generations affected
    - ≥ 1 relative diagnosed < age 50
    - 1 should be a 1st-degree relative of the other 2
    - Familial adenomatous polyposis must be excluded
    - **Revised Bethesda guidelines**
    - Colorectal carcinoma (CRC) diagnosed prior to age 50
    - Presence of synchronous or metachronous CRC or other Lynch-associated tumor, regardless of age
    - CRC with histologic features suggestive of microsatellite instability in patient < age 60
    - CRC diagnosed in ≥ 1 first-degree relative with a Lynch-associated tumor, with 1 of the cancers diagnosed prior to age 50
    - CRC diagnosed in ≥ 2 first-degree or second-degree relatives with Lynch-associated tumors, regardless of age
  - Neither of these guidelines is foolproof; hence, many studies recommend testing all CRCs for Lynch syndrome

CLINICAL DIAGNOSIS AND MANAGEMENT OF FAMILIAL/HEREDITARY TUMOR SYNDROMES

Features That Suggest the Presence of a Familial Cancer Predisposition

In Individual Patient	In Patient's Family
Age at diagnosis younger than usual	1 first-degree relative with same or a related tumor and 1 of the individual features listed
Associated with other genetic traits	≥ 2 first-degree relatives with neoplasms in same site
Neoplasms with rare morphological features	≥ 2 first-degree relatives with neoplasm types belonging to a known familial cancer syndrome
Associated with congenital defects	≥ 2 first-degree relatives with rare tumors
Multiple primary neoplasms within same organ	≥ 2 relatives in 2 generations with tumors of the same site or etiologically related sites
Multiple primary neoplasms within different organs and tissues	
Bilateral primary neoplasms in paired organs or lobes	
Multifocal neoplasms within same organ or tissue	
Neoplasms occurring in gender that is not usually affected	
Associated with an inherited precursor lesion	
Associated with another rare disease	
Associated with cutaneous lesions known to be related to cancer susceptibility disorders	

Future Perspectives

- Progress of recent years in understanding pathogenesis of familial tumor syndromes is expected to continue to improve patient screening
  - Also become, in the long term, a catalyst for development of new therapeutic options for surgically untreatable tumors
- With the fast-moving field, a new syndrome is frequently identified
- Awareness of possible syndromes when dealing with patients is critical for proper patient management
- Hereditary cancer syndromes in children and adolescents are becoming more recognized in the field of pediatric hematology/oncology
- Recently, germline mutations of *DICER1* have been identified in patients with rare neoplasms, suggesting existence of a discovered syndrome involving cancer predisposition
  - Familial pleuropulmonary blastoma tumor predisposition (*DICER1*) syndrome
  - Additional manifestations of syndrome have been identified, including cystic nephroma, medulloepithelioma, Sertoli-Leydig cell tumor, and others
- Importance of learning about them for the practicing physicians
- Of particular use for identification of genetic testing resources and regularly updated clinical management information for many of these disorders
- There are now a number of additional online resources available that provide more comprehensive information about these conditions
  - GeneTests website, a resource to those seeing individuals with genetic disorders: http://www.genetests.org/
- Pathologist plays a crucial role; important for surgical pathologists to be aware of specific pathology findings that suggest a possible tumor syndrome

SELECTED REFERENCES

1. Curtin K et al: Familial risk of childhood cancer and tumors in the li-fraumeni spectrum in the utah population database: Implications for genetic evaluation in pediatric practice. Int J Cancer. 133(10):2444-53, 2013
2. Dahia PL: Novel hereditary forms of pheochromocytomas and paragangliomas. Front Horm Res. 41:79-91, 2013
3. Drost M et al: Genetic screens to identify pathogenic gene variants in the common cancer predisposition Lynch syndrome. Proc Natl Acad Sci U S A. 110(23):9403-8, 2013
4. Hazewinkel Y et al: Extracolonic cancer risk in patients with serrated polyposis syndrome and their first-degree relatives. Fam Cancer. Epub ahead of print, 2013
5. Kalkan E et al: Endocrine tumors associated with neurofibromatosis type 1, peutz-jeghers syndrome and other familial neoplasia syndromes. Front Horm Res. 41:166-81, 2013
6. Lolkema MP et al: Ethical, legal, and counseling challenges surrounding the return of genetic results in oncology. J Clin Oncol. 31(15):1842-8, 2013
7. Przybycin CG et al: Hereditary syndromes with associated renal neoplasia: a practical guide to histologic recognition in renal tumor resection specimens. Adv Anat Pathol. 20(4):245-63, 2013
8. Schiffman JD et al: Update on pediatric cancer predisposition syndromes. Pediatr Blood Cancer. 60(8):1247-52, 2013
9. Shuch B et al: Germline PTEN mutation Cowden syndrome: An underappreciated form of hereditary kidney cancer. J Urol. Epub ahead of print, 2013
10. Ward RL et al: Population-based molecular screening for lynch syndrome: implications for personalized medicine. J Clin Oncol. 31(20):2554-62, 2013
11. Mishra N et al: Identification of patients at risk for hereditary colorectal cancer. Clin Colon Rectal Surg. 25(2):67-82, 2012
12. Laury AR et al: Thyroid pathology in PTEN-hamartoma tumor syndrome: characteristic findings of a distinct entity. Thyroid. 21(2):135-44, 2011
13. Nosé V: Familial thyroid cancer: a review. Mod Pathol. 24 Suppl 2:S19-33, 2011
14. Zhang Y et al: Endocrine tumors as part of inherited tumor syndromes. Adv Anat Pathol. 18(3):206-18, 2011
15. Dotto J et al: Familial thyroid carcinoma: a diagnostic algorithm. Adv Anat Pathol. 15(6):332-49, 2008

Clinical Features

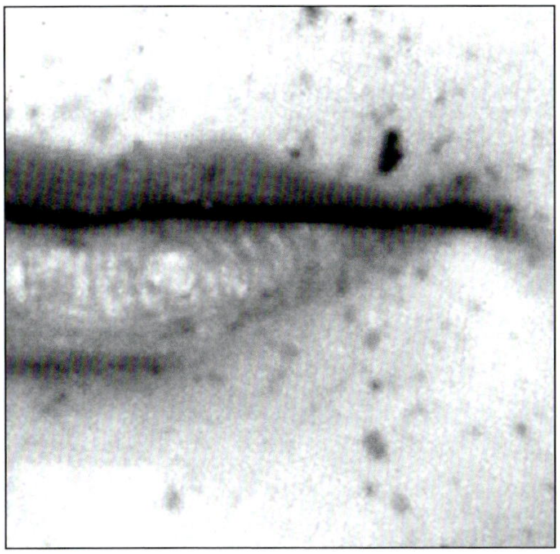

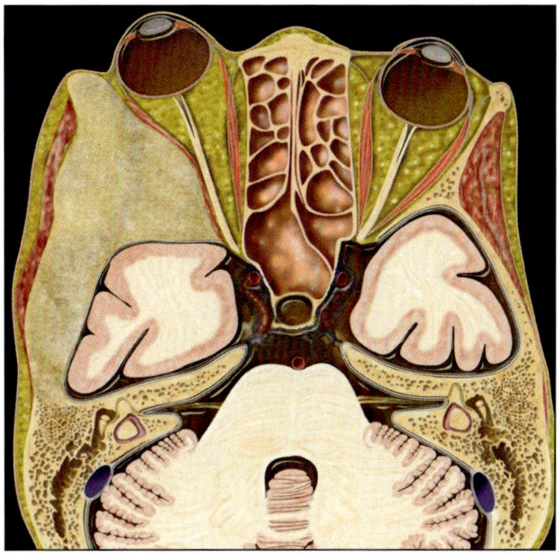

(Left) *Pigmented skin lesions are present in Carney complex and also in McCune-Albright, Peutz-Jeghers, Birt-Hogg-Dubé, neurofibromatosis, and PTEN-hamartoma tumor syndromes. (Courtesy J. Carney, MD, PhD.)* ***(Right)*** *McCune-Albright syndrome consists of a triad of polyostotic fibrous dysplasia, pigmented skin lesions, and sexual precocity. These patients may develop hyperplasia and adenomas of endocrine glands.*

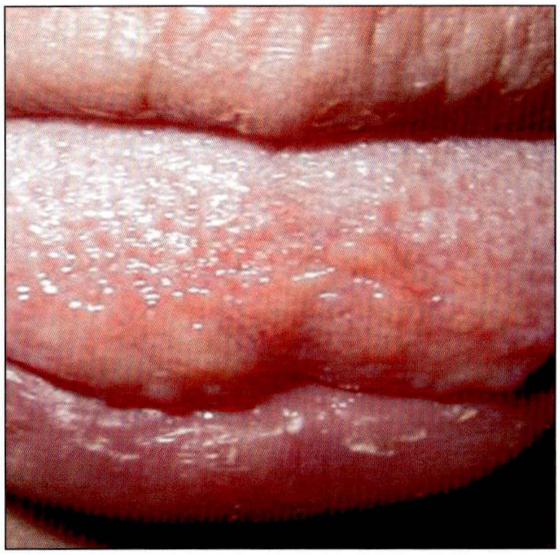

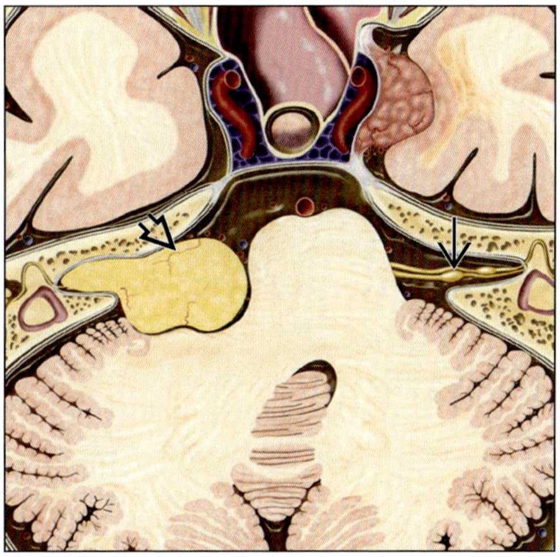

(Left) *Patients with multiple endocrine neoplasia 2B (MEN2B) develop medullary thyroid carcinoma, pheochromocytoma, and present with multiple neuromas of the tongue &/ or ganglioneuromatosis of the intestine, a marfanoid habitus, &/or medullated corneal nerve fibers.* ***(Right)*** *Bilateral vestibular schwannomas involving the vestibular branch of CN8 are pathognomonic of NF2. They present as a cerebellopontine angle mass → and may be multiple →.*

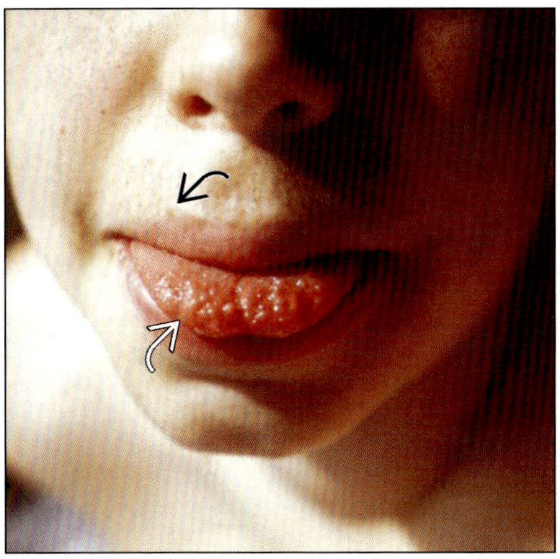

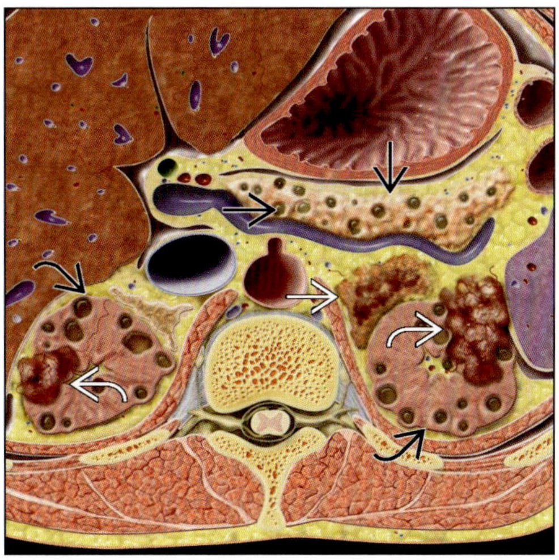

(Left) *Patients with MEN2B may present with multiple neuromas of the tongue → and lip &/or pigmented skin lesions →.* ***(Right)*** *The presence of multiple lesions, including multiple and bilateral tumors, is a characteristic feature of inherited tumor syndromes. Graphic representation of abdominal lesions seen in patients with von Hippel-Lindau syndrome shows the bilateral and multiple renal cysts →, renal tumors →, pancreatic cysts →, and adrenal pheochromocytoma →.*

Syndromes

ATAXIA-TELANGIECTASIA SYNDROME

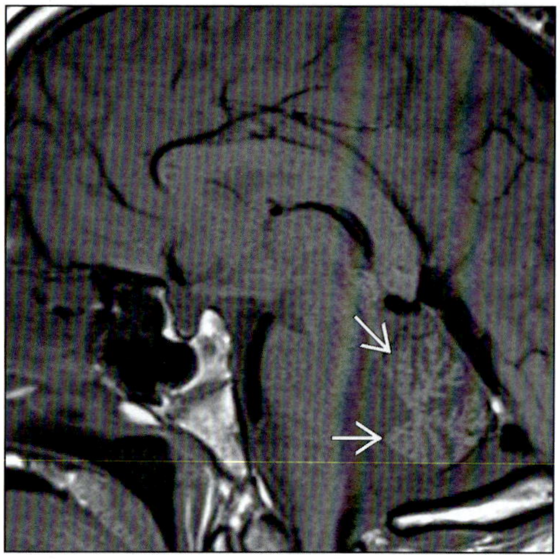

Cerebellar atrophy is a hallmark of ataxia-telangiectasia, particularly in the vermis ➔. However, this may not be evident in MR until late childhood.

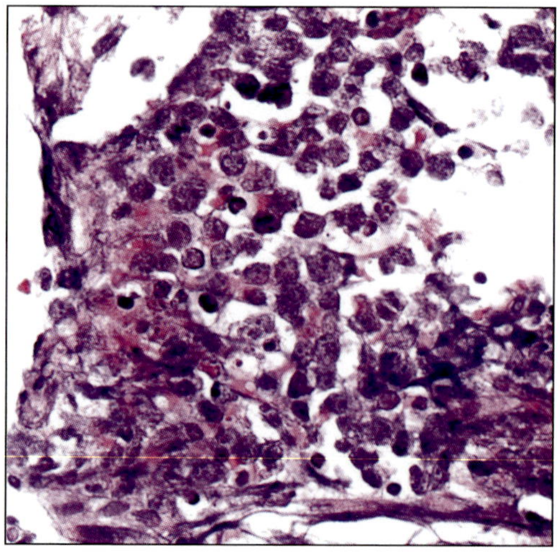

This diffuse large B-cell lymphoma developed in an ataxia-telangiectasia (AT) patient. AT patients have an increased predisposition to various cancers, particularly of B- and T-cell lineage.

TERMINOLOGY

Abbreviations

- Ataxia-telangiectasia (AT)
- Ataxia-telangiectasia mutated (*ATM*) gene

EPIDEMIOLOGY

Incidence

- 1 per 40,000-100,000
- Occurs in all geographic regions with variable local prevalence

Gender

- Similar frequency in males and females

CLINICAL IMPLICATIONS

Clinical Presentation

- Ataxia of gait, stance, and trunk most frequent
  - Progresses to affect extremities and eye movements
- Dysarthria
- Late cerebellar tremor in variant AT rather than profound ataxia

Imaging Findings

- Atrophy of cerebellar vermis and hemispheres in older children (not evident in early childhood)

GENETICS

Autosomal Recessive Disease

- Caused by germline inactivation of ataxia-telangiectasia mutated (*ATM*) gene
- Chromosomal region 11q22-23
- Encodes for ~ 300 kDa serine/threonine protein kinase with sequence homology to PI3K family
  - Predominantly a nuclear protein
  - Major function is regulation of DNA repair secondary to double-strand DNA breaks
  - Normally in the form of inactive dimers
  - Activated ATM protein monomers recruited to areas of DNA damage
  - MRN (MRE11A/RAD50/NBS1) complex required for optimal activation of ATM in areas of double-stranded DNA breaks
  - Several protein kinases (e.g., CHK2) and p53 key substrates phosphorylated by ATM
  - Other functions include regulation of cell cycle, apoptosis, telomere maintenance, response to oxidative stress, mitochondrial homeostasis, insulin signaling
- In classic AT, ATM is almost completely absent secondary to severe/truncating mutations

Heterozygous Carriers of *ATM* Mutations Predisposed to Cancers

- Contributes to small subset of familial breast and ovarian cancer

CLINICAL IMPLICATIONS AND ANCILLARY TESTS

Hypersensitivity to Ionizing Radiation

- Most characteristic biologic feature

↑ α-Fetoprotein in Serum

- Useful biomarker
- Rising serum levels typical
- Not a feature of other ataxia and immunodeficiency syndromes in differential diagnosis

Early Diagnosis

- Allows genetic counseling and avoidance of extended medical work-ups

NONNEOPLASTIC MANIFESTATIONS

Central Nervous System Degeneration

- Progressive ataxia starts early (6-18 months of age)
  - Wheelchair bound by 1st decade of life
  - Cerebellar atrophy, particularly vermis
  - Extensive Purkinje and granule cell loss
  - Cell loss in inferior olives (retrograde)
  - Ectopic Purkinje cells may be found in molecular layer
  - Peripheral nervous system may also be affected and contribute to symptoms
- Mental deficiency
- Posterior spinal column dysfunction

Skin and Eye

- Telangiectasias
  - Involve bulbar conjunctivae and eventually bridge of nose
  - Appear between ages 2 and 8 years
- Seborrheic dermatitis common
- Cutaneous granulomas
- Café au lait spots
- Gray hair, skin atrophy

Deficiency of Cellular Immunity

- Hypoplasia of thymus, tonsil, and adenoids
- Lymphopenia
- ↓ IgA, IgE, IgG2

Respiratory Infections and Bronchiectasis

- Important cause of death in AT in addition to cancer

Endocrine Abnormalities

- Hypogonadism/infertility
- Insulin resistance/type 2 diabetes
- Short stature

ASSOCIATED NEOPLASMS

Hematolymphoid Malignancies

- Predominant neoplasms affecting AT patients (> 100x risk compared to general population)
- T-cell and B-cell lineage
- Myeloid leukemia very uncommon

Solid Tumors

- More evident as patients are living longer
- Ovarian carcinoma, breast carcinoma, thyroid carcinoma, salivary gland tumors, gastric carcinoma, melanoma, and leiomyomas/leiomyosarcomas may develop

CANCER RISK MANAGEMENT

Lifetime Cancer Risk

- 30% in AT patients
- Avoid x-ray-based tests if possible given characteristic radiosensitivity of AT

DIFFERENTIAL DIAGNOSIS

AT-Like Disorder

- Usually caused by hypomorphic mutations in *ATM* or mutations in genes encoding related proteins (e.g., *MRE11A*)
  - Missense or splice-site rather than truncating mutations in *ATM* more common than in classic AT
  - Milder phenotype

Nijmegen Breakage Syndrome (NBS)

- Caused by mutations in *NBS1*
  - Encodes for another component of MRN protein complex
- Patients also demonstrate immunodeficiency, radiosensitivity, and cancer predisposition
- Microcephaly and mental retardation, but lack progressive ataxia and telangiectasias

Disorders Associated With Defects in DNA Single-Strand Break (SSB) Repair

- Ataxia with oculomotor apraxia types 1 and 2, spinocerebellar ataxia with axonal neuropathy type 1
- Neurodegenerative syndromes and neurologic features overlap with AT
- No manifestations outside of nervous system

SELECTED REFERENCES

1. Shiloh Y et al: The ATM protein kinase: regulating the cellular response to genotoxic stress, and more. Nat Rev Mol Cell Biol. 14(4):197-210, 2013
2. Hoche F et al: Neurodegeneration in ataxia telangiectasia: what is new? What is evident? Neuropediatrics. 43(3):119-29, 2012
3. McKinnon PJ: ATM and the molecular pathogenesis of ataxia telangiectasia. Annu Rev Pathol. 7:303-21, 2012
4. Chiam LY et al: Cutaneous granulomas in ataxia telangiectasia and other primary immunodeficiencies: reflection of inappropriate immune regulation? Dermatology. 223(1):13-9, 2011
5. Vogel CA et al: Chronic noninfectious necrotizing granulomas in a child with Nijmegen breakage syndrome. Pediatr Dermatol. 27(3):285-9, 2010
6. Lavin MF: Ataxia-telangiectasia: from a rare disorder to a paradigm for cell signalling and cancer. Nat Rev Mol Cell Biol. 9(10):759-69, 2008
7. Thorstenson YR et al: Contributions of ATM mutations to familial breast and ovarian cancer. Cancer Res. 63(12):3325-33, 2003

BASAL CELL NEVUS SYNDROME/GORLIN SYNDROME

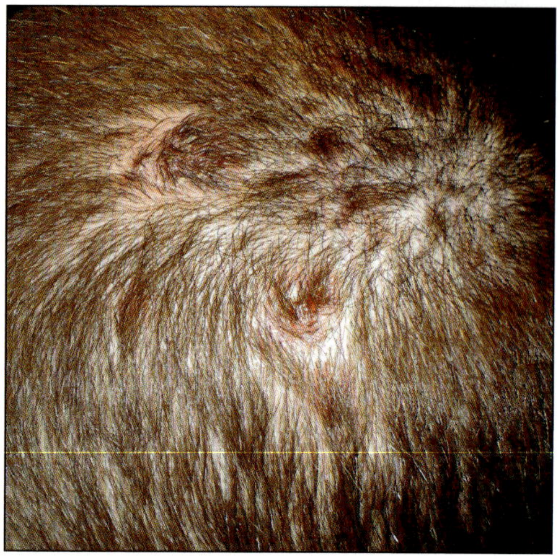

Multiple crusted pink plaques on the scalp represent basal cell carcinomas in this patient with Gorlin syndrome. (Courtesy K. Hoffmann, MD.)

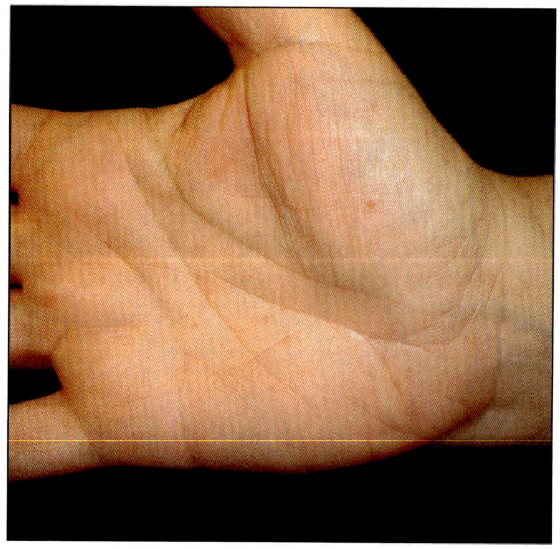

Multiple pink 1-2 mm depressions are shown on the palm, consistent with palmar pitting characteristic of Gorlin syndrome. (Courtesy K. Hoffmann, MD.)

TERMINOLOGY

Synonyms

- Nevoid basal cell carcinoma syndrome
- Basal cell carcinoma nevus syndrome
- Gorlin-Goltz syndrome

EPIDEMIOLOGY

Age at Presentation

- From birth (may not be detected until later)
  - Bony abnormalities
- 1st decade
  - Jaw cysts (of mandible/maxilla)
- 2nd decade
  - Palmoplantar pitting
- Childhood but more often late puberty/adulthood
  - Basal cell carcinomas (sometimes resembling skin tags)

Incidence

- ~ 1 in 19,000 births

GENETICS

Inheritance

- Autosomal dominant

PTCH1 Gene

- Mutations in this gene found in ~ 60-75% of those tested
- *PTCH1*
  - Located on chromosome 9q
  - Part of sonic hedgehog pathway
  - *PTCH1* encodes patched protein
  - Patched protein inhibits smoothened
  - Mutated *PTCH1* leads to disinhibition of smoothened and tumor growth
- No clear genotype/phenotype correlation

CLINICAL IMPLICATIONS AND IMAGING FINDINGS

Clinical Findings

- Triggers that should prompt evaluation for Gorlin syndrome
  - Keratocystic odontogenic tumor if age < 20 years old
  - Basal cell carcinoma if age < 20 years old
  - Palmar or plantar pits
  - Lamellar calcification of falx cerebri
  - Medulloblastoma, desmoplastic
- Characteristic facies
  - Frontal bossing
  - Hypoplastic maxilla
  - Broad nasal root (and hypertelorism)

Imaging Findings

- Head
  - Calcification of
    - Falx, tentorium cerebelli, sella turcica
  - Jaw cysts
    - Panorex (digital if possible)
  - Cleft lip/palate
- Trunk
  - Ribs
    - Bifid, missing, splayed
  - Spine
    - Scoliosis, vertebral anomalies
- Long bones
  - Bone cysts
- Hands/feet
  - Flame-shaped lucencies

BASAL CELL NEVUS SYNDROME/GORLIN SYNDROME

ASSOCIATED NEOPLASMS

Skin

- Basal cell carcinoma
  - May look like skin tags in children
  - Often sun-exposed skin
  - May be non-sun-exposed areas
  - Typical clinical morphology
    - Pearly, pink, telangiectatic papules or nodules
    - Erythematous, scaly, thin macules or plaques
    - May be eroded/ulcerated
  - All histopathologic subtypes
    - Superficial multicentric with buds of basaloid islands off epidermal base
    - Nodular with islands of basaloid cells with peripheral palisading in dermis
    - May be pigmented
    - Micronodular, morpheaform, infiltrative, infundibulocystic, etc.
- Palmoplantar pits
  - Several millimeters in diameter
  - Pink in color
  - Histopathology: Basaloid proliferation
- Epidermal inclusion cyst/milium

Musculoskeletal

- Odontogenic keratocyst
  - May become secondarily infected
  - Thin capsule with lining of stratified squamous epithelium
  - Sites
    - Mandibular molar/ramus (~ 40%)
    - Mandibular canine/incisor (~ 20%)
    - Maxillary molar tuberosity (~ 10%)

Central Nervous System

- Medulloblastoma
  - Especially desmoplastic
- Meningioma
  - May be consequence of radiation treatment of medulloblastoma

Genitourinary

- Ovarian fibroma/fibrosarcoma

Cardiac

- Fibroma

CANCER RISK MANAGEMENT

Multidisciplinary Care

- Dermatology, surgery, dental/oral medicine, orthopaedics, ophthalmology, neurology, genetics
- Regular skin examinations necessary
  - Every 6 months to 1 year (every 4 months in adults)
- Medulloblastoma
  - Baseline MR of brain with contrast and epilepsy protocol
    - Annually until age 8
- Minimize ionizing radiation exposure, as it can induce basal cell carcinomas
  - Consider MR over serial CT scans
- Treatments/interventions to prevent new basal cell carcinomas
  - Oral retinoids
  - Sun avoidance/sun protection
- *PTCH1* gene testing: Not mandatory for diagnosis
  - Scenarios in which testing is recommended
    - Prenatal testing if known mutation within family
    - Cases highly suspicious for Gorlin syndrome but not yet meeting criteria
    - Predictive testing for patients with affected family member

DIFFERENTIAL DIAGNOSIS

Early Onset Basal Cell Carcinomas (Sporadic)

- Increasingly, patients < age 40 are developing basal cell carcinoma
  - May be linked to tanning
- No other stigmata of Gorlin syndrome

Bazex-Dupré-Christol Syndrome

- Similarities to Gorlin syndrome
  - Multiple basal cell carcinomas (may have earlier onset than in Gorlin syndrome)
  - Milia
- Distinguishing features from Gorlin syndrome
  - X-linked dominant inheritance
  - Hypotrichosis
  - Follicular atrophoderma
  - Hypohidrosis

Rombo Syndrome

- Reported in 1 large Swedish family
- Similarities to Gorlin syndrome
  - Multiple basal cell carcinomas
  - Milia
- Distinguishing features from Gorlin syndrome
  - Multiple trichoepitheliomas
  - Atrophoderma vermiculata
  - Acral cyanosis

Brooke-Spiegler Syndrome

- Multiple facial papules, often clustered on central face (previously termed multiple trichoepitheliomas)
- Papulonodules may predominate on scalp (previously termed cylindromatosis)
- Histopathology
  - Trichoepithelioma (not basal cell carcinomas)
    - Basaloid islands, often with advanced follicular differentiation (e.g., horn cysts)
    - Peripheral palisading
    - Clefts between fibrotic stroma and unaffected dermis
  - Cylindroma
    - Jigsaw puzzle arrangement of islands with ductal differentiation surrounded by thickened basement membrane
  - Spiradenoma
    - Blue islands in dermis with alternating pattern of light and dark cells

BASAL CELL NEVUS SYNDROME/GORLIN SYNDROME

Familial Multiple Basaloid Follicular Hamartomas

- Multiple facial papules
- Presenting in childhood
- Histopathology
  - Basaloid follicular hamartoma (not basal cell carcinoma)
    - Interconnecting cells with squamoid appearance with interspersed horn cysts, mucinous stroma
    - CK20(+) cells present

Generalized Basaloid Follicular Hamartoma Syndrome

- Reported in 1 large North Carolina family
- Similarities to Gorlin syndrome
  - Palmoplantar pitting
- Distinguishing features from Gorlin syndrome
  - No basal cell carcinomas
  - No jaw cysts
  - Multiple basaloid follicular hamartomas
    - Depicted in this syndrome as buds of basaloid islands arranged around 1 follicle or small cystic structure

Hereditary Infundibulocystic Basal Cell Carcinoma

- Distinguishing features from Gorlin syndrome
  - Multiple small papules on central face
  - Absence of palmar pits
  - No jaw cysts
  - Histopathology shows infundibulocystic basal cell carcinoma
    - Squamoid, ramifying appearance superficially, often with more typical nodular basal cell carcinoma at base

Other Syndromes With Basal Cell Carcinoma

- Defective DNA repair syndromes (e.g., xeroderma pigmentosum)

CRITERIA FOR DIAGNOSIS

Major Criteria

- Basal cell carcinoma
  - 1 if patient < 20 years of age
  - 2 or more if patient > 20 years of age
- Palmoplantar pitting
  - 3 or more
- Odontogenic keratocyst
  - Patient age: < 20 years
- Calcification of falx cerebri
  - Sometimes the tentorium cerebelli or sella turcica
  - Patient age: < 20 years
- Family history of Gorlin syndrome
- Medulloblastoma (primitive neuroectodermal tumor)
  - Patient age: ≤ 2 years

Minor Criteria

- Tumors
  - Cardiac fibroma
  - Ovarian fibroma
  - Lymphomesenteric cysts
- Skeletal/developmental abnormalities
  - Bifid/fused/splayed/missing rib
  - Bifid/wedged/fused vertebra, kyphoscoliosis
  - Short 4th metacarpal, postaxial polydactyly
  - Macrocephaly
  - Cleft lip/palate
- Ocular abnormalities
  - Strabismus
  - Congenital cataract
  - Hypertelorism
  - Glaucoma
  - Coloboma

Number of Criteria Needed

- 2 major, **or**
- 1 major and 2 minor, **or**
- 1 major and molecular confirmation

SELECTED REFERENCES

1. Sartip K et al: Neuroimaging of nevoid basal cell carcinoma syndrome (NBCCS) in children. Pediatr Radiol. 43(5):620-7, 2013
2. Abuzahra F et al: Multiple familial and pigmented basal cell carcinomas in early childhood - Bazex-Dupré-Christol syndrome. J Eur Acad Dermatol Venereol. 26(1):117-21, 2012
3. Castori M et al: Genetic skin diseases predisposing to basal cell carcinoma. Eur J Dermatol. 22(3):299-309, 2012
4. Bree AF et al: Consensus statement from the first international colloquium on basal cell nevus syndrome (BCNS). Am J Med Genet A. 155A(9):2091-7, 2011
5. Parren LJ et al: Hereditary tumour syndromes featuring basal cell carcinomas. Br J Dermatol. 165(1):30-4, 2011
6. Tom WL et al: Features of basal cell carcinomas in basal cell nevus syndrome. Am J Med Genet A. 155A(9):2098-104, 2011
7. Tiodorovic-Zivkovic D et al: Clinical and dermatoscopic findings in Bazex-Dupré-Christol and Gorlin-Goltz syndromes. J Am Acad Dermatol. 63(4):722-4, 2010
8. Wheeler CE Jr et al: Autosomal dominantly inherited generalized basaloid follicular hamartoma syndrome: report of a new disease in a North Carolina family. J Am Acad Dermatol. 43(2 Pt 1):189-206, 2000
9. Requena L et al: Multiple hereditary infundibulocystic basal cell carcinomas: a genodermatosis different from nevoid basal cell carcinoma syndrome. Arch Dermatol. 135(10):1227-35, 1999
10. Hahn H et al: Mutations of the human homolog of Drosophila patched in the nevoid basal cell carcinoma syndrome. Cell. 85(6):841-51, 1996
11. Shanley S et al: Nevoid basal cell carcinoma syndrome: review of 118 affected individuals. Am J Med Genet. 50(3):282-90, 1994
12. Evans DG et al: Complications of the naevoid basal cell carcinoma syndrome: results of a population based study. J Med Genet. 30(6):460-4, 1993
13. Brownstein MH: Basaloid follicular hamartoma: solitary and multiple types. J Am Acad Dermatol. 27(2 Pt 1):237-40, 1992
14. Michaëlsson G et al: The Rombo syndrome: a familial disorder with vermiculate atrophoderma, milia, hypotrichosis, trichoepitheliomas, basal cell carcinomas and peripheral vasodilation with cyanosis. Acta Derm Venereol. 61(6):497-503, 1981

Graphic, Clinical, Imaging, and Microscopic Features

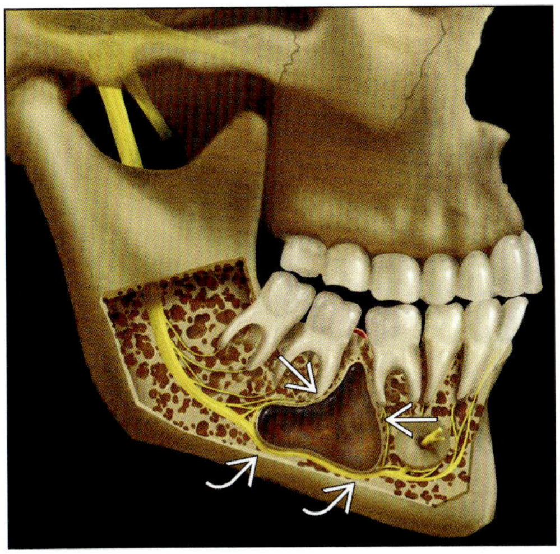

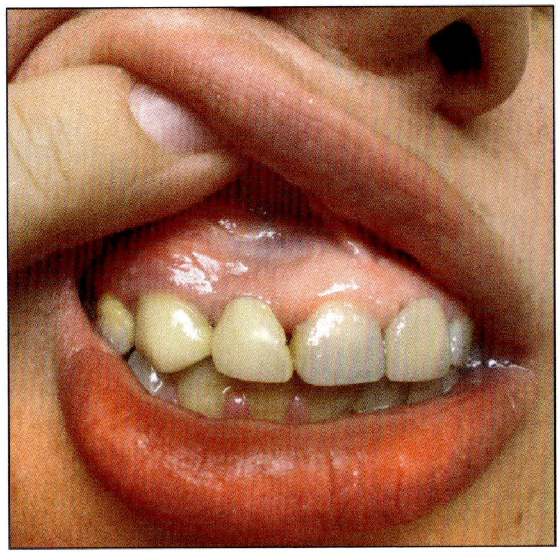

(Left) *Lateral graphic of the mandible (buccal cortex removed) illustrates features of a classic keratocystic odontogenic tumor , splaying roots of the 1st and 2nd molar teeth, displacing the inferior alveolar nerve .* ***(Right)*** *This patient with Gorlin syndrome had multiple basal cell carcinomas of the skin as well as several odontogenic jaw cysts. The photograph shows a scar from where 1 of the jaw cysts was surgically excised. (Courtesy K. Hoffmann, MD.)*

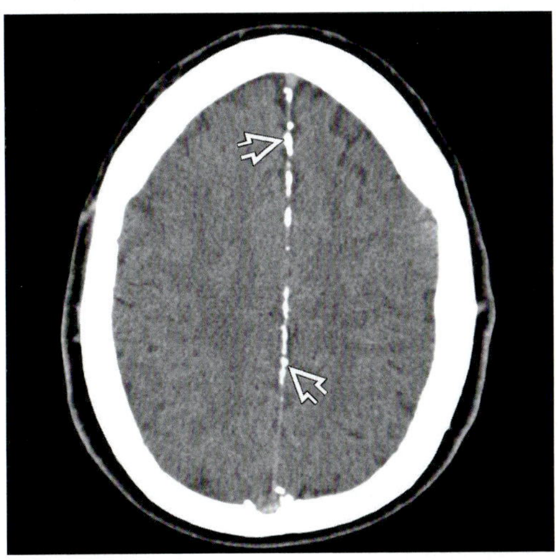

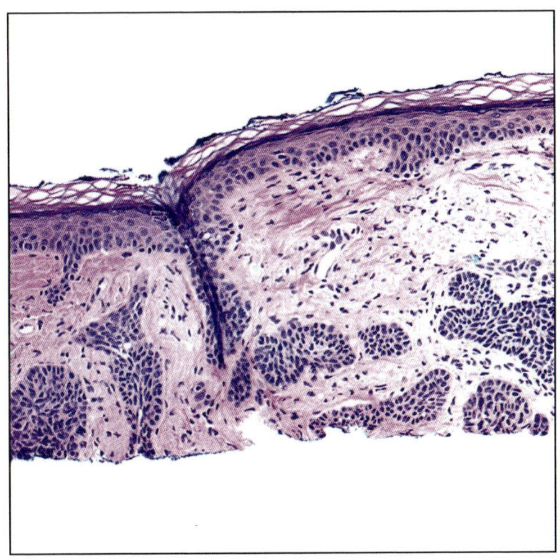

(Left) *Axial nonenhanced CT shows beaded calcification of the falx cerebri . Basal cell nevus syndrome should be suspected when multiple jaw cysts &/or precocious dural calcification is detected. Dural calcification is unusual in patients < 10 years of age.* ***(Right)*** *This is a typical basal cell carcinoma, with islands of basaloid epithelium that have peripheral palisading situated in a myxoid stroma.*

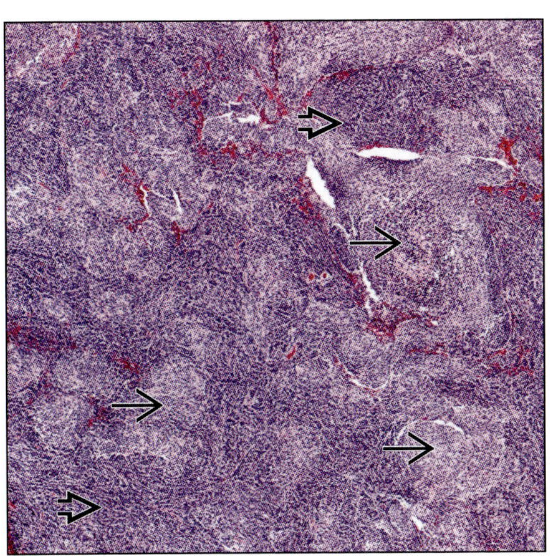

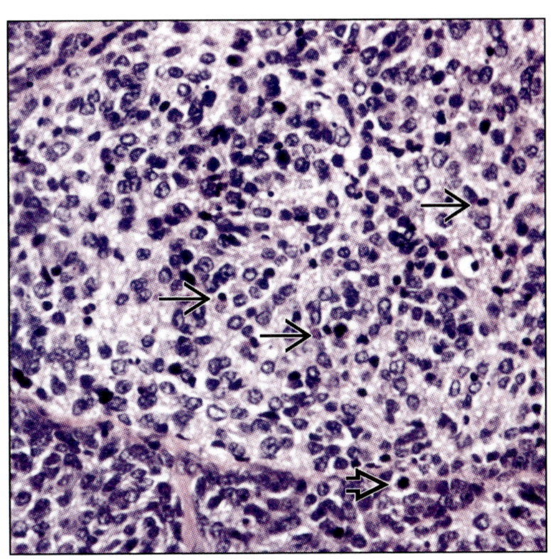

(Left) *H&E shows a low-power view of nodular/desmoplastic medulloblastoma with hypocellular nodules against a background of increased cellularity , giving the appearance of "pale islands." (Courtesy A. Polydorides, MD, PhD.)* ***(Right)*** *This high-power view of nodular/desmoplastic medulloblastoma shows prominent apoptoses within nodules, mitoses , and occasional cytologic atypia within extranodular areas. (Courtesy A. Polydorides, MD, PhD.)*

BECKWITH-WIEDEMANN SYNDROME

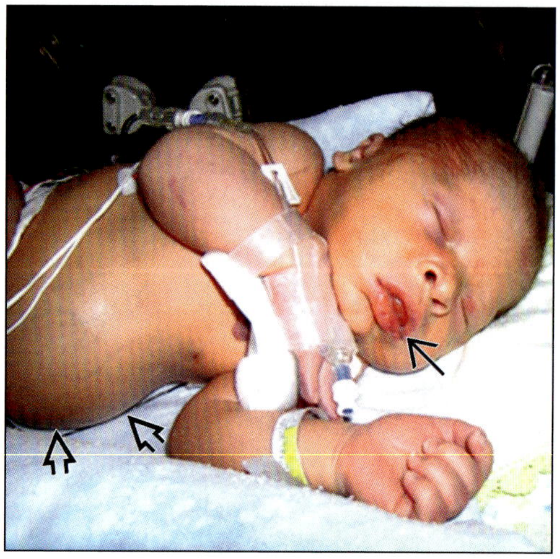

A term infant with Beckwith-Wiedemann syndrome has a protuberant abdomen ⇨, secondary to enlarged liver and kidneys, and a large mouth with macroglossia →. (Courtesy J. Byrne, MD.)

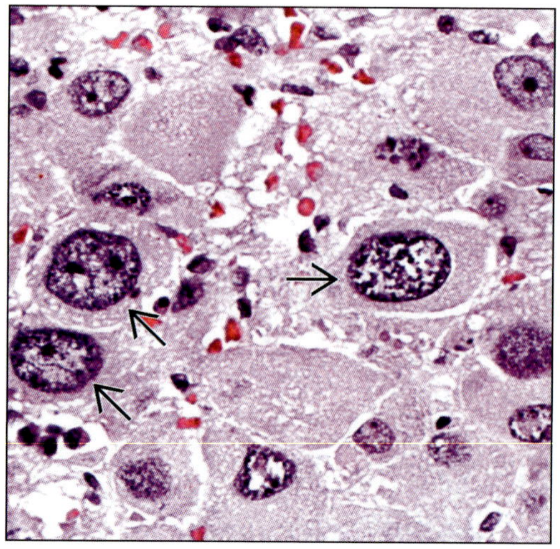

Photomicrograph shows adrenal cortical cytomegaly, a characteristic finding in Beckwith-Wiedemann syndrome. There are large polyhedral cells with hyperchromatic nuclei →. (Courtesy E. Klatt, MD.)

TERMINOLOGY

Abbreviations
- Beckwith-Wiedemann syndrome (BWS)

Synonyms
- Wiedemann-Beckwith syndrome

Definitions
- Disorder of growth regulation
- Predisposition to embryonal tumors

EPIDEMIOLOGY

Incidence
- ~ 1 in 14,000

Gender
- M:F = 1:1
  - Exception is monozygotic twins
    - F:M = 3:1

Ethnicity Relationship
- All ethnicities

Age Range
- Increased growth
  - In utero
  - 1st few years of life
- Associated malignancies
  - Generally present by 8 years

Other
- Associated with assisted reproduction
  - Risk is 1 in 4,000 for in vitro fertilization

CLINICAL IMPLICATIONS

Clinical Presentation
- Highly variable presentation
  - Ranges from mild to severe
- Somatic overgrowth
  - Classic triad
    - Exomphalos
    - Gigantism
    - Macroglossia (can cause abnormal feeding/breathing/speech)
  - Initial increased growth
    - In utero
    - Through 1st few years of life
    - Height and weight are often above 90th percentile for age in initial years of life
    - Normalizes by childhood
  - Overgrowth may be unilateral (hemihyperplasia)
  - Visceromegaly can involve
    - Liver
    - Spleen
    - Pancreas
    - Adrenals
    - Kidneys: May be associated with renal medullary dysplasia, nephrocalcinosis, or medullary sponge kidney
    - Heart
- Characteristic facies in early childhood (often normal by adulthood)
  - Prominent eyes
  - Midfacial hypoplasia
  - Macroglossia
  - Prominent mandible
  - Anterior earlobe creases
  - Posterior helical pits
  - Nevus flammeus may be present
- Abdominal wall defects
  - Umbilical hernia
  - Omphalocele

- Diastasis recti

Clinical Risk Factors

- Pathologic factors and risk
  - Associated with assisted reproduction
- Prognostic factors and risk
  - Worse prognosis with perinatal hypoglycemia
    - Hypoglycemia in 30-50% of BWS
  - Higher risk of tumor development with
    - Hemihyperplasia
    - Nephromegaly
    - Nephrogenic rests
- Risk of malignancy
  - Estimated at 7.5%
  - Range: 4-21%

Imaging Findings

- Ultrasonographic findings
  - Ultrasound can also detect large kidneys, large abdominal circumference, omphalocele, and polyhydramnios from obstructed swallowing
  - 3D/4D ultrasound can delineate facial features in utero; protuberant tongue or hepatomegaly may be detected

GENETICS

Inheritance

- Sporadic in ~ 85%
- Familial in ~ 15%
  - Heterogeneous transmission
    - Sometimes autosomal dominant maternal transmission

Molecular Pathology

- Involves chromosome 11p15.5 in ~ 80% of cases
  - *IGF2* and *KCNQ1OT1* are normally expressed from paternal allele
    - *KCNQ1OT1*-associated imprinting center (IC2) is usually methylated on maternal allele
  - *H19*, *CDKN1C*, and *KCNQ1* are normally expressed from maternal allele
    - *H19*-associated imprinting center (IC1) is usually methylated on paternal allele
- Different molecular pathology is associated with different clinical phenotypes
  - Epigenetic
    - Altered methylation: Loss of methylation at IC2 occurs in 50%; gain of methylation occurs at IC1 in 10%
    - Loss of methylation at IC2 is associated with decreased risk of renal findings compared with gain of methylation at IC1
  - Genetic
    - Microdeletion
    - *CDKN1C* mutation
    - Uniparental disomy of 11p15.5 (~ 10-20% of cases; usually paternal allele) is associated with high risk of Wilms tumor
    - Duplication, inversion, translocation of 11p15 in < 1% of cases

ASSOCIATED NEOPLASMS

Embryonal Tumors/Malignancies

- Wilms tumor (nephroblastoma)
  - ~ 60% of all tumors in BWS
  - Histopathology: Often characterized by 3 elements
    - Blastema (embryological structure related to kidney development)
    - Mesenchyme (may be composed of striated muscle, bone, cartilage, fat, fibroblastic tissue)
    - Epithelium
- Adrenal cytomegaly
  - Hyperplastic adrenal glands
  - Characteristic cytology
    - Large, polyhedral cells with eosinophilic granular cytoplasm and enlarged nuclei
- Adrenal cortical carcinoma
  - Cells with eosinophilic cytoplasm
  - Often with numerous mitoses and invasive growth pattern
- Hepatoblastoma
  - High levels of α-fetoprotein (100,000-300,000 μg/mL)
  - Different histologic variants
    - Epithelial (fetal pattern)
    - Embryonal and fetal pattern
    - Macrotrabecular pattern
    - Small cell undifferentiated pattern
    - Mixed epithelial and mesenchymal pattern ± teratoid features
- Rhabdomyosarcoma
  - Subtypes reported
    - Embryonal: Dense foci of rhabdomyoblasts with areas of loose, myxoid stroma
    - Alveolar: Small blue cells in aggregates floating in spaces lined by fibrous septae
- Neuroblastoma
  - Round blue cells, sometimes forming rosettes

CANCER RISK MANAGEMENT

Tumor Surveillance Protocol

- Abdominal ultrasound
  - Every 3-4 months
  - Until age 8
- α-fetoprotein assay
  - Every 3-4 months
  - Until age 4

DIFFERENTIAL DIAGNOSIS

Maternal Diabetes Mellitus

- Can cause macrosomia in fetus
- May be associated with polyhydramnios
- Omphalocele is uncommon

Isolated Hemihyperplasia

- May be associated with Wilms tumor &/or alterations on 11p15
- Diagnosis of exclusion

BECKWITH-WIEDEMANN SYNDROME

Isolated Omphalocele
- May be associated with normal growth or growth restriction

Simpson-Golabi-Behmel Syndrome
- X-linked recessive
- Mutations in *GPC3* or *CXORF5*
- High mortality in infancy
- Macrocephaly, coarse face, macroglossia, polydactyly, heart defects
- Increased risk of tumors
  - Wilms tumor
  - Hepatoblastoma
  - Neuroblastoma
  - Gonadoblastoma
  - Hepatocellular carcinoma

Sotos Syndrome
- Autosomal dominant, mutation in *NSD1*
- Overgrowth, advanced bone age, mental retardation
- Characteristic facies
  - High forehead
  - Inverted pear-shaped head
  - Sparse frontal hair
  - Pointed chin
- Cardiac/renal anomalies
- Increased risk of tumors
  - Examples
    - Teratoma
    - Neuroblastoma
    - Acute lymphoblastic leukemia
    - Wilms tumor

Perlman Syndrome
- Autosomal recessive
- Mutation in *DIS3L2*
- Similarities to BWS
  - Macroglossia
  - Overgrowth
  - Neonatal hypoglycemia

Hemihypoplasia
- Underdevelopment of 1 side of body
  - Relative to underdeveloped side, normal side may be misdiagnosed as being hyperplastic

Syndromic Wilms Tumor
- Syndromes related to *WT1* mutation
  - Examples
    - WAGR (Wilms tumor, aniridia, genitourinary anomalies, mental retardation) syndrome
    - Denys-Drash syndrome (gonadal dysgenesis, nephropathy, Wilms tumor)
    - Frasier syndrome (pseudohermaphroditism, glomerulonephropathy, gonadoblastoma, rarely Wilms tumor)
    - Genitourinary anomalies syndrome (abnormal external genitalia, Wilms tumor)

Nonsyndromic Wilms Tumor
- Wilms tumor not associated with any syndrome (e.g., BWS, WAGR syndrome, Denys-Drash syndrome, Frasier syndrome)

CRITERIA FOR DIAGNOSIS

Major Findings
- Abdominal wall defects
  - Omphalocele
  - Umbilical hernia
- Macroglossia
- Macrosomia
  - Height to weight ratio > 97th percentile
- Anterior ear lobe creases &/or posterior helical pits
- Visceromegaly
- Embryonal tumor in childhood
- Hemihyperplasia
- Cytomegaly of adrenal fetal cortex, usually diffuse and bilateral
- Renal abnormalities
  - Medullary dysplasia
  - Abnormality of medullary sponge kidney
- Positive family history of BWS
- Cleft palate

Minor Findings
- Pregnancy-related findings
  - Polyhydramnios
  - Enlarged placenta
  - Thickened umbilical cord
  - Premature onset of labor/delivery
  - Preeclampsia
- Neonatal hypoglycemia
- Nevus flammeus
- Cardiomegaly/cardiomyopathy/other abnormalities
- Characteristic facies
- Diastasis recti
- Advanced bone age

Criteria Based on Findings
- 3 major or 1 minor + 2 major findings support BWS diagnosis

SELECTED REFERENCES

1. Chen CP: Prenatal findings and the genetic diagnosis of fetal overgrowth disorders: Simpson-Golabi-Behmel syndrome, Sotos syndrome, and Beckwith-Wiedemann syndrome. Taiwan J Obstet Gynecol. 51(2):186-91, 2012
2. Mussa A et al: Nephrological findings and genotype-phenotype correlation in Beckwith-Wiedemann syndrome. Pediatr Nephrol. 27(3):397-406, 2012
3. Weksberg R et al: Beckwith-Wiedemann syndrome. Eur J Hum Genet. 18(1):8-14, 2010
4. Wangler MF et al: Inheritance pattern of Beckwith-Wiedemann syndrome is heterogeneous in 291 families with an affected proband. Am J Med Genet A. 137(1):16-21, 2005
5. Halliday J et al: Beckwith-Wiedemann syndrome and IVF: a case-control study. Am J Hum Genet. 75(3):526-8, 2004
6. Smith AC et al: Association of alveolar rhabdomyosarcoma with the Beckwith-Wiedemann syndrome. Pediatr Dev Pathol. 4(6):550-8, 2001

Gross and Microscopic Features

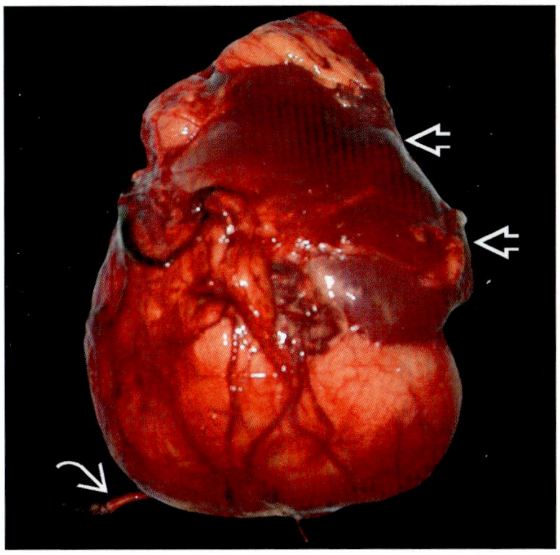

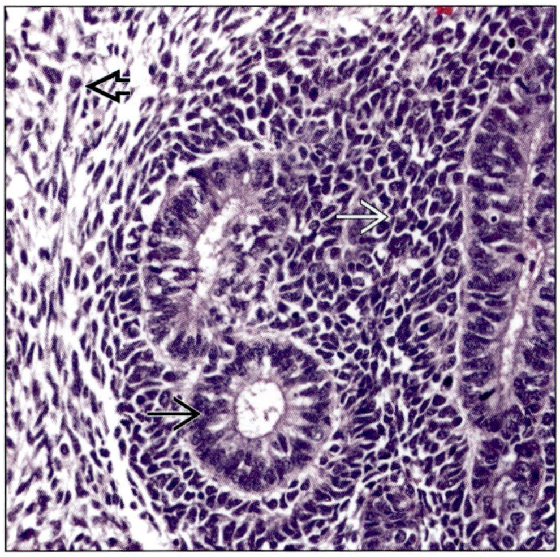

(Left) *Total nephrectomy specimen from a Beckwith-Wiedemann syndrome patient with Wilms tumor shows an area of relatively intact residual kidney* ➡ *and ureter* ➡*. Wilms tumors often weigh > 500 g. (Courtesy L. Erickson, PA.)* ***(Right)*** *Typical triphasic morphology of Wilms tumor is shown. Note the blastemal* ➡*, epithelial* ➡*, and stromal* ➡ *components. (Courtesy A. Putnam, MD.)*

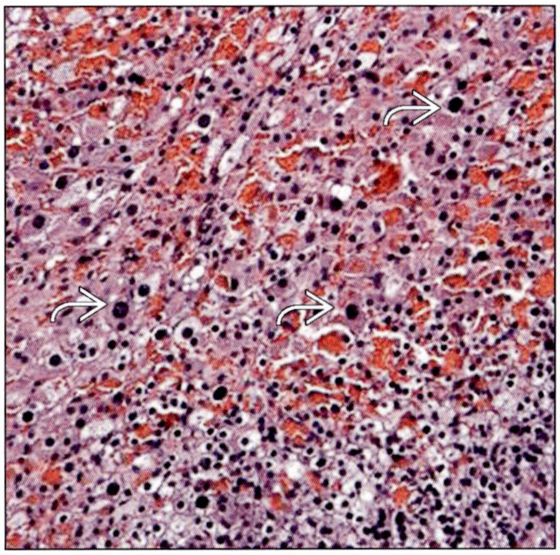

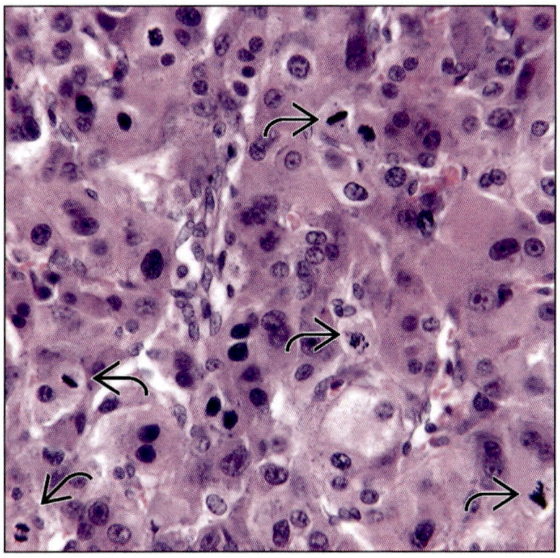

(Left) *Adrenal cortical cytomegaly is usually present in children with Beckwith-Wiedemann syndrome. The adrenal cortical cells are composed of a mixture of small cells and large polyhedral cells with markedly enlarged nuclei* ➡*.* ***(Right)*** *Adrenal cortical carcinoma in a child with Beckwith-Wiedemann syndrome shows that the tumor is composed of large cells with nuclear pleomorphism, prominent nucleoli, and numerous mitotic figures* ➡*.*

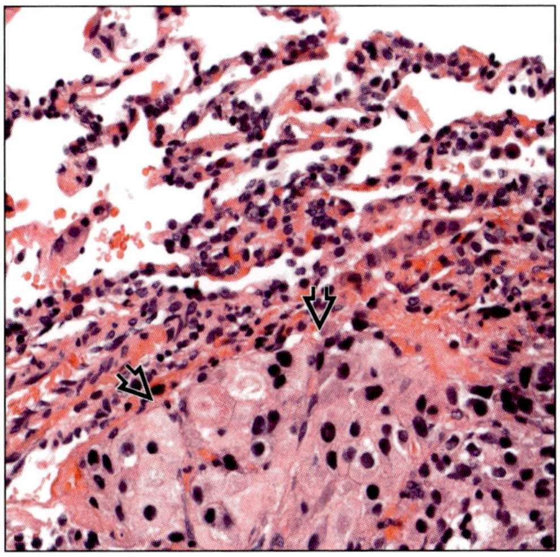

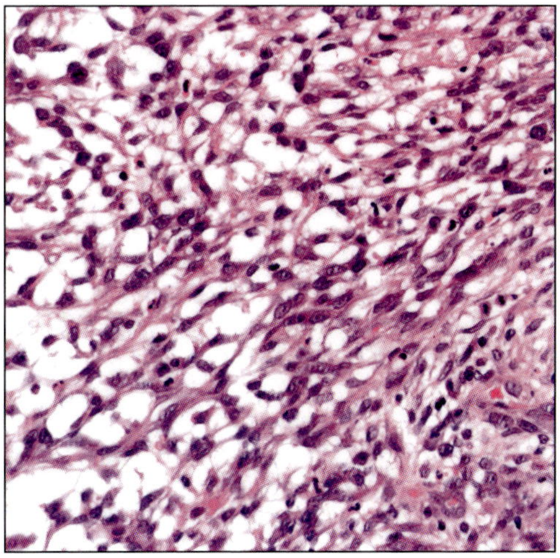

(Left) *This is a metastatic adrenal cortical carcinoma* ➡ *to the lung in a 6-month-old child with Beckwith-Wiedemann syndrome.* ***(Right)*** *The cells of this embryonal rhabdomyosarcoma have ovoid or spindled nuclei and moderate amounts of eosinophilic cytoplasm. Nuclear atypia is mild to moderate. The prominent myxoid stroma, a common feature, imparts a reticular or filigree pattern in this part of the tumor. (Courtesy C. Fisher, MD.)*

BIRT-HOGG-DUBÉ SYNDROME

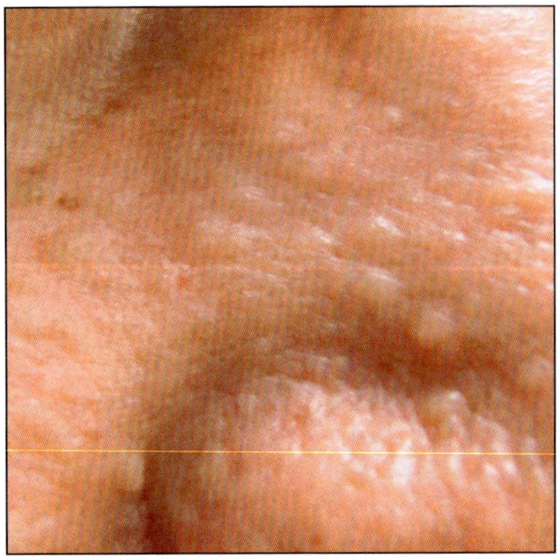

Smooth, skin-colored to slightly hypopigmented papules are seen on the cheek and nose in a patient with Birt-Hogg-Dubé syndrome. (Courtesy B. Goldberg, MD.)

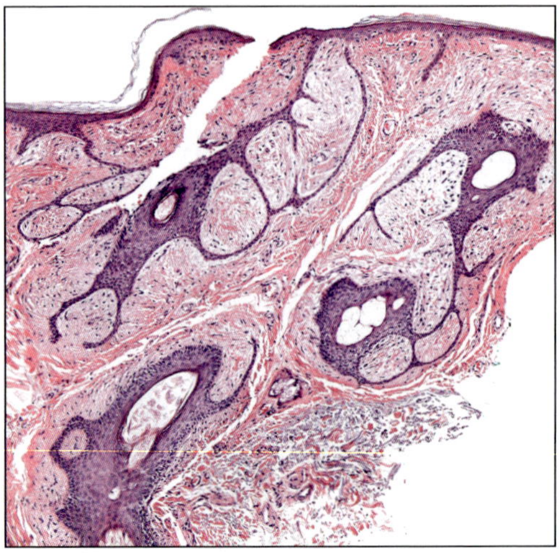

This fibrofolliculoma shows characteristic reticulated, lace-like, thin strands of epithelium extending away from hair follicles. The reticulated epithelium is embedded in a loose stroma.

TERMINOLOGY

Abbreviations

- Birt-Hogg-Dubé syndrome (BHDS)

Synonyms

- Hornstein-Knickerberg syndrome

EPIDEMIOLOGY

Age Range

- Cutaneous lesions tend to present after age 30
- Pulmonary cysts generally present by age 20
- Renal cell carcinoma generally occurs after age 50

GENETICS

Inheritance

- Autosomal dominant

Gene Defect

- Caused by mutations in gene coding for folliculin (*FLCN*)
  - *FLCN* mutation in ~ 85% of families with BHDS
  - Exact role of folliculin unknown
    - May be involved in WNT, mTOR, &/or AKT signaling
    - May have role in determining polarity in cilia

CLINICAL IMPLICATIONS AND ANCILLARY TESTS

Clinical Presentation

- Cutaneous
  - Papules
    - Multiple
    - Smooth
    - Skin-colored to white
    - Occur in adulthood
  - Sites
    - Face/ears
    - Neck
    - Sometimes upper trunk
  - In ~ 80% of adult patients with BHDS
- Pulmonary
  - Cysts
    - Rupture can lead to pneumothorax
  - In ~ 80% of adult patients with BHDS
  - Multiple cysts usually detectable on CT scan
    - Tend to affect middle and lower lobes toward mediastinum
    - Often intimately associated with interlobular septae or visceral pleura
- Renal tumors
  - Present in adulthood
  - In ~ 15-30% of patients with BHDS

Imaging Findings

- CT scan of chest
  - Pulmonary cysts
    - Middle lobe
    - Lower lobe
    - Associated with septae/pleura

ASSOCIATED NEOPLASMS

Cutaneous

- Fibrofolliculoma/trichodiscoma
  - Most experts now consider fibrofolliculoma and trichodiscoma a histologic spectrum of the same entity
    - On step sectioning, most tumors showing features of trichodiscoma have foci compatible with fibrofolliculoma
  - Fibrofolliculoma (as originally described)

- Interconnecting epithelial strands, forming lace-like patterns, extending from hair follicles
- Epithelial strands embedded in loose stroma

○ Trichodiscoma (as originally described)
- Loose stroma
- Often with hair follicle at 1 border

- Skin tag (acrochordon)
  - Some (but not all) skin tags in BHDS have microscopic features of fibrofolliculoma/trichodiscoma on step sectioning
- Perifollicular fibroma
  - Some experts consider perifollicular fibroma equivalent to angiofibroma or fibrofolliculoma/trichodiscoma
    - Supported by microscopic findings of perifollicular fibroma and fibrofolliculoma in same tumor
  - Formerly associated with Hornstein-Knickenberg syndrome
    - Perifollicular fibromas and GI polyps
    - Currently, this syndrome considered synonymous with BHDS
- Angiofibroma
  - Histopathology
    - Stellate fibroblasts
    - Fibrotic stroma
    - Sometimes with concentric fibrosis around vessels/follicles
- Rare reports of
  - Lipoma
  - Leiomyoma
  - Dermatofibrosarcoma protuberans
  - Leiomyosarcoma
  - Malignant melanoma

Renal

- Renal cell carcinoma
  - Previously, chromophobe or oncocytic subtypes considered overrepresented in BHDS
  - Recent studies suggest that any histologic subtype is possible
  - Risk of development is 15% by age 70
- Renal cysts

Pulmonary

- Pulmonary cysts
  - Rupture can lead to (recurrent) pneumothorax in ~ 30% of patients
    - When ruptured, may be misdiagnosed as blebs or bullae or other cystic air space disease
  - When intact
    - Cysts lined by friable, cuboidal, nonatypical pneumocytes
    - Pneumocytes resemble type II pneumocytes
  - Cyst wall may connect to
    - Interlobular septae
    - Pleura

Thyroid

- Nodules
- Cysts
- Carcinoma

Colorectal

- Some families may be at increased risk of colon carcinoma

Parotid

- Oncocytoma

Rarely Reported Neoplasms

- Squamous cell carcinoma of head/neck
- Hodgkin disease
- Uterine cancer
- Prostate cancer
- Breast cancer
- Squamous cell carcinoma of cervix
- Rhabdomyoma
- Adrenal mass

CANCER RISK MANAGEMENT

Renal Cell Carcinoma

- Some experts recommend screening with annual MR
  - From age 20
- Annual ultrasound is alternative to MR

Colorectal Carcinoma

- Colonoscopy
  - Especially in families in which colon cancer seems overrepresented

DIFFERENTIAL DIAGNOSIS

Familial Multiple Discoid Fibromas

- Facial/ear papules
  - Multiple
  - Variable size
  - With surface telangiectasias
  - Histopathology
    - Features similar to trichodiscoma
    - No evidence of interconnecting epithelial strands
    - Some authors suggest the term "discoid fibroma" to avoid confusion with trichodiscoma and BHDS
- Age
  - Facial/ear papules develop in childhood
- No association with renal carcinoma
- Very low risk of pneumothorax
- Genetics
  - Absence of *FLCN* mutation
  - Mutations in folliculin-interacting protein 1 (*FNIP1*)
  - Autosomal dominant inheritance

Tuberous Sclerosis

- Facial papules
  - Tendency to cluster on central face
  - Multiple
  - Pink-red to skin colored
  - Histopathology
    - Angiofibroma/fibrous papule
- Other skin findings
  - Hypomelanotic macules
  - "Confetti" macules
  - Periungual fibromas

- Shagreen patch (connective tissue nevus)
- Other associated neoplasms
  - Brain
    - Cortical tubers
    - Subependymal nodules
    - Subependymal giant cell astrocytoma
  - Retina
    - Hamartomas
    - Achromic patch
  - Renal
    - Angiomyolipoma
    - Cysts
  - Cardiac rhabdomyoma
  - Pulmonary lymphangioleiomyomatosis
  - Hamartomatous rectal polyps
- Genetics
  - *TSC1* and *TSC2* mutations
    - Encode hamartin and tuberin, part of mTOR pathway
  - Autosomal dominant inheritance

Cowden Syndrome

- Facial/ear papules
  - Multiple
  - Verrucous to smooth
  - Skin colored to pink-yellow
  - Histopathology
    - Trichilemmoma: Lobules of pale cells bordered by peripheral palisading and thickened basement membrane
- Oral papillomatosis
- Acral keratoses
- Other skin lesions include tumor of the follicular infundibulum, sclerotic fibroma
- Other associated neoplasms
  - Breast carcinoma
  - Thyroid carcinoma
- Genetics
  - *PTEN* mutation
  - Autosomal dominant inheritance

Brooke-Spiegler Syndrome

- Autosomal dominant inheritance
- *CYLD* mutation
- Multiple trichoepitheliomas, spiradenomas, cylindromas

Lymphangioleiomyomatosis

- Can lead to recurrent pneumothorax
- Renal angiomyolipomas
- Tends to affect women

Pulmonary Endometriosis

- Women
- Median age: 36 years
- Often present with pleural pain, shortness of breath
- Sometimes with history of pelvic endometriosis
- Histopathology
  - Proliferative or secretory endometrium

DIAGNOSIS

Criteria

- Patients should fulfill 1 major or 2 minor criteria for diagnosis
- Major criteria
  - At least 5 fibrofolliculomas/trichodiscomas
    - At least 1 histologically confirmed
    - Adult-onset
  - *FLCN* mutation
- Minor criteria
  - Multiple lung cysts
    - Bilateral
    - Basal location
    - No other apparent cause
    - ± spontaneous pneumothorax
  - Renal cell carcinoma
    - Early onset (< age 50)
    - **Or** multifocal/bilateral carcinoma
    - **Or** mixed chromophobe/oncocytic histology
  - 1st-degree relative with BHDS

SELECTED REFERENCES

1. Furuya M et al: Birt-Hogg-Dube syndrome: clinicopathological features of the lung. J Clin Pathol. 66(3):178-86, 2013
2. The Fourth Birt-Hogg-Dubé Symposium, Cincinnati, USA, 28(th)-30 (th) March, 2012. Fam Cancer. 12(1):133-40, 2013
3. Vernooij M et al: Birt-Hogg-Dubé syndrome and the skin. Fam Cancer. Epub ahead of print, 2013
4. Happle R: Hornstein-Birt-Hogg-Dubé syndrome: a renaming and reconsideration. Am J Med Genet A. 158A(6):1247-51, 2012
5. Shvartsbeyn M et al: Perifollicular fibroma in Birt-Hogg-Dubé syndrome: an association revisited. J Cutan Pathol. 39(7):675-9, 2012
6. Tobino K et al: Differentiation between Birt-Hogg-Dubé syndrome and lymphangioleiomyomatosis: quantitative analysis of pulmonary cysts on computed tomography of the chest in 66 females. Eur J Radiol. 81(6):1340-6, 2012
7. Agarwal PP et al: Thoracic CT findings in Birt-Hogg-Dube syndrome. AJR Am J Roentgenol. 196(2):349-52, 2011
8. Houweling AC et al: Renal cancer and pneumothorax risk in Birt-Hogg-Dubé syndrome; an analysis of 115 FLCN mutation carriers from 35 BHD families. Br J Cancer. 105(12):1912-9, 2011
9. Kluger N et al: Birt-Hogg-Dubé syndrome: clinical and genetic studies of 10 French families. Br J Dermatol. 162(3):527-37, 2010
10. Menko FH et al: Birt-Hogg-Dubé syndrome: diagnosis and management. Lancet Oncol. 10(12):1199-206, 2009
11. Misago N et al: Fibrofolliculoma/trichodiscoma and fibrous papule (perifollicular fibroma/angiofibroma): a revaluation of the histopathological and immunohistochemical features. J Cutan Pathol. 36(9):943-51, 2009
12. Leter EM et al: Birt-Hogg-Dubé syndrome: clinical and genetic studies of 20 families. J Invest Dermatol. 128(1):45-9, 2008
13. Toro JR et al: BHD mutations, clinical and molecular genetic investigations of Birt-Hogg-Dubé syndrome: a new series of 50 families and a review of published reports. J Med Genet. 45(6):321-31, 2008

Gross and Microscopic Features

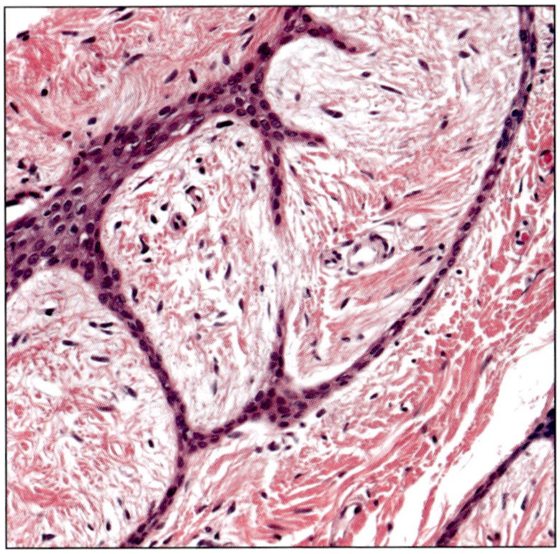

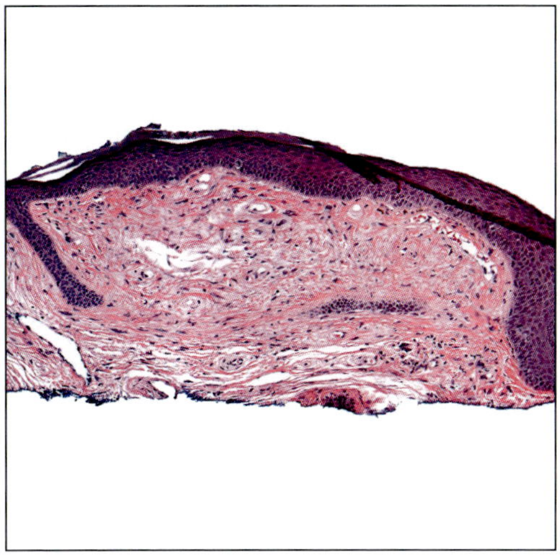

(Left) *This is a high-magnification view of a typical fibrofolliculoma, with a loose stroma in which there are reticulated, thin strands of epithelium.* ***(Right)*** *This lesion, previously termed trichodiscoma, has the same loose stroma as fibrofolliculoma, but absent reticulated strands of epithelium, often with a hair follicle bordering the loose stroma. On step sections, reticulated epithelium is often present, evidence that fibrofolliculoma and trichodiscoma are the same lesion.*

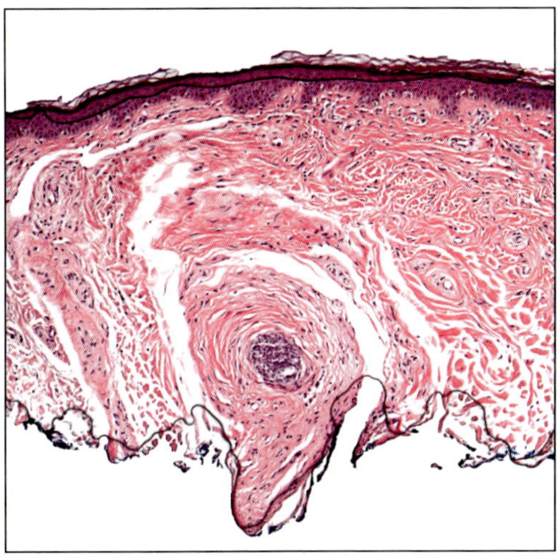

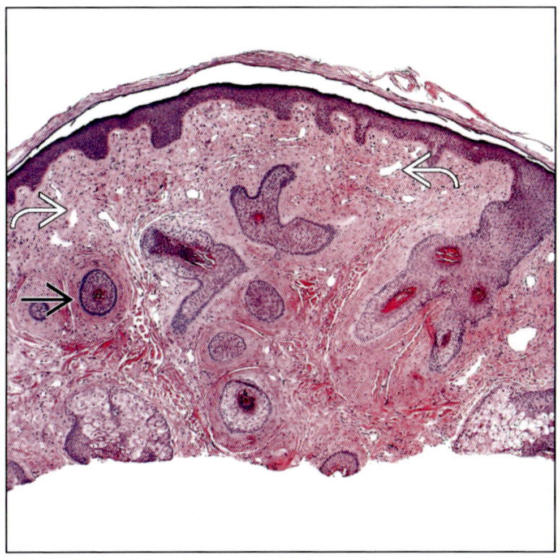

(Left) *This perifollicular fibroma (PFF) has the same loose stroma as in fibrofolliculoma/trichodiscoma. The stroma is concentric around hair follicle epithelium, with clefting from the surrounding normal dermis. On step sections, some PFFs show changes of fibrofolliculoma, suggesting they are related lesions.* ***(Right)*** *Angiofibroma (fibrous papule) has ectatic thin-walled vessels ➔ and dense collagenous stroma; there may be perifollicular fibrosis →. (Courtesy S. Billings, MD.)*

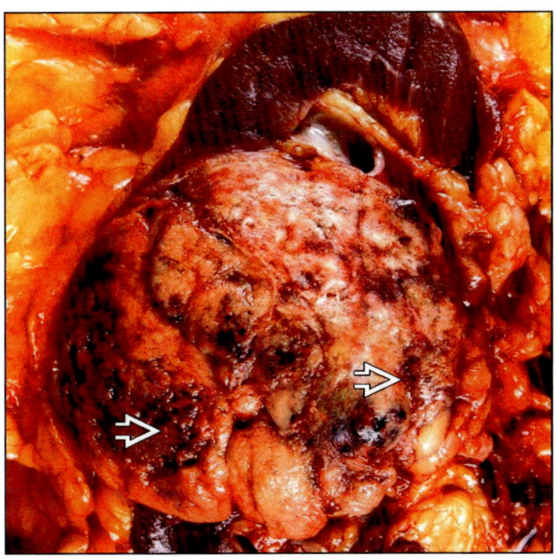

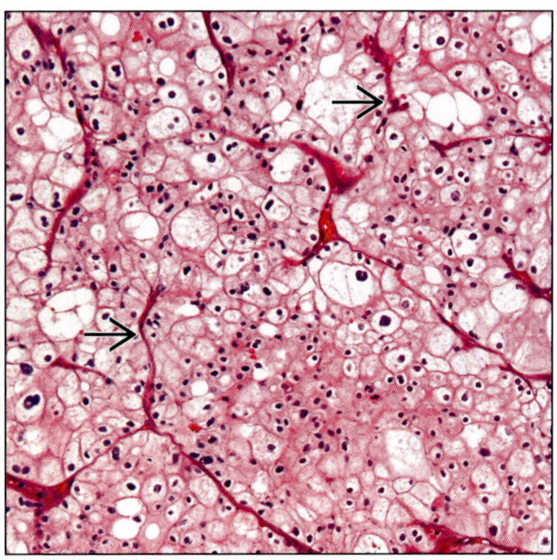

(Left) *Chromophobe renal cell carcinoma is typically well circumscribed, with a tan-gray, multilobulated cut surface. Hemorrhage and necrosis ➔ are grossly identified in > 1/4 of cases. (Courtesy S. Tickoo, MD.)* ***(Right)*** *Typically, a chromophobe renal cell carcinoma shows solid sheets of clear and eosinophilic cells, separated by thin and incomplete vascular septations → that do not completely encircle cell nests. (Courtesy S. Tickoo, MD.)*

BLOOM SYNDROME

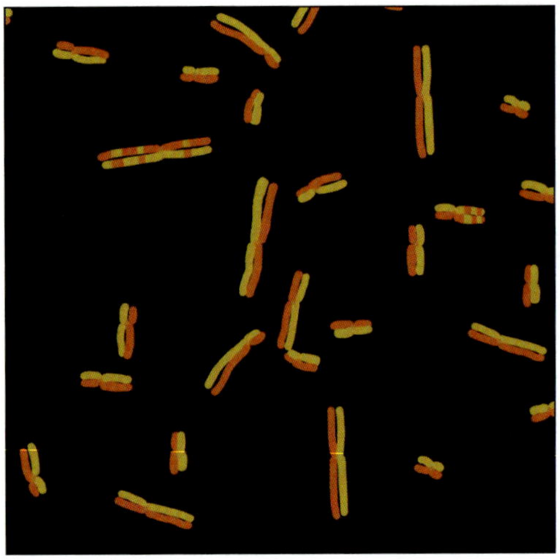

This image depicts the results of sister chromatid exchange (SCE) analysis performed on cells from an unaffected patient. Note that only a few SCEs are present in this control patient.

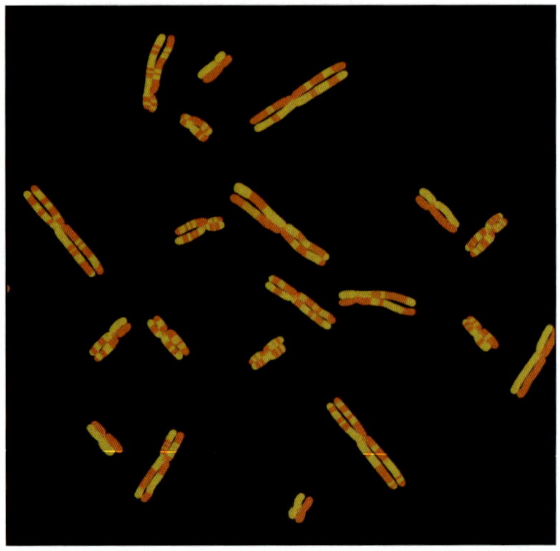

This image depicts the results of SCE analysis performed on cells from a Bloom syndrome patient. Note the markedly increased number of SCEs.

TERMINOLOGY

Abbreviations

- Bloom syndrome (BSyn)

Synonyms

- Bloom-Torre-Machacek syndrome
- Congenital telangiectatic erythema

Definition

- Rare autosomal recessive disorder resulting from mutations in the *BLM* gene; 1st described by dermatologist Dr. David Bloom in 1954

EPIDEMIOLOGY

Incidence

- Exceedingly rare (265 reported cases from 222 families in the Bloom Syndrome Registry as of 2009)
- Parental consanguinity common
- Cases have been described in North and South America, Europe, Asia, Africa, and Australia
- ~ 1/4 of people with BSyn are of Jewish descent, particularly Central and Eastern European (Ashkenazi) Jewish background
  - Seen in 1 in 48,000 live births in this population
- ~ 3/4 of people with BSyn are of non-Jewish background
  - Founder mutations have been described in many human populations, including
    - Japanese
    - European (Italian, Portuguese)
    - Brazilian
    - North American (including Spanish American)

ETIOLOGY/PATHOGENESIS

Molecular Pathogenesis

- Caused by biallelic mutations in the *BLM* gene, located at 15q26.1 (most commonly homozygous; less frequently compound heterozygous)
  - Described mutations include missense, nonsense, insertions/deletions, and splicing defects due to intron mutations
- *BLM* is a tumor-suppressor gene and belongs to family of RecQ DNA helicases
  - RecQ helicases are important for repair of DNA damage
  - Protein product (BLM) permits unwinding of DNA in order to resolve disruptive structures that have developed during replication
  - Mutations in other RecQ helicase genes result in additional DNA repair deficiency syndromes
    - Werner syndrome (*WRN* gene on chromosome 8)
    - Rothmund-Thomson syndrome (*RECQL4* gene on chromosome 8)

Immunodeficiency

- Pathogenesis of immunodeficiency is not well characterized
  - Hypogammaglobulinemia
  - Decreased or absent delayed hypersensitivity
  - Abnormal functioning of $\alpha\beta$ T cells

CLINICAL FEATURES

Consistent Features

- Short stature and microcephaly due to growth retardation, pre- and postnatal, otherwise normal proportions
- Paucity of subcutaneous fat in infancy and childhood
- High predisposition to hematolymphoid and epithelial neoplasms

Variable Features
- Photosensitivity with development of erythema or telangiectasias in sun-exposed areas
- Patchy areas of hyper- and hypopigmentation
- Characteristic facies (long, narrow face with malar hypoplasia, small mandible, and prominent nose)
- Affected males experience infertility and affected females undergo early menopause
- Average intelligence; some patients with learning disabilities
- High-pitched voice
- Diarrhea and vomiting at an early age
- Immunodeficiency leading to recurrent infections
- Increased risk of chronic obstructive lung disease and diabetes mellitus (adult-onset type)

ANCILLARY TESTS

Confirmation of Diagnosis
- Cytogenetic testing
  - Diagnostic test: Evaluation for increased number of sister chromatid exchanges (SCE) in any cell (typically peripheral blood lymphocytes)
    - Cells are cultured for 2 cell cycles in a medium containing bromodeoxyuridine (BrDu) and arrested at metaphase
    - Upon fluorescence-plus-Giemsa coloration, differential staining of the 2 sister chromatids is apparent (1 appears dark, 1 appears light)
    - In BSyn, sister chromatids show an increased number of exchanges (at least 10x increase compared to control)
  - Increase in random chromosome breakage seen on metaphase spread including chromatid gaps, breaks and rearrangements, chromatid interchange configurations such as quadriradial interchange configuration, telomeric associations, anaphase bridges, and lagging chromosomal fragments
- Molecular testing
  - Targeted mutation analysis (e.g., evaluation for blmAsh [c.2207_2212del6ins7] in patients of Ashkenazi Jewish descent)
  - Sequence analysis of entire coding region
  - Deletion/duplication analysis

Prenatal Testing
- Can be performed via SCE analysis or by specific mutation testing if familial mutation is known (chorionic villous sampling or amniocentesis)

ASSOCIATED NEOPLASMS

Increased Cancer Risk
- Up to 50% of patients with BSyn will develop a malignancy
  - ~ 10% have ≥ 2 primary cancers, with fewer numbers reported to have 3, 4, or even 5 primary neoplasms
- Mean age of cancer diagnosis: ~ 24 years
- Hematolymphoid malignancies predominant in first 2 decades of life
- Carcinomas predominant after first 2 decades of life
- Increased cancer incidence shortens overall lifespan

Hematolymphoid Malignancies
- Leukemia (both acute myeloid leukemia and acute lymphoblastic leukemia)
  - There may be preferential occurrence of monosomy 7 (-7) and deletion of long arm of chromosome 7 (del[7q]) in myelodysplastic syndrome/acute myeloid leukemia in BSyn patients
- Lymphoma (predominantly non-Hodgkin lymphoma, less frequently Hodgkin lymphoma)

Carcinomas
- Arise in varied sites including skin, head, neck, lung, uterus, breast, and gastrointestinal tract (including esophagus [both squamous cell carcinoma and adenocarcinoma], stomach, and colon)

Rare Tumor Types
- Medulloblastoma, Wilms tumor, osteogenic sarcoma

Carriers
- *BLM* mutation carriers do not have an increased cancer risk

CANCER RISK MANAGEMENT

Patients With BSyn
- Markedly increased risk of a variety of malignancies, which occur earlier compared to general population, necessitates careful and broad cancer surveillance throughout patient's life
- Exposure to radiation or DNA-damaging chemicals should be avoided

SELECTED REFERENCES

1. Amor-Guéret: Bloom's Syndrome. Orphanet encyclopedia, September 2013. http://www.orpha.net/data/patho/GB/uk-Bloomsyndrome.pdf. Accessed September 17, 2013
2. Weil Cornell Medical College: The Bloom's Syndrome Registry. http://weill.cornell.edu/bsr. Accessed September 17, 2013
3. Seif AE: Pediatric leukemia predisposition syndromes: clues to understanding leukemogenesis. Cancer Genet. 204(5):227-44, 2011
4. German J et al: Syndrome-causing mutations of the BLM gene in persons in the Bloom's Syndrome Registry. Hum Mutat. 28(8):743-53, 2007
5. German J: Bloom's syndrome. XX. The first 100 cancers. Cancer Genet Cytogenet. 93(1):100-6, 1997
6. German J et al: Bloom syndrome: an analysis of consanguineous families assigns the locus mutated to chromosome band 15q26.1. Proc Natl Acad Sci U S A. 91(14):6669-73, 1994
7. Chaganti RS et al: A manyfold increase in sister chromatid exchanges in Bloom's syndrome lymphocytes. Proc Natl Acad Sci U S A. 71(11):4508-12, 1974
8. Bloom D: Congenital telangiectatic erythema resembling lupus erythematosus in dwarfs; probably a syndrome entity. AMA Am J Dis Child. 88(6):754-8, 1954

CARNEY COMPLEX INCLUDING LAMB SYNDROME

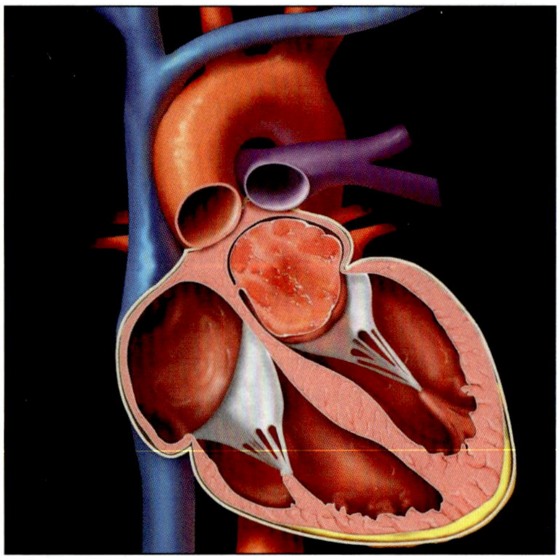

Myxoid lesions associated with Carney complex (CNC) are located in different sites, including skin, heart, and breast. Cardiac myxomas may occur in any chamber and at any age.

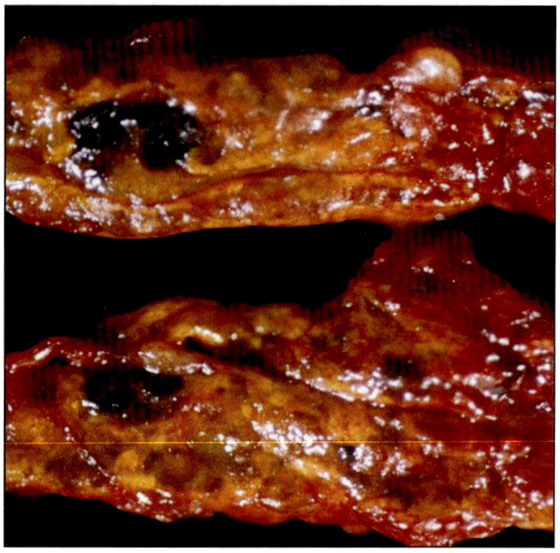

Gross findings of PPNAD include decreased, normal, or slightly increased weight, presence of small black-brown and yellow nodules, atrophy of the cortex, and loss of normal zonation.

TERMINOLOGY

Abbreviations

- Carney complex (CNC)
- Lentigines, atrial myxomas, mucocutaneous myxomas, and blue nevi syndrome (LAMB)

Synonyms

- Nevi, atrial myxoma, myxoid neurofibroma, and ephelides (NAME) syndrome
- Carney syndrome

Definitions

- Multiple neoplasia syndrome featuring cardiac, endocrine, cutaneous, and neural tumors, as well as variety of pigmented lesions of skin and mucosae
- CNC may simultaneously involve multiple endocrine glands, as in classic multiple endocrine neoplasia syndromes 1 and 2

EPIDEMIOLOGY

Age Range

- Mean age at diagnosis is 10-20 years

Gender

- M = F

Incidence

- > 400 patients have been diagnosed with CNC
- Cardiac myxomas are most common primary cardiac tumor and occur in 7 per 10,000 individuals

ETIOLOGY/PATHOGENESIS

Etiology

- Autosomal dominant disorder characterized by complex of myxomas, spotty pigmentation, and endocrine overactivity
    - Several patients described in earlier years under acronyms NAME and LAMB probably had CNC
    - CNC is not only multiple neoplasia syndrome but also causes variety of pigmented lesions of skin and mucosae
- Genetic mutation in *PRKAR1A* gene (17q22-24) and chromosome 2p16
    - *PRKAR1A* encodes regulatory R1 α-subunit of protein kinase A

CLINICAL IMPLICATIONS

Clinical Presentation

- Skin
    - Multiple facial lentigines and mucosal labial pigmentation
    - Subcutaneous myxoid neurofibromas
    - Epithelioid blue nevus
- Endocrine organs
    - Adrenal
        - Primary pigmented nodular adrenocortical disease (PPNAD)
        - Cushing syndrome
    - Thyroid
        - Thyroid nodules
    - Pituitary adenoma
        - Acromegaly/gigantism or galactorrhea, depending on tumor type
- Heart
    - Atrial myxomas are most common primary tumor of heart
    - Majority of tumors arise from left atrial septum near fossa ovalis
    - Lesions arising from right atrium or in young adults are more likely to be associated with familial syndrome
    - May present with tumor emboli
- Testis

- Large cell calcifying Sertoli cell tumor (LCCSCT), often bilateral
- Gastrointestinal tract
  - Psammomatous melanotic schwannoma in esophagus and stomach
- Psammomatous melanotic schwannomas
- Breast ductal adenoma
- Osteochondromyxoma

Treatment

- Depends on main pathology
  - Bilateral adrenalectomy
  - Removal of cardiac myxomas
  - Surgery with removal of testicular tumors
  - Surgery with removal of other tumors

Prognosis

- Most tumors associated with CNC are slow growing with no malignant potential
- Sudden death due to cardiac myxoma may occur
  - Decreased lifespan expected
- Complications of Cushing syndrome

MACROSCOPIC FINDINGS

Atrial Myxoma

- Mobile, pedunculated, ball-shaped mass

PPNAD

- Small to normal-sized adrenal glands
- Multiple bilateral, small cortical nodules (0.1-0.3 cm)
  - May be pigmented, brown, or black; some may be pale to bright yellow

Large Cell Calcifying Sertoli Cell Tumor

- Ranges in size from microscopic to large tumor replacing entire testis
- Usually multicentric, bilateral, and calcified

Psammomatous Melanotic Schwannoma

- Black, multiple nodules that occur simultaneously or asynchronously at different sites

MICROSCOPIC FINDINGS

Histologic Features

- Atrial myxoma
  - Composed of plump, stellate, or spindled cells arranged in cords and primitive-appearing vessels in loose, myxoid stroma
    - Stroma often contains hemorrhage or hemosiderin with variable numbers of inflammatory cells
  - Heterologous elements such as glands or extramedullary hematopoiesis can be found in small minority of cases (2%)
- PPNAD
  - Nodules composed of cells with compact eosinophilic cytoplasm, with abundant brown granular pigment (lipofuscin)
  - Cell nuclei are vesicular and may contain prominent nucleoli
  - Intervening cortical tissue is atrophic
- Large cell calcifying Sertoli cell tumor
  - Tumor has ill-defined periphery
  - Multiple cellular arrangement patterns of distribution: Usually solid or trabecular
  - Large tumor cells with abundant granular and eosinophilic cytoplasm
  - Laminated calcospherites are characteristic
    - May be only few or multiple, and often with confluence
  - Mitoses are rare
  - Neutrophilic infiltration is usually present
- Pituitary adenoma
  - Adenoma with solid growth pattern
  - Round and polygonal cells with granular eosinophilic cytoplasm and round to oval nuclei
  - Usually growth hormone (GH) &/or prolactin-producing tumors
- Psammomatous melanotic schwannoma
  - Peripheral nerve sheath tumor affecting posterior spinal nerve roots, alimentary tract, bone, and skin
  - Spindle and epithelioid cells intermixed with melanin, psammoma bodies, and adipose tissue
  - ~ 10% are malignant and metastasize

DIAGNOSIS

Criteria

- Definite diagnosis of CNC is given if 2 or more major manifestations are present
- **Major diagnostic criteria for CNC**
  - Spotty skin pigmentation with typical distribution on such sites as the lips, conjunctiva and inner or outer canthi, or vaginal and penile mucosa
  - Myxoma (cutaneous and mucosal)
  - Cardiac myxoma
  - Breast myxomatosis or fat-suppressed MR imaging findings are suggestive
  - PPNAD or paradoxical positive response of urinary glucocorticosteroid excretion to dexamethasone administration during Liddle test
  - Acromegaly due to GH-producing adenoma
  - Large cell calcifying Sertoli cell tumor
  - Thyroid carcinoma or multiple adenomatous nodules in young patient
  - Psammomatous melanotic schwannomas
  - Blue nevus, epithelioid blue nevus
  - Breast ductal adenoma
  - Osteochondromyxoma
- **Supplementary criteria**
  - Affected 1st-degree relative
  - Inactivating mutation of *PRKAR1A* gene
- **Cutaneous manifestations constitute 3 of the major disease manifestations**
  - Cutaneous or mucosal myxoma
  - Blue nevi (multiple) or epithelioid blue nevus
- **Findings suggestive of, or possibly associated with CNC, but not diagnostic**
  - Intense freckling (without darkly pigmented spots or typical distribution)
  - Multiple blue nevi of common type

CARNEY COMPLEX INCLUDING LAMB SYNDROME

  - Café au lait spots or other birthmarks
  - Elevated IGF1 levels, abnormal GTT, or paradoxical GH response to TRH testing in absence of clinical acromegaly
  - Cardiomyopathy
  - Pilonidal sinus
  - History of Cushing syndrome, acromegaly, or sudden death in extended family
  - Multiple skin tags or other skin lesions, including lipomas and angiofibromas
  - Colonic polyps (usually in association with acromegaly)
  - Hyperprolactinemia (usually mild and almost always combined with clinical or subclinical acromegaly)
  - Single, benign thyroid nodule in young patient; multiple thyroid nodules in older patient (detected on ultrasound)
  - Family history of carcinoma, particularly of thyroid, colon, pancreas, and ovary; other multiple benign or malignant tumors
  - Relationship between cutaneous and noncutaneous manifestations of CNC appears to be essential clue to molecular etiology
  - > 1/2 of CNC patients present with both characteristic dermatological and endocrine signs
    - Significant number of patients present with skin lesions that are only suggestive, not characteristic, of CNC
- **Classification based on both dermatological and endocrine markers has subgrouped CNC patients as**
  - Multisymptomatic (with extensive endocrine and skin signs)
  - Intermediate (with few dermatological and endocrine manifestations)
  - Paucisymptomatic (with isolated PPNAD and no cutaneous signs)

Diagnostic Criteria for Clinical Diagnosis

- Patient must have ≥ 2 of the following
  - Spotty skin pigmentation with a typical distribution (often vermillion border of lips, conjunctiva and ocular canthi, vaginal or penile mucosa)
  - Myxoma (cutaneous: Often on the eyelid, external ear, nipple)
  - Cardiac myxoma
  - Breast myxomatosis or fat-suppressed MR findings suggestive of this diagnosis
  - Acromegaly due to GH-producing adenoma (somatotropinoma)
  - PPNAD or paradoxical positive response of urinary glucocorticosteroid to dexamethasone administration during diagnostic test for Cushing syndrome
  - Thyroid carcinoma or multiple hypoechoic nodules on thyroid ultrasonography in a young patient
  - LCCSCT of testis or characteristic calcification on testicular ultrasonography
  - Psammomatous melanotic schwannoma
  - Blue nevus, epithelioid blue nevus (multiple)
  - Breast ductal adenoma, or mammary tumor with intraductal papilloma
  - Osteochondromyxoma of bone
  - Additionally, criteria is satisfied by a patient meeting only 1 of these criteria, but having either
    - Affected 1st-degree relative or
    - Inactivating mutation of the *PRKAR1A* gene

Similar Clinical and Pathological Features

- Peutz-Jeghers syndrome (PJS), with which it shares mucosal lentiginosis and unusual gonadal tumor, and large cell calcifying Sertoli cell tumor
- McCune-Albright syndrome: Sporadic condition also characterized by multiple endocrine and nonendocrine tumors

ANCILLARY TESTS

Immunohistochemistry

- Atrial myxoma
  - Cells stain positive for CD34, CD31, and S100
  - Calretinin is positive in 74-100% of cases and can be useful to distinguish this lesion from myxoid thrombus
- PPNAD
  - Increased expression of glucocorticoid receptor
- Large cell calcifying Sertoli cell tumor
  - Positive for vimentin, inhibin-α, NSE, S100, desmin, and smooth muscle actin
  - Negative for α-fetoprotein, HCG, PLAP, podoplanin, OCT3/4, and cytokeratin (may be focally positive)

Molecular Genetics

- Genetic heterogeneity with ≥ 2 main loci for candidate genes
  - Chromosome 2 locus at 2p15-16
  - Mutations of *PRKAR1A* gene on chromosome 17 (17q22-24)

DIFFERENTIAL DIAGNOSIS

Other Syndromes

- Share clinical features and molecular pathways with several other familial lentiginosis syndromes, such as
  - McCune-Albright syndrome
  - Peutz-Jeghers syndrome
  - LEOPARD (multiple lentigines, electrocardiographic conduction abnormalities, ocular hypertelorism, pulmonic stenosis, abnormal genitalia, retardation of growth, and sensorineural deafness)
  - Noonan syndrome
  - PTEN-hamartoma tumor syndromes (e.g., Cowden disease [CD] and Bannayan-Ruvalcaba-Riley syndrome [BRRS])
  - In all of these conditions, skin lesions accompany underlying endocrine &/or other abnormalities, and, similarly to CNC, are considered important diagnostic sign

McCune-Albright Syndrome

- Probably the closest to CNC in terms of molecular pathway link

- Patients have characteristic lesions that affect predominantly 3 systems: Skin, endocrine system, and skeleton
- Café au lait spots in McCune-Albright syndrome patients are similar to those observed in CNC
  - Tend to be more intensely pigmented
- Caused by post-zygotic activating mutations of *GNAS1*

Peutz-Jeghers Syndrome

- Autosomal dominant familial lentiginosis syndrome characterized by melanocytic macules of lips, buccal mucosa, and digits, multiple gastrointestinal hamartomatous polyps, and increased risk of various neoplasms
- Lentigines observed in Peutz-Jeghers syndrome patients show similar density and distribution to those in CNC patients
- Peutz-Jeghers syndrome was first mapped to chromosome 19p13.3, and gene-encoding serine threonine kinase 11 (*STK11* a.k.a. *LKB1*) was found to be mutated in most patients

LEOPARD

- Multiple **l**entigines, **e**lectrocardiographic conduction abnormalities, **o**cular hypertelorism, **p**ulmonic stenosis, **a**bnormal genitalia, **r**etardation of growth, and sensorineural **d**eafness

Cowden Disease and Bannayan-Ruvalcaba-Riley Syndrome (PTEN-Hamartoma Tumor Syndromes)

- Cowden disease and BRRS share clinical characteristics, such as mucocutaneous lesions, hamartomatous polyps of gastrointestinal tract, and increased risk of developing neoplasms
- Both conditions are caused by mutations in *PTEN* gene
  - *PTEN* is located on 10q23.31 and encodes phosphatidylinositol-3,4,5-triphosphate 3-phosphatase
    - Tumor suppressor gene that has been found mutated in a number of tumors
- Thyroid is usually affected by numerous adenomatous nodules, follicular adenomas, and follicular carcinoma
  - Findings are similar to those familial syndromes characterized by predominance of nonthyroidal tumors
    - PTEN-hamartoma tumor syndrome, Carney complex, Werner syndrome, and Pendred syndrome

SELECTED REFERENCES

1. Courcoutsakis NA et al: The complex of myxomas, spotty skin pigmentation and endocrine overactivity (Carney complex): imaging findings with clinical and pathological correlation. Insights Imaging. 4(1):119-33, 2013
2. Miettinen M et al: Immunohistochemical loss of succinate dehydrogenase subunit A (SDHA) in gastrointestinal stromal tumors (GISTs) signals SDHA germline mutation. Am J Surg Pathol. 37(2):234-40, 2013
3. Yazdan P et al: Epithelioid and fusiform blue nevus of chronically sun-damaged skin, an entity distinct from the epithelioid blue nevus of the Carney complex. Am J Surg Pathol. 37(1):81-8, 2013
4. Bertherat J: Adrenocortical cancer in Carney complex: a paradigm of endocrine tumor progression or an association of genetic predisposing factors? J Clin Endocrinol Metab. 97(2):387-90, 2012
5. Gill AJ: Succinate dehydrogenase (SDH) and mitochondrial driven neoplasia. Pathology. 44(4):285-92, 2012
6. Gourgari E et al: Large-cell calcifying Sertoli cell tumors of the testes in pediatrics. Curr Opin Pediatr. 24(4):518-22, 2012
7. Kacerovska D et al: Spectrum of cutaneous and soft tissue lesions in two Carney complex patients-adnexal induction versus authentic adnexal neoplasms. Am J Dermatopathol. 34(7):729-36, 2012
8. Martucci F et al: Familial isolated pituitary adenomas: An emerging clinical entity. J Endocrinol Invest. 35(11):1003-14, 2012
9. Park KU et al: Novel Mutation in PRKAR1A in Carney Complex. Korean J Pathol. 46(6):595-600, 2012
10. Patronas Y et al: In vitro studies of novel PRKAR1A mutants that extend the predicted RIα protein sequence into the 3'-untranslated open reading frame: proteasomal degradation leads to RIα haploinsufficiency and Carney complex. J Clin Endocrinol Metab. 97(3):E496-502, 2012
11. Pringle DR et al: Thyroid-specific ablation of the Carney complex gene, PRKAR1A, results in hyperthyroidism and follicular thyroid cancer. Endocr Relat Cancer. 19(3):435-46, 2012
12. Rodriguez FJ et al: Genetic predisposition to peripheral nerve neoplasia: diagnostic criteria and pathogenesis of neurofibromatoses, Carney complex, and related syndromes. Acta Neuropathol. 123(3):349-67, 2012
13. Son EJ et al: Familial follicular cell-derived thyroid carcinoma. Front Endocrinol (Lausanne). 3:61, 2012
14. Libé R et al: Frequent phosphodiesterase 11A gene (PDE11A) defects in patients with Carney complex (CNC) caused by PRKAR1A mutations: PDE11A may contribute to adrenal and testicular tumors in CNC as a modifier of the phenotype. J Clin Endocrinol Metab. 96(1):E208-14, 2011
15. Yin Z et al: Differential role of PKA catalytic subunits in mediating phenotypes caused by knockout of the Carney complex gene Prkar1a. Mol Endocrinol. 25(10):1786-93, 2011
16. Almeida MQ et al: Carney complex and other conditions associated with micronodular adrenal hyperplasias. Best Pract Res Clin Endocrinol Metab. 24(6):907-14, 2010
17. Rothenbuhler A et al: Clinical and molecular genetics of Carney complex. Best Pract Res Clin Endocrinol Metab. 24(3):389-99, 2010
18. Alevizaki M et al: Multiple endocrine neoplasias: advances and challenges for the future. J Intern Med. 266(1):1-4, 2009
19. Mantovani G et al: Analysis of GNAS1 and PRKAR1A gene mutations in human cardiac myxomas not associated with multiple endocrine disorders. J Endocrinol Invest. 32(6):501-4, 2009
20. Stratakis CA et al: The triad of paragangliomas, gastric stromal tumours and pulmonary chondromas (Carney triad), and the dyad of paragangliomas and gastric stromal sarcomas (Carney-Stratakis syndrome): molecular genetics and clinical implications. J Intern Med. 266(1):43-52, 2009
21. Horvath A et al: Large deletions of the PRKAR1A gene in Carney complex. Clin Cancer Res. 14(2):388-95, 2008

CARNEY COMPLEX INCLUDING LAMB SYNDROME

Tumors and Lesions Associated With Carney Complex

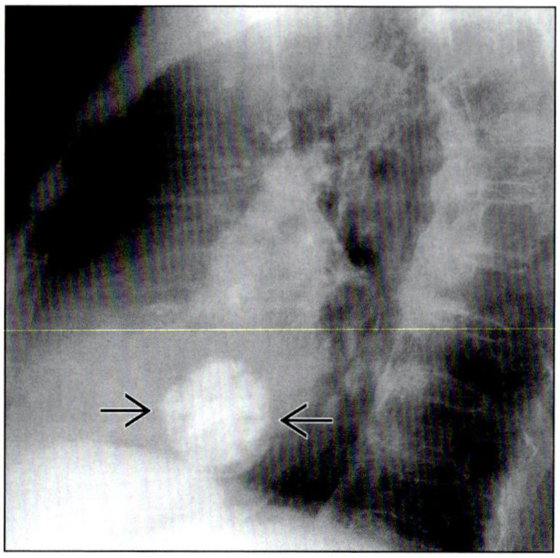

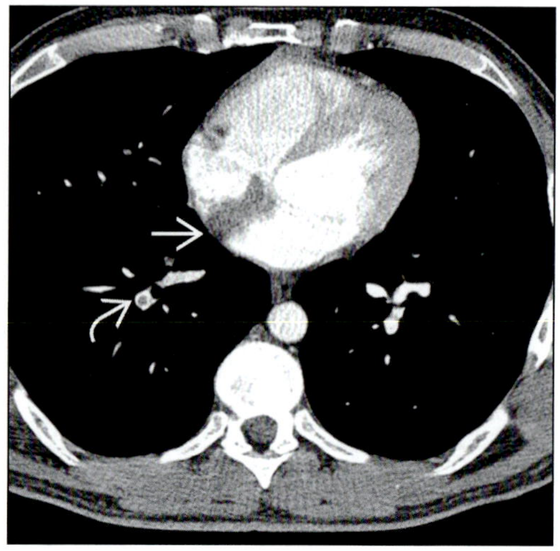

(Left) *Lateral radiograph shows densely calcified left atrial myxoma →. This patient had multiple transient ischemic attacks, a clinical feature associated with cardiac myxoma.* ***(Right)*** *Axial CECT shows myxoma involving the interarterial septum and extending into the right atrium →. A tumor embolism is seen in a right lower lobe pulmonary artery branch →. The tumor is of decreased density compared to contrasted heart chambers and has a different density than adipose tissue.*

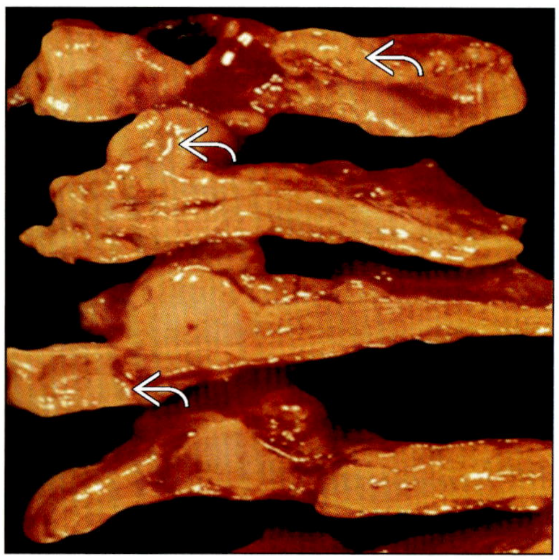

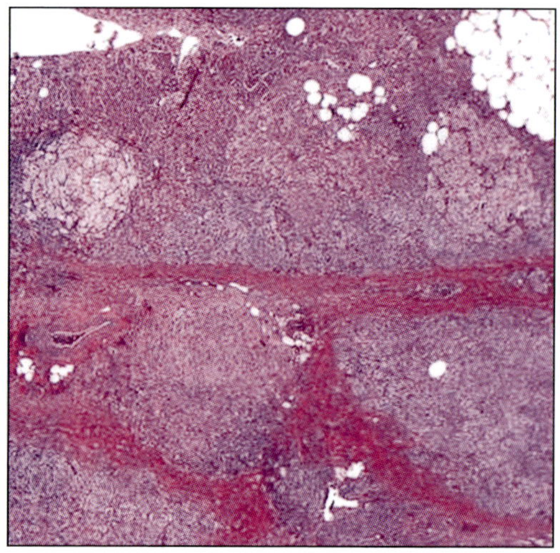

(Left) *Gross cross section of an adrenal gland from a patient with Cushing syndrome, CNC, and primary pigmented nodular adrenocortical disease (PPNAD) shows presence of small, nonpigmented nodules →, most of which cannot be appreciated grossly.* ***(Right)*** *On low-power magnification, the normal adrenal gland architecture is replaced by multiple nodules, most of which are unencapsulated but some have a thin fibrous capsule. There is lipomatous metaplasia and the adjacent adrenal is atrophic.*

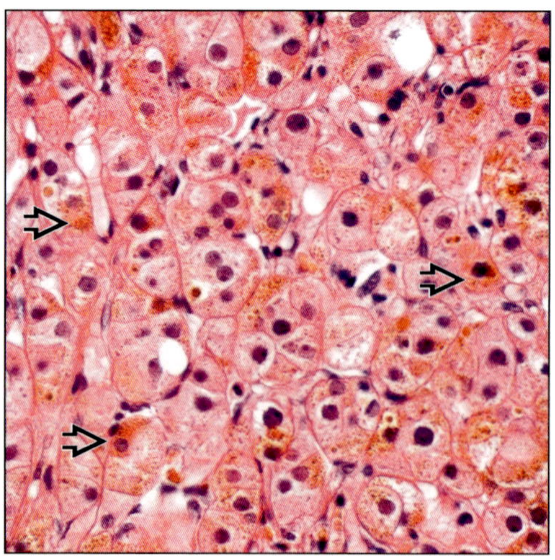

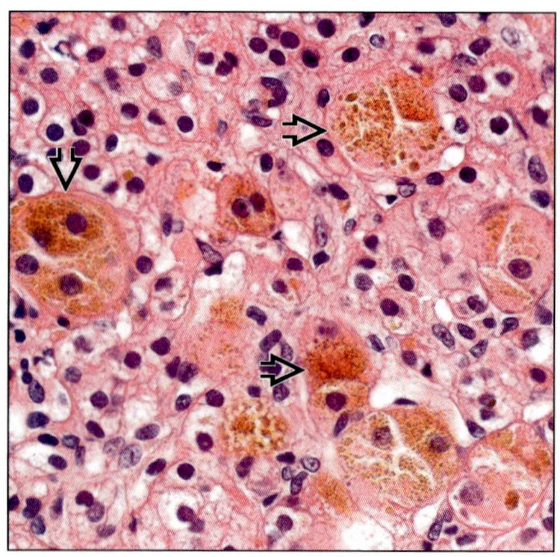

(Left) *In PPNAD, there is loss of zonation of the adrenal cortex, which has multiple small cortical nodules composed of enlarged globular cortical cells with granular and eosinophilic cytoplasm. Note a variable amount of lipochrome pigment deposition →.* ***(Right)*** *The adrenal cortex shows loss of zonation and atrophy of cortex adjacent to nodules in PPNAD. The nodules are composed of enlarged globular cortical cells with granular eosinophilic cytoplasm with lipochrome pigment →.*

Tumors Associated With Carney Complex

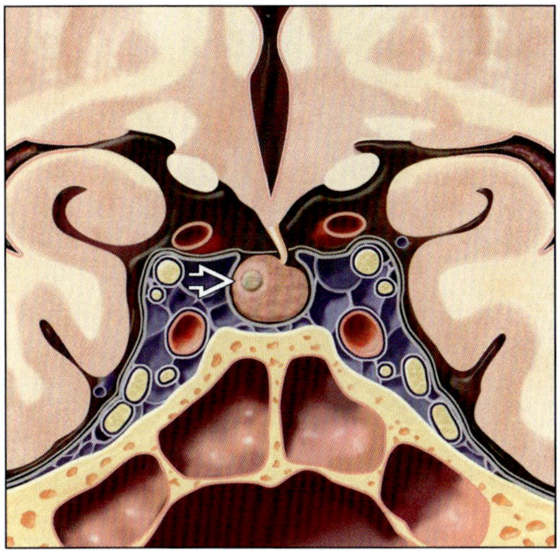

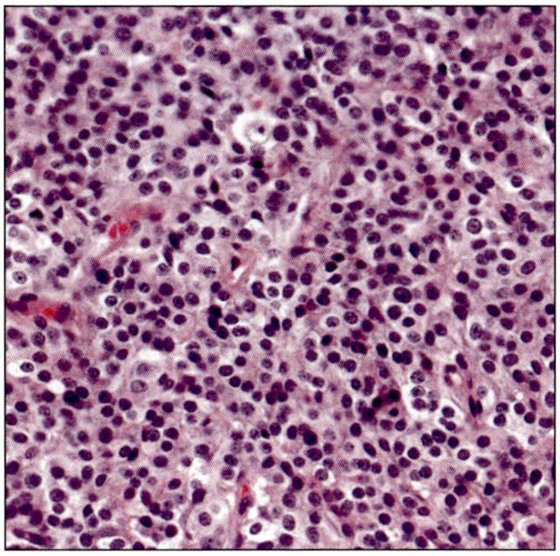

(Left) *Pituitary adenomas, microadenomas ➡, or macroadenomas, which are usually GH-producing adenomas, are some of the findings in Carney complex.* ***(Right)*** *Photomicrograph shows a sparsely granulated somatotroph adenoma composed of chromophobic cells. The nuclei can be centrally located but also tend to be eccentric, pushed to the cell periphery, and indented by the fibrous bodies.*

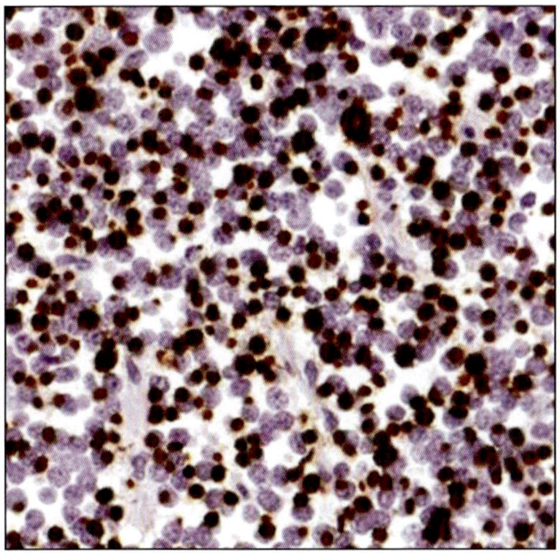

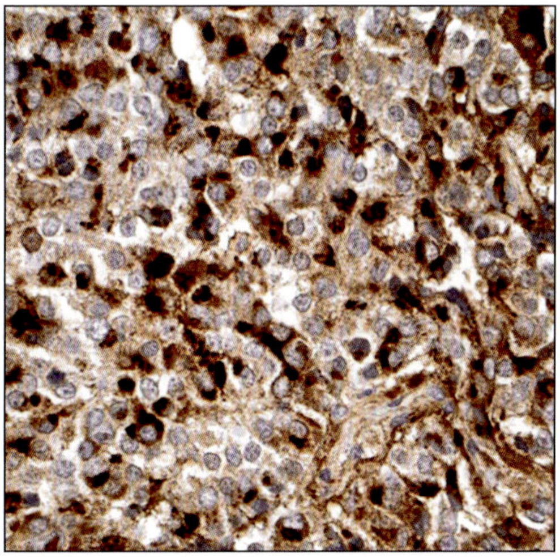

(Left) *CAM5.2 reveals diffuse paranuclear keratin aggresomes (fibrous bodies) in sparsely granulated somatotroph adenomas. Occasional fibrous bodies can be seen in aggressive acidophil stem cell adenomas as well as in intermediate-type somatotroph adenomas.* ***(Right)*** *GH in a densely granulated somatotroph adenoma shows numerous GH-containing cytoplasmic secretory granules that correlate with the cytoplasmic eosinophilic appearance on H&E.*

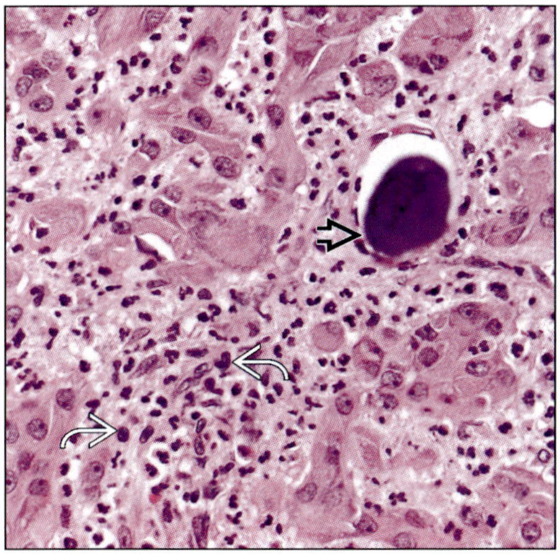

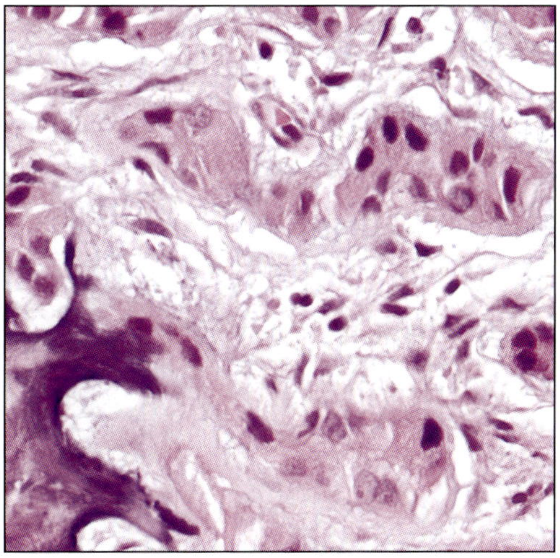

(Left) *Large cell calcifying Sertoli cell tumor (LCCSCT) shows cords and small nests of large epithelioid cells embedded in a fibrous background with dense neutrophilic infiltrate. A psammoma body ➡ is also seen. The neutrophilic background is an important diagnostic feature ➡.* ***(Right)*** *LCCSCT is shown with nests of large epithelioid cells with abundant eosinophilic cytoplasm. A large area of calcification is seen in the loose fibromyxoid stroma.*

COSTELLO SYNDROME

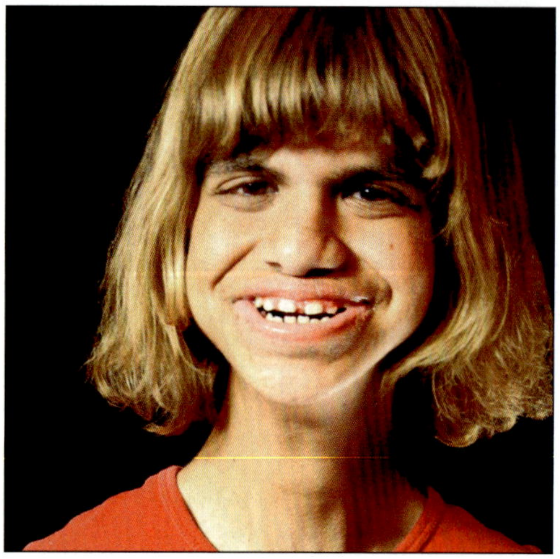

This young girl with Costello syndrome has the characteristic facies, with thick lips, a large mouth, and prominent epicanthal folds.

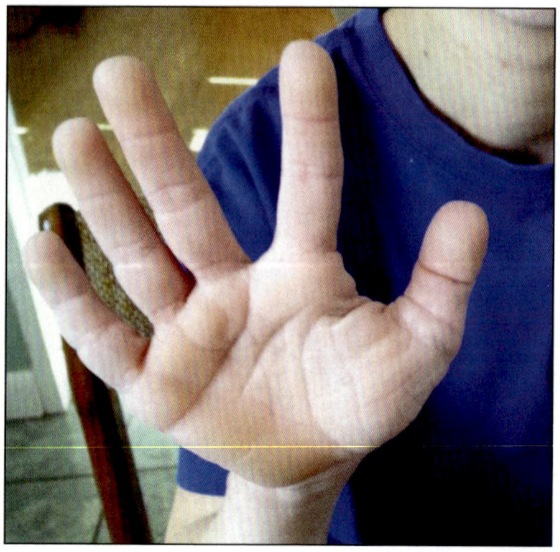

This is a hand of a patient with Costello syndrome. Deep palmar creases and ulnar deviation are apparent.

TERMINOLOGY

Synonym

- Facio-cutaneous skeletal syndrome

Definitions

- Syndrome of delayed development, intellectual impairment, heart defects, loose skin, flexible joints
- Cumulative incidence of cancer ~ 15% by age 20

EPIDEMIOLOGY

Incidence/Prevalence

- Very rare; several hundred reported cases
- Estimated prevalence: 1 in 300,000 to 1 in 1.25 million

GENETICS

HRAS Mutation in 80-90%

- H-Ras protein is relevant to cell growth/turnover
  - H-Ras is overactive in Costello syndrome
  - Most common mutation is p.G12S

Inheritance

- Autosomal dominant transmission
- Almost all reported cases secondary to new mutation (no prior history in family members)

CLINICAL IMPLICATIONS AND ANCILLARY TESTS

Clinical Presentation

- May be large for gestational age, secondary to edema
- Characteristic, coarse facies
  - Large mouth, thick lips, low-set ears, epicanthal folds, depressed nasal bridge, anteverted nostrils
- Curly or sparse, fine hair
- Redundant skin over neck, hands
- Deep palmoplantar creases
- Palmoplantar keratoderma
- Difficulty feeding, slow growth, short stature
  - Failure to thrive
- Hypotonia, joint laxity, ulnar deviation (splayed fingers)
- Tight Achilles tendons
- Chiari I malformation
- Skeletal malformations
  - Short stature, relative macrocephaly, kyphoscoliosis, positional foot deformity
- Dental issues
- Vision problems (e.g., nystagmus)
- Cardiovascular system complications (e.g., hypertrophy, pulmonic stenosis, arrhythmia, aortic dilation)

ASSOCIATED NEOPLASMS

Skin Papillomas

- Tendency to be perinasal/perioral/perianal
- May be present in young children or absent until > 10 years of age

Rhabdomyosarcoma

- 19 of 268 patients (7%) in 1 review
  - 9 embryonal, 1 alveolar, 1 mixed histology, 1 pleomorphic, 1 spindle cell type, 6 unclassified
- Median age: 2.3 years

Bladder Carcinoma (Urothelial Carcinoma)

- 4 of 268 patients (1.4%) in 1 review
  - 3/4 with transitional cell carcinoma
  - 1/4 with low-grade papillary bladder carcinoma

Neuroblastoma

- 5 of 268 patients (1.9%) in 1 review

- 4/5 with ganglioneuroblastoma
- Mean age: 13.5 years

Fibrosarcoma

- 1 of 268 patients (0.4%) in 1 review

CANCER RISK MANAGEMENT

Rhabdomyosarcoma

- Abdominal/pelvic ultrasound: Every 3-4 months until age 8 years

Transitional Cell Carcinoma

- Annual urinalysis, beginning at 10 years of age

DIFFERENTIAL DIAGNOSIS

Cardiofaciocutaneous Syndrome

- Associated cancers/tumors
  - Acute lymphoblastic leukemia, non-Hodgkin lymphoma, hepatoblastoma, embryonal rhabdomyosarcoma
- Autosomal dominant
  - Germline mutations in *BRAF*, *MEK1*, *MEK2*

Noonan Syndrome

- Associated cancers/tumors
  - Neuroblastoma (8 of 1,051 patients in 1 review)
  - Acute lymphoblastic leukemia (8 of 1,051 patients in 1 review)
  - Low-grade glioma (6 of 1,051 patients in 1 review)
  - Rhabdomyosarcoma (6 of 1,051 patients in 1 review)
- By 20 years of age, ~ 4% cumulative incidence of cancer
- Autosomal dominant
  - Germline mutations in *PTPN11*, *SOS1*, *KRAS*, *NRAS*, *RAF1*, *BRAF*, *SHOC2*, or *MEK1* in 70-75%
- Short stature, developmental delay, congenital heart defects

LEOPARD Syndrome (Noonan Syndrome With Multiple Lentigines)

- Associated tumors overlap with Costello syndrome
- Autosomal dominant, germline mutations in *PTPN11*, *BRAF*, *RAF1*

DIAGNOSTIC FEATURES

Frequency of Major Features

- Short stature (97%), abnormal palmar creases (99%), loose skin (94%)
- Characteristic facies (98%), thick lips (95%)
- Dysphagia/feeding difficulty/gastrostomy tube (95%)
- Developmental delay/mental retardation (100%)

Frequency of Unique Features

- Congenital heart defects (65%)
  - Examples: Pulmonic stenosis (20%), hypertrophic cardiomyopathy (40%), atrial tachycardia (30%)
- Benign (44%), malignant (16%) tumors
- Stretchy skin with hyperpigmentation
- Kyphoscoliosis, engaging personality, normal head circumference

Frequency of Other Features

- Polyhydramnios (62%), birth weight > 50%, hernias (50%), vision: Ptosis, strabismus

SELECTED REFERENCES

1. McCormick EM et al: Assessing genotype-phenotype correlation in Costello syndrome using a severity score. Genet Med. 15(7):554-7, 2013
2. Gripp KW et al: Costello syndrome: a Ras/mitogen activated protein kinase pathway syndrome (rasopathy) resulting from HRAS germline mutations. Genet Med. 14(3):285-92, 2012
3. Kratz CP et al: Cancer in Noonan, Costello, cardiofaciocutaneous and LEOPARD syndromes. Am J Med Genet C Semin Med Genet. 157C(2):83-9, 2011
4. Rauen KA et al: Molecular aspects, clinical aspects and possible treatment modalities for Costello syndrome: Proceedings from the 1st International Costello Syndrome Research Symposium 2007. Am J Med Genet A. 146A(9):1205-17, 2008

IMAGE GALLERY

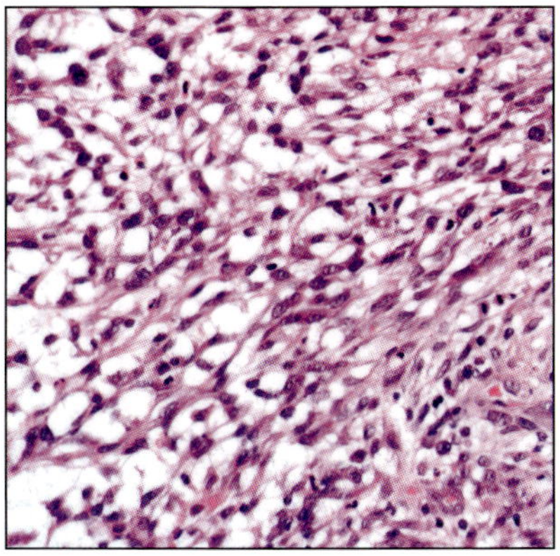

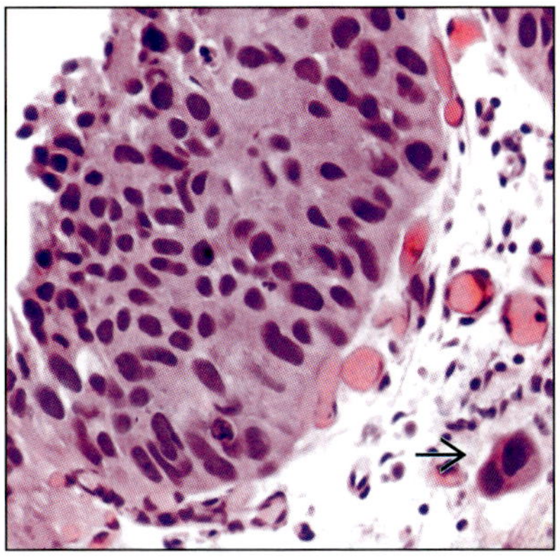

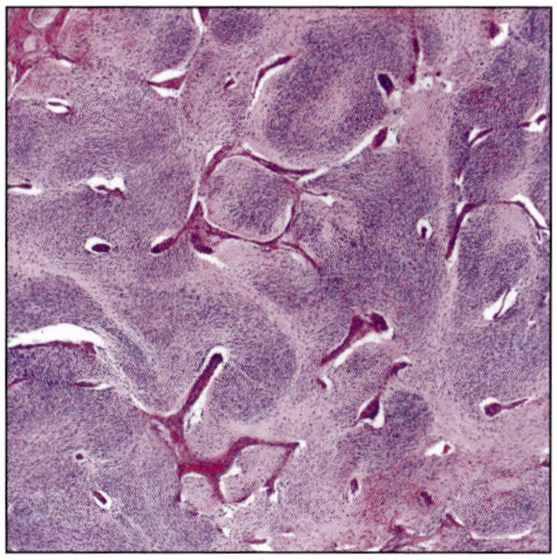

(Left) *This embryonal rhabdomyosarcoma has ovoid/spindled nuclei with eosinophilic cytoplasm set in a myxoid stroma that imparts a filigree pattern. (Courtesy C. Fisher, MD.)* ***(Center)*** *In this urothelial carcinoma in situ with microinvasion, the small cluster of neoplastic cells ⇨ focally invades the lamina propria (p.T1). (Courtesy S. Tickoo, MD.)* ***(Right)*** *This is a low-power view of a poorly differentiated neuroblastoma. (Courtesy J. Comstock, MD.)*

DENYS-DRASH SYNDROME

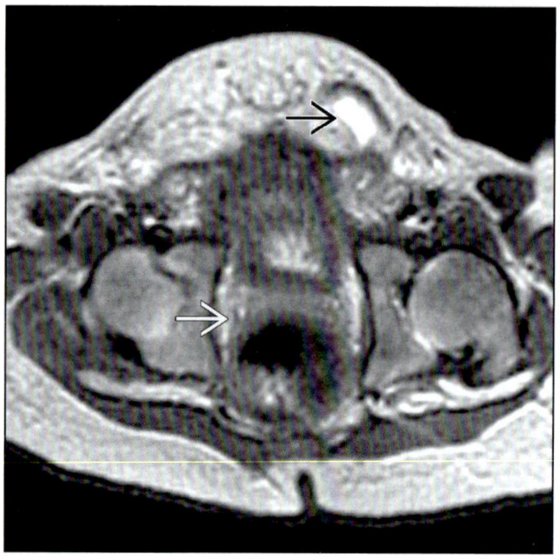

Axial T2WI MR of a baby shows presence of an undescended testis in the right inguinal area ⇒. A vagina is also demonstrated ➡, however, confirming internal genital organs of both sexes.

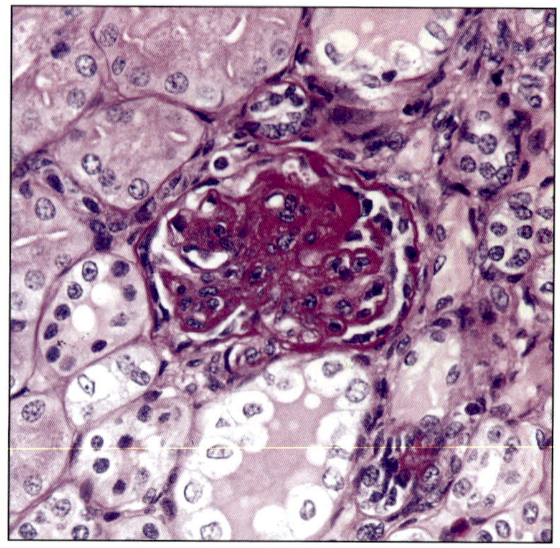

PAS stain shows glomeruli with mesangial sclerosis characterized by an increase in matrix deposits. Diffuse mesangial sclerosis is a primary feature of DDS seen in ~ 95% of patients. (Courtesy S. Meehan, MD.)

TERMINOLOGY

Abbreviations

- Denys-Drash syndrome (DDS)

Definition

- Disorder characterized by ambiguous genitalia or pseudohermaphroditism, early-onset nephrotic syndrome, and ↑ risk for Wilms tumor (WT)

EPIDEMIOLOGY

Incidence

- Very rare, ~ 200 cases reported

Gender

- Karyotype
  - Most tested are male (46, XY)
    - Including > 80% of patients with ambiguous external genitalia and > 60% of patients with female external genitalia
  - Few female karyotype probably due to underdiagnosis of DDS in both genotypic and phenotypic females with nephropathy
- External genitalia
  - Male: 13%
  - Female: 42% (most are male with pseudohermaphrodism)
  - Ambiguous: 43%

Age

- Onset of nephropathy
  - Range: 1 month to 17 years
  - Average: 1.4 years
- Onset of WT
  - Range: 1 month to 13 years
  - Average: 1.6 years

GENETICS

WT1

- Located at Chr 11p13
- Transcript critical in early and late stages of genitourinary development
- DDS is caused by germline point mutation in zinc finger region of *WT1*
  - C to T transition missense mutation at amino acid 394 in exon 9 involving 3rd zinc finger of *WT1* most common
  - Also G to A transition at +5 of splice donor site within intron 9

GENITALIA

External Genitalia

- Most are male with pseudohermaphrodism having external female or ambiguous genitalia

Internal Genitalia

- Most have **dysgenic gonads**
  - "Streak gonads" composed of fibrous tissue without epithelial structures
  - Immature, infantile, or rudimentary gonads
  - Wolffian structures present in phenotypic female
  - Both wolffian and müllerian structures present
- May also have both testicular and ovarian tissues present or ovotestis (true hermaphrodites)
- Only in few cases is internal genitalia appropriate to external genitalia

RENAL FEATURES

Nephrotic Syndrome

- Present in 95% of cases, a primary feature of DDS
- Early onset that progresses rapidly to end-stage renal disease (ESRD)

DENYS-DRASH SYNDROME

- Presents usually in 1st year of life
- Microscopic features: **Diffuse mesangial sclerosis**
  - Fibrillar expansion in mesangial matrix
  - No mesangial cell proliferation
  - Podocyte hypertrophy with vacuolations
  - Glomerular basement membrane thickening due to subepithelial apposition of thin layers of basal lamina
  - Tubular dilations, which may contain casts
  - Tubulointerstitial inflammation and fibrosis
  - Fully developed lesion shows glomerular basement membrane thickening and massive enlargement of mesangial areas
  - Mesangial sclerosis may eventually contract glomerular tuft into a sclerotic mass within Bowman space
  - Focal mesangial sclerosis may also occur in a smaller subset
- Nuclear expression of WT1 in podocytes absent or decreased, suggesting decreased binding capacity of mutated protein

ASSOCIATED NEOPLASMS

Wilms Tumor

- Malignant immature tumor of nephrogenic blastemal cell origin that may differentiate into epithelial or mesenchymal cells recapitulating renal embryogenesis
- Present in 74% of DDS patients
- Age of onset similar to that of nephropathy
- May also present as an abdominal mass
- ~ 20% of WTs are bilateral
- No distinct histologic features from sporadic WT cases

Gonadal Malignancies

- ~ 4% of DDS patients develop gonadal malignancies
- Most common is gonadoblastoma, a tumor composed of seminomatous/dysgerminomatous elements and immature sex cord-stromal elements
- Juvenile granulosa cell tumor also reported

OTHER ASSOCIATED FINDINGS

Structural and Functional Abnormalities

- Overall present in 10% of DDS
- Can be an isolated abnormality (e.g., hernia, contractures) or multiple abnormalities (e.g., cleft palate, mental retardation, nystagmus)
- Renal abnormalities include unilateral hydronephrosis, renal pelvis or ureter duplication, double kidney and horseshoe kidney

CANCER RISK MANAGEMENT

Wilms Tumor

- Bilateral nephrectomy for children with ESRD suggested
- For DDS children on dialysis, unilateral nephrectomy suggested, followed later by contralateral nephrectomy at time of kidney transplantation

Gonadal Malignancies

- Elective gonadectomy proposed

PROGNOSIS

Outcome

- With limited cases followed, 32% of patients alive with age range of 3 months to 21 years
- 38% of patients died at an average age of 2 years (range: 1 month to 7.5 years)
- Most common cause of death is renal failure (80%) followed by sepsis (3.5%)
- < 2% of patients died from WT

DIFFERENTIAL DIAGNOSIS

WT, Aniridia, Genitourinary Abnormalities, and Mental Retardation (WAGR) Syndrome

- Rarely, aniridia and retardation may occur in DDS
- WT and genitourinary abnormalities in absence of nephropathy in DDS (~ 5%) can make distinction difficult
  - Diagnosis of DDS made if external genitalia are female and internal genitalia show both wolffian and müllerian structures or karyotype is male

Frasier Syndrome

- Phenotype: Ambiguous genitalia, streak gonads, and segmental glomerulosclerosis
- Nephropathy similar but usually of a later age of onset

Diffuse Mesangial Sclerosis

- Rare occurrence as isolated finding (nephropathy) without other phenotypic features seen in DDS

Nephrotic Syndrome in Infants

- Consider congenital nephrosis, idiopathic nephrosis, diffuse mesangial proliferation, minimal change or focal segmental sclerosis, and isolated diffuse mesangial sclerosis

SELECTED REFERENCES

1. Niaudet P et al: WT1 and glomerular diseases. Pediatr Nephrol. 21(11):1653-60, 2006
2. Breslow NE et al: End stage renal disease in patients with Wilms tumor: results from the National Wilms Tumor Study Group and the United States Renal Data System. J Urol. 174(5):1972-5, 2005
3. Royer-Pokora B et al: Twenty-four new cases of WT1 germline mutations and review of the literature: genotype/phenotype correlations for Wilms tumor development. Am J Med Genet A. 127A(3):249-57, 2004
4. Yang AH et al: The dysregulated glomerular cell growth in Denys-Drash syndrome. Virchows Arch. 445(3):305-14, 2004
5. McTaggart SJ et al: Clinical spectrum of Denys-Drash and Frasier syndrome. Pediatr Nephrol. 16(4):335-9, 2001
6. Mueller RF: The Denys-Drash syndrome. J Med Genet. 31(6):471-7, 1994

Microscopic Features

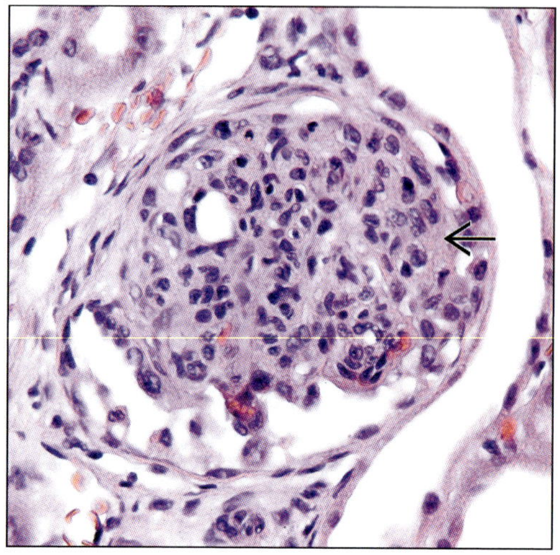

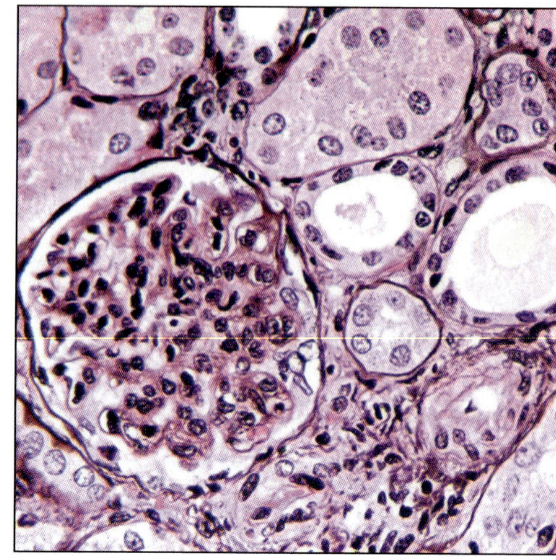

(Left) *High-power view shows a glomerulus in DDS with early mesangial sclerosis shown by an increase in matrix deposits* →*. (Courtesy S. Meehan, MD.)* ***(Right)*** *Silver stain shows a glomerulus with an early increase in mesangial matrix deposition. Glomerular capillary loops are open. Mesangial sclerosis eventually causes rapid decline in glomerular filtration rate and progresses to ESRD. Nephropathy and its complications are the most common cause of death in DDS. (Courtesy S. Meehan, MD.)*

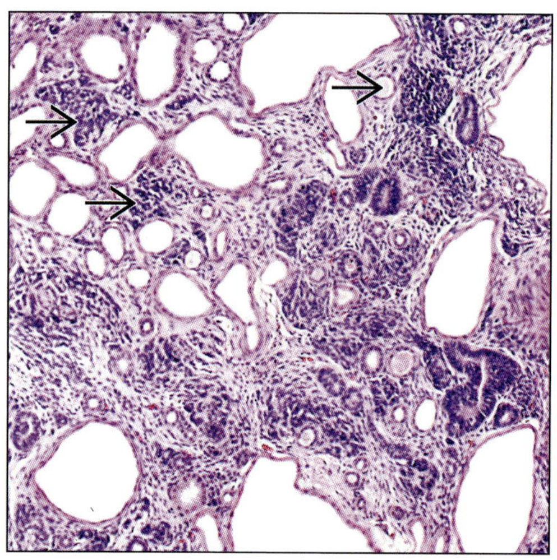

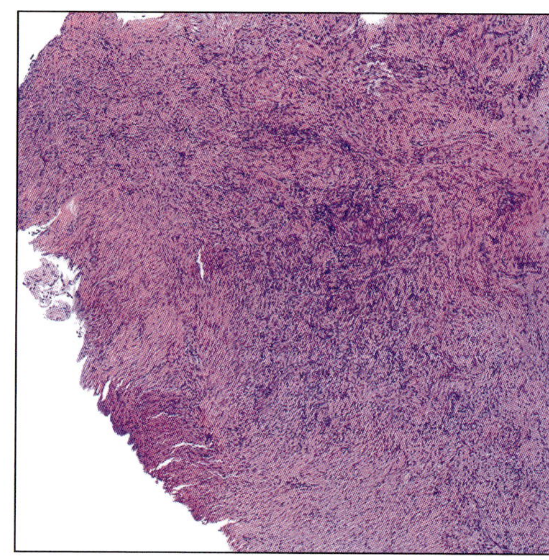

(Left) *H&E of kidney from a DDS patient shows multiple nephrogenic rests* →*. Nephrogenic rests are considered to be precursors of WT. DDS increases the risk for WT, which is encountered in 74% of patients. (Courtesy S. Meehan, MD.)* ***(Right)*** *H&E shows a dysgenetic gonad in DDS, composed purely of ovarian-type stroma without any epithelial cells ("streak gonad"). The majority of patients with DDS are karyotypically male (46, XY) and most have female or ambiguous external genitalia.*

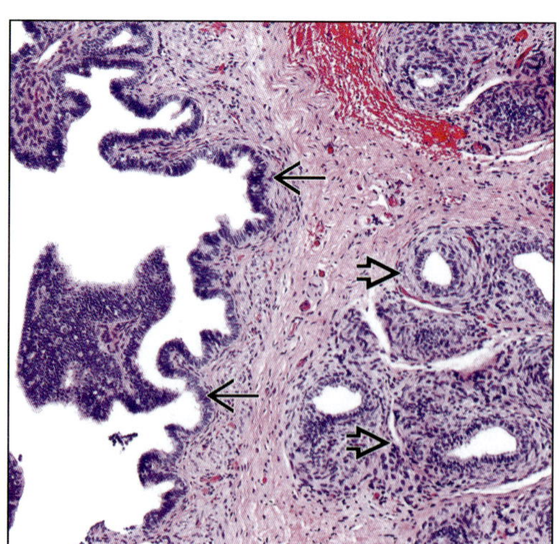

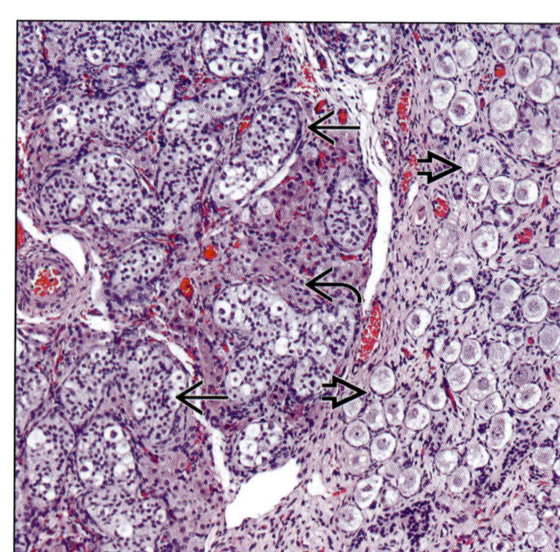

(Left) *H&E shows a dysgenetic gonad containing both müllerian-type structure (fallopian tube)* → *and wolffian-type structure (epididymis/ductuli efferentes)* ⇨*.* ***(Right)*** *H&E shows an ovotestis containing both testicular and ovarian elements. Seminiferous tubules* → *containing mostly Sertoli cells are present. In addition, ovarian follicles are clustered nearby* ⇨*. Note the presence of intersitial steroid-producing cells* ↪*. Ovotestis increases the risk for the development of gonadoblastoma.*

Associated Neoplasms

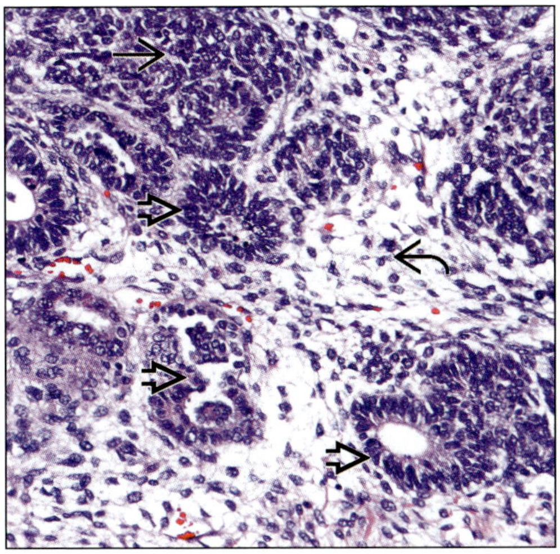

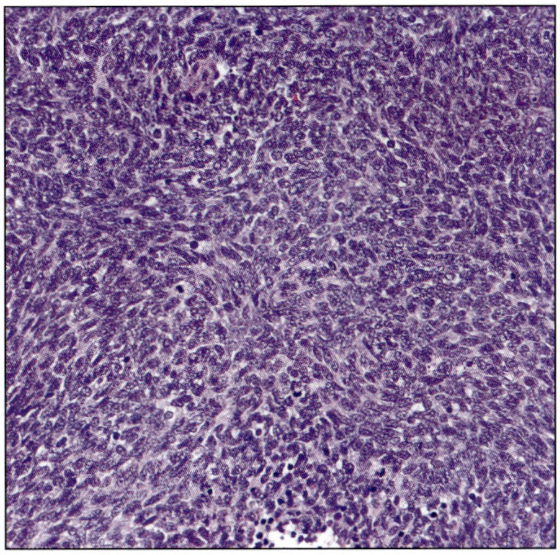

(Left) *H&E shows WT with classic triphasic histology consisting of blastemal cells ➔, epithelial cells ➔, and stromal cells ➔. WT may also have biphasic or uniphasic histology. Although DDS has a high risk for WT, only a small subset of patients will die from this malignancy.* ***(Right)*** *Low-power view shows WT consisting purely of blastemal cells. These are tightly packed primitive cells with high nuclear to cytoplasmic ratio, giving the appearance of small round blue cells.*

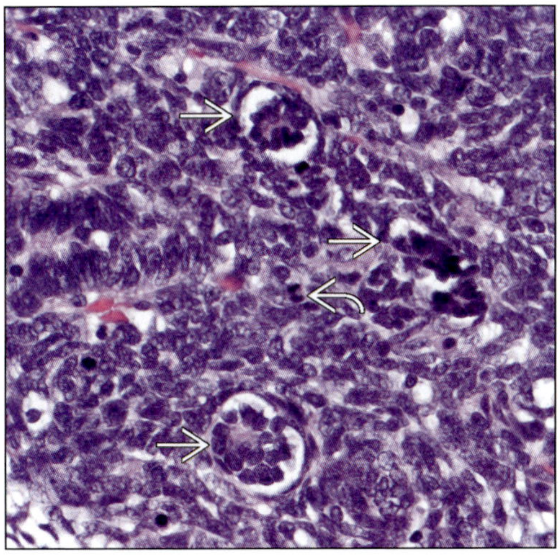

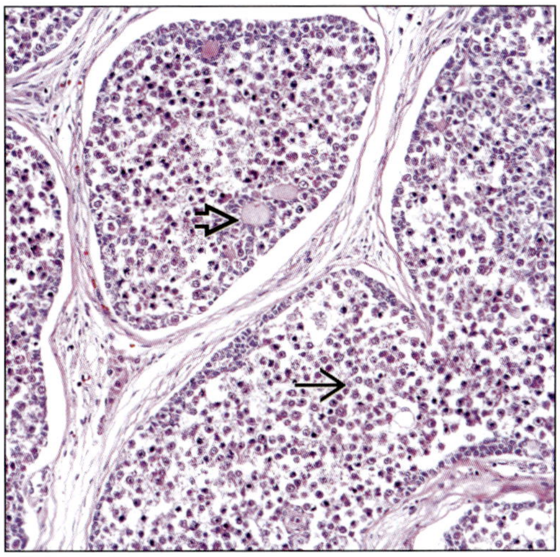

(Left) *H&E shows WT containing some glomeruloid epithelial structures ➔ admixed with blastemal cells. Note presence of mitosis ➔. WT is a primitive neoplasm that recapitulates renal embryogenesis.* ***(Right)*** *Gonadoblastoma is characterized by nests containing large seminomatous germ cells ➔ located in the center, and sex cord-stromal cells forming Call-Exner-like structures ➔ at the periphery of the nests. (Courtesy S. Shen, MD, PhD.)*

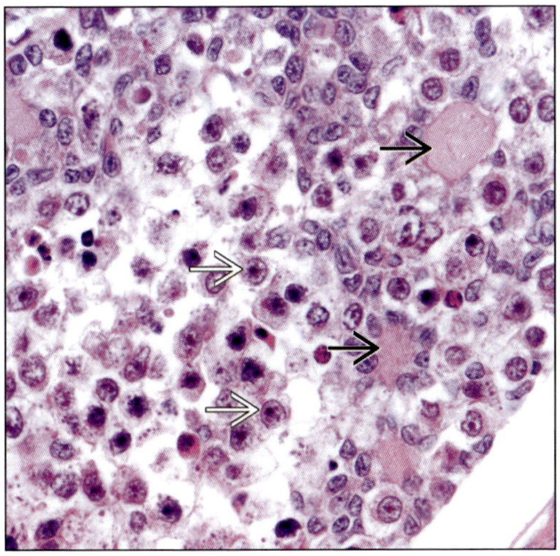

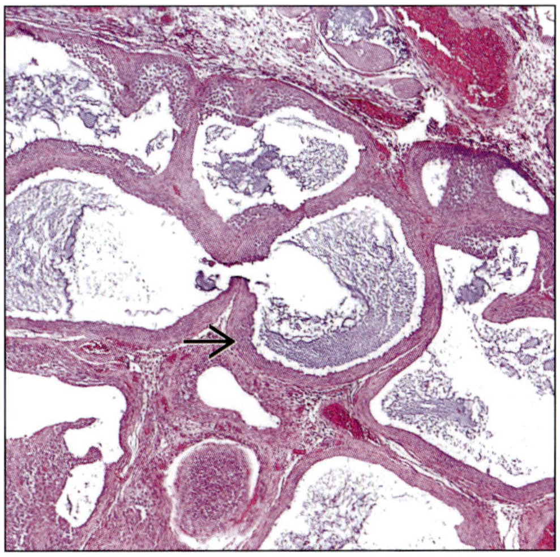

(Left) *Gonadoblastoma shows smaller sex cord-stromal cells forming Call-Exner body-like structures ➔ and large seminomatous cells with abundant clear cytoplasm and prominent nucleoli ➔. Gonadoblastoma usually occurs in dysgenetic gonads such as in DDS. (Courtesy S. Shen, MD, PhD.)* ***(Right)*** *Juvenile granulosa cell tumor is composed of multicystic follicular spaces lined by multilayers of granulosa cells ➔ containing basophilic fluid. (Courtesy S. Shen, MD, PhD.)*

DYSKERATOSIS CONGENITA

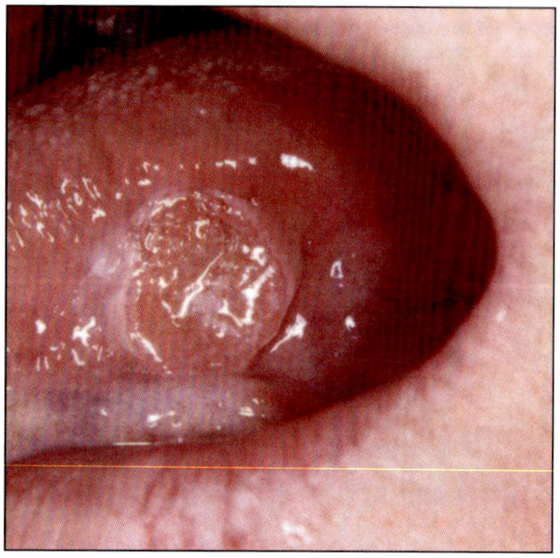

Squamous cell carcinoma on the posterior lateral border of the tongue presents as an exophytic, firm, indurated mass with rolled borders. (Courtesy S. Müller, DMD.)

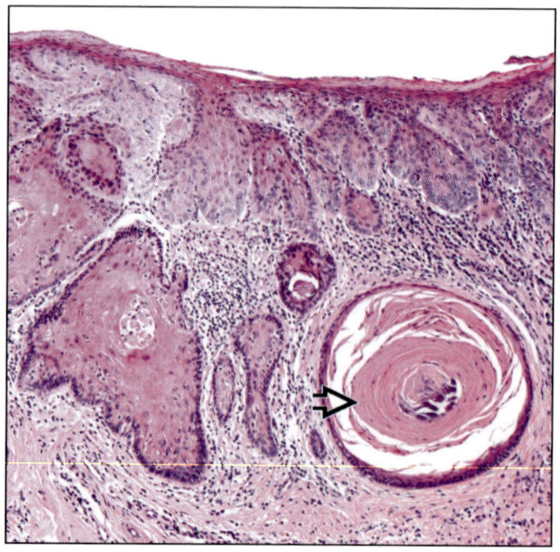

Well-differentiated squamous cell carcinoma extends from the overlying epithelium into the lamina propria with keratin pearl formation ➲. (Courtesy S. Müller, DMD.)

TERMINOLOGY

Definition

- Syndrome with 3 characteristic features
  - Oral leukoplakia
  - Abnormal nails
  - Reticulate hyperpigmentation
- Secondary to defective telomere maintenance

Synonyms

- Zinsser-Cole-Engman syndrome
- Hoyeraal-Hreidarsson syndrome
- Revesz syndrome

EPIDEMIOLOGY

Prevalence

- ~ 1 in 1 million
- ~ 500 reported cases in literature from 1910-2008

Gender

- Male predominance for X-linked form

Natural History

- Phenotype variable
  - Severely affected patients may die early from bone marrow failure
- Median overall survival age: 42 years

Age of Onset

- Variable, but classically
  - 1st decade
    - Skin hyperpigmentation
    - Oral leukoplakia
    - Nail changes
  - 2nd decade
    - Bone marrow failure
  - Median age: 29 years for development of cancer

GENETICS

Germline Mutations

- *TERT, TERC, DKC1, TINF2* genes; documented in ~ 50% of cases
  - These function in maintaining telomeres
  - *TERT* and *TERC* encode telomerase, which maintains telomere length; telomerase is a ribonucleoprotein with 2 components
    - *TERC* encodes RNA component of telomerase
    - *TERT* encodes telomerase reverse transcriptase enzyme
    - *TERT* and *TERC* mutations also described in cases of idiopathic pulmonary fibrosis &/or aplastic anemia
  - *DKC1* encodes dyskerin, which stabilizes telomerase complex
    - Dyskerin: 58 kD nucleolar protein, associates with small nucleolar RNAs
    - Dyskerin binds to telomerase RNA
  - *TINF2* is related to shelterin complex, which helps protect telomeres
    - Shelterin made of 6 proteins
    - Shelterin protects telomere ends from destruction &/or DNA repair
- Other genes (also involved in telomere maintenance)
  - *NOLA2* (encodes NOP10), *NOLA3* (encodes NHP2), *RTEL1, CTC1, TCAB1, WRAP53*
- Patients with dyskeratosis congenita have short telomeres
  - Exception is subset of dyskeratosis congenita with mutations in *USB1* (*C16orf57*)
    - This subset has overlapping features with poikiloderma with neutropenia and Rothmund-Thomson syndrome
- Telomeres are noncoding sequences at chromosome ends
  - Telomeres become shorter with each cell division

- Telomerase adds genetic repeat TTAGGG to 3' end of DNA after replication, to prevent shortening of telomeres
- Rapidly dividing cells are most at risk for telomere shortening; these cells (germ cells, stem cells) have telomerase
- Cells with shortened telomeres become apoptotic through p53 pathway

- Genetic anticipation
  - Disease presents at a progressively earlier age in subsequent generations
  - Seen in families with *TERC* mutations

Inheritance

- X-linked recessive
  - When secondary to *DKC1* mutations, located on X chromosome
- Autosomal dominant
  - When secondary to *TERC* or *TINF2* mutations
- Autosomal dominant or recessive
  - When secondary to *TERT* mutations
- Autosomal recessive
  - When secondary to *CTC1, WRAP53, NHP2, NOP10*

CLINICAL IMPLICATIONS AND ANCILLARY TESTS

Clinical Presentation

- Variable severity: Ranges from mild skin findings with normal bone marrow to early bone marrow failure and death
  - Hoyeraal-Hreidarsson syndrome more severe
    - Cerebellar hypoplasia
    - Microcephaly
    - Severe immunodeficiency
    - Aplastic anemia
    - Enteropathy
    - Intrauterine growth retardation
    - Developmental delay
  - Revesz syndrome
    - Bilateral exudative retinopathy
    - Developmental delay
    - Oral leukoplakia, abnormal nails, reticulate hyperpigmentation
    - Cerebellar hypoplasia
    - Bone marrow hypoplasia
  - Phenotypic variability correlated with genotype
    - *TINF2* mutations cause severe disease with early death; age of onset often < 5 years, aplastic anemia often before 10 years
    - Disease secondary to *TERC* mutations less severe than *DKC1* mutations, but bone marrow failure may present earlier with *TERC* mutations
    - Cancer more common in disease secondary to *TERT* and *TERC* mutations (may be because patients with *TERT* and *TERC* mutations live longer)
    - Cancer less common in disease secondary to *TINF2* mutations
- Classic triad
  - Appears in 1st decade
  - Oral leukoplakia (~ 80% of cases)
  - Abnormal nails (~ 90% of cases)
  - Reticulate hyperpigmentation (~ 90% of cases)
- Associations (% generally based on London registry)
  - Bone marrow
    - Failure (~ 85%): Most common cause of death by 3rd decade (~ 60-70%), presents in 2nd decade
    - Aplastic anemia (in up to 86% of patients)
    - Myelodysplastic syndrome
    - Leukemia
    - Immunologic abnormalities may be the initial presentation (i.e., lymphopenia, low B-cell counts, hypogammaglobulinemia, decreased T-cell function)
  - Cancers of head/neck/skin/anogenital region (52/552 patients on literature review)
    - Lead to mortality in up to 60%
    - Cumulative incidence of cancer 40-50% by age 50
    - Head/neck squamous cell carcinoma: 40% of patients on review
  - Pulmonary fibrosis (~ 20%)
    - Leads to mortality in ~ 10-15%
  - Narrow/blocked tear ducts causing epiphora (~ 30%)
  - Mental retardation (~ 25%)
  - Short stature (~ 20%)
  - Dental problems
    - Extensive caries (~ 17%)
  - Esophageal stricture (~ 17%)
  - Alopecia
  - Premature graying (~ 16%)
  - Palmoplantar keratoderma
  - Osteoporosis, avascular necrosis (hip/shoulder) (~ 5%)
  - Liver disease (~ 7%)
  - Cerebellar hypoplasia (~ 7%)
  - Hypogonadism (~ 6%)
  - Microcephaly (~ 6%)
  - Urethral stenosis (~ 5%)
  - Deafness (~ 1%)

Management

- Bone marrow failure
  - Consider treatment if Hgb < 8 g/dL, PLT < 30,000/mm^3, neutrophils below 1,000/mm^3
  - Mainstay of treatment: Stem cell transplantation
- Less severe cases: Treatment options
  - Anabolic steroid oxymetholone
  - Granulocyte-macrophage colony-stimulating factor
  - Granulocyte colony-stimulating factor &/or erythropoietin
- Prevent pulmonary fibrosis
  - Avoid busulfan and other agents associated with fibrosis

ASSOCIATED NEOPLASMS

Based on 552 Reported Cases of Dyskeratosis Congenita

- Squamous cell carcinoma of head/neck (especially tongue)
  - 24 cases in 22 patients

DYSKERATOSIS CONGENITA

  - Metachronous cancers documented
- Skin cancer
  - 8 cases
- Anorectal carcinoma
  - 6 cases
- Gastric carcinoma
  - 2 adenocarcinoma (2 unspecified)
- Lung carcinoma
  - 2 bronchial, 1 adenocarcinoma, 1 unspecified
- Esophageal carcinoma
  - 3 cases
- Hodgkin lymphoma
  - 3 cases
- Colorectal carcinoma
  - 2 adenocarcinomas (1 unspecified)
- Other
  - 2 pancreatic adenomas, 2 liver adenomas, 1 retinoblastoma, 1 cervical squamous cell carcinoma, 1 non-Hodgkin lymphoma

CANCER RISK MANAGEMENT

Prevention
- Avoid radiotherapy
- Avoid smoking
- Limit sun exposure, use sunscreen/sun protection

Leukemia
- CBC annually (or more often if abnormal)
- Consider annual bone marrow aspirate after baseline examination

Squamous Cell Carcinoma (Head/Neck, Anogenital)
- Monthly self examination (oral/head/neck)
- Annual skin examination by oncology &/or dermatology
- Biannual dental examination
- Annual gynecologic examination

DIFFERENTIAL DIAGNOSIS

Isolated Aplastic Anemia
- Can be secondary to mutations in telomere maintenance genes like dyskeratosis congenita
- Other features of dyskeratosis congenita absent

Fanconi Anemia
- Pigmentary changes
- Short stature
- Eye abnormalities
- CNS malformations, developmental delay
- Urogenital/cardiac/gastrointestinal/oral abnormalities
- Acute myeloid leukemia and other hematologic malignancies
- Solid tumors, including Wilms tumor and squamous cell carcinoma (head/neck, gynecologic)

Other Inherited Bone Marrow Failure Syndromes
- Diamond-Blackfan anemia
- Shwachman-Diamond syndrome
- Severe congenital neutropenia
- Amegakaryocytic thrombocytopenia
- Thrombocytopenia absent radii

Idiopathic Pulmonary Fibrosis
- Can be secondary to mutations in telomere maintenance genes like dyskeratosis congenita
- Other features of dyskeratosis congenita absent

CRITERIA FOR DIAGNOSIS

Suggested Criteria
- 2 of 4 major with at least 2 minor
- Major criteria
  - Oral leukoplakia
  - Nail dystrophy
  - Reticulate hyperpigmentation
  - Bone marrow failure
- Minor criteria
  - Epiphora
  - Short stature
  - Dental caries/loss
  - Premature hair loss/graying
  - Hyperhidrosis
  - Intrauterine growth retardation
  - Pulmonary disease
  - Liver disease
  - Esophageal stricture
  - Hypogonadism, undescended testes, urethral stricture/phimosis
  - Osteoporosis, aseptic necrosis, scoliosis
  - Mental retardation, developmental delay
  - Microcephaly, cerebellar hypoplasia, ataxia, deafness
  - Malignancy

SELECTED REFERENCES

1. Alter BP et al: Telomere length is associated with disease severity and declines with age in dyskeratosis congenita. Haematologica. 97(3):353-9, 2012
2. Dokal I: Dyskeratosis congenita. Hematology Am Soc Hematol Educ Program. 2011:480-6, 2011
3. Jyonouchi S et al: Dyskeratosis congenita: a combined immunodeficiency with broad clinical spectrum--a single-center pediatric experience. Pediatr Allergy Immunol. 22(3):313-9, 2011
4. Mason PJ et al: The genetics of dyskeratosis congenita. Cancer Genet. 204(12):635-45, 2011
5. Alter BP et al: Cancer in dyskeratosis congenita. Blood. 113(26):6549-57, 2009
6. Savage SA et al: Dyskeratosis congenita: the first NIH clinical research workshop. Pediatr Blood Cancer. 53(3):520-3, 2009
7. Vulliamy T et al: Dyskeratosis congenita. Semin Hematol. 43(3):157-66, 2006

Microscopic Features

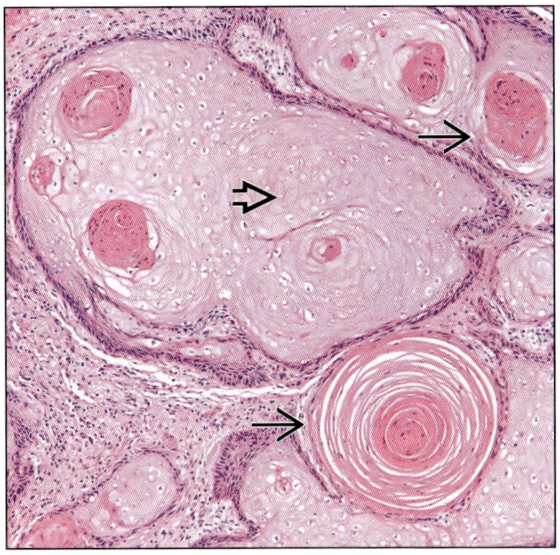

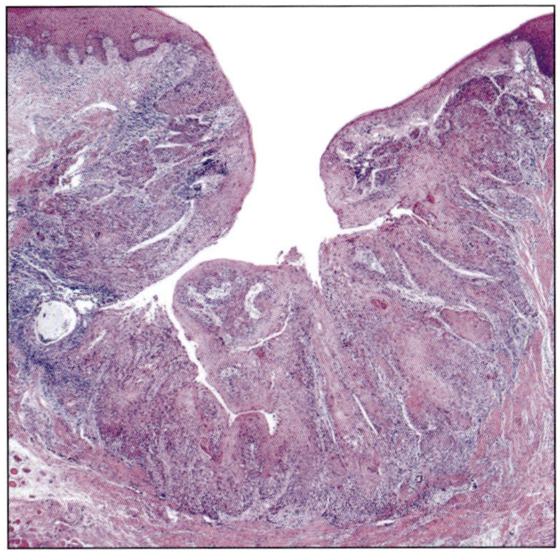

(Left) Hematoxylin & eosin shows well-differentiated squamous cell carcinoma. Note the extensive keratin pearls → and large, pale, eosinophilic carcinoma cells ⇨. (Courtesy S. Owens, MD.) **(Right)** This invasive squamous cell carcinoma has a broad, pushing border and is adjacent to mucosal epithelium with little cytologic atypia. (Courtesy S. Müller, DMD.)

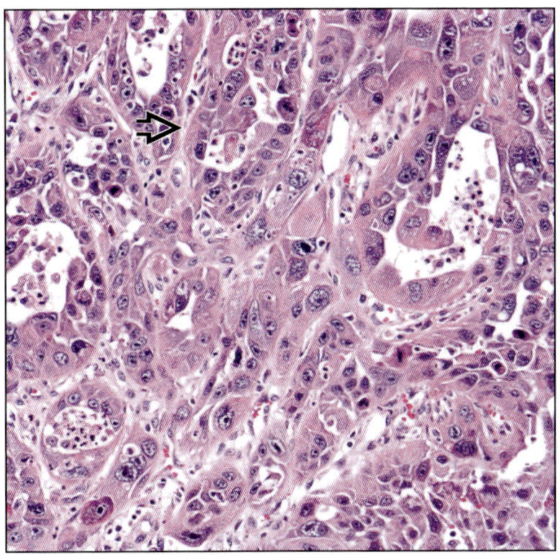

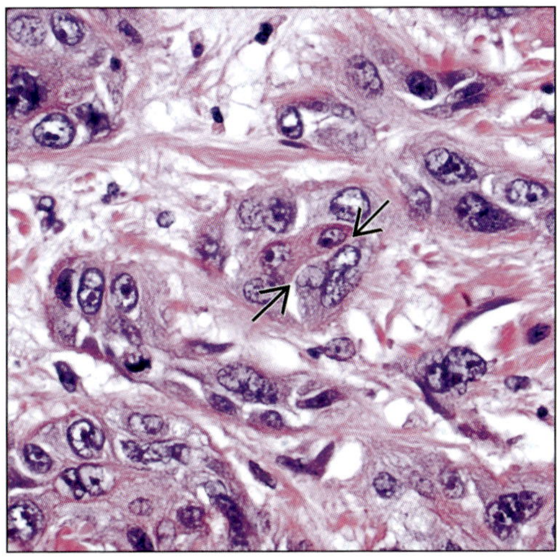

(Left) This squamous cell carcinoma of the lower lip has an acantholytic appearance characterized by tumor nests with a pseudoglandular architecture ⇨. (Courtesy S. Müller, DMD.) **(Right)** There are few features to distinguish this poorly differentiated squamous cell carcinoma from other poorly differentiated neoplasms. When present, intercellular bridges (desmosomes) → can be helpful. (Courtesy S. Owens, MD.)

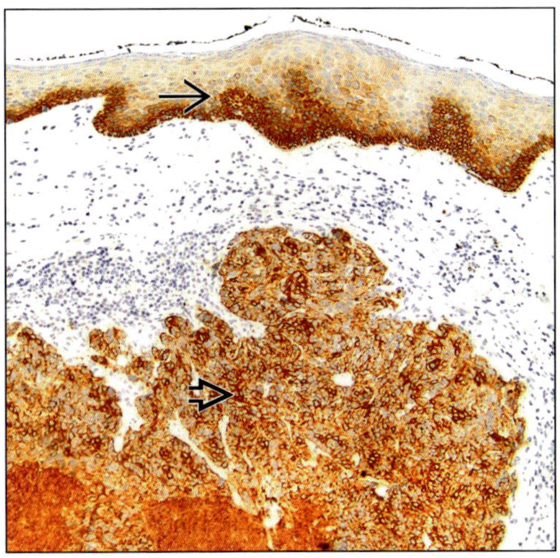

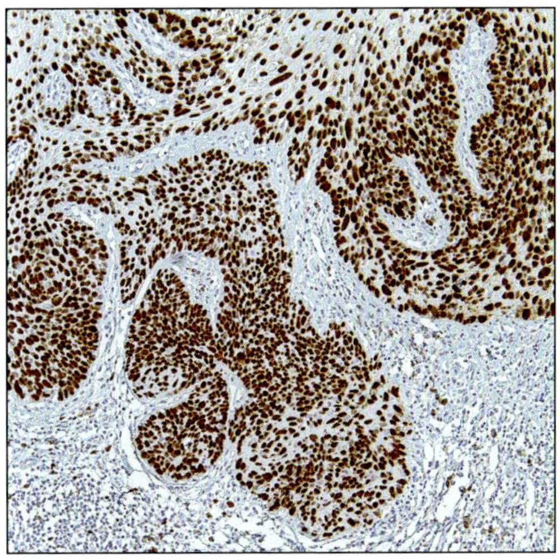

(Left) CK5/6 stains a squamous cell carcinoma beneath normal squamous mucosa. Note the positivity of the normal squamous cells → as well as the carcinoma ⇨. (Courtesy S. Owens, MD.) **(Right)** Positive p63 nuclear staining in this invasive squamous carcinoma nest differentiates squamous cell carcinoma (positive) from other possible neoplasms, including adenocarcinoma and neuroendocrine tumors (negative) in the anal canal. (Courtesy S. Owens, MD.)

FAMILIAL ACUTE MYELOID LEUKEMIA

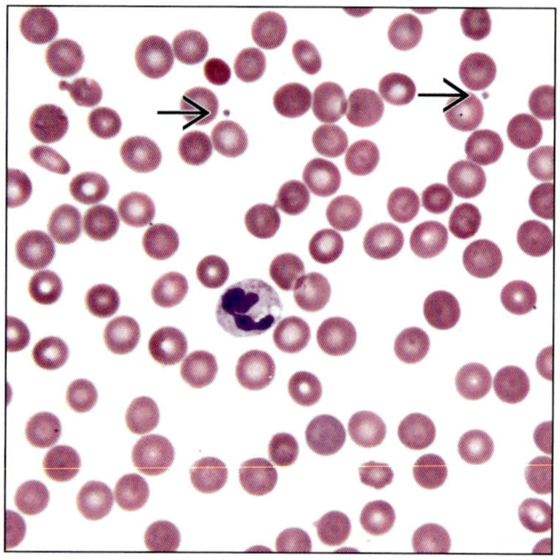

Peripheral blood smear shows thrombocytopenia with 2 platelets ⇒ per high-powered field. Thrombocytopenia is characteristic of familial platelet disorder with propensity to acute myeloid leukemia (FPD/AML).

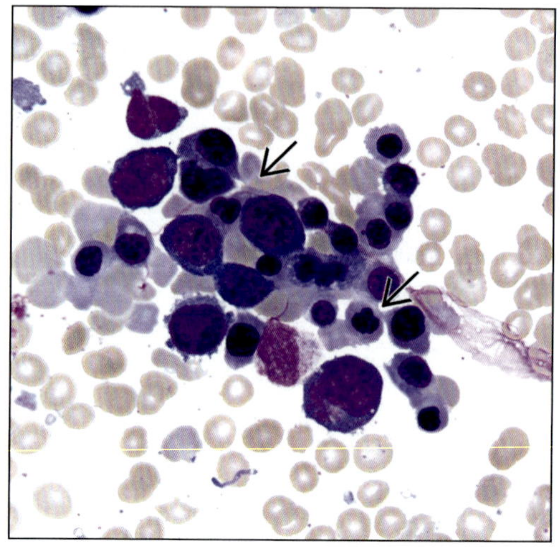

Bone marrow aspirate smear shows erythroid precursors with dysplastic changes ⇒. Dysplasia in 1 or more myeloid lineages is morphologic hallmark of myelodysplastic syndromes (MDS).

TERMINOLOGY

Abbreviations

- Myelodysplastic syndromes (MDS)
- Acute myeloid leukemia (AML)

Definitions

- MDS: Heterogeneous group of clonal hematopoietic stem cell disorders characterized by ineffective hematopoiesis, clinical cytopenia(s), dysplasia in 1 or more myeloid lineages, and increased risk of evolution to AML
- AML: Heterogeneous group of clonal hematopoietic neoplasms characterized by ≥ 20% blasts or blast equivalents in peripheral blood or bone marrow
  - Exceptions include AML with specific recurrent genetic abnormalities (t[15;17], t[8;21], inv[16]/t[16;16]) or acute erythroid leukemia
- Familial MDS/AML is defined as > 1 first- or second-degree relative with MDS/AML; some cases are genetically defined but most familial clusters are of unknown etiology
- Familial MDS/AML syndromes with defined genetic lesions include
  - **Familial platelet disorder with propensity to develop acute myeloid leukemia (FPD/AML)**
    - Rare AD disease characterized by *RUNX1* mutation, platelet dysfunction, clinical thrombocytopenia, and increased risk of MDS/AML (incidence of MDS/AML in affected patients is > 40%; no specific subtype)
  - **Familial *CEBPA* mutation**
    - Rare AD disease characterized by AML ± maturation including frequent Auer rods, aberrant CD7 expression, and no abnormalities detected on conventional cytogenetic analysis (near-complete penetrance)
  - **Familial *GATA2* mutation**
    - Rare AD disease characterized by MDS/AML and poor clinical outcome (highly penetrant; no specific MDS/AML subtype)
  - **Recently described *GATA2* mutation in MonoMAC syndrome**
    - MonoMAC syndrome (a.k.a. DCML deficiency) is an inherited (AD transmission) or sporadic immunodeficiency
    - Characterized by disseminated nontuberculous mycobacterial infections (typically *Mycobacterium avium* complex [MAC]), human papillomavirus (HPV) infections, primary alveolar proteinosis, opportunistic fungal infections, profound monocytopenia, decreased/absent NK and B cells, decreased circulating/tissue dendritic cells
    - Predisposition to MDS/AML in 50% of patients (few myelodysplastic/myeloproliferative overlap cases also reported)
  - **Recently described *GATA2* mutation in Emberger syndrome**
    - Inherited (AD transmission with incomplete penetrance) or sporadic disorder
    - Characterized by primary lymphedema secondary to lymphatic hypoplasia and predisposition to MDS/AML
    - Patients may also have immune dysfunction as evidenced by disseminated cutaneous warts, as well as sensorineural deafness
  - Other well-defined syndromes with variable predisposition to MDS/AML include
    - **Bone marrow failure syndromes**: Congenital amegakaryocytic thrombocytopenia, Diamond-Blackfan anemia, dyskeratosis congenita, severe congenital neutropenia, Shwachman-Diamond syndrome
    - **DNA damage repair deficiency syndromes**: RecQ helicase deficiencies (Bloom syndrome, Rothmund-Thomson syndrome, Werner syndrome); Fanconi anemia

- **Cell cycle and cell differentiation defects**: Neurofibromatosis type 1, Noonan syndrome, and Noonan-like syndrome (juvenile myelomonocytic leukemia)
- **Li-Fraumeni syndrome**
- In most cases, gene defects underlying these syndromes do not appear to be responsible for sporadic cases of MDS/AML

EPIDEMIOLOGY

Mutations in *RUNX1*, *CEBPA*, and *GATA2*

- All are rare; reports of different entities range from 5 to > 20 affected families

GENETICS

General Points

- Underlying genetic cause of many clusters of familial MDS/AML have not yet been elucidated
- Given variable penetrance and latency periods, single germline mutations that have been described likely predispose to MDS/AML by rendering families highly susceptible to additional, somatic mutations

Transcription Factor Mutations

- *RUNX1* mutation in FPD/AML
  - Runt-related transcription factor 1 (*RUNX1*), a.k.a. acute myeloid leukemia 1 (*AML1*), a.k.a. core-binding factor subunit α-2 (*CBFA2*)
    - *RUNX1* (21q22.3) encodes α-subunit of core binding factor transcription factor, which plays a role in normal hematopoiesis and myeloid differentiation
    - Number of *RUNX1* mutations have been described in FPD/AML (large intragenic deletions, Runt domain mutations) and tend to be specific to families; mutational heterogeneity may be reason for variable phenotype
    - *RUNX1* mutations/translocations also occur in sporadic cases of MDS/AML
- *CEBPA* mutation
  - CCAAT/enhancer binding protein α (*CEBPA*)
    - *CEBPA* (19q13.1) encodes a transcription factor (C/EBPα) that can act as a homodimer or a heterodimer with C/EBPβ and C/EBPγ and plays a role in myeloid differentiation
    - *CEBPA* mutations also occur in sporadic cases of AML
    - *CEBPA* point mutations are commonly biallelic (2 acquired in sporadic AML, 1 germline and 1 acquired in familial AML) manifesting as a dominant-negative N-terminal mutation and a C-terminal mutation (in familial AML, germline mutation is always N-terminal mutation)
- *GATA2* mutation
  - GATA binding protein 2 (*GATA2*)
    - *GATA2* (3q21.3) encodes a member of the GATA family of zinc-finger transcription factors (named for promoter consensus sequence to which they bind) and plays a role in hematopoiesis and other nonhematopoietic processes
    - > 30 mutations in *GATA2* have been described in sporadic and familial MDS/AML, MonoMAC and Emberger (e.g., missense, nonsense, frameshift, small and large deletions)
    - Aberrant activation or overexpression of *GATA2* has also been described in de novo AML
    - 3 mutations have been seen in multiple families with varying phenotypes
    - C.1-200_871 + 527del (Met1_Ser290del) has been described in familial MonoMAC and in familial MDS (1 MonoMAC patient also demonstrated unilateral lymphedema)
    - C.1061 C > T (Thr354Met) has been described in familial MonoMAC, familial MDS, and familial MDS/AML (no evidence of lymphedema in these patients)
    - C.1187 G > A (Arg398Gln) has been described in familial MonoMAC and familial MDS and familial AML (no evidence of lymphedema in these patients)
    - *GATA2* has been shown to play a role in lymphatic vasculature development
    - Lymphedema may occur secondary to significant *GATA2* gene abnormalities (nonsense or frameshift mutations, partial or complete deletions) causing haploinsufficiency, as have been described in Emberger syndrome and de novo MDS/AML with lymphedema

Additionally Reported Genetic Abnormalities

- **Telomere maintenance mutations**: Telomerase reverse transcriptase *(TERT)* and telomerase RNA component *(TERC)* mutations have been described in 5 families with MDS/AML (most also with aplastic anemia [AA]) but lacking phenotypic characteristics of bone marrow failure syndrome dyskeratosis congenita (variable penetrance; no specific MDS/AML subtype)
  - Telomerase is a ribonuclease that maintains telomere length by addition of telomere repeat TTAGGG
    - *TERT* (5p15.33) encodes reverse transcriptase protein component of telomerase (hTERT)
    - *TERC* (3q26) encodes RNA component (hTR), which provides template for telomere repeat
  - Mutations in *TERT* and *TERC* underlie a subset of dyskeratosis congenital cases and have been described in de novo MDS, idiopathic pulmonary fibrosis (familial and sporadic), and AA; *TERT* mutations have been described in de novo AML
- **Aplastic anemia/myelodysplasia with *SRP72* mutations**: Case report of AD transmission of heterozygous *SRP72* mutations in 2 families with AA &/or MDS
- **Monosomy 7**: Described in families with early onset of MDS (pathogenesis is poorly understood)
  - Apparently AD inheritance pattern
  - Occurs in sporadic MDS/AML as well as in syndromic MDS/AML

- Children with early onset MDS and monosomy 7 may represent children with MDS/AML-predisposition syndrome that is otherwise phenotypically silent
- Alternatively, these families may have as of yet unidentified gene mutation(s) rendering affected members vulnerable to loss of a chromosome 7

CLINICAL IMPLICATIONS AND ANCILLARY TESTS

Familial vs. Sporadic MDS/AML

- Younger age of presentation in familial MDS/AML
- Relatives of AML patients < 21 years old at diagnosis have 6.5x increase risk of MDS/AML and 3x risk of any myeloid malignancy

FPD/AML

- Patients often present with mild to moderate bleeding
- Platelet aggregation study shows impaired response to collagen and absent 2nd wave of epinephrine-induced aggregation; decreased aggregation with arachidonate is also seen (author observation)
- Subset of affected patients (over 40%) develop MDS/AML at a younger age than sporadic AML (median age 33)

CEBPA Mutation

- Eosinophilia common
- Favorable prognosis of AML, even with relapse
- Wide range in age of onset (as young as 4 to over 35), consistent with evidence of secondary mutations in addition to germline mutations in affected families

GATA2 Mutation

- In families with *GATA2* mutations and early onset MDS/AML alone, prognosis is poor
- In MonoMAC patients, some morphologic features of MDS are different than those commonly observed in de novo MDS
  - Frequent marrow hypocellularity, frequent marrow fibrosis, presence of CD56-positive plasma cells, consistent trilineage dysplasia, and frequent hemophagocytic histiocytes
- No clear genotype-phenotype correlations

ASSOCIATED NEOPLASMS

FPD/AML

- Increased risk for T-acute lymphoblastic leukemia
- No increased risk for other non-myeloid neoplasms

MonoMAC

- Reported malignancies (some due to HPV infection): Vulvar carcinoma, metastatic melanoma, cervical carcinoma, Bowen disease of vulva, Epstein-Barr virus-positive leiomyosarcoma

CANCER RISK MANAGEMENT

Stem Cell Transplantation

- Genetic screening is advised when evaluating relatives as potential donors for patients undergoing allogeneic stem cell transplantation

SELECTED REFERENCES

1. Pasquet M et al: High frequency of GATA2 mutations in patients with mild chronic neutropenia evolving to MonoMac syndrome, myelodysplasia, and acute myeloid leukemia. Blood. 121(5):822-9, 2013
2. Bodor C et al: Germ-line GATA2 p.THR354MET mutation in familial myelodysplastic syndrome with acquired monosomy 7 and ASXL1 mutation demonstrating rapid onset and poor survival. Haematologica. 97(6):890-4, 2012
3. Goldin LR et al: Familial aggregation of acute myeloid leukemia and myelodysplastic syndromes. J Clin Oncol. 30(2):179-83, 2012
4. Holme H et al: Marked genetic heterogeneity in familial myelodysplasia/acute myeloid leukaemia. Br J Haematol. 158(2):242-8, 2012
5. Kazenwadel J et al: Loss-of-function germline GATA2 mutations in patients with MDS/AML or MonoMAC syndrome and primary lymphedema reveal a key role for GATA2 in the lymphatic vasculature. Blood. 119(5):1283-91, 2012
6. Kirwan M et al: Exome sequencing identifies autosomal-dominant SRP72 mutations associated with familial aplasia and myelodysplasia. Am J Hum Genet. 90(5):888-92, 2012
7. Bigley V et al: The human syndrome of dendritic cell, monocyte, B and NK lymphoid deficiency. J Exp Med. 208(2):227-34, 2011
8. Calvo KR et al: Myelodysplasia in autosomal dominant and sporadic monocytopenia immunodeficiency syndrome: diagnostic features and clinical implications. Haematologica. 96(8):1221-5, 2011
9. Dickinson RE et al: Exome sequencing identifies GATA-2 mutation as the cause of dendritic cell, monocyte, B and NK lymphoid deficiency. Blood. 118(10):2656-8, 2011
10. Hahn CN et al: Heritable GATA2 mutations associated with familial myelodysplastic syndrome and acute myeloid leukemia. Nat Genet. 43(10):1012-7, 2011
11. Hsu AP et al: Mutations in GATA2 are associated with the autosomal dominant and sporadic monocytopenia and mycobacterial infection (MonoMAC) syndrome. Blood. 118(10):2653-5, 2011
12. Ostergaard P et al: Mutations in GATA2 cause primary lymphedema associated with a predisposition to acute myeloid leukemia (Emberger syndrome). Nat Genet. 43(10):929-31, 2011
13. Vinh DC et al: Autosomal dominant and sporadic monocytopenia with susceptibility to mycobacteria, fungi, papillomaviruses, and myelodysplasia. Blood. 115(8):1519-29, 2010
14. Kirwan M et al: Defining the pathogenic role of telomerase mutations in myelodysplastic syndrome and acute myeloid leukemia. Hum Mutat. 30(11):1567-73, 2009
15. Owen C et al: Familial myelodysplasia and acute myeloid leukaemia--a review. Br J Haematol. 140(2):123-32, 2008
16. Smith ML et al: Mutation of CEBPA in familial acute myeloid leukemia. N Engl J Med. 351(23):2403-7, 2004
17. Song WJ et al: Haploinsufficiency of CBFA2 causes familial thrombocytopenia with propensity to develop acute myelogenous leukaemia. Nat Genet. 23(2):166-75, 1999
18. Weiss HJ et al: A familialdefect in platelet function associated with imapired release of adenosine diphosphate. N Engl J Med. 281(23):1264-70, 1969

Microscopic Features and Cytogenetics

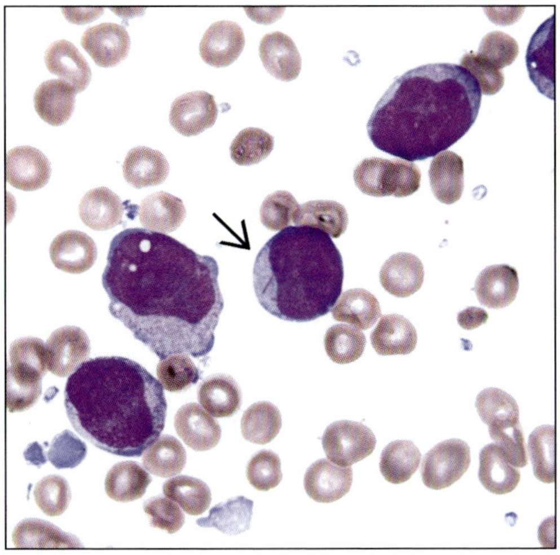

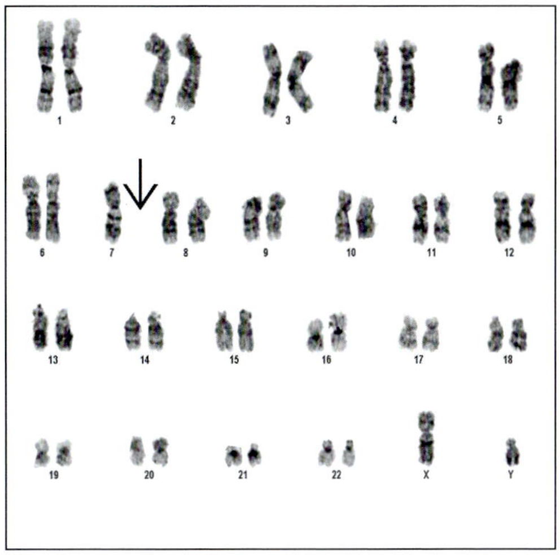

(Left) *Aspirate smear from a patient with AML shows intermediate-sized blasts with slightly irregular nuclear contours, fine chromatin, and distinct nucleoli, and 1 cell with distinct Auer rods ⇨. Auer rods are frequently seen in AML with CEBPA mutation.* ***(Right)*** *Patients with familial MDS/AML may also have cytogenetic abnormalities, frequently monosomy 7 ⇨, as depicted in this karyotype. (Courtesy P. Dal Cin, PhD.)*

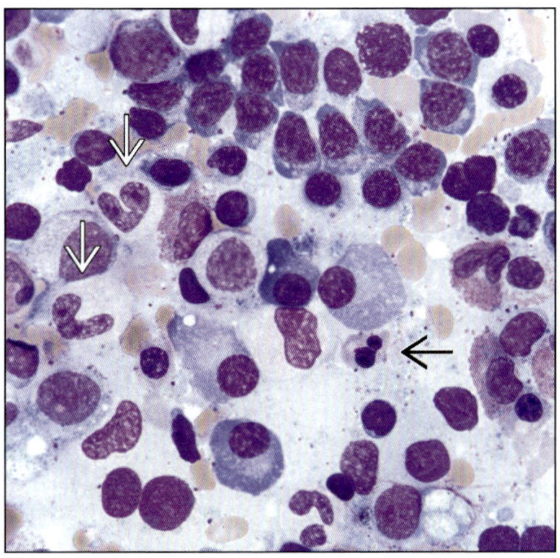

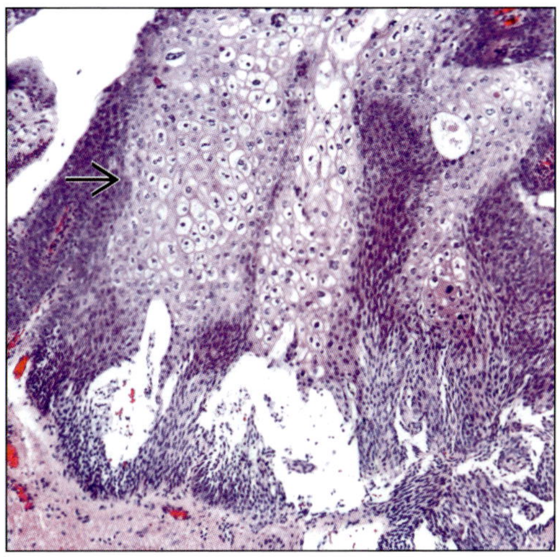

(Left) *Bone marrow aspirate smear from a 26-year-old man with MonoMAC syndrome shows erythroid hyperplasia, ↑ plasma cells and myelodysplasia in the erythroid (nuclear budding) ⇨, and myeloid (hypogranularity) ➡ lineages.* ***(Right)*** *Koilocytes (large squamous cells with pyknotic nuclei and abundant clear cytoplasm) ⇨ are present in this urethral condyloma biopsy from a 26-year-old man with MonoMAC syndrome. HPV infection is common in MonoMAC.*

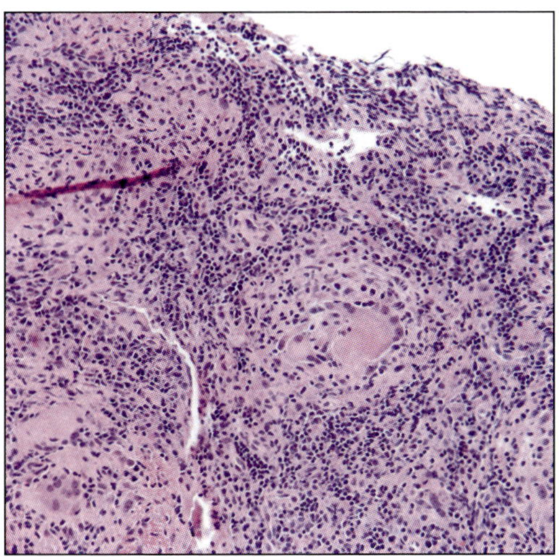

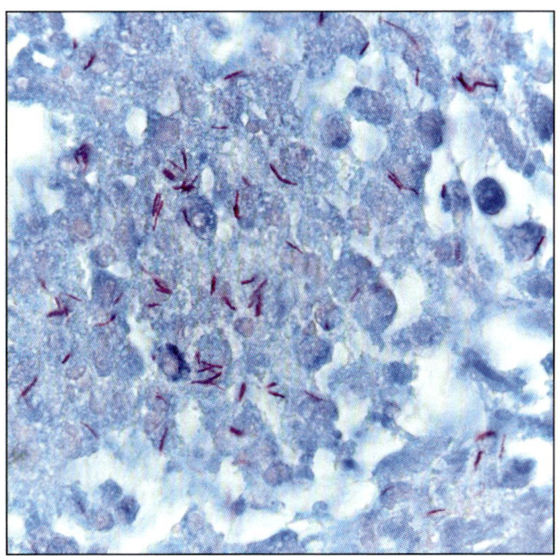

(Left) *Thoracic lymph node biopsy from a 26-year-old man with MonoMAC syndrome shows nonnecrotizing granulomatous inflammation. Necrosis was identified in other sections.* ***(Right)*** *High-magnification view of acid-fast bacilli stain from a lymph node of a 26-year-old man with MonoMAC syndrome shows that numerous red-staining mycobacterial organisms are present. PCR studies identified the species as Mycobacterium kansasii.*

FAMILIAL ADENOMATOUS POLYPOSIS

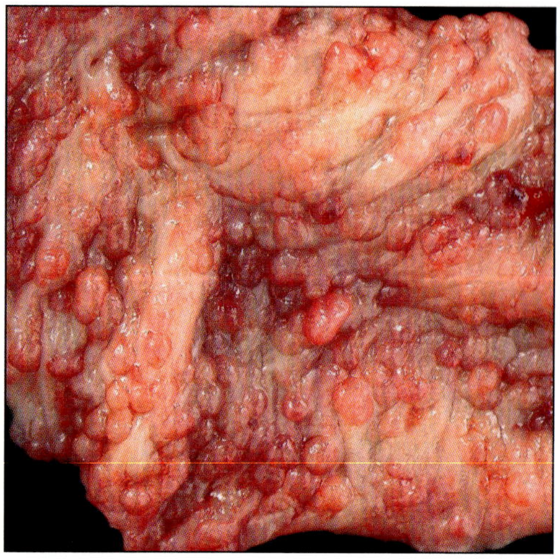

Gross photo of the colon from a patient with familial adenomatous polyposis (FAP) shows hundreds of small sessile polyps carpeting the mucosal surface. (Courtesy A. Polydorides, MD.)

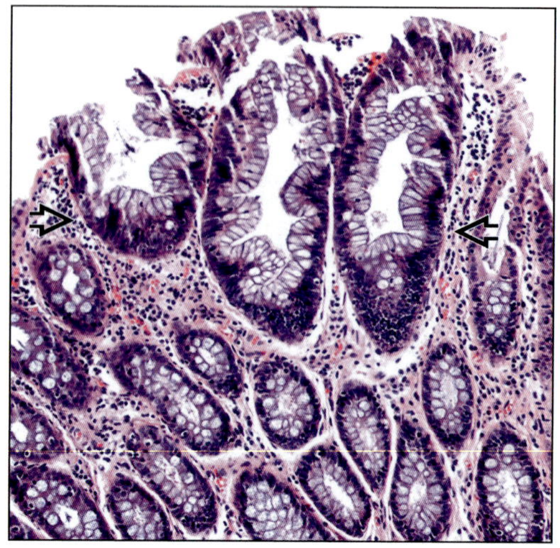

Photomicrograph shows 3 adenomatous crypts ➡ that stand out from the adjacent normal mucosa. Microscopic foci like this are common in the flat colonic mucosa of FAP patients.

TERMINOLOGY

Abbreviations

- Familial adenomatous polyposis (FAP)
- Attenuated familial adenomatous polyposis (AFAP)
- Congenital hypertrophy of retinal pigment epithelium (CHRPE)
- Colorectal carcinoma (CRC)

Synonyms

- Adenomatous polyposis coli (APC), familial polyposis coli, Gardner syndrome, Turcot syndrome, Crail syndrome, Bussey-Gardner polyposis

EPIDEMIOLOGY

Age Range

- 1st adenomas detected between ages 10 and 20 years
- Mean age of diagnosis: 34-36 years if not in a known kindred undergoing screening
- Mean age of CRC: 40-42 years, but can occur in teenagers

Incidence

- 0.003-0.015% of population
- Most common genetic polyposis syndrome
  - FAP accounts for < 1% of all CRCs

Natural History

- Adenomas increase in size and number with age
  - Polyp count and patient age predict cancer risk
  - As in sporadic adenomas, only a small percentage progress to cancer
- AFAP: Fewer adenomas at a later onset (~ 15 years later than FAP)
  - Upper GI lesions almost always present, but extraintestinal manifestations rare
  - Lower risk of developing CRC
  - Phenotype identical to *MYH*-associated polyposis, which is autosomal recessive
    - Requires genetic testing to differentiate the 2

Gender

- M = F

GENETICS

Germline Mutation in *APC* Gene

- Tumor suppressor gene that downregulates β-catenin (Wnt signaling pathway)
  - Controls cell cycle and stabilizes microtubules
- Located on chromosome 5q21-22
- Specific *APC* mutations correlate with phenotypes
  - AFAP associated with mutations at 3' and 5' ends of *APC* gene, whereas CHRPEs, osteomas, desmoids, and epidermal cysts are associated with mutations in middle of gene
  - Hot spot for severe polyposis phenotype at codon 1309
    - More polyps and earlier onset of CRC in families with mutations near this hot spot
- 30-40% of FAP cases arise de novo (no family history)
  - Cause of these spontaneous mutations unknown
- *APC* I1307K mutation
  - Autosomal dominant mutation that imparts a 10-20% lifetime CRC risk
  - No polyposis or extracolonic manifestations
  - Affects 6% of Ashkenazi Jews
  - Renders *APC* gene susceptible to further mutations that lead to CRC

CLINICAL IMPLICATIONS

Clinical Presentation

- Rectal bleeding, diarrhea, colicky abdominal pain, mucous discharge, intussusception

- Rarely, severe electrolyte depletion can occur with diffuse polyposis
- Acute pancreatitis due to adenoma obstructing ampulla/pancreatic duct

Imaging Findings

- Polyps can be detected in both upper GI and lower GI locations, especially with fluoroscopic-guided barium enema
- Osteomas of jaw in Gardner syndrome can be identified on radiographs
- Desmoid tumors in Gardner syndrome can be identified on CT

MACROSCOPIC FINDINGS

General Features

- Diagnostic criteria for FAP (any of the following)
  - ≥ 100 colorectal adenomas (classical FAP)
  - < 100 colorectal adenomas in AFAP
  - Germline *APC* mutation
  - Family history of FAP plus at least 1 of the following
    - Epidermoid cyst, osteoma, desmoid

Endoscopic Findings

- Hundreds of small sessile adenomas carpet the colon
  - Similar location as in sporadic adenomas with predilection for rectosigmoid
  - Some larger pedunculated polyps
  - May have rectal sparing in AFAP
- CRC distribution follows adenomas (70-80% left-sided)
  - Often multiple CRCs, either synchronous or metachronous

Specimen Handling

- Total resection
  - Aside from taking sections of all large polyps to look for invasive carcinoma, face-down sections of the flat mucosa can be taken to show unicryptal adenomas that are pathognomonic of FAP (so-called Bussey section)

MICROSCOPIC FINDINGS

General Features

- Colonic adenomas look identical to sporadic counterparts
- Presence of unicryptal adenomas in flat mucosa diagnostic of FAP

ASSOCIATED NEOPLASMS

Other GI (Extracolonic Lesions)

- Small intestine
  - Mostly duodenal/ampullary adenomas
    - Possible cocarcinogenic effect of bile
    - 10-15 years later than colonic adenomas but 30 years earlier than general population
    - 50-100% of FAP patients have these on routine screening (50-100%)
    - Cumulative cancer risk: 2-10%
    - Common cause of death in patients who have had a prophylactic colectomy (20%)
- Stomach
  - Mostly fundic gland polyps (40-60%)
    - More numerous, occurring at a younger age, and more likely to have dysplasia (up to 25%) than sporadic
  - Antral adenomas (6%)
  - Gastric cancer is rare, but cases have been reported
- Liver
  - Increasing rate of hepatoblastomas in male infants
  - Rare hepatic adenomas and hepatocellular carcinomas
  - Rare malignant embryonal tumor
- Pancreas
  - Adenocarcinoma
  - Rare reports of intraductal mucinous neoplasms
- Biliary tract
  - Adenocarcinoma and dysplasia of bile ducts and gallbladder

Extraintestinal Manifestations

- Soft tissue (10-30% of FAP patients)
  - Fibromatosis (desmoid tumors)
    - Locally aggressive (even fatal) but "benign" tumors: Do not metastasize
    - 2nd most common cause of death in FAP patients (after CRC)
    - Unencapsulated
    - Hereditary desmoid disease: Rare *APC* mutation that causes multiple desmoids and other extraintestinal manifestations without colonic disease
    - Most common in small bowel mesentery
    - Often post surgery/trauma
    - Hormones may affect growth (pregnancy, estrogen); tamoxifen sometimes used for treatment
- Bones
  - Multiple osteomas of the skull, long bones, and mandible
- Teeth (70-80% of FAP patients)
  - Impaction, supernumerary/absent, abnormal roots
- Eye (75-90% of FAP patients)
  - Congenital hypertrophy of retinal pigment epithelium (CHRPE)
    - Pigmented fundus lesion
    - Earliest manifestation of FAP; can be seen in young infants
- Skin
  - Multiple epidermal inclusion cysts of face and scalp
  - Lipomas, fibromas, sebaceous cysts
- Endocrine system
  - Papillary thyroid carcinoma, cribriform morular variant, in women
  - Adrenal cortical neoplasms
  - Pancreatic islet cell neoplasms
  - Rare reports of parathyroid and pituitary adenomas
- Brain (Turcot syndrome)
  - Hereditary CRC & brain tumor
    - FAP patients: Medulloblastomas

FAMILIAL ADENOMATOUS POLYPOSIS

Variants of FAP		
Variant	**Phenotype**	**Comment**
Attenuated familial adenomatous polyposis (AFAP)	Fewer adenomas and later age of onset, lower risk of colorectal carcinoma (CRC)	Need to exclude autosomal recessive *MYH*-associated polyposis
Gardner syndrome	FAP with extraintestinal manifestations (desmoids, osteomas, epidermoid cysts)	Significant mortality from extraintestinal lesions, especially after colectomy
Turcot syndrome	FAP with medulloblastoma	CRC with glioma is likely Lynch syndrome, not FAP

Extraintestinal Features in FAP	
Benign Lesions	**Malignant Lesions**
CHRPE (75-90%)	Papillary thyroid cancer (2-3%)
Epidermoid cysts (50%)	Brain tumor (medulloblastoma) (< 1%)
Osteoma (50-90%)	Hepatoblastoma (1%)
Desmoid tumor (10-30%)	Hepatocellular carcinoma (< 1%)
Supernumerary teeth (70-80%)	Pancreatic adenocarcinoma (2%)
Adrenal adenomas (7-13%)	Pancreatic islet cell neoplasms (rare)
Lipomas and fibromas (prevalence unknown)	Adrenal cortical carcinoma (rare)
Juvenile angiofibroma (prevalence unknown)	Biliary tract adenocarcinoma (rare)

    - Lynch patients: Gliomas
- Head and neck
  - Nasopharyngeal angiofibroma

CANCER RISK MANAGEMENT

Surgery

- Prophylactic colectomy with ileoanal pouch anastomosis is surgical treatment of choice
- Goal is to do this when patient is in their teens (if diagnosis can be established this early)
- Patients will still require surveillance of pouch to remove adenomas
- Upper endoscopy with biopsy of gastric and duodenal polyps
  - Most duodenal/ampullary adenomas can be excised endoscopically, but some may require a Whipple procedure
- Surgical excision of desmoids (when possible)

Medical Management

- Chemoprevention of polyps with indomethacin and other NSAIDs
- Medical treatment of desmoids includes hormonal therapy, imatinib, and NSAIDs

Genetic Testing

- Protein truncation test (PTT)
  - Looks for abnormally shortened APC protein in exon 15
- Gene sequencing
  - *APC* gene is very large; hence, sequencing is difficult
    - Sequencing is done to try and predict phenotype of affected family members (likelihood of desmoids or severe phenotype)
  - Latest techniques are about 95% sensitive in detecting mutations in classic FAP, < 30% in AFAP
    - Important to test for *MYH*-associated polyposis if these tests are negative
  - Multiplex ligation probe amplification (MLPA) is used to look for large deletions and duplications
- Sequencing of exons 1-14 coupled with PTT of exon 15 is one commonly used testing strategy
  - If PTT is positive, then exon 15 can be sequenced

SELECTED REFERENCES

1. Patel SG et al: Familial colon cancer syndromes: an update of a rapidly evolving field. Curr Gastroenterol Rep. 14(5):428-38, 2012
2. Burger B et al: Prevalence of skin lesions in familial adenomatous polyposis: a marker for presymptomatic diagnosis? Oncologist. 16(12):1698-705, 2011
3. Claes K et al: The genetics of familial adenomatous polyposis (FAP) and MutYH-associated polyposis (MAP). Acta Gastroenterol Belg. 74(3):421-6, 2011
4. Aretz S: The differential diagnosis and surveillance of hereditary gastrointestinal polyposis syndromes. Dtsch Arztebl Int. 107(10):163-73, 2010
5. Half E et al: Familial adenomatous polyposis. Orphanet J Rare Dis. 4:22, 2009
6. Vasen HF et al: Guidelines for the clinical management of familial adenomatous polyposis (FAP). Gut. 57(5):704-13, 2008
7. Nieuwenhuis MH et al: Correlations between mutation site in APC and phenotype of familial adenomatous polyposis (FAP): a review of the literature. Crit Rev Oncol Hematol. 61(2):153-61, 2007
8. Bussey HJ: Familial polyposis coli and hepatocellular neoplasms. Hepatology. 12(1):175-6, 1990
9. Bodmer WF et al: Localization of the gene for familial adenomatous polyposis on chromosome 5. Nature. 328(6131):614-6, 1987

Gross, Microscopic, and Genetic Features

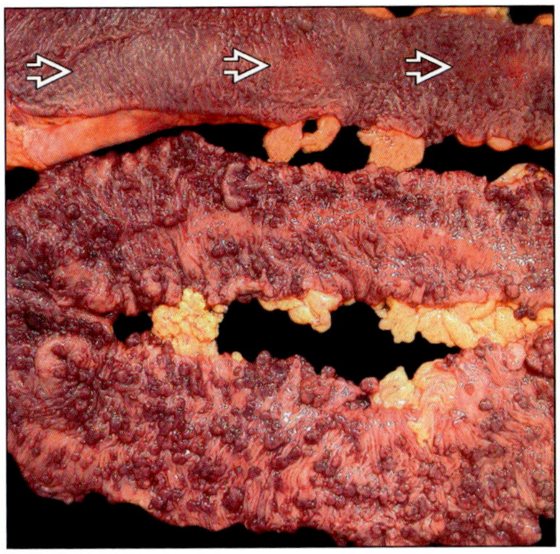

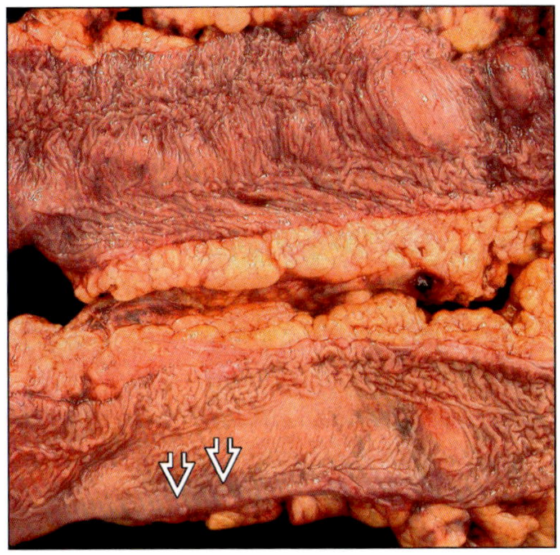

(Left) *Gross photo shows a colectomy specimen from a case of familial adenomatous polyposis with rectal sparing. Polyps carpet the more proximal mucosa, but the rectal mucosa at the top ➡ is flattened and atrophic. (Courtesy A. Polydorides, MD.)* **(Right)** *Gross photograph shows a colectomy specimen from a case of attenuated familial adenomatous polyposis with only a few colonic polyps ➡. (Courtesy A. Polydorides, MD.)*

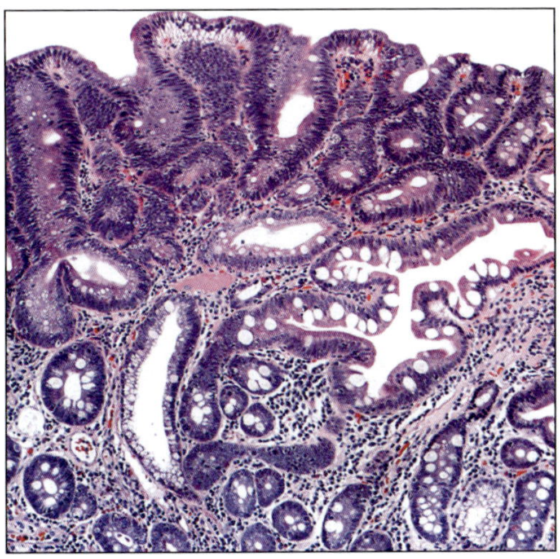

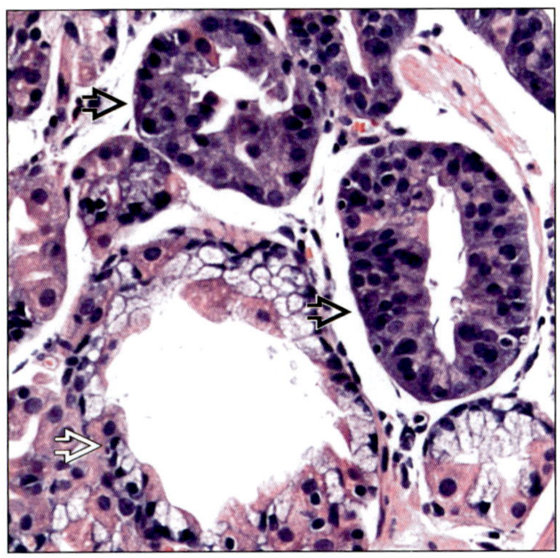

(Left) *This medium-power view shows a duodenal adenoma in a patient with familial adenomatous polyposis. Note low-grade dysplasia involving the surface epithelium. (Courtesy A. Polydorides, MD.)* **(Right)** *This high-power view of a fundic gland polyp shows low-grade dysplasia ⇨. The nondysplastic epithelium shows dilated oxyntic glands typical of a fundic gland polyp ➡.*

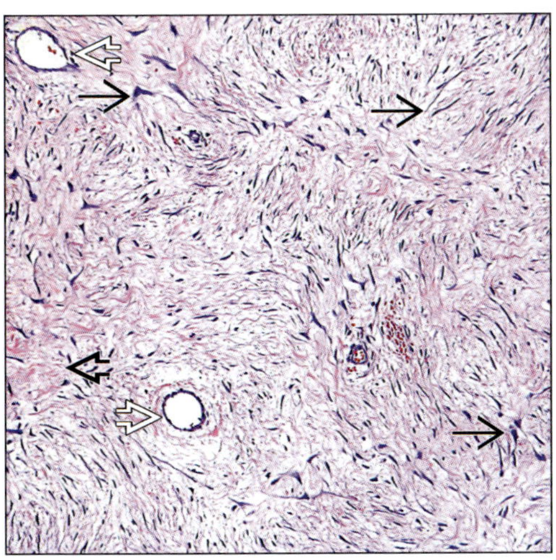

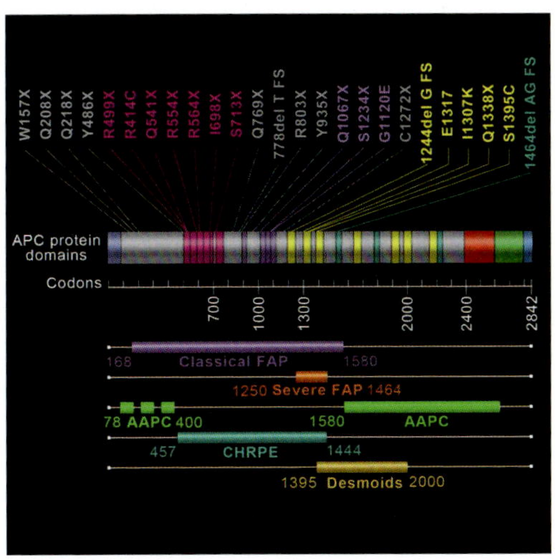

(Left) *This medium-power view of a mesenteric fibromatosis (desmoid tumor) shows spindle cells →, collagen ⇨, and evenly spaced blood vessels ➡. (Courtesy A. Polydorides, MD.)* **(Right)** *This drawing shows the location of various mutations along the APC gene and what phenotypic abnormalities have been associated with each mutation site.*

FAMILIAL CHORDOMA

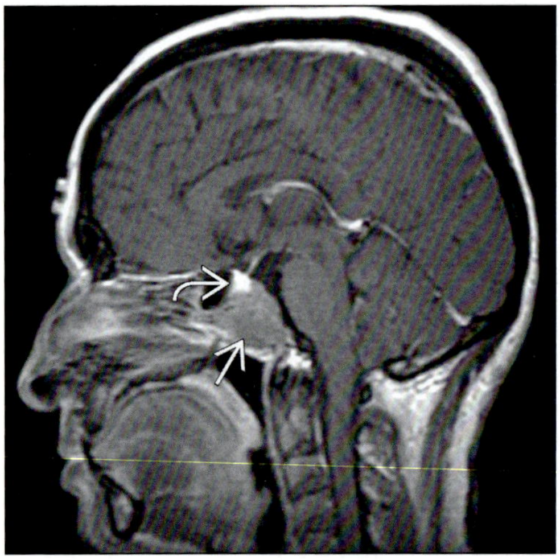

Sagittal T1WI C+ MR shows a classic expansile chordoma ➡ of the clivus. Note the adjacent pituitary gland ➦. Given the delicate location, symptoms are common.

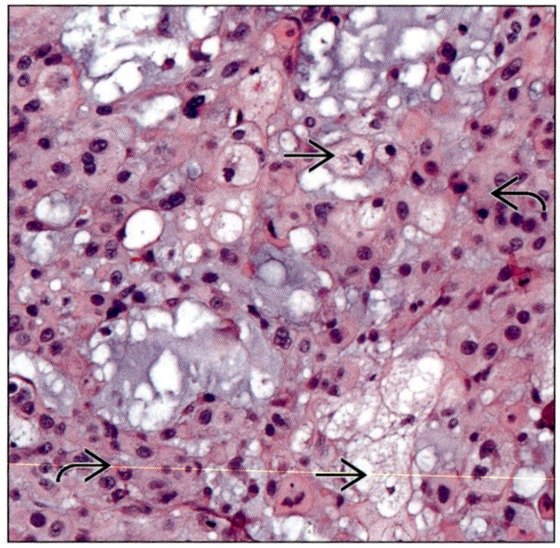

This image shows the classic histology for a conventional chordoma: A mixture of eosinophilic cells ➦ and bubbly physaliferous cells ➡ within a blue myxoid matrix.

TERMINOLOGY

Definitions

- Chordoma occurring in at least 2 blood relatives

EPIDEMIOLOGY

Incidence

- Extremely rare with few families reported so far

Age

- Wide age range reported (30-50 years most common)
- Very rare in people < 10 years

Gender

- M:F = 2:1

Site

- Most familial chordomas appear to arise in sacrococcygeal (~ 50%) and clival (~ 45%) locations

GENETICS

Currently Under Active Investigation

- Familial Chordoma Study (National Institute of Health)

Inheritance Pattern

- Possible autosomal dominant inheritance pattern
  - Male-to-male transmission reported in some families

Genetic Alterations

- Similar to sporadic cases
  - Duplication of region on chromosome 6q27 containing T-brachyury gene
  - Reports of loss of heterozygosity of 7q33
  - Possible tumor suppressor gene locus at 1p36

Other Associations

- Chordoma presenting in infancy can also be seen in tuberous sclerosis complex (TSC)
  - Autosomal dominant disease
  - Mutation of *TSC1* on 9q34 and *TSC2* on 16p13.3

ASSOCIATED NEOPLASMS

Chordoma

- Etiology
  - Thought to arise from notochordal remnants
  - Supported by characteristic midline location
- Clinical presentation
  - Cranial tumors
    - Headache
    - Visual complaints (e.g., diplopia)
    - Other cranial nerve defects
    - Evidence of pituitary dysfunction
    - May present as a nasal polyp
  - Sacrococcygeal tumors
    - Longstanding lower back pain
    - Regional neurogenic issues (bladder dysfunction, constipation)
  - Nonsacrococcygeal spinal tumors
    - Symptoms related to compression of spinal cord or spinal nerve roots
    - Lumbar vertebrae may show compression fractures
- Imaging findings
  - Cranial tumors
    - Consistent involvement of midline structures
    - Destructive lesion in clivus, sphenooccipital region, or hypophyseal region
    - Mass effect on adjacent brain tissue
    - May show calcific densities
  - Sacrococcygeal tumors
    - Lytic, destructive bone tumor
    - Often shows anterior soft tissue extension

- Nonsacrococcygeal spinal tumors
  - Predominantly lytic; some sclerotic
  - Most localized to vertebral bodies
- Macroscopic findings
  - Soft, lobulated, translucent tissue
  - May appear mucoid
  - Sacrococcygeal chordomas that show anterior soft tissue extension are often covered by periosteum
  - Recurrent tumors in any location generally show multiple nodules
- Microscopic findings
  - All tumors characteristically lobulated
  - Conventional chordoma
    - Cells with clear to eosinophilic cytoplasm
    - Heavily vacuolated physaliferous cells
    - Typically prominent myxoid stroma
  - Chondroid chordoma
    - Contain areas of chondroid matrix or frank cartilage in addition to more conventional areas
    - Almost all occur in skull base
  - Dedifferentiated chordoma
    - Defined as a high-grade sarcoma arising in association with or at site of a previously documented chordoma
    - Dedifferentiated areas usually show up in recurrent tumors
    - Most occur in sacrococcygeal region
- Immunophenotype
  - Strong nuclear expression of brachyury
  - Generally strong expression of cytokeratin &/or epithelial membrane antigen (EMA)
  - Variable expression of S100

Astrocytoma, Pilocytic

- 2 cases have been reported in association with familial chordoma

CANCER RISK MANAGEMENT

Screening

- No current screening protocol in place
- Detection of T-brachyury gene duplication may confer susceptibility to chordoma development
- MR of entire craniospinal axis at the time a family aggregation is identified

Treatment

- Complete resection with wide tumor-free margins is mainstay of therapy
  - Depending on site, only incomplete resection may be possible
- Radiation therapy is debatable but does not appear to be effective
- Most chemotherapies are ineffective
  - Recent discoveries of overexpression of tyrosine kinases and transcriptional regulators in chordomas raise possible utility of tyrosine kinase inhibitors (TKI) and other drugs

Prognosis

- Indolent but locally aggressive
  - Most morbidity is due to local recurrence
  - Most mortality is due to local extension of tumor (brain, upper respiratory tract, genitourinary/gastrointestinal tracts)
- Metastases in up to 30% of cases
  - Skin, lungs, other bones
- Age < 40 may be good prognostic factor
- Chondroid chordoma may have better survival rate than conventional chordoma (controversial)

SELECTED REFERENCES

1. Bydon M et al: Novel therapeutic targets in chordoma. Expert Opin Ther Targets. 16(11):1139-43, 2012
2. Gagliardi F et al: Current therapeutic options and novel molecular markers in skull base chordomas. Neurosurg Rev. 35(1):1-13; discussion 13-4, 2012
3. Walcott BP et al: Chordoma: current concepts, management, and future directions. Lancet Oncol. 13(2):e69-76, 2012
4. Yang XR et al: T (brachyury) gene duplication confers major susceptibility to familial chordoma. Nat Genet. 41(11):1176-8, 2009
5. Hallor KH et al: Frequent deletion of the CDKN2A locus in chordoma: analysis of chromosomal imbalances using array comparative genomic hybridisation. Br J Cancer. 98(2):434-42, 2008
6. Chugh R et al: Chordoma: the nonsarcoma primary bone tumor. Oncologist. 12(11):1344-50, 2007
7. Bhadra AK et al: Familial chordoma. A report of two cases. J Bone Joint Surg Br. 88(5):634-6, 2006
8. Larizza L et al: Update on the cytogenetics and molecular genetics of chordoma. Hered Cancer Clin Pract. 3(1):29-41, 2005
9. Yang X' et al: Corroboration of a familial chordoma locus on chromosome 7q and evidence of genetic heterogeneity using single nucleotide polymorphisms (SNPs). Int J Cancer. 116(3):487-91, 2005
10. Lee-Jones L et al: Sacrococcygeal chordomas in patients with tuberous sclerosis complex show somatic loss of TSC1 or TSC2. Genes Chromosomes Cancer. 41(1):80-5, 2004
11. Kelley MJ et al: Familial chordoma, a tumor of notochordal remnants, is linked to chromosome 7q33. Am J Hum Genet. 69(2):454-60, 2001
12. Miozzo M et al: A tumor suppressor locus in familial and sporadic chordoma maps to 1p36. Int J Cancer. 87(1):68-72, 2000
13. Dalprà L et al: First cytogenetic study of a recurrent familial chordoma of the clivus. Int J Cancer. 81(1):24-30, 1999
14. Stepanek J et al: Familial chordoma with probable autosomal dominant inheritance. Am J Med Genet. 75(3):335-6, 1998
15. Eisenberg MB et al: Loss of heterozygosity in the retinoblastoma tumor suppressor gene in skull base chordomas and chondrosarcomas. Surg Neurol. 47(2):156-60; discussion 160-1, 1997
16. Butler MG et al: Cytogenetic, telomere, and telomerase studies in five surgically managed lumbosacral chordomas. Cancer Genet Cytogenet. 85(1):51-7, 1995
17. Coffin CM et al: Chordoma in childhood and adolescence. A clinicopathologic analysis of 12 cases. Arch Pathol Lab Med. 117(9):927-33, 1993

FAMILIAL CHRONIC LYMPHOCYTIC LEUKEMIA

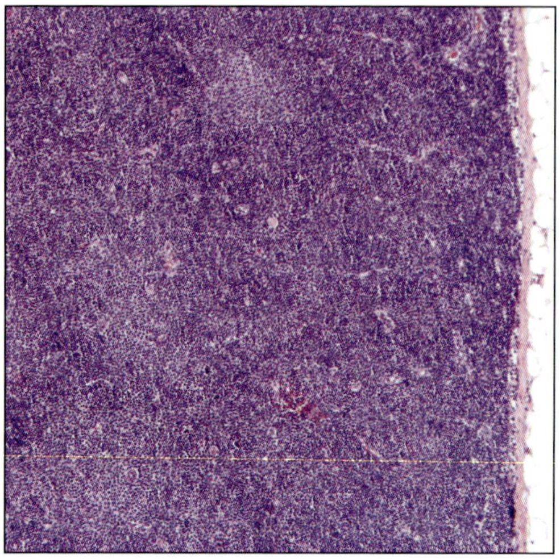

CLL/SLL involves a lymph node with proliferation centers. Note the vaguely nodular, irregularly distributed, pale-staining areas in a dark background of small cells. (Courtesy L. J. Medeiros, MD.)

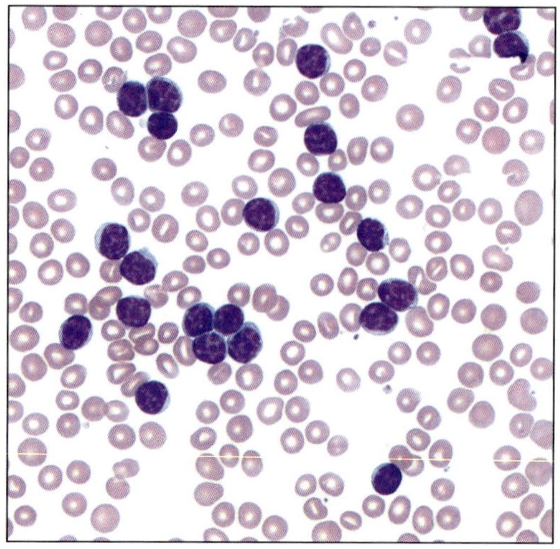

CLL in the peripheral blood. Marked lymphocytosis is seen; lymphocytes have scant cytoplasm, clumped "soccer ball" chromatin, round nuclei, and indistinct nucleoli. (Courtesy C. Bueso-Ramos, MD.)

TERMINOLOGY

Abbreviations

- Chronic lymphocytic leukemia (CLL)/small lymphocytic leukemia (SLL)

Definitions

- CLL/SLL: Neoplasm of mature B cells occurring in peripheral blood/bone marrow &/or nodal/extranodal tissues (hereafter referred to as CLL)
- Monoclonal B-cell lymphocytosis (MBL): Monoclonal or oligoclonal expansion of B cells, often with a CLL-like phenotype, detected at less than $5x10^9$ cells/liter in peripheral blood and without evidence of extramedullary tissue involvement
- Familial CLL: Occurrence of CLL in a relative of a patient with CLL (more strict definitions define familial CLL as occurrence of CLL in ≥ 2 first-degree relatives)

EPIDEMIOLOGY

Incidence and Risk

- Age-adjusted incidence rate of sporadic CLL/SLL in USA is 4.3 per 100,000 persons per year (2006-2010 SEER data) with a median age at diagnosis of 71 years
- 13% of CLL patients report family member with lymphoproliferative disorder
- 6-9% of CLL patients report family member with CLL
- Population-based studies demonstrate 1st-degree relatives of CLL patients have 8.5x relative risk for CLL
- Some studies indicate lower mean age at diagnosis in familial CLL whereas others do not find difference in age of onset between sporadic and familial CLL
- Incidence of MBL ↑ in unaffected relatives in CLL families (overall rate of 17% vs. 3-5% in general population)

ETIOLOGY/PATHOGENESIS

Environmental

- No consistent environmental risk has been identified through epidemiological studies
- Geographic variation is marked, with highest incidence in Caucasian populations of North America/Europe
  - Familial aggregation could reflect at least partial contribution of a common environmental factor
  - Alternatively, incidence of CLL in Asian populations is similar regardless of country of residence (United States vs. countries in Asia), suggesting genetic rather than environmental predisposition

Genetic

- Genetic basis of familial predisposition to CLL is poorly understood
- Some factors suggest that CLL is a genetically heterogeneous disease
  - Only a small number of family members (often only 2) are affected in CLL families
  - Linkage studies performed in high-risk CLL families have identified few regions of interest but have not identified germline gene mutations
- Familial risk may be secondary to multiple varied susceptibility loci, each conferring small relative risks
  - Genome-wide association studies have identified multiple single nucleotide polymorphisms (SNPs) at 22 susceptibility loci to date
    - 2q13, 2q37.1, 6p25.3, 11q24.1, 15q23, 19q13.32, 2q37.3, 8q24.21, 15q21.3, 16q24.1,15q25.2, 6p21.3, 6p21.31,10q23.31, 18q21.33, 11p15.5, 4q25, 2q33.1, 9p21.3, 18q21.32, 15q15.1, and 2p22.2
  - Coinheritance of several of these low-risk variants may contribute to familial predisposition for CLL
- Some studies indicate evidence of anticipation in familial CLL whereas others do not

- No evidence that CCG- or CAG-trinucleotide repeat instability is molecular basis for anticipation in familial CLL (if it truly occurs)

CLINICAL IMPLICATIONS

Comparison of Sporadic and Familial CLL

- Large study showed no adverse prognosis in patients with familial CLL vs. sporadic CLL
  - No significant difference in stage at diagnosis or 10-year overall survival
  - No significant difference in need for treatment
- Small studies have suggested differences in familial and sporadic CLL, but findings require further investigation/confirmation
  - Higher frequency of mutated immunoglobulin heavy-chain variable genes in familial CLL
  - Higher frequency of deletion 13q in familial CLL
  - Higher frequency of deletion 11q in sporadic CLL
  - Higher serum levels of B-lymphocyte stimulator (a.k.a. B-cell activating factor) in familial CLL
- No difference in expression of CD23, CD38, or ζ-chain-associated protein kinase-70 (ZAP-70) between familial and sporadic CLL
- No difference in serum levels of β-2 microglobulin between familial and sporadic CLL

ASSOCIATED NEOPLASMS

Familial CLL

- Relative of a patient with CLL has a 2.6x relative risk for developing any lymphoproliferative disorder (absolute risk is very low)
  - Increased risk is for other (mostly indolent) B-cell non-Hodgkin lymphomas, particularly lymphoplasmacytic lymphoma and hairy cell leukemia
  - Not influenced by gender, type of relative, or age at diagnosis
- Risk of Hodgkin lymphoma variable in different studies
- No increased risk of aggressive B-cell or T-cell lymphomas or plasma cell myeloma

CANCER RISK MANAGEMENT

MBL

- Natural history of progression of MBL to CLL in CLL families is unknown
- Currently, no intervention is advised if a family member is found to have MBL by peripheral blood flow cytometry

CLL

- Screening of asymptomatic relatives is not recommended at this time given low absolute risk of development of lymphoproliferative disorder

Stem Cell Transplantation

- Screening for MBL/CLL may be advised when evaluating 1st-degree relatives as potential donors for patients with CLL undergoing allogeneic stem cell transplantation

SELECTED REFERENCES

1. Berndt SI et al: Genome-wide association study identifies multiple risk loci for chronic lymphocytic leukemia. Nat Genet. 45(8):868-76, 2013
2. Slager SL et al: Common variants within 6p21.31 locus are associated with chronic lymphocytic leukaemia and, potentially, other non-Hodgkin lymphoma subtypes. Br J Haematol. 159(5):572-6, 2012
3. Slager SL et al: Common variation at 6p21.31 (BAK1) influences the risk of chronic lymphocytic leukemia. Blood. 120(4):843-6, 2012
4. Crowther-Swanepoel D et al: Common genetic variation at 15q25.2 impacts on chronic lymphocytic leukaemia risk. Br J Haematol. 154(2):229-33, 2011
5. Slager SL et al: Genome-wide association study identifies a novel susceptibility locus at 6p21.3 among familial CLL. Blood. 117(6):1911-6, 2011
6. Crowther-Swanepoel D et al: Common variants at 2q37.3, 8q24.21, 15q21.3 and 16q24.1 influence chronic lymphocytic leukemia risk. Nat Genet. 42(2):132-6, 2010
7. Goldin LR et al: Common occurrence of monoclonal B-cell lymphocytosis among members of high-risk CLL families. Br J Haematol. 151(2):152-8, 2010
8. Goldin LR et al: Familial Aspects of Chronic Lymphocytic Leukemia, Monoclonal B-Cell Lymphocytosis (MBL), and Related Lymphomas. European J Clin Med Oncol. 2(1):119-126, 2010
9. Setlur SR et al: Comparison of familial and sporadic chronic lymphocytic leukaemia using high resolution array comparative genomic hybridization. Br J Haematol. 151(4):336-45, 2010
10. Goldin LR et al: Elevated risk of chronic lymphocytic leukemia and other indolent non-Hodgkin's lymphomas among relatives of patients with chronic lymphocytic leukemia. Haematologica. 94(5):647-53, 2009
11. Brown JR: Inherited predisposition to chronic lymphocytic leukemia. Expert Rev Hematol. 1(1):51-61, 2008
12. Di Bernardo MC et al: A genome-wide association study identifies six susceptibility loci for chronic lymphocytic leukemia. Nat Genet. 40(10):1204-10, 2008
13. Auer RL et al: Trinucleotide repeat dynamic mutation identifying susceptibility in familial and sporadic chronic lymphocytic leukaemia. Br J Haematol. 136(1):73-9, 2007
14. Sellick GS et al: A high-density SNP genome-wide linkage search of 206 families identifies susceptibility loci for chronic lymphocytic leukemia. Blood. 110(9):3326-33, 2007
15. Capalbo S et al: Increased risk of lymphoproliferative disorders in relatives of patients with B-cell chronic lymphocytic leukemia: relevance of the degree of familial linkage. Eur J Haematol. 65(2):114-7, 2000
16. Yuille MR et al: Familial chronic lymphocytic leukaemia: a survey and review of published studies. Br J Haematol. 109(4):794-9, 2000

FAMILIAL GASTROINTESTINAL STROMAL TUMOR

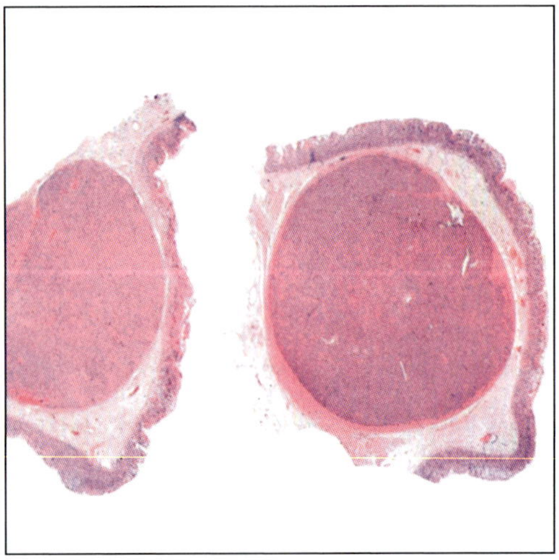

Low-power view shows 2 epithelioid gastrointestinal stromal tumors (GISTs) from a patient with Carney triad. These patients often have multinodular or multifocal gastric GISTs.

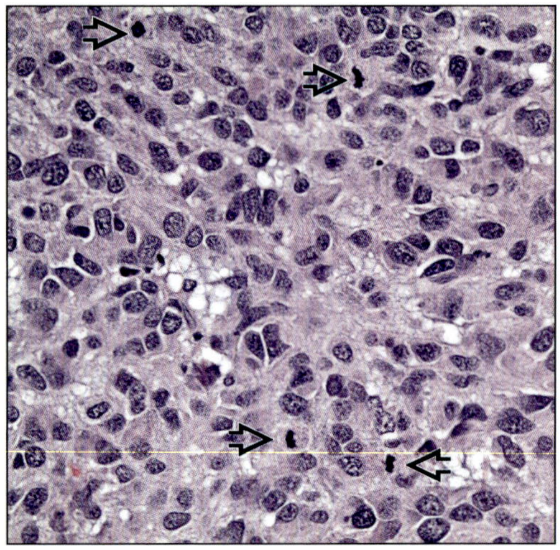

This high-power view shows an epithelioid pediatric-type GIST from a patient with Carney-Stratakis syndrome. Despite the numerous mitoses ➢, these lesions have a relatively good prognosis.

TERMINOLOGY

Abbreviations

- Gastrointestinal stromal tumor (GIST)
- Familial GIST (FGIST)

EPIDEMIOLOGY

Incidence

- Most common mesenchymal tumor arising in gut
  - 6.8 cases per million per year in USA, 14.5 cases per million per year in Sweden
    - Vast majority are sporadic, not familial
- Sporadic GISTs are typically seen in middle-aged to older patients
- Familial GISTs tend to occur in younger patients and there are often synchronous or metachronous tumors

SYNDROMES/GENETICS

Germline Mutations of *KIT*

- Patients have multiple GISTs, hyperpigmentation, urticaria pigmentosa, and dysphagia
- Autosomal dominant
- Most mutations are in exon 11
  - Mutations in other exons tend not to be associated with hyperpigmentation

Germline Mutations of Platelet-Derived Growth Factor Receptor Alpha (*PDGFRA)*

- GISTs are typically epithelioid or mixed
- Patients have multiple GISTs **without** hyperpigmentation, urticaria pigmentosa, and dysphagia
  - 1 kindred also had large hands associated with multiple GISTs, and intestinal neurofibromatosis
  - 1 patient from a different kindred with a unique *PDGFRA* mutation also had multiple lipomas and fibrous tumors of small bowel

Carney-Stratakis Syndrome

- Germline mutations in succinate dehydrogenase (SDH) complex B, C, and D subunits
- Patients have dyad of GISTs and paragangliomas
  - Autosomal dominant
  - GISTs are typically epithelioid or mixed, and are often multinodular
    - Histologically, these tumors appear malignant with high mitotic rate and increased cellularity, but they often behave in a benign fashion
    - May have lymph node metastases, but still have a good prognosis
    - Respond to sunitinib much more than imatinib
  - Dyad GISTs are wild type for *KIT* and *PDGFRA* mutations (also referred to as pediatric GISTs)
    - Loss of SDH immmunostaining may be used to screen for tumors with *SDH* mutation

Carney Triad

- Gastric GISTs, paragangliomas, and pulmonary chondromas
  - Also may have adrenal cortical adenomas and esophageal leiomyomas
  - GISTs are typically epithelioid or mixed, and are often multinodular
  - Histologically, these GISTs appear malignant with high mitotic rate and increased cellularity, but they often behave in a benign fashion
    - Up to 29% have reported lymph node metastasis (nonsyndromic adult GISTs rarely spread to lymph nodes)
    - Even with these metastases, patients still have an excellent prognosis
    - Respond to sunitinib much more than imatinib
- 85% of patients are young females

Genetic Syndromes Associated With GIST			
Syndrome/Disease	**Gene Affected**	**Associated Lesions**	**Pattern of Inheritance**
Carney-Stratakis syndrome	Succinate dehydrogenase (*SDH*), subunits B, C, and D	Paragangliomas, epithelioid GISTs	Autosomal dominant
Carney triad	Unknown	Pulmonary chondromas, paragangliomas, epithelioid GISTs, adrenal cortical adenomas, esophageal leiomyomas	Female predominance raised question of X-linked trait, but ~ 15% of patients are male; now thought not to be familial
Neurofibromatosis type 1	*NF1*	Café au lait spots, neurofibromas, neuroendocrine neoplasms of gut, malignant peripheral nerve sheath tumors, GISTs, gliomas, pheochromocytomas, rhabdomyosarcomas, leukemias	Autosomal dominant
Familial GIST syndrome	*KIT*	GISTs, hyperpigmentation, dysphagia, urticaria pigmentosa/systemic mastocytosis, nevi	Autosomal dominant
Familial GIST syndrome	*PDGFRA*	GISTs, large hands, small intestinal fibrous tumors	Autosomal dominant

- Originally thought to be an X-linked trait as all of the 1st reported patients were all women, but now not thought to be familial
- Genetic defect unknown
    - Losses of chromosome 1p have been found in tumors (not germline)
    - Immunostains for SDH subunits may be negative, but germline mutations are not found in Carney triad patients

Neurofibromatosis Type 1 (NF1)

- May have multiple small intestinal GISTs (as well as the usual neurogenic tumors and other stigmata of NF1)
    - NF1 patients 150x more likely than the general population to get GISTs
- Autosomal dominant due to mutation in *NF1* (tumor suppressor gene)
- GISTs in NF1 often wild type for *KIT* and *PDGFRA*
    - Overall good prognosis and respond to sunitinib much better than imatinib

CLINICAL IMPLICATIONS AND ANCILLARY TESTS

Unique Features of Syndromic GISTs

- Presence of synchronous or metachronous stromal tumors or tumors in young patients should alert pathologist to possibility of familial syndromes
    - Epithelioid or mixed histology gastric tumors in young people should prompt work-up for paragangliomas and pulmonary chondromas
        - Immunostains for SDH subunits may be helpful to triage germline sequencing
        - Germline sequencing of *PDGFRA* may also be helpful if family history is positive and no paragangliomas are found
    - Multiple small bowel GISTs should raise the question of NF1
    - Presence of multiple GISTs in patients with hyperpigmented skin should prompt germline *KIT* sequencing

SELECTED REFERENCES

1. Otto C et al: Multifocal gastric gastrointestinal stromal tumors (GISTs) with lymph node metastases in children and young adults: a comparative clinical and histomorphological study of three cases including a new case of Carney triad. Diagn Pathol. 6:52, 2011
2. Zhang L et al: Gastric stromal tumors in Carney triad are different clinically, pathologically, and behaviorally from sporadic gastric gastrointestinal stromal tumors: findings in 104 cases. Am J Surg Pathol. 34(1):53-64, 2010
3. Thalheimer A et al: Familial gastrointestinal stromal tumors caused by the novel KIT exon 17 germline mutation N822Y. Am J Surg Pathol. 32(10):1560-5, 2008
4. Antonescu CR: Gastrointestinal stromal tumor (GIST) pathogenesis, familial GIST, and animal models. Semin Diagn Pathol. 23(2):63-9, 2006
5. de Raedt T et al: Intestinal neurofibromatosis is a subtype of familial GIST and results from a dominant activating mutation in PDGFRA. Gastroenterology. 131(6):1907-12, 2006
6. O'Riain C et al: Gastrointestinal stromal tumors: insights from a new familial GIST kindred with unusual genetic and pathologic features. Am J Surg Pathol. 29(12):1680-3, 2005
7. Yantiss RK et al: Multiple gastrointestinal stromal tumors in type I neurofibromatosis: a pathologic and molecular study. Mod Pathol. 18(4):475-84, 2005
8. Chompret A et al: PDGFRA germline mutation in a family with multiple cases of gastrointestinal stromal tumor. Gastroenterology. 126(1):318-21, 2004
9. Robson ME et al: Pleomorphic characteristics of a germ-line KIT mutation in a large kindred with gastrointestinal stromal tumors, hyperpigmentation, and dysphagia. Clin Cancer Res. 10(4):1250-4, 2004
10. Maeyama H et al: Familial gastrointestinal stromal tumor with hyperpigmentation: association with a germline mutation of the c-kit gene. Gastroenterology. 120(1):210-5, 2001

FAMILIAL HODGKIN LYMPHOMA

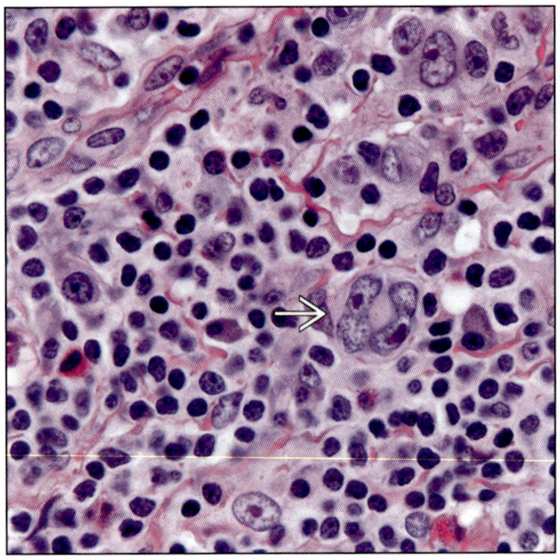

Lymph node biopsy from a patient with NSCHL demonstrates a diagnostic (bilobed) Reed-Sternberg cell ➔ in a background of reactive small lymphocytes, eosinophils, plasma cells, and histiocytes.

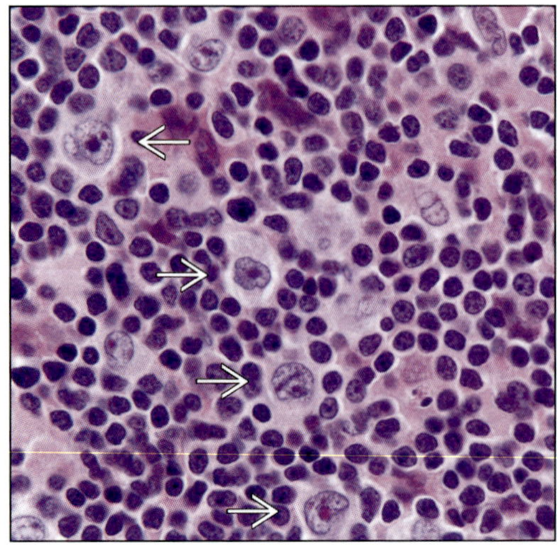

Lymph node biopsy from a patient with NLPHL demonstrates neoplastic lymphocyte-predominant (LP) cells ➔ in a background of reactive small lymphocytes and histiocytes.

TERMINOLOGY

Abbreviations

- Hodgkin lymphoma (HL) is classified into 2 categories
  - Classical Hodgkin lymphoma (CHL), which is composed of 4 subtypes
    - Nodular sclerosis classical Hodgkin lymphoma (NSCHL)
    - Mixed cellularity classical Hodgkin lymphoma (MCCHL)
    - Lymphocyte-rich classical Hodgkin lymphoma (LRCHL)
    - Lymphocyte-depleted classical Hodgkin lymphoma (LDCHL)
  - Nodular lymphocyte-predominant Hodgkin lymphoma (NLPHL)

Definitions

- CHL: Lymphoid neoplasm composed of neoplastic Hodgkin and Reed-Sternberg (HRS) cells in reactive inflammatory background (95% of HL)
  - Bilobed Reed-Sternberg cells and mononuclear Hodgkin cells display large eosinophilic nucleoli; express CD30 and CD15 (variable); do not express CD45 or uniform CD20
  - 4 subtypes (NSCHL, MCCHL, LRCHL, and LDCHL) demonstrate distinct morphologic and clinical features
  - NSCHL (70% CHL)
    - HRS and inflammatory cells form nodules surrounded by fibrous bands
    - Peak incidence age: 15-34 years
    - Often arises in mediastinum or cervical lymph nodes
  - MCCHL (20-25% CHL)
    - HRS and inflammatory cells form diffuse or interfollicular pattern
    - Median age of presentation: 38 years
    - Often arises in cervical or supraclavicular lymph nodes (mediastinum uncommon)
  - LRCHL (4-5% CHL)
    - HRS cells are surrounded by small, reactive lymphocytes (eosinophils and neutrophils rare) in a nodular or diffuse pattern
    - Median age of presentation: 43 years
    - Often arises in peripheral lymph nodes (mediastinum uncommon)
  - LDCHL (< 1% CHL)
    - HRS cells may be scant, frequent, or pleomorphic in a variably fibrotic background depleted of small lymphocytes
    - Typically presents in 4th decade
    - Often arises in retroperitoneal or abdominal lymph nodes
- NLPHL: Lymphoid neoplasm composed of neoplastic lymphocyte-predominant (LP) cells in reactive inflammatory background (5% of HL)
  - LP cells are large with multilobated "popcorn" nuclei; express CD20 and CD45; do not express CD30 and CD15
  - LP cells are confined within follicular dendritic cell meshworks, resulting in a nodular appearance at low magnification
  - Most common in 30-50 year age group
  - Typically presents in peripheral lymph nodes
- Familial Hodgkin lymphoma is defined as ≥ 2 first- or second-degree relatives with HL (either CHL or NLPHL)

EPIDEMIOLOGY

Incidence

- Age-adjusted incidence rate of sporadic HL in USA is 2.8 per 100,000 persons per year (2006-2010 SEER data)
- Familial HL is rare but well recognized
  - Incidence is difficult to determine

- Majority of studies (case series, twin study, population registry studies) represent CHL (± subtyping), with examples including
  - Grufferman et al (1977): Siblings of young adults with HL have ~ 7x excess risk of developing HL, and show strong gender concordance
  - Kerzin-Storrar et al (1983): 4x excess of HL cases among 1st- and 2nd-degree relatives with HL (predominantly MCCHL)
  - Chakravarti et al (1986): Concordance for histological types of HL between affected relatives (out of 34 cases, 23 pairs concordant for NSCHL and 4 pairs concordant for MCCHL)
  - Mack et al (1995): HL found in 10 of 179 pairs of monozygotic twins (0.1 cases would have been expected based on national age-specific incidence rates); no concordant HL found in 187 pairs of dizygotic twins
  - Goldin et al (2004): 2.5-3.5x relative risk of HL in relatives of patients with HL, higher in males vs. females and in siblings vs. parents/offspring
- Few studies have evaluated NLPHL independently
  - Saarinen et al (2013): 19x relative risk of NLPHL in 1st-degree relatives of patients with NLPHL, most prominent in female relatives of young patients

Inheritance Pattern

- Uncertain; some studies suggest autosomal recessive pattern of inheritance

ETIOLOGY/PATHOGENESIS

Environmental/Infectious

- CHL in general
  - Some clinical and morphologic/genetic characteristics of NSCHL suggest at least partial contribution of common environmental factor
    - Young age at presentation
    - Increasing risk at higher levels of economic development
    - mRNA gene-expression profile similar to that of tissue repair
  - CHL can be associated with Epstein-Barr virus (EBV), particularly in
    - Immunocompromised patients (HIV infection)
    - Resource-poor populations
    - Children or in older populations (e.g., 50 years or older)
    - Males
  - Some studies have described geographic clustering (localized increased incidence of HL described in New York state, UK, Israel)
- Familial HL
  - Excess risk in young adults and in siblings (as described in some studies) could suggest that a common environmental exposure or prolonged close contact at an early age may contribute to risk of familial HL

Genetic

- Genetic basis of familial predisposition to HL is poorly understood
- Some studies have identified underlying immunodeficiency in family members of patients with HL
- Susceptibility gene(s) may predispose host to develop HL (in some cases, possibly in response to an environmental agent such as EBV)
  - Correlation between major histocompatibility complex (MHC)/human leukocyte antigen (HLA) loci and HL
    - Numerous HLA loci have been implicated in susceptibility to HL, e.g., individuals carrying HLA-A*01 allele have an ↑ risk of developing EBV(+) CHL and individuals carrying HLA-A*02 allele have a ↓ risk of developing EBV(+) CHL
  - Genome-wide linkage analysis
    - Studies of CHL families have suggested susceptibility genes on chromosome 4p and possibly additional regions on chromosomes 2 and 11
  - Genome-wide association studies
    - Study of patients with CHL identified 3 susceptibility loci at 2p16.1 (*REL*), 8q24.21 (*PVT1*), and 10p14 (*GATA3*) and confirmed a strong HLA association
    - Study of patients with CHL identified 2 loci in MHC region (1 adjacent to *MICB*, 1 at *HLA-DRA*) regardless of EBV status, and confirmed association between EBV(+) CHL and genetic variants within class I HLA region
    - Study of patients with NSCHL identified risk loci at 6p21.32
- Evaluation of familial chromosomal abnormalities/gene mutations
  - Chromosomal analysis revealed inherited translocation [t(2;3)(q11.2;p21.21)] in a family with multiple affected members (NSCHL), resulting in disruption of *KLHDC8B* and loss of protein expression
    - 5' untranslated region (UTR) variant that reduces *KLHDC8B* translation was found in 3 additional CHL families
    - In vitro, reduced expression of protein product (which participates in cytokinesis) results in ↑ binucleated cell formation
    - *KLHDC8B*-associated variations were not detected in multiple NLPHL families by direct sequencing of all exons, exon-intron boundaries, and 5' UTR
  - Whole exome sequencing and linkage studies revealed truncating germline mutation in *NPAT* gene in a family of 4 cousins with NLPHL

CLINICAL IMPLICATIONS

Clinical Features

- Male patients have higher familial risks vs. female patients

FAMILIAL HODGKIN LYMPHOMA

- Risk of HL is higher in relatives of HL patients with early age of onset compared to late age of onset
- Siblings of patients with HL have a higher risk of developing HL compared to parents or offspring
  - Relative risk is highest in brother pairs and sister pairs

Comparison to Sporadic HL

- Patients with familial HL present at earlier age of onset compared to patients with sporadic HL
- No specific laboratory or morphologic features distinguish familial HL from sporadic HL

Mortality

- 5-year and 10-year mortality is similar for patients with HL ± family history of HL

ASSOCIATED NEOPLASMS

Familial HL

- Relative of patient with HL
  - 1.65x relative risk of development of any lymphoproliferative disorder
  - 2.11x relative risk of development of chronic lymphocytic leukemia

Familial NLPHL

- Relative of patient with NLPHL
  - Registry-based standardized incidence risk of 1.9 for all non-Hodgkin lymphoma
  - Registry-based standardized incidence risk of 5.3 for CHL

CANCER RISK MANAGEMENT

Familial HL

- Overall, familial HL appears to comprise 4.5% of all HL cases
- No consensus guidelines on screening of asymptomatic relatives of patients with HL

SELECTED REFERENCES

1. Saarinen S et al: High familial risk in nodular lymphocyte-predominant Hodgkin lymphoma. J Clin Oncol. 31(7):938-43, 2013
2. Cozen W et al: A genome-wide meta-analysis of nodular sclerosing Hodgkin lymphoma identifies risk loci at 6p21.32. Blood. 119(2):469-75, 2012
3. Urayama KY et al: Genome-wide association study of classical Hodgkin lymphoma and Epstein-Barr virus status-defined subgroups. J Natl Cancer Inst. 104(3):240-53, 2012
4. Saarinen S et al: Analysis of KLHDC8B in familial nodular lymphocyte predominant Hodgkin lymphoma. Br J Haematol. 154(3):413-5, 2011
5. Saarinen S et al: Exome sequencing reveals germline NPAT mutation as a candidate risk factor for Hodgkin lymphoma. Blood. 118(3):493-8, 2011
6. Enciso-Mora V et al: A genome-wide association study of Hodgkin's lymphoma identifies new susceptibility loci at 2p16.1 (REL), 8q24.21 and 10p14 (GATA3). Nat Genet. 42(12):1126-30, 2010
7. Hjalgrim H et al: HLA-A alleles and infectious mononucleosis suggest a critical role for cytotoxic T-cell response in EBV-related Hodgkin lymphoma. Proc Natl Acad Sci U S A. 107(14):6400-5, 2010
8. Anderson LA et al: Survival patterns among lymphoma patients with a family history of lymphoma. J Clin Oncol. 26(30):4958-65, 2008
9. Niens M et al: HLA-A*02 is associated with a reduced risk and HLA-A*01 with an increased risk of developing EBV+ Hodgkin lymphoma. Blood. 110(9):3310-5, 2007
10. Diepstra A et al: Association with HLA class I in Epstein-Barr-virus-positive and with HLA class III in Epstein-Barr-virus-negative Hodgkin's lymphoma. Lancet. 365(9478):2216-24, 2005
11. Goldin LR et al: A genome screen of families at high risk for Hodgkin lymphoma: evidence for a susceptibility gene on chromosome 4. J Med Genet. 2005 Jul;42(7):595-601. Erratum in: J Med Genet. 42(12):952, 2005
12. Osborne J et al: Germline mutations and polymorphisms in the NFKBIA gene in Hodgkin lymphoma. Int J Cancer. 116(4):646-51, 2005
13. Cartwright RA et al: Epidemiology of Hodgkin's disease: a review. Hematol Oncol. 22(1):11-26, 2004
14. Goldin LR et al: Familial aggregation of Hodgkin lymphoma and related tumors. Cancer. 100(9):1902-8, 2004
15. Westergaard T et al: Birth order, sibship size and risk of Hodgkin's disease in children and young adults: a population-based study of 31 million person-years. Int J Cancer. 72(6):977-81, 1997
16. Mack TM et al: Concordance for Hodgkin's disease in identical twins suggesting genetic susceptibility to the young-adult form of the disease. N Engl J Med. 332(7):413-8, 1995
17. Merk K et al: Immune deficiency in family members of patients with Hodgkin's disease. Cancer. 66(9):1938-43, 1990
18. Cimino G et al: Immune-deficiency in Hodgkin's disease (HD): a study of patients and healthy relatives in families with multiple cases. Eur J Cancer Clin Oncol. 24(10):1595-601, 1988
19. Chakravarti A et al: Etiological heterogeneity in Hodgkin's disease: HLA linked and unlinked determinants of susceptibility independent of histological concordance. Genet Epidemiol. 3(6):407-15, 1986
20. Hors J et al: HLA and susceptibility to Hodgkin's disease. Immunol Rev. 70:167-92, 1983
21. Kerzin-Storrar L et al: Incidence of familial Hodgkin's disease. Br J Cancer. 47(5):707-12, 1983
22. Haim N et al: Malignant lymphoma in first-degree blood relatives. Cancer. 49(10):2197-200, 1982
23. Grufferman S et al: Hodgkin's disease in siblings. N Engl J Med. 296(5):248-50, 1977
24. Razis DV et al: Familial Hodgkin's disease: its significance and implications. Ann Intern Med. 51:933-71, 1959

Microscopic Features

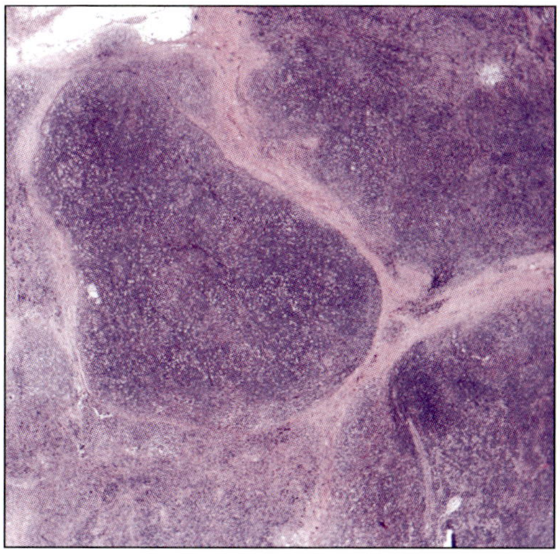

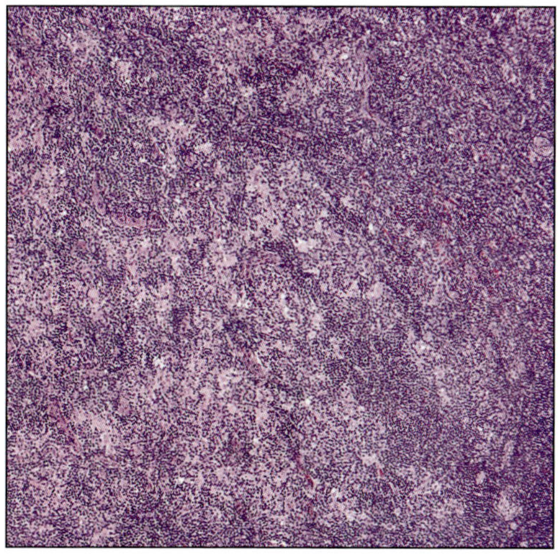

(Left) *Lymph node biopsy from a patient with NSCHL shows effacement of lymph node architecture by neoplastic nodules surrounded by dense fibrous bands. (Courtesy C. Yin, MD.)* ***(Right)*** *Lymph node biopsy from a patient with NLPHL shows a large nodule with a "moth-eaten" pattern due to the presence of admixed larger cells in a background of small lymphocytes. (Courtesy P. Lin, MD.)*

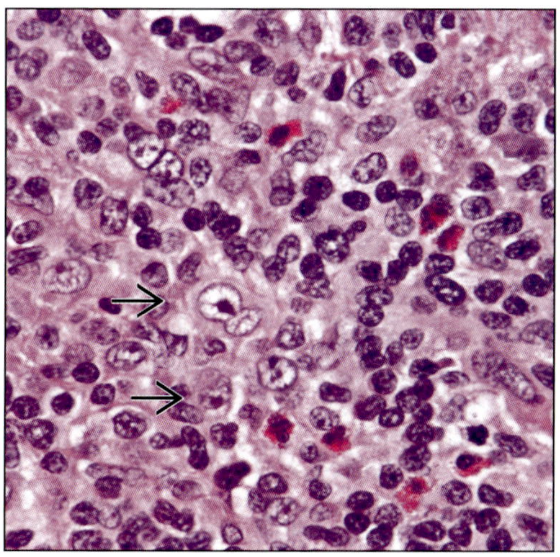

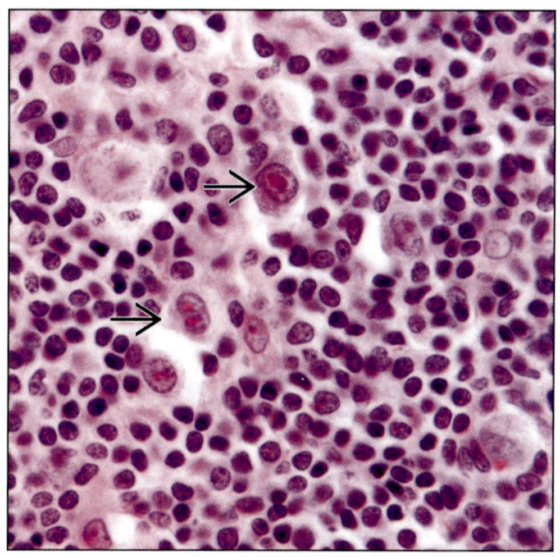

(Left) *Lymph node biopsy from a patient with MCCHL shows a few scattered Hodgkin cells → in a background of small lymphocytes, eosinophils, and histiocytes. (Courtesy L. J. Medeiros, MD.)* ***(Right)*** *Lymph node biopsy from a patient with LRCHL (nodular variant) shows HRS cells → in a background of numerous small lymphocytes. Note absence of eosinophils and plasma cells. (Courtesy L. J. Medeiros, MD.)*

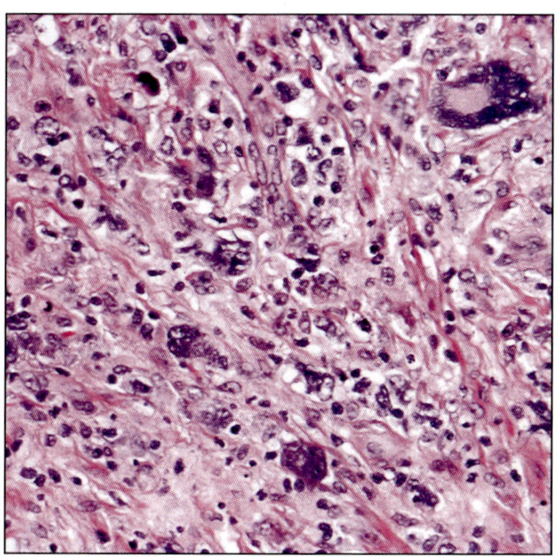

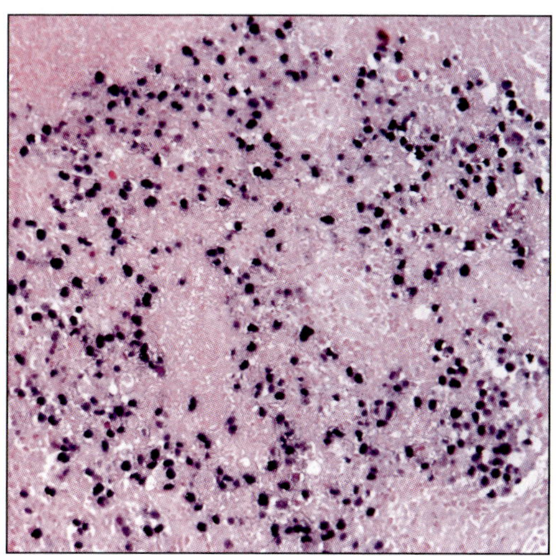

(Left) *Lymph node biopsy from a patient with LDCHL shows several highly pleomorphic HRS cells. The background shows stromal elements and depletion of small lymphocytes. (Courtesy L. J. Medeiros, MD.)* ***(Right)*** *Lymph node biopsy from a patient with NSCHL (syncytial variant) showing numerous cells positive for expression of EBV-encoded RNA (EBER) by in situ hybridization. Approximately 20% of cases of NSCHL are EBER(+). (Courtesy L. J. Medeiros, MD.)*

FAMILIAL ISOLATED HYPERPARATHYROIDISM

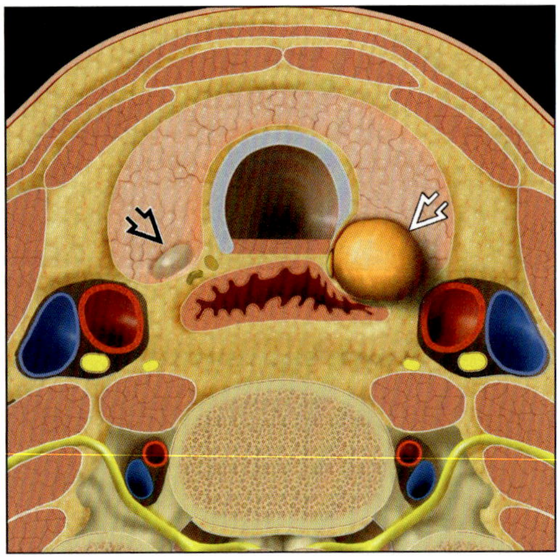

Graphic shows both an enlarged parathyroid gland ➡ (due to adenoma) and a normal-sized parathyroid gland ➡. This helps differentiate this from hyperplasia, which usually shows enlargement of all glands.

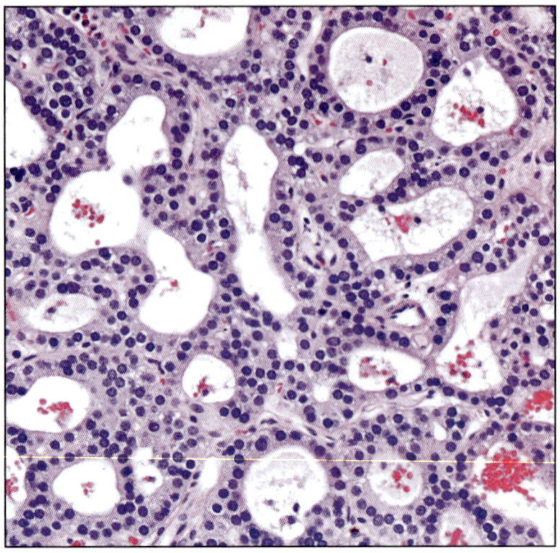

In addition to a solid and nodular growth pattern, a variety of different growth patterns can be seen within an individual gland and among glands in an individual. This parathyroid gland has a follicular growth pattern.

TERMINOLOGY

Abbreviations

- Familial isolated hyperparathyroidism (FIHP)
- Familial isolated primary hyperparathyroidism (FIPHT)
- Parathyroid hormone (PTH)

Definitions

- Familial isolated hyperparathyroidism is defined as hereditary primary hyperparathyroidism without the association of other diseases or tumors
- FIHP is an inherited condition characterized by overactivity of parathyroid glands
  - 1 or more overactive parathyroid gland releases excess parathyroid hormone, which causes hypercalcemia
- Parathyroid hormone stimulates removal of calcium from bone and the absorption of calcium from the diet
  - Production of excess PTH is caused by the parathyroid glands
- FIHP is mainly due to 4-gland hyperplasia or single-gland adenoma

EPIDEMIOLOGY

Age Range

- Age at which familial isolated hyperparathyroidism is diagnosed varies from childhood to adulthood

Gender

- F ~ M

Incidence

- 90% of hyperparathyroidism cases are sporadic
- 10% of hyperparathyroidism cases are familial
  - In 1% of cases of familial primary hyperparathyroidism (e.g., FIHP), parathyroid is the only endocrine organ involved
  - Remainder of cases are associated with MEN1, MEN2, HPT-JT, and familial hypocalciuric hypercalcemia

GENETICS

Autosomal Dominant

- Mutations in parafibromin gene *CDC73* (also *HRPT2*) on chromosome 1q25 have been found in a small proportion of FIHP cases
- FIHP phenotypes have been associated with mutant multiple endocrine neoplasia 1 (*MEN1*) and calcium sensing receptor (*CASR*) genotypes
- Genomic screen of 7 familial hyperparathyroidism families has identified a suggestive 1.7 Mb region on chromosome 2
- For majority of cases of FIHP, genetic cause is unknown

CLINICAL IMPLICATIONS AND ANCILLARY TESTS

Clinical Presentation

- 1st indication of condition is elevated calcium levels identified through a routine blood test
  - Even though the affected individual may not yet have signs or symptoms of hyperparathyroidism or hypercalcemia
- Because the production of excess PTH is caused by abnormalities of parathyroid glands, FIHP is considered a form of primary hyperparathyroidism
- Typically, only 1 of the 4 parathyroid glands is affected, but in some people, > 1 gland develops a tumor
  - Tumors are usually adenomas

- Rarely, people with FIHP develop parathyroid carcinoma
- Disruption of normal calcium balance resulting from overactive parathyroid glands causes many of the common signs and symptoms of familial isolated hyperparathyroidism
  - Kidney stones
  - Nausea
  - Vomiting
  - Hypertension
  - Weakness
  - Fatigue
  - Osteoporosis
- In contrast to sporadic primary hyperparathyroidism, FIHP is characterized by earlier onset of disease, higher incidence of multiglandular involvement, and higher recurrence rate

Treatment

- Parathyroid surgery is treatment of choice, especially when disorder is complicated by symptomatic hypercalcemia, bone loss or fractures, and hypercalciuria and nephrolithiasis
- Subtotal parathyroidectomy is recommended for multiglandular involvement

ASSOCIATED CONDITIONS

Parathyroid Hyperplasia

- 4-gland hyperplasia is often seen in familial isolated hyperparathyroidism
- Hyperplasia may be either chief cell or oxyphil cell variants

Parathyroid Adenoma

- Common occurrence in familial isolated hyperparathyroidism

Parathyroid Carcinoma

- Exceedingly rare in patients with FIHP
- Accounts for < 1% of all cases of FIHP
- Patients with the *CDC73* (also *HRPT2*) mutation have a greater risk of developing carcinoma

CANCER RISK MANAGEMENT

Screening and Guidelines

- There are no published guidelines on surveillance
- Based on phenotype, annual screening with serum calcium, phosphorous, and parathyroid hormone levels
- Every 1-2 years, reassessment of renal status
- Annual palpation of thyroid and parathyroid glands is recommended beginning at age 10-12 years
  - Adenomas and carcinomas have been reported in adolescents

DIAGNOSIS

Clinical

- Familial isolated hyperparathyroidism is essentially a diagnosis of exclusion
- Clinical picture is of familial primary hyperparathyroidism in absence of sufficient clinical, radiological, or biochemical evidence for diagnoses of
  - Multiple endocrine neoplasia type 1 (MEN1)
  - Multiple endocrine neoplasia type 2A (MEN2A)
  - Hyperparathyroidism-jaw tumor syndrome
  - Familial benign hypocalciuric hypercalcemia

Laboratory Tests

- Elevated PTH in context of hypercalcemia in a patient with no renal disease

Genetic Tests

- *CDC73* (also *HRPT2)* mutations
  - Tumor suppressor gene located on chromosome 1q25, which encodes the 531 amino acid protein parafibromin
  - Almost all mutations in this gene inactivate parafibromin expression or function
  - Relatively high incidence of parathyroid carcinoma is described in patients with *CDC73* mutations
  - Studies report *CDC73* mutations in 0-5.3% of all cases of FIHP
- *MEN1* mutations
  - According to current studies, *MEN1* mutations have been reported in up to 17.6% of unrelated FIHP families
- *CASR* mutations
  - Located on chromosome 3q
  - Current studies show up to 11.8% detection rate of *CASR* mutations in FIHP families

Surgical Procedures

- Parathyroidectomy

DIFFERENTIAL DIAGNOSIS

Sporadic Parathyroid Adenomas

- Predisposing factors poorly understood; possible association with prior ionizing radiation
- Later onset of disease than FIHP
- Lower incidence of multiglandular involvement than FIHP
- Lower recurrence rate than FIHP

Multiple Endocrine Neoplasia Type 1

- Autosomal dominant familial tumor syndrome in which patients develop tumors of the parathyroid glands, enteropancreatic neuroendocrine system, pituitary gland, and skin
- Primary hyperparathyroidism, caused by an adenoma or hyperplasia, is the 1st manifestation of MEN1 in > 90% of patients
- Parathyroid adenomas occur in ~ 90% of MEN1 patients
  - Cause hyperparathyroidism and hypercalcemia

FAMILIAL ISOLATED HYPERPARATHYROIDISM

Differential Diagnosis of Familial Isolated Hyperparathyroidism (FIPH)		
Syndrome	**Clinical Characteristics**	**Pathological Features**
Sporadic parathyroid adenomas	No associated findings; later occurrence, low recurrence rate	Parathyroid adenoma
Multiple endocrine neoplasia type 1 (MEN1)	> 95% of patients with MEN1 develop hyperparathyroidism	Majority are parathyroid adenoma
Multiple endocrine neoplasia type 2A (MEN2A)	Parathyroid tumors may be present in up to 50% of patients with MEN2A	Usually all 4 glands are enlarged; hyperplasia or adenoma
Hyperparathyroidism-jaw tumor syndrome (HPT-JT)	Associated with fibroosseous tumors of the jaw, and with renal and endometrial tumors	Parathyroid adenoma or carcinoma
Familial benign hypocalciuric hypercalcemia (FBHH)	Difficult to distinguish from FIPH	Normal parathyroid size, weight, and histology

- Patients with MEN1 inherit a mutation in tumor suppressor gene *MEN1* on chromosome 11q13

Multiple Endocrine Neoplasia Type 2A

- Rare familial tumor syndrome caused by the *RET* proto-oncogene
- Parathyroid tumors are found in 35-50% of affected family members
- Virtually all patients develop medullary thyroid carcinoma
- ~ 50% of patients develop pheochromocytomas, which are bilateral in 60-80% of cases

Hyperparathyroidism-Jaw Tumor Syndrome

- Autosomal dominant disorder characterized by adenomatous or carcinomatous parathyroid tumors, fibroosseus tumors of jaw bones, renal tumors and cysts, and uterine tumors
  - Penetrance of each of these phenotypic features is variable
- Gene responsible for HPT-JT is tumor suppressor gene *CDC73* (formerly *HRPT2*) located on chromosome 1q25

Familial Benign Hypocalciuric Hypercalcemia (FBHH)

- Most difficult of familial hyperparathyroidism syndromes to distinguish clinically from FIHP
- Usually caused by heterozygous inactivating mutations of *CASR* on chromosome 3q
- Characteristic features include
  - Mild to moderate hypercalcemia with nonsuppressed PTH
  - Relative hypocalciuria while hypercalcemic
  - Almost 100% penetrance of gene for hypercalcemia since birth
  - Persistence of hypercalcemia following subtotal parathyroidectomy
  - Normal parathyroid size, weight, and histology at surgery
- Atypical presentations with severe hypercalcemia, hypercalciuria, normocalcemia following parathyroidectomy, and pancreatitis have all been described
- General recommendation is that if FBHH is suspected, kindred should be investigated to resolve diagnostic uncertainty

SELECTED REFERENCES

1. Mackenzie-Feder J et al: Primary hyperparathyroidism: an overview. Int J Endocrinol. 2011:251410, 2011
2. Pepe J et al: Sporadic and hereditary primary hyperparathyroidism. J Endocrinol Invest. 34(7 Suppl):40-4, 2011
3. Kandil E et al: Familial isolated primary hyperparathyroidism with double adenoma. South Med J. 103(3):236-8, 2010
4. Hannan FM et al: Familial isolated primary hyperparathyroidism caused by mutations of the MEN1 gene. Nat Clin Pract Endocrinol Metab. 4(1):53-8, 2008
5. Masi G et al: Clinical, genetic, and histopathologic investigation of CDC73-related familial hyperparathyroidism. Endocr Relat Cancer. 15(4):1115-26, 2008
6. Cetani F et al: Genetic analyses in familial isolated hyperparathyroidism: implication for clinical assessment and surgical management. Clin Endocrinol (Oxf). 64(2):146-52, 2006
7. Guarnieri V et al: Diagnosis of parathyroid tumors in familial isolated hyperparathyroidism with HRPT2 mutation: implications for cancer surveillance. J Clin Endocrinol Metab. 91(8):2827-32, 2006
8. Mizusawa N et al: Genetic analyses in patients with familial isolated hyperparathyroidism and hyperparathyroidism-jaw tumour syndrome. Clin Endocrinol (Oxf). 65(1):9-16, 2006
9. Warner JV et al: Familial isolated hyperparathyroidism is linked to a 1.7 Mb region on chromosome 2p13.3-14. J Med Genet. 43(3):e12, 2006
10. Simonds WF et al: Familial isolated hyperparathyroidism is rarely caused by germline mutation in HRPT2, the gene for the hyperparathyroidism-jaw tumor syndrome. J Clin Endocrinol Metab. 89(1):96-102, 2004
11. Simonds WF et al: Familial isolated hyperparathyroidism: clinical and genetic characteristics of 36 kindreds. Medicine (Baltimore). 81(1):1-26, 2002
12. Yoshimoto K et al: Familial isolated primary hyperparathyroidism with parathyroid carcinomas: clinical and molecular features. Clin Endocrinol (Oxf). 48(1):67-72, 1998
13. Wassif WS et al: Familial isolated primary hyperparathyroidism. Clin Endocrinol (Oxf). 42(4):441-3, 1995

Diagrammatic and Microscopic Features

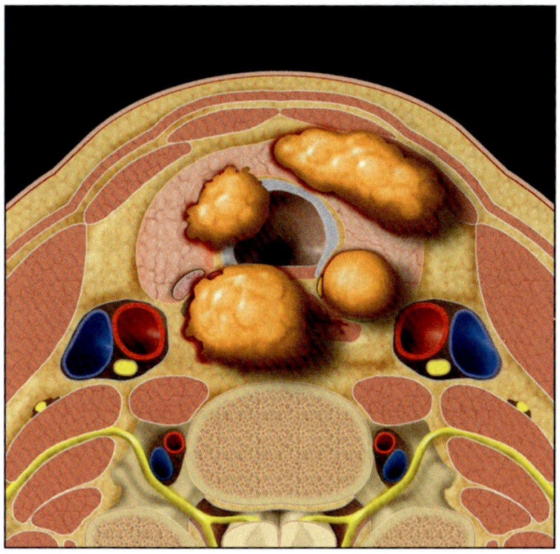

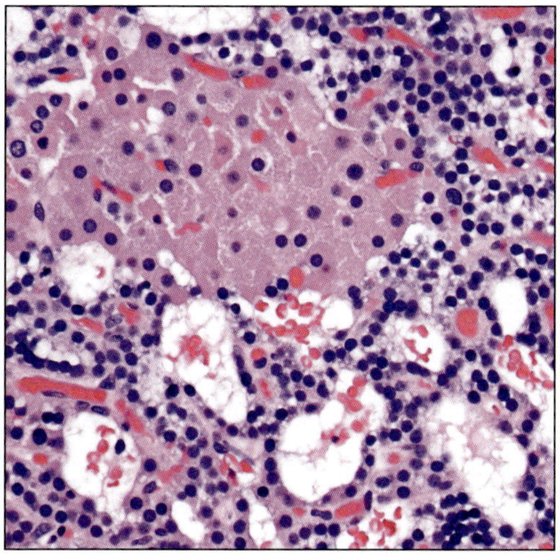

(Left) *Asymmetric hyperplasia or pseudoadenomatous variant of hyperplasia with marked variation in size of each parathyroid gland can be confused with adenoma.* ***(Right)*** *This example of parathyroid hyperplasia shows chief cells in a microfollicular pattern mixed with nodules of oncocytic cells, a common pattern in parathyroid hyperplasia. The nuclei of parathyroid cells are round with dense chromatin.*

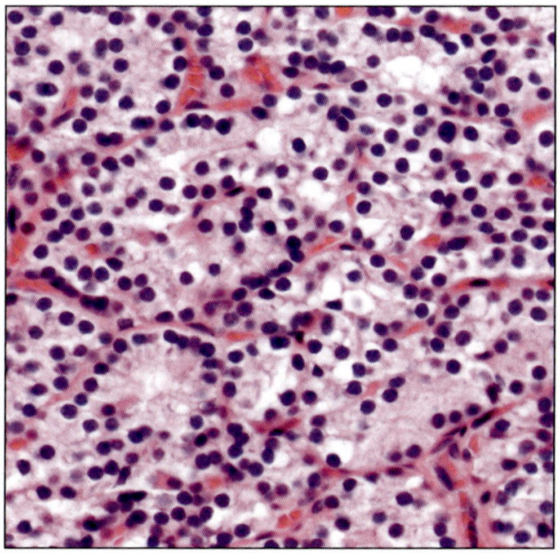

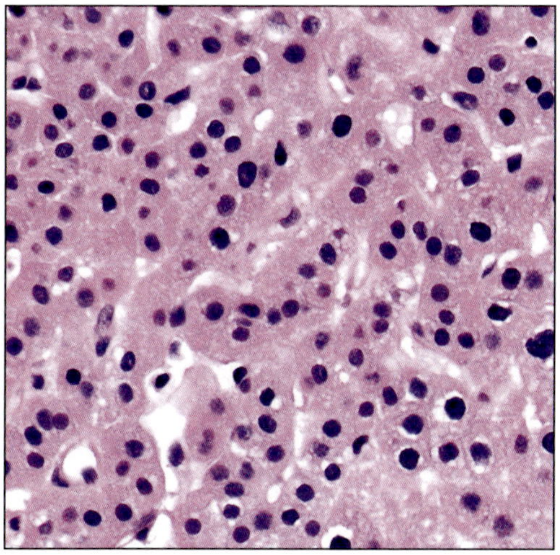

(Left) *Parathyroid chief cells are the predominant cell type in parathyroid hyperplasia. Parathyroid cells have small amounts of cytoplasm and small dense nuclei.* ***(Right)*** *This hyperplastic parathyroid shows prominent parathyroid oxyphil cells. The nuclei are mildly pleomorphic, but markedly increased nuclear to cytoplasmic ratios and mitotic figures are not identified.*

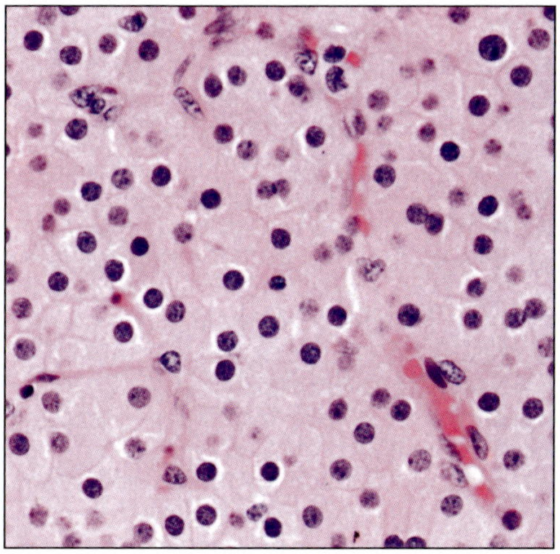

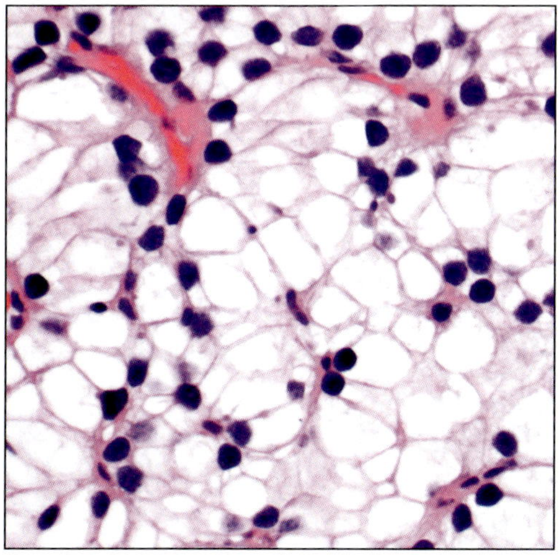

(Left) *This parathyroid shows prominent oxyphil cells, which are not typically present in the normal parathyroid in children but develop with increasing age. Oxyphil cells can form small nodules in the normal parathyroid glands of older adults and should not be mistaken for parathyroid disease.* ***(Right)*** *Foci of clear cells are identified in this hyperplastic parathyroid. Note the characteristically well-defined cytoplasmic membranes of parathyroid cells.*

FAMILIAL NON-HODGKIN LYMPHOMA

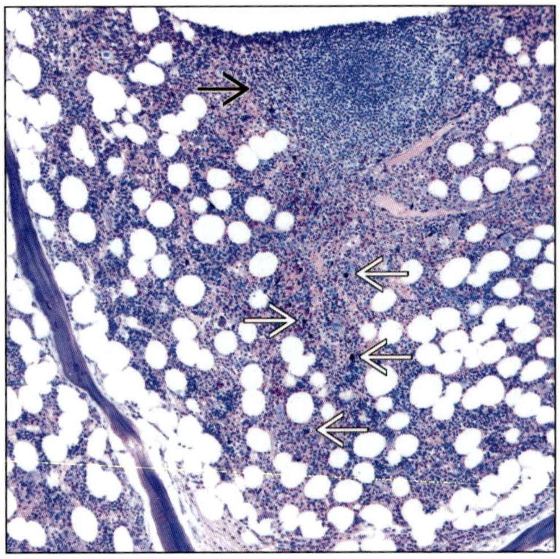

Giemsa stain of a bone marrow biopsy from a WM patient shows morphologic evidence of LPL (discrete lymphoid nodule ⇒ and many dark purple mast cells ➡). WM/LPL can occur in familial clusters.

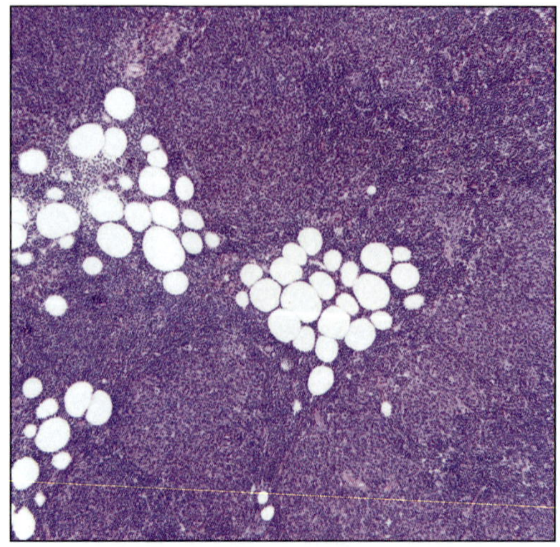

Lymph node biopsy from a patient with follicular lymphoma (FL) shows multiple lymphoid nodules extending into extranodal adipose tissue. Risk of FL is increased 4x in relatives of patients with FL.

TERMINOLOGY

Abbreviations

- Non-Hodgkin lymphoma (NHL)

Definitions

- NHL is umbrella term to describe mature B-, T- and natural killer (NK)-cell neoplasms and consists of > 45 distinct entities
- Familial NHL is defined as ≥ 2 first-degree relatives with NHL (any subtype)

EPIDEMIOLOGY

NHL

- Age-adjusted incidence rate of all NHL in USA is 19.7 per 100,000 persons per year (2006-2010 SEER data)
- Median age at diagnosis: 66 years of age

Familial NHL

- Rare (< 5% of NHL cases are associated with familial clusters)

Risks

- Relatives are at highest risk of developing the same lymphoma subtype as the proband, although other subtypes can also occur
- Including all subtypes, family history of lymphoma is associated with 1.5-4x relative risk of developing lymphoma (based on various epidemiological studies)
- Studies incorporating classification information show that risk is increased for some subtypes
  - Relatives of patients with Waldenström macroglobulinemia/lymphoplasmacytic lymphoma (WM/LPL) demonstrate 20x increased risk of WM/LPL
    - 5x increased risk for monoclonal gammopathy of undetermined significance
    - 3x increased risk for chronic lymphocytic leukemia (CLL) or any NHL
  - Relatives of patients with diffuse large B-cell lymphoma (DLBCL) demonstrate 10x increased risk of DLBCL
  - Relatives of patients with CLL demonstrate 8.5x increased risk of CLL
    - 2.6x increased risk for any NHL (particularly hairy cell leukemia and WM/LPL)
  - Relatives of patients with follicular lymphoma (FL) demonstrate 4x increased risk of FL
  - Relatives of patients with multiple myeloma (MM) demonstrate 1.7x increased risk of MM
  - Reports of familial mantle cell lymphoma are rare

ETIOLOGY/PATHOGENESIS

Genetics

- Linkage mapping studies in NHL families have not identified germline gene mutations
- Evidence of highly penetrant genes has not been found in twin studies
- Familial risk may be secondary to multiple, varied susceptibility loci, each conferring small relative risks
  - Genetic susceptibility studies have identified loci associated with increased susceptibility to NHL, including areas involved in immune function regulation, inflammation, oxidative stress, metabolism, and DNA repair
    - Genome-wide association studies have identified single nucleotide polymorphisms (SNPs) at > 20 susceptibility loci in familial CLL
    - Polymorphisms in *IL10* and *BCL2* have been found specifically in familial NHL cases
    - Possible association of SNPs within the 6p21.31 locus with mantle cell lymphoma and T-cell lymphoma has been described

Environmental Exposures

- Viral exposure may account for some familial clustering of specific subtypes
  - Human T-cell lymphotrophic virus type 1 (HTLV-1) in families with adult T-cell leukemia/lymphoma (Japan, Caribbean)
  - Epstein-Barr virus (EBV) in families with Burkitt lymphoma (Africa)
- Risk of developing WM/LPL is increased in context of parental gastric carcinoma, raising the possibility of association with *H. pylori* infection

Immune Function

- Patients with autoimmune disorders or other immune-related conditions (some of which may be hereditary) are at increased risk for lymphoma
  - Congential immunodeficiency syndromes such as ataxia-telangiectasia, Bruton agammaglobulinemia, Chediak-Higashi syndrome, common variable immunodeficiency, and Wiskott-Aldrich syndrome are known to be associated with development of lymphoma
  - Autoimmune disorders are associated with increased risk of WM/LPL (both sporadic and familial)

CLINICAL IMPLICATIONS

Familial NHL Vs. Sporadic NHL

- Family history of NHL is associated with younger age at diagnosis
- Some studies find differences in risk based on gender (M > F) or type of relation (highest in siblings) whereas others do not find significant differences in these areas
- No differences in site or nodal vs. extranodal presentation in familial vs. sporadic NHL
- No differences in histologic subtype in familial vs. sporadic NHL
- No differences in survival, 5-year mortality, or 10-year mortality in familial NHL vs. sporadic NHL
  - In small sample, breakdown by lymphoma type showed worse 5-year mortality for patients with T-cell or anaplastic lymphoma and family history of NHL vs. sporadic T-cell or anaplastic lymphoma, but equivalent 5-year mortality for low- and high-grade B-cell lymphomas
- Retrospective study demonstrated that familial WM is associated with inferior treatment outcomes compared to sporadic WM

ASSOCIATED NEOPLASMS

WM/LPL Families

- No increased risk of myeloid neoplasms or solid tumors

CANCER RISK MANAGEMENT

Cancer Screening

- Currently, screening of asymptomatic relatives of patients with NHL is not recommended given the low absolute risk of developing lymphoproliferative disorder

SELECTED REFERENCES

1. Kristinsson SY et al: Familial aggregation of lymphoplasmacytic lymphoma/Waldenstrom macroglobulinemia with solid tumors and myeloid malignancies. Acta Haematol. 127(3):173-7, 2012
2. Slager SL et al: Common variants within 6p21.31 locus are associated with chronic lymphocytic leukaemia and, potentially, other non-Hodgkin lymphoma subtypes. Br J Haematol. 159(5):572-6, 2012
3. Treon SP et al: Familial disease predisposition impacts treatment outcome in patients with Waldenstrom macroglobulinemia. Clin Lymphoma Myeloma Leuk. 12(6):433-7, 2012
4. Goldin LR et al: Highly increased familial risks for specific lymphoma subtypes. Br J Haematol. 146(1):91-4, 2009
5. Liang XS et al: Common genetic variants in candidate genes and risk of familial lymphoid malignancies. Br J Haematol. 146(4):418-23, 2009
6. Anderson LA et al: Survival patterns among lymphoma patients with a family history of lymphoma. J Clin Oncol. 26(30):4958-65, 2008
7. Brown JR et al: Prevalence of familial malignancy in a prospectively screened cohort of patients with lymphoproliferative disorders. Br J Haematol. 143(3):361-8, 2008
8. Kristinsson SY et al: Risk of lymphoproliferative disorders among first-degree relatives of lymphoplasmacytic lymphoma/Waldenstrom macroglobulinemia patients: a population-based study in Sweden. Blood. 112(8):3052-6, 2008
9. Goldin LR et al: Family studies in chronic lymphocytic leukaemia and other lymphoproliferative tumours. Br J Haematol. 139(5):774-9, 2007
10. Skibola CF et al: Genetic susceptibility to lymphoma. Haematologica. 92(7):960-9, 2007
11. Wang SS et al: Common genetic variants in proinflammatory and other immunoregulatory genes and risk for non-Hodgkin lymphoma. Cancer Res. 66(19):9771-80, 2006
12. Altieri A et al: Familial aggregation of lymphoplasmacytic lymphoma with non-Hodgkin lymphoma and other neoplasms. Leukemia. 19(12):2342-3, 2005
13. Tort F et al: Familial lymphoid neoplasms in patients with mantle cell lymphoma. Haematologica. 89(3):314-9, 2004
14. Vachon CM et al: Clinical characteristics of familial vs. sporadic non-Hodgkin lymphoma in patients diagnosed at the Mayo Clinic (1986-2000). Leuk Lymphoma. 45(5):929-35, 2004

FAMILIAL NONMEDULLARY THYROID CARCINOMA

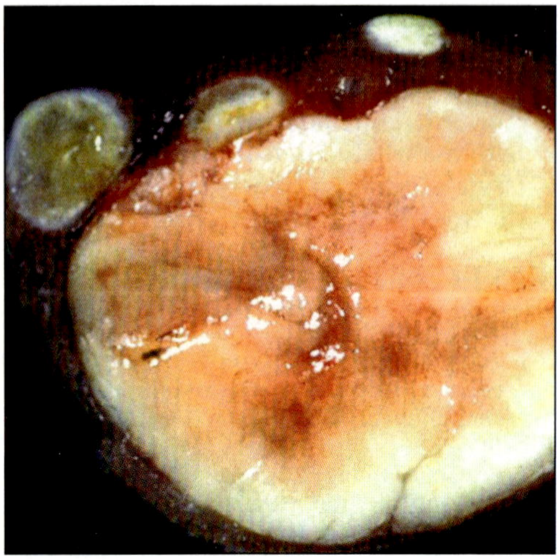

Gross cut surface from a thyroid of a young patient with PTEN-hamartoma tumor syndrome shows multiple well-circumscribed gray-white nodules compressing a small amount of uninvolved thyroid.

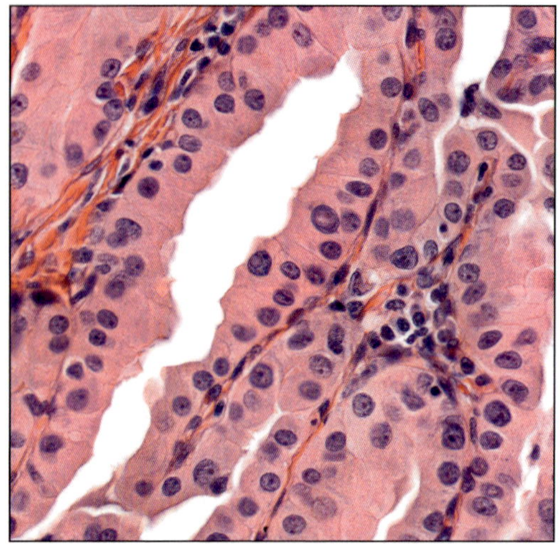

This histopathological picture of a thyroid from a patient with familial nonmedullary thyroid carcinoma shows a thyroid carcinoma with oxyphilia, an unusual type of thyroid cancer.

TERMINOLOGY

Familial Follicular Cell-Derived Carcinoma or Familial Nonmedullary Thyroid Carcinoma (FNMTC)

- Familial nonmedullary thyroid carcinoma or familial follicular cell tumors derived from thyroid follicular cells can be subdivided into 2 subgroups
- **Familial tumor syndromes characterized by predominance of nonthyroidal tumors**
  - **PTEN-hamartoma tumor syndrome (PHTS)**
    - Cowden syndrome (CS) and Bannayan-Riley-Ruvalcaba syndrome (BRRS) are major entities comprising PHTS
  - **Familial adenomatous polyposis (FAP):** Characterized by hundreds of adenomatous colonic polyps that develop during early adulthood
    - Develop diverse tumors
  - **Carney complex**: Consists of myxomas, spotty pigmentation, and endocrine overactivity
  - **Werner syndrome**: Rare premature-aging syndrome that begins in 3rd decade
  - **Pendred syndrome**: Most common hereditary syndrome associated with bilateral sensorineural deafness
    - Also called deaf-mutism and goiter
- **Familial tumor syndromes characterized by predominance of nonmedullary thyroid carcinoma**
  - Characterized by 3 or more 1st-degree relatives with follicular-derived nonmedullary thyroid carcinoma and occurs regardless of presence of another familial syndrome
  - **Pure familial papillary thyroid carcinoma (PTC) ± oxyphilia**: Mapped to chromosomal region 19p13
  - **FNMTC type 1**: Mapped to chromosome 2q21
  - **FPTC with papillary renal cell carcinoma**: Mapped to chromosomal region 1q21
  - **Familial PTC with multinodular goiter**: Mapped to chromosomal region 14q
  - Others

EPIDEMIOLOGY

Syndromes Characterized by Predominance of Nonthyroidal Tumors and Syndromes With a Predominance of Nonmedullary Thyroid Carcinoma (NMTC)

- Criterion of FNMTC families is that ≥ 3 first-degree family members are affected with NMTC
- Benign thyroid lesions such as multinodular hyperplasia (MNG) and follicular thyroid adenoma are associated with FNMTC
  - Personal or family history of benign thyroid conditions is present in ~ 45% of patients with FNMTC
- Age range at which each affected individual is diagnosed is broad; but usually < 35 years
- F:M reported ratio varies from 2:1 to 12:1

GENETICS

Syndromes Characterized by Predominance of Nonthyroidal Tumors

- PHTS
  - Caused by germline mutations of *PTEN* gene and inherited in autosomal dominant fashion
  - *PTEN* (phosphatase and tensin homolog deleted on chromosome 10) is tumor suppressor gene located on 10q23.3
  - > 90% of PHTS patients manifest a phenotype by 20 years of age
- Familial adenomatous polyposis (FAP)

  - Inherited autosomal dominant syndrome caused by germline mutations in adenomatous polyposis coli (*APC*) gene on chromosome 5q21
- Carney complex
  - Autosomal dominant condition
    - Most cases are classified as type 1 and are associated with mutation to protein kinase A regulatory subunit type 1-α (*PRKAR1A*) gene, probable tumor suppressor gene on chromosome 17q22-24
    - Type 2 patients have mutation on chromosome 2p16, which may be regulator of genomic stability
- Werner syndrome
  - Autosomal recessive disease caused by mutations in *WRN* gene on chromosome 8p11-p12
- Pendred syndrome
  - Autosomal recessive trait, result of mutations in *SLC26A4* (*PDS*) gene, which encodes protein pendrin and is located on chromosome 7q21-34

Syndromes With Predominance of Nonmedullary Thyroid Carcinoma

- Although NMTC is mostly sporadic, evidence for a familial form, which is not associated with other Mendelian cancer syndromes, is well documented
- To date, no FNMTC predisposing genes have been identified
- Linkage analyses have mapped 6 different chromosomal regions that may harbor FNMTC susceptibility genes
  - 6 potential regions for harboring an FNMTC gene have been identified: MNG1 (14q32), TCO (19p13.2), FPTC/PRN (1q21), NMTC1 (2q21), FTEN (8p23.1-p22), and the telomere-telomerase complex
- Important genes reported to have been excluded are *RET, TRK, MET, APC, PTEN,* and *TSHR*
- Based on current evidence, FNMTC is likely to represent a polygenic mode of inheritance
- Putative susceptibility genes identified appear to account for only a minority of FNMTCs
- Identification of genes for FNMTC could be utilized in the screening, management, and surveillance of NMTC

Pure Familial PTC ± Oxyphilia

- "Thyroid carcinoma with oxyphilia" locus (TCO; MIM 603386) was mapped to chromosome 19p13.2 in a French family with an unusual form of NMTC with cell oxyphilia
- Speculated that TCO locus is associated only with this unique form of FNMTC with cell oxyphilia
- There are suggestions that TCO might be a tumor suppressor gene
- TCO locus may account for FNMTC in a minority of cases
- Rare type of thyroid cancer with distinct morphology

FPTC With Papillary Renal Cell Carcinoma

- Locus predisposing to FNMTC was identified on chromosome 1p13.2-1q22 in a USA family with recurrent PTC and papillary renal neoplasia (PRN) (FPTC/PRN or PRN1; MIM 605642)
- To date, no further families with a PTC and PRN association have been reported
- 2 studies that performed linkage analysis on a total of 29 FNMTC families (without PRN) did not find an association between FNMTC and FPTC/PRN locus
  - These findings suggest that FPTC/PRN locus may harbor a susceptibility gene for a unique FNMTC phenotype where PTC is associated with PRN

FNMTC Type 1

- Susceptibility locus named "nonmedullary thyroid carcinoma 1" was mapped to chromosome 2q21 in a large Tasmanian family with high frequency of PTC (NMTC1; MIM 606240)
- Extensive genome-wide scan followed by haplotype analysis revealed that the majority of subjects with PTC shared a common haplotype on chromosome 2q21
- Studies suggested that the 2q21 locus, NMTC1 locus, has a more significant association with familial PTC follicular variant (FV) than with familial PTC
  - NMTC locus is also associated with some oxyphilic tumors

FPTC With Multinodular Goiter (MNG)

- MNG susceptibility locus (MNG1; MIM 138800) was mapped to chromosome 14q32 in a large Canadian family with MNG and low occurrence of NMTC
- Additional studies failed to find linkage between the MNG1 locus and FNMTC
  - MNG1 locus has shown evidence of linkage only to FNMTC in original Canadian kindred with multiple MNGs
  - Linkage analyses in a further 124 families have failed to confirm an association between MNG1 and FNMTC
- Therefore, this locus may not be involved in FNMTC, or it may account for only a minority of FNMTC cases with MNG

Other Possible Candidates

- FTEN: Mapped to chromosome 8p23.1-p22
  - Linkage to the 8q23.1-p22 locus was confirmed in a family with 11 cases of benign thyroid disease and 5 cases of carcinoma
- Telomere-telomerase complex
  - Study of the telomere-telomerase complex in a series of patients with FNMTC revealed significantly shorter telomere lengths, higher telomerase reverse transcriptase (*TERT*) gene amplification, and *TERT* mRNA expression in patients with FPTC when compared with sporadic PTCs
    - This study did not report any mutations of *TERT* gene or the telomerase RNA component

FAMILIAL NONMEDULLARY THYROID CARCINOMA

CLINICAL IMPLICATIONS AND ANCILLARY TESTS

Syndromes Characterized by Predominance of Nonthyroidal Tumors

- Diagnosis of thyroid cancer is usually in younger patients than their sporadic counterpart
- Multifocal and bilateral PTC
- FNMTC is 1 component of a defined cancer susceptibility syndrome with preponderance of nonthyroidal tumors

Syndromes With Predominance of Nonmedullary Thyroid Carcinoma

- FNMTC is a clinical entity characterized by an earlier age of onset, more frequent multifocal and bilateral disease, and recurrence compared with its sporadic NMTC
- Familial cases of PTC are reportedly more aggressive than their sporadic counterparts
- 10x increase in risk of thyroid cancer in relatives of patients with thyroid cancer

ASSOCIATED NEOPLASMS

Syndromes Characterized by Predominance of Nonthyroidal Tumors

- Thyroid carcinoma is usually bilateral and multifocal
- **FAP**
  - **FAP, GI manifestations**: Colonic polyps, colonic adenocarcinoma, duodenal/ampullary adenomas, fundic gland polyps, liver lesions
  - **FAP, extraintestinal manifestations**: Desmoid tumors, osteomas, congenital hypertrophy of retinal pigmented epithelium, brain tumors, and papillary thyroid carcinoma cribriform morular variant
- **PHTS**: Breast carcinoma, endometrial carcinoma, renal carcinoma, and multiple other tumors including papillary and follicular thyroid carcinoma
- **Carney complex**: Multiple facial lentigines, myxomas, epithelioid blue nevus, neurofibromas, primary pigmented adrenal cortical nodular disease, atrial myxomas
  - Less common: Large cell calcifying Sertoli cell tumor, psammomatous melanotic schwannoma, and multiple thyroid nodules and follicular adenoma
- **Werner syndrome**: Multiple malignancies occurring at a younger age such as melanoma, soft tissue sarcoma, osteosarcoma, and thyroid carcinoma

Syndromes With Predominance of Nonmedullary Thyroid Carcinoma

- Thyroid carcinoma usually bilateral and multifocal
- Papillary renal cell carcinoma in association with familial PTC/PRN

CANCER RISK MANAGEMENT

Screening

- Family history of individuals with FNMTC should be reviewed carefully to rule out syndromes characterized by a predominance of nonthyroidal tumors and risk of renal cancer
- If a familial predisposition exists, annual screening of thyroid by ultrasound and physical examination
  - Screening should start no later than an age 10 years younger than that of youngest relative diagnosed with either benign or malignant thyroid tumors
- Renal imaging is recommended for individuals from families with history of renal cell carcinoma
- Surveillance for other cancers according to their syndromes
  - Screening for other tumors is advised by the American Cancer Society

Treatment

- Because FNMT is more aggressive and has higher rates of intrathyroidal spread and recurrence than the sporadic tumors, total thyroidectomy and neck dissection is recommended

Prophylactic Surgery

- Role of prophylactic surgery in most of these conditions is still undefined

SELECTED REFERENCES

1. Mazeh H et al: In patients with thyroid cancer of follicular cell origin, a family history of nonmedullary thyroid cancer in one first-degree relative is associated with more aggressive disease. Thyroid. 22(1):3-8, 2012
2. Laury AR et al: Thyroid pathology in PTEN-hamartoma tumor syndrome: characteristic findings of a distinct entity. Thyroid. 21(2):135-44, 2011
3. Moses W et al: Prevalence, clinicopathologic features, and somatic genetic mutation profile in familial versus sporadic nonmedullary thyroid cancer. Thyroid. 21(4):367-71, 2011
4. Nosé V: Familial thyroid cancer: a review. Mod Pathol. 24 Suppl 2:S19-33, 2011
5. Smith JR et al: Thyroid nodules and cancer in children with PTEN hamartoma tumor syndrome. J Clin Endocrinol Metab. 96(1):34-7, 2011
6. Bonora E et al: Genetic predisposition to familial nonmedullary thyroid cancer: An update of molecular findings and state-of-the-art studies. J Oncol. 2010:385206, 2010
7. Khan A et al: Familial nonmedullary thyroid cancer: a review of the genetics. Thyroid. 20(7):795-801, 2010
8. Nosé V: Familial follicular cell tumors: classification and morphological characteristics. Endocr Pathol. 21(4):219-26, 2010
9. Nosé V: Thyroid cancer of follicular cell origin in inherited tumor syndromes. Adv Anat Pathol. 17(6):428-36, 2010
10. Suh I et al: Distinct loci on chromosome 1q21 and 6q22 predispose to familial nonmedullary thyroid cancer: a SNP array-based linkage analysis of 38 families. Surgery. 146(6):1073-80, 2009
11. Dotto J et al: Familial thyroid carcinoma: a diagnostic algorithm. Adv Anat Pathol. 15(6):332-49, 2008
12. Nosé V: Familial non-medullary thyroid carcinoma: an update. Endocr Pathol. 19(4):226-40, 2008

Microscopic Features

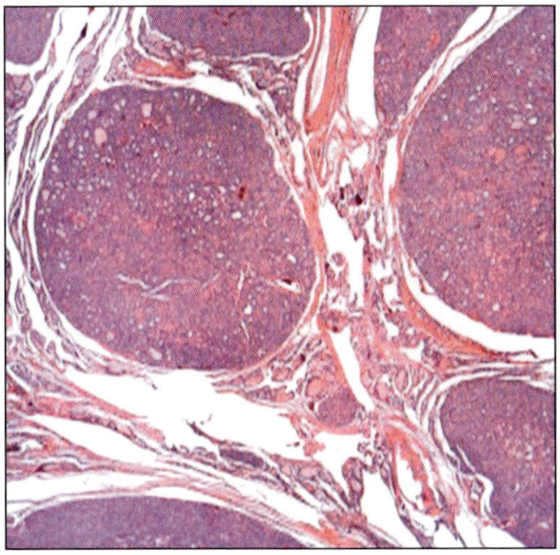

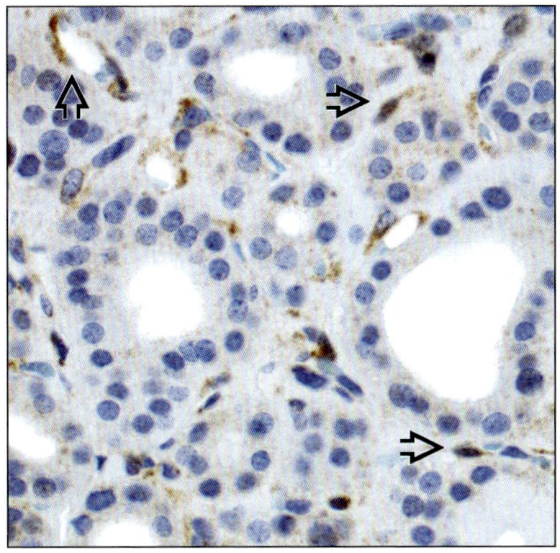

(Left) *This photomicrograph from an 18-year-old woman with PHTS shows multiple well-circumscribed, nonencapsulated adenomatous nodules surrounded by a small residual compressed thyroid parenchyma.* ***(Right)*** *Immunohistochemistry for PTEN in an adenomatous nodule of a patient with PHTS shows loss of staining of the follicular cells with preservation of staining of the endothelial cells ⇨.*

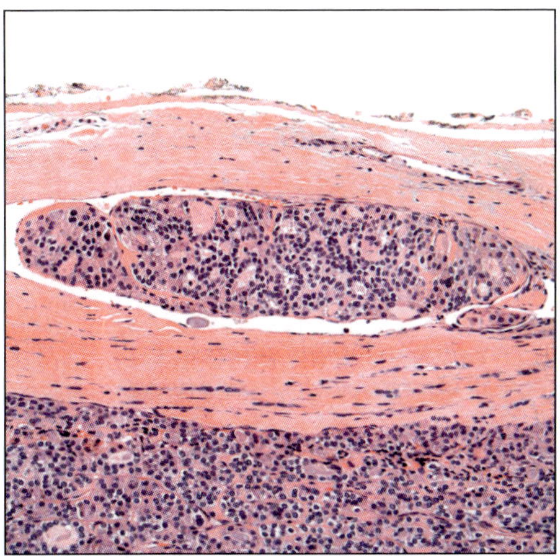

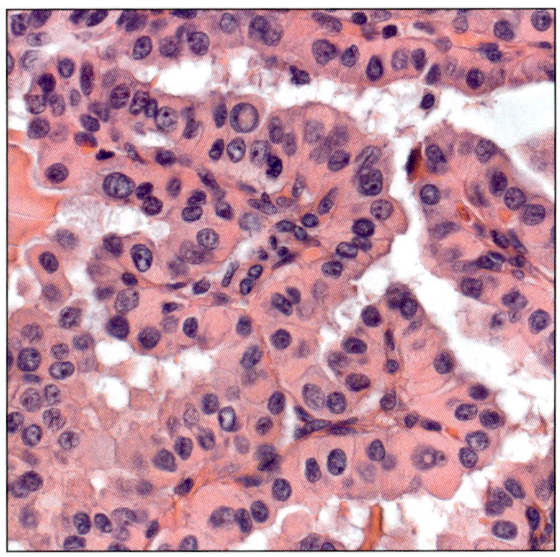

(Left) *This image in a follicular thyroid carcinoma in a patient with PTEN-hamartoma tumor syndrome shows a characteristic vascular invasion. The thyroid from this patient also had multiple adenomatous nodules and a papillary carcinoma.* ***(Right)*** *Papillary thyroid carcinoma with oxyphilia is also usually present in other family members with this familial syndrome. This tumor is characterized by large cells with granular cytoplasm and with the nuclear features of papillary thyroid carcinoma.*

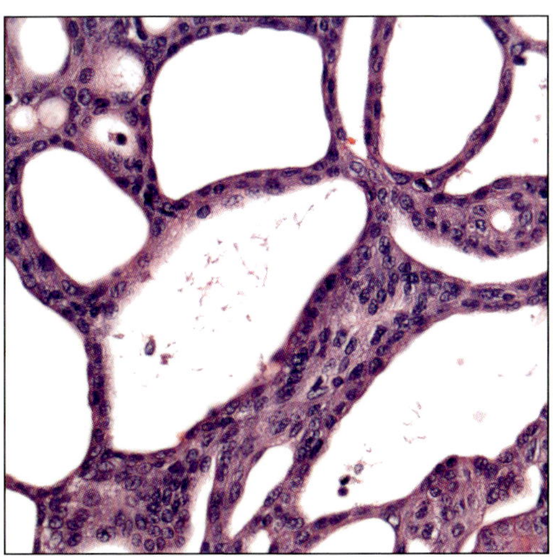

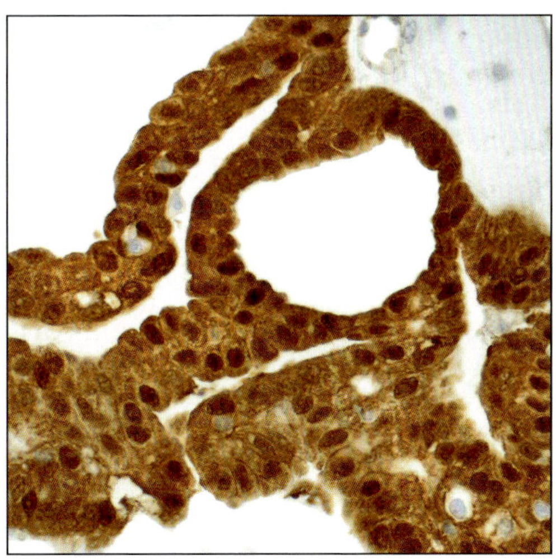

(Left) *This photomicrograph shows the characteristic appearance of the cribriform morular variant of papillary thyroid carcinoma, which is present in about 12% of patients with familial adenomatous polyposis (FAP). Nuclear features of papillary carcinoma and colloid are absent.* ***(Right)*** *There is strong nuclear and cytoplasmic staining for β-catenin in cribriform morular variant carcinoma, which distinguishes these tumors from other variants of papillary thyroid carcinoma that are negative.*

FAMILIAL PLASMA CELL MYELOMA

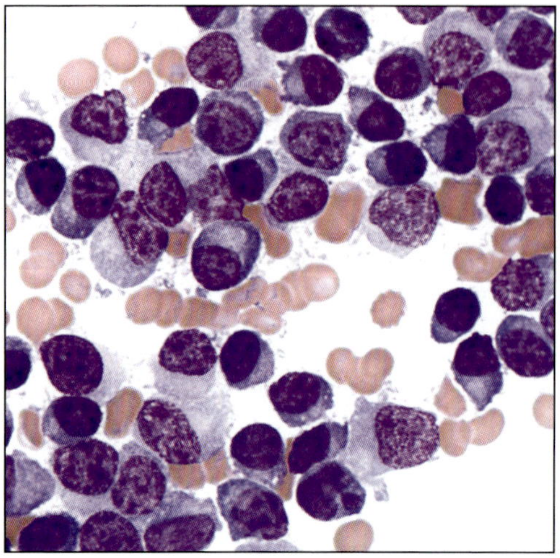

A diagnosis of MM requires identification of a clonal plasma cell population in the bone marrow even when the immunologic or radiographic studies strongly support the presence of disease.

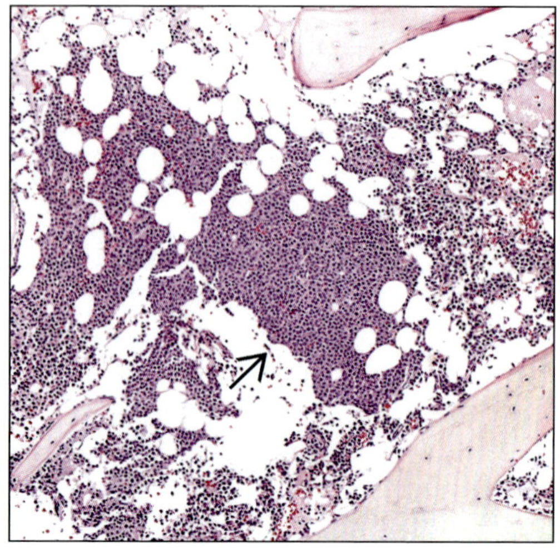

Homogeneous sheets ⇒ of plasma cells displacing normal bone marrow stroma indicate MM. Infiltrates may be widely spaced and irregularly distributed with considerable areas of bone marrow sparing.

TERMINOLOGY

Abbreviations

- Monoclonal gammopathy of undetermined significance (MGUS)

Definitions

- Occurrence of MM in > 1 family member
  - More than expected due to rarity of disease
  - Multiple myeloma (MM): Classified as plasma cell myeloma (PCM) in 2008 WHO classification of plasma cell neoplasms

EPIDEMIOLOGY

Incidence

- 20,000 cases of MM diagnosed in USA in 2008
  - Multivariate analysis of SEER data (1973-1998)
    - Main effect on incidence of MM is race
    - Sex, age, year of diagnosis, and geographic area are not as important
- African Americans diagnosed with MGUS and MM 2-3x more than European Americans
  - African Americans have fewer IgH translocations
- > 100 cases of familial MM have been reported
  - Effects of genetic factors, environmental factors, or both are currently being studied
- 40% of 1st-degree relatives of patients with MM have cancer
  - 10% are hematologic neoplasms

ETIOLOGY

Genetic/Environmental

- Hypothesis that 1st "hit" is germline and inherited; 2nd "hit" is somatic and environmental
  - Environmental factors linked to familial MM
    - Many family members are born and raised in rural areas
    - Increased exposure to pesticides, insecticides, herbicides
    - MM develops in some spouses of MM patients
  - MGUS is precursor lesion to MM
    - Asymptomatic, premalignant condition
    - Progression to MM of 1% per year

Putative Autosomal Dominant Transmission of MM

- Families with probable myeloma syndrome
- Dominant allele is on a non-sex-determining chromosome
  - Affects females and males
  - Does not skip generations
- Significant association with other malignancies
  - High frequency of breast cancer in some studies
  - Increased incidence of lymphoma, leukemia, pancreatic cancer, melanoma, and prostate cancer
- Genotypically and phenotypically heterogeneous
  - Genetic causes may overlap with those for other hematopoietic and solid tumor malignancies
  - Genetic differences vary between MM families

Genetics

- Genome-wide association study
  - Single nucleotide polymorphism at 3p22.1 (rs1052501), *ULK4* gene
    - C allele associated with 30% increased risk of MGUS and 40% increased risk of MM
- Potential myeloma-prone germ-line mutations
  - Germline *CDKN2A* mutation in melanoma-prone family
    - Mutation associated with development of MM in 1 family member
- Sequencing studies have identified novel loci in MM DNA

- Mutations involving key genes, i.e., histone methylation, NF-K/β pathway
- Single nucleotide polymorphisms in MM
  - Involve genes in target pathways, i.e., DNA repair, immune response
  - Need additional studies to verify and examine familial associations
- Genetic variations found in some MM patients
  - Different IL-10 promoter region haplotypes lead to significantly different IL-10 genotypes
  - Genetic differences in benzene metabolism

Role of Immune-Mediated Conditions

- Hyperresponsive B cells in families with MGUS/MM
  - Increased IgA, IgG, or IgM production after pokeweed mitogen stimulation in vitro
    - Suggests role in familial monoclonal gammopathy
- Hyperphosphorylated autoantigen targets of paraproteins more prevalent in familial MGUS/MM
  - Possible role in development of MGUS/MM by chronic antigen stimulation
  - Paratarg-7 (P-7)
    - Target of 15% of IgA and IgG paraproteins; 11% of IgM paraproteins
    - Hyperphosphorylation of protein is inherited in a dominant manner
    - Carrier of P-7 is at increased risk of developing MGUS/MM (odds ratio = 6.5)
  - P-8, encoded by *ATG13* gene
    - Hyperphosphorylation of protein is inherited in a dominant manner
- Patients with giant cell arteritis and polymyalgia rheumatica have
  - Increased risk of MM (odds ratio = 7.8 and 1.9, respectively)
  - Increased risk of MGUS (odds ratio = 11.3 and 2.9, respectively)

CLINICAL IMPLICATIONS

Familial Aggregation of MM

- Family-, case-, and population-based studies
  - Primarily white populations examined
  - Families of MGUS probands have increased
    - Relative risk for MGUS of 2.6-3.3%
    - Relative risk for MM of 2.0-2.9%
    - 1st-degree relatives have 2-4x increased risk of lymphoproliferative disorders
  - Families of MM probands have increased
    - Relative risk for MGUS of 2.0-2.4%
    - Relative risk for MM of 2.1-3.7%
    - 1st-degree relatives have relative risk for MM of 5.64
    - Standard incidence ratio for MM in offspring is 3.33 (2.1-5.0) in Swedish study
- African Americans or people of African descent
  - Scant data
    - Rare study supports role for genetic factors

Familial MM or Myeloma Syndrome

- Rare disorder
  - Increased risk of MM in 1st-degree relatives of patients with MM
- Excess cases of solid and hematologic cancers
  - Important to document extended family pedigrees
  - Examine both genetic factors and environmental exposure

ASSOCIATED NEOPLASMS

Familial MM

- Breast cancer, pancreatic cancer, melanoma, bladder or prostate cancer, lymphoma, and leukemia may be part of syndrome

MGUS or MM

- Increased risk of chronic lymphocytic leukemia
- Increased risk of acute lymphoblastic leukemia (MM)

CANCER RISK MANAGEMENT

Myeloma Susceptibility Loci Testing

- Linkage analysis studies of family members
  - Find markers specific to familial disease
  - Monitor at-risk family members

Test for M-Component in Family Members

- MGUS is single best marker of familial disease

SELECTED REFERENCES

1. Baker A et al: Uncovering the biology of multiple myeloma among African Americans: a comprehensive genomics approach. Blood. 121(16):3147-52, 2013
2. Greenberg AJ et al: Single-nucleotide polymorphism rs1052501 associated with monoclonal gammopathy of undetermined significance and multiple myeloma. Leukemia. 27(2):515-6, 2013
3. Greenberg AJ et al: Familial monoclonal gammopathy of undetermined significance and multiple myeloma: epidemiology, risk factors, and biological characteristics. Blood. 119(23):5359-66, 2012
4. Broderick P et al: Common variation at 3p22.1 and 7p15.3 influences multiple myeloma risk. Nat Genet. 44(1):58-61, 2011
5. Lindqvist EK et al: Personal and family history of immune-related conditions increase the risk of plasma cell disorders: a population-based study. Blood. 118(24):6284-91, 2011
6. Coleman EA et al: Initial report of a family registry of multiple myeloma. Cancer Nurs. 32(6):456-64, 2009
7. Kristinsson SY et al: Patterns of hematologic malignancies and solid tumors among 37,838 first-degree relatives of 13,896 patients with multiple myeloma in Sweden. Int J Cancer. 125(9):2147-50, 2009
8. Landgren O et al: Risk of plasma cell and lymphoproliferative disorders among 14621 first-degree relatives of 4458 patients with monoclonal gammopathy of undetermined significance in Sweden. Blood. 114(4):791-5, 2009
9. Vachon CM et al: Increased risk of monoclonal gammopathy in first-degree relatives of patients with multiple myeloma or monoclonal gammopathy of undetermined significance. Blood. 114(4):785-90, 2009
10. Lynch HT et al: Familial myeloma. N Engl J Med. 359(2):152-7, 2008
11. Lynch HT et al: Phenotypic heterogeneity in multiple myeloma families. J Clin Oncol. 23(4):685-93, 2005

FAMILIAL TESTICULAR TUMOR

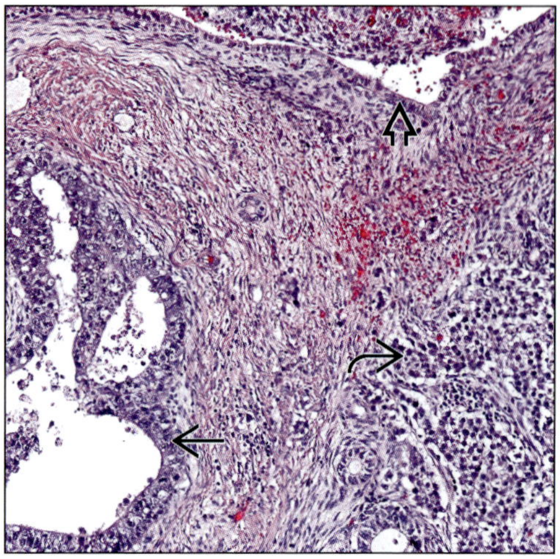

Image shows mixed TGCT that consists of seminoma ⮳, embryonal carcinoma →, and mature teratoma ⇨. In young adults, mixed TGCT is the 2nd most common testicular tumor after pure seminoma.

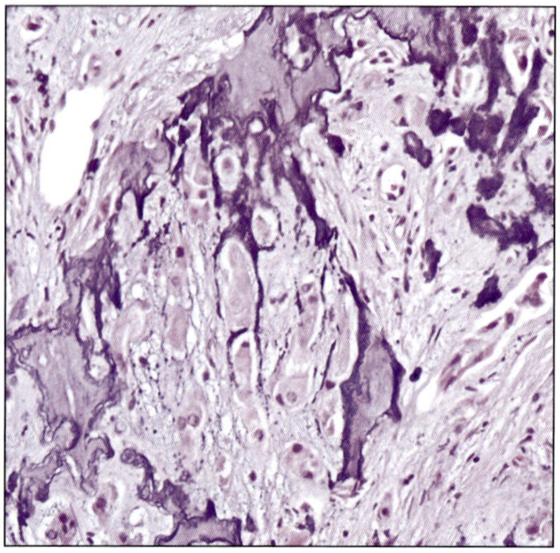

Large-cell calcifying Sertoli cell tumor shows distinctive large cells with abundant eosinophilic cytoplasm & calcifications; it is associated with Carney complex & Peutz-Jeghers syndrome. (Courtesy S. Shen, MD.)

FAMILIAL TESTICULAR GERM CELL TUMORS

Terminology

- Abbreviations
  - Testicular germ cell tumor (TGCT)
  - Familial testicular germ cell tumor (FTGCT)
  - Hereditary testicular germ cell tumor (HTGCT)
- Definitions
  - **FTGCT**
    - Affected individuals from families with ≥ 2 cases of TGCT
  - **HTGCT**
    - FTGCT with consistent passage of susceptibility gene via Mendelian inheritance
    - No definitive human susceptibility gene identified so far
    - Existence not yet firmly established

Epidemiology

- Incidence
  - In USA, there will be 7,920 cases of testicular cancers estimated in 2013
  - Incidence increased 3-6% annually since the 1970s
  - 95% of testicular tumors are TGCT
  - ~ 1.5% of patients with TGCT reported positive family history of TGCT
    - ~ 120 FTGCT cases per year
- Age range
  - 3 distinct age groups of TGCT
    - Mostly young adults between 20 and 35 years (pure and mixed germ-cell tumor [GCT])
    - Neonates and infants (mostly pure teratoma and yolk sac tumor)
    - Older men (spermatocytic seminoma)
  - Most reported FTGCT cases under 1st group
  - Diagnosis of FTGCT is 2-3 years younger than in usual TGCT

Risk Factors for TGCT

- Family history, prior TGCT, cryptorchidism, and testicular microlithiasis
- Syndromic associations such as Klinefelter syndrome (47 XXY) and XY gonadal genesis
- Testicular microlithiasis more common in FTGCT family members
- Incidence of cryptorchidism similar in FTGCT and sporadic TGCT

Family History as Risk for TGCT

- 4-6x ↑ risk of TGCT in sons of affected individuals
- 8-10x ↑ risk of TGCT in siblings of affected individuals
  - Represent highest familial risk for any human cancers
  - Higher risk among brothers suggests recessive or X-linked inheritance
- 88% of FTGCT have 2 affected individuals; highest incidence is up to 5 members
  - Indicates very low penetrance for HTGCT
- Risk in twins: 37x higher for dizygotic, 76x higher for monozygotic
- Also ↑ risk of ovarian GCT in female family members (**familial ovarian GCT**)
  - TGCT 15x ↑ than ovarian GCT

Genetic Factors

- Several candidate genes reported
- Most either showed conflicting results or needed further investigations
- *KITLG*, *SPRY4*, and *BAK1* confirmed by genome-wide association studies

Clinical Implications

- Bilaterally in FTGCT slightly ↑ at 6.5-9.8% vs. 2.8% in TGCT with negative family history
- Clinical behavior of FTGCT likely similar to usual TGCT, which is dependent on stage, specific GCT component, and treatment type

FAMILIAL TESTICULAR TUMOR

Genes Implicated in Familial Testicular Germ Cell Tumors

Genomic Region	Gene
Xq27	Unknown
2p23	Unknown
3p12	Unknown
3q26	Unknown
12p13-q21	Possible *KITLG*
18q21-23	Unknown
4q12	*KIT*
5q31.3	*DND1*
Yq11.2	Y *gr/gr*
2q31.2	*PDE11A*
12q22	*KITLG*
5q31.3	*SPRY4*
6p21.3-p21.2	*BAK1*

Pathological Findings

- Similar to usual TGCT in younger adult patients
  - TGCT in this age group associated with intratubular germ cell neoplasia (ITGCN)
- Seminoma and nonseminoma diagnosis at 1:1 ratio in FTGCT

FAMILIAL SEX CORD-STROMAL TUMORS

Terminology

- Abbreviations
  - Sex cord-stromal tumors (SCST)
  - Familial sex cord-stromal tumors (FSCST)

Epidemiology

- < 5% of testicular tumors
- Most SCST are sporadic
- FSCST very rarely encountered in Peutz-Jeghers syndrome and Carney complex

Syndromic Associations

- **Large cell calcifying Sertoli cell tumor** (LCCSCT) and **Sertoli cell tumor** associated with Peutz-Jeghers syndrome and Carney complex; LCCSCT a component of Carney complex
  - Carney complex caused by inherited mutation in *PRKAR1A*
    - Autosomal dominant inheritance characterized by cardiac or cutaneous myxomas, lentiginosis, endocrine tumors or overactivity, and schwannoma
    - 1/3 develop LCCSCT within 1st decade and in almost all adult males
    - Clinical testing available for *PRKAR1A*, detecting ~ 55% mutation
  - Peutz-Jeghers syndrome caused by inherited mutation in *STK11*
    - Autosomal dominant inheritance characterized by gastrointestinal polyposis and oral pigmentations
- **Juvenile granulosa cell tumor** associated with sex chromosomal abnormalities, ambiguous genitalia, and ipsilateral cryptorchidism

Clinical Implications

- LCCSCT is benign
- Juvenile granulosa cell tumor mostly have indolent behavior

Pathologic Findings

- Similar to usual SCST

SELECTED REFERENCES

1. Banks KC et al: 10 rare tumors that warrant a genetics referral. Fam Cancer. 12(1):1-18, 2013
2. Gallagher DJ et al: Genitourinary cancer predisposition syndromes. Hematol Oncol Clin North Am. 24(5):861-83, 2010
3. Greene MH et al: Familial testicular germ cell tumors in adults: 2010 summary of genetic risk factors and clinical phenotype. Endocr Relat Cancer. 17(2):R109-21, 2010
4. Giambartolomei C et al: A mini-review of familial ovarian germ cell tumors: an additional manifestation of the familial testicular germ cell tumor syndrome. Cancer Epidemiol. 33(1):31-6, 2009
5. Mai PL et al: Younger age-at-diagnosis for familial malignant testicular germ cell tumor. Fam Cancer. 8(4):451-6, 2009
6. Mueller CM et al: Constitutional cytogenetic analysis in men with hereditary testicular germ cell tumor: no evidence of disease-related abnormalities. Cancer Epidemiol Biomarkers Prev. 16(12):2791-4, 2007
7. Gundy S et al: Increased predisposition to cancer in brothers and offspring of testicular tumor patients. Pathol Oncol Res. 10(4):197-203, 2004
8. Lutke Holzik MF et al: Genetic predisposition to testicular germ-cell tumours. Lancet Oncol. 5(6):363-71, 2004
9. Lutke Holzik MF et al: Syndromic aspects of testicular carcinoma. Cancer. 97(4):984-92, 2003
10. Dong C et al: Familial testicular cancer and second primary cancers in testicular cancer patients by histological type. Eur J Cancer. 37(15):1878-85, 2001

FAMILIAL UVEAL MELANOMA

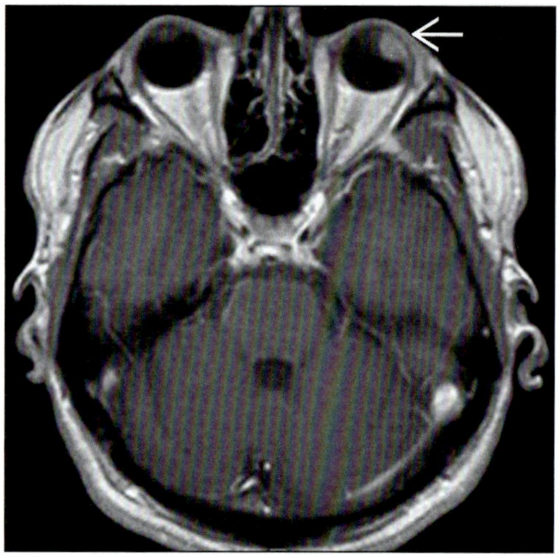

Axial T1-weighted MR image post-contrast demonstrates a well-circumscribed intraocular mass centered in the uveal tract ➡. Histologic examination confirmed the diagnosis of melanoma.

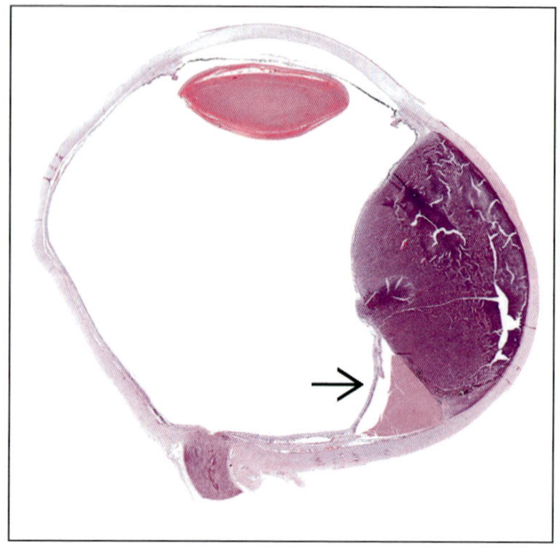

Uveal melanomas arise predominantly in the choroid and form well-circumscribed masses. Serous detachment of overlying/adjacent retina is common ➡.

TERMINOLOGY

Description

- Malignant intraocular neoplasm with melanocytic differentiation arising in choroid, ciliary body, or iris

EPIDEMIOLOGY

Uveal Melanoma

- Most frequent primary intraocular neoplasm in adults
- Annual incidence: 5-6 per 1 million in United States
  - Predominantly disease of adults (mean age ~ 60 years)
  - Predilection for whites, light-colored eyes; no gender predilection

Familial Uveal Melanoma

- Families with multiple members with uveal melanoma very rare (< 1%)
- If cancers other than uveal melanoma are considered, familial predisposition for uveal melanoma is much higher (~ 10%)

GENETICS

BAP1-Associated Tumor Predisposition Syndrome

- Autosomal dominant syndrome associated with mutations in *BRCA1*-associated protein 1 (*BAP1*) located in chromosome region 3p21.1
- Encodes for a nuclear ubiquitin carboxy-terminal hydroxylase
  - Binds *BRCA1* and *ASXL1*
  - Plays role in DNA damage response, apoptosis, senescence, chromatin modulation/stem cell biology, and regulation of cell cycle
- Inactivating somatic mutations in 1/2 of uveal melanomas, particularly when metastatic
- Inactivating somatic mutations in a small subset of lung and breast cancers
- Monosomy 3 (containing *BAP1*) strongly associated with metastatic risk in uveal melanoma
- Germline mutations associated with increased risk in families for uveal melanoma, cutaneous melanoma, malignant mesothelioma, renal cell carcinoma, and other cancers
  - Frequent epithelioid/rhabdoid cytology
- Protein loss may be identified by immunohistochemistry in tumor tissues

CDKN2A

- Encodes tumor suppressors *p14ARF* and *P16*
- Best known high-risk melanoma susceptibility gene
- Germline mutations strongly associated with cutaneous melanoma, but rare in uveal melanoma (< 1% of patients)

GNAQ and *GNA11*

- Somatic mutations frequent in uveal melanoma
  - Early genetic events leading to MAPK pathway activation
- Germline mutations not a feature of familial uveal melanoma

BRAF

- Somatic mutations frequent in cutaneous melanoma but very rare in uveal melanoma
- Germline mutations associated with cardiofaciocutaneous syndrome but not with melanoma predisposition

ASSOCIATED NEOPLASMS

Uveal Melanoma

- High propensity for metastases (~ 50%), particularly the liver
- Composed of 3 main cell types in various proportions

- Spindle A: Narrow nuclei, inconspicuous nucleoli
- Spindle B: Oval, plump nuclei with prominent nucleoli
- Epithelioid: Abundant cytoplasm, prominent nucleoli, associated with poor prognosis

- Gene expression profiles
  - Class 1: Low metastatic risk
  - Class 2: High metastatic risk, frequent monosomy 3
- Other prognostic factors include tumor size, extracellular matrix patterns (i.e., vascular mimicry), mitotic activity, extraocular extension, necrosis, and lymphocytic infiltrates

Cutaneous Melanoma and Atypical Melanocytic Lesions

- Melanocytic *BAP1*-mutated atypical intradermal tumors (MBAIT) or nevoid melanoma-like melanocytic proliferations (NEMMP)
  - Terms proposed for a subset of tumors with spitzoid features and high prevalence of somatic *BRAF* (V600E) mutation in patients with germline *BAP1* mutations
    - Terminology not uniformly accepted
  - Combined somatic *BAP1* and *BRAF* mutations also found in a subset of atypical Spitz tumors/nevi

Astrocytoma

- Melanoma-astrocytoma predisposition recognized in rare families
- Associated with *CDKN2A* mutations, particularly when exons coding for *p14ARF* are involved
- Astrocytomas pathologically high grade (i.e., glioblastomas)

Mesothelioma

- Genetic factors important
  - Some patients develop mesothelioma after short exposure to asbestos whereas others do not, even after heavy exposure
- Recognized component of *BAP1*-associated tumor predisposition syndrome
- *BAP1* mutations also occur is sporadic mesothelioma (up to 60%)
  - More frequent in tumors with epithelioid morphology

Renal Cell Carcinoma

- Recognized component of *BAP1*-associated tumor predisposition syndrome
  - Clear cell histology
- Somatic *BAP1* mutations in 8-14% of clear cell renal carcinomas

Others

- Meningioma, lung adenocarcinoma, neuroendocrine carcinoma, paraganglioma

CANCER RISK MANAGEMENT

Uveal Melanoma Families

- Members with uveal melanomas and other possibly related cancers (e.g., cutaneous melanomas and mesotheliomas) should be screened for *BAP1* mutations
- Ophthalmologic and dermatologic exams; avoid environmental insults (e.g., sun exposure)

SELECTED REFERENCES

1. Hawkes JE et al: Lack of GNAQ and GNA11 germ-line mutations in familial melanoma pedigrees with uveal melanoma or blue nevi. Front Oncol. 3:160, 2013
2. Murali R et al: Tumours associated with BAP1 mutations. Pathology. 45(2):116-26, 2013
3. Popova T et al: Germline BAP1 Mutations Predispose to Renal Cell Carcinomas. Am J Hum Genet. Epub ahead of print, 2013
4. Carbone M et al: BAP1 cancer syndrome: malignant mesothelioma, uveal and cutaneous melanoma, and MBAITs. J Transl Med. 10:179, 2012
5. Abdel-Rahman MH et al: Cancer family history characterization in an unselected cohort of 121 patients with uveal melanoma. Fam Cancer. 9(3):431-8, 2010
6. Harbour JW et al: Frequent mutation of BAP1 in metastasizing uveal melanomas. Science. 330(6009):1410-3, 2010
7. Goldstein AM et al: High-risk melanoma susceptibility genes and pancreatic cancer, neural system tumors, and uveal melanoma across GenoMEL. Cancer Res. 66(20):9818-28, 2006

IMAGE GALLERY

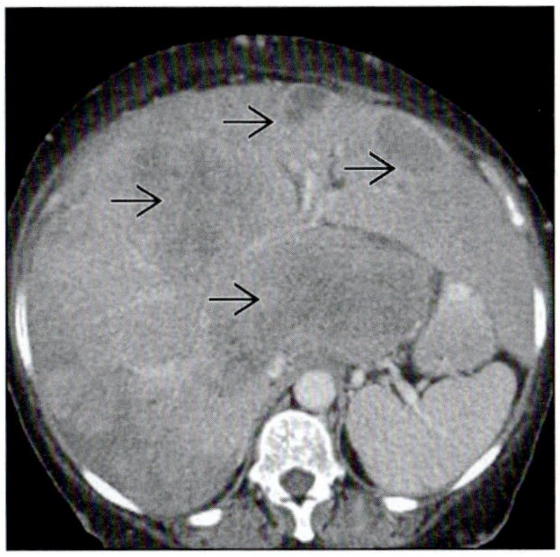

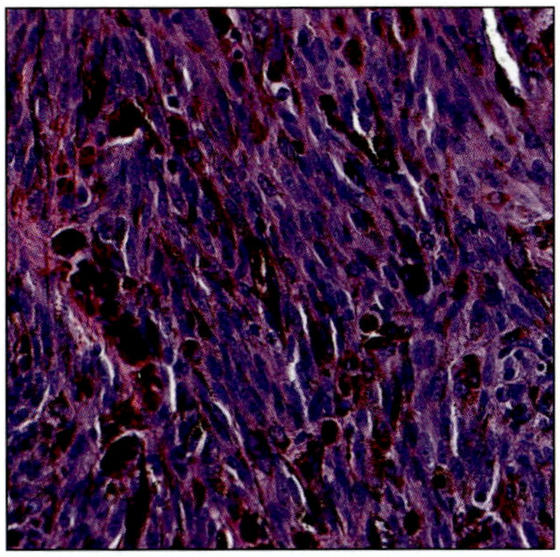

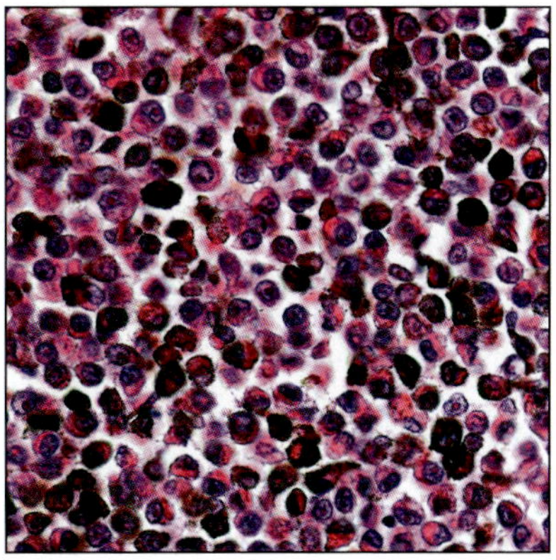

(Left) *The majority of patients with metastatic uveal melanoma have hepatic involvement* ⇨*, as demonstrated in this abdominal CT scan.* ***(Center)*** *Most uveal melanomas are characterized by spindle cells. Melanotic pigment is variable.* ***(Right)*** *The presence of epithelioid cells in uveal melanoma is a negative prognostic factor and is associated with class 2 (high-risk) tumors and BAP1 mutations. These cells contain ample cytoplasm, round nuclei and macronuclei.*

FAMILIAL WILMS TUMOR

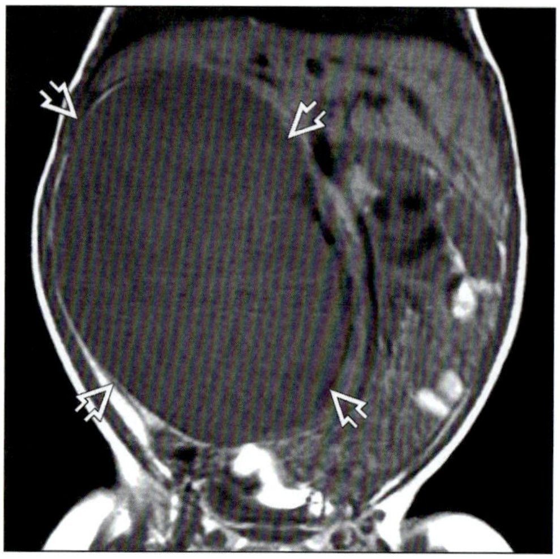

Coronal T1WI MR shows a huge, homogeneous mass occupying the right flank ⊳, displacing the bowel and liver. This Wilms tumor compresses the vena cava along the left margin of the mass, without venous invasion.

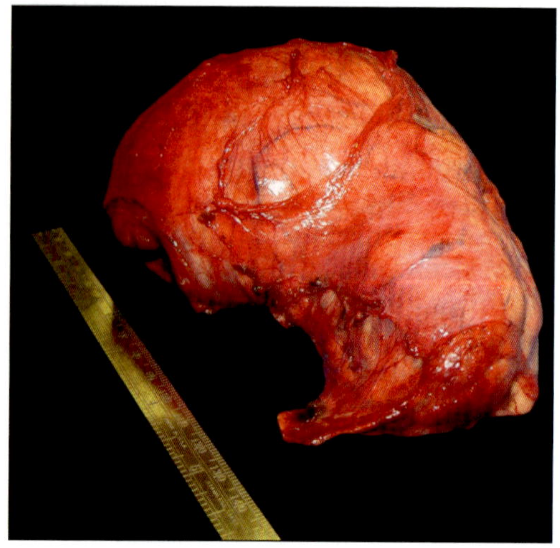

Gross image shows a very large WT replacing the kidney that was eventually resected from a patient after several rounds of chemotherapy were given to shrink the mass.

TERMINOLOGY

Abbreviations

- Wilms tumor (WT)
- Familial Wilms tumor (FWT)

Definitions

- WT: Malignant embryonic neoplasm arising from undifferentiated renal mesenchyme that exhibits triphasic histology of blastemal, epithelial, and stromal elements
- FWT: Individuals affected by renal WT with positive family history of WT
  - Familial predisposition occurs outside the context of congenital anomalies, genetic syndromes, or *WT1* mutation
- WT-associated syndromes are grouped separately

Synonyms

- Familial nephroblastoma

EPIDEMIOLOGY

Incidence

- WT diagnosed in 1 in 10,000 Caucasian children and comprises ~ 85% of childhood renal malignancies
  - Majority of WT are sporadic (up to 99%)
  - FWT comprises ~ 2% of cases
    - Very rare cases of familial extrarenal WT cases have been reported

Age Range

- Sporadic WT
  - Average age of diagnosis for unilateral tumors: 42-47 months
  - Average age of diagnosis for bilateral tumors: 30-33 months
  - ~ 80% of cases diagnosed before 15 years of age
- FWT
  - Younger patients than in sporadic WT
  - Average age of diagnosis for unilateral tumors: ~ 35 months
  - Average age of diagnosis for bilateral tumors: ~ 16 months

Gender

- Males and females equally affected
- No gender bias in obligate carrier parents of children with WT

Site

- Sporadic WT
  - Bilateral involvement in 5-10% of cases
- FWT
  - Higher chance for bilateral involvement seen in ~ 16% of cases

ETIOLOGY/PATHOGENESIS

Genetics

- Etiology of WT is heterogeneous and may vary in sporadic, familial, and WT-associated syndrome settings
- Sporadic WT
  - *WT1* at Chr 11p13 acts as a tumor suppressor gene and is inactivated in individuals with constitutional WT
    - *WT1* is a member of zinc finger transcription factors and encodes a 449-amino acid protein containing 4 zinger motifs and a regulatory domain
    - Most mutations in WT are deletions or truncation mutations
- FWT
  - *WT1* mutation occurs **rarely** in FWT
    - Considered not the predisposition gene in most WT families
  - 2 FWT genes mapped

- *FWT1* at Chr 17q12-q21
- *FWT2* at Chr 19q13.4
- Specific genes in these 2 regions have not yet been identified
- Lack of linkage in some families to *FWT1* and *FWT2* suggests the existence of at least 1 additional FWT gene

  - WT predisposition suggested as result of an autosomal dominant allele that is incompletely penetrant (25-60% penetrance)
  - Other WT genes
    - Mutations in *P53* and β-catenin observed in 5% and 15% of WT cases, respectively
    - Other genes at Chr 16q, Chr 1p, and Chr 7p
    - Alterations are mainly somatic

CLINICAL IMPLICATIONS

Clinical Risk Factors

- Positive family history
  - Majority of affected families have 2-3 members with WT
  - Hallmark of FWT: Affected individuals are either siblings or cousins, related through an unaffected obligate carrier

Clinical Presentation

- Most commonly, abdominal mass detected by parents
- Abdominal pain, gross hematuria, fever, or hypertension
- FWT rarely presents with features of genetic syndromes associated with WT (e.g., Wilms tumor; aniridia, genitourinary anomalies, and mental retardation [WAGR]; Denys-Drash, Perlman, Beckwith-Wiedemann syndromes)

Prognosis

- Similar for WT in sporadic, familial, and WT-associated syndromes settings
- High cure rate for WT; estimated survival of 90% for localized disease and 70% for advanced disease

Treatment

- Similar therapeutic approach for WT in sporadic, familial, and WT-associated syndromes setting
- Children Oncology Group (COG) and National Wilms Tumor Study (NWTS) advocate primary tumor resection & further chemotherapy &/or radiotherapy determined by stage and histology (favorable or unfavorable)

MACROSCOPIC FINDINGS

General Features

- Majority of WT are unicentric and solitary but with higher chance for bilaterality in familial setting
- Tumor macroscopic findings similar for WT in sporadic, familial, and WT-associated syndromes setting
  - Cut surface usually shows homogeneous pale gray-tan appearance
  - May vary in consistency depending on proportion of components; firmer and fleshier with predominance of stromal component

MICROSCOPIC FINDINGS

General Features

- Tumor histologic findings similar for WT in sporadic, familial, and WT-associated syndromes setting
  - Characterized by triphasic histology consisting of variable admixture of undifferentiated blastemal cells, epithelial cells, and stromal cells
  - Monophasic or biphasic WT may also occur
  - Blastemal cells
    - Tightly packed small cells with high nuclear:cytoplasmic ratio, overlapping nuclei, even chromatin, and brisk mitotic activity
  - Epithelial cells
    - From primitive to well-differentiated tubules and glomeruloid bodies resembling those found in normal kidneys
  - Stromal cells
    - Most are undifferentiated spindle cells or have muscle or fibroblastic differentiations
    - Occasionally may contain ganglion cells, neuroglia, bone, cartilage, or fat cells
- Immunohistochemistry
  - Nuclear immunoreactivity for WT1 of blastemal and epithelial cells
  - CK7 positivity in epithelial cells
  - Pax-2 often positive
  - Blastemal cells usually negative for pankeratin and vimentin

CANCER RISK MANAGEMENT

Screening for WT

- Clinical and genetic testing and surveillance for WT recommended for children in families with FWT
- Screening for FWT similar with other conditions considered high (> 20%) or moderate (5-20%) risks for WT, such as WAGR, Denys-Drash, Perlman, and Beckwith-Wiedemann syndromes
  - Regular ultrasound ~ every 3 months

SELECTED REFERENCES

1. Huff V: Wilms' tumours: about tumour suppressor genes, an oncogene and a chameleon gene. Nat Rev Cancer. 11(2):111-21, 2011
2. Scott RH et al: Syndromes and constitutional chromosomal abnormalities associated with Wilms tumour. J Med Genet. 43(9):705-15, 2006
3. Ruteshouser EC et al: Familial Wilms tumor. Am J Med Genet C Semin Med Genet. 129C(1):29-34, 2004
4. Dome JS et al: Recent advances in Wilms tumor genetics. Curr Opin Pediatr. 14(1):5-11, 2002
5. Breslow NE et al: Familial Wilms' tumor: a descriptive study. Med Pediatr Oncol. 27(5):398-403, 1996

FANCONI ANEMIA

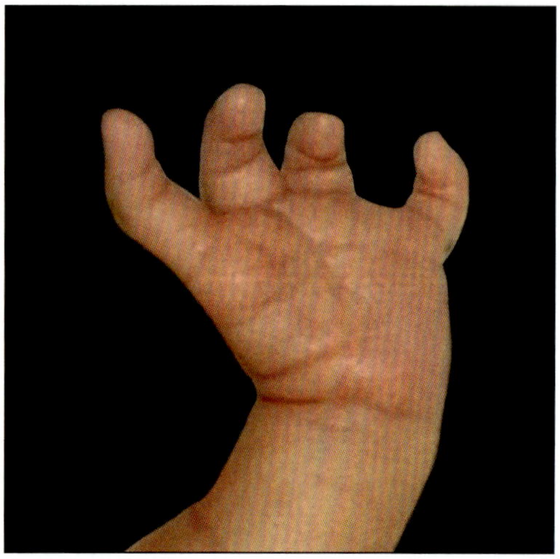

Clinical photograph of a hand of a child with Fanconi anemia (FA) shows the dramatic "classic" finding of an absent or hypoplastic thumb. (Courtesy C. Clericuzio, MD.)

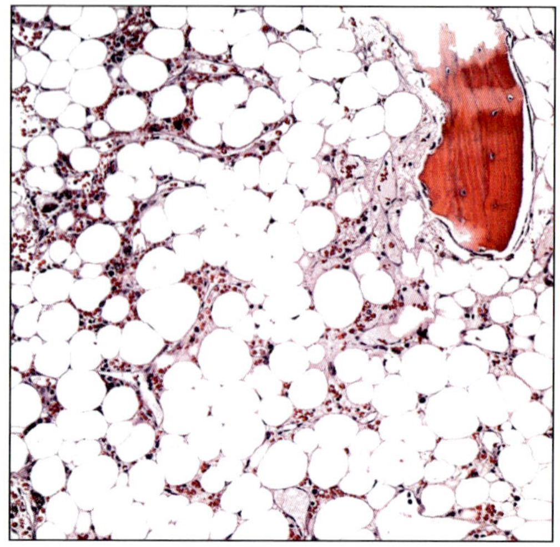

Bone marrow biopsy from a patient with FA shows marked hypocellularity with trilineage hematopoietic failure. Stromal elements, lymphocytes, and plasma cells remain. (Courtesy D. Czuchlewski, MD.)

TERMINOLOGY

Abbreviations

- Fanconi anemia (FA)

Definition

- Described by pediatrician Dr. Guido Fanconi in 1972
- 1 of several DNA damage repair deficiency syndromes including ataxia-telangiectasia, Bloom syndrome, Cockayne syndrome, Nijmegen breakage syndrome, Rothmund-Thomson syndrome, trichothiodystrophy, Werner syndrome, and xeroderma pigmentosum
- FA is a clinically and genetically heterogeneous inherited disorder characterized by
  - Autosomal or X-linked recessive pattern of inheritance
  - Congenital abnormalities in majority of patients
    - Low birth weight/short stature
    - Classic finding of hypoplastic or absent thumbs &/or radii
    - Pigmentation abnormalities
    - Renal malformations
    - Duodenal atresia or other gastrointestinal malformations
    - Microcephaly &/or microphthalmia
    - Congenital heart disease
    - Ear abnormalities/deafness
    - Hypogonadism
    - Neurologic abnormalities
    - Endocrine dysfunction
    - 25-40% of patients are phenotypically normal
  - Bone marrow failure presenting in 1st decade of life
    - Pancytopenia with marrow aplasia (patients present with sequelae such as anemia, bleeding, and easy bruising)
    - By 5th decade, cumulative incidence of bone marrow failure is 90%
  - Increased risk of hematologic neoplasms and solid tumors

EPIDEMIOLOGY

Incidence

- 4-7 patients per 1 million births
- Most cases are autosomal recessive in inheritance
  - Mutations affecting *FANCB* are X-linked recessive
- Increased incidence of FA in the Ashkenazi Jewish population due to specific *FANCC* mutations (IVS4 + 4A > T) (carrier frequency of 1.1%)
- Heterozygote frequency is 1 in 300
- Accounts for ~ 20% of cases of childhood aplastic anemia

ETIOLOGY/PATHOGENESIS

Molecular Pathogenesis

- Biallelic mutation in any of (at least) 13 separate genes composing the Fanconi anemia pathway
- Collectively, proteins encoded by these genes serve to sense DNA damage and initiate DNA repair
- FA pathway proteins fall into 3 separate groups, encoded by the following genes
  - Fanconi anemia core complex
    - *FANCA, FANCB, FANCC, FANCE, FANCF, FANCG, FANCL, FANCM*
    - *FANCA* is the most frequently mutated gene in this complex (mutations account for ~ 65% of FA cases)
  - ID complex
    - *FANCI, FANCD2*
  - Downstream effectors
    - *FANCJ, FANCN* (a.k.a. *BRIP1* and *PALB2*, respectively)
    - *FANCD1* (a.k.a. *BRCA2*)
- Functional interactions of FA proteins
  - Core complex detects DNA damage and ubiquitinates the ID complex proteins

- ID complex colocalizes at site of DNA damage with FA downstream effectors and other DNA repair proteins, including
  - RAD51 protein, which binds and promotes accurate DNA repair via homologous recombination
  - BRCA1 protein, which binds to facilitate repair and mediate cell cycle checkpoint control
- Genotype-phenotype correlations
  - Some *FANCC* mutations predispose to early-onset bone marrow failure
  - Incidence of acute myeloid leukemia (AML) and severe cytopenias is higher in patients with some *FANCG* and *FANCA* mutations
  - Patients with biallelic inactivating mutations in *FANCD1* have a 97% cumulative incidence of midline brain tumors, Wilms tumor, and AML by age 6

ANCILLARY TESTS

Confirmation of Diagnosis

- Cytogenetic testing
  - Diagnostic test: Chromosomal breakage (typically tests peripheral blood lymphocytes)
  - Cannot detect FA carriers with this test
- Molecular testing
  - Sequence analysis and targeted mutation analysis (nontargeted approach difficult given number of large genes that would require evaluation)
  - Carrier and prenatal testing can be performed by specific mutation testing if familial mutation is known

Evaluation for Hematologic Malignancy

- Bone marrow biopsy: Morphologic evaluation is gold standard for diagnosis of myelodysplastic syndrome (MDS)
- Cytogenetic analysis: Clonal amplification of chromosome 3q26-q29 often precedes progression to MDS/AML

ASSOCIATED NEOPLASMS

Hematologic Neoplasms

- By age 45, cumulative incidence of hematologic malignancy is 25%; median diagnosis age: 11-14 years
- Predominantly myeloid malignancies (600x increased risk of AML; 5,000x increased risk of MDS)
  - In ~ 25% of cases, leukemia (or cancer) diagnosis precedes recognition of underlying FA

Solid Tumors

- Squamous cell carcinoma (head, neck, esophagus, anogenital), hepatocellular carcinoma, brain tumors
- By 5th decade, 30% cumulative incidence

Breast Cancer Risk

- Heterozygous mutations in downstream effectors *FANCJ* (a.k.a. *BRIP1*), *FANCN* (a.k.a. *PALB2*), *FANCD1* (a.k.a. *BRCA2*) confer breast cancer susceptibility

CANCER RISK MANAGEMENT

Patients With FA

- Increased surveillance for commonly associated neoplasms
- Exposure to radiation or DNA-damaging chemicals should be avoided
  - Special protocols required for patients undergoing stem cell transplantation

SELECTED REFERENCES

1. Knoch J et al: Rare hereditary diseases with defects in DNA-repair. Eur J Dermatol. 22(4):443-55, 2012
2. Seif AE: Pediatric leukemia predisposition syndromes: clues to understanding leukemogenesis. Cancer Genet. 204(5):227-44, 2011
3. Green AM et al: Fanconi anemia. Hematol Oncol Clin North Am. 23(2):193-214, 2009
4. Moldovan GL et al: How the fanconi anemia pathway guards the genome. Annu Rev Genet. 43:223-49, 2009
5. Pinto FO et al: Diagnosis of Fanconi anemia in patients with bone marrow failure. Haematologica. 94(4):487-95, 2009

IMAGE GALLERY

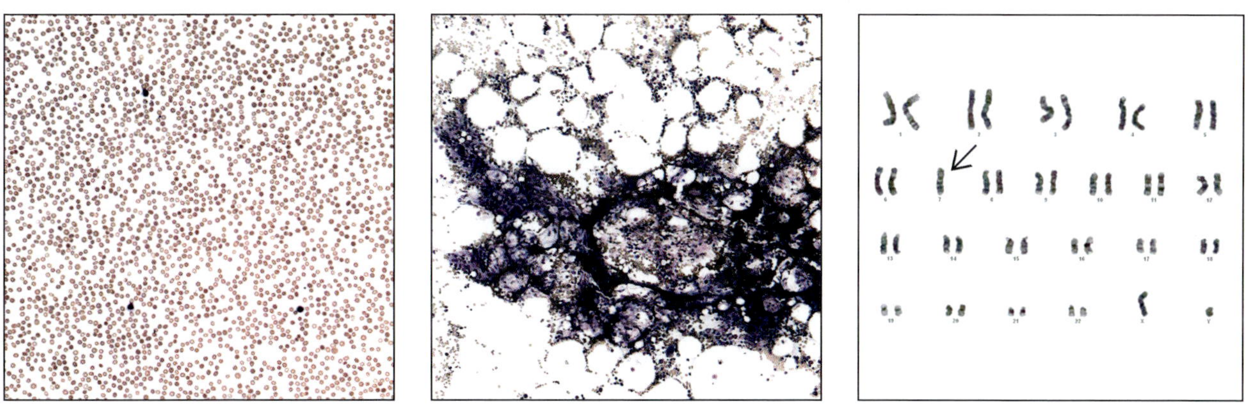

(Left) *Peripheral blood shows mildly macrocytic RBCs and profound leukopenia and thrombocytopenia, typical of FA presentation. (Courtesy D. Czuchlewski, MD.)* ***(Center)*** *Bone marrow aspirate from a child with FA shows bone marrow failure with essentially empty spicules. (Courtesy D. Czuchlewski, MD.)* ***(Right)*** *FA patients are at high risk of myelodysplastic syndrome/acute myeloid leukemia. Progression may be accompanied by clonal cytogenetic abnormalities, frequently monosomy 7 ⇒. (Courtesy D. Czuchlewski, MD.)*

HEREDITARY BREAST/OVARIAN CANCER SYNDROME: BRCA1

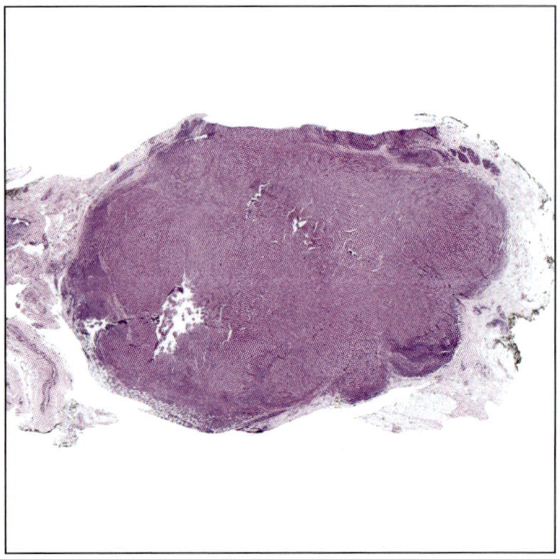

The majority of BRCA1 cancers are poorly differentiated, negative for hormone receptors, and cluster with basal-like carcinomas. However, 20-30% are ER positive and are of luminal B carcinoma type.

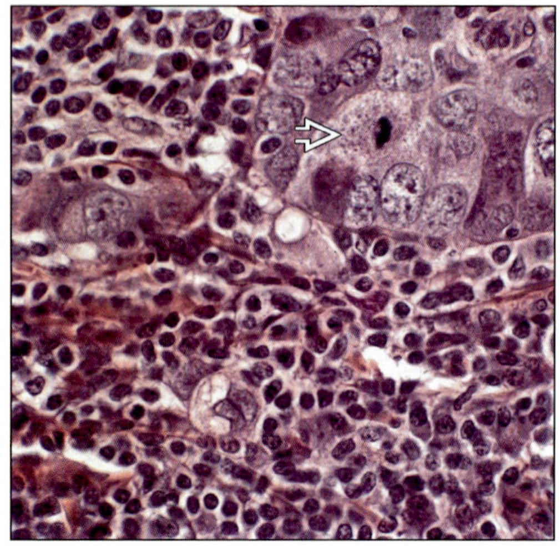

Hallmarks of BRCA1 cancers are a solid (syncytial) growth pattern, a high mitotic rate ⮚, and an associated dense lymphoplasmacytic infiltrate, which are features of medullary carcinoma.

TERMINOLOGY

Synonyms

- BRCA1 syndrome
- Breast cancer 1 syndrome
- Early-onset breast/ovarian cancer syndrome
- Online Mendelian Inheritance in Man (OMIM) #113705

Definitions

- Hereditary breast &/or ovarian cancers resulting from inheritance of a germline mutation in *BRCA1*
  - Early-onset and multiple primary breast tumors
  - Family history of breast or ovarian cancer

EPIDEMIOLOGY

Population Incidence

- 0.1-0.3% of individuals
  - Slightly less common than *BRCA2* mutations
- Specific mutations are found at increased frequency in ethnic populations
  - Finns, French Canadians, and many others
  - Ashkenazi Jewish population
    - ~ 1% (1 in 40)
    - 185delAG and 5382insC
    - There is also a common *BRCA2* mutation

Modifiers of Risk

- Parity decreases risk of breast cancer
- Low-dose ionizing radiation to chest before age 20 increases risk
- Mutations in other genes
  - None yet well defined
  - Genome-wide association studies (GWAS) are investigating possible associations

Cancer Incidence

- ~ 2% of all breast cancers are related to *BRCA1* germline mutations
- ~ 50% of all cancers related to a germline mutation are due to *BRCA1* germline mutations

GENETICS

BRCA1 Gene

- Located on 17q21
- Large 81 kb gene
  - Does not share sequence homology with *BRCA2* or other genes
- 23 coding exons
- Transcript 7,094 base pairs
  - Protein 1,863 amino acids (210 kDa)
  - No sequence homology with other proteins
- Autosomal dominant inheritance
  - De novo mutations are rare
- More than 1,000 different mutations identified
  - Majority are small deletions or insertions
    - Results in frameshift mutations, nonsense mutations, or splice site alterations
    - Protein may be truncated or absent
    - Less common are full-length proteins with missense mutations
  - Inactivating mutations impair conservative DNA repair and genomic stability functions

Protein Function

- Central role in DNA repair, cell cycle control, transcriptional regulation, as well as many other functions
- Regulation of repair of DNA damage
  - Repair of DNA double-stranded breaks by homologous recombination
    - Cells that lack BRCA1 rely on other less reliable mechanisms for DNA repair

        - Increases replication errors and genomic instability
    - Chromosomal instability contributes to tumor formation
        - *BRCA1* defects are postulated to be initiating oncogenic event
- Cell cycle regulation, checkpoint control
    - Accumulating DNA abnormalities enable mutations in genes essential to cell cycle checkpoint activation
- Transcriptional regulation
    - Required for transactivation of the estrogen receptor promoter
    - May explain why ~ 90% of *BRCA1*-related cancers are estrogen receptor negative
- Also functional in chromatin remodeling and protein ubiquitination

CLINICAL IMPLICATIONS AND ANCILLARY TESTS

Population to Be Tested

- American Society of Clinical Oncology recommends that patients with > 10% mutation risk undergo testing
    - 85% of mutation carriers will be detected using a 10% cut-off
- National Institute for Health and Clinical Excellence in United Kingdom recommends testing individuals with > 20% risk of having a mutation
- Counseling should occur before testing to ensure patient is aware of implications for self and family

Clinical Criteria

- Personal history of breast cancer in a woman < 40 years of age
    - Risk increased if cancer is negative for estrogen receptor
        - Risk is 35% for women < 30 if cancer is poorly differentiated and estrogen receptor negative
- Breast cancer in 1st-degree relatives (mother, sister, daughter)
    - Risk increased if cancer diagnosed at young age
    - Risk increased if individuals have multiple cancers
- Risk increased if ovarian cancers are also present in family
- Risk increased if a relative has known mutation

Calculating Risk

- There are multiple models to predict probability of an individual carrying a germline *BRCA1* or *BRCA2* mutation
    - Empiric models
        - Do not make assumptions about genetic risks (e.g., mutation frequency, mode of inheritance, penetrance)
        - Examples include Penn II model, Myriad II (Frank model), and National Cancer Institute model
    - Genetic risk prediction models
        - Make assumptions about the number of genes and allele frequencies
        - Include information about relationships among individuals in a kindred
        - Accuracy depends on validity of assumptions
        - Examples include BRCAPRO and the Breast and Ovarian Analysis of Disease Incidence and Carrier Estimation Algorithm (BOADICEA)
        - BRCAPRO available at http://www4.utsouthwestern.edu/breasthealth/cagene/
        - BOADICEA available at http://astor.som.jhmi.edu/BayesMendel/brcapro.html

Genetic Testing

- Full sequencing required to detect all mutations
- Additional testing required to detect deletions and amplifications
    - 18% of genetic changes are not detected by standard analysis
- All testing is performed by Myriad Genetics in USA

Interpretation of Results

- Mutation associated with breast cancer risk in other families
    - Patient classified as having BRCA1 syndrome
    - Testing of additional family members should be considered
- Mutation linked to a relative with breast cancer
    - Testing of additional individuals in family may be helpful to establish linkage
- Mutation known to be benign or have low clinical significance
    - Mutations that do not change amino acid type
    - Mutations known to occur in individuals without cancer
- Variant of uncertain significance (VUS)
    - Not yet linked to an individual with breast cancer
    - Detected in 7% of individuals (> 1,500 identified)
    - More frequent in populations of non-European origin as fewer individuals have been studied

Immunoperoxidase Studies

- Majority of *BRCA1*-associated carcinomas are negative for hormone receptors and HER2 (triple-negative breast carcinoma [TNBC])
    - These cancers group with basal-like carcinomas by gene expression profiling
    - There is an 80% overlap between TNBC and basal-like carcinomas
- Identifying a cancer as TNBC increases likelihood that a cancer is associated with *BRCA1*
    - However, > 10% of *BRCA1*-associated cancers are not basal-like cancers

ASSOCIATED NEOPLASMS

Female Breast Cancer

- Risk
    - 40-90% by age 70
        - Varies by mutation
        - May be modified by mutations in additional genes
- Macroscopic findings

- Carcinomas typically have pushing borders that are evident grossly and microscopically
- Histology
  - Predominantly high-grade, poorly differentiated carcinomas
    - Dense lymphocytic infiltrate (predominantly T cell)
    - High nuclear grade, syncytial pattern
    - Foci of geographic tumor necrosis
    - High proliferative index
  - Medullary features (syncytial growth pattern, lymphocytic infiltrate)
    - 13% fulfill criteria for medullary carcinoma
    - 60% have medullary features
  - 70-80% negative for estrogen receptor, progesterone receptor, and HER2
    - > 95% poorly differentiated
    - *TP53* mutations common (> 90%); ~ 55% positive by immunohistochemistry
    - 50-80% positive for CK5/6, CK14, or EGFR
    - BRCA1 regulates the expression of estrogen receptor
  - 20-30% positive for estrogen receptor and negative for HER2
    - ~ 45% poorly differentiated
    - ~ 50% positive by immunohistochemistry for p53
    - < 20% positive for CK5/6, CK14, or EGFR
    - Majority show loss of wild-type *BRCA1* allele
  - Majority (~ 90%) classified as basal-like carcinoma according to mRNA expression profiling
    - ~ 15% of basal-like carcinomas are related to germline *BRCA1* mutations
    - ER-positive subset are classified as luminal B

Male Breast Cancer

- 1.8% lifetime risk (compared to 0.07% risk in general population)
  - < 4% of male breast cancer cases associated with *BRCA1*
  - Lower than risk associated with *BRCA2*

Ovarian, Fallopian Tube, and Peritoneal Carcinoma

- 40-50% lifetime risk
- 60-85% involve fimbriated end of fallopian tube
- Serous tubal intraepithelial carcinoma (80%) and endometrioid tubal carcinoma (20%) are found in ~ 8% of prophylactic surgeries
  - Entire tube should be examined microscopically
    - Immunohistochemical studies for p53 and MIB-1 (Ki-67) can be helpful to identify early neoplasia
  - If no invasion is seen, risk of recurrence in peritoneum is 4-5%

Other Cancers

- Prostate: Relative risk = 1.8% (age < 65)
  - Risk of prostate cancer may vary depending on location of *BRCA1* mutation
- Pancreas: Relative risk = 2.3% (age < 65)
- Cervix: Relative risk = 2.6% (age < 65)
- Uterus: Relative risk = 2.6% (age < 65)

CANCER RISK MANAGEMENT

Chemoprevention

- Oral contraceptives
  - Reduces risk of ovarian cancer by 50%
  - Breast cancer risk may be increased by some types of oral contraceptives (results of studies have not been consistent)
- Tamoxifen
  - Reduces risk
    - Evidence derives from observed 50% reduction in risk of contralateral cancer among mutation carriers treated with tamoxifen
  - Protective effect observed in *BRCA1* and *BRCA2* carriers
    - *BRCA1* carriers appear to benefit despite predilection to develop ER negative tumor for reasons that remain unclear

Screening

- Mammography
  - Should begin at age 10 years younger than youngest affected person in family
  - May have limited sensitivity because young women often have dense breast tissue
- Magnetic resonance (MR) imaging
  - MR detects cancer due to blood flow and is more sensitive for detecting cancers in dense breasts

Prophylactic Surgery

- Bilateral mastectomy reduces breast cancer risk by 97%
  - However, not all breast tissue can be removed and achieve acceptable cosmetic results
  - Greatest benefit for patients before a diagnosis of cancer
- Bilateral salpingo-oophorectomy reduces breast and ovarian cancer risk
  - Breast cancer risk reduced by 50%
    - Mechanism not well understood but may be due to decreased estrogen production
  - Ovarian and fallopian tube cancer risk reduced by 70-96%
    - There remains a 4-5% risk of papillary serous carcinoma of peritoneum

SELECTED REFERENCES

1. Crum CP et al: The oviduct and ovarian cancer: causality, clinical implications, and "targeted prevention". Clin Obstet Gynecol. 55(1):24-35, 2012
2. Kaplan JS et al: Pathologic features and immunophenotype of estrogen receptor-positive breast cancers in BRCA1 mutation carriers. Am J Surg Pathol. 36(10):1483-8, 2012
3. Schneegans SM et al: Validation of three BRCA1/2 mutation-carrier probability models Myriad, BRCAPRO and BOADICEA in a population-based series of 183 German families. Fam Cancer. 11(2):181-8, 2012
4. Vargas AC et al: Phenotype-genotype correlation in familial breast cancer. J Mammary Gland Biol Neoplasia. 16(1):27-40, 2011
5. Amir E et al: Assessing women at high risk of breast cancer: a review of risk assessment models. J Natl Cancer Inst. 102(10):680-91, 2010

BRCA1-Related Cancers

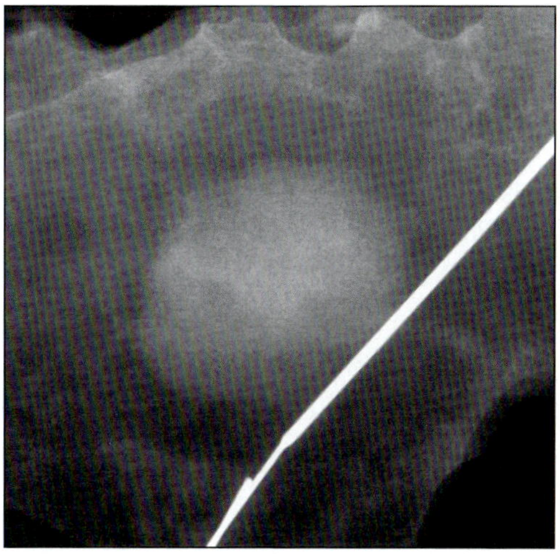
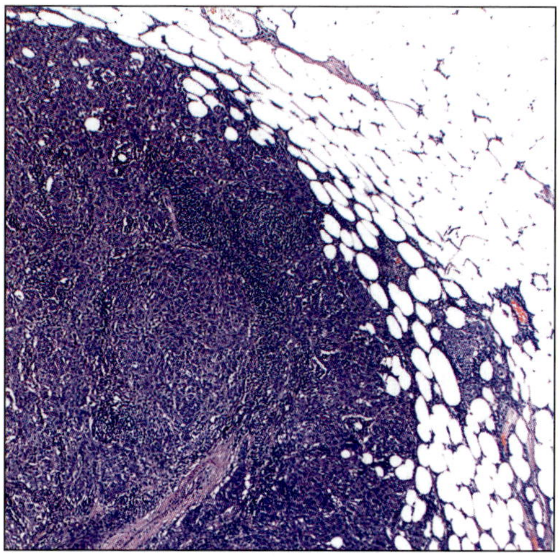

(Left) *BRCA1-related invasive carcinomas often present as circumscribed masses that may be mistaken for benign lesions. Associated calcifications are unusual. Young women often have dense breast tissue that can obscure masses and make detection difficult. In addition, cancers grow rapidly and can present in the interval between screening.* ***(Right)*** *The typical BRCA1-related carcinoma has a solid growth pattern, a dense T-cell rich lymphocytic infiltrate, and a pushing border.*

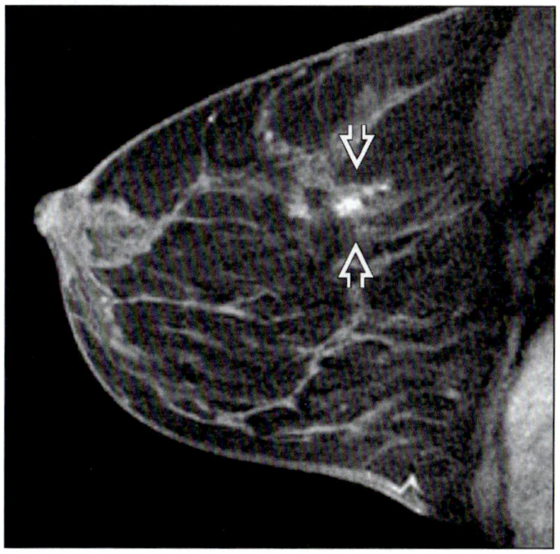
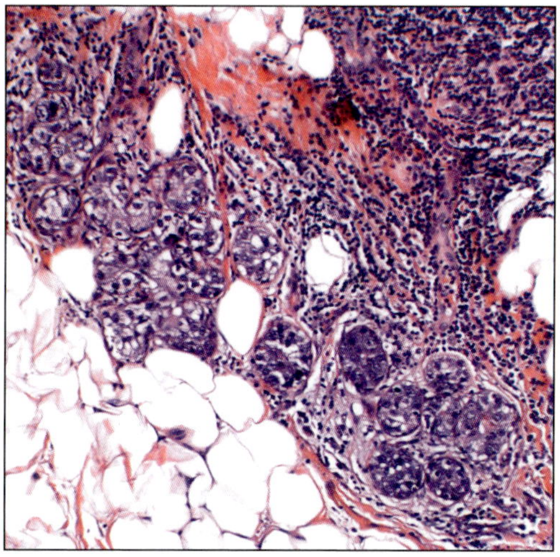

(Left) *Screening by MR is an option for young women. MR detects cancers by vascular uptake, which is not affected by dense breast tissue. A common MR finding for DCIS is linear clumped enhancement ➡.* ***(Right)*** *The DCIS associated with BRCA1 cancers can be limited in extent and difficult to detect. In this case, the cells in this lobule are highly atypical and are associated with a dense lymphocytic infiltrate. The cells were negative for estrogen and progesterone receptors and HER2.*

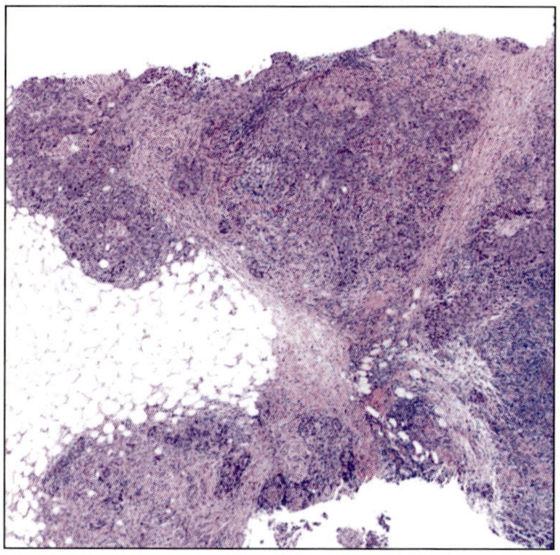
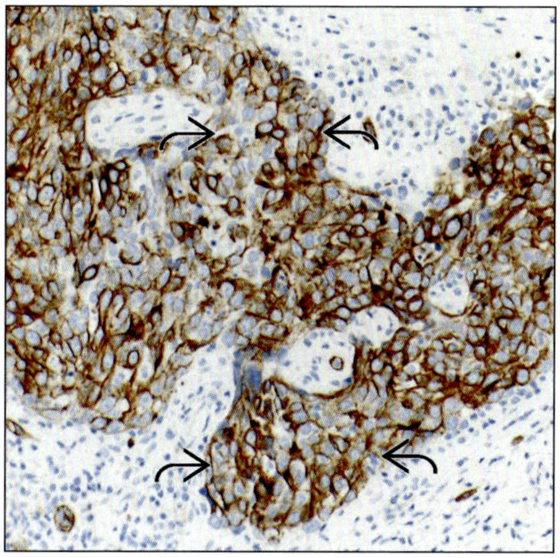

(Left) *This needle core biopsy from a palpable breast mass in a 34-year-old woman with a positive family history of breast cancer shows a poorly differentiated cancer with a high proliferative rate and a brisk inflammatory response. Subsequent genetic testing revealed a BRCA1 mutation.* ***(Right)*** *BRCA1-associated cancers are usually negative for ER, PR, and HER2. Tumor cells often show strong cytoplasmic expression of basal cytokeratin CK5/6 ↪, consistent with a basal-like carcinoma.*

HEREDITARY BREAST/OVARIAN CANCER SYNDROME: BRCA2

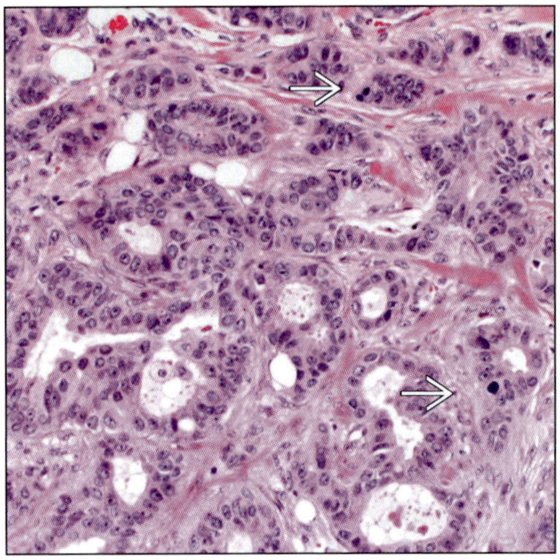

Breast cancers associated with BRCA2 are generally moderately to poorly differentiated with a high mitotic rate ➔. Unlike BRCA1-associated cancers, they do not have a characteristic appearance.

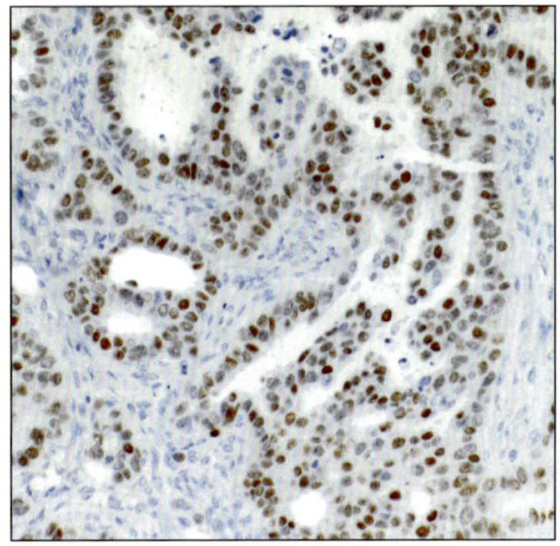

BRCA2-associated breast cancers, in contrast to BRCA1 cancers, usually express hormone receptors (as seen here for estrogen receptor). HER2 overexpression is very rare in either type of cancer.

TERMINOLOGY

Synonyms

- BRCA2 syndrome
- Breast cancer 2 syndrome
- Early-onset breast-ovarian cancer syndrome
- Online Mendelian Inheritance in Man (OMIM) I #600185

Definitions

- Hereditary breast &/or ovarian cancers resulting from inheritance of a germline mutation in *BRCA2*
  - Early-onset and multiple primary breast tumors
  - Family history of breast or ovarian cancer

EPIDEMIOLOGY

Population Incidence

- 0.1-0.7% of individuals
  - Slightly more common than *BRCA1* mutations
- Specific mutations are found at increased frequency in ethnic populations
  - Ashkenazi Jewish population
    - ~ 1-3% of individuals
    - 6174delT
    - There are also 2 common *BRCA1* mutations
  - Icelandic population
    - 0.6% of individuals
    - 999del5 detected in 38% of males and 10.4% of females with breast cancer
    - *BRCA2* mutations found in 90% of families with male and female breast cancer

Modifiers of Risk

- Parity may increase risk (whereas it decreases risk for *BRCA1* carriers)
- Low-dose ionizing radiation to chest before age 20 increases risk
- Mutations in other genes
  - None yet well defined
  - Genome-wide association studies (GWAS) are investigating possible associations

Cancer Incidence

- ~ 2% of all breast cancers are related to *BRCA2* germline mutations
  - ~ 50% of all breast cancers related to a germline mutation are due to *BRCA2*
- ~ 7% of ovarian cancers are related to *BRCA2* germline mutations
  - ~ 27% of ovarian cancers due to a germline mutation are related to *BRCA2*

GENETICS

BRCA2 Gene

- Located on 13q13.1
- Large 84 kb gene
  - Does not share sequence homology with *BRCA1* or other genes
- 27 coding exons
- Transcript is 10,930 base pairs
  - Protein is 3,418 amino acids (390 kDa)
- Autosomal dominant inheritance
  - De novo mutations are rare
- > 1,000 different mutations identified
  - Majority are small deletions or insertions
    - Results in frameshift mutations, nonsense mutations, or splice site alterations
    - Protein may be truncated or absent
    - Less common are full-length proteins with missense mutations
  - Inactivating mutations impair conservative DNA repair and genomic stability functions
- Central portion of gene designated "ovarian cancer cluster region"

- Mutations in this region are 2x as likely to be associated with ovarian cancer as are mutations in 5′ or 3′ region
- Risk of breast cancer associated with mutation in this region is lower

Protein Function

- Central role in DNA repair, transcription, gametogenesis, and centrosome duplication
- Regulation of repair of DNA damage
  - Repair of DNA double-stranded breaks through homologous recombination

CLINICAL IMPLICATIONS AND ANCILLARY TESTS

Population to be Tested

- American Society of Clinical Oncology recommends that patients with > 10% mutation risk undergo testing
  - 85% of mutation carriers will be detected using this 10% cut-off
- National Institute for Health and Clinical Excellence in United Kingdom recommends testing individuals with > 20% mutation risk
- Counseling should occur before testing to ensure patients are aware of implications for themselves and their families

Clinical Criteria

- Personal history of breast cancer in women < 40 years of age
- Breast cancer in 1st-degree relatives (mother, sister, daughter)
  - Risk increased if cancer diagnosed at young age
  - Risk increased if individuals have multiple cancers
- Risk increased if a male with breast cancer is in the family
- Risk increased if ovarian cancers are also present in the family
- Risk increased if a relative has a known mutation

Calculating Risk

- There are multiple models to predict probability of an individual carrying a germline *BRCA2* or *BRCA2* mutation
  - Empiric models
    - Do not make assumptions about genetic risks (e.g., mutation frequency, mode of inheritance, penetrance)
    - Examples include Penn II model, Myriad II (Frank) model, and National Cancer Institute model
  - Genetic risk prediction models
    - Make assumptions about number of genes and allele frequencies
    - Include information about relationships among individuals in a kindred
    - Accuracy depends on validity of assumptions
    - Examples include BRCAPRO and the Breast and Ovarian Analysis of Disease Incidence and Carrier Estimation Algorithm (BOADICEA)
      - BRCAPRO available at http://www4.utsouthwestern.edu/breasthealth/cagene/
      - BOADICEA available at http://astor.som.jhmi.edu/BayesMendel/brcapro.html

Genetic Testing

- Full sequencing required to detect all mutations
- Additional testing required to detect large deletions and amplifications
  - 18% of genetic changes are not detected by standard testing
- All testing is performed by Myriad Genetics in USA
- Targeted mutation analysis may be population or family specific
  - Individuals of some ethnic backgrounds are at higher risk for certain mutations
  - Specific mutation may be sought if there is an affected relative with a known mutation

Interpretation of Results

- Mutation associated with breast cancer in other families
  - Patient classified as having BRCA2 syndrome
  - Testing of additional family members should be considered
- Mutation linked to a relative with breast cancer
  - Testing of additional individuals in family may be helpful to establish definite linkage
- Mutation known to be benign or have low clinical significance
  - Mutations that do not change amino acid type
  - Mutations known to occur in individuals without cancer
- Variant of uncertain significance (VUS)
  - Not yet linked to an individual with breast cancer
  - Detected in 7% of individuals (> 1,500 identified)
  - More frequent in populations of non-European ancestry

ASSOCIATED NEOPLASMS

Female Breast Cancer

- Risk
  - ~ 45% lifetime risk
    - Varies by mutation
    - May be modified by mutations in additional genes
- Histology
  - Moderately to poorly differentiated
  - No specific histologic type
    - Pushing margins
    - Lack of tubule formation
    - Some studies have suggested a higher incidence of tubulolobular and pleomorphic lobular carcinomas
    - Other series have not shown significant differences between *BRCA2* carcinomas and sporadic carcinomas
- Majority are positive for estrogen receptor
  - HER2 overexpression is rare (< 5%), lower than the incidence in sporadic breast cancer

- *TP53* mutations (30-65%) are less common than in *BRCA1*-associated cancers (> 90%)
- Majority classified as luminal B by gene expression profiling

Male Breast Cancer

- Risk
  - ~ 7% lifetime risk (compared to 0.07% in general population)
  - 8-16% of male breast cancers are in individuals with *BRCA2* mutations
    - 60-75% chance that *BRCA2* mutation exists in families with ≥ male with breast cancer
    - Association with *BRCA1* is less common (< 4% of all male breast cancers)

Ovarian, Fallopian Tube, and Peritoneal Carcinoma

- ~ 11-18% lifetime risk
  - Risk for ovarian cancer lower than that observed in *BRCA1* mutation carriers (40-50% lifetime risk)
- Age
  - Average onset is 55-58 years compared to 63 years in general population
  - Young women (< 40 years) with ovarian/tubal/peritoneal carcinoma are unlikely to have a *BRCA1* or *BRCA2* mutation
    - These women tend to have borderline tumors and cancers of more favorable histologic types
- Fallopian tube
  - Serous tubal intraepithelial carcinoma (80%) and endometrioid tubal carcinoma (20%) are found in ~ 5-7% of prophylactic salpingo-oophorectomies
    - 60-85% involve fimbriated end of fallopian tube
    - Entire tube should be examined microscopically
    - Immunohistochemical studies for p53 and MIB-1 (Ki-67) can be helpful
- Ovary
  - Carcinomas are usually high-grade serous carcinomas
    - Only ~ 2% of tumors are mucinous or borderline
    - Endometrioid, clear cell, and papillary carcinomas occur but are rare
- Primary peritoneal carcinoma
  - Women have ~ 4% risk after bilateral prophylactic salpingo-oophorectomy

Other Cancers

- Prostate: Relative risk is 4.6%
  - 1-2% of cancers diagnosed before age 65
  - Increased prostate cancer risk is not a consistent finding across all studies
- Pancreas, gall bladder, & bile duct: Relative risk is 3.5%
  - Presence of pancreatic cancer in a breast cancer family may be predictor of a *BRCA2* mutation
- Gastrointestinal
  - Stomach: Relative risk is 2.6%
  - As with *BRCA1*, initial reports of increased colon cancer risk have generally not been replicated

CANCER RISK MANAGEMENT

Chemoprevention

- Oral contraceptives
  - Reduces risk of ovarian cancer by 50%
  - Breast cancer risk may be increased by some types of oral contraceptives; results of studies have not been consistent
- Tamoxifen
  - Reduces risk
    - Evidence derives from observed 50% reduction in risk of contralateral cancer among mutation carriers treated with tamoxifen

Screening

- Mammography
  - Should begin at 10 years younger than youngest affected family member
  - May have limited sensitivity as young women often have dense breast tissue
- Magnetic resonance (MR) imaging
  - MR detects cancers due to blood flow and is more sensitive in detecting cancer in dense breasts
  - Highly sensitive but not very specific; false-positive results are frequent

Prophylactic Surgery

- Bilateral mastectomy reduces breast cancer risk by 97%
  - However, not all breast tissue can be removed and achieve acceptable cosmetic results
  - Greatest benefit for patients before a diagnosis of cancer
    - After cancer has been diagnosed, there may be no benefit if distant metastases are present
- Bilateral salpingo-oophorectomy reduces breast and ovarian cancer risk
  - Breast cancer reduced by 50%
    - Mechanism not well understood but may be due to decreased estrogen production
  - Ovarian and fallopian tube cancer reduced by 70-96%
    - There remains a 4% risk of papillary serous carcinoma of peritoneum

SELECTED REFERENCES

1. Fakkert IE et al: Breast cancer incidence after risk-reducing salpingo-oophorectomy in BRCA1 and BRCA2 mutation carriers. Cancer Prev Res (Phila). 5(11):1291-7, 2012
2. Iqbal J et al: The incidence of pancreatic cancer in BRCA1 and BRCA2 mutation carriers. Br J Cancer. 107(12):2005-9, 2012
3. Lynch HT et al: Hereditary breast cancer: practical pursuit for clinical translation. Ann Surg Oncol. 19(6):1723-31, 2012
4. Rhiem K et al: The risk of contralateral breast cancer in patients from BRCA1/2 negative high risk families as compared to patients from BRCA1 or BRCA2 positive families: a retrospective cohort study. Breast Cancer Res. 14(6):R156, 2012

BRCA2-Related Carcinomas

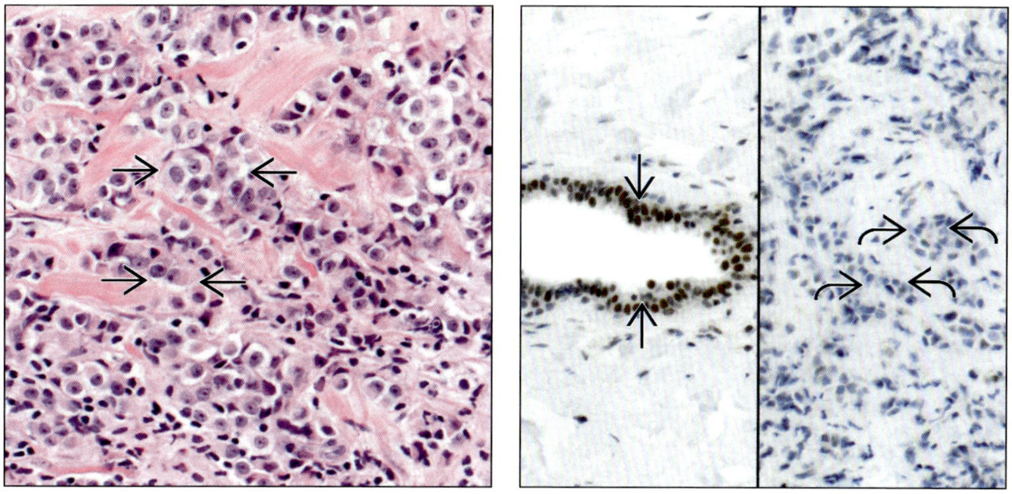

(Left) A 70-year-old man was discovered to be a carrier of a BRCA2 mutation after 2 of his daughters were diagnosed with ovarian cancer. He subsequently developed an invasive high-grade lobular carcinoma →. (Right) Tumors arising in BRCA2 mutation carriers exhibit allelic loss of the remaining wild-type BRCA2 gene in their cancer and possible loss of BRCA2 expression. The normal ducts show expression of BRCA2 protein by IHC → whereas the tumor has lost reactivity ↷.

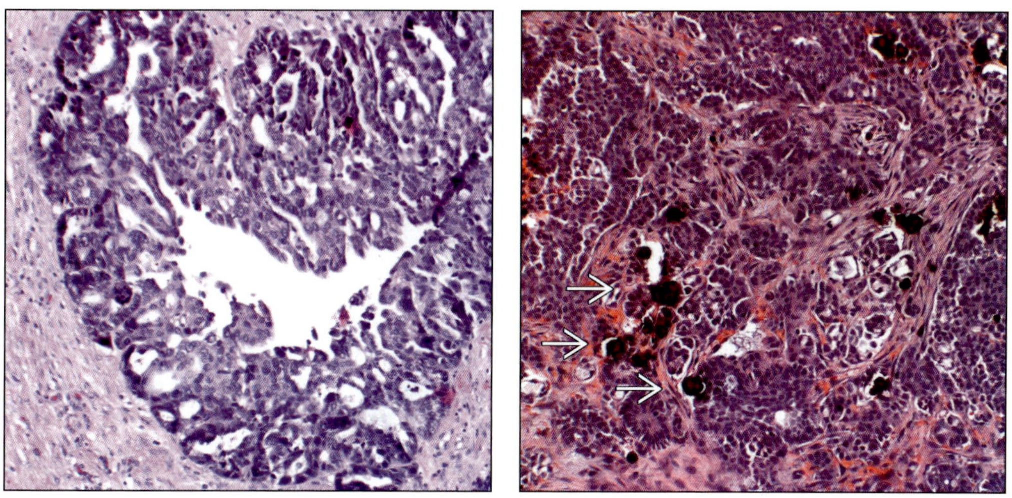

(Left) Germline BRCA2 mutations increase the risk of fallopian tube cancers. A high incidence of early neoplastic lesions are found at the fimbriated ends of the tubes. (Right) About 7% of ovarian carcinomas are due to BRCA2 mutations. The majority are high-grade serous carcinomas with psammoma body calcifications →. Other types such as endometrioid, clear cell, and papillary occur but are unusual. After oophorectomy, ~ 4% of women develop primary peritoneal carcinomas.

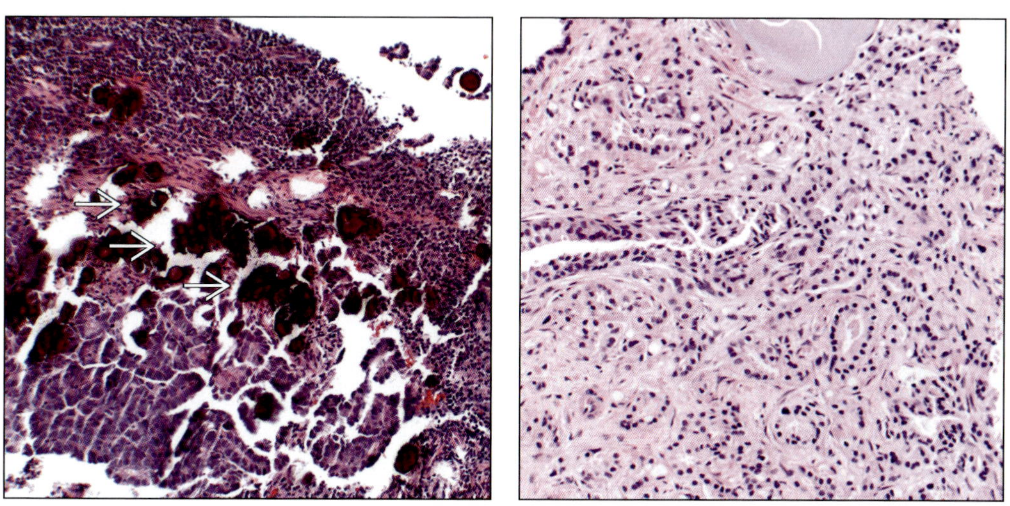

(Left) It may be difficult to distinguish metastases from primary carcinomas in women at high risk for both breast and ovarian cancers. In this core needle biopsy of a breast mass, the papillary architecture and psammoma bodies → favor metastatic ovarian serous carcinoma. A metastasis was confirmed by positivity for pax-8 and WT1. (Right) BRCA2 germline mutations also increase the risk of other types of cancers, such as early onset (before age 55) prostate cancer, as seen here.

HEREDITARY DIFFUSE GASTRIC CANCER

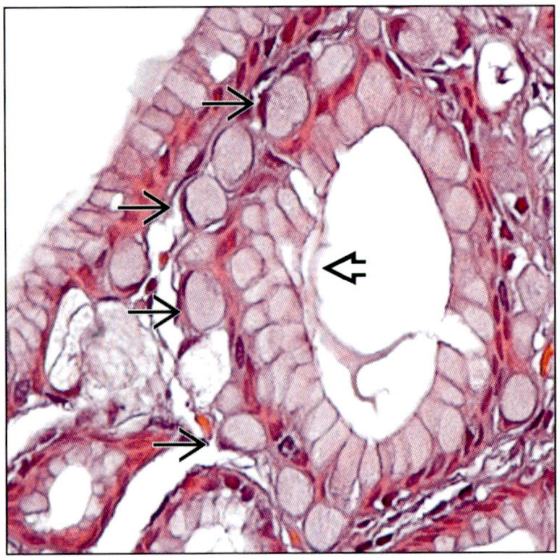

This high-power image shows signet ring cells ➙ surrounding a benign gastric gland ⇨. This signet ring cell carcinoma in situ is diagnostic of hereditary diffuse gastric cancer (HDGC). (Courtesy F. Carneiro, MD.)

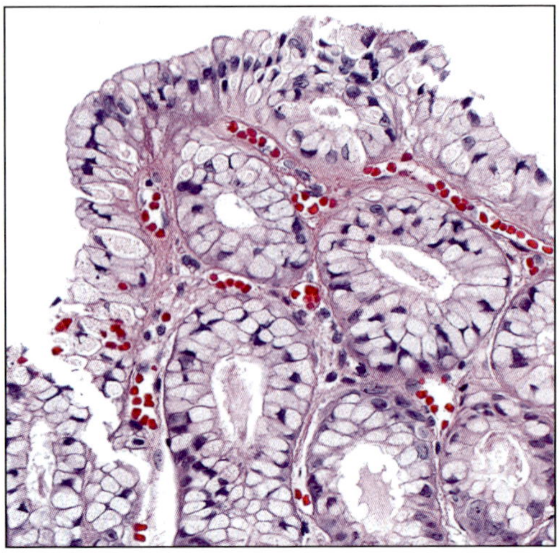

This high-power view shows disorganized gastric surface epithelium with vacuolated cells. This vacuolization is often seen in hereditary diffuse gastric cancer and has been called globoid change.

TERMINOLOGY

Abbreviations

- Hereditary diffuse gastric cancer (HDGC)

EPIDEMIOLOGY

Prevalence

- 10% of gastric cancers have familial clustering
  - Of these, 1-3% represent HDGC
- 1st described in Maori families from New Zealand, but syndrome is seen in all ethnic groups
  - Large clusters in New Zealand and Canada
  - Asian countries with high incidence of sporadic gastric carcinoma seem to have low incidence of HDGC
    - Reason for this is unknown

GENETICS

E-Cadherin/*CDH1* Gene

- Mutation in *CDH1* gene in 30-40% of patients who fit clinical definition of HDGC
  - Autosomal dominant
    - Cumulative risk of gastric cancer at age 80 years is 67% for men and 83% for women
    - Lifetime risk of lobular breast carcinoma in women is 39-60%
    - Increased risk of prostate cancer in men
    - Increased risk of signet ring cell colorectal cancer in both men and women
  - Cell-cell adhesion protein that acts as tumor suppressor gene
    - Mutations typically cause truncation of protein and loss of function
  - 2nd hit that inactivates good copy of the gene appears to be promoter methylation
    - May be important mechanism in sporadic diffuse gastric cancer
    - May be "drugable" target

MICROSCOPIC FINDINGS

Endoscopic Biopsies

- Classic lesion is the presence of signet ring cell carcinoma in situ
  - Signet ring cells within basement membrane of glands with pagetoid spread
  - May also see vacuolization of foveolar epithelium, called globoid change
    - Globoid change by itself is not specific for HDGC
- 1 study has shown that immunohistochemical staining for E-cadherin is negative in 77% of signet ring cell carcinoma foci in HDGC (some foci do stain positively)
- If unsure about pathology, best to have case reviewed by a pathologist who has experience with HDGC cases

Resection Specimens

- Multiple foci of signet ring cell carcinoma
  - Some studies suggest most tumors are found at antral transition zone; others refute this, finding most lesions in fundus and body
  - Some patients have hundreds of small in situ lesions whereas others have only 1 or 2
    - May need to take hundreds of sections to find small in situ lesions
    - May be easier to identify these subtle changes with PAS stain
    - There are documented cases of patients with *CDH1* mutations whose prophylactic gastrectomy specimen did not show any carcinoma despite totally embedding entire stomach

CLINICAL IMPLICATIONS AND ANCILLARY TESTS

Major Clinical Criteria

- 2 or more cases of gastric cancer in 1st- or 2nd-degree relatives with ≥ 1 diffuse gastric cancer in a patient < 50 years of age
- 3 or more cases of gastric cancer in 1st- or 2nd-degree relatives at any age with at least 1 documented case of diffuse gastric cancer
- Only 30-40% of cases that fulfill these 2 major criteria will have *CDH1* mutation, suggesting other genes may cause a similar syndrome

Minor or Additional Clinical Criteria

- Diffuse gastric cancer in patient < 40 years of age without family history
- Diffuse gastric cancer and lobular breast cancer in 1 patient, or 1 patient with diffuse gastric cancer and family member with lobular breast cancer or signet ring colon cancer
- Patients who fulfill these clinical criteria should undergo sequencing of their *CDH1* gene
  - Some variability among experts regarding these clinical criteria as some would test a single patient < 45 years with diffuse gastric cancer and no family history
  - > 100 mutations have been reported that lead to HDGC, so entire gene must be sequenced
  - ≥ 1 group of physicians recommends waiting until 16 years to test children of affected families

ASSOCIATED NEOPLASMS

Lobular Carcinoma of Breast

- Strong evidence that suggests association with HDGC

Signet Ring Cell Carcinoma of Colon

- Both sexes
- Uncommon tumor should raise question of Lynch syndrome or HDGC

Prostatic Adenocarcinoma

- Weak evidence that suggests association with HDGC
  - Likely unrelated given frequency of prostate cancer

CANCER RISK MANAGEMENT

Endoscopic Surveillance

- Early lesions are not evident endoscopically
  - Not very effective as number of biopsies needed to ensure adequate sampling is too high
    - 1 study found over 1,750 mucosal biopsies would be needed to have a 90% chance of finding an in situ lesion
  - Up to 25% of patients who test positive for *CDH1* mutation refuse gastrectomy
    - Offered endoscopy with biopsy every 6 months

Prophylactic Total Gastrectomy

- Treatment of choice to prevent gastric cancer
  - Procedure has low mortality rate but high morbidity
  - In New Zealand, recommended after age 20 in known carriers
    - Others recommend gastrectomy 5 years earlier than earliest known cancer in individual family
    - Risk of advanced disease is < 1% at age 20 years, 4% at age 30 years, but between 21% and 46% at age 50 years

SELECTED REFERENCES

1. Benusiglio PR et al: Cleft lip, cleft palate, hereditary diffuse gastric cancer and germline mutations in CDH1. Int J Cancer. 132(10):2470, 2013
2. Carneiro F: Hereditary gastric cancer. Pathologe. 33 Suppl 2:231-4, 2012
3. Fujita H et al: Endoscopic surveillance of patients with hereditary diffuse gastric cancer: biopsy recommendations after topographic distribution of cancer foci in a series of 10 CDH1-mutated gastrectomies. Am J Surg Pathol. 36(11):1709-17, 2012
4. Seevaratnam R et al: A systematic review of the indications for genetic testing and prophylactic gastrectomy among patients with hereditary diffuse gastric cancer. Gastric Cancer. 15 Suppl 1:S153-63, 2012
5. Mastoraki A et al: Prophylactic total gastrectomy for hereditary diffuse gastric cancer. Review of the literature. Surg Oncol. 20(4):e223-6, 2011
6. Pandalai PK et al: Prophylactic total gastrectomy for individuals with germline CDH1 mutation. Surgery. 149(3):347-55, 2011
7. Carneiro F et al: Pathology and genetics of familial gastric cancer. Int J Surg Pathol. 18(3 Suppl):33S-36S, 2010
8. Guilford P et al: Hereditary diffuse gastric cancer: translation of CDH1 germline mutations into clinical practice. Gastric Cancer. 13(1):1-10, 2010
9. Lee AF et al: Periodic acid-schiff is superior to hematoxylin and eosin for screening prophylactic gastrectomies from CDH1 mutation carriers. Am J Surg Pathol. 34(7):1007-13, 2010
10. Lynch HT et al: Hereditary diffuse gastric cancer: lifesaving total gastrectomy for CDH1 mutation carriers. J Med Genet. 47(7):433-5, 2010
11. Oliveira C et al: Hereditary gastric cancer. Best Pract Res Clin Gastroenterol. 23(2):147-57, 2009
12. Oliveira C et al: Quantification of epigenetic and genetic 2nd hits in CDH1 during hereditary diffuse gastric cancer syndrome progression. Gastroenterology. 136(7):2137-48, 2009
13. Barber ME et al: Histopathological and molecular analysis of gastrectomy specimens from hereditary diffuse gastric cancer patients has implications for endoscopic surveillance of individuals at risk. J Pathol. 216(3):286-94, 2008
14. Rogers WM et al: Risk-reducing total gastrectomy for germline mutations in E-cadherin (CDH1): pathologic findings with clinical implications. Am J Surg Pathol. 32(6):799-809, 2008
15. Masciari S et al: Germline E-cadherin mutations in familial lobular breast cancer. J Med Genet. 44(11):726-31, 2007

HEREDITARY HYPERPARATHYROIDISM-JAW TUMOR SYNDROME

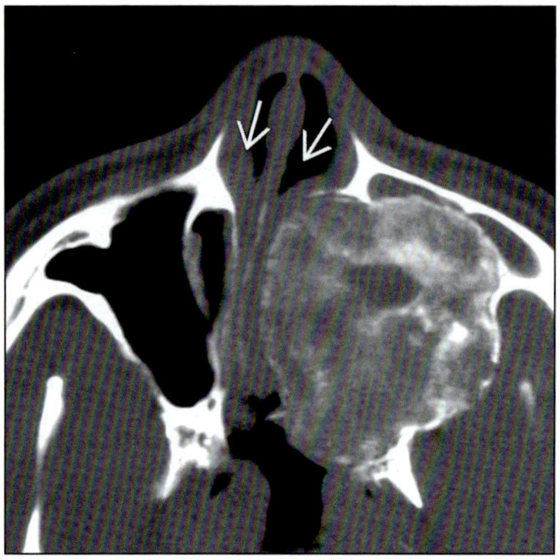

Axial bone CT shows a large, well-demarcated left maxillary ossifying fibroma with mixed calcific and soft tissue density components. Note that the mass obstructs both sides of the nose ➔.

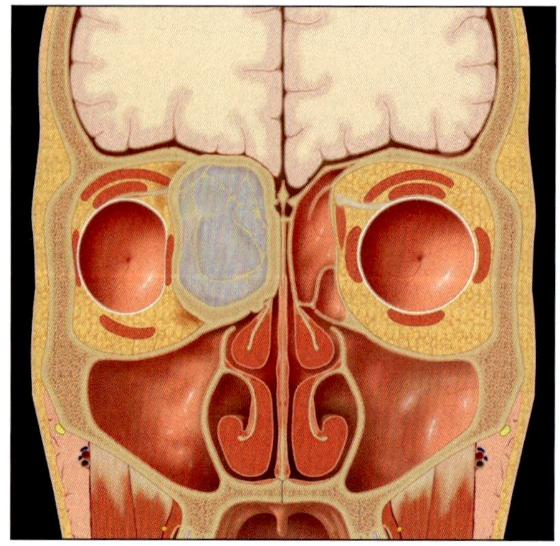

Nonossifying fibroma shows a large, well-demarcated maxillary mass with mixed calcification and fibrosis. Note that the mass obstructs 1 side of the nose and compresses the eye.

TERMINOLOGY

Abbreviations

- Hyperparathyroidism (HPT)
- Hyperparathyroidism-jaw tumor (HPT-JT) syndrome

Synonyms

- Familial isolated hyperparathyroidism (FI-HPT)
- Familial cystic parathyroid adenomatosis
- Familial primary hyperparathyroidism with multiple ossifying jaw fibromas

Definitions

- Autosomal dominant disorder characterized by parathyroid hyperplasia, adenoma, or carcinoma, ossifying fibromas of jaw bones, hamartomas, renal cysts, and tumors including Wilms tumor, resulting from inactivating mutations in *HRPT2* gene
  - 15% of HPT-JT develop parathyroid carcinoma

EPIDEMIOLOGY

Incidence

- Currently unknown
- 1st described in 1990; to date, ~ 40 affected families have been reported
- Primary hyperparathyroidism is a common endocrine syndrome, but > 90% are sporadic
- 10% of HPT are familial and include
  - HPT-JT
  - FI-HPT
  - Familial hypocalciuric hypercalcemia
  - Multiple endocrine neoplasia (MEN) syndromes

GENETICS

Molecular Genetics

- Most cases are due to inactivating mutation of *HRPT2* tumor suppressor gene on 1q25-q31
  - Germline inactivating mutation of *HRPT2* gene can be demonstrated in > 1/2 of cases
- Somatic mutation of *HRPT2* is uncommon in sporadic parathyroid adenomas
- In contrast, mutations of *HRPT2* are frequently seen in apparently sporadic cases of parathyroid carcinoma
  - Some 20% of patients with apparently sporadic parathyroid cancer may harbor germline *HRPT2* mutations, suggesting that such cases may in fact represent undiagnosed HPT-JT
  - Recent studies suggest that dysregulation of several microRNAs may contribute to the pathogenesis of parathyroid cancers harboring *HRPT2* mutation
- Germline *HRPT2* mutation is a rare cause of familial isolated primary hyperparathyroidism, but in some cases, genetic cause remains unknown
- *HRPT2* gene encodes the protein parafibromin, which consists of 531 amino acids and has weak homology to yeast protein Cdc73p
  - Mutations in *HRPT2* are scattered throughout coding region, and most are predicted to cause inactivation of protein product
  - Parafibromin is also thought to either promote or inhibit cell growth and proliferation depending on signals within cell
  - Parafibromin is found throughout the body and is likely involved in gene transcription
  - In human cell lines, endogenous parafibromin represses expression of *MYC* proto-oncogene
  - Parafibromin appears to be essential/vital for progression of mammalian embryonic development
  - Homozygous parafibromin null mice die in utero, and conditional knockout of parafibromin in adult mice results in cachexia and death

- Germline *HRPT2* inactivating mutation in HPT-JT syndrome-associated parathyroid adenoma or hyperplasia, and increased risk of parathyroid carcinoma
- Germline *HRPT2* mutations have been identified in subset of patients with mutation-positive carcinomas (consider genetic testing in patients with parathyroid carcinoma)
- Somatic *HRPT2* mutations common in sporadic parathyroid carcinomas and rare in sporadic adenomas

ETIOLOGY/PATHOGENESIS

Mutations of *HRPT2* Gene on 1q25-q31

- Mutations of the parafibromin gene *HRPT2* have been found in > 1/2 of families with HPT-JT
  - Encodes protein parafibromin
    - These mutations were predicted to inactivate parafibromin protein
- Germline *HRPT2* mutations have been identified in subset of patients with mutation-positive carcinomas thought to be sporadic
  - *HRPT2* gene was 1st implicated in development of sporadic parathyroid carcinoma

CLINICAL IMPLICATIONS AND ANCILLARY TESTS

Image Findings

- Ossifying fibroma
  - Radiography: Well-demarcated, expansile mass with central soft tissue density area surrounded by ossified rim
  - Bone scan: Increased uptake by affected bones

Clinical Presentation

- **Hyperparathyroidism**
  - Develops in late adolescence in 80% of patients
  - More aggressive course with severe hypercalcemia and higher incidence of parathyroid carcinoma
- **Jaw tumors**
  - Well-demarcated osseous lesion (ossifying fibroma) of mandible or maxilla
- Other features reported include renal cysts, Wilms tumor, and papillary thyroid carcinoma

Serologic Testing

- Blood test measuring ionized calcium and intact parathormone (iPTH)

Treatment

- **Medical therapy**
  - Calcimimetics are useful for patients with primary hyperparathyroidism who are poor surgical candidates or have nonlocalizable tumors or inoperable disease
- **Surgery**
  - Cornerstone of treatment for primary hyperparathyroidism
    - Surgical approach in HPT-JT is controversial because of increased risk of parathyroid cancer, but subtotal parathyroidectomy with close postoperative biochemical monitoring for recurrence is currently recommended over prophylactic total parathyroidectomy
    - Subtotal parathyroidectomy is indicated in familial syndromes such as MEN1 and familial isolated primary hyperparathyroidism (FIHP)
    - En bloc resection is recommended as primary treatment for parathyroid carcinoma
    - Bilateral neck exploration with excision of adenoma is classic approach, although minimally invasive surgery guided by noninvasive imaging and intraoperative PTH monitoring is gaining favor in nonfamilial cases

Prognosis

- Majority of patients with adenoma can be cured by surgery
- Guarded, once parathyroid carcinoma is confirmed

ASSOCIATED NEOPLASMS

Parathyroid

- Parathyroid involvement may include parathyroid hyperplasia, parathyroid adenomas, cystic parathyroid adenomas, and carcinomas
- **Hyperparathyroidism**
  - Familial disease usually involves multiple glands
  - **Hyperplasia**
    - Parathyroid hyperplasia may be chief cell or oxyphil cell hyperplasia
  - **Parathyroid adenomas** may be multiple
    - Familial cases with histopathological features similar to those observed in sporadic cases
    - Parathyroid adenomas affect 1 or more glands
    - Mean age at diagnosis is 32 years
  - **Parathyroid carcinoma**
    - Higher incidence of parathyroid carcinoma in HPT-JT
    - Parathyroid carcinoma is present in ~ 15% of families with HPT-JT
    - Invasive growth
    - Capsular invasion beyond thickened capsule
    - Thick fibrous bands present
    - Invasion of vessels outside thickened capsule and perineural invasion
    - Cellular monotony is common, but occasional tumors have pronounced pleomorphism
    - Macronucleoli
    - Increased Ki-67 proliferative index and mitosis
    - Presence of necrosis
    - Should always be considered when evaluating parathyroid pathology in patients with HPT-JT
- Familial disease is typically multigland whereas sporadic HPT tends to only affect 1 gland
- Parathyroid adenomas associated with HPT-JT syndrome are usually negative for immunoexpression of parafibromin

HEREDITARY HYPERPARATHYROIDISM-JAW TUMOR SYNDROME

- Lack of parafibromin staining offers promise as a marker of parathyroid malignancy

Ossifying Fibroma of Jaw

- Present in ~ 30% of affected family members
- Gross pathology shows classic appearance of tumor with central pink-yellow area of fibrous tissue surrounded by pale yellow, dense, peripheral ossified tissue
- Microscopically, tumor is densely cellular fibrous and ossifies beginning at periphery
- Tumor composed of dense, relatively avascular fibroblast-rich stroma and irregular spicules of woven bone with osteoblastic rimming
- No malignant predisposition

Renal Diseases

- Renal cysts
  - Multiple cysts
  - Polycystic renal disease
- Renal hamartomas
- Renal cortical adenomas
- Renal failure

Wilms Tumor

- Has occasionally been reported in families with HPT-JT, including occurrences in adults

Other Associated Malignant Neoplasms

- Papillary renal cell carcinoma
- Mixed epithelial stromal tumor of kidney
- Testicular germ cell tumor
- Prostate carcinoma
- Pancreatic carcinoma
- Thyroid carcinoma with oncocytic cells
- Uterine adenosarcoma

Other Associated Benign Diseases

- Benign uterine diseases
- Leiomyomas
- Adenomyosis
- Endometrial hyperplasia

CANCER RISK MANAGEMENT

Screening

- No definitive guidelines for surveillance
- Annual screening with serum calcium, phosphorus, and parathormone levels should begin at 10-12 years of age
- If test results are abnormal, imaging of parathyroid glands is indicated
- If HPT-JT is diagnosed, family members should undergo molecular testing and imaging studies
- Strong association with *HRPT2* mutation and familial and sporadic parathyroid cancer
- Screening for subclinical jaw lesions is indicated as an adjunct to determining who has inherited HPT-JT
- Subset of patients positive for somatic mutation of *HRPT2* were also positive for a germline mutation of the same gene
  - Suggests that a subset of patients with apparent sporadic carcinoma carried germline mutations of *HRPT2* and might have HPT-JT or a forme fruste of the syndrome
    - Patients with carcinoma, therefore, should have jaw and kidney imaging studies
- Baseline evaluation of renal function test with reassessment every 1-2 years is suggested
- Imaging evaluation of renal masses or cysts is suggested

SELECTED REFERENCES

1. Bricaire L et al: Frequent large germline HRPT2 deletions in a French National cohort of patients with primary hyperparathyroidism. J Clin Endocrinol Metab. 98(2):E403-8, 2013
2. Kutcher MR et al: Hyperparathyroidism-jaw tumor syndrome. Head Neck. 35(6):E175-7, 2013
3. Cavaco BM et al: Identification of de novo germline mutations in the HRPT2 gene in two apparently sporadic cases with challenging parathyroid tumor diagnoses. Endocr Pathol. 22(1):44-52, 2011
4. Cetani F et al: Molecular pathogenesis of primary hyperparathyroidism. J Endocrinol Invest. 34(7 Suppl):35-9, 2011
5. Frank-Raue K et al: [Hereditary variants of primary hyperparathyroidism--MEN1, MEN2, HPT-JT, FHH, FIHPT.] Dtsch Med Wochenschr. 136(38):1889-94, 2011
6. Frank-Raue K et al: CDC73-related hereditary hyperparathyroidism: five new mutations and the clinical spectrum. Eur J Endocrinol. 165(3):477-83, 2011
7. Pepe J et al: Sporadic and hereditary primary hyperparathyroidism. J Endocrinol Invest. 34(7 Suppl):40-4, 2011
8. Lin L et al: Nuclear localization of the parafibromin tumor suppressor protein implicated in the hyperparathyroidism-jaw tumor syndrome enhances its proapoptotic function. Mol Cancer Res. 5(2):183-93, 2007
9. Yamashita Y et al: A case of hyperparathyroidism-jaw tumour syndrome found in the treatment of an ossifying fibroma in the maxillary bone. Int J Oral Maxillofac Surg. 36(4):365-9, 2007
10. Gill AJ et al: Loss of nuclear expression of parafibromin distinguishes parathyroid carcinomas and hyperparathyroidism-jaw tumor (HPT-JT) syndrome-related adenomas from sporadic parathyroid adenomas and hyperplasias. Am J Surg Pathol. 30(9):1140-9, 2006
11. Howell VM et al: Rapid mutation screening for HRPT2 and MEN1 mutations associated with familial and sporadic primary hyperparathyroidism. J Mol Diagn. 8(5):559-66, 2006
12. Mizusawa N et al: Genetic analyses in patients with familial isolated hyperparathyroidism and hyperparathyroidism-jaw tumour syndrome. Clin Endocrinol (Oxf). 65(1):9-16, 2006
13. VanderWalde LH et al: Surgical approach to the patient with familial hyperparathyroidism. Curr Treat Options Oncol. 7(4):326-33, 2006

Gross and Microscopic Features

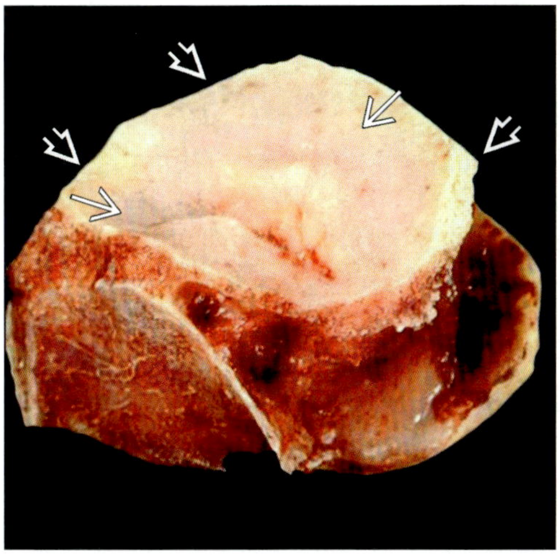

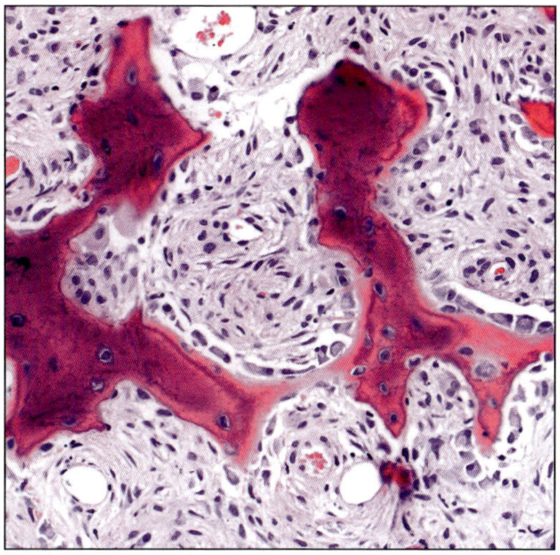

(Left) *Gross image shows the classic appearance of an ossifying fibroma with central pink-yellow area of fibrous tissue ➔ surrounded by pale yellow, dense, peripheral ossified tissue ➔.* ***(Right)*** *Typical ossifying fibroma exhibits a dense, avascular, fibroblast-rich stroma and irregular spicules of woven bone with osteoblastic rimming.*

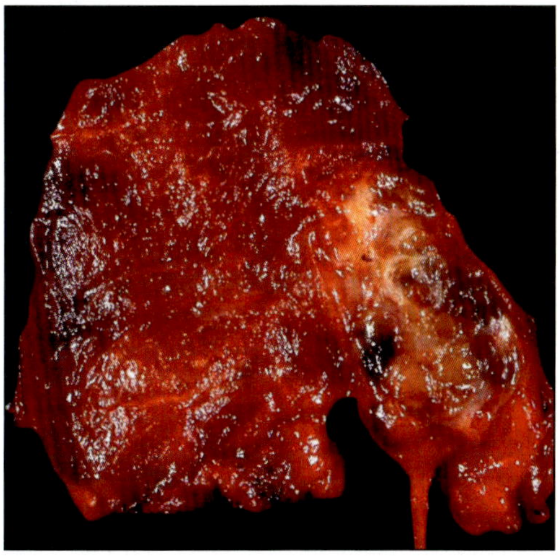

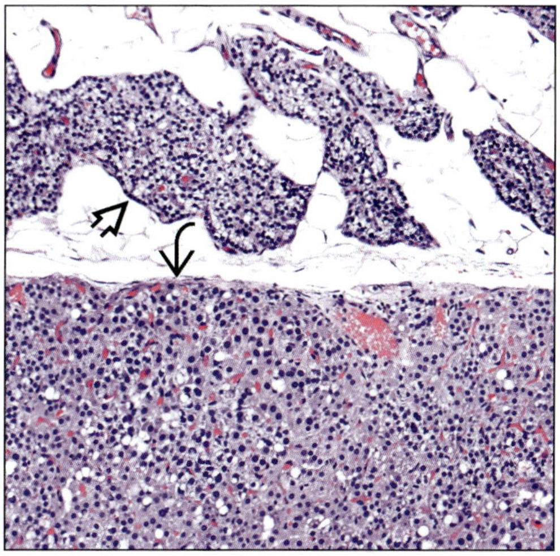

(Left) *Gross photograph shows a large parathyroid adenoma that had grown down into the mediastinum. Parathyroid carcinomas are generally larger than adenomas, but they can show overlap in size. Parathyroid carcinomas, unlike adenomas, show unequivocal invasion.* ***(Right)*** *Chief cell parathyroid adenoma ➔ shows a rim of normal parathyroid tissue ➔. Parathyroid adenomas are often composed of chief cells or mixtures of cell types, but can be composed of oncocytic or clear cells.*

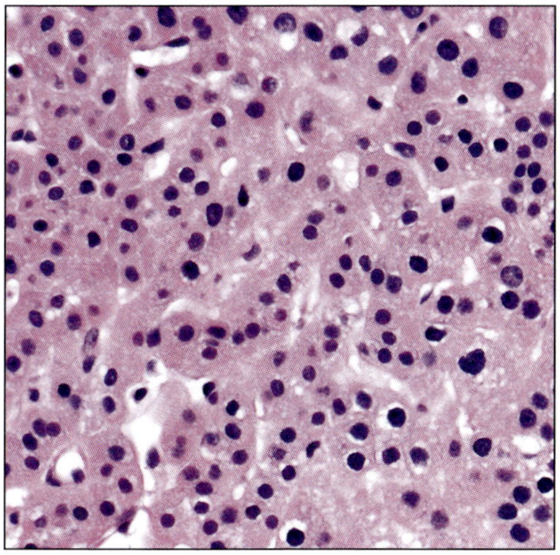

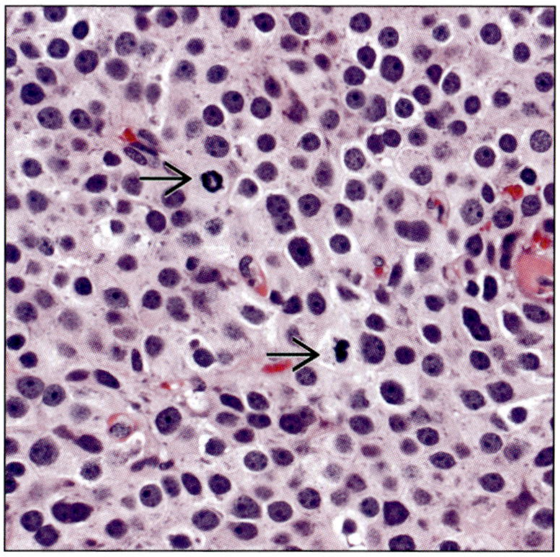

(Left) *Oxyphil cells (10-20 μm in diameter) are larger than chief cells (10 μm in diameter) and have abundant eosinophilic granular cytoplasm. Oxyphil cell adenomas comprise ~ 3-6% of parathyroid adenomas.* ***(Right)*** *Oxyphilic parathyroid carcinoma shows multiple mitotic figures ➔, which can be seen in both parathyroid adenomas and carcinomas but are more common in carcinomas.*

HEREDITARY LEIOMYOMATOSIS AND RENAL CELL CARCINOMA

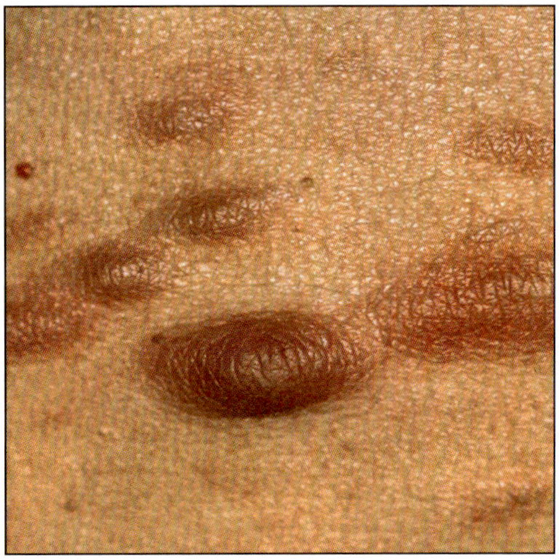

This photograph shows a cluster of leiomyomas in the skin. The nodules are reddish-brown and can be painful. Multiple cutaneous leiomyomas are the most prominent feature of HLRCC. (Courtesy C. Ko, MD.)

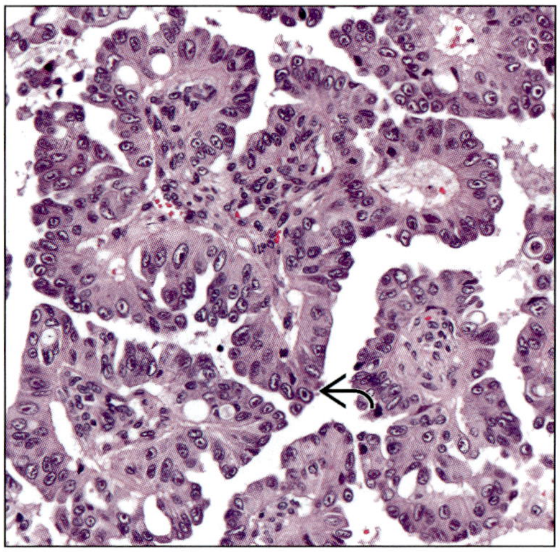

H&E shows RCC in HLRCC with papillary architecture. This RCC is characterized by high-grade nuclei with a large inclusion-like nucleolus ➔ producing a cytomegalovirus inclusion-like appearance.

TERMINOLOGY

Abbreviations

- Hereditary leiomyomatosis and renal cell carcinoma (HLRCC)

Synonyms

- Multiple cutaneous and uterine leiomyomatosis syndrome
- Reed syndrome

Definitions

- Autosomal inherited disorder characterized by development of multiple cutaneous and uterine smooth muscle tumors and renal cell carcinoma (RCC) linked to fumarate hydratase *(FH)* mutation

EPIDEMIOLOGY

Age Range

- Smooth muscle tumors and RCC develop at younger age in patients with HLRCC than in those with sporadic onset
  - Males: By age 35, nearly all will have cutaneous leiomyomas
  - Females: By age 45, risk for cutaneous leiomyomas is > 70%
    - Uterine leiomyomas: Mean age at diagnosis: 30 years (range: 18-53 years)
- Median age of patients with RCC: 42-44 years
  - Younger than in sporadic RCCs with papillary or tubulopapillary architectures

Gender

- Risk of disease is greater in men vs. women
  - However, number of cutaneous tumors is more numerous in women
  - Renal tumor: M:F = 1.1:1

Incidence

- Rare; *FH* mutation predisposing to HLRCC has been described in ~ 180 families worldwide

CLINICAL IMPLICATIONS

Clinical Presentation

- Most patients initially present with multiple skin lesions due to smooth muscle tumors
  - Usually multiple, involving limbs and trunk
  - Sometimes itchy, painful; can be disfiguring
- Gynecologic symptoms at reproductive age due to uterine smooth muscle tumors
  - Metrorrhagia, menorrhagia, pelvic pain, and fertility problems

GENETICS

FH Mutation

- FH in chromosome 1q42-1q44
- Mutation found in 76-100% of families with clinical manifestation of HLRCC
- Heterozygous germline mutation
  - Majority are missense (~ 58%); nonsense (~ 11%) or frameshift (~ 18%) mutations
  - Splice site mutations, in-frame deletions or insertions, exon 7 duplications, exon 1 deletions, and whole gene deletion also reported
- Mutations of 2 alleles seen in associated tumors ("2-hit" hypothesis)
  - *FH* suggested as a tumor suppressor gene
- > 100 different *FH* germline mutations have been reported
- *FH* gene encodes an enzyme in Krebs cycle that catalyzes hydration of fumarate to L-malate
  - Mutation causes accumulation of fumarate and succinate

- Mutation causes aberrant stabilization and overexpression of hypoxia inducible factor 1 (HIF1) transcription factor
  - HIF1 regulates transcription of genes important for vascularization, glucose transport, and glycolysis, all of which are important for tumor growth
  - Somewhat similar mechanism with inactivation of *VHL* in hereditary clear cell RCC, which causes nondegradation and accumulation of HIF1
- Unrelated biallelic mutations of *FH* result in **fumarate hydratase (FH) deficiency (fumaric aciduria)**
  - Rare recessive syndrome with severe neurological symptoms, muscle hypotonia, and microcephaly
  - Marked decrease in FH activity results in metabolic crises and infant death
  - Symptoms not seen in HLRCC
  - Unclear why manifestations are completely different

Comparative Genomic Hybridization

- 27% of HLRCC renal tumors show gains in Chr 2, 7, and 17 and losses in 13q12.3-q21.1, 14, 18, and X
  - Gains in Chr 7 and 17 are common in sporadic papillary renal cell carcinoma

CLINICAL IMPLICATIONS AND ANCILLARY TESTS

FH Mutation Testing

- Usually by direct sequencing of *FH* coding region
  - Reveals genetic alterations in ~ 90% of families suspected for HLRCC
- If clinically highly suspicious and initial test is negative, additional methods such as multiplex ligation probe amplification (MLPA) are recommended

ASSOCIATED NEOPLASMS

Smooth Muscle Tumors

- **Cutaneous leiomyomas (piloleiomyomas)**
  - With age, eventually up to 100% of men and 80% of women will develop them
  - Originate from hair follicle arrector pili muscles
  - Size range: 2 mm to 4 cm
  - Vast majority are benign, with rare reports of leiomyosarcoma
  - Histologic hallmark of inclusion-like orangeophilic nucleolus with perinuclear clearing
- **Uterine smooth muscle tumors**
  - With age, up to 77% of women will develop uterine leiomyomas
  - Usually multiple (up to 20)
  - Size range: 1-8.5 cm
  - Grossly shows firm, solid, white-tan, whorled cut surface; similar in appearance to sporadic tumors
  - Mostly benign (leiomyomas)
    - Fascicles of spindle cells with elongated, blunt-edged nuclei
    - Can show increased atypia, multinucleation, &/or mitotic activity (up to 6 per HPF)
    - Histologic hallmark of nuclei with inclusion-like orangeophilic nucleolus with perinuclear clearing
  - Uterine leiomyosarcomas have been reported in 6 cases from HLRCC families

RCC

- Risk of developing RCC is lower and often manifests later than smooth muscle tumors
  - Seen in ~ 20-25% of *FH* mutation-positive families
- 6.5x greater risk than general population; higher in younger patients
  - Risk is 230x greater in patients 15-29 years old and 45x increase in patients 30-44 years old
  - Youngest patient reported was 11 years old
- When symptomatic, patients with renal tumor present with back pain, fatigue, and weight loss; discovery after work-up for suspicion of HLRCC after cutaneous lesion manifestation is not uncommon
- Usually involves 1 person in *FH* mutation-positive family
- **Macroscopy**
  - Tumors are predominantly unilateral and solitary, unlike other RCCs in hereditary setting
- **Microscopy**
  - Most RCCs in HLRCC were previously classified as papillary RCC (PRCC) type 2 and collecting duct carcinoma (CDC) but now considered as a different type of RCC
  - Exhibit features different from papillary RCC and CDC; possibly a distinct subtype of RCC
    - Variable architecture that includes papillary (most common), tubulopapillary, tubular, solid, and mixed
    - Papillae are thick with abundant collagen
    - Cells are large, high grade with abundant eosinophilic cytoplasm
    - Nuclei pseudostratification is common and may resemble rosettes
    - Mitoses common (2-6/10 HPF)
    - May have focal clear cell area
    - Histologic hallmark of nuclei with inclusion-like orangeophilic nucleolus with perinuclear clearing, resembling cytomegalovirus cytopathic change
    - Nuclear features are widespread, detected in almost all cells, including in foci of clear cells if present
  - Mucicarmine stain is negative for mucin, unlike in CDC
- Immunohistochemistry
  - CK7(-), unlike in PRCC
  - CD10(-), CK20(-), and TFE3(-)
  - HMWK (34bE12)(-), unlike in CDC
- Aggressive, most present with higher stage (≥ pT3a)
  - Frequent metastasis to lymph nodes and involvement of adrenal glands
  - Most aggressive RCC among hereditary renal tumors
- Rare reports of concurrent clear cell RCC in bilateral cases; unclear if associated or incidental

Other Tumors

- Rarely reported

HEREDITARY LEIOMYOMATOSIS AND RENAL CELL CARCINOMA

Lehtonen Modified Criteria for Diagnosis of HLRCC	
Major Criterion	**Minor Criteria**
Presence of multiple cutaneous leiomyomas (histopathologically confirmed) indicates high likelihood of HLRCC	HLRCC can be suspected when an individual meets ≥ 2 of the following criteria
	Surgical treatment of severely symptomatic uterine leiomyomas before age 40
	Type 2 papillary or collecting duct renal cell carcinoma before age 40
	1st-degree family member who meets criteria for number 1 or 2
	Occurrence of severely symptomatic uterine leiomyomas before age 40 in 2nd-degree paternal family members may also be relevant

- Adrenal gland adenomas, breast tumor, bladder tumor, brain tumor, lymphoid malignancy, basal cell carcinomas, thyroid tumors, ovarian cystadenomas

CANCER RISK MANAGEMENT

Diagnosis

- Proposed practical criteria for diagnosis
- If clinical features are suggestive, genetic counseling and molecular testing should be performed for
  - Individual with multiple cutaneous leiomyomas, ≥ 1 histologically confirmed
  - Individual with leiomyoma and family history of HLRCC
  - Individual with ≥ 1 tubulopapillary RCCs showing large inclusion-like nucleolus and perinucleolar clearing
- All family members of a person with germline *FH* mutation should be tested

Surveillance

- Currently, no consensus
  - Lifelong clinical surveillance warranted in individuals who are at risk
  - No established standard for age of surveillance for RCC, but ideally should start at earliest age due to aggressive nature
    - For renal tumors, baseline renal ultrasound and abdominal CT scan with contrast or MR at age 20 years, then annual MR or semiannual ultrasound
    - For uterine tumors, annual gynecologic ultrasound at age 20 years
    - Dermatologic examination for lesions suspicious for cutaneous leiomyomas

Treatment

- Smooth muscle tumors
  - Surgical excision for solitary skin tumors
  - Myomectomy desired for smaller uterine tumors to retain fertility
- Renal cell carcinomas
  - Radical surgery preferred, even if small in size because of its aggressive nature
    - This approach is in contrast to renal tumors in other hereditary settings that are usually observed until a certain size is reached
  - Chemotherapy using inhibitors for HIF1-activated targets is being tried
    - LDHA inhibition has been shown to cause increase apoptosis in FH-deficient cells in xenograft mouse model, suggesting a possible therapeutic strategy

SELECTED REFERENCES

1. Sanz-Ortega J et al: Morphologic and molecular characteristics of uterine leiomyomas in hereditary leiomyomatosis and renal cancer (HLRCC) syndrome. Am J Surg Pathol. 37(1):74-80, 2013
2. Tolvanen J et al: Strong family history of uterine leiomyomatosis warrants fumarate hydratase mutation screening. Hum Reprod. 27(6):1865-9, 2012
3. Gardie B et al: Novel FH mutations in families with hereditary leiomyomatosis and renal cell cancer (HLRCC) and patients with isolated type 2 papillary renal cell carcinoma. J Med Genet. 48(4):226-34, 2011
4. Garg K et al: Morphologic features of uterine leiomyomas associated with hereditary leiomyomatosis and renal cell carcinoma syndrome: a case report. Am J Surg Pathol. 35(8):1235-7, 2011
5. Lehtonen HJ: Hereditary leiomyomatosis and renal cell cancer: update on clinical and molecular characteristics. Fam Cancer. 10(2):397-411, 2011
6. Smit DL et al: Hereditary leiomyomatosis and renal cell cancer in families referred for fumarate hydratase germline mutation analysis. Clin Genet. 79(1):49-59, 2011
7. Alrashdi I et al: Hereditary leiomyomatosis and renal cell carcinoma: very early diagnosis of renal cancer in a paediatric patient. Fam Cancer. 9(2):239-43, 2010
8. Ashrafian H et al: Expression profiling in progressive stages of fumarate-hydratase deficiency: the contribution of metabolic changes to tumorigenesis. Cancer Res. 70(22):9153-65, 2010
9. Koski TA et al: Array comparative genomic hybridization identifies a distinct DNA copy number profile in renal cell cancer associated with hereditary leiomyomatosis and renal cell cancer. Genes Chromosomes Cancer. 48(7):544-51, 2009
10. Lehtonen HJ et al: Conventional renal cancer in a patient with fumarate hydratase mutation. Hum Pathol. 38(5):793-6, 2007
11. Merino MJ et al: The morphologic spectrum of kidney tumors in hereditary leiomyomatosis and renal cell carcinoma (HLRCC) syndrome. Am J Surg Pathol. 31(10):1578-85, 2007
12. Sudarshan S et al: HIF and fumarate hydratase in renal cancer. Br J Cancer. 96(3):403-7, 2007
13. Wei MH et al: Novel mutations in FH and expansion of the spectrum of phenotypes expressed in families with hereditary leiomyomatosis and renal cell cancer. J Med Genet. 43(1):18-27, 2006

Tumors in HLRCC

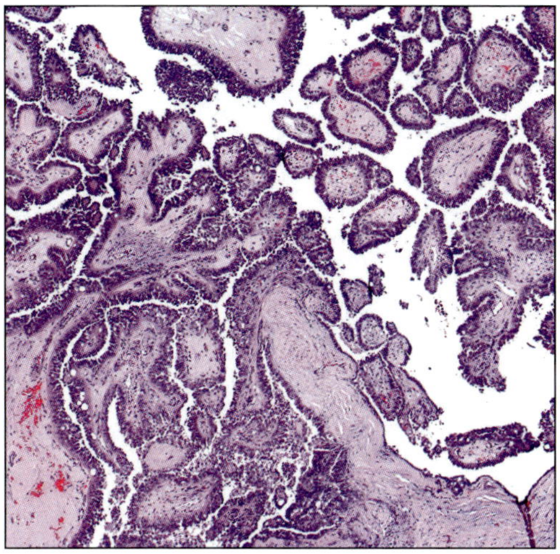

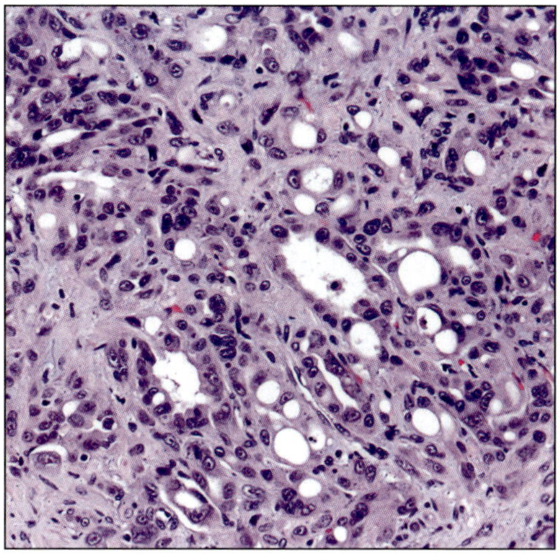

(Left) *Low-power view shows RCC in HLRCC with predominant papillary architecture. These RCCs were previously classified as papillary RCC type 2 (eosinophilic type) or collecting duct carcinoma and are now considered to be distinct. The neoplastic papillae have thick stalks and are lined by stratified high-grade tumor cells with eosinophilic cytoplasm.* ***(Right)*** *H&E shows RCC in HLRCC exhibiting tubular growth. The cells in the tubules and papillae have similar cytologic features.*

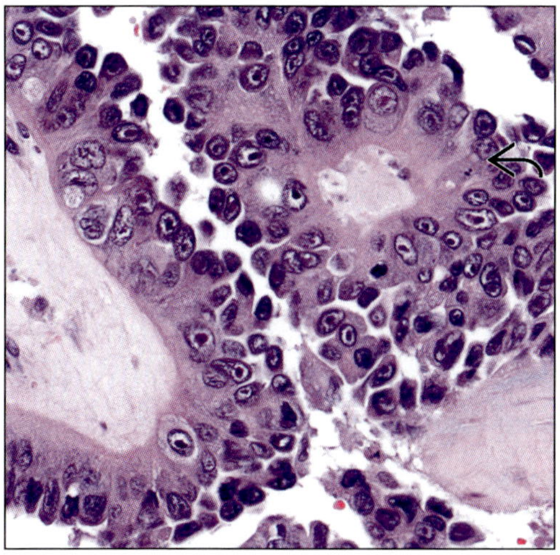

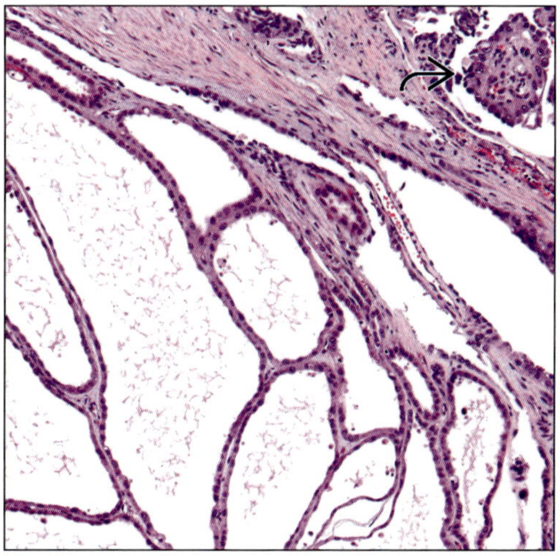

(Left) *Hallmark of RCC is the presence of large nuclei with inclusion-like orangeophilic nucleolus and perinucleolar clearing, resembling cytomegalovirus cytopathic change. This feature is seen diffusely in the tumor. Nuclear stratification is common, and nuclei may form pseudorosettes ⮫.* ***(Right)*** *Low-power view shows RCC in HLRCC with focal tubulocystic area adjacent to a papillary structure ⮫. Both papillae and tubulocystic areas exhibit similar characteristic nuclear features.*

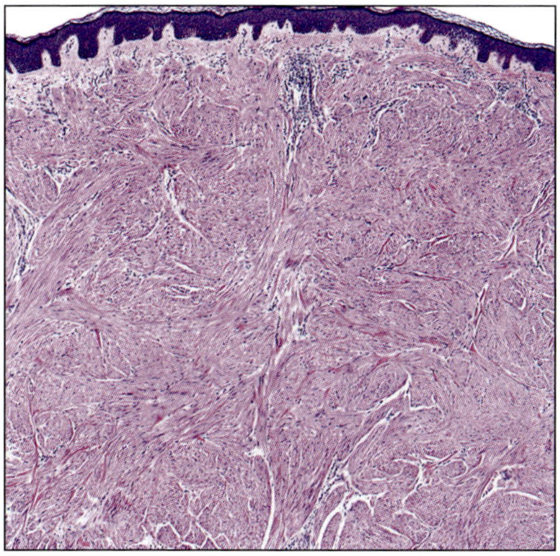

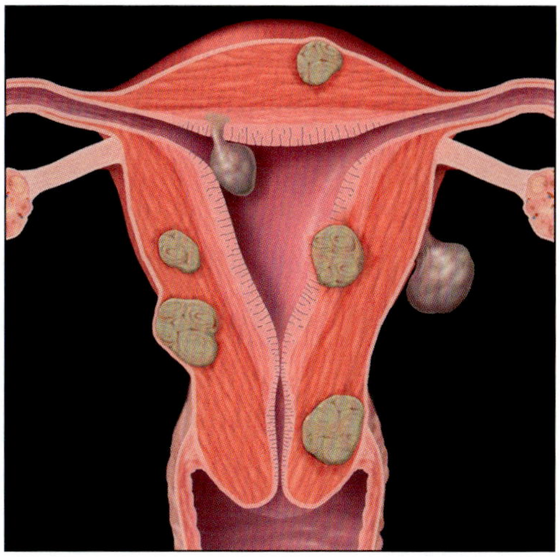

(Left) *H&E shows cutaneous leiomyoma consisting of fascicles of smooth muscle cells. These lesions are thought to arise from pili erector muscle of the skin. Eventually, up to 100% of men and 80% of women with HLRCC will develop cutaneous leiomyomas. (Courtesy C. Ko, MD.)* ***(Right)*** *Graphic image shows uterus in HLRCC with leiomyomas at submucosal, intramural, and subserosal sites. HLRCC patients are at high risk for early onset, multiple, atypical, &/or cellular leiomyomas.*

HEREDITARY MULTIPLE EXOSTOSIS

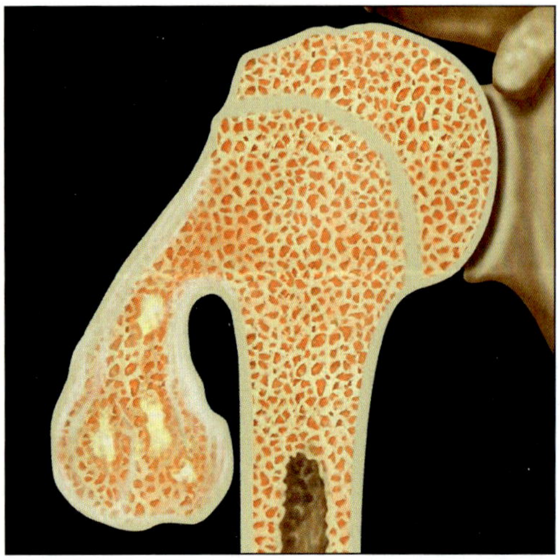

Osteochondroma arising from the proximal femur is shown. The osteochondromas grow in a direction away from the joint. The cartilaginous cap is irregular with areas of thick cartilage alternating with thinner areas.

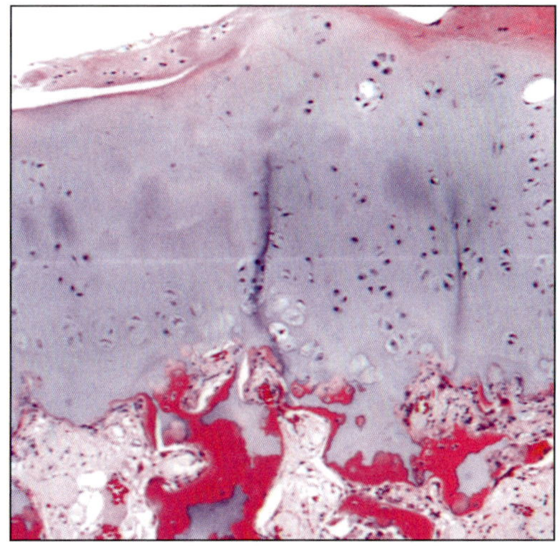

The cartilaginous cap of osteochondromas is composed of hyaline cartilage with cellularity comparable with an actively growing skeleton. The cartilage undergoes endochondral ossification.

TERMINOLOGY

Abbreviations

- Hereditary multiple exostosis (HME)
- Multiple hereditary osteochondromatosis (MHO)

Synonyms

- Multiple cartilaginous exostoses

Definitions

- HME is characterized by multiple exostoses
- Autosomal dominant condition caused by mutations in 1 of the *EXT* genes
- ≥ 2 osteochondromas of juxtaepiphyseal region of long bones are required for diagnosis

EPIDEMIOLOGY

Age Range

- Median age at diagnosis is 3 years
- Nearly all affected individuals are identified by age 12
- Most patients are in their 2nd decade of life at time of diagnosis

Site

- Typically arises in appendicular skeleton
  - Distal femur, proximal tibia, proximal humerus
- Can involve flat bones, such as ilium and scapula

Gender

- Male predominance

Incidence

- Prevalence ranges from 0.9 to 2 per 100,000 live births
- Sporadic osteochondromas are ≥ 6x more common than MHO

ETIOLOGY/PATHOGENESIS

Histogenesis

- Mutation in 1 of the *EXT* genes detected in 85-90% of cases
- *EXT1* (8q24.11-q24.13)
  - > 80 different mutations in *EXT1*
  - Accounts for 50-76% of families with hereditary multiple exostosis
- *EXT2* (11p11-p12)
  - 21-50% of families have mutation in *EXT2*
- *EXT3* (19p)
  - Rare
- De novo mutations
  - In ~ 10% of affected individuals

Molecular Genetics

- Germline alterations in *EXT1* (located at 8q24) and *EXT2* (located at 11p11-p12) are involved in hereditary multiple osteochondromas
  - Loss of wild-type alleles has been reported in MHO and rare cases of sporadic osteochondroma
- Most of these mutations are predicted to result in truncated or nonfunctional protein
- No definitive proof of linkage to *EXT3* gene (located on 19p)
- Contiguous gene deletion syndromes
  - Deletion of *EXT1* and *TRPS1* genes: Langer-Giedion syndrome
    - Multiple osteochondromas with craniofacial dysmorphism and mental retardation
  - Deletion of *EXT2* and *ALX4*: Potocki-Shaffer syndrome
    - Multiple osteochondromas, enlarged parietal foramina, craniofacial dysostosis, and mental retardation
- Function of gene products of *EXT1* and *EXT2*

- Proteins exostosin-1 (*EXT1* gene) and exostosin-2 (*EXT2* gene) are localized to endoplasmic reticulum and catalyze heparan sulphate polymerization
  - These 2 proteins are hypothesized to be essential for fibroblast growth factor and Indian hedgehog signaling within normal growth plate

CLINICAL IMPLICATIONS

Clinical Presentation

- HME is characterized by multiple osteochondromas near diaphyses of the extremities, ribs, scapulae that undergo ossification
- Disorder can be associated with mild short stature
- HME can be diagnosed at birth
- 60% have positive family history of multiple osteochondromas
- Multiple slowly enlarging firm lesions present for many years
- Arises from surface of bone

Diagnosis

- Presence of multiple exostoses in an individual (average: 6)
- *EXT1* phenotype is more severe than that associated with *EXT2*
  - Patients with *EXT1* mutations have more exostoses, more limb malalignment, and more pelvic and flat bone involvement than *EXT2* mutations
- Family history

Prognosis

- Malignant transformation of osteochondroma to chondrosarcoma occurs in 0.5-5% of MHO patients
  - Rarely, osteosarcoma and dedifferentiated chondrosarcoma have also been reported
- Patients may show deformities of forearm, inequality in limb length, varus or valgus angulation of knee, deformity of ankle, and disproportionate short stature

Associated Malignant and Benign Neoplasms

- < 5% malignant transformation to chondrosarcoma or other sarcomas
  - Chondrosarcoma has predilection for proximal femur or axial skeleton
    - Seldom occurs before age 10 and rare after 50
- Osteochondromas and multiple exostosis

Cancer Risk Management

- Treated successfully with low morbidity
- Baseline radiographs of pelvis and shoulder

MACROSCOPIC FINDINGS

General Features

- Generally similar to sporadic osteochondroma
- Arises from surface of bone
- Outer layer consists of thin sheath of fibrous tissue that overlies pearly gray-white cartilaginous cap
  - Cartilaginous cap is of varying thickness
  - Ranging from < 2.5 to several cm in depth
  - Base of cartilage cap undergoes enchondral ossification and merges with areas that have appearance of cancellous bone

MICROSCOPIC FINDINGS

General Features

- Overall architecture recapitulates that of disorganized growth plate
- Chondrocytes exhibit minimal cytologic atypia and no mitotic activity
- Peripheral cap of hyaline cartilage
  - Cellularity of cartilage decreases from deep to superficial layer
  - Chondrocytes are arranged in vague columns
- Newly formed trabeculae at base of cartilage mimics primary spongiosa of normal growth plate

SELECTED REFERENCES

1. Huegel J et al: Perichondrium phenotype and border function are regulated by Ext1 and heparan sulfate in developing long bones: a mechanism likely deranged in Hereditary Multiple Exostoses. Dev Biol. 377(1):100-12, 2013

IMAGE GALLERY

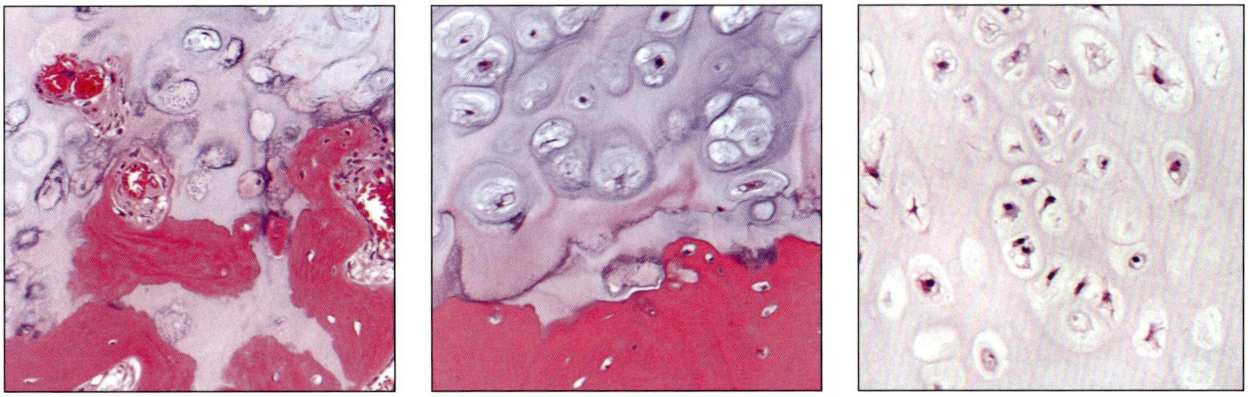

*(**Left**) The overall architecture of an osteochondroma recapitulates that of a disorganized growth plate. The cartilage undergoes endochondral ossification. (**Center**) The cartilaginous cap of an osteochondroma is composed of hyaline cartilage. The cellularity of cartilage decreases from deep to superficial layer. (**Right**) The columns of chondrocytes mimic the zone of hypertrophy of the growth plate.*

HEREDITARY CUTANEOUS MELANOMA

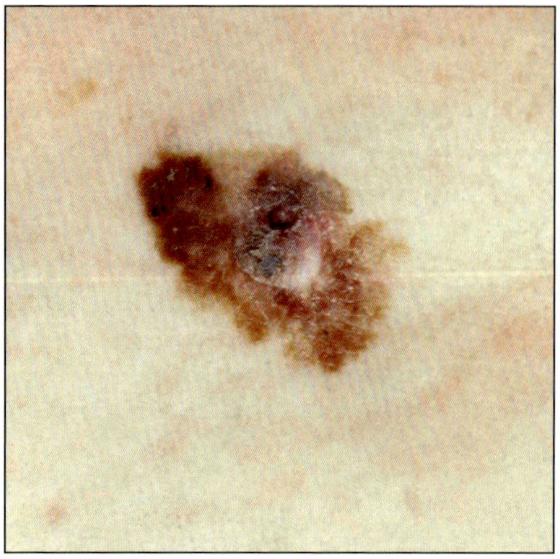

Clinical photograph shows a large melanoma with variegated color, jagged border, and irregular surface, all of which are concerning clinical signs. (Courtesy J. Hall, MD.)

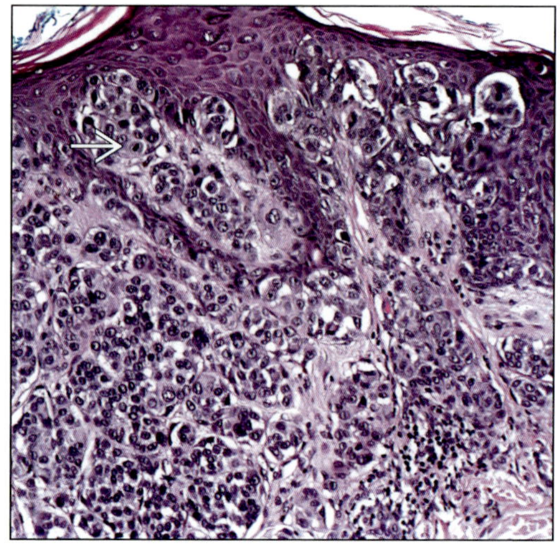

This melanoma from the back of a 16-year-old girl is composed of atypical epithelioid cells with several mitotic figures ➡. (Courtesy C. Cockerell, MD.)

TERMINOLOGY

Definition of Hereditary Cutaneous Melanoma

- ≥ 3 blood relatives with cutaneous melanoma in areas with high sun exposure
- ≥ 2 blood relatives with cutaneous melanoma in areas with low sun exposure

EPIDEMIOLOGY

Incidence of Hereditary Cutaneous Melanoma

- 5-7% of cutaneous melanoma patients are from high-risk families
  - In individuals with multiple relatives with cutaneous melanoma
    - Percentage increases to ~ 54%
  - In individuals with multiple primary cutaneous melanomas
    - Percentage increases to ~ 15%

Hereditary vs. Sporadic Cutaneous Melanoma

- Most cutaneous melanoma is sporadic
  - Likely secondary to somatic mutations
    - May be induced by ultraviolet light, especially with intermittent sun exposure and sunburn
- Up to 10% of cases of cutaneous melanoma
  - Secondary to germline mutations
  - Mutations are currently detectable in up to 40% of families with suspected hereditary cutaneous melanoma

Age

- Mean age at presentation with cutaneous melanoma: 34 years

GENETICS

CDKN2A Mutations (Tumor Suppressor Gene on 9p21)

- In 20-40% of cutaneous melanoma kindreds; present in 0.2-2% of all cutaneous melanoma patients
  - Melanoma penetrance
    - 30% by age 50 years
    - 67% by age 80 years
  - Lifetime risk of cutaneous melanoma
    - 53% in Europe
    - 75% in United States
    - 91% in Australia
- Risk of *CDKN2A* mutation carriage
  - ~ 50% risk if relative with known *CDKN2A* mutation
  - 50% risk if 3 or more relatives with cutaneous melanoma
  - 45% risk if 1 relative with multiple cutaneous melanomas
  - 20-45% risk if 2 or more relatives with cutaneous melanoma
  - 10-20% risk if multiple primary cutaneous melanomas and no family history of cutaneous melanoma
  - ~ 20% risk if affected by cutaneous melanoma and pancreatic cancer
  - < 1% if early onset of 1 cutaneous melanoma
- Mutations are generally inactivating
  - Often missense leading to loss of function of p16INK4A
  - Sometimes affect both p16INK4A and p14ARF
  - Less commonly, deletions, insertions, and splice site mutations affect p14ARF alone
- Gene transcripts of *CDKN2A*
  - p16INK4A
    - Part of retinoblastoma pathway
    - Physiologic targets include CDK4 and CDK6

- Thought to cause senescence in melanocytes and melanocytic nevi
- p14ARF
  - Part of p53 pathway
  - Function is to block HDM2-mediated degradation of p53

Linkage to 1p36 and 1p22

- 1p36
  - Multiple cutaneous melanomas and dysplastic nevi may be seen

CDK4 Mutations (Oncogene on 12q14)

- CDK4 functions in retinoblastoma pathway
- Mutations in exon 2, codon 24 disrupts binding to p16INK4A

BAP1 Mutations

- Associated with ocular melanoma
- Rarely, kindreds with ocular melanoma also have increased risk of cutaneous melanoma
- Unusually, may be seen in hereditary cutaneous melanoma kindreds
- Cutaneous melanomas
  - Uniquely nevoid

Genes With Low Associated Risk of Cutaneous Melanoma

- *MC1R* (melanocortin-1 receptor gene)
  - Risk of cutaneous melanoma
    - Increased 2-4x
  - Can alter risk of cutaneous melanoma for *CDKN2A* mutation carriers
  - Associated with red hair, Fitzpatrick skin type I, freckling
  - Associated with *BRAF*-mutant cutaneous melanomas
- Other genes with low associated risk of cutaneous melanoma
  - Many of these genes found in genome-wide association studies
  - Examples include
    - *OCA2, TYR, TYRP1, TPCN2, ASIP, GSTM1, VDR*
- Genes associated with other hereditary syndromes, with slightly increased risk of cutaneous melanoma
  - *BRCA1, BRCA2*
  - *P53*
  - *RB1*
  - *WRN*
  - *PTEN*

Inheritance

- Autosomal dominant

Genotype-Phenotype Correlation

- *CDKN2A* mutations
  - Also associated with pancreatic cancer
    - Increased lifetime risk of 11-25%
  - Mutations in p14ARF function
    - Associated with astrocytoma

CLINICAL IMPLICATIONS AND ANCILLARY TESTS

Clinical Presentation

- Familial atypical multiple mole-melanoma syndrome
  - Mutations in *CDKN2A* and *CDK4* genes may be found
  - Increased risk of cutaneous melanoma and pancreatic cancer
- Xeroderma pigmentosum
  - Mutations in *XPA, XPB/ERCC3, XPC, XPD/ERCC2, XPE/DDB1, XPF/ERCC4, XPG/ERCC5, POLH*
  - Sun sensitivity (can be extreme)
  - High risk of cutaneous melanoma, basal cell carcinoma, and squamous cell carcinoma
- Examples of other syndromes with occasional development of cutaneous melanoma
  - Hereditary breast and ovarian cancer syndrome
    - *BRCA1* and *BRCA2* mutations
    - Increased risk of breast and ovarian cancers
    - Risk of cutaneous melanoma appears to be increased in patients < age 65
  - Li-Fraumeni syndrome
    - Mutations in *P53*
    - Most common cancers include osteosarcoma, other sarcomas, leukemia, breast cancer, adrenal cortical carcinoma, and brain cancer
    - Increased risk of cutaneous melanoma, but exact quantification of risk is unknown
  - Hereditary retinoblastoma
    - *RB1* mutations
    - Increased risk of retinoblastoma, osteosarcoma, cutaneous melanoma, and other sarcomas
  - Werner syndrome
    - Mutations in *WRN*
    - Premature aging with increased risk of cancer, including cutaneous melanoma

Clinical Risk Factors

- Cutaneous melanoma in 1 first-degree relative
  - 2.5-3x increased risk of cutaneous melanoma than general population
- Cutaneous melanoma in a parent and a sibling
  - 9x increased risk of cutaneous melanoma than general population
- *CDKN2A* mutation carrier
  - 75-100x greater risk of cutaneous melanoma than general population
- Degree/amount of sun exposure
  - Presence of extensive sun damage to skin
  - Prior history of skin cancers
- Geographic location
- Number of nevi, especially if > 50
  - Number of nevi with atypical features
    - Size > 6 mm, irregular/ill-defined borders, irregular color
- Very fair skin with inability to tan
- Presence of many freckles
- Hair color, especially red or blonde
- Eye color, especially blue
- Genetic mutations and modifier genes

HEREDITARY CUTANEOUS MELANOMA

ASSOCIATED NEOPLASMS

Malignant Melanoma

- Cutaneous
- Ocular (uveal tract)
  - Increased risk only in certain families (linked to 9p12.32)
  - No increased risk in families with *CDKN2A* mutations

Dysplastic Melanocytic Nevi (Atypical Melanocytic Nevi, Clark Nevi)

- Originally described in kindreds with increased risk of cutaneous melanoma
- Subsequently described in individuals with no increased risk of cutaneous melanoma
- Controversial on many levels
  - Definition not universal
    - Clinical vs. histopathologic: Clinically atypical nevi are not necessarily histopathologically atypical, and vice versa
- Clinically dysplastic melanocytic nevi
  - Size > 6 mm
  - Irregular color
  - Irregular borders
  - Asymmetric
  - History of change
  - Presence of elevated and flat (papular and macular) components
- Histopathologic criteria for dysplastic melanocytic nevi
  - Include cytologic and architectural criteria
  - Cytologic criteria
    - Nuclear size
    - Pleomorphism
  - Architectural features
    - Single melanocytes vs. nests
    - Nest size
    - Distribution of nests
    - Bridging of rete
    - Pagetoid scatter
    - Fibroplasia, sometimes lamellar
    - Extension of junctional component past dermal component
    - Lymphocytic infiltrate

Pancreatic Cancer

- Average age is 5.8 years younger than patients affected by sporadic pancreatic cancer

Astrocytoma

- Linked to mutations in *CDKN2A* (p14ARF)

Breast Carcinoma

- Possible 4x increased risk in families with *CDKN2A* mutations

CANCER RISK MANAGEMENT

Photoprotection

- Sunscreen, sun protective clothing, avoidance of sunburn

Skin Examination

- Head-to-toe examination (including scalp and genitalia)
  - Baseline at age 10 years
  - Repeat every 6-12 months
  - May increase frequency during puberty or pregnancy
  - May use dermoscopy or other modalities
  - Monthly self-examination of skin
- Baseline photography may be helpful

Suspicious Lesions

- Prompt excision and histopathologic evaluation

Education

- On photoprotection and characteristics of melanoma

Pancreatic Cancer Surveillance

- Multimodal screening
  - Endoscopic ultrasound, computed tomography, endoscopic retrograde cholangiopancreatography, and magnetic resonance imaging

SELECTED REFERENCES

1. Njauw CN et al: Germline BAP1 inactivation is preferentially associated with metastatic ocular melanoma and cutaneous-ocular melanoma families. PLoS One. 7(4):e35295, 2012
2. Abdel-Rahman MH et al: Melanoma candidate genes CDKN2A/p16/INK4A, p14ARF, and CDK4 sequencing in patients with uveal melanoma with relative high-risk for hereditary cancer predisposition. Melanoma Res. 21(3):175-9, 2011
3. Bonadies DC et al: Hereditary melanoma. Curr Probl Cancer. 35(4):162-72, 2011
4. Bartsch DK et al: Clinical and genetic analysis of 18 pancreatic carcinoma/melanoma-prone families. Clin Genet. 77(4):333-41, 2010
5. Gemmel C et al: Pancreatic cancer screening: state of the art. Expert Rev Gastroenterol Hepatol. 3(1):89-96, 2009
6. Kannengiesser C et al: Functional, structural, and genetic evaluation of 20 CDKN2A germ line mutations identified in melanoma-prone families or patients. Hum Mutat. 30(4):564-74, 2009
7. Udayakumar D et al: Melanoma genetics: an update on risk-associated genes. Hematol Oncol Clin North Am. 23(3):415-29, vii, 2009
8. Gudbjartsson DF et al: ASIP and TYR pigmentation variants associate with cutaneous melanoma and basal cell carcinoma. Nat Genet. 2008 Jul;40(7):886-91. Epub 2008 May 18. Erratum in: Nat Genet. 40(8):1029, 2008
9. Begg CB et al: Lifetime risk of melanoma in CDKN2A mutation carriers in a population-based sample. J Natl Cancer Inst. 97(20):1507-15, 2005
10. Parker JF et al: Pancreatic carcinoma surveillance in patients with familial melanoma. Arch Dermatol. 139(8):1019-25, 2003
11. Bishop DT et al: Geographical variation in the penetrance of CDKN2A mutations for melanoma. J Natl Cancer Inst. 94(12):894-903, 2002
12. Box NF et al: MC1R genotype modifies risk of melanoma in families segregating CDKN2A mutations. Am J Hum Genet. 69(4):765-73, 2001

Associated Lesions

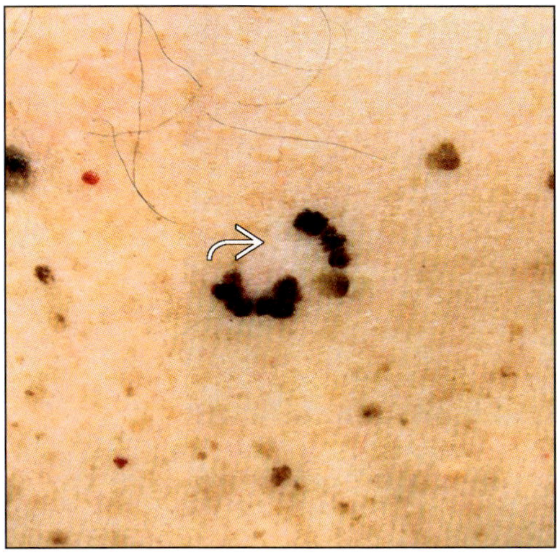
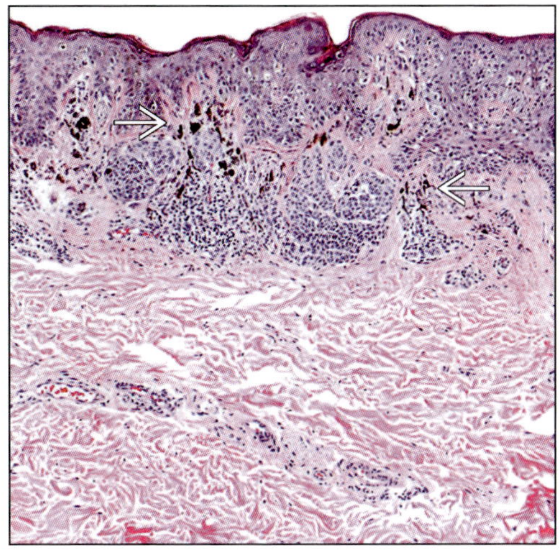

(Left) *Clinical photograph of a melanoma, superficial spreading type, shows darkly pigmented areas surrounding a central area of regression* ↪. *(Courtesy J. Wu, MD.)* **(Right)** *This melanoma is composed of large melanocytes with mild dermal inflammation and scattered melanophages* ➡. *(Courtesy S. Dadras, MD.)*

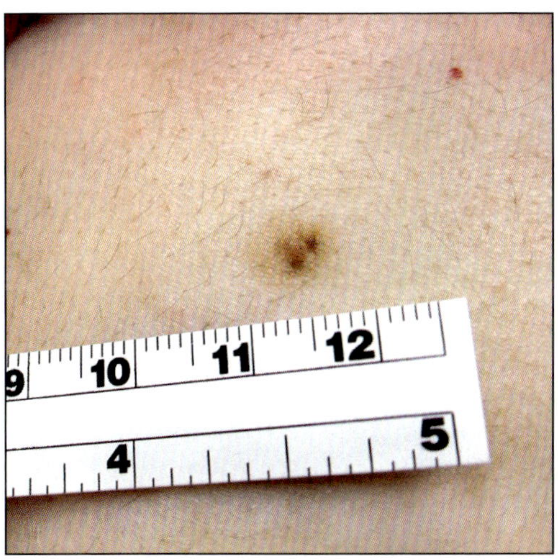

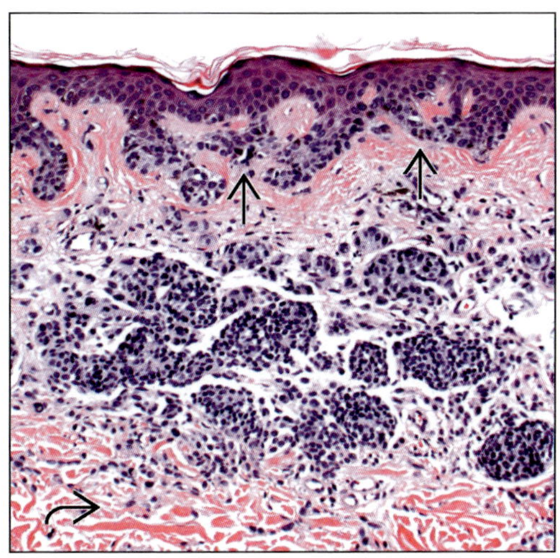

(Left) *This is a multicolored, irregularly bordered, asymmetric melanocytic nevus that mimics a melanoma. (Courtesy J. Hall, MD.)* **(Right)** *Mildly atypical compound melanocytic nevus shows a proliferation of small nests and a few single cells along the dermal-epidermal junction with focal bridging across rete ridges* →. *The dermal component is composed of small, relatively uniform-appearing cells that show dispersion (maturation) with dermal descent* ↪. *(Courtesy D. Cassarino, MD.)*

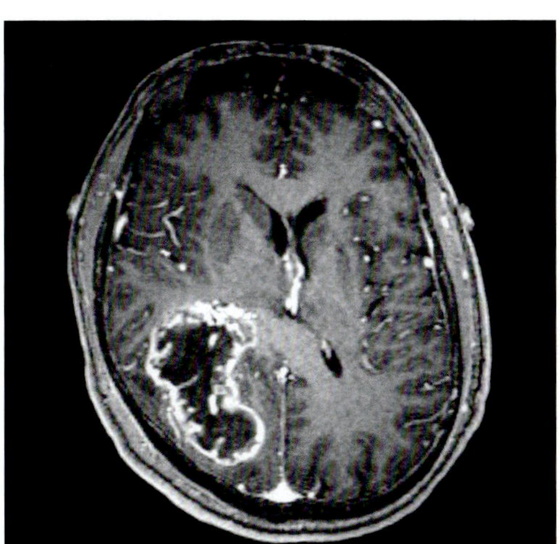
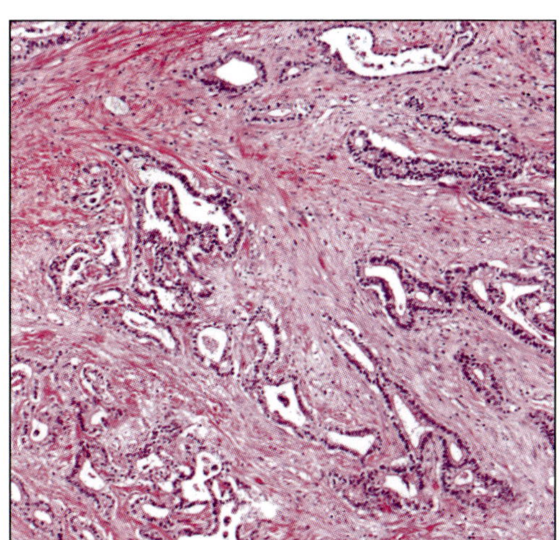

(Left) *Glioblastoma multiforme typically has an irregular, contrast-enhancing rim around a dark, necrotic center. (Courtesy P. Burger, MD.)* **(Right)** *Ductal pancreatic adenocarcinoma typically features small to medium-sized glands with haphazard growth embedded in a dense desmoplastic stroma. (Courtesy M. Mino-Kenudson, MD.)*

HEREDITARY NEUROBLASTOMA

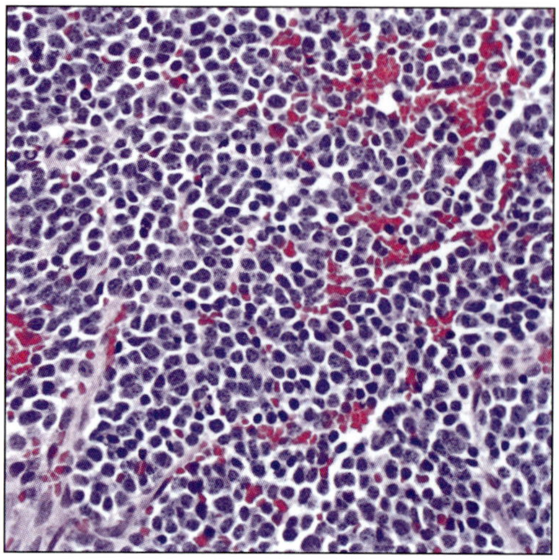

Undifferentiated neuroblastoma shows cells with scant cytoplasm with round and hyperchromatic nuclei. The differential diagnosis should include other small blue round cell tumors.

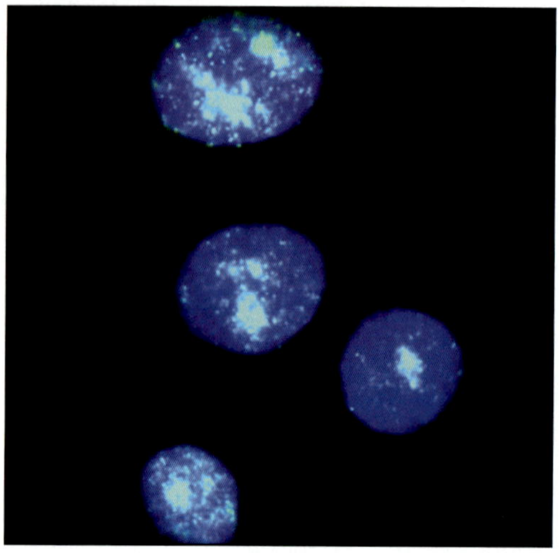

Fluorescence in situ hybridization (FISH) of this neuroblastoma shows marked amplification of MYCN, demonstrated by numerous green dots in the neuroblastoma cells.

TERMINOLOGY

Abbreviations

- Neuroblastoma (NB)
- Ganglioneuroblastoma (GNB)

Definitions

- Malignant tumor derived from primordial neural crest cells that usually presents in childhood
  - NB is less differentiated
  - GNB is moderately differentiated, showing variable cytodifferentiation into ganglion cells

EPIDEMIOLOGY

Incidence

- Hereditary NB is rare
- Prevalence of NB in the general population 1:7,500 to 1:10,000
- Inherited cases represent ~ 2-3.5% of new cases
- Overall risk to siblings is ~ 0.2%
- Familial NBs are thought to have an earlier median age at diagnosis than those with sporadic NB
- Age at diagnosis in other 40% is extremely variable
- Most cases (> 60%) of hereditary NB are diagnosed before 1 year of age

GENETICS

Genetic Changes

- NB harbors a variety of genetic changes
  - Gain of genetic material from 17q
  - Loss of heterozygosity at 1p36 and 11q
  - Mutations on *PHOX2B*
  - High frequency of *MYCN* (N-myc) amplification
  - Anaplastic lymphoma kinase (*ALK*) is a frequent target of genetic alteration in advanced NB

Heterogeneous Etiology

- Autosomal dominant
- Mutations on *PHOX2B* on 4p12
- *ALK* mutations
- *MYCN* amplification
- Potential susceptibility loci at 16p12-p31, 4p16,2p21-p25.1, 12p12.1-p13.33
  - Suggests a possible oligogenic model in which 2 loci have a synergistic effect on NB

PHOX2B

- Heterozygous mutations in *PHOX2B* found in 1 of 8 families cosegregating for NB
- *PHOX2B* found as a candidate gene because of reported increased risk of NB individuals with congenital central hypoventilation syndrome (due to de novo *PHOX2B* mutations)
  - Patients with this syndrome have increased risk (5-10%) of NB, GNB, or ganglioneuroma

ALK

- *ALK* locus, centromeric to the *MYCN* locus, was identified as a recurrent target of copy number gain and gene amplification
- Germline mutations in *ALK* gene explain most hereditary NBs
  - Activating mutations can also be somatically acquired
- DNA sequencing of *ALK* revealed 8 novel missense mutations in up to ~ 35% of NB
- Heritable mutations of *ALK* are main cause of familial NB
- Germline or acquired activation of this cell-surface kinase is a tractable therapeutic target for this lethal pediatric malignancy

CLINICAL IMPLICATIONS AND ANCILLARY TESTS

Clinically Relevant Pathologic Features

- Gross appearance
  - Cystic degeneration and calcification can be seen
- Microscopy
  - Small round blue cells with very scant cytoplasm
  - Homer Wright rosettes or pseudorosettes
  - Ganglionic differentiation
- Mitotic-karyorrhectic index (MKI), applicable for stroma-poor tumors
  - Count of cells undergoing mitosis or karyorrhexis (per 5,000 cells)
- Adverse factors
  - Older age at diagnosis
  - Advanced stage of disease (except IV-S)
  - High histologic grade of tumor
  - Diploid DNA value
  - *MYCN* oncogene amplification
  - Cytogenetic abnormalities of chromosomes 1 and 17
  - Pattern of urinary catecholamine excretion
  - Increased levels of ferritin NSE, LDH, creatine kinase BB, or chromogranin-A
  - Abnormalities in ganglioside composition
  - Lack of high-affinity nerve growth factor receptors

ASSOCIATED NEOPLASMS

Neuroblastoma

- Patients with familial NB have a 20% risk of developing bilateral adrenal and multifocal primary NBs

Ganglioneuroma

- Patients with familial NB have increased risk of developing benign tumors as ganglioneuromas

CANCER RISK MANAGEMENT

Screening

- Urinary catecholamines
  - NB could be detected by screening at age of 6 months
    - Evidence of improvement in survival of children with screen-detected NB
    - Associated with favorable biological features
    - Lack of *MYCN* amplification
- Urinary homovanillic acid and vanillylmandelic acid
  - Increased in > 95% of cases of NB
  - Due to clinical heterogeneity of hereditary NB and possibility of a later age at presentation, a prolonged period of time screening may be necessary
- Lactate dehydrogenase
  - > 1,500 IU/L associated with worse clinical outcome
- Ferritin
  - > 142 ng/mL associated with worse clinical outcome
- Neuron-specific enolase (NSE)
  - > 100 ng/mL associated with worse clinical outcome

High Importance of Cytogenetics

- *MYCN* amplification is associated with worse prognosis
- Loss of heterozygosity of 1p and 11q associated with worse prognosis
- Activating mutations of *ALK* receptor tyrosine kinase confer sensitivity to ALK inhibition with small molecules, providing a molecular rationale for targeted therapy of this disease

Prognosis

- 5-year survival based on stage at time of diagnosis
  - Stage I: > 90%
  - Stage II: 70-80%
  - Stage III: 40-70%
  - Stage IV
    - < 1 year old: > 60%
    - 1-2 years old: 20%
    - > 2 years old: 10%
  - Stage IV-S: > 80%

SELECTED REFERENCES

1. Suganuma R et al: Peripheral neuroblastic tumors with genotype-phenotype discordance: a report from the Children's Oncology Group and the International Neuroblastoma Pathology Committee. Pediatr Blood Cancer. 60(3):363-70, 2013
2. Carpenter EL et al: Targeting ALK in neuroblastoma--preclinical and clinical advancements. Nat Rev Clin Oncol. 9(7):391-9, 2012
3. Fisher JP et al: Neonatal neuroblastoma. Semin Fetal Neonatal Med. 17(4):207-15, 2012
4. Deyell RJ et al: Advances in the understanding of constitutional and somatic genomic alterations in neuroblastoma. Cancer Genet. 204(3):113-21, 2011
5. Ogawa S et al: Oncogenic mutations of ALK in neuroblastoma. Cancer Sci. 102(2):302-8, 2011
6. Janoueix-Lerosey I et al: [ALK, a key gene in the pathogenesis of neuroblastoma.] Med Sci (Paris). 25(4):330-2, 2009
7. Krona C et al: Analysis of neuroblastoma tumour progression; loss of PHOX2B on 4p13 and 17q gain are early events in neuroblastoma tumourigenesis. Int J Oncol. 32(3):575-83, 2008
8. Mossé YP et al: Identification of ALK as a major familial neuroblastoma predisposition gene. Nature. 455(7215):930-5, 2008
9. Raabe EH et al: Prevalence and functional consequence of PHOX2B mutations in neuroblastoma. Oncogene. 27(4):469-76, 2008
10. Shimada A et al: Expression of KIT and PDGFR is associated with a good prognosis in neuroblastoma. Pediatr Blood Cancer. 50(2):213-7, 2008
11. Attiyeh EF et al: Chromosome 1p and 11q deletions and outcome in neuroblastoma. N Engl J Med. 353(21):2243-53, 2005
12. Bourdeaut F et al: Germline mutations of the paired-like homeobox 2B (PHOX2B) gene in neuroblastoma. Cancer Lett. 228(1-2):51-8, 2005
13. Claviez A et al: Low occurrence of familial neuroblastomas and ganglioneuromas in five consecutive GPOH neuroblastoma treatment studies. Eur J Cancer. 40(18):2760-5, 2004
14. De Preter K et al: No evidence for involvement of SDHD in neuroblastoma pathogenesis. BMC Cancer. 4:55, 2004

Imaging, Microscopic, and Gross Features

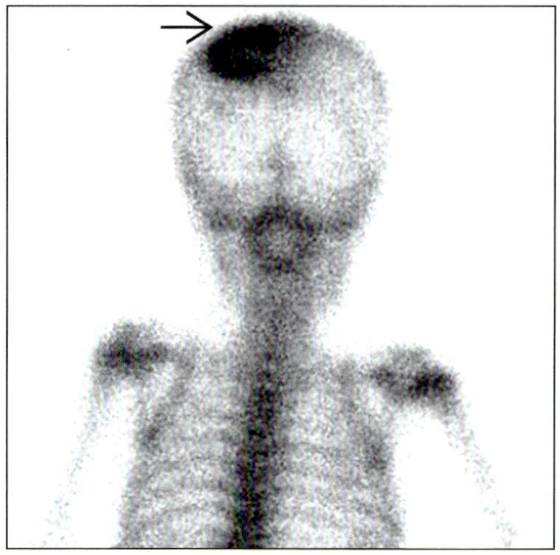

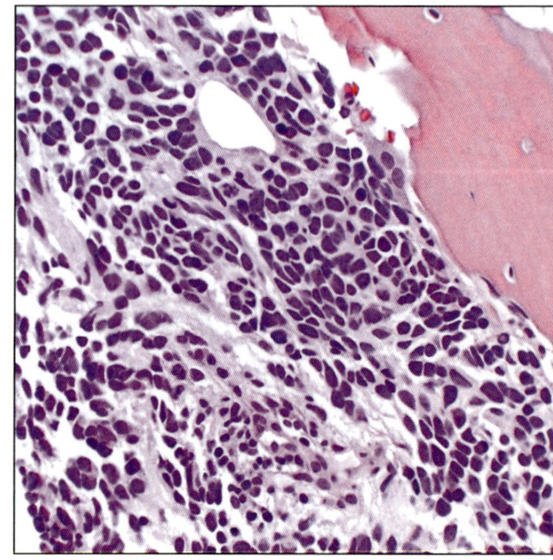

(Left) *Posterior bone scan shows calvarial metastasis* → *of a neuroblastoma in a small child.* ***(Right)*** *This is a focus of metastatic neuroblastoma in a core biopsy specimen of bone. The marrow has been extensively replaced by sheets of metastatic small round cell tumor and shows no areas with normal trilineage hematopoiesis.*

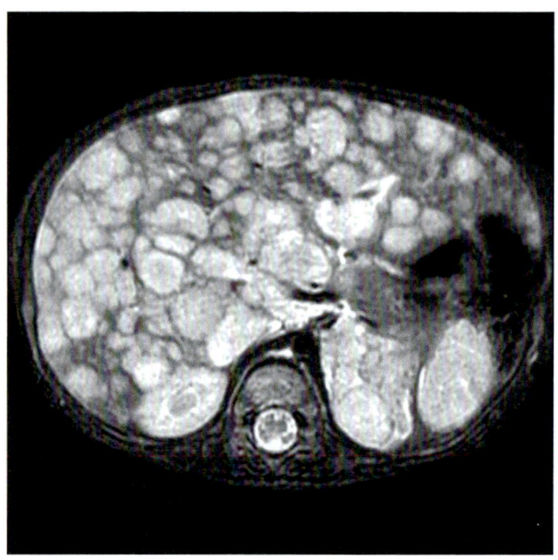

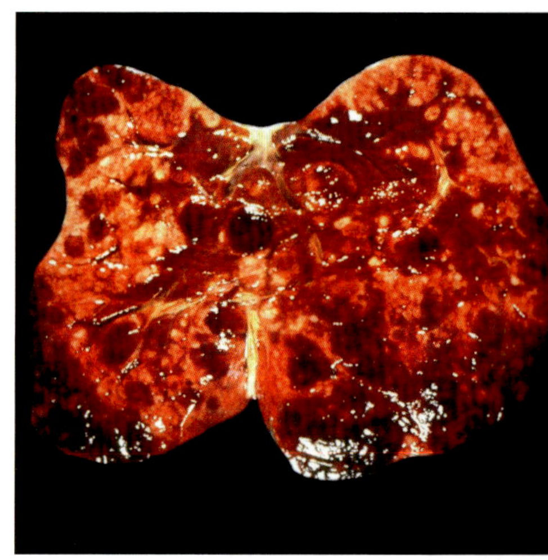

(Left) *Axial T2-weighted MR shows a left adrenal mass, which proved to be a neuroblastoma. It was widely metastatic; the liver was filled with multiple high-signal nodular lesions, with little normal remaining hepatic parenchyma.* ***(Right)*** *This specimen of a liver shows diffuse involvement and extensive replacement by multiple deposits of metastatic neuroblastoma. There are several foci of hemorrhage.*

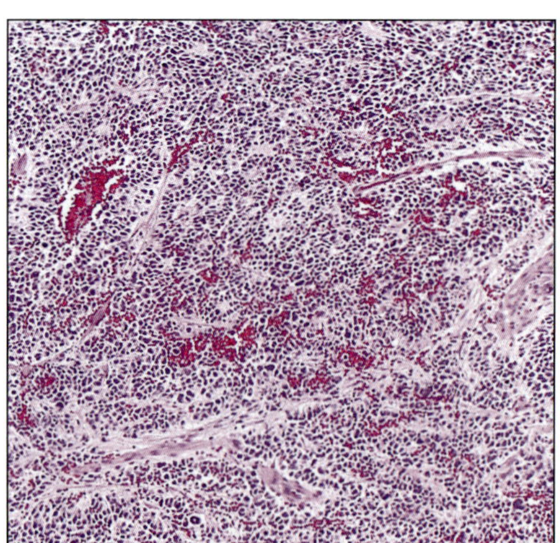

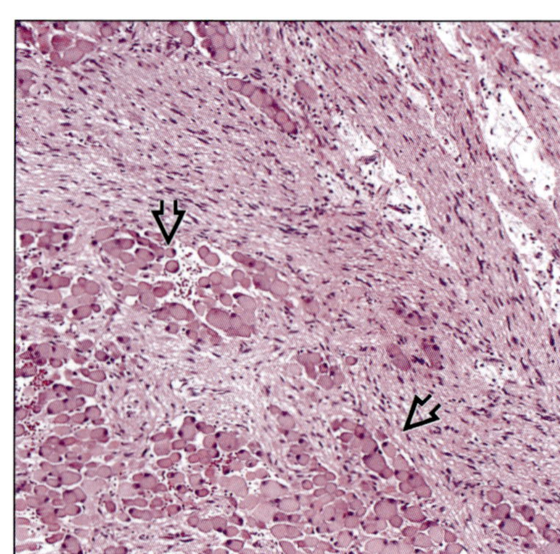

(Left) *Schwannian stroma in an NB is often present as thin septa composed of spindled cells, sometimes with wavy nuclei. The Schwann cell component can be demonstrated by immunohistochemistry for S100 protein.* ***(Right)*** *The neuroblastomatous component of this intermixed ganglioneuroblastoma (GNB) is predominantly mature ganglion cells* ⇨*. The ganglion cells are present in clusters in this tumor, differing from the pattern in maturing GNB in which they are present as single cells.*

Microscopic Features and Ancillary Tests

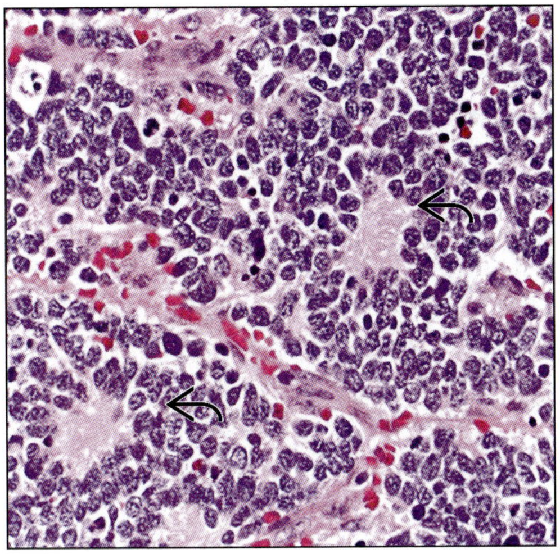

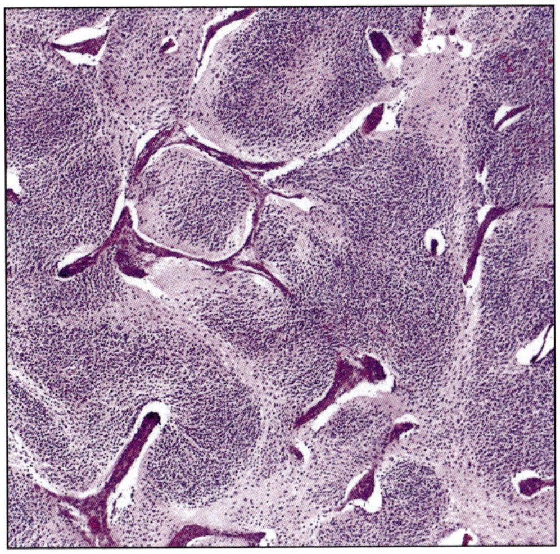

(Left) *Homer Wright rosettes ➔ are composed of neuroblasts surrounding a central core of neurites (cytoplasmic processes). These can be found in varying numbers in poorly differentiated NBs but are not wholly specific. Small foci of schwannian stroma are also seen.* ***(Right)*** *Low-power view of a poorly differentiated neuroblastoma shows thin septa composed of schwannian stroma. Pale, eosinophilic neuropil is seen in places between the nodules or nests of neuroblastoma cells.*

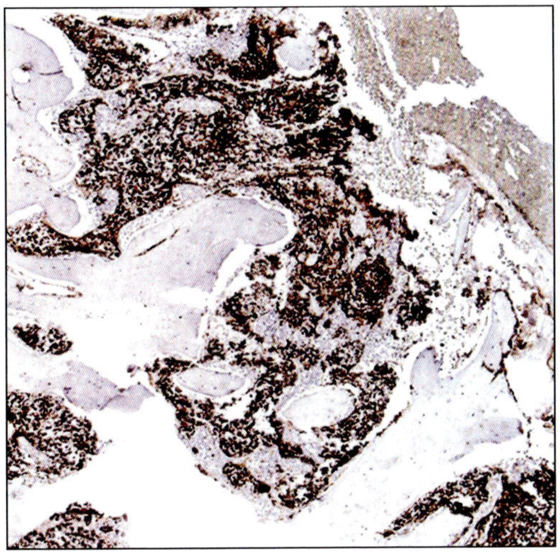

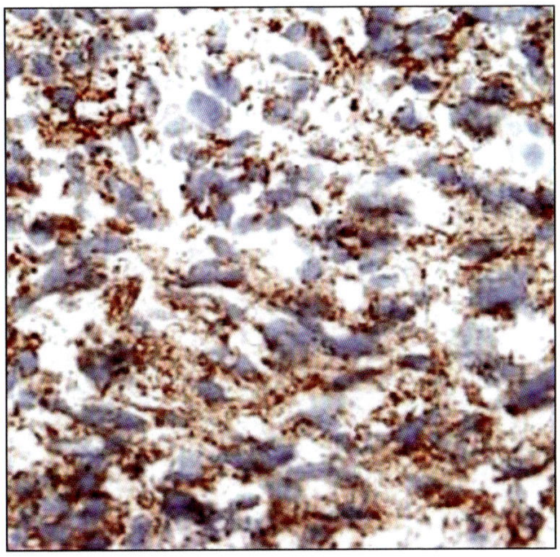

(Left) *In this bone marrow trephine specimen, there is diffuse immunoreactivity for neuroblastoma antigen (NB84) in metastatic deposits of neuroblastoma that extend between bony trabeculae.* ***(Right)*** *Synaptophysin immunostain shows granular pattern. Although synaptophysin is not specific, it can be used for differential diagnosis of other small round blue cell tumors like lymphoma, rhabdomyosarcoma, or Ewing sarcoma. NBs are also positive for chromogranin and CD56.*

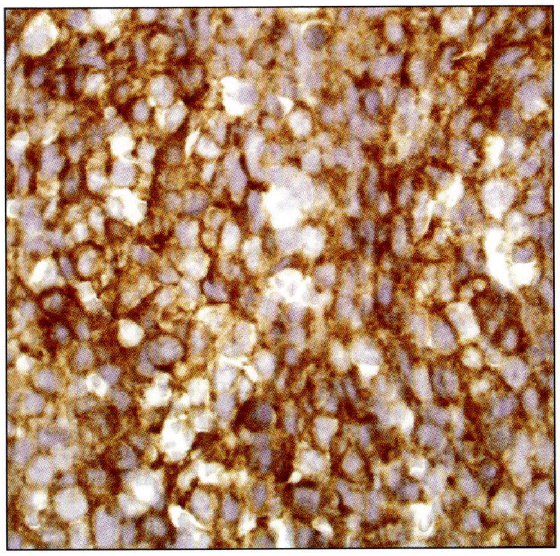

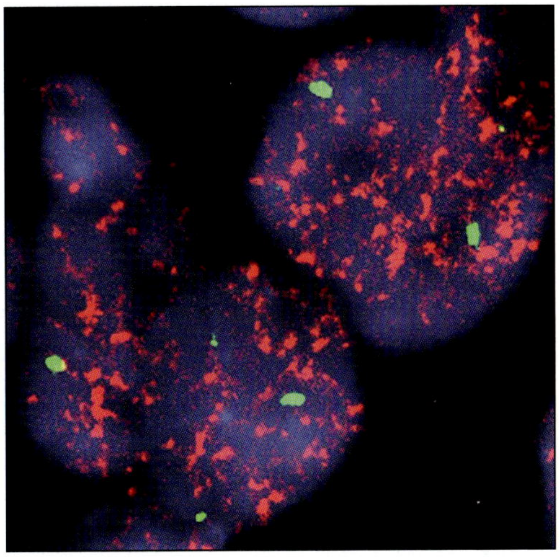

(Left) *Immunohistochemical staining for ALK1 in neuroblastoma shows strong membranous staining. Activating mutations in ALK gene have been reported in neuroblastoma and provide a potential therapeutic target.* ***(Right)*** *FISH of a neuroblastoma shows marked amplification of MYCN demonstrated by numerous red dots. This finding predicts poor prognosis, although the amount of amplification does not relate to outcome.*

HEREDITARY PANCREATIC CANCER SYNDROME

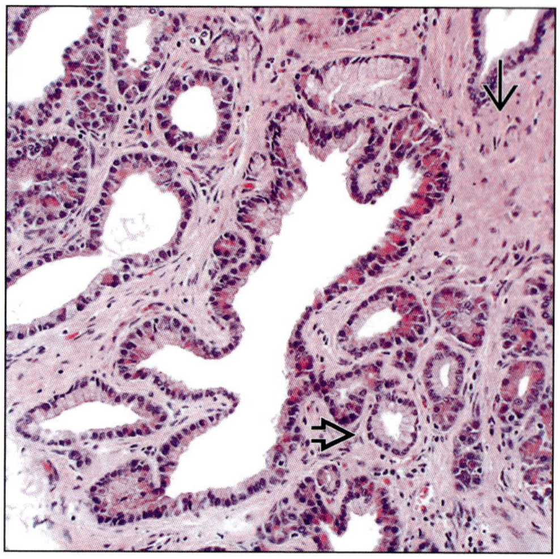

This medium-power image from a patient with hereditary pancreatitis shows chronic pancreatitis with scar → and atrophy of the acinar units ⇨. (Courtesy M. Bronner, MD.)

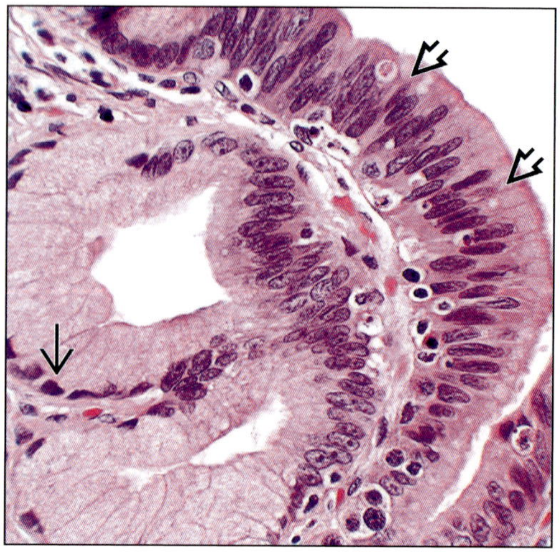

This image shows PanIN-2 from a patient with hereditary pancreatitis. Note the enlarged nuclei on the surface ⇨ compared to the bland nuclei →. (Courtesy M. Bronner, MD.)

TERMINOLOGY

Abbreviations

- Familial pancreatic cancer (FPC)
- Familial atypical multiple mole melanoma syndrome (FAMMM)
- Hereditary pancreas cancer syndromes (HPCS)

Definitions

- FPC is defined as a group of families with 2 or more close relatives with pancreatic cancer, but who do not fulfill criteria of any other cancer syndromes
- HPCS are well-defined syndromes that have an increased risk of pancreatic neoplasms
  - Multiple endocrine neoplasia type 1 (MEN1), von Hippel-Lindau disease, neurofibromatosis type 1, tuberous sclerosis, hereditary breast and ovarian, FAMMM, Peutz-Jeghers, and hereditary pancreatitis are all HPCS

EPIDEMIOLOGY

Prevalence

- Up to 10% of pancreatic carcinomas have a familial component
  - Known genetic syndromes account for < 20% of this group
    - **Most causes of FPC are still unknown**
    - Mutations in *ATM* and *PALLD* genes have been identified in small kindreds of FPC patients
  - The more family members affected, the higher the relative risk of pancreatic cancer to individuals within that family
  - Cigarette smoking is a synergistic environmental cofactor

GENETICS

Autosomal Dominant

- Although most genes/syndromes have yet to be defined, those that have been identified tend to be autosomal dominant with 60-80% penetrance
- Carcinomas tend to occur at an earlier age in each successive generation and also increase in aggressiveness

ETIOLOGY/PATHOGENESIS

Histogenesis

- Given the wide variety of genes and syndromes involved, there is not much consistency in what has been described
  - Patients with hereditary pancreatitis and FAMMM seem to develop multifocal pancreatic intraepithelial neoplasias (PanINs) as precursor lesions
  - Patients with other forms of FPC develop multiple intraductal papillary mucinous neoplasms
- Invasive carcinomas arise an average of 12 years earlier in familial cases compared to sporadic cases, and they have a worse prognosis

CANCER RISK MANAGEMENT

Surveillance

- No clear-cut agreement on the best method to follow in patients at risk for FPC
  - Endoscopic ultrasound (with fine-needle aspiration of lesions, if present) and MR cholangiopancreatography are thought to be the 2 best modalities for initial screening
  - There is little agreement on the age at which screening should start

Hereditary Pancreatic Cancer Syndromes

Syndrome	Gene(s)	Tumor(s)
MEN1	*MEN1*	Pancreatic endocrine neoplasms
von Hippel-Lindau (VHL) disease	*VHL*	Serous cystadenomas, pancreatic endocrine neoplasms
Tuberous sclerosis (TSC)	*TSC1, TSC2*	Pancreatic endocrine neoplasms (*TSC2* mutations)
Hereditary breast and ovarian cancer syndrome	*BRCA2, PALB2, BRCA1*	Adenocarcinoma
Familial atypical multiple mole melanoma syndrome	*P16/CDKN2A*	Adenocarcinoma
Peutz-Jeghers syndrome	*STK11*	Adenocarcinoma
Lynch syndrome	*MLH1, PMS2, MSH2, MSH6*	Adenocarcinoma
Hereditary pancreatitis	*PRSS1, PRSS2, SPINK1, CFTR*	Adenocarcinoma
Familial adenomatous polyposis	*APC, MYH*	Adenocarcinoma (ampullary)

Relative Risk of Pancreatic Cancer

Risk Factor	Relative Risk (%)
Family history: 1 first-degree relative affected	1.5-1.75
Family History: 2 first-degree relatives affected	6
Family history: 3 first-degree relatives affected	14-32
Cigarette smoking and family history of pancreatic cancer	3.7-8.2
Hereditary breast and ovarian cancer	4-13
Familial atypical multiple mole melanoma	13-22
Peutz-Jeghers syndrome	36-132
Hereditary pancreatitis	53-87
Lynch syndrome	4.5
Familial adenomatous polyposis	4.5
Diabetes > 20 years	2

    - For patients with Peutz-Jeghers syndrome, screening is recommended to start between 25 and 30 whereas 35 years is the recommended starting age for hereditary pancreatitis and 40-50 years for FPC (10 years prior to the youngest family member's age at diagnosis of cancer)
- There is no agreement on minimal findings that should prompt surgical intervention

Surgery

- Patients with lesions showing high-grade dysplasia/ PanIN-2-3 are offered total pancreatectomy, but this is a very morbid procedure

SELECTED REFERENCES

1. Canto MI et al: International Cancer of the Pancreas Screening (CAPS) Consortium summit on the management of patients with increased risk for familial pancreatic cancer. Gut. 62(3):339-47, 2013
2. Potjer TP et al: Variation in precursor lesions of pancreatic cancer among high-risk groups. Clin Cancer Res. 19(2):442-9, 2013
3. Bartsch DK et al: Familial pancreatic cancer--current knowledge. Nat Rev Gastroenterol Hepatol. 9(8):445-53, 2012
4. Canto MI et al: Frequent detection of pancreatic lesions in asymptomatic high-risk individuals. Gastroenterology. 142(4):796-804; quiz e14-5, 2012
5. Roberts NJ et al: ATM mutations in patients with hereditary pancreatic cancer. Cancer Discov. 2(1):41-6, 2012
6. Sakorafas GH et al: Individuals at high-risk for pancreatic cancer development: management options and the role of surgery. Surg Oncol. 21(2):e49-58, 2012
7. Segura PP et al: Hereditary pancreatic cancer: molecular bases and their application in diagnosis and clinical management: a guideline of the TTD group. Clin Transl Oncol. 14(8):553-63, 2012
8. Solomon S et al: Inherited pancreatic cancer syndromes. Cancer J. 18(6):485-91, 2012
9. Solomon S, Whitcomb DC, LaRusch J. PRSS1-Related Hereditary Pancreatitis. 1993-2013, 2012
10. Brentnall TA: Pancreatic cancer surveillance: learning as we go. Am J Gastroenterol. 106(5):955-6, 2011
11. Matsubayashi H et al: Risk factors of familial pancreatic cancer in Japan: current smoking and recent onset of diabetes. Pancreas. 40(6):974-8, 2011
12. Hruban RH et al: Update on familial pancreatic cancer. Adv Surg. 44:293-311, 2010
13. Maisonneuve P et al: Epidemiology of pancreatic cancer: an update. Dig Dis. 28(4-5):645-56, 2010
14. Shi C et al: Familial pancreatic cancer. Arch Pathol Lab Med. 133(3):365-74, 2009
15. Shi C et al: Increased prevalence of precursor lesions in familial pancreatic cancer patients. Clin Cancer Res. 15(24):7737-7743, 2009

HEREDITARY PAPILLARY RENAL CELL CARCINOMA

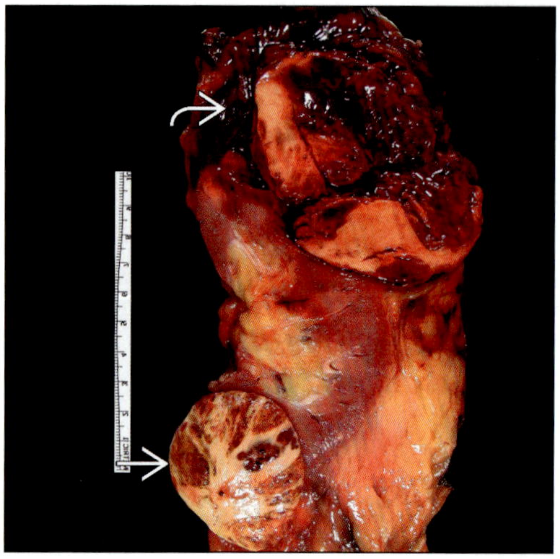

Kidney shows multifocal PRCCs. Upper pole PRCC ➔ is dark red-brown due to diffuse hemorrhage, and lower pole PRCC ➔ has yellow discoloration due to histiocytic infiltrates. These changes are common in PRCC.

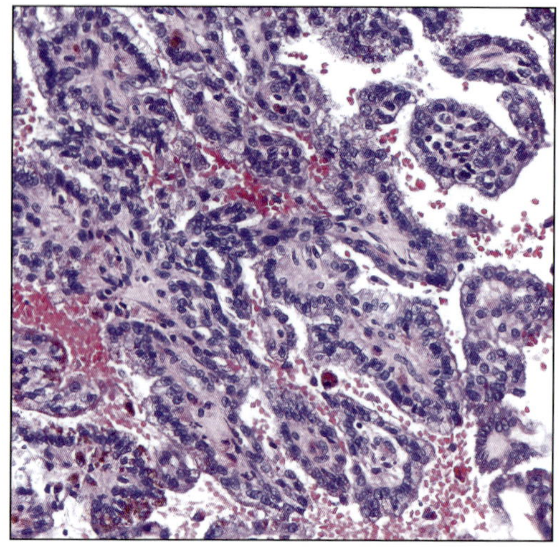

PRCC type 1 shows well-formed papillae lined by cuboidal cells with amphophilic cytoplasm. Nuclei are usually low grade. Note hemosiderin pigment-laden histiocytes and red blood cells from hemorrhage.

TERMINOLOGY

Abbreviations

- Hereditary papillary renal cell carcinoma (HPRCC)
- Papillary renal cell carcinoma (PRCC)

Definitions

- Autosomal dominant hereditary disease characterized by development of multiple type 1 PRCCs related to germline *MET (c-MET)* mutation

EPIDEMIOLOGY

Age Range

- PRCC typically develops between 45 and 63 years
  - Somewhat late onset for hereditary renal cancer syndrome; however, tumor development as early as 2nd or 3rd decade may occur

Gender

- More common in men (M:F = 2.4:1)

Ethnicity Relationship

- No known ethnic relationship
  - Most cases encountered in Caucasian families; possibly biased by general population ethnic distribution

Incidence

- Rare, only ~ 30 families with *MET* mutation described worldwide
  - 1 study did not find *MET* mutation in 59 clinic-based PRCC cases, including a subset with bilateral &/or multifocal tumors
  - PRCC represents 5% of familial renal cancers in National Institute of Health (NIH) database
- Vast majority of PRCC are sporadic tumors; 2nd most common type of renal epithelial tumor
  - *MET* mutation also rarely detected in some PRCC type 1 without known family history of PRCC type 1

ETIOLOGY/PATHOGENESIS

Genetics

- Mutation in *MET* proto-oncogene
  - Gene located in Chr 7q31.1-34
  - MET is receptor for hepatocyte growth factor (HGF) or scatter factor (SF)
  - Most are germline missense mutations
  - Mutation occurs in glycine-rich subdomain adjacent to ATP binding site or in activation loop of tyrosine kinase domain
    - Results in constitutive activation of receptor
  - MET overexpression is frequently observed in HPRCC
    - Suggested as potential therapeutic target
  - Penetrance suggested to be high
- HPRCC cytogenetics
  - Chr +7 detected in HPRCC tumors; similar to sporadic tumors
  - No Chr -3p detected

CLINICAL IMPLICATIONS

Clinical Presentation

- Diagnosis in index patients from families with HPRCC not different from sporadic PRCCs
  - Renal cancers often detected incidentally
  - When symptomatic, may present with hematuria, abdominal pain, &/or mass
  - Suspicion for HPRCC raised by history of multiple family members with renal cancers
  - Subsequent radiologic screening may identify affected family members with asymptomatic renal cancers

- Renal cancers can be lethal if not detected and treated at early stage
- Estimated prevalence of renal tumors is 1,100-1,300 microscopic papillary tumors in a kidney

CLINICAL IMPLICATIONS AND ANCILLARY TESTS

MET Proto-Oncogene Mutation Screening

- Not advocated to be performed in every case of PRCC because HPRCC is rare
  - 1 study screened 59 patients with PRCC that included 22% with bilateral &/or multifocal tumors and no *MET* mutation was identified
- Testing should be performed only if there is clinical suspicion of the disease
  - Unusually young age of onset, positive family history, bilateral &/or multifocal PRCCs
- Testing can be performed on blood samples (lymphocytes)

ASSOCIATED NEOPLASMS

PRCC Type 1

- **Macroscopy**
  - Bilateral and multifocal tumors in > 80% of cases of HPRCC
  - Reported number of PRCCs ranges from 1-26
  - HPRCC tumors have similar gross appearance to sporadic PRCC
    - Well circumscribed with fibrous pseudocapsule
    - Hemorrhages are common and cause red or dark brown discoloration
    - Intratumoral collections of histiocytes may produce yellow streaks or contrasts
- **Microscopy**
  - Predominant histology of PRCC type 1 in HPRCC is similar to those in sporadic type
    - Papillary architecture with fibrovascular core that occasionally contains foamy histiocytes
    - May also have tubular or tubulopapillary architecture; may impart solid appearance when predominant
    - Tumor cells are small with scant to modest amount of basophilic or amphophilic cytoplasm
  - Admixed areas of clear cells present in > 90% of tumors, more common than in sporadic PRCCs
    - Amount of clear cells varies from 1-70%
    - PRCC lacks delicate vasculature in clear cell RCC
    - Electron microscopy detects intracytoplasmic lipid and glycogen, unlike in usual PRCC cells
- **Immunohistochemistry**
  - AMACR(+), CK7(+), and EMA(+)
- Suggested to be more aggressive than sporadic PRCC
  - Patients typically survive into 7th decade of life

PRCC Type 2

- HPRCC with mixture of PRCC types 1 and 2 reported; association not established as in type 1
- Suggested that some PRCC type 1 classified before 1997 are perhaps type 2

Papillary Adenoma

- Small (≤ 5 mm) tumor nodule in renal parenchyma with papillary, tubular, or tubulopapillary architectures
- Similar cytology to PRCC type 1
  - Distinguished from PRCC type 1 by size criteria
- Like PRCC, multiple adenomas are present in kidney
- Similar genetic and immunophenotypic profiles to PRCC type 1
- Benign tumor with no metastatic potential

Other Tumors

- No known extrarenal manifestations, in contrast to most other hereditary renal cancer syndromes

CANCER RISK MANAGEMENT

Management

- Observation can be performed for smaller tumors
  - No standard size cut-off for therapeutic intervention; some follows 3 cm as cut-off, similar to criterion used for VHL disease
- Nephron-sparing surgery prioritized to preserve renal function
- Radical surgery if tumor is large or kidney is extensively involved
- Treatment with *MET* inhibitors (e.g., SK1363089 or ARQ197) in phase 2 trials shows promising results

Surveillance

- Lifelong clinical surveillance of affected family members should be performed
- Baseline radiographic examination of kidneys to detect asymptomatic tumor
- Regular follow-up to detect new tumor and careful monitoring for progression of smaller tumors

SELECTED REFERENCES

1. Wadt KA et al: Novel germline c-MET mutation in a family with hereditary papillary renal carcinoma. Fam Cancer. 11(3):535-7, 2012
2. Bellon SF et al: c-Met inhibitors with novel binding mode show activity against several hereditary papillary renal cell carcinoma-related mutations. J Biol Chem. 283(5):2675-83, 2008
3. Schmidt LS et al: Early onset hereditary papillary renal carcinoma: germline missense mutations in the tyrosine kinase domain of the met proto-oncogene. J Urol. 172(4 Pt 1):1256-61, 2004
4. Lindor NM et al: Papillary renal cell carcinoma: analysis of germline mutations in the MET proto-oncogene in a clinic-based population. Genet Test. 5(2):101-6, 2001
5. Lubensky IA et al: Hereditary and sporadic papillary renal carcinomas with c-met mutations share a distinct morphological phenotype. Am J Pathol. 155(2):517-26, 1999
6. Schmidt L et al: Germline and somatic mutations in the tyrosine kinase domain of the MET proto-oncogene in papillary renal carcinomas. Nat Genet. 16(1):68-73, 1997

HEREDITARY PARAGANGLIOMA/PHEOCHROMOCYTOMA SYNDROMES

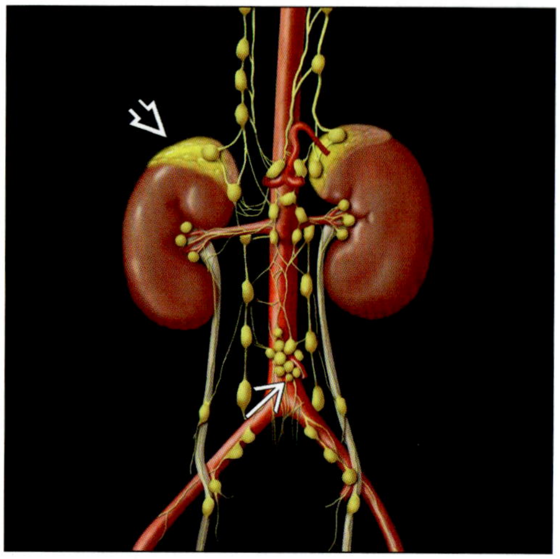

Graphic shows paraganglia and neuroendocrine tissues symmetrically distributed along the paravertebral axis in the abdomen, including the organ of Zuckerkandl ➔ and the adrenal medulla ⇒.

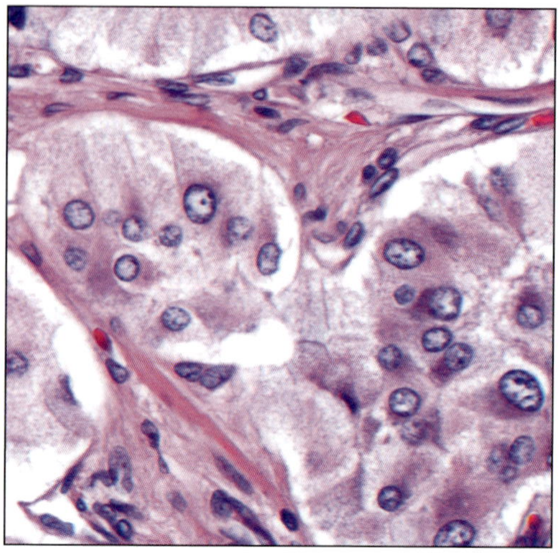

This pheochromocytoma (PCC) has the characteristic alveolar pattern (zellballen) with variably sized nests of tumor cells surrounded by thin-walled vessels and thin bands of fibrous tissue.

TERMINOLOGY

Abbreviations

- Hereditary paraganglioma/pheochromocytoma (PGL/PCC) syndromes
- Paraganglioma (PGL)
- Pheochromocytoma (PCC)

Definitions

- PCCs and PGLs are neuroendocrine tumors that arise in adrenal medulla or extraadrenal sympathetic and parasympathetic paraganglia
  - Occur sporadically or as part of different hereditary tumor syndromes
  - Tumors arising within adrenal medulla are known as PCCs; histologically identical tumors arising elsewhere are termed PGLs
- Hereditary PGL/PCC syndromes are characterized by presence of PGL &/or PCC that occur as part of a familial syndrome
  - > 30% of PCCs and PGLs are currently believed to be caused by germline mutations and several novel susceptibility genes have recently been discovered
  - *RET*, *VHL*, *NF1*, *SDHA*, *SDHB*, *SDHC*, *SDHD*, *SDHAF2*, *KIF1Bβ*, *TMEM127*, and *MAX* have been associated with hereditary PCC or PGL
- Hereditary PGL/PCC syndromes should be considered in all individuals with PGL or PCC with the following findings
  - Multiple tumors, including bilateral tumors
  - Multifocal with multiple synchronous or metachronous tumors
  - Early onset (age < 40 years)
  - Family history of such tumors
- Familial PGL/PCC syndrome is term restricted to tumors from germline mutations in *SDHx* genes
- Simplex cases: Many individuals with a hereditary PGL/PCC syndrome may present with solitary tumor of head or neck, thorax, abdomen, adrenal, or pelvis and no family history of the disorder
- In PGL/PCC that appear to be sporadic based on the absence of a family history, rate of occult germline mutation is said to be ~ 12% and ranges from 7.5-24%

Syndromes Characterized by Susceptibility to PCC and PGL

- Most tumors were known to be associated with multiple endocrine neoplasia type 2 (MEN2), von Hippel-Lindau disease (VHL), and neurofibromatosis type 1 (NF1)
- More recently, mutations in genes encoding different subunits of succinate dehydrogenase (SDH) complex have been linked to familial PGL/PCC syndrome (PGL1, 2, 3, and 4)
- Small fraction is associated with other syndromes (e.g., Carney triad, Carney-Stratakis syndrome, MEN1)
- Several other genes have recently been added to the list (associated with unknown hereditary PGL/PCC)
  - Kinesin family member 1B *(KIF1B)*
  - EGL-9 homolog 1 (*EGLN1*), also termed *PHD2*
  - Transmembrane protein 127 *(TMEM127)*
  - *MYC*-associated factor X *(MAX)*

GENETICS

MEN2

- Autosomal dominant syndrome caused by mutation of *RET* proto-oncogene
- Activating *RET* mutation predisposes to PCC, which is often bilateral and recurrent
  - Low risk of malignancy
- MEN2 prevalence is estimated at 1:30,000
- MEN2 often suspected on basis of family history; individuals with PCC infrequently present as simplex cases

- Clinically, can be divided into 3 types: MEN2A (55% of all cases), MEN2B (5-10%), and familial medullary thyroid carcinoma (FMTC, 35-40%)
- MEN2A and MEN2B patients have almost 100% risk of developing medullary thyroid carcinoma
- ~ 50% of individuals with MEN2A and MEN2B develop PCC
- Subtype FMTC has medullary thyroid carcinoma as its only feature

Familial PGL/PCC Syndromes

- Germline mutations in *SDHx* genes give rise to familial PGL/PCC syndrome, sometimes only referred to as familial PGL
- Prevalence of PGL/PCC syndrome is unknown, but a review of ~ 13% of all PGL/PCC cases gives an estimate of 1:50,000 to 1:20,000; majority represented by PGL1 and PGL4
- Associated with germline mutations in genes encoding subunits of SDH enzyme complex in context of familial PGL syndromes; PGL1, PGL2, PGL3, and PGL4 caused by mutations in *SDHD*, *SDHAF2*, *SDHC*, and *SDHB* genes, respectively
  - PGL2 is caused by mutations in *SDHAF2/SDH5*, which encodes for a molecule that is an accessory to the function of the SDH enzyme and its SDHA subunit
- Mutations were recently found in SDHA subunit in a limited number of patients with PGL &/or PCC
- *SDHB* mutations in particular may also predispose to thyroid and renal cancer, and possibly other tumors
  - Patients harboring *SDHB* mutation are at increased risk of malignancy
- **Genotype-phenotype correlation**
  - People with *SDHB*, *SDHD*, and *SDHC* mutations can develop PCCs or PGLs anywhere in paraganglia
    - Genotype-phenotype correlations guiding diagnostic testing and patient care
    - Germline mutations in *SDHB* are strongly associated with extraadrenal sympathetic PGL
    - Chromaffin tumors in people with germline *SDHB* mutations are 6x more likely to be extraadrenal than chromaffin tumors in general
    - PGL in people with germline *SDHB* mutation are more likely to become malignant than sporadic PGL or in those with germline *SDHD* and *SDHC* mutations
    - *SDHB* mutations also predict shorter survival
    - Up to 50% of people with malignant extraadrenal PGL have a germline *SDHB* mutation PGL
    - People with a germline *SDHD* mutation are more likely to develop head and neck and abdominal PGL compared with people with a germline *SDHB* mutation
    - Germline *SDHC* mutations appear to be primarily associated with head and neck PGL

von Hippel-Lindau Syndrome (VHL)

- Autosomal dominant disorder caused by mutation of *VHL*
- Features include retinal angiomas, central nervous system hemangioblastomas, clear cell renal cell carcinoma, pancreatic endocrine tumors, endolymphatic sac tumors, renal, pancreatic and epididymal cysts, and PCCs
- Occurs in ~ 1/36,000 individuals
- ~ 10-26% of VHL patients develop PCC or PGL, but risk varies between families
  - Frequency of PCC in individuals with VHL is 10-20%
- Mean age of onset of PCC in VHL is ~ 30 years
  - PCCs occur in only 6-9% of individuals with VHL type 1
  - Prevalence of PCC rises to 40-59% in individuals with VHL type 2
  - In type 2C VHL, PCCs are sole manifestation of the syndrome (simplex cases)
- VHL mutations predispose to unilateral or bilateral PCCs and, much less frequently, to sympathetic or parasympathetic PGLs
  - ~ 50% of PCCs are bilateral
- PCCs in VHL secrete primarily norepinephrine and normetanephrine
- ~ 5% Of VHL-related catecholamine secreting tumors become malignant, most commonly extraadrenal sympathetic PGL
  - Only 3% displayed malignant tumors
  - Bilateral PCC was seen in 44% of the patients
  - Mean age at diagnosis of PGL/PCC is 29 years
  - PCC or PGL is 1st manifestation of VHL disease in 30-55% of cases
  - VHL can be distinguished from other hereditary PGL/ PCC syndromes clinically

NF1

- Autosomal dominant disorder caused by mutation of *NF1*
- Major features of NF1 include neurofibromas, café au lait spots, iris hamartomas, and axillary and inguinal freckling
- Gastrointestinal stromal tumors (GISTs) and carcinoid tumors may also occur
- PCCs and PGLs are not among most common manifestations of NF1 but occur in 0.1-5.7% of patients
- PCCs occur in 20-50% of individuals with NF1 and hypertension
- NF1-associated PCCs and PGLs typically have characteristics similar to those of sporadic tumors, with a relatively late mean age of onset and ~ 10% risk of malignancy
- Up to 84% of PCC are unilateral
- Extraadrenal sympathetic PGL can occur
- 95% of patients with NF1 had PCC and 6% had PGL; all PGLs were sympathetic
- 14% of patients displayed bilateral PCC
- 9% developed malignant disease

Carney Triad (CT)

- Rare multitumoral syndrome of unknown etiology
  - Some SDH-deficient GISTs are driven by classical SDH mutations, but precise mechanisms of tumorigenesis in those associated with Carney triad remain unknown

HEREDITARY PARAGANGLIOMA/PHEOCHROMOCYTOMA SYNDROMES

- Usually occurs in young women
- Neoplasms affect stomach, lungs, paraganglionic system, adrenal cortex, and esophagus
  - Triad: Gastric stromal tumor, PGL, and pulmonary chondroma
  - PCC, adrenal cortical adenoma, and esophageal leiomyoma are also associated
  - Multifocal tumors develop in affected organs
- Mean age at presentation with PGL/PCC is 28 years
- 92% present with PGL, including both sympathetic and parasympathetic tumors, and ~ 16% present with PCC
- Multiple PGLs are found in 22% of patients and bilateral PCC in 3%
- Metastasis occurs in 11% of patients

Carney-Stratakis Syndrome

- Mutations in *SDHB*, *SDHC*, and *SDHD* can give rise to Carney-Stratakis syndrome, characterized by dyad of PGLs and GISTs
- 100% of patients had PGL and 1 patient also presented with unilateral PCC, with a mean age of 33 years at presentation
- PGLs occur in head and neck, thorax, and abdomen
- Multiple PGLs, which could be both sympathetic and parasympathetic, were seen in 73% of patients
- None of the tumors were malignant

MEN1

- Caused by mutations in *MEN1* gene
- *MEN1* gene is a 10-exon gene that encodes 610-amino acid protein, menin
- Mutation spectrum
  - > 1,300 different mutations of *MEN1* gene have been characterized
  - Penetrance of *MEN1* is high: 45% by age 30, 82% by age 50, 96% by age 70
  - Spread over entire coding and intronic sequence
    - > 60% truncating mutation, 20% missense mutation, 10% frame deletions or insertions, 10% others
  - Most are inactivating
- Function is unknown; may act as regulator of gene transcription, cell proliferation, apoptosis, and genome stability
- No cases of PGL and only 7 cases of PCC in MEN1 syndrome have been reported in the literature
  - Reported tumors were unilateral in all cases and malignant in 1 case

Other Genes Involved in PGL/PCC

- Several other genes have recently been added to the list (associated with unknown hereditary PGL/PCC)
  - Kinesin family member 1B (*KIF1B*); EGL-9 homolog 1 (*EGLN1*), also termed *PHD2*; transmembrane protein 127 (*TMEM127*); and *MYC*-associated factor X (*MAX*)
- No specific syndrome has been attributed yet, but patients with germline *KIF1Bβ* mutations seem to be predisposed to at least PCCs and neuroblastomas
  - Ganglioneuroma, leiomyosarcoma, and lung adenocarcinoma have also been reported in a family with *KIF1Bβ* mutations
- Only 1 PGL patient, suffering from recurrent PGL and erythrocytosis, has been reported to have a germline mutation in *EGLN1*
  - Presentation with sympathetic PGL and a recurrent tumor was diagnosed 3 years later, but no metastases have been reported
- So far, no specific syndrome has been described for *TMEM127*
  - *TMEM127* mutations were identified in 2% of the cases considered sporadic, all of which had PCC
  - 96% of patients have PCC and 39% have bilateral PCC
- *MAX* mutations segregate with disease in families with PCC, but no specific syndrome has been described yet
  - Usually bilateral tumors, early age of onset, &/or familial antecedents with the disease
  - Notably, 25% of patients showed metastasis at diagnosis, suggesting that *MAX* mutations are associated with high risk of malignancy
  - So far, no studies on PGLs have been reported

CLINICAL IMPLICATIONS AND ANCILLARY TESTS

Immunohistochemistry

- SDHA and SDHB are important surrogate markers to triage patients for genetic testing
  - Identifying the ~ 15% of PGL/PCC associated with mitochondrial complex 2 dysfunction, immunohistochemistry for SDHB is a vital tool for triaging genetic testing
    - Yield is particularly high in extraadrenal PCC/PGL
- SDHB immunoexpression is lost in PGL and PCC with *SDHA*, *SDHB*, *SDHC*, and *SDHD* mutation
- SDHA protein is lost when *SDHA* is mutated
- Endothelial cells and sustentacular cells serve as intrinsic positive controls
- Any PGL/PCC should be considered potentially hereditary until this possibility is excluded
- High rate of malignant behavior of *SDHB* mutated PGL/PCC is emphasized and recognition of *SDHB* mutation should lead to more aggressive surgery and surveillance
  - Particularly if compared to tumors arising in MEN2 and VHL syndrome
    - More commonly bilateral but have a low risk of metastasis

Diagnosis/Testing

- **Molecular genetics**
  - Diagnosis/testing
    - Diagnosis based on physical examination, family history, imaging studies, biochemical testing, and molecular genetic testing
    - *SDHD*, *SDHC*, and *SDHB*: 3 nuclear genes responsible for hereditary PGL/PCC syndromes, encode 3 of 4 subunits of mitochondrial enzyme succinate dehydrogenase (SDH)

  - 4th nuclear gene, *SDHAF2* (a.k.a. *SDH5*) encodes a protein that appears to be required for flavination of another SDH subunit, SDHA
  - Molecular genetic testing for disease-causing variants in *SDHD, SDHC,* and *SDHB* is clinically available
- MEN1 mutational analysis should be undertaken in
  - Index case with ≥ 2 MEN1-associated endocrine tumors
  - Asymptomatic 1st-degree relative
  - 1st-degree relative of *MEN1* mutation carrier
  - In patient with suspicious or atypical MEN1
  - Genetic counseling useful for individuals and families with nonclassic MEN1 presentations

ASSOCIATED NEOPLASMS

MEN2

- MEN2A: Characterized by medullary thyroid carcinoma, PCC, and hyperparathyroidism
- MEN2B: Lacks hyperparathyroidism but includes mucocutaneous neuromas &/or diffuse ganglioneuromatosis of gastroenteric mucosa, slender body habitus, joint laxity, and skeletal malformations

Familial PGL/PCC Syndromes

- *SDHB* mutations in particular may predispose to thyroid and renal cancer, and possibly other tumors
- GIST

VHL Syndrome

- Retinal angiomas, central nervous system hemangioblastomas, clear cell renal cell carcinoma, pancreatic endocrine tumors, endolymphatic sac tumors, renal, pancreatic, and epididymal cysts, and PCCs

NF1

- Neurofibromas, café au lait spots, iris hamartomas, and axillary and inguinal freckling
- Optic nerve glioma, duodenal neuroendocrine tumors, bone lesions

Carney Triad

- Extraadrenal sympathetic PGL, gastric stromal sarcoma, and pulmonary chondroma

Carney-Stratakis Syndrome

- Association of PGLs and GISTs (dyad)

Other Genes Involved In PGL/PCC

- Ganglioneuroma, leiomyosarcoma, and lung adenocarcinoma have also been reported in a family with *KIF1Bβ* mutations

CANCER RISK MANAGEMENT

RET-Associated PGL/PCC

- Activating mutations predispose to PCCs, which are often bilateral (63%), and only 3% are malignant
- PGL are rare in MEN2

VHL-Associated PGL/PCC

- *VHL* mutations predispose to unilateral or bilateral PCCs: Bilateral in 44%, and only 3% were malignant
- In VHL patients with PGL/PCC, 90% had PCC and 19% had PGL

NF1-Associated PGL/PCC

- PCCs and PGLs not among most common tumors in NF1; occur in up to 6% of patients with NF1
- NF1-associated tumors with similar characteristics as sporadic tumors
- ~ 10% are malignant

SDHx-Associated PGL/PCC

- Prevalence of PGL/PCC in this syndrome is unknown, but presently represent ~ 15% of all PGL/PCC
  - 92% are PGL
- Frequently parasympathetic, multifocal in > 55%
- PGL1 (*SDHD*)
  - Mutations in *SDHD* (*PGL1*) demonstrate parent-of origin effects and generally cause disease only when mutation is inherited from father
  - Individual who inherits *SDHD* mutation from his/her mother has low but not negligible risk of developing disease
  - Individual who inherits *SDHD* mutation from his/her father is at high risk of manifesting PGL and, to lesser extent, PCCs
- PGL2 (*SDHAF2*)
  - All parasympathetic PGL and no metastases
- PGL3 (*SDHC*)
  - Rare and associated with parasympathetic PGL (93%); 17% multiple
- PGL4 (*SDHB*)
  - Malignancy associated with *SDHB* mutation
  - Higher morbidity and mortality than mutations in other *SDHx* genes
  - 78% are PGL, 25% are unilateral PCC

Genetic Counseling

- Hereditary PGL/PCC syndromes are inherited in autosomal dominant manner
- Mutations in *SDHD* (PGL1) demonstrate parent-of origin effects and generally cause disease only when mutation is inherited from father
- Each child of individual with hereditary PGL/PCC syndrome has 50% chance of inheriting disease-causing mutation
- Individual who inherits *SDHD* mutation from his/her mother has low but not negligible risk of developing disease
- Individual who inherits *SDHD* mutation from his/her father is at high risk of manifesting PGL and, to lesser extent, PCC
- Prenatal testing for pregnancies at increased risk is possible for families in which disease-causing mutation is known

Patient Evaluation

- Includes detailed family history, including specific knowledge of any relatives with unexplained or incompletely explained sudden death

HEREDITARY PARAGANGLIOMA/PHEOCHROMOCYTOMA SYNDROMES

- Personal medical history for following symptoms of catecholamine excess: Sustained or paroxysmal elevations in blood pressure, headache, episodic profuse sweating, palpitations, pallor, and anxiety
  - Paroxysmal symptoms that may be triggered by changes in body position, increases in intraabdominal pressure, some medications, exercise, or micturition in case of urinary bladder PGLs
    - Urinary bladder PGLs may also be accompanied by painless hematuria
- Head and neck PGLs may present as enlarging masses that are asymptomatic or associated with symptoms of mass effects from size and location of tumors
  - Associated symptoms may include unilateral hearing loss, pulsatile tinnitus, cough, hoarseness of voice, pharyngeal fullness, swallowing difficulty, pain, and problems with tongue motion
- Physical examination directed toward signs suggestive of PGL/PCC
  - Sympathetic PGLs and PCCs: Documentation of elevated blood pressure, tachyarrhythmias or other arrhythmias, and palpable abdominal masses
  - Head and neck PGLs: Head and neck masses

SELECTED REFERENCES

1. Dahia PL: Novel hereditary forms of pheochromocytomas and paragangliomas. Front Horm Res. 41:79-91, 2013
2. Dwight T et al: Familial SDHA mutation associated with pituitary adenoma and pheochromocytoma/paraganglioma. J Clin Endocrinol Metab. 98(6):E1103-8, 2013
3. Elston MS et al: Novel mutation in the TMEM127 gene associated with phaeochromocytoma. Intern Med J. 43(4):449-51, 2013
4. Jafri M et al: Evaluation of SDHB, SDHD and VHL gene susceptibility testing in the assessment of individuals with non-syndromic phaeochromocytoma, paraganglioma and head and neck paraganglioma. Clin Endocrinol (Oxf). 78(6):898-906, 2013
5. Mete O et al: Precursor lesions of endocrine system neoplasms. Pathology. 45(3):316-30, 2013
6. Toledo RA et al: In vivo and in vitro oncogenic effects of HIF2A mutations in pheochromocytomas and paragangliomas. Endocr Relat Cancer. 20(3):349-59, 2013
7. Boguszewski CL et al: Genetic studies in a coexistence of acromegaly, pheochromocytoma, gastrointestinal stromal tumor (GIST) and thyroid follicular adenoma. Arq Bras Endocrinol Metabol. 56(8):507-12, 2012
8. Burnichon N et al: MAX mutations cause hereditary and sporadic pheochromocytoma and paraganglioma. Clin Cancer Res. 18(10):2828-37, 2012
9. Grogan RH et al: Bilateral adrenal medullary hyperplasia associated with an SDHB mutation. J Clin Oncol. 29(8):e200-2, 2011
10. Janeway KA et al: Defects in succinate dehydrogenase in gastrointestinal stromal tumors lacking KIT and PDGFRA mutations. Proc Natl Acad Sci U S A. 108(1):314-8, 2011
11. Jiang S et al: Minireview: the busy road to pheochromocytomas and paragangliomas has a new member, TMEM127. Endocrinology. 152(6):2133-40, 2011
12. Barontini M et al: VHL disease. Best Pract Res Clin Endocrinol Metab. 24(3):401-13, 2010
13. Qin Y et al: Germline mutations in TMEM127 confer susceptibility to pheochromocytoma. Nat Genet. 42(3):229-33, 2010
14. Yao L et al: Spectrum and prevalence of FP/TMEM127 gene mutations in pheochromocytomas and paragangliomas. JAMA. 304(23):2611-9, 2010
15. Yeh IT et al: A germline mutation of the KIF1B beta gene on 1p36 in a family with neural and nonneural tumors. Hum Genet. 124(3):279-85, 2008
16. Recasens M et al: Asymptomatic bilateral adrenal pheochromocytoma in a patient with a germline V804M mutation in the RET proto-oncogene. Clin Endocrinol (Oxf). 67(1):29-33, 2007
17. van Nederveen FH et al: Precursor lesions of the adrenal gland. Pathobiology. 74(5):285-90, 2007
18. Benn DE et al: Clinical presentation and penetrance of pheochromocytoma/paraganglioma syndromes. J Clin Endocrinol Metab. 91(3):827-36, 2006
19. Dahia PL: Evolving concepts in pheochromocytoma and paraganglioma. Curr Opin Oncol. 18(1):1-8, 2006
20. McNicol AM: Histopathology and immunohistochemistry of adrenal medullary tumors and paragangliomas. Endocr Pathol. 17(4):329-36, 2006
21. Valdés G et al: Association of adrenal medullar and cortical nodular hyperplasia: a report of two cases with clinical and morpho-functional considerations. Endocrine. 30(3):389-96, 2006
22. Arum SM et al: A RET mutation with decreased penetrance in the family of a patient with a "sporadic" pheochromocytoma. Endocrine. 28(2):193-8, 2005
23. Dahia PL et al: A HIF1alpha regulatory loop links hypoxia and mitochondrial signals in pheochromocytomas. PLoS Genet. 1(1):72-80, 2005
24. Dahia PL et al: Novel pheochromocytoma susceptibility loci identified by integrative genomics. Cancer Res. 65(21):9651-8, 2005
25. Eisenhofer G et al: Malignant pheochromocytoma: current status and initiatives for future progress. Endocr Relat Cancer. 11(3):423-36, 2004

Diagrammatic Features of Paraganglia and Paraganglioma

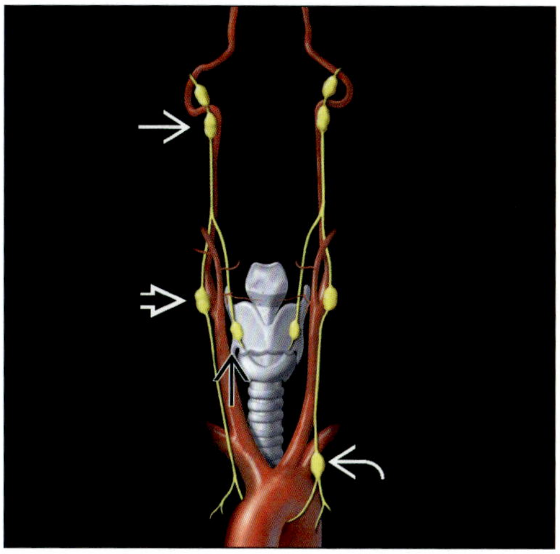

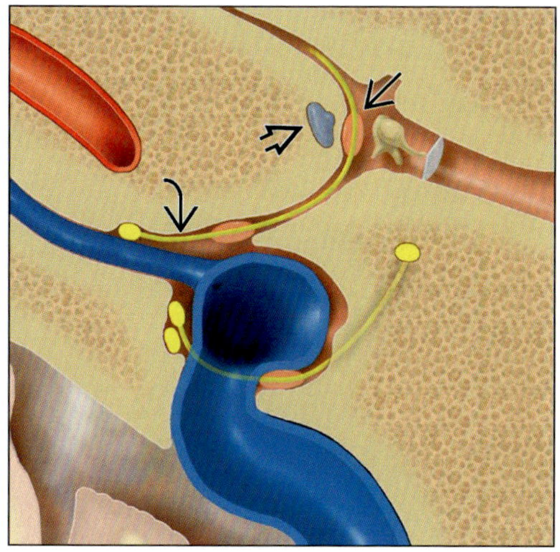

(Left) *Graphic shows paraganglia in head, neck, and upper thorax that are associated with arteries or cranial nerves. They include aortic and carotid bodies and jugulotympanic, vagal, and laryngeal paraganglia.* ***(Right)*** *Axial graphic shows glomus bodies along the course of the inferior tympanic nerve (branch of Jacobsen) on the cochlear promontory. Glomus tympanicum tumors arise from this normal cellular collection. Also note the cochlea.*

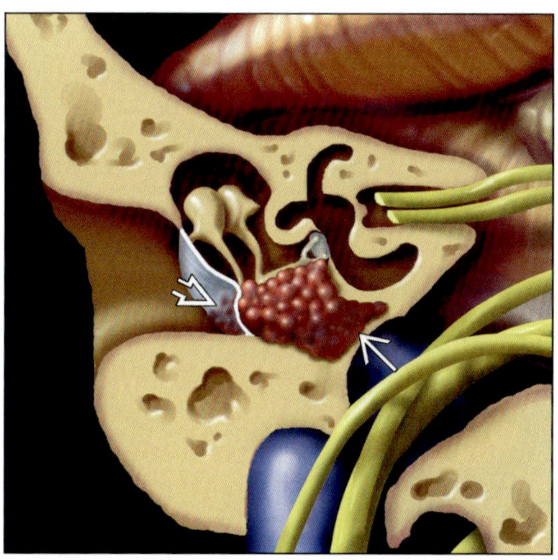

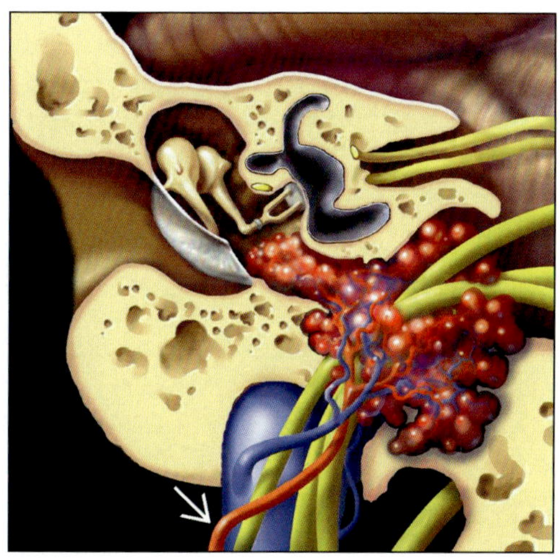

(Left) *Graphic shows a vascular glomus tympanicum PGL pedunculating off the cochlear promontory into the inferior middle ear cavity. The bony floor of the middle ear cavity is intact. The pulsatile tumor mass is behind the lower tympanic membrane.* ***(Right)*** *A glomus jugulare paraganglioma is centered in the jugular foramen with superolateral extension into the middle ear. The main arterial supply for this vascular tumor is the ascending pharyngeal artery.*

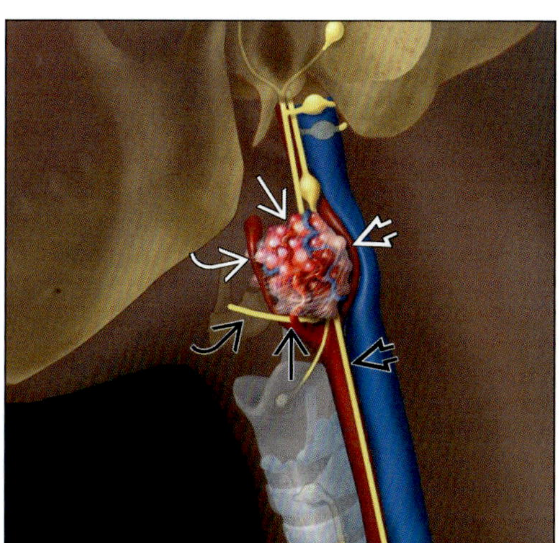

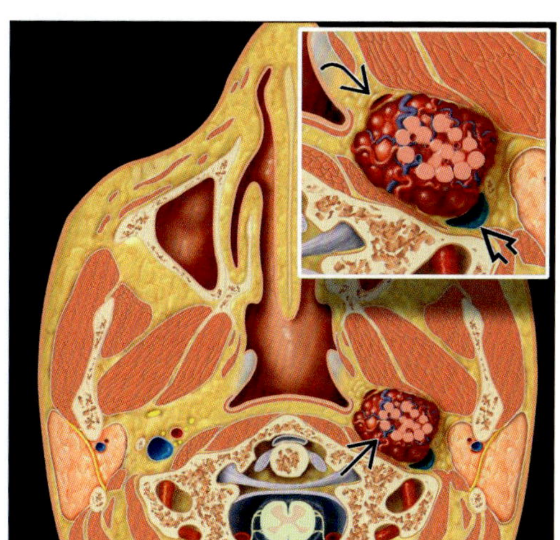

(Left) *Lateral graphic depicts a carotid body paraganglioma at the carotid bifurcation, splaying the ICA and ECA. The main arterial feeder is the ascending pharyngeal artery. The vagus and hypoglossal nerves are in close proximity.* ***(Right)*** *Axial graphic depicts a glomus vagale paraganglioma, located in the nasopharyngeal carotid space. The mass is seen interposed between and displacing the internal carotid artery and jugular vein (inset).*

Pheochromocytoma

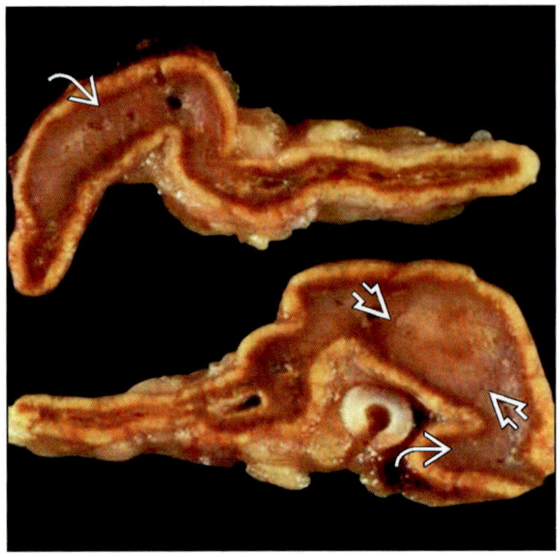

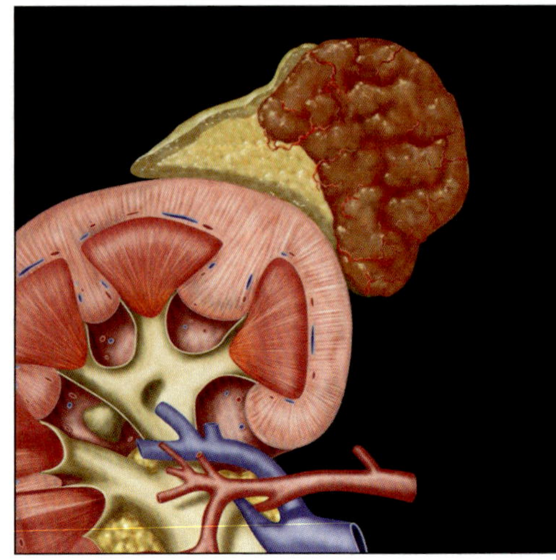

(Left) *Cross section of the adrenal from a patient with multiple endocrine neoplasia type 2A (MEN2A) reveals diffuse medullary expansion, and a well-defined nodule representing a pheochromocytoma (PCC).* ***(Right)*** *This graphic shows a MEN2-associated PCC and associated adrenal medullary hyperplasia, which is characteristically present in adrenal glands of MEN2 patients.*

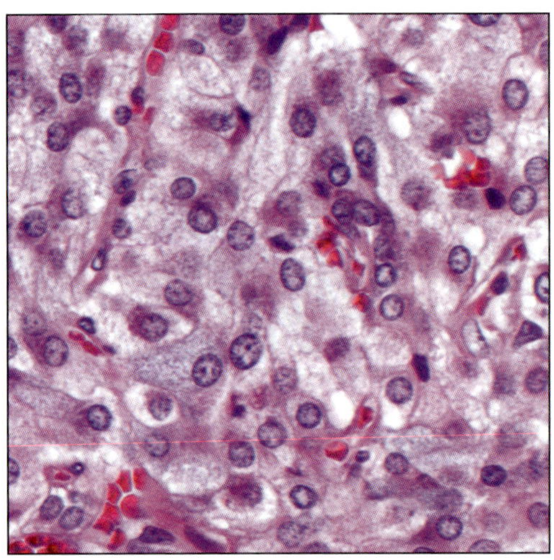

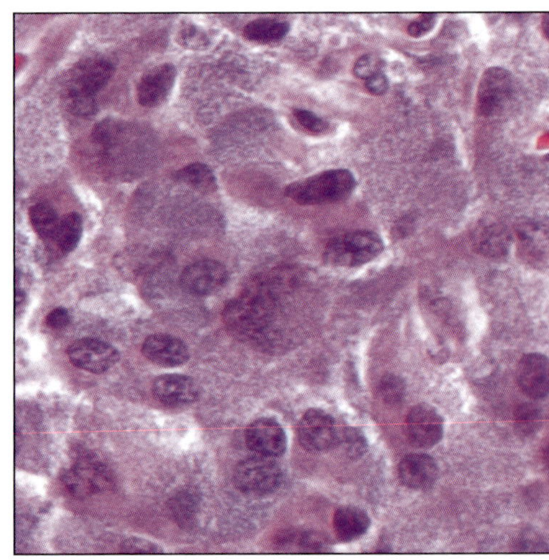

(Left) *Some PCCs show a mosaic-like pattern of cells that have amphophilic to slightly eosinophilic cytoplasm mixed with scattered often large cells with granular basophilic cytoplasm.* ***(Right)*** *Some PCCs show a mosaic-like pattern of often large cells with granular basophilic cytoplasm admixed with cells that have amphophilic to slightly eosinophilic cytoplasm.*

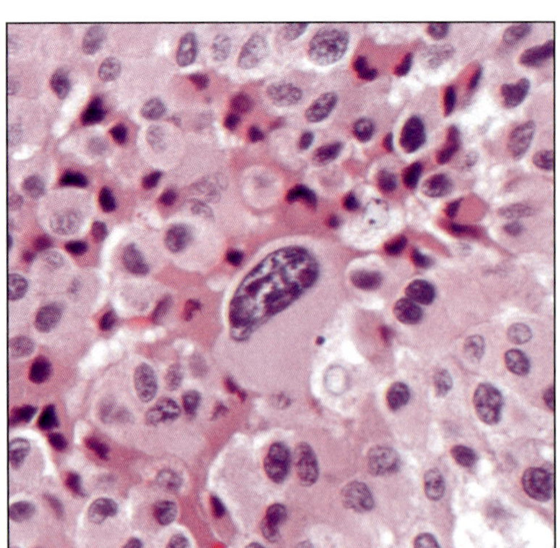

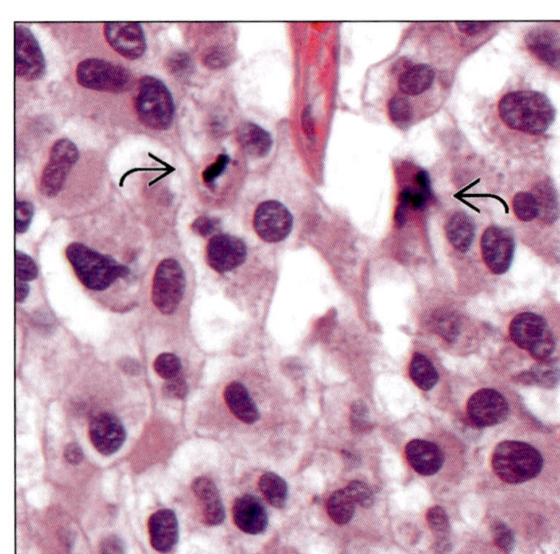

(Left) *Some PCCs lack the organoid pattern and instead may show a diffuse growth pattern. Such PCCs are formed by small cells with ample eosinophilic cytoplasm with occasional bizarre cells.* ***(Right)*** *This tumor from a patient with hereditary familial paraganglioma (PGL) syndrome has a solid, patternless component with large sheets of tumor cells. There is cellular pleomorphism and mitoses.*

Paraganglioma

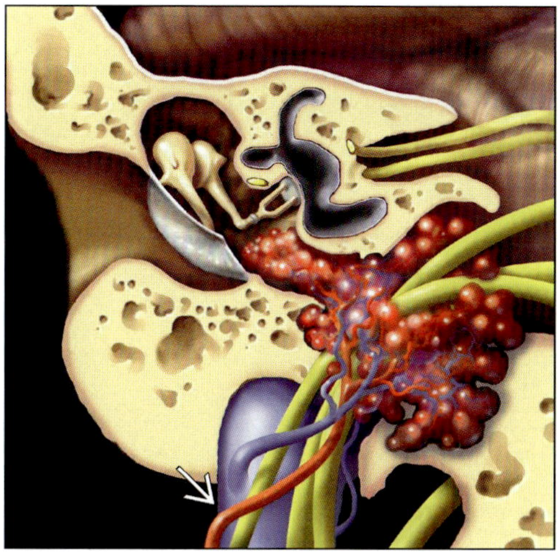

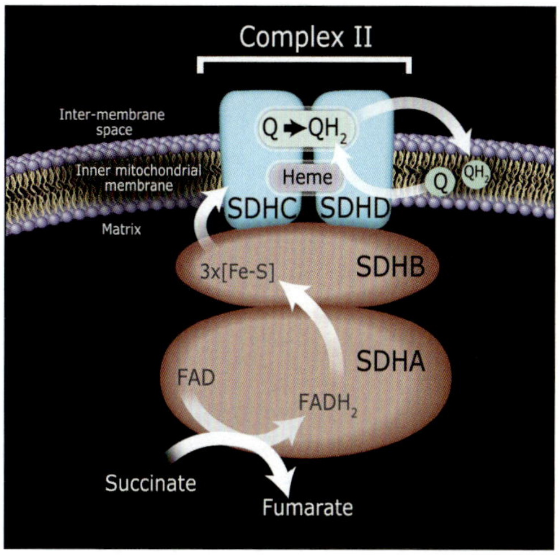

(Left) *Coronal graphic shows glomus jugulare PGL centered in the jugular foramen with superolateral extension into the middle ear. The ascending parapharyngeal artery* ➔ *is feeding this vascular tumor.* ***(Right)*** *Graphic of part of the mitochondrial respiratory chain complex II shows the relationship between the succinate ubiquinone oxidoreductase subunits (SDHA → SDHD). Inactivating mutations result in hereditary PGL.*

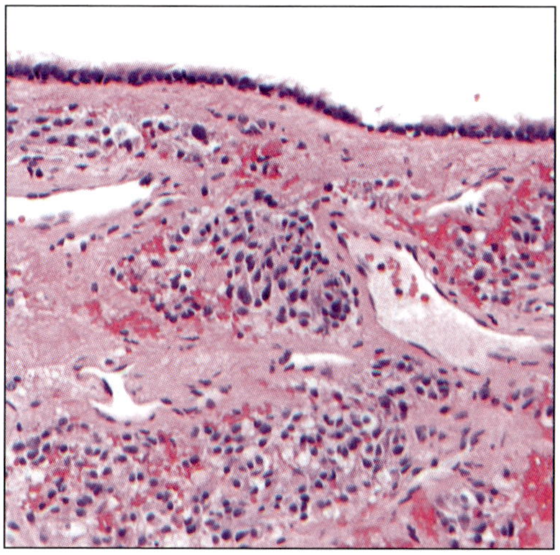

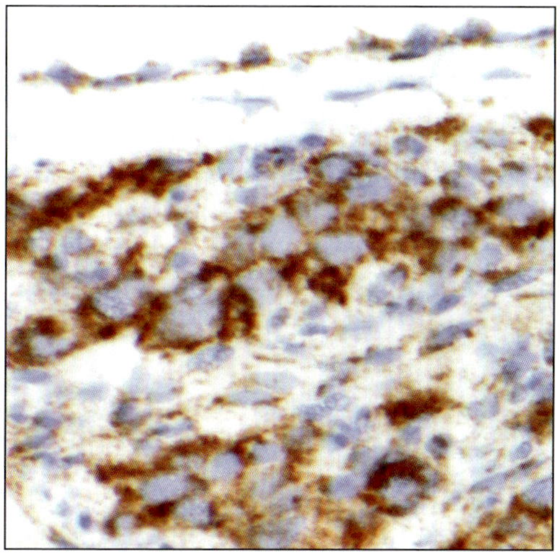

(Left) *This highly vascular glomus jugulare PGL is underneath an intact mucosa and shows groups of neoplastic cells interspersed between the vascular channels.* ***(Right)*** *SDHB immunostaining reveals maintenance of immunoreactivity in a PGL in a MEN2-associated hereditary PGL patient, without SDHB or SDHD mutation. The staining is coarsely granular as the protein is localized in the mitochondria.*

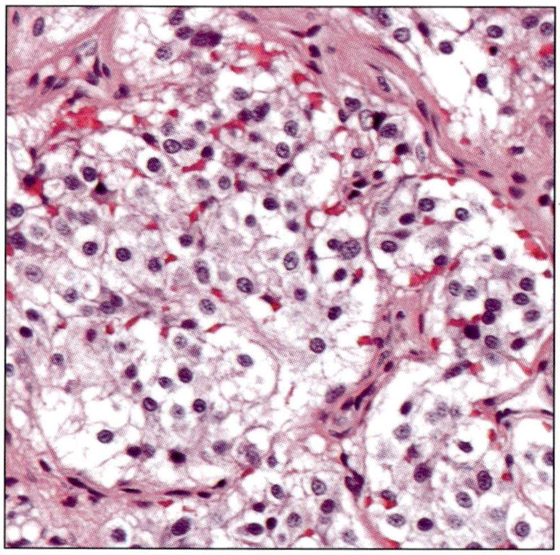

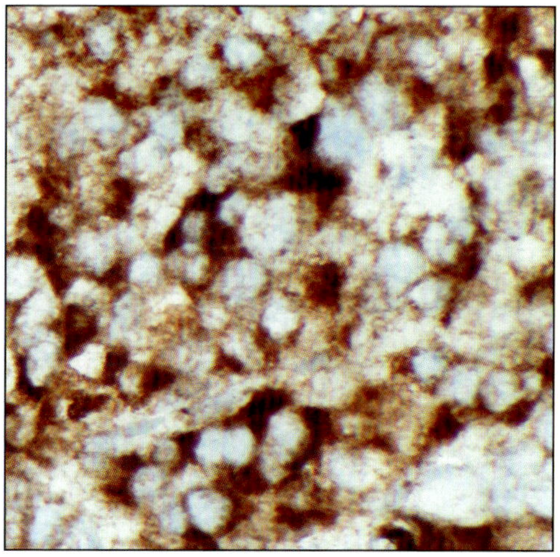

(Left) *This picture shows a PGL with the characteristic alveolar patterns with variably sized nests of tumor cells surrounded by thin-walled vessels. This tumor has a solid component with large sheets of tumor cells.* ***(Right)*** *PCCs and other PGLs without mutations of SDHx genes show immunoreactivity of tumor cell cytoplasm for SDHB protein. The immunoreactivity is granular because the protein is localized to mitochondria.*

HEREDITARY PROSTATE CANCER

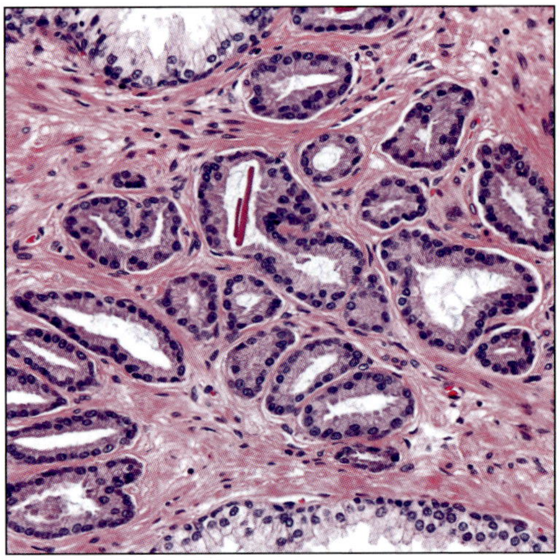

H&E shows Gleason 3 + 3 = 6 prostate cancer. Majority of prostate cancers are diagnosed as low-grade, organ-confined disease with an indolent course.

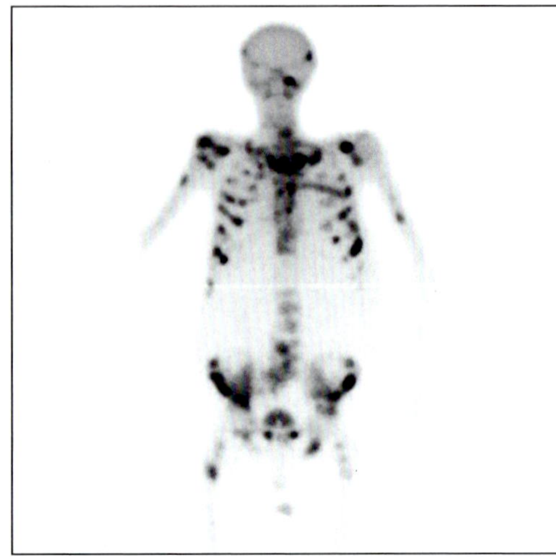

Anterior bone scan shows multiple bony metastases with relative sparing of distal appendicular skeleton. Only < 5% of prostate cancer are diagnosed with metastasis.

TERMINOLOGY

Abbreviations

- Sporadic prostate cancer (SPC)
- Familial prostate cancer (FPC)
- Hereditary prostate cancer (HPC)

Definitions

- **FPC**
  - Affected individuals with ≥ 1 first-degree relative who also has prostate cancer
- **HPC**
  - Subtype of FPC with consistent passage of susceptibility gene via Mendelian inheritance
  - Despite strong evidence for existence of prostate cancer susceptibility genes, no definitive example has been identified so far
  - Clinical criteria for diagnosis of HPC proposed by Carter et al
    - Family with prostate cancer in ≥ 3 first-degree relatives
    - Family with prostate cancer in 3 successive generations from paternal or maternal side
    - Family with 2 first-degree relatives with prostate cancer at age ≤ 55 years
    - Diagnosis of HPC requires any 1 of these 3 criteria

EPIDEMIOLOGY

Incidence

- Prostate cancer is leading cause of cancer mortality and 2nd cause of cancer morbidity in men in the USA
  - Estimated that there will be 238,590 prostate cancer diagnosed in the USA in 2013
- ~ 5-10% of prostate cancer patients can be accounted for by genetic susceptibility
- Identification of true prevalence of FPCs or HPCs difficult due to the very high occurrence rate of prostate cancer

Family History as Risk Factor

- ~ 10-15% of prostate cancer patients have at least 1 relative who also has prostate cancer
- Risk is greater for men with affected brothers than for men with affected fathers
- Risk ↑ with number of relatives affected
  - Risk is higher with first-degree than with second-degree relatives affected
  - Risk is higher with 2 than with 1 first-degree relative affected
- Concordance between monozygotic twins of 27% vs. 7% between dizygotic twins

Age Range

- Peak occurrence of prostate cancer overall is at 65-75 years and median age is 67 years
  - HPC diagnosed ~ 6 to 7 years earlier than SPC
  - Estimated that prostate cancer attributable to high-risk susceptibility alleles is 43% for men diagnosed ≤ 55 years, 34% for men ≤ 70 years, and 9% for men ≤ 85 years old

ETIOLOGY/PATHOGENESIS

Risk Factors

- Major risk factors for prostate cancer are age, ethnicity (black), and family history

Genetics

- Several candidate genes proposed, with *BRCA2* so far being the most consistently replicated in studies
- *BRCA2*-associated prostate cancer
  - **Hereditary breast and ovarian cancer syndrome (HBOC)**

Prostate Cancer Family History Effects on Lifetime Risk

Family History	Relative Risk (%)	Absolute Risk (%)
Negative	1	8
Father with prostate cancer at age ≥ 60 years	1.5	12
1 brother with prostate cancer at age ≥ 60 years	2	15
Father with prostate cancer at age < 60 years	2.5	20
1 brother with prostate cancer at age < 60 years	3	25
2 affected male relatives*	4	30
≥ 3 affected male relatives	5	35-45

Father and brother, 2 brothers, a brother and a maternal grandfather or uncle, or a father and a paternal grandfather or uncle; from Bratt O et al.

Predisposition to Prostate Cancer in Patients With Positive Family History

Locus	Gene	Attributable Risk (%)	Age
1q23-q25 (HPC1)	*RNASEL*	4-13	Early
1q42.2-43 (PCAP)	*PCTA-1*	40-50	Early
8q24	Unknown	-	-
8q24	HapC	11-31	-
8q24	*POU5F1P1*	21	-
13q12	*BRCA2*	5%	Early
17p11 (HPC2)	*ELAC2*	0.5-4	Early
Xq27-28 (HPCX)	Unknown	16	-

    - Caused by inherited mutation in *BRCA2,* and manifests clinically with mutation in the other allele (Knudson "2-hit" hypothesis)
    - In women, mutations confer up to 87% lifetime risk of breast cancer and up to 54% risk of ovarian cancer
    - In men, mutations confer 7% risk of breast cancer
    - Also increase risk for prostate cancer, pancreatic cancer, and melanoma
  - *BRCA2* carriers have cumulative risk for prostate cancer of 16% vs. 3.8% for noncarriers
  - Seems to contribute to a very small minority of prostate cancer risk with prevalence rate of only < 1%
- Other candidate genes
  - Studies show conflicting results

CLINICAL IMPLICATIONS

Clinical Presentation

- Pre-radical prostatectomy PSA level higher in HPC than in FPC and SPC
- Clinical features and long-term oncological outcomes are similar post-radical prostatectomy in patients with FPC, HPC, and SPC
- Some studies suggest BRCA-associated prostate cancers have a more aggressive phenotype

PATHOLOGICAL FEATURES

Gross and Microscopic Features

- So far, no differences have been described in gross or microscopic features of tumors in FPC, HPC, and SPC
- Multifocality, a common trait for familial tumors in general, is frequent in sporadic prostate cancers

CANCER RISK MANAGEMENT

BRCA2 Mutation

- In men not selected for family history, *BRCA2* contributes to a very small minority of prostate cancer risk (< 1%)
- Unclear benefit of screening for this mutation in men

SELECTED REFERENCES

1. Banks KC et al: 10 rare tumors that warrant a genetics referral. Fam Cancer. 12(1):1-18, 2013
2. Alvarez-Cubero MJ et al: Genetic analysis of the principal genes related to prostate cancer: A review. Urol Oncol. Epub ahead of print, 2012
3. Bambury RM et al: Prostate cancer: germline prediction for a commonly variable malignancy. BJU Int. 110(11 Pt C):E809-18, 2012
4. Colloca G et al: The evolving role of familial history for prostate cancer. Acta Oncol. 50(1):14-24, 2011
5. Gallagher DJ et al: Genitourinary cancer predisposition syndromes. Hematol Oncol Clin North Am. 24(5):861-83, 2010
6. Kiemeney LA et al: Screening for prostate cancer in Dutch hereditary prostate cancer families. Int J Cancer. 122(4):871-6, 2008
7. Siddiqui SA et al: Impact of familial and hereditary prostate cancer on cancer specific survival after radical retropubic prostatectomy. J Urol. 176(3):1118-21, 2006
8. Bratt O et al: Hereditary prostate cancer: clinical characteristics and survival. J Urol. 167(6):2423-6, 2002
9. Bratt O: Hereditary prostate cancer: clinical aspects. J Urol. 168(3):906-13, 2002

HEREDITARY RENAL EPITHELIAL TUMORS, OTHERS

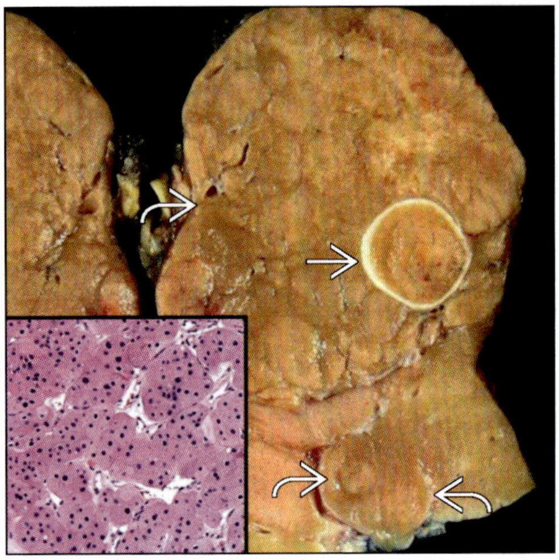

Kidney shows multiple renal oncocytomas (ROs) ➡. A possible 4th tumor is present encased within the larger RO ➡. RO is characterized by tumor cells with abundant eosinophilic cytoplasm and uniform round nuclei (inset).

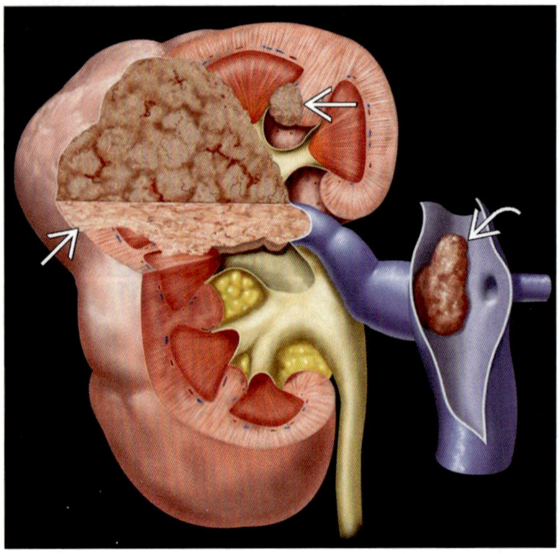

Graphic shows heterogeneous, vascular, expansile RCC from the renal cortex, invading the renal vein and IVC ➡. Tumor is multicentric ➡, as is the case in up to 5% of sporadic RCCs (and higher for familial cases).

TERMINOLOGY

Abbreviations

- Clear cell renal cell carcinoma (CCRCC)
- Papillary renal cell carcinoma (PRCC)
- Chromophobe renal cell carcinoma (CHRCC)
- Renal oncocytoma (RO)

Definitions

- **Familial renal tumor**
  - Families with ≥ 2 members within 2 generations with renal tumor and no evidence of known hereditary renal tumor syndrome
  - Reported mostly in CCRCC and also in ROs, PRCC, and CHRCC

FAMILIAL RENAL ONCOCYTOMA

Definition

- Familial renal tumor with affected individuals predisposed to develop bilateral and multifocal ROs

General Features

- Rare, described in ~ 30 families
- Between 2 and 4 affected family members
- Patient age: 38-83 years old (median: 49, mean: 55)
  - Younger onset than in sporadic renal oncocytoma
- More common in males (M:F = 4:1)
- Partial or complete loss of Chr 1 most frequent
  - Chromosomal changes less frequently observed compared to sporadic ROs
- Most ROs detected incidentally or by screening of affected family members
- For unclear reason, some patients develop renal insufficiency that progresses into end-stage kidney disease
- Some affected individuals have pulmonary cysts; association unclear

Renal Tumor

- Has benign outcome; no reported malignant transformation
- Not known if affected individuals have predisposition for renal oncocytosis or hybrid oncocytic tumor

CONSTITUTIONAL CHROMOSOME 3 TRANSLOCATION

Definition

- Hereditary renal tumor characterized by Chr 3 translocation and predisposition for CCRCC

Synonym

- Familial non-VHL, nonpapillary, CCRCC

General Features

- Rare, so far 13 different constitutional translocations identified
  - 7 translocations associated with familial disease
    - t(3;8)(p14;q24), t(2;3)(q35;q21), t(3;6)(q12;q15), t(2;3)(q33;q21), t(1;3)(q32;q13.3), t(3;8)(p13;q24), and t(3;8)(p14;q24.1)
    - Candidate genes: *FHIT*, *TRC8*, *DIRC1*, *DIRC2*, *DIRC3*, *HSPBAP1*, *LSAMP*, *NORE1*, *KCNIP4*, and *FBXW7*
- Affected individuals predisposed to multifocal and bilateral CCRCC
- Lifetime risk in some families: > 80%; however, in absence of family history, Chr 3 translocation carriers are not at high risk of developing CCRCC
- Between 2 and 5 affected family members
- Patient age: 9-92 years old (median: 54, mean: 53)
  - Younger onset than sporadic CCRCC
- M:F = 1.8:1
- "3-hit" model of tumorigenesis proposed
  - Germline Chr 3 translocation

- Nondisjunctional loss of derivative chromosome carrying 3p segment
  - Somatic mutation in remaining 3p allele of ≥ 1 CCRCC tumor suppressor gene (e.g., *VHL*)
- No known extrarenal manifestations, including those encountered in VHL
  - Few affected individuals (3%) also developed breast cancer
- Annual surveillance not recommended unless there is personal or family history of clear cell RCC &/or tumor suppressor gene mutation

Renal Tumor

- CCRCC

FAMILIAL CLEAR CELL RCC

Definition

- Familial renal tumor with predisposition for clear cell RCC and with no identifiable genetic factor

General Features

- Currently, a diagnosis of exclusion of other hereditary causes of CCRCC
  - Exclude von Hippel-Lindau disease, chromosome 3 translocation, Birt-Hogg-Dubé syndrome, and tuberous sclerosis complex
- Rare, so far ~ 70 families with familial CCRCC reported with no identifiable genetic factor
- Perhaps has a multigenic inheritance mechanism
- More common in males (M:F = 1.9:1)
- Later onset, compared to other familial renal tumors
  - 1 family member develops CCRCC between 50 to 70 years
- Most patients present with solitary tumor
- Suggested management dependent on size to renal tumor; observation if < 3 cm (similar to VHL patients)
  - Conservative surgery, such as partial nephrectomy or enucleation if amenable

Renal Tumor

- CCRCC

HEREDITARY HYPERPARATHYROIDISM-JAW TUMOR SYNDROME

Definition

- Hereditary autosomal dominant disorder characterized by functional parathyroid neoplasm and ossifying fibroma of jaw with increased risk for renal and uterine tumors

General Features

- Very rare; largest study involved 19 affected family members
  - Patient age range: 3-63 years old
- Autosomal dominant inheritance
- Tumor suppressor gene identified as *CDC73* or *HRPT2* located at Chr 1q25-31 and encodes for parafibromin protein
- No germline mutations in *MEN1*
- Parathyroid neoplasm often functional parathyroid adenoma that can be multifocal
  - ~ 15% may have parathyroid carcinoma
- ~ 75% may have uterine neoplasm, such as adenofibromas, leiomyomas or adenomyosis, or adenosarcomas
- ~ 15% may have renal tumors
- Patients may also have renal hamartomas or polycystic kidney disease

Renal Tumor

- PRCC
- Wilms tumor
- Renal cortical adenoma
- Benign epithelial cysts

PAPILLARY THYROID CARCINOMA WITH ASSOCIATED NEOPLASIA

Definition

- Inherited renal tumor syndrome characterized by papillary thyroid cancer, nodular thyroid disease, and renal tumor

General Features

- Rare, ~ 5% of papillary thyroid carcinoma overall has familial association
- Autosomal dominant inheritance with age-dependent penetrance
- Women more affected than men
- Linked to Chr 1q21
- Specific gene not yet identified; potential candidates include *NRAS* and *NTRK1*
- No germline mutations in *MET* proto-oncogene present

Renal Tumor

- PRCC
- Multifocal papillary adenomas
- Renal oncocytoma reported in 1 patient

FAMILIAL NONCLEAR CELL RCC

General Features

- Familial renal tumor with no identifiable genetic factor, also described with PRCC and CHRCC
- 1 report from NIH of 68 affected individuals with familial renal tumor included
  - 54% CCRCC (familial CCRCC)
  - 16% RO (familial RO)
  - 12% PRCC
  - 4% CHRCC

SELECTED REFERENCES

1. Shuch B et al: The surgical approach to multifocal renal cancers: hereditary syndromes, ipsilateral multifocality, and bilateral tumors. Urol Clin North Am. 39(2):133-48, v, 2012

HEREDITARY RENAL EPITHELIAL TUMORS, OTHERS

Hereditary or Familial Renal Tumor Syndromes

Syndrome	Gene	Chromosome	Gene Product	Renal Tumor
von Hippel-Lindau	*VHL*	3p25-26	pVHL	Clear cell RCC and clear cell tumorlets
Hereditary papillary RCC	*MET*	7q31	MET	Papillary RCC type 1
Hereditary leiomyomatosis and renal cancer	*FH*	1q42-43	Fumarate hydratase	Papillary RCC, NOS (mostly classified as papillary RCC type 2 previously)
Birt-Hogg-Dubé	*FLCN* or *BHD*	17p11.2	Folliculin	Hybrid oncocytic tumor, renal oncocytoma, renal oncocytosis, chromophobe RCC, and clear cell RCC
Familial oncocytoma	Unknown	Unknown	Unknown	Renal oncocytoma (association with renal oncocytosis or hybrid oncocytic tumor not known)
Tuberous sclerosis	*TSC1*	9q34	Hamartin	Angiomyolipoma, clear cell RCC, benign epithelial cyst, and renal oncocytoma
	TSC2	16p13.3	Tuberin	
Succinate dehydrogenase B-associated hereditary paraganglioma/ pheochromocytoma	*SDHB*	1p36	SDHB	RCC, NOS (mostly classified as renal oncocytoma previously)
Constitutional chromosome 3 translocation	Unknown; candidate genes: *FHIT, TRC8, DIRC1, DIRC2, DIRC3, HSPBAP1, LSAMP, NORE1, KCNIP4,* and *FBXW7*	Unknown	Unknown	Clear cell RCC
Familial clear cell RCC	Unknown	Unknown	Unknown	Clear cell RCC
Hereditary hyperparathyroidism-jaw tumor syndrome	*CDC73* or *HRPT2*	1q25-31	Parafibromin	Papillary RCC, Wilms tumor, cortical adenoma, and benign epithelial cyst
Papillary thyroid carcinoma with associated neoplasia	Unknown; potential candidate genes: *NRAS* and *NTRK1*	1q21	Unknown	Papillary RCC and papillary adenoma; possibly renal oncocytoma

2. Singer EA et al: Outcomes of patients with surgically treated bilateral renal masses and a minimum of 10 years of followup. J Urol. 188(6):2084-8, 2012
3. Verine J et al: Hereditary renal cancer syndromes: an update of a systematic review. Eur Urol. 58(5):701-10, 2010
4. Woodward ER et al: Population-based survey of cancer risks in chromosome 3 translocation carriers. Genes Chromosomes Cancer. 49(1):52-8, 2010
5. Kuiper RP et al: The tumor suppressor gene FBXW7 is disrupted by a constitutional t(3;4)(q21;q31) in a patient with renal cell cancer. Cancer Genet Cytogenet. 195(2):105-11, 2009
6. Linehan WM et al: Hereditary kidney cancer: unique opportunity for disease-based therapy. Cancer. 115(10 Suppl):2252-61, 2009
7. Newey PJ et al: Parafibromin--functional insights. J Intern Med. 266(1):84-98, 2009
8. Woodward ER et al: Familial non-VHL clear cell (conventional) renal cell carcinoma: clinical features, segregation analysis, and mutation analysis of FLCN. Clin Cancer Res. 14(18):5925-30, 2008
9. Zbar B et al: Familial renal carcinoma: clinical evaluation, clinical subtypes and risk of renal carcinoma development. J Urol. 177(2):461-5; discussion 465, 2007
10. Eleveld MJ et al: Molecular analysis of a familial case of renal cell cancer and a t(3;6)(q12;q15). Genes Chromosomes Cancer. 31(1):23-32, 2001
11. Junker K et al: Familial and sporadic renal oncocytomas--a comparative molecular-genetic analysis. Eur Urol. 40(3):330-6, 2001
12. Podolski J et al: Characterization of a familial RCC-associated t(2;3)(q33;q21) chromosome translocation. J Hum Genet. 46(12):685-93, 2001
13. Haven CJ et al: A genotypic and histopathological study of a large Dutch kindred with hyperparathyroidism-jaw tumor syndrome. J Clin Endocrinol Metab. 85(4):1449-54, 2000
14. Malchoff CD et al: Papillary thyroid carcinoma associated with papillary renal neoplasia: genetic linkage analysis of a distinct heritable tumor syndrome. J Clin Endocrinol Metab. 85(5):1758-64, 2000
15. Malchoff CD et al: Familial papillary thyroid carcinoma is genetically distinct from familial adenomatous polyposis coli. Thyroid. 9(3):247-52, 1999
16. Bodmer D et al: An alternative route for multistep tumorigenesis in a novel case of hereditary renal cell cancer and a t(2;3)(q35;q21) chromosome translocation. Am J Hum Genet. 62(6):1475-83, 1998
17. Weirich G et al: Familial renal oncocytoma: clinicopathological study of 5 families. J Urol. 160(2):335-40, 1998
18. Cohen AJ et al: Hereditary renal-cell carcinoma associated with a chromosomal translocation. N Engl J Med. 301(11):592-5, 1979

Associated Neoplasms

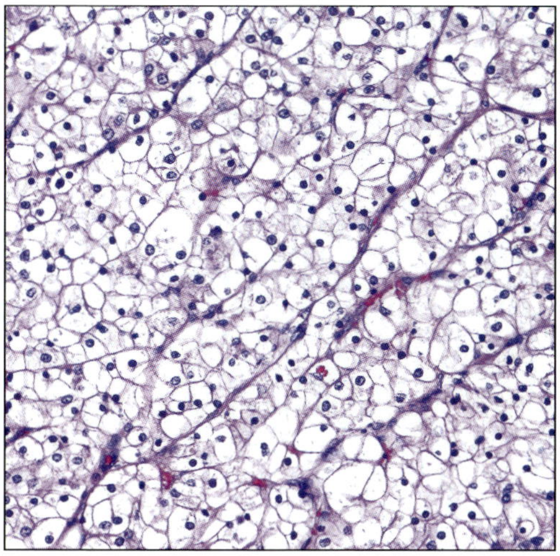
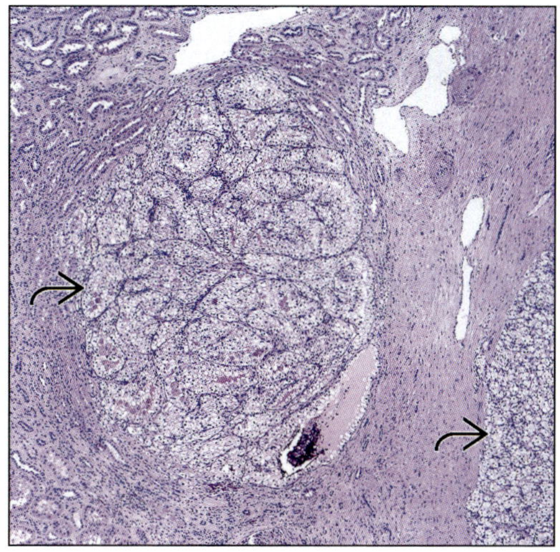

(Left) *CCRCC typically shows tumor cells with optically clear cytoplasm because of lipid and glycogen contents. Tumor cells are arranged in solid nests separated by intricate meshwork of delicate vasculatures imparting a chicken-wire appearance.* ***(Right)*** *Kidney section shows multiple small CCRCCs. Multifocal and bilateral CCRCCs are common in hereditary RCCs such as VHL and in constitutional Chr 3 translocation patients. Familial CCRCC tends to present with solitary tumor.*

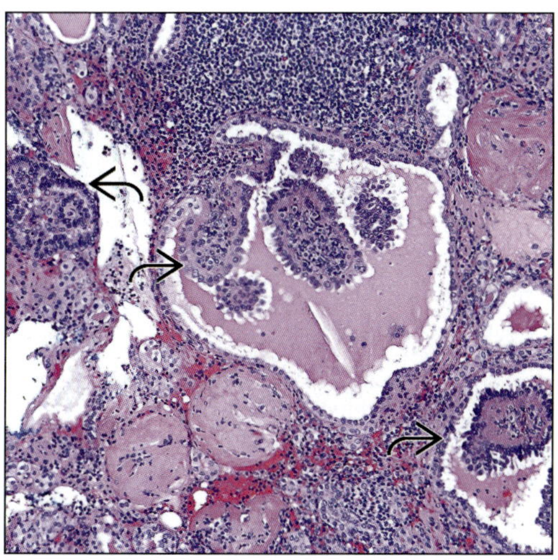
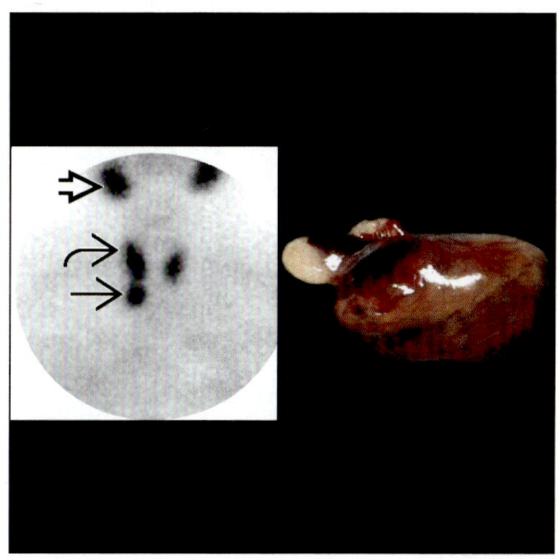

(Left) *Kidney with multiple papillary adenomas (PAs) is seen in papillary thyroid carcinoma with associated neoplasia. PAs exhibit simple papillae lined by small cuboidal cells with low-grade nuclei. Cytology resembles PRCC type 1 cells and is distinguished only by size (> 5 mm).* ***(Right)*** *Tc-99m MIBI shows parathyroid adenoma inferior to the inferior pole of the right thyroid lobe. Activity is also evident in salivary glands. Gross specimen shows encapsulated brown-tan parathyroid adenoma.*

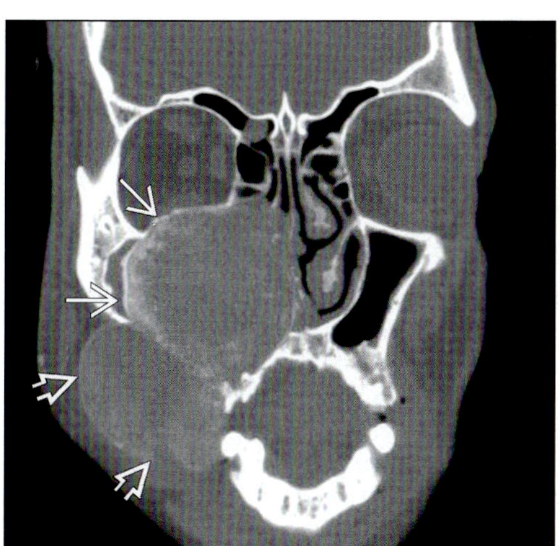
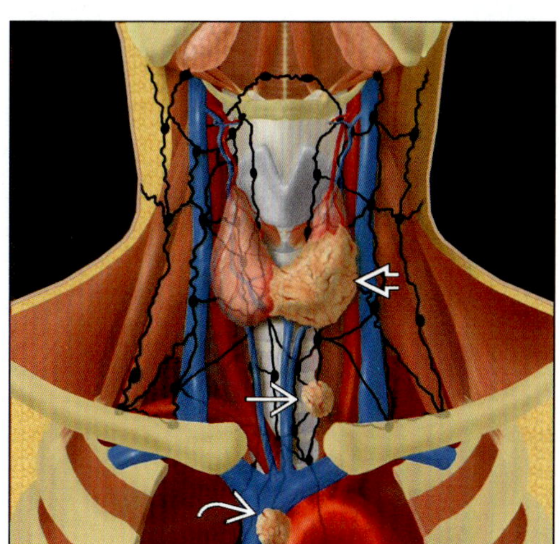

(Left) *Coronal bone CT demonstrates a very large, bilobed, ossifying fibroma with a large maxillary antral portion and smaller component extending into the buccal space. Peripheral ossification of the maxillary component is noted.* ***(Right)*** *Coronal graphic illustrates a left thyroid lobe differentiated thyroid carcinoma with metastatic nodal disease in the left paratracheal chain and superior mediastinum.*

HEREDITARY RETINOBLASTOMA

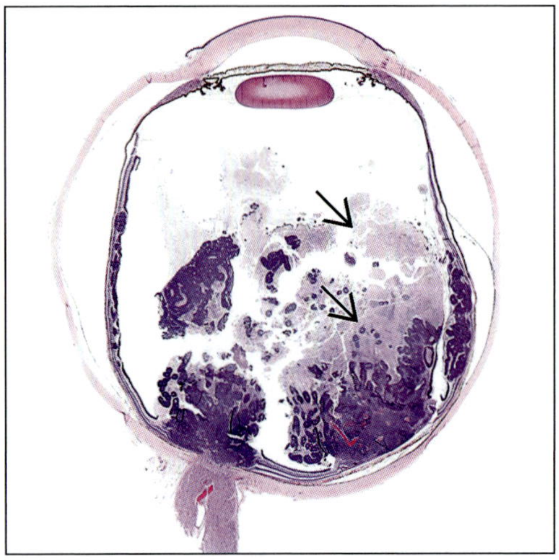

Retinoblastoma is a proliferative tumor with frequent necrosis ⇒, centered in the retina. It is the main tumor developing in patients with germline RB1 mutations.

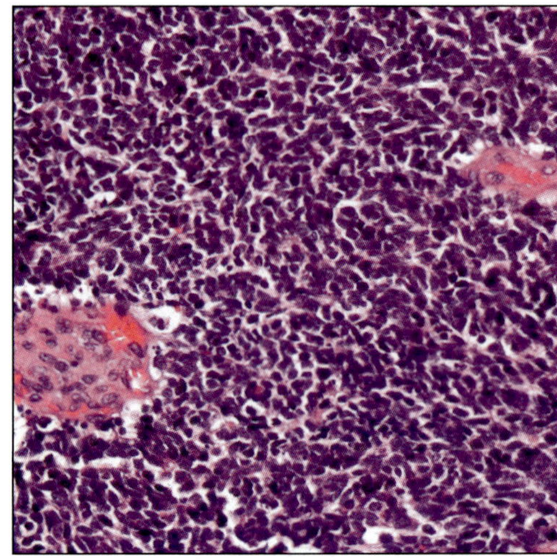

Retinoblastoma is histologically a round blue cell tumor, highly cellular, and composed of sheets or nests of proliferative neoplastic cells.

TERMINOLOGY

Definition

- Familial cancer syndrome with predisposition for retinoblastoma development, often multiple, and other cancers resulting from germline mutations in tumor suppressor gene *RB1*

EPIDEMIOLOGY

Retinoblastoma

- Most common intraocular malignancy in children
  - Incidence: 1 in 15,000-34,000 births
  - No gender or ethnic predilection

GENETICS

Germline Mutations in *RB1* Gene

- Located at chromosomal region 13q14
- 5-10% of retinoblastomas inherited in autosomal dominant fashion
- Autosomal dominant inheritance with high penetrance
  - 60-80% of carriers develop retinoblastomas
- *RB1* encodes for ubiquitously expressed nuclear protein
  - Important role in cell cycle control, cellular differentiation, and survival
  - Undergoes phosphorylation in cell cycle-dependent fashion
  - Regulator of restriction (R) point of cell cycle
    - Unphosphorylated (active) in G_0 → hypophosphorylated in G_1 → hyperphosphorylated (inactive) as cell passes through R point → dephosphorylated (reactivated) by PP1 phosphatase at M/G_1 transition
- 13q-deletion syndrome (< 5% of retinoblastomas)
  - Retinoblastoma in association with moderate growth and mental retardation, facial abnormalities, microphthalmia, cardiac anomalies, anal atresia, colobomas, cataracts, and muscle hypotonia
- Germline *RB1* mutations in 25% of retinoblastoma patients without family history (i.e., new mutations)
  - Progeny may be affected
- Polymorphisms in other genes may affect risk for retinoblastoma development (e.g., *MDM2*, *MDM4*)

Somatic Mutations in *RB1*

- Reported in sarcomas, small cell lung carcinoma, bladder carcinoma, and breast carcinoma
- Promoter hypermethylation (epigenetic inactivation) in astrocytomas and lymphoma subsets

Knudson "2-Hit" Hypothesis

- Model for classic tumor suppressor genes
- 2 inactivating mutations required for tumor development
- 1st mutation may be either somatic (sporadic) or germinal (inherited)
- 2nd mutation is sporadic

CLINICAL IMPLICATIONS AND ANCILLARY TESTS

Presentation and Complications

- Earlier age of presentation for hereditary retinoblastoma
  - Mean age at presentation of sporadic retinoblastoma: 18-24 months
  - Mean age at presentation of hereditary retinoblastoma: 12 months
- Sporadic retinoblastoma is usually unilateral whereas hereditary retinoblastoma is often bilateral (~ 60%)
- Increased risk for 2nd primary tumors, particularly craniofacial locations

- ~ 70% of 2nd primaries develop in irradiation field or at boundary
  - Median age of presentation: 13 years for craniofacial location, but risk continues through life
  - Risk highest for patients receiving external beam radiotherapy in 1st year of life
  - Addition of chemotherapy also increases risk
  - Extent of resection important prognostic factor
- 2nd primary tumors are leading cause of death in hereditary retinoblastoma patients in developed countries
  - Higher risk of 2nd primary malignancies in patients with recurrent nonsense *RB1* mutations compared with low penetrance mutations in some studies
  - No significant increase in mortality due to nonneoplastic disorders

MICROSCOPIC FINDINGS

Retinoblastoma

- Small round blue cell tumor
  - Evidence of retinoblastic differentiation: Flexner-Wintersteiner rosettes and fleurettes
  - Homer Wright (neuroblastic) rosettes may also be present
  - Necrosis and calcifications common
  - May invade optic nerve and secondarily brain and CSF

ASSOCIATED NEOPLASMS

Retinoma/Retinocytoma

- Composed entirely of photoreceptor differentiation
  - Lacks mitotic activity and necrosis
- Usually benign, but may develop malignant transformation into retinoblastoma
- Inactivation of both *RB1* gene copies, but lacks additional alterations typical of retinoblastoma

Pineoblastoma/CNS PNET

- Part of "trilateral" retinoblastoma syndrome (bilateral retinoblastoma + pineoblastoma or suprasellar PNET)
- Occurs in < 1% of patients with retinoblastoma
- Intracranial tumor frequently (~ 80%) in pineal region = pineoblastoma ("3rd eye")

Soft Tissue and Bone Sarcomas

- Susceptibility secondary to germline predisposition (i.e., *RB1* mutations) and radiation therapy
- Encompass ~ 1/2 of 2nd cancers in survivors of hereditary retinoblastoma
- Bone sarcomas: Osteosarcoma (most common), chondrosarcoma and Ewing sarcoma
- Soft tissue tumors
  - Pathologic subtypes include leiomyosarcoma, fibrosarcoma, rhabdomyosarcoma, pleomorphic sarcoma, liposarcoma/lipomatous tumors
    - Leiomyosarcoma most common pathology in some studies
    - Majority of leiomyosarcomas in women are uterine (i.e., outside of radiation field)
    - Most of nonleiomyosarcoma soft tissue tumors in radiation field

Others

- Melanoma of skin; carcinomas of bladder, lung, upper respiratory tract, and skin; tumors of the central nervous system/meningiomas

SELECTED REFERENCES

1. Maccarthy A et al: Second and subsequent tumours among 1927 retinoblastoma patients diagnosed in Britain 1951-2004. Br J Cancer. 108(12):2455-63, 2013
2. Rodjan F et al: Second cranio-facial malignancies in hereditary retinoblastoma survivors previously treated with radiation therapy: clinic and radiologic characteristics and survival outcomes. Eur J Cancer. 49(8):1939-47, 2013
3. de Oliveira Reis AH et al: Influence of MDM2 and MDM4 on development and survival in hereditary retinoblastoma. Pediatr Blood Cancer. 59(1):39-43, 2012
4. Dommering CJ et al: RB1 mutations and second primary malignancies after hereditary retinoblastoma. Fam Cancer. 11(2):225-33, 2012
5. Kleinerman RA et al: Sarcomas in hereditary retinoblastoma. Clin Sarcoma Res. 2(1):15, 2012
6. Yu CL et al: Cause-specific mortality in long-term survivors of retinoblastoma. J Natl Cancer Inst. 101(8):581-91, 2009
7. Antoneli CB et al: Trilateral retinoblastoma. Pediatr Blood Cancer. 48(3):306-10, 2007

IMAGE GALLERY

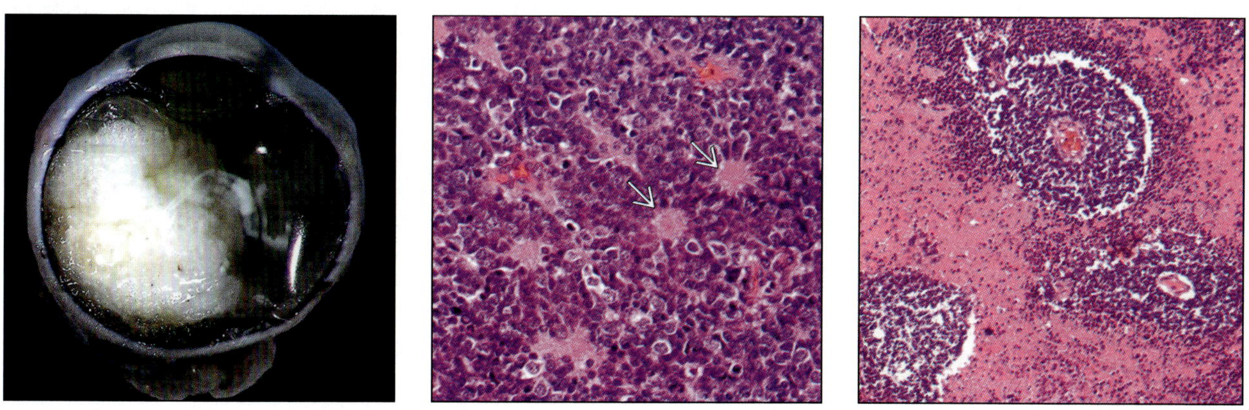

(Left) *Retinoblastomas may form large masses and occupy a significant intraocular volume. They classically demonstrate a white reflection on ophthalmologic exam, leading to the classic sign known as leukocoria.* ***(Center)*** *Homer Wright rosettes* ▶ *are characterized by an acellular delicate eosinophilic core and may be encountered in retinoblastomas, although they are not specific.* ***(Right)*** *In keeping with their high-grade nature, retinoblastomas are frequently necrotic.*

HOWEL-EVANS SYNDROME/KERATOSIS PALMARES AND PLANTARES WITH ESOPHAGEAL CANCER

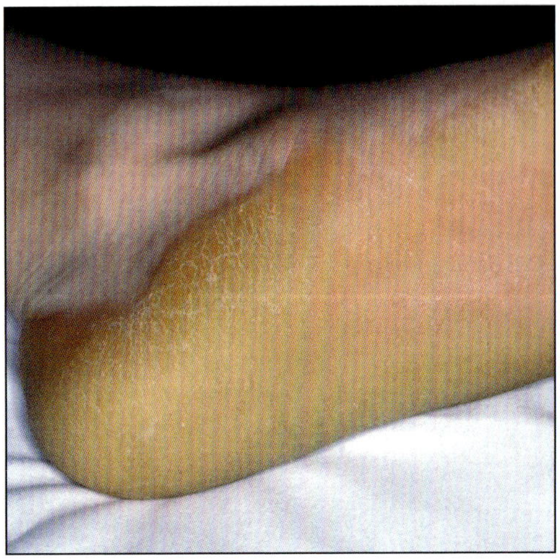

Clinical photograph shows plantar keratoderma. The histopathology of keratoderma is characterized by marked hyperkeratosis. (Courtesy L. Milstone, MD.)

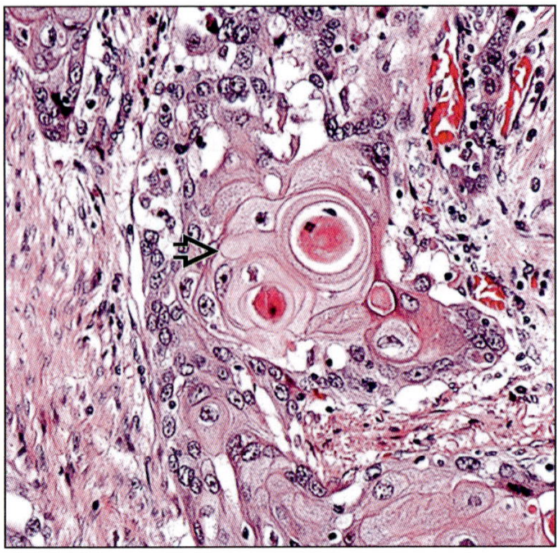

Hematoxylin & eosin shows squamous cell carcinoma (SCC) of the esophagus. It has the same features as SCC elsewhere. Note the abnormal keratinization in the keratin "pearl" ⮚. (Courtesy E. Montgomery, MD.)

TERMINOLOGY

Synonyms

- Tylosis with esophageal cancer
- Tylosis-esophageal cancer, tylosis esophageal cancer
- Focal nonepidermolytic palmoplantar keratoderma with carcinoma of esophagus
- Tylosis = palmoplantar keratoderma

EPIDEMIOLOGY

Incidence

- Unclear
- Originally described in 2 United Kingdom families in 1958
  - These 2 families possibly related
- Also described in other countries (e.g., North America, India, Germany)

GENETICS

Inheritance

- Autosomal dominant
- Linkage to chromosome 17q25
  - Missense mutations in *RHBDF2* gene

CLINICAL IMPLICATIONS AND ANCILLARY TESTS

Cutaneous Findings

- Palmoplantar keratoderma
  - Distribution
    - May affect palms only, soles only, or both
    - May be accentuated on weight-bearing areas of soles
    - May be exacerbated by friction
    - May be diffuse
  - Age at presentation
    - Typically between ages 6 and 12 (type A)
    - Early childhood presentation (before age 5) termed type B, with more benign course
    - Rarely present at birth
  - Worsens with friction
    - e.g., heavy footwear
    - e.g., manual labor
  - May or may not be associated with hyperhidrosis
- Squamous cell carcinoma
  - May develop in areas of tylosis
  - Often presents as ulcerated area
- Rare findings
  - Follicular papules on body
  - Sparse hair

Gastrointestinal Symptoms/Findings

- Gastroesophageal reflux disease
- Esophageal ulcers
  - Ulcers
  - Strictures
- Esophageal squamous cell carcinoma

Oral Findings

- Mucosa
  - Oral leukoplakia
- Teeth
  - Premature loss
  - Poor dental enamel

ASSOCIATED NEOPLASMS

Esophageal Cancer

- United Kingdom kindreds
  - Developed at mean age of 45
  - Estimated 95% chance of carcinoma by age 65
- American kindred
  - Developed later (6th, 7th decades)

HOWEL-EVANS SYNDROME/KERATOSIS PALMARES AND PLANTARES WITH ESOPHAGEAL CANCER

CANCER RISK MANAGEMENT

Esophageal Cancer

- No clear guidelines
- Estimated 70% of those with palmoplantar keratoderma ultimately develop esophageal carcinoma
- Screening has been recommended from age 20

Bronchial Cancer

- Unclear prevalence (much lower than esophageal cancer)
- No clear screening guidelines

Squamous Cell Carcinoma of the Skin

- Unclear prevalence
- Frequent skin examination
- Biopsy of any ulcerated areas

DIFFERENTIAL DIAGNOSIS

Focal Palmoplantar and Oral Mucosa Hyperkeratosis Syndrome

- Inheritance
  - Autosomal dominant
- Clinical findings
  - Palmoplantar keratoderma
  - Oral leukoplakia of gingiva
- Associations
  - No association with esophageal cancer

Acquired Tylosis as Paraneoplastic Phenomenon

- Acquired later in life (not inherited)
- Clinical findings
  - Palmoplantar keratoderma
  - Internal carcinoma
    - e.g., bronchogenic
- Family history
  - Negative for esophageal/bronchogenic cancer or tylosis

Dyskeratosis Congenita

- Inheritance
  - Often X-linked recessive
- Genetics
  - Often mutation in *DKC1* gene that encodes dyskerin
- Clinical findings
  - Oral leukoplakia
  - Palmoplantar keratoderma
  - Nail dystrophy
  - Reticulated hyperpigmentation of skin
  - Bone marrow failure
- Associations
  - Increased risk of squamous cell carcinoma of
    - Oropharynx
    - Esophagus
    - Bronchus
    - Rectum
    - Cervix/vagina
  - Increased risk of
    - Myelodysplasia, acute myelogenous leukemia
    - Hodgkin disease
    - Gastrointestinal adenocarcinomas

Hidrotic Ectodermal Dysplasia

- Inheritance
  - Autosomal recessive
- Genetics
  - Mutation in *GJB6* gene that encodes connexin 30
- Clinical findings
  - Alopecia
  - Nail dystrophy
  - Clubbing of fingers
  - Palmoplantar keratoderma

Pachyonychia Congenita

- Inheritance
  - Autosomal dominant
- Genetics
  - Secondary to mutations in *KRT6/16/17* genes
- Clinical findings
  - Palmoplantar keratoderma
  - Thickened nails
  - Oral leukoplakia
  - Some types associated with steatocystoma multiplex

Other Palmoplantar Keratodermas

- Inherited but isolated (no other findings)
  - Examples
    - Unna-Thost syndrome
    - Vörner syndrome
- Inherited and associated with other specific findings
  - Examples
    - Richner-Hanhart syndrome (oculocutaneous tyrosinemia)
    - Olmsted syndrome (mutilating with periorificial plaques)
    - Carvajal syndrome (cardiomyopathy)

SELECTED REFERENCES

1. Blaydon DC et al: RHBDF2 mutations are associated with tylosis, a familial esophageal cancer syndrome. Am J Hum Genet. 90(2):340-6, 2012
2. Grundmann JU et al: Lung carcinoma with congenital plantar keratoderma as a variant of Clarke-Howel-Evans syndrome. Int J Dermatol. 42(6):461-3, 2003
3. Simon M et al: [The Clark-Howel-Evans-McConnell syndrome. Observations in one family over 5 generations.] Hautarzt. 48(11):800-5, 1997
4. Kelsell DP et al: Close mapping of the focal non-epidermolytic palmoplantar keratoderma (PPK) locus associated with oesophageal cancer (TOC). Hum Mol Genet. 5(6):857-60, 1996
5. Stevens HP et al: Linkage of an American pedigree with palmoplantar keratoderma and malignancy (palmoplantar ectodermal dysplasia type III) to 17q24. Literature survey and proposed updated classification of the keratodermas. Arch Dermatol. 132(6):640-51, 1996
6. Yesudian P et al: Genetic tylosis with malignancy: a study of a South Indian pedigree. Br J Dermatol. 102(5):597-600, 1980
7. Howel-Evans W et al: Carcinoma of the oesophagus with keratosis palmaris et plantaris (tylosis): a study of two families. Q J Med. 27(107):413-29, 1958

JUVENILE POLYPOSIS SYNDROME

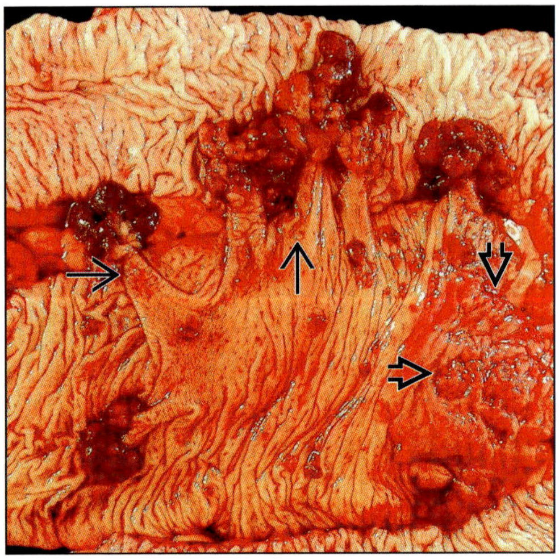

Gross photograph shows multiple juvenile polyps. The larger polyps ➔ are pedunculated and multilobulated whereas the smaller ones are sessile and smooth ➲. (Courtesy A. Srivastava, MD.)

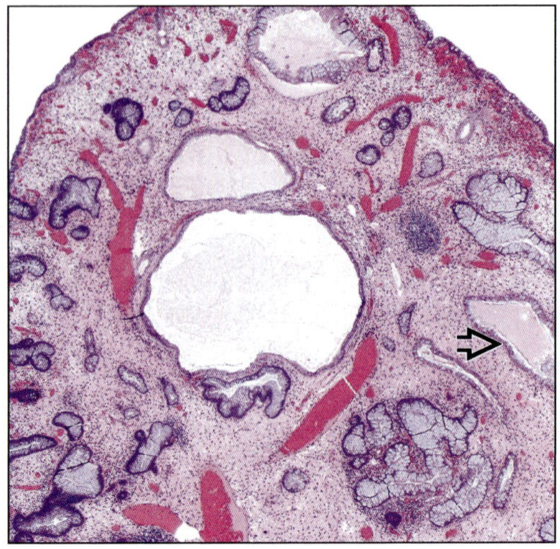

Juvenile polyps have marked stromal expansion and cystically dilated crypts. The stroma is edematous and inflamed whereas the cysts are filled with inspissated mucin ➲. (Courtesy A. Srivastava, MD.)

TERMINOLOGY

Abbreviations

- Juvenile polyp (JP)
- Juvenile polyposis syndrome (JPS)

Definitions

- Hamartomatous polyp
  - May occur sporadically (most juvenile polyps are nonsyndromic)
    - 90% of all polyps found in children
    - 20-50% may have > 1 polyp
    - No increase in cancer risk in sporadic JP
  - May be manifestation of inherited familial polyposis syndrome
    - Patients with JPS have increased risk of colorectal carcinoma
- Diagnostic criteria for JPS (any 1 of the following 3)
  - > 5 juvenile polyps (most patients have 50-200)
  - Presence of at least 1 JP outside of colon
  - Any number of polyps in patient with positive family history

EPIDEMIOLOGY

Incidence

- 1 in 100,000 worldwide

Age

- Typically presents in 1st decade of life

Inheritance

- 75% of cases show autosomal dominant inheritance
- 25% of cases appear de novo in patients without family history

GENETICS

Specific Mutations

- Germline mutations in *SMAD4 (DPC4)* gene on 18q21 present in 20-30% of JPS patients
  - Exon 9 deletion is most common abnormality
  - Patients with *SMAD4* germline mutations are more likely to have polyps in upper gastrointestinal tract and positive family history
  - Significant proportion with *SMAD4* mutation may also have hereditary hemorrhagic telangiectasia
    - Recent study found that 81% of JPS patients with *SMAD4* mutations had hereditary hemorrhagic telangiectasia and another 14% were suspected of having it
- Germline mutations in *BMPR1A* gene on 10q23 present in similar proportion of JPS cases (20-30%)
- Germline mutations in *ENG* may also lead to JPS in unknown proportion of patients
  - Data suggest early childhood onset of polyps with *ENG* mutations
  - Also associated with hereditary hemorrhagic telangiectasia similar to *SMAD4* mutations
- All 3 genes involved with transforming growth factor-β (TGF-β) pathway
- Older literature suggests *PTEN* mutations were also found in juvenile polyposis, but recent studies suggest these cases are better classified as Cowden/*PTEN*-hamartoma tumor syndrome instead of JPS

CLINICAL IMPLICATIONS

Presentation

- Hematochezia
- Anemia
- Diarrhea
- Prolapse

JUVENILE POLYPOSIS SYNDROME

Juvenile Polyposis Coli
- Most common inherited form
- Present clinically in 1st decade of life
- Polyps confined to colon

Generalized Juvenile Polyposis
- Diffuse involvement of gastrointestinal tract
- Colon, stomach, and small intestine involved

Gastric Juvenile Polyposis
- Rare form of disease
- Polyps confined to stomach
- Patients may present with protein-losing enteropathy and mimic Cronkhite-Canada syndrome

Juvenile Polyposis of Infancy
- Rare
- Usually associated with death in infancy due to protein-losing enteropathy
- Initially thought to be autosomal recessive due to lack of family history, but recent studies have found large de novo chromosome 10 deletions containing both the *BMPR1A* and *PTEN* genes in affected individuals

Associated Manifestations
- Present in 2/3 of JPS patients
  - Hydrocephalus and mental retardation
  - Pulmonary arteriovenous malformation
  - Cleft palate and polydactyly
  - Malrotation of gut
  - Meckel diverticulum

ASSOCIATED NEOPLASMS

Colorectal Adenocarcinoma
- Mean age of developing cancer reported to be between 35 and 43 years
- Risk of developing colon cancer increases to 68% at age 60

Gastric Adenocarcinoma
- Associated with *SMAD4* mutations and severe gastric polyposis

Small Intestinal and Pancreatic Adenocarcinoma
- Rare reports of duodenal, ampullary, and pancreatic adenocarcinoma in patients with JPS

CANCER RISK MANAGEMENT

Genetic Testing
- Direct sequencing of *SMAD4* and *BMPR1A* will identify about 40-50% of cases
- Multiplex ligation probe-dependent amplification (MLPA) can pick up another 4-5% of cases by identifying large deletions and duplications in either *SMAD4* or *BMPR1A*

Screening
- In suspected patients, endoscopic screening generally starts at ~ age 15 and consists of upper and lower endoscopy as well as small bowel imaging with either capsule endoscopy or MR enterography
- In known JPS patients, screening endoscopy should be done annually

Surgery
- If patients are symptomatic or endoscopic surveillance is not feasible due to number of polyps, then surgery may be needed
- Patients who develop dysplasia or have a high prevalence of colon cancer in their families typically have a total colectomy
  - Continued surveillance is still required after colectomy to remove polyps in rectal cuff

MACROSCOPIC FINDINGS

Gross Features
- Most patients have > 50 polyps
- Most polyps are pedunculated (> 2/3)
- Sessile polyps are infrequent, usually smaller in size, and often with smooth surface
- Size is variable, but most measure ~ 1.0 cm in greatest dimension
- Larger lesions are multilobulated and show surface ulceration
- Gross appearance may resemble adenomas
- Cut surface in larger polyps is soft, gelatinous due to mucin-filled cysts

MICROSCOPIC FINDINGS

Histologic Features
- Epithelial component in colonic polyps
  - Surface erosion or ulceration
  - Granulation tissue cap may be present
  - Markedly dilated cysts
    - Cysts filled with mucin or distended with crypt abscesses
    - Epithelium lining cysts is of variable height and may be completely flattened
  - Hyperplastic regenerative changes may be present
  - Random sections from grossly normal mucosa in colectomy specimens may show early "incipient" JP with cystically dilated and inflamed crypts
  - Dysplasia or carcinoma may be present
  - Crypt:stroma ratio in polyps is higher in patients with *SMAD4* mutations as compared to those with *BMPR1A* mutations
- Stromal component in colonic polyps
  - Marked expansion of lamina propria
  - Loose edematous and inflamed (neutrophils or lymphoid follicles) stroma
    - Degree of inflammation is variable
    - Mucin extravasation from ruptured cysts accentuates inflammatory response
  - Hemorrhage and hemosiderin deposits present in larger polyps with torsion injury
  - Smooth muscle proliferation may be present in larger pedunculated polyps
    - Must distinguish from Peutz-Jeghers polyp

JUVENILE POLYPOSIS SYNDROME

  - Ganglioneuromas have been described previously, but these cases were probably *PTEN*-hamartoma/ Cowden syndrome, not JPS
  - Polyps from patients with *BMPR1A* have been reported to have a higher stroma:crypt ratio than those from patients with *SMAD4* mutations
- Gastric polyps
  - Cystic epithelial component lined by foveolar-type epithelium
  - Variable degree of inflammation
  - Polyps resemble hyperplastic polyps or those seen in Cronkhite-Canada syndrome
    - Difficult to separate various hamartomatous gastric polyps without clinical information
- Dysplasia and carcinoma
  - Not present in sporadic juvenile polyps
  - May be present in larger (> 1 cm) polyps in syndromic patients
    - Pathologist must be wary of overinterpreting reactive atypia due to inflammation
  - Prevalence of dysplasia ranges from 8-20%
  - Higher incidence of dysplastic change present in polyps with villous architecture
  - JPS patients may have adenomas as well as juvenile polyps
  - Adenocarcinomas are more common in distal colon and rectum
  - Carcinoma involving stomach or small bowel is rare
- Differential diagnosis
  - Inflammatory polyposis
    - Small polyps are identical to inflammatory pseudopolyps
    - Biopsies of flat mucosa to rule out idiopathic inflammatory bowel disease may be warranted in some cases
  - Peutz-Jeghers polyposis (PJP)
    - Pedunculated juvenile polyps with prolapse-type changes may mimic those seen in PJP
    - Lobules in PJP are separated by compact smooth muscle bundles, unlike disarrayed proliferation seen in some juvenile polyps
    - Epithelial component in PJP is arranged in distinct lobular configuration
    - Mucocutaneous manifestations typical of PJP not seen in juvenile polyposis
  - PTEN-hamartoma tumor syndrome/Cowden syndrome
    - Polyps may be indistinguishable, but stroma in Cowden more fibrotic and less inflamed
  - Cronkhite-Canada syndrome (CCS)
    - Polyps may be very similar to JPS
    - Ectodermal manifestations (onychodystrophy, alopecia, hyperpigmentation) diagnostic of CCS
  - Hereditary mixed polyposis syndrome
    - Patients get juvenile polyps, serrated polyps, and adenomas
    - Easily confused with JPS since patients with JPS often have adenomas
    - Autosomal dominant inheritance
    - Increased risk of colon cancer
    - No extraintestinal manifestations

SELECTED REFERENCES

1. Drut R: The mucosa beyond the polyps in juvenile polyposis. Fetal Pediatr Pathol. 31(1):6-10, 2012
2. Jasperson KW: Genetic testing by cancer site: colon (polyposis syndromes). Cancer J. 18(4):328-33, 2012
3. Latchford AR et al: Juvenile polyposis syndrome: a study of genotype, phenotype, and long-term outcome. Dis Colon Rectum. 55(10):1038-43, 2012
4. O'Malley M et al: The prevalence of hereditary hemorrhagic telangiectasia in juvenile polyposis syndrome. Dis Colon Rectum. 55(8):886-92, 2012
5. Patel SG et al: Familial colon cancer syndromes: an update of a rapidly evolving field. Curr Gastroenterol Rep. 14(5):428-38, 2012
6. Schwenter F et al: Juvenile polyposis, hereditary hemorrhagic telangiectasia, and early onset colorectal cancer in patients with SMAD4 mutation. J Gastroenterol. 47(7):795-804, 2012
7. Stadler ZK et al: Juvenile polyposis syndrome presenting with familial gastric cancer and massive gastric polyposis. J Clin Oncol. 30(25):e229-32, 2012
8. Tam B et al: The real face of juvenile polyposis syndrome. J Gastrointest Oncol. 3(4):362-8, 2012
9. Williams JC et al: Combined juvenile polyposis and hereditary hemorrhagic telangiectasia. Proc (Bayl Univ Med Cent). 25(4):360-4, 2012
10. Arber N et al: Small bowel polyposis syndromes. Curr Gastroenterol Rep. 13(5):435-41, 2011
11. Brosens LA et al: Juvenile polyposis syndrome. World J Gastroenterol. 17(44):4839-44, 2011
12. Hood B et al: Juvenile polyps and juvenile polyp syndromes in children: a clinical and endoscopic survey. Clin Pediatr (Phila). 50(10):910-5, 2011
13. van Hattem WA et al: Histologic variations in juvenile polyp phenotype correlate with genetic defect underlying juvenile polyposis. Am J Surg Pathol. 35(4):530-6, 2011
14. Aretz S: The differential diagnosis and surveillance of hereditary gastrointestinal polyposis syndromes. Dtsch Arztebl Int. 107(10):163-73, 2010
15. Lam-Himlin D et al: Morphologic characterization of syndromic gastric polyps. Am J Surg Pathol. 34(11):1656-62, 2010
16. Chen HM et al: Genetics of the hamartomatous polyposis syndromes: a molecular review. Int J Colorectal Dis. 24(8):865-74, 2009
17. Gammon A et al: Hamartomatous polyposis syndromes. Best Pract Res Clin Gastroenterol. 23(2):219-31, 2009
18. Calva D et al: Hamartomatous polyposis syndromes. Surg Clin North Am. 88(4):779-817, vii, 2008

Microscopic Features

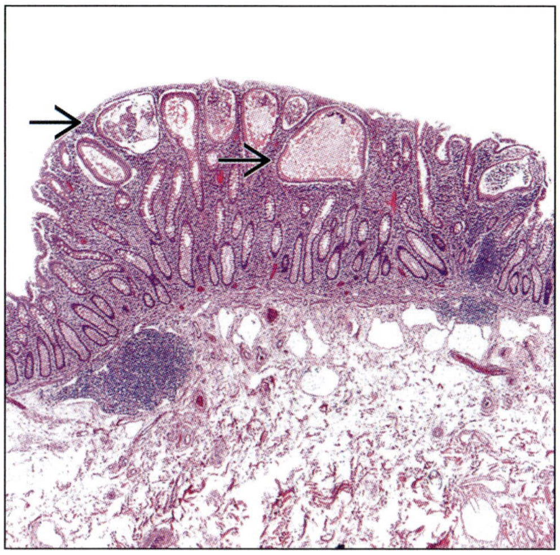

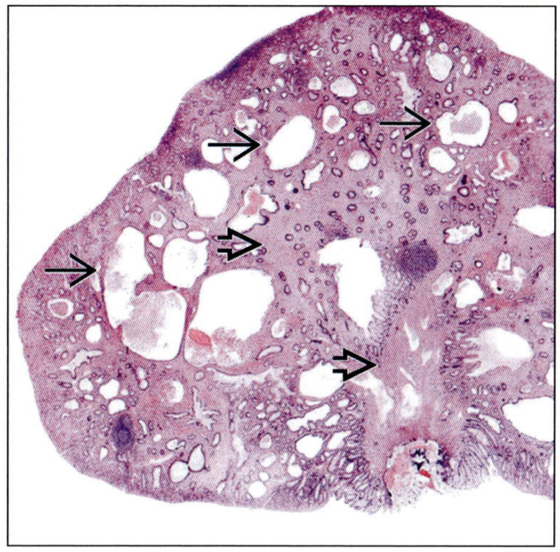

(Left) *This low-power view shows a small juvenile polyp from a resection specimen. There is cystic dilatation of glands → without much in the way of stroma.* ***(Right)*** *This low-power view of a larger juvenile polyp shows the overall lobular growth pattern with an ulcerated surface. This polyp has abundant stroma ⇨ as well as cystically dilated glands →.*

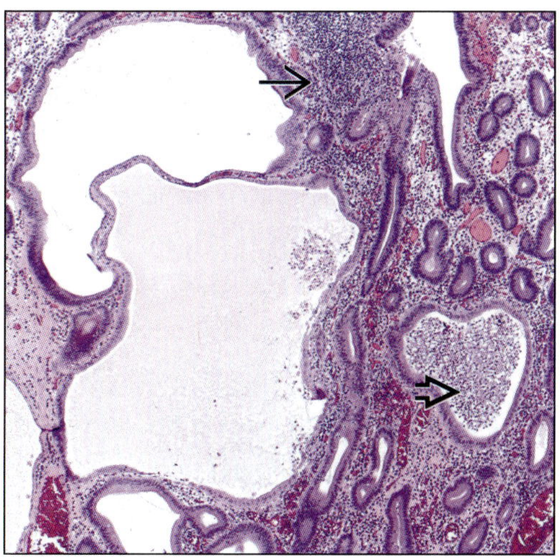

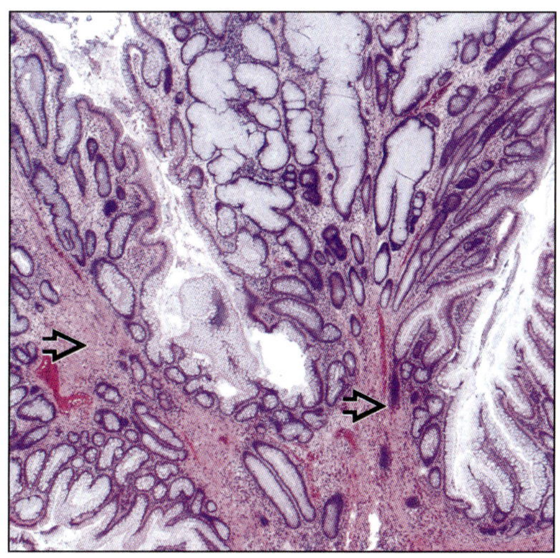

(Left) *Hematoxylin & eosin shows a juvenile polyp with marked cystic change and crypt abscess formation ⇨. The stromal inflammation in such polyps may be in the form of neutrophils, lymphoid follicles →, or both. (Courtesy A. Srivastava, MD.)* ***(Right)*** *Larger pedunculated juvenile polyps may undergo prolapse and show a prominent smooth muscle proliferation ⇨ that may be mistaken for a Peutz-Jeghers polyp. (Courtesy A. Srivastava, MD.)*

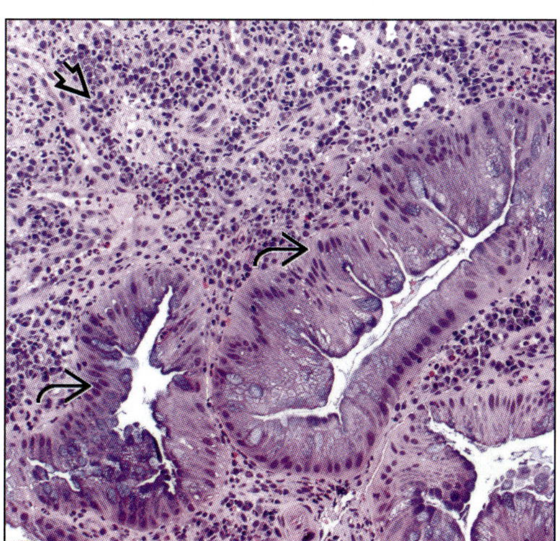

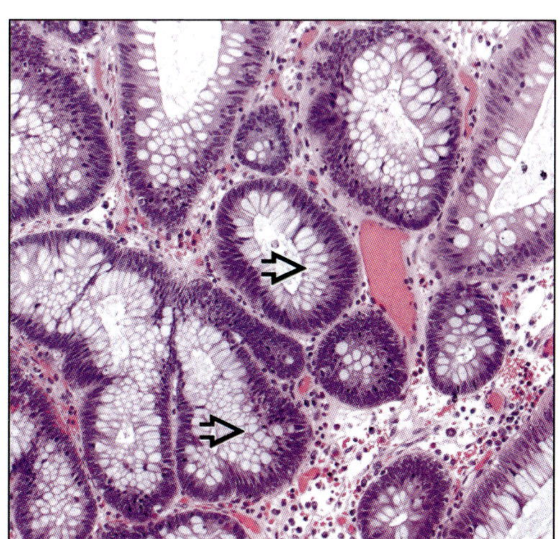

(Left) *Regenerative changes in juvenile polyps may mimic serrated or adenomatous polyps. Prominent hyperplastic regenerative change ↪ is present in this juvenile polyp with inflamed granulation tissue ⇨ on the surface. (Courtesy A. Srivastava, MD.)* ***(Right)*** *Adenoma-like regenerative changes ⇨ are seen in this sporadic juvenile polyp in a 4-year-old child. Juvenile polyps in syndromic patients may harbor truly dysplastic foci or even carcinoma. (Courtesy A. Srivastava, MD.)*

LI-FRAUMENI SYNDROME/LI-FRAUMENI-LIKE SYNDROME

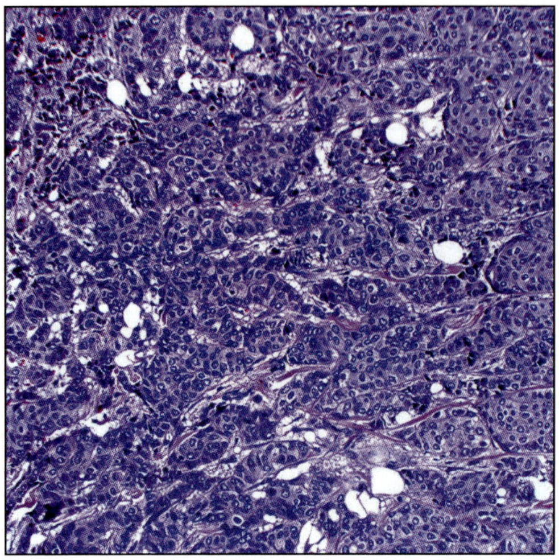

Breast cancer is the most common malignancy associated with LFS and occurs at a median age of 33 years. The majority are poorly differentiated but positive for hormone receptors.

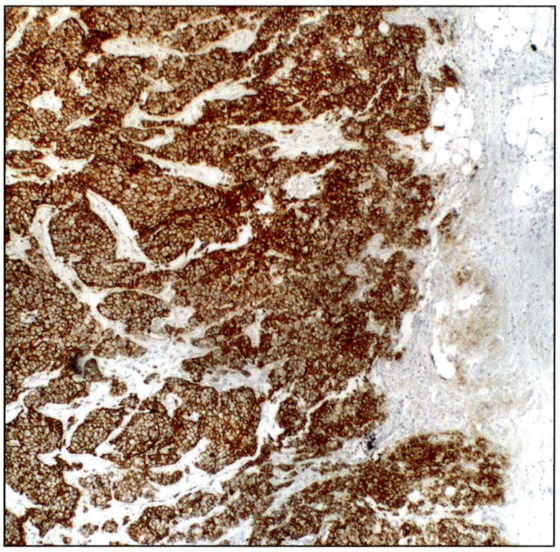

Over 1/2 of breast carcinomas occurring in women with LFS overexpress HER2. This is much higher than breast cancers in general (~ 20%).

TERMINOLOGY

Abbreviations

- Li-Fraumeni Syndrome (LFS)
- Li-Fraumeni-Like (LFL) syndrome

Synonyms

- LFS
  - Sarcoma family syndrome of Li and Fraumeni
  - Sarcoma, breast, leukemia, and adrenal gland (SBLA) syndrome
  - Online Mendelian Inheritance in Man (OMIM) #151623

Definitions

- LFS
  - Constellation of tumor types occurring in patients and kindreds
    - 0-10 years: Brain tumors, adrenal cortical carcinomas, soft tissue sarcomas, and leukemia
    - 11-20 years: Bone sarcomas
    - > 20 years: Breast cancers and brain tumors
  - Autosomal dominant inheritance
  - Classic LFS criteria
    - Individual (proband) diagnosed with sarcoma before age 45
    - 1st-degree relative with any cancer before age 45
    - 1st- or 2nd-degree relative with any cancer before age 45, or sarcoma at any age
  - ~ 70-80% of individuals with classic LFS criteria carry a germline *TP53* mutation
- LFL syndrome
  - Birch definition requires following 3 criteria
    - Patient diagnosed with any childhood cancer or sarcoma, brain tumor, or adrenal cortical carcinoma before age 45
    - 1st- or 2nd-degree relative with sarcoma, leukemia, breast cancer, brain tumor, or adrenal cortical carcinoma, or leukemia at any age
    - 1st- or 2nd-degree relative with any cancer diagnosed before age 60
  - Eeles definition
    - 2 first- or second-degree relatives with sarcoma, leukemia, breast cancer, brain tumor, or adrenal cortical carcinoma at any age
  - ~ 40% of individuals with LFL carry a germline *TP53* mutation

EPIDEMIOLOGY

Population Incidence

- *TP53* germline mutations
  - 1/5,000 to 1/25,000 individuals
  - A population in southeastern Brazil has 1/300 incidence
    - Due to specific mutation *R337H* (*c.1010G* > A, *p.Arg337His*)
    - Lifetime risk of ~ 50-60% for cancer
    - High incidence of childhood adrenal cortical carcinomas
    - Also increased risk for thyroid cancer and renal cancer; these cancers are not typical of LFS in other kindreds

Incidence Among Women With Breast Carcinoma

- *TP53* germline mutations are associated with ~ 1% of breast carcinomas in women < 40 years of age
- Responsible for ~ 3% of all breast cancers due to a germline mutation

Modifiers of Risk

- Increased sensitivity to ionizing radiation
- Radiation exposure may increase risk of malignancy

GENETICS

TP53 Gene

- Located on 17p13.1
  - 20 kb, 11 coding exons, 393 amino acids
- Belongs to a family of growth-regulating genes
- Autosomal dominant inheritance
  - Lifetime risk higher and age of onset earlier in women than in men
- Types of germline *TP53* mutations
  - Majority of cases (~ 75%) are missense mutations
    - Most are within central DNA binding domain: 85% in exons 5 through 8
    - Altered protein can have a dominant-negative effect: Abnormal protein interferes with function of wild-type protein
    - Unlike other recessive germline tumor suppressor genes, 2/3 of tumors in individuals with missense mutations retain the wild-type allele
    - Retention likely due to lower selective pressure to lose wild-type protein
  - Minority of cases are null mutations
    - May be due to nonsense mutations, splice mutations, deletions, or insertions
    - Results in nonfunctional protein
    - Loss of wild-type allele is necessary to alter normal *P53* function
    - Acts like other recessive tumor-suppressor genes: Majority of tumors exhibit loss of the wild-type allele
- 535 germline mutations in 532 families have been reported
  - *TP53* Mutation Database is maintained by the International Agency for Research on Cancer (IARC) and is updated each year

Function of TP53 Protein

- Central role in cell cycle control, DNA replication, DNA repair, and apoptosis
  - Binds to double-stranded DNA
  - Transactivation function for promoter sequences
- Activated in response to various stress signals
- Loss of function is thought to suppress a mechanism of protection against accumulation of genetic alterations
  - Cell cycle arrest allows repair of genetic damage prior to DNA replication and fixation of mutations
  - Terminally damaged cells undergo apoptosis

Li-Fraumeni-Like Syndrome

- Individuals who fulfill some but not all criteria for LFS
- ~ 20-40% carry germline *TP53* mutations
- Others due to mutations in *BRCA2*, Fanconi genes (*BRIP1*, *PALB2*, and *RAD51C*), and DNA mismatch repair genes
- In the past, some cases of LFL were attributed to *CHEK2* germline mutations
  - Most common tumor associated with *CHEK2* is early-onset breast carcinoma
  - Full spectrum of tumors associated with LFS is not seen

CLINICAL IMPLICATIONS AND ANCILLARY TESTS

Population to be Screened

- When strict criteria are met, *TP53* mutations are found in 60-80%
- If less strict criteria are used (LFL), *TP53* mutations are found in 15-35%

Chompret Criteria for Screening

- Individual (proband) must have 1 of the following tumors before age 46: Soft tissue sarcoma, osteosarcoma, premenopausal breast cancer, brain tumor, adrenal cortical carcinoma, leukemia, or lepidic pattern of lung adenocarcinoma, and at least 1 of 3 criteria listed below
  - At least 1 first- or second-degree relative with an LFS tumor before age 56 or with multiple tumors
    - Breast cancer is not included if proband has breast cancer
  - Proband has multiple tumors (not including breast cancers), 2 of which belong to LFS tumors and 1st of which occurred before age 46
  - Proband has adrenal cortical carcinoma or choroid plexus tumor, irrespective of family history
- 30% of individuals fulfilling these criteria have a germline *TP53* mutation

Genetic Testing

- DNA sequencing is gold standard for identifying *TP53* mutations
- Sequence analysis of exons 2 through 11 detects ~ 95% of mutations
- Deletions of the gene, promoter region, or exon 1 may be present in ~ 1% of families
- Duplications, inversions, large deletions, and mutations in noncoding regions may not be detected by standard sequence analysis

Immunohistochemistry for p53

- TP53 protein degrades rapidly and has 20-minute half-life
  - Some mutant forms of p53 cannot transcriptionally activate MDM2
  - Loss of this negative feedback loop results in p53 accumulation
- Immunohistochemistry does not detect normal levels of p53 in nontumor cells
  - Increased p53 protein is also not seen in normal cells of individuals with germline mutations
- Many antibodies to p53 are available
  - Target different epitopes on the protein
  - May detect only wild-type protein, mutant protein, or both
- Increased p53 protein is only associated with ~ 2/3 of mutations
  - Some mutant forms of p53 have half-lives of up to 4 hours
  - Strong diffuse (> 10-20%) immunoreactivity is a specific, but not sensitive, test for p53 mutations
- Weak &/or focal p53 positivity may be present when mutations are absent

LI-FRAUMENI SYNDROME/LI-FRAUMENI-LIKE SYNDROME

- Results of immunohistochemistry for p53 have not been reported for tumors in LFS kindreds

ASSOCIATED NEOPLASMS: *TP53*

Any Tumor

- < 20% of affected individuals develop a cancer in childhood
- > 90% of affected individuals develop some type of tumor by age 70
  - 80% are breast, sarcoma, brain, or adrenal tumors
  - 7-20% of individuals with multiple primary tumors have LFS
- Risk for malignancy is 100x greater than for unaffected individuals
- Penetrance varies with type of mutation
- Individuals with cancer have greater risk of developing 2nd cancer
  - 15% have 2 cancers, 4% have 3 cancers, 2% have 4 cancers
  - Increased risk if 1st cancer occurred at early age
  - Radiation treatment for 1st cancer may elevate risk
  - Usually occurs 6-12 years after 1st cancer

Breast Cancer

- Most common malignancy in LFS (~ 33% of total)
- Increased risk for females starts at age 20 and continues into adulthood
  - 6% of women diagnosed before age 31 have a germline *TP53* mutation
- ~ 55% of women will develop breast cancer by age 45 (average age at diagnosis is 33)
  - ~ 100% lifetime risk for women
  - ~ 2% per year will develop subsequent contralateral breast cancer
    - Overall, 25% will have multiple breast cancers
  - Breast cancer in men has not been reported
- ~ 55% of invasive carcinomas are positive for hormone receptors and HER2
  - This pattern is present in < 20% of sporadic breast carcinomas
  - Least common pattern is negativity for both hormone receptors and HER2 (present in ~ 5%)
- Increased incidence of phyllodes tumor reported in LFS compared with general population

Soft Tissue Sarcoma

- 2nd most common malignancy in this syndrome (~ 20% of total)
  - Many types: Only Ewing sarcoma has not been associated with LFS
- Most commonly develop in childhood (< 10 years of age)
  - 5-10% of children with sarcomas have a germline *TP53* mutation
- Rhabdomyosarcoma most common in individuals < 5 years of age
  - 9% of individuals with this sarcoma have LFS

Osteosarcoma

- ~ 15% of LFS tumors
  - 2-3% of persons with osteosarcoma have LFS
- Most commonly develop during adolescence
- 10% of individuals with an osteosarcoma diagnosed before age 20 have a germline *TP53* mutation

Brain Tumors

- Often develop in childhood
  - 2-10% of children with brain tumors have LFS
- Smaller 2nd peak in incidence in 4th-5th decades
- Glioblastomas are most common type (13%)
  - Also astrocytomas and medulloblastomas
- Choroid plexus tumors in children are characteristic

Adrenal Cortical Carcinoma

- 80% of children with this carcinoma have LFS
  - Median age of onset is 3 years
  - Some are due to de novo mutations
- Cases in adults usually occur before 50 years of age

Hematologic Malignancies

- Include both lymphoma and leukemia

Other Cancers

- Lung cancer (lepidic pattern)
- Gastrointestinal cancers (colon, gastric, pancreatic)

CANCER RISK MANAGEMENT

Screening

- In USA, National Comprehensive Cancer Network (NCCN) has published screening guidelines
  - Children and adults should have yearly comprehensive physical examinations including skin and neurological assessment
  - Breast cancer
    - Breast self-exam (BSE) training and regular monthly BSE starting at age 18
    - Clinical breast exam, starting at age 20-25 years (or 5-10 years before earliest breast cancer in family, whichever 1st), 2x per year
    - Annual mammogram &/or MR when clinical breast exams start
    - Prophylactic mastectomy can be considered
  - Men and women should be screened for colorectal cancer every 2-5 years starting at age 25
  - Organ targeted surveillance may be performed depending on pattern of cancers in specific families

SELECTED REFERENCES

1. IARC TP53 Database. World Health Organization. http://p53.iarc.fr. Accessed January 31, 2012
2. Mai PL et al: Li-Fraumeni syndrome: report of a clinical research workshop and creation of a research consortium. Cancer Genet. 205(10):479-87, 2012
3. Masciari S et al: Breast cancer phenotype in women with TP53 germline mutations: a Li-Fraumeni syndrome consortium effort. Breast Cancer Res Treat. 133(3):1125-30, 2012

Tumors Associated With Li-Fraumeni Syndrome

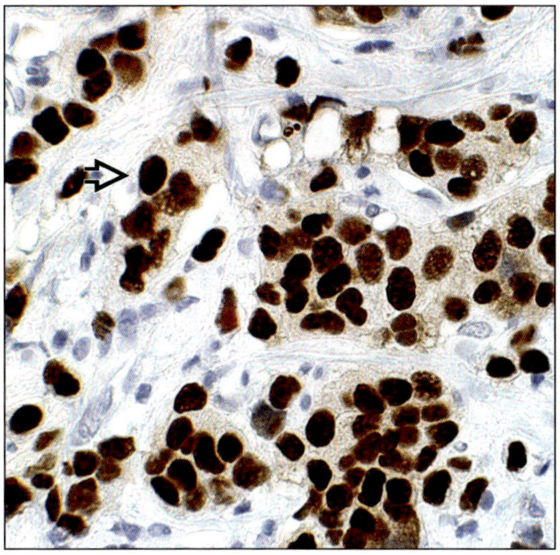
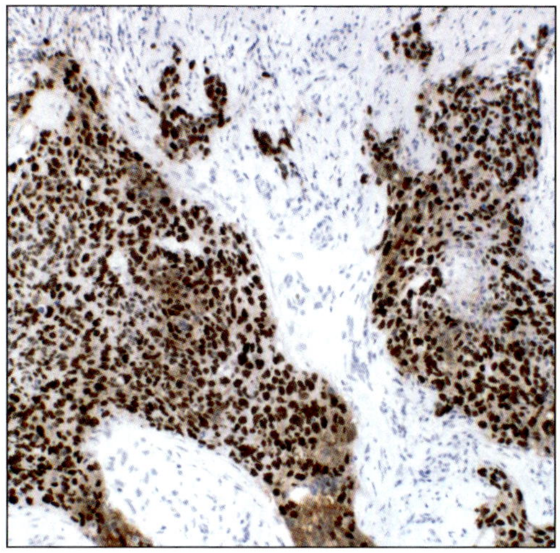

(Left) *The majority of breast carcinomas associated with Li-Fraumeni syndrome (LFS) are positive for ER ⇨ and PR.* ***(Right)*** *Immunohistochemical studies for p53 detect mutant forms that do not undergo normal degradation, allowing the protein to accumulate in the nucleus. Mutant forms that do undergo degradation or mutations that result in a truncated protein will not be detected. Overall, immunohistochemistry probably detects ~ 2/3 of tumors with mutations.*

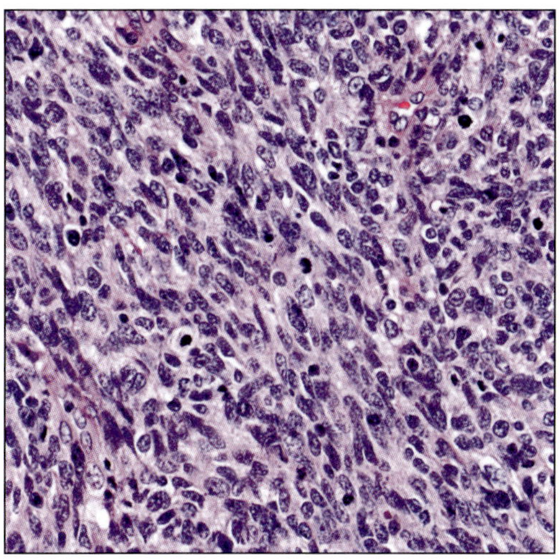
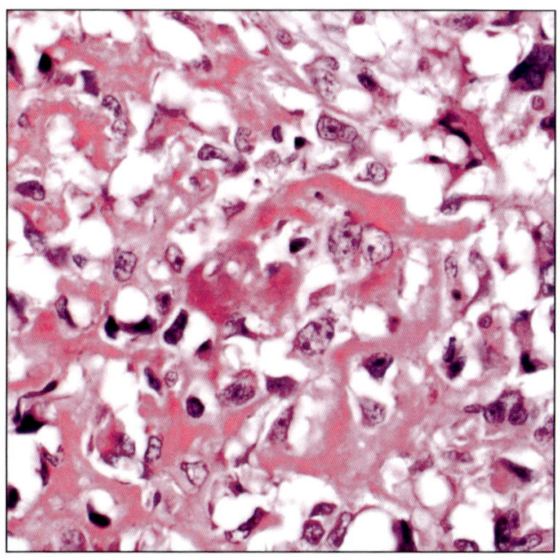

(Left) *Soft tissue sarcomas are the 2nd most common type of tumor associated with LFS (~ 20%). All types (except Ewing sarcoma) occur. Rhabdomyosarcoma (seen here) is most common in affected children < 5 years of age. Overall, 9% of individuals with this tumor have a germline TP53 mutation.* ***(Right)*** *Approximately 15% of tumors associated with LFS are osteosarcomas. These are the most common type of tumor to be diagnosed in adolescents with this syndrome.*

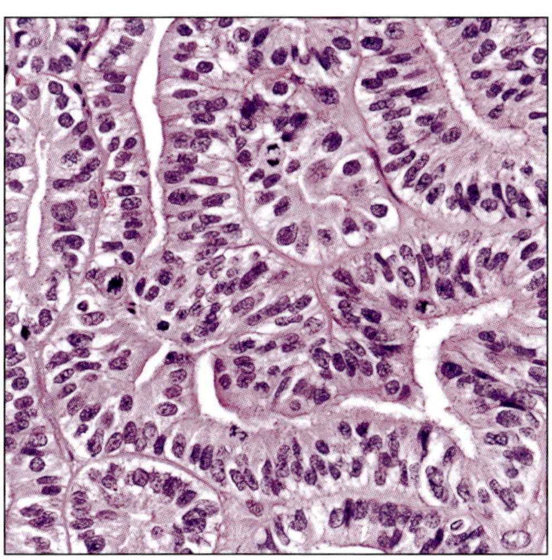
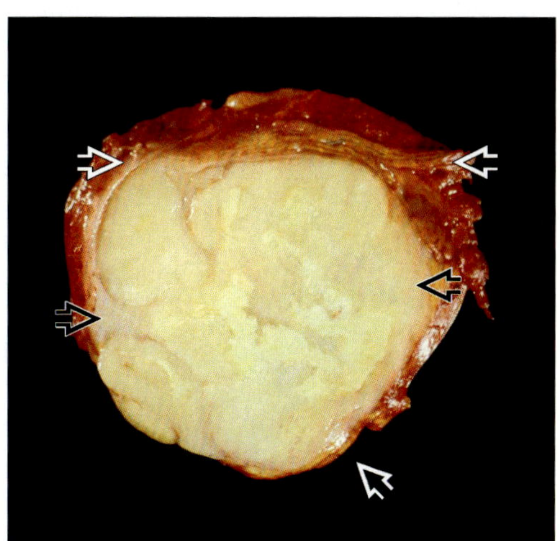

(Left) *There are 2 peaks for brain tumors in LFS: Childhood and in the 4th and 5th decades. Choroid plexus carcinomas, such as this example, are frequently seen in children. (Courtesy P. Burger, MD.)* ***(Right)*** *This adrenal cortical carcinoma ⇨ displaces the normal adrenal gland ➡. In 80% of children with this tumor, a germline TP53 mutation will be present. Mutations at codons 152, 158, and 337 are particularly common. A few cases are due to de novo mutations.*

LYNCH SYNDROME

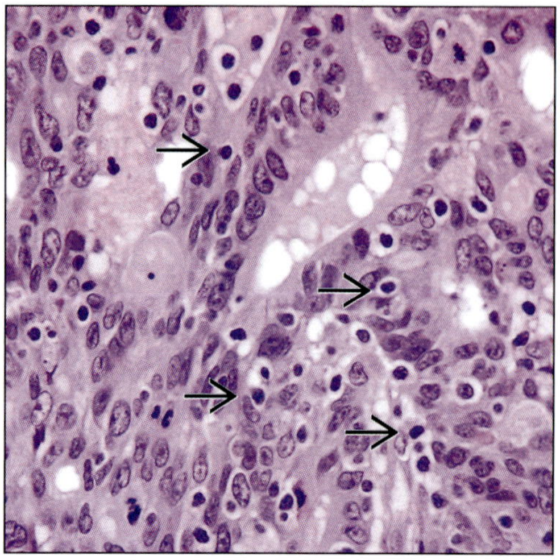

Colon cancer from a Lynch syndrome patient shows a large number of tumor-infiltrating lymphocytes (TILs) ➔. These TILs are often seen in Lynch syndrome cancers.

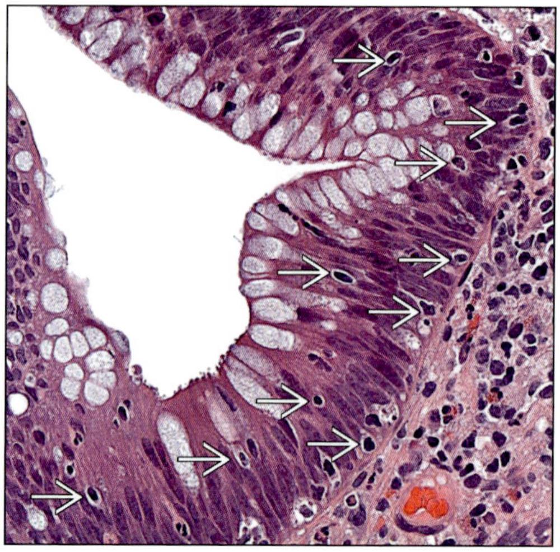

This Lynch syndrome adenoma has a large number of adenoma-infiltrating lymphocytes ➔. Although not specific, these lymphocytes are a marker of Lynch syndrome.

TERMINOLOGY

Synonyms

- Hereditary nonpolyposis colorectal cancer (HNPCC) (old term for Lynch syndrome)

EPIDEMIOLOGY

Prevalence

- Lynch syndrome is most common heritable cause of cancer
- ~ 3% of all colorectal cancers (CRCs)

GENETICS

Lynch Syndrome

- Autosomal dominant
- Mutations in genes coding for mismatch repair proteins (MLH1, PMS2, MSH2, MSH6)
  - Mutation in *EPCAM* (a gene immediately adjacent to *MSH2*) leads to epigenetic silencing of *MSH2*
    - Immunostains for MSH2 and MSH6 will be negative, implying an *MSH2* mutation, but sequencing will not find *MSH2* mutation

Constitutional Mismatch Repair-Deficiency (CMMR-D) Syndrome

- Autosomal recessive (very rare)
  - Patient inherits a mutated copy of mismatch repair gene from each parent (biallelic mutation)
- Early childhood cancers (lymphoma/leukemia plus Lynch-associated solid tumors)
  - Café au lait spots similar to neurofibromatosis type 1

CLINICAL IMPLICATIONS AND ANCILLARY TESTS

Clinical Features

- Multiple epithelial cancers occur at average age of ~ 20 years younger than expected
- Several guidelines have been proposed to help identify patients who should be tested for Lynch syndrome
  - Amsterdam criteria II
    - At least 3 relatives with a Lynch-associated cancer
    - 2 or more successive generations affected
    - 1 or more relatives diagnosed before age 50
    - 1 should be a 1st-degree relative of the other 2
    - Familial adenomatous polyposis must be excluded
  - Revised Bethesda guidelines
    - CRC diagnosed prior to age 50
    - Presence of synchronous or metachronous CRC or other Lynch-associated tumor, regardless of age
    - CRC with histologic features suggestive of microsatellite instability (MSI) in patients < age 60
    - CRC diagnosed in 1 or more 1st-degree relatives with a Lynch-associated tumor, with 1 of the cancers diagnosed prior to age 50
    - CRC diagnosed in 2 or more 1st-degree or 2nd-degree relatives with Lynch-associated tumors, regardless of age
- Neither of these guidelines is foolproof; hence, many studies recommend testing all CRCs for Lynch syndrome

Immunohistochemistry (IHC)

- Immunostains for MLH1, PMS2, MSH2, and MSH6 have become fairly routine
  - 5-10% false-negative rate, as protein may be antigenic but still not function due to mutation
  - Advantage of IHC over microsatellite instability (MSI-H) testing is that IHC reveals which gene is mutated

Correlations Between Mutations and Immunohistochemistry		
Mutation/DNA Abnormality	IHC Staining Pattern	Additional Testing/Results
MLH1	Negative stains for MLH1 and PMS2	*BRAF* wild type, negative for methylation, sequence *MLH1*
MSH2	Negative stains for MSH2 and MSH6	Sequence *MSH2*; if normal, look for *EPCAM* mutation
MSH6	Negative stain for MSH6	Sequence *MSH6*
PMS2	Negative stain for PMS2	Sequence *PMS2*
EPCAM	Negative stains for MSH2 and MSH6	After *MSH2* sequence is normal, sequence *EPCAM*, possible IHC for EPCAM

Microsatellite Instability

- Mutations in proofreading genes lead to replication errors in DNA
  - These replication errors can be detected in short DNA repeats called microsatellites
  - ~ 95% of all Lynch syndrome colorectal cancers have MSI-H
    - Can be tested easily using formalin-fixed paraffin-embedded tissue
    - Need both normal and neoplastic tissue for comparison
- MSI-H is also seen in 10-15% of sporadic colon cancers (not specific for Lynch syndrome)
  - Sporadic tumors often have *BRAF V600E* mutations &/or methylation of *MLH1*
    - Neither of these are present in Lynch tumors

ASSOCIATED NEOPLASMS

Gastrointestinal Tract Tumors

- Colorectal cancer
  - 80% lifetime risk
  - Histologic features are often characteristic
    - Increased numbers of tumor-infiltrating lymphocytes and a Crohn-like reaction around edge of tumor
    - More likely to be well or poorly differentiated
    - More likely to have mucinous differentiation and lack dirty necrosis
    - More often right sided
    - More likely to have a circumscribed growth pattern and to exhibit histologic heterogeneity
- Adenocarcinoma of stomach, small bowel, appendix, ampulla, and biliary tree
  - May share some of histologic features listed above for colon cancers

Nongastrointestinal Tract Tumors

- Endometrium
  - 40-60% lifetime risk
  - Endometrioid carcinomas with mucinous differentiation, histologic heterogeneity, dedifferentiation, and increased host response
- Ovaries
  - 4-12% lifetime risk
  - Clear cell and endometrioid carcinomas
- Adrenal
  - As many as 5% of adrenal cortical carcinomas may be associated with Lynch syndrome
- Prostate
  - Lynch patients have 2x the risk of prostate cancer as general population
- Kidney, ureters, bladder
  - Urothelial carcinomas
    - *MSH2* mutations may selectively increase risk of bladder cancers compared to other mismatch repair gene mutations
- Skin
  - Sebaceous neoplasms and multiple keratoacanthomas = Muir-Torre syndrome
  - Café au lait spots in CMMR-D syndrome
- Brain
  - Glioblastoma in Turcot syndrome variant of Lynch syndrome
- Leukemia/lymphoma
  - Occurs in patients with CMMR-D

CANCER RISK MANAGEMENT

Surveillance Endoscopy

- Every 1-2 years starting between ages 20 and 25

Surgery

- Prophylactic colectomy is an option, but most patients opt for colonoscopic surveillance

SELECTED REFERENCES

1. Capper D et al: BRAF V600E-specific immunohistochemistry for the exclusion of Lynch syndrome in MSI-H colorectal cancer. Int J Cancer. 133(7):1624-30, 2013
2. Hitchins MP: The role of epigenetics in Lynch syndrome. Fam Cancer. 12(2):189-205, 2013
3. Shia J et al: Lynch syndrome-associated neoplasms: a discussion on histopathology and immunohistochemistry. Fam Cancer. 12(2):241-60, 2013
4. Shi C et al: Molecular testing in colorectal cancer: diagnosis of Lynch syndrome and personalized cancer medicine. Am J Clin Pathol. 137(6):847-59, 2012
5. Greenson JK et al: Pathologic predictors of microsatellite instability in colorectal cancer. Am J Surg Pathol. 33(1):126-33, 2009
6. Polydorides AD et al: Adenoma-infiltrating lymphocytes (AILs) are a potential marker of hereditary nonpolyposis colorectal cancer. Am J Surg Pathol. 32(11):1661-6, 2008
7. Greenson JK et al: Phenotype of microsatellite unstable colorectal carcinomas: Well-differentiated and focally mucinous tumors and the absence of dirty necrosis correlate with microsatellite instability. Am J Surg Pathol. 27(5):563-70, 2003

LYNCH SYNDROME

Microscopic Features and Molecular Tests

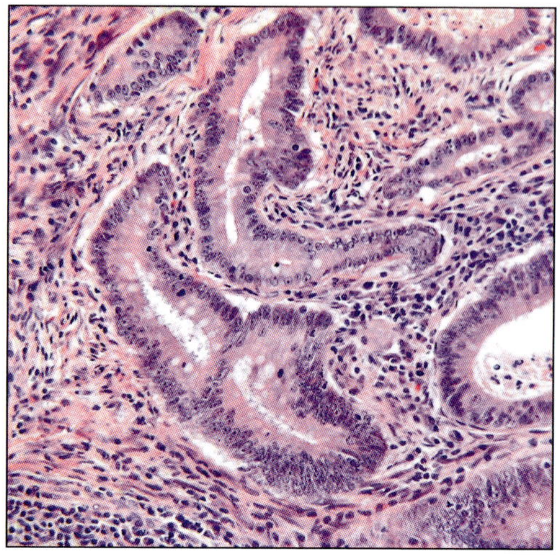

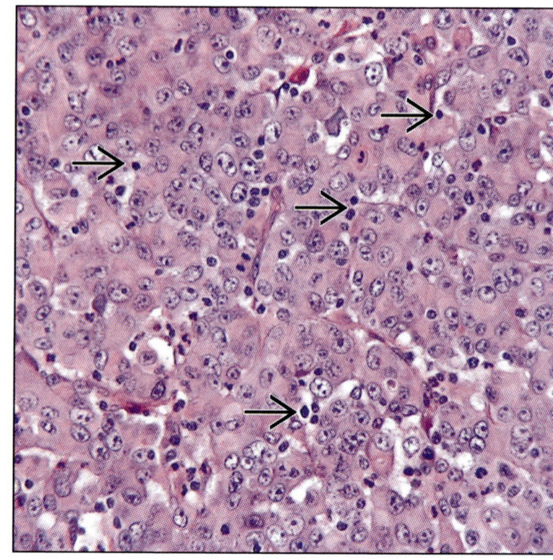

(Left) *Lynch syndrome tumor shows well-differentiated adenoma-like glands. Increased numbers of tumor-infiltrating lymphocytes and a Crohn-like reaction around edge of tumor suggest Lynch syndrome. The Lynch-associated tumors are likely to be circumscribed and to exhibit histologic heterogeneity.* ***(Right)*** *Poorly differentiated colon cancer from Lynch syndrome patient shows large numbers of tumor-infiltrating lymphocytes →.*

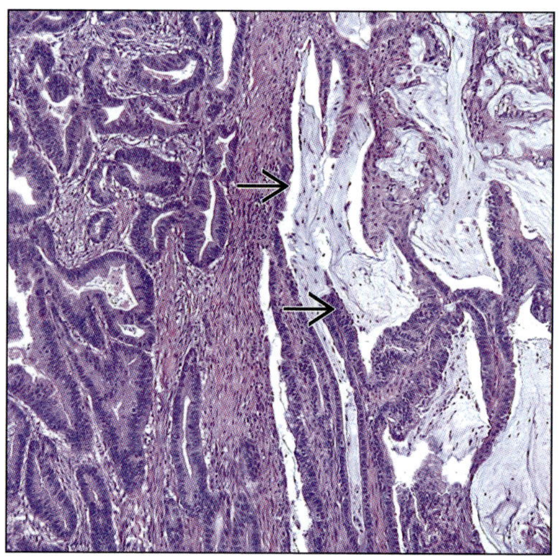

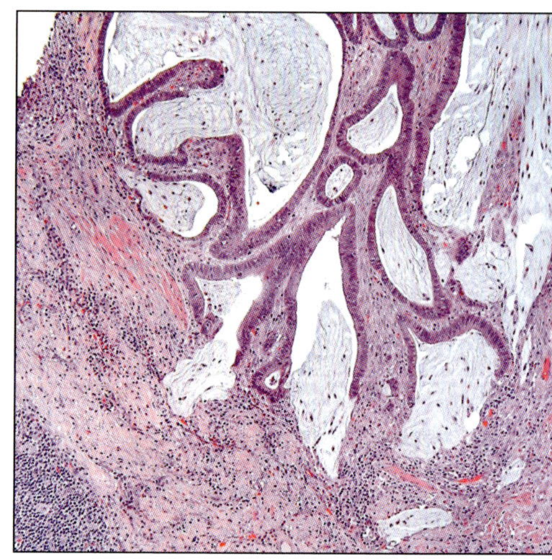

(Left) *Well-differentiated Lynch syndrome colon cancer shows mucinous differentiation → on the right. Even focal mucinous differentiation can be a tip-off that the patient may have Lynch syndrome.* ***(Right)*** *Well-differentiated Lynch syndrome colon cancer shows mucinous differentiation. Lynch syndrome-associated tumors are more likely to have mucinous differentiation and lack dirty necrosis.*

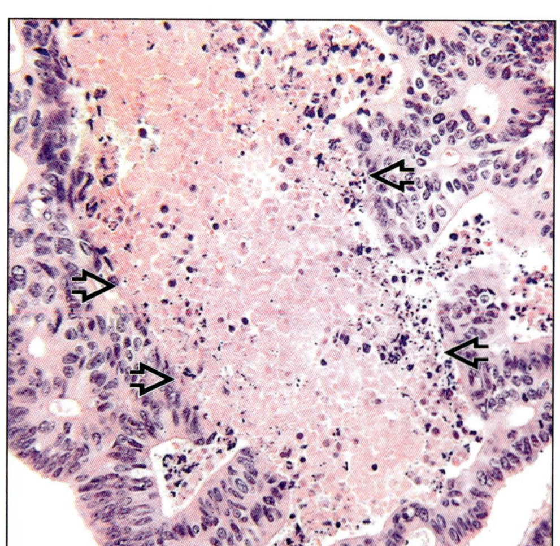

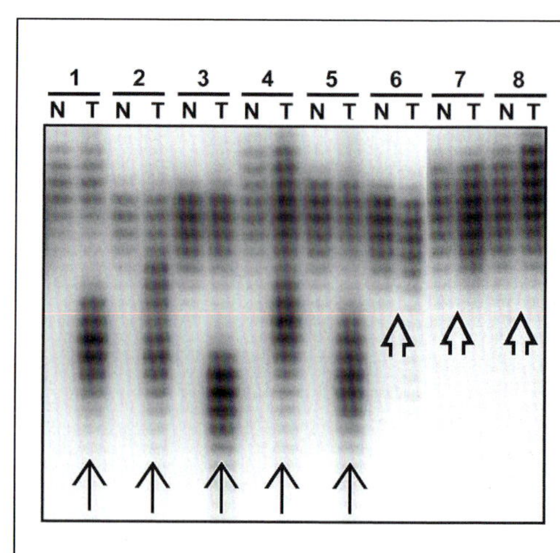

(Left) *Image shows the typical appearance of microsatellite stable (MSS), non-Lynch syndrome colon cancer with abundant dirty necrosis ⇨. Dirty necrosis is much more common in non-Lynch microsatellite stable tumors.* ***(Right)*** *PCR gel electrophoresis shows extra bands in the tumor lanes of specimens 1, 2, 3, 4, and 5 →, indicating microsatellite instability. Note identical patterns in normal and tumor samples in specimens 6, 7, and 8 ⇨, indicating microsatellite stability. (Courtesy S. Gruber, MD.)*

Microscopic Features and Molecular Tests

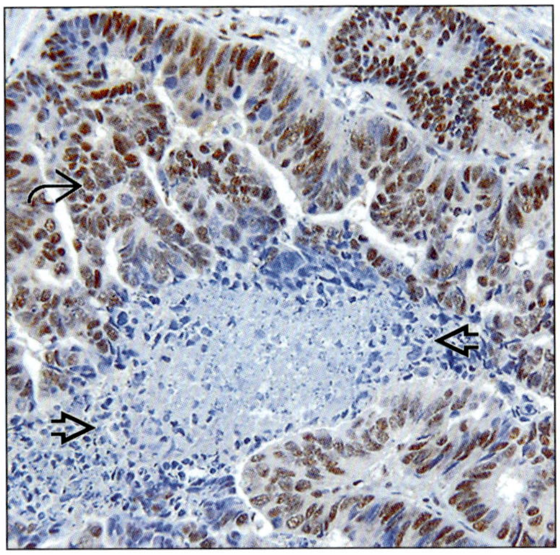

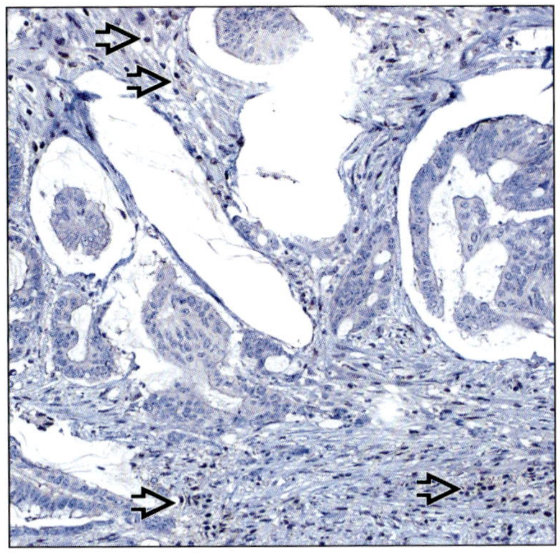

*(**Left**) This MSS colorectal carcinoma shows strong nuclear staining ⮫ for MLH1. Note the dirty necrosis ➯ typical of MSS carcinomas. Immunostains for PMS2, MSH2, and MSH6 were also positive. (**Right**) Immunohistochemical stain for PMS2 shows nuclear staining for PMS2 in inflammatory cells ➯ but no staining in the tumor cells. Stains for MLH1, MSH2, and MSH6 were positive in the tumor. This patient had a mutation in PMS2.*

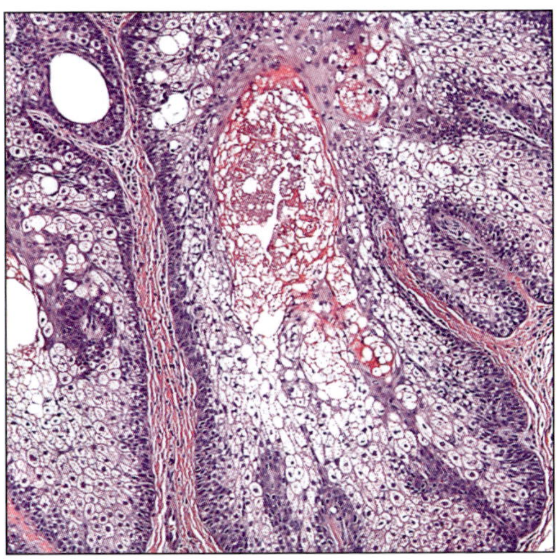

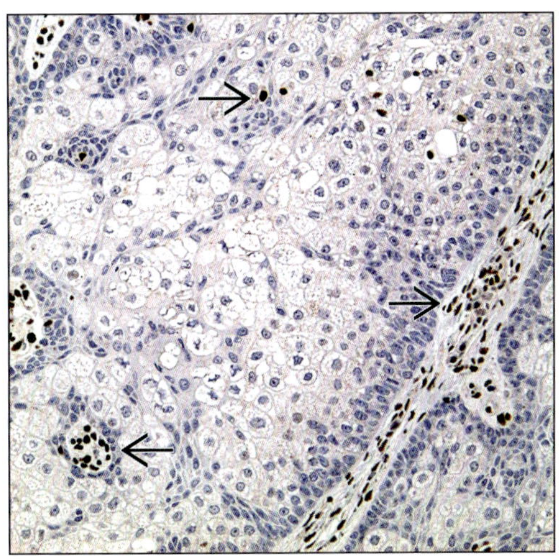

*(**Left**) Medium-power view shows a sebaceous adenoma, a type of neoplasm seen in patients with Muir-Torre syndrome, a variant of Lynch syndrome. (**Right**) Immunostain for MSH2 shows positive nuclear staining in lymphocytes ➔ but negative staining in the nuclei of the sebaceous adenoma, indicative of a deficient mismatch repair protein in the neoplastic cells. This is consistent with Muir-Torre syndrome due to an MSH2 mutation.*

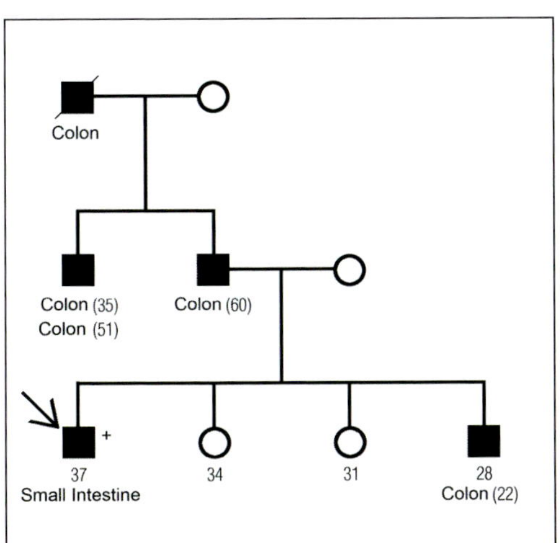

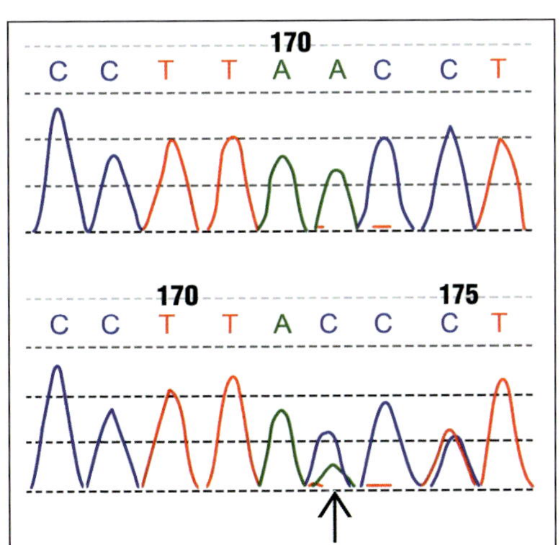

*(**Left**) This pedigree shows a family with Lynch syndrome and a patient ➔ whose DNA is sequenced in the next image. Note the autosomal dominant inheritance pattern. The age of cancer onset is younger in successive generations. (**Right**) This DNA sequencing chromatograph from the patient in the previous pedigree chart shows a frame-shift mutation ➔ in MSH2.*

MELANOMA/PANCREATIC CARCINOMA SYNDROME

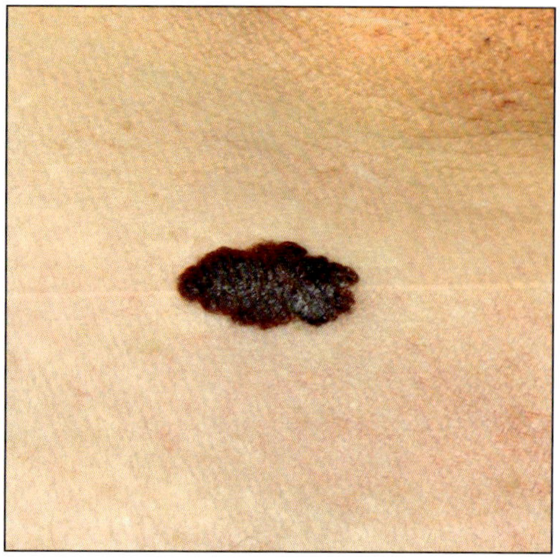

Clinical photograph of a nodular-type melanoma shows a darkly pigmented elevated lesion with irregular borders on the chest. (Courtesy J. Wu, MD.)

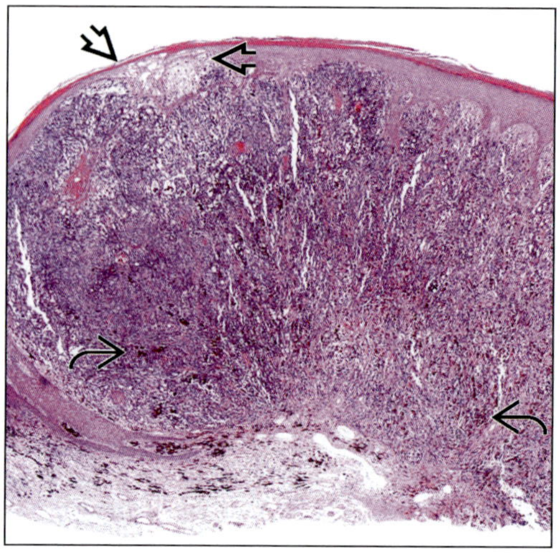

Low-power examination of a nodular melanoma shows a large, expansile dermal nodule with irregular pigmentation ➙ and areas of epidermal thinning and necrosis ➙. (Courtesy S. Dadras, MD.)

TERMINOLOGY

Definition

- Hereditary melanoma
  - In geographic areas with high sun exposure: ≥ 3 affected blood relatives
  - In geographic areas with lower sun exposure: ≥ 2 affected blood relatives

EPIDEMIOLOGY

Incidence of Hereditary Cutaneous Melanoma

- 5-7% of cutaneous melanoma patients are from high-risk families

Incidence of Hereditary Pancreatic Cancer

- Considered to be low (1-3%), but possibly up to 10% of pancreatic cancer has a familial basis

GENETICS

CDKN2A Mutations

- Splice sites or ankyrin repeats 3 and 4 tend to be affected
- Lifetime risk of melanoma: ~ 75%
- Lifetime risk of pancreatic cancer may be close to 20%
- Mutations are generally inactivating

Inheritance

- Generally autosomal dominant

CLINICAL IMPLICATIONS AND ANCILLARY TESTS

Clinical Presentation

- Familial atypical multiple mole-melanoma syndrome
  - Increased risk of cutaneous melanoma and pancreatic cancer
  - Patients may have > 100 atypical melanocytic nevi
- Some kindreds have cutaneous melanoma and pancreatic cancer without increased numbers of atypical melanocytic nevi

Clinical Risk Factors

- Number of relatives affected by melanoma or pancreatic cancer
- *CDKN2A* mutation carrier
- Number of nevi, especially if > 50
- Very fair skin with inability to tan
- Presence of many freckles
- Hair color, especially red or blonde
- Eye color, especially blue
- Degree/amount of sun exposure
  - Presence of extensively sun-damaged skin

ASSOCIATED NEOPLASMS

Malignant Melanoma

- Cutaneous

Dysplastic Melanocytic Nevi (Atypical Melanocytic Nevi, Clark Nevi)

- Originally described in kindreds with increased risk of cutaneous melanoma
- Subsequently described in individuals with no increased risk of cutaneous melanoma
- Clinically dysplastic melanocytic nevi
  - Size often > 6 mm, irregular color, irregular borders, asymmetric, may have history of change, may have elevated (papular) and flat (macular) components
- Histopathologic criteria for dysplastic melanocytic nevi
  - Atypical cytology &/or disordered architecture
    - Single melanocytes, irregular nests, bridged rete, pagetoid scatter, fibroplasia

Pancreatic Cancer

- Cumulative lifetime risk: 11-17%
- Average age is 5.8 years younger than patients affected by sporadic pancreatic cancer

Breast Cancer

- Risk is higher in kindreds without multiple atypical melanocytic nevi

CANCER RISK MANAGEMENT

Photoprotection

- Sunscreen, sun protective clothing, avoidance of sunburn

Avoidance of Other Carcinogens

- Cigarette smoking increases pancreatic cancer risk

Skin Examination

- Head-to-toe examination (including scalp and genitalia)
  - Baseline at age 10 years
  - Repeat every 6-12 months
  - May increase frequency during puberty or pregnancy
  - May use dermoscopy
  - Monthly self-examination of skin
- Baseline photography may be helpful

Suspicious Lesions

- Prompt excision and histopathologic evaluation

Education

- On photoprotection and characteristics of melanoma

Pancreatic Cancer

- Suggested age to initiate screening
  - 10 years before youngest age of diagnosis of pancreatic cancer in a given family **or** age 50 years
- Screening is controversial
  - Multimodal screening
    - Endoscopic ultrasound
    - Computed tomography, magnetic resonance imaging
    - Endoscopic retrograde cholangiopancreatography

DIFFERENTIAL DIAGNOSIS

Disorders With Chronic Pancreatic Inflammation

- Familial pancreatic cancer
  - Generally not associated with melanoma
  - Families with ≥ 2 first-degree relatives with confirmed exocrine pancreatic cancer
  - Exclusion of other inherited tumor syndromes with associated pancreatic cancer
    - Examples includes melanoma/pancreatic carcinoma syndrome, hereditary breast and ovarian cancer, hereditary pancreatitis
  - Mutations in *BRCA2*, *PALB2*, and *ATM* in some families
- Hereditary pancreatitis
- Cystic fibrosis

Other Hereditary Tumor Syndromes With Increased Risk of Pancreatic Cancer

- Peutz-Jeghers syndrome
- Hereditary breast and ovarian cancers
- Li-Fraumeni syndrome
- Hereditary nonpolyposis colorectal carcinoma
- Familial adenomatous polyposis

Hereditary Multiple Melanoma

- Some kindreds with hereditary melanoma have no associated risk of pancreatic cancer

SELECTED REFERENCES

1. Bartsch DK et al: Familial pancreatic cancer--current knowledge. Nat Rev Gastroenterol Hepatol. 9(8):445-53, 2012
2. Bartsch DK et al: Clinical and genetic analysis of 18 pancreatic carcinoma/melanoma-prone families. Clin Genet. 77(4):333-41, 2010
3. Gemmel C et al: Pancreatic cancer screening: state of the art. Expert Rev Gastroenterol Hepatol. 3(1):89-96, 2009

IMAGE GALLERY

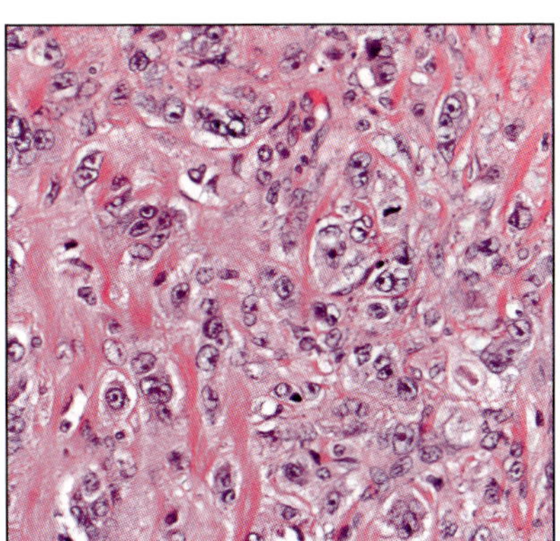

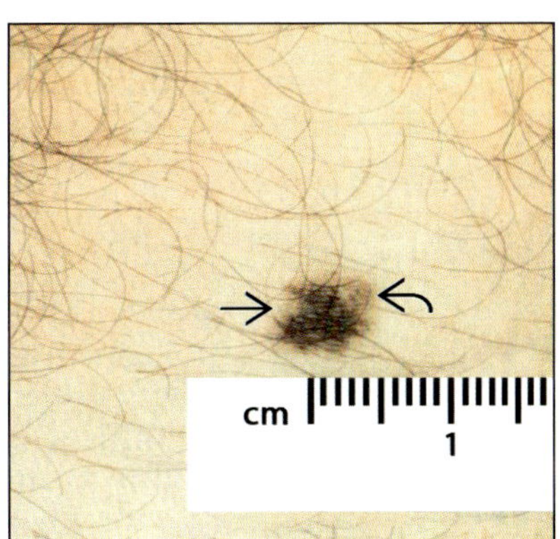

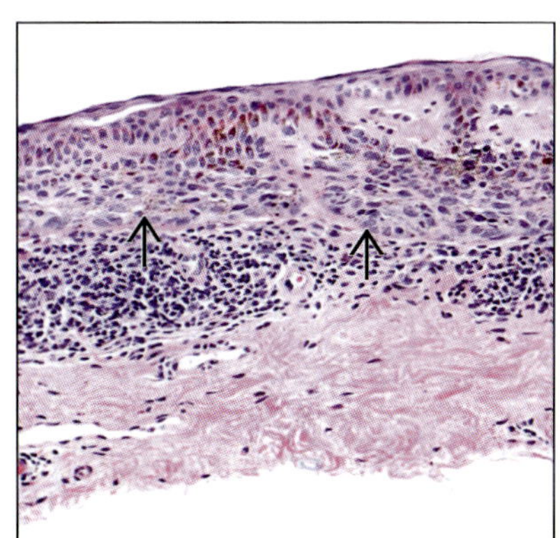

(Left) *This poorly differentiated pancreatic adenocarcinoma is composed of single and clustered tumor cells. (Courtesy M. Mino-Kenudson, MD.)* ***(Center)*** *Clinical photograph of an atypical compound nevus shows a central papular area ➔ surrounded by an irregular macular periphery ➔. (Courtesy P. Duray, MD.)* ***(Right)*** *Severely atypical compound nevus exhibits a junctional proliferation of atypical melanocytes ➔, with fused rete ridges. (Courtesy S. Dadras, MD.)*

MULTIPLE ENDOCRINE NEOPLASIA TYPE 1

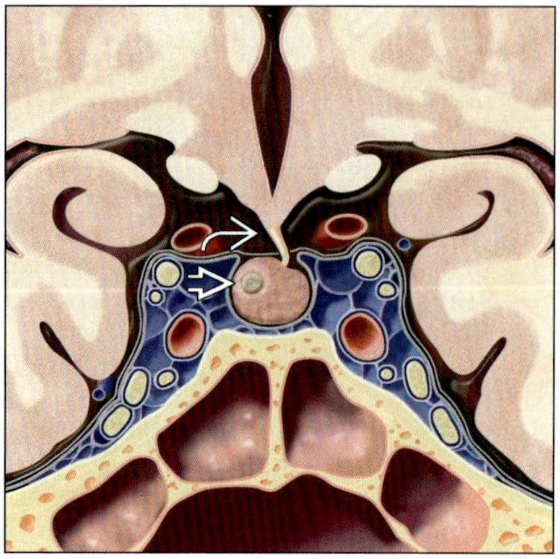

Over 30% of MEN1 patients develop pituitary adenoma. Coronal graphic shows a small microadenoma ➡ that enlarges the right side of the pituitary gland and deviates the infundibulum toward the left ➡.

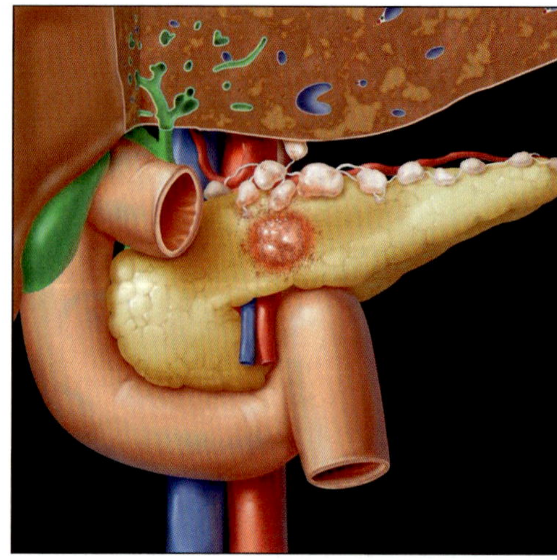

Graphic shows a small hypervascular lesion in the pancreatic body with regional lymph node metastases. Pancreatic gastrinomas and insulinomas are commonly observed in MEN1 patients.

TERMINOLOGY

Abbreviations

- Multiple endocrine neoplasia type 1 (MEN1)

Synonyms

- Wermer syndrome
- Multiple endocrine adenomatosis type 1

Definitions

- Rare autosomal dominant disease resulting in proliferative lesions of multiple endocrine organs involving mainly parathyroid, endocrine pancreas/duodenum, and pituitary glands

EPIDEMIOLOGY

Etiology

- Caused by mutations in *MEN1* gene

Pathogenesis

- *MEN1* gene is a 10 exon gene that encodes 610-amino acid protein menin
- Function is unknown; may act as regulator of gene transcription, cell proliferation, apoptosis, and genome stability

Incidence

- 1:20,000-50,000

Age

- Penetrance increases with age

Gender

- 1:1 sex distribution

GENETICS

MEN1 Gene

- Located on chromosome 11q13
- Consists of 10 exons and encodes menin

Mutation Spectrum

- > 1,300 different mutations of *MEN1* gene have been characterized
- Penetrance of *MEN1* mutations is high: 45% by age 30, 82% by age 50, 96% by age 70
- Spread over entire coding and intronic sequence
  - > 60% truncating mutation, 20% missense mutation, 10% in frame deletions or insertions, 10% others
- Most are inactivating mutations, consistent with those expected in tumor suppressor gene
  - Precise role of menin in tumor suppression remains elusive
- Clinical recommendation cannot be based on genotype
  - Truncating mutations: Increased risk of pancreatic endocrine tumor
  - Frameshift mutations in exon 2: Increased incidence of pituitary tumor
- 5-25% of patients with MEN1 may not harbor germline mutation in *MEN1* gene-coding region
  - Whole or partial deletions or mutations in promoter region

Testing

- *MEN1* mutational analysis should be undertaken in
  - Index case with 2 or more MEN1-associated endocrine tumors
  - Asymptomatic 1st-degree relative
  - 1st-degree relative of *MEN1* mutation carrier
  - Patients with suspicious or atypical MEN1
- Genetic counseling useful for individuals and families with nonclassic MEN1 presentations

- Testing should be undertaken as soon as possible, even before the age of 5

ASSOCIATED NEOPLASMS

Presentation

- **Hyperparathyroidism (HPT)**
  - Present in > 90% of MEN1 patients
    - Occurs at younger ages (19 years) than sporadic counterpart (50 years)
  - Percentage of patients who develop biochemical evidence of hyperparathyroidism increases with age
    - 43% and 94% at age 20 and 50 years, respectively
  - Most are asymptomatic, severe cases with "moans, groans, bones, and stones" as hallmarks of hypercalcemia
  - Multiglandular disorder
  - High recurrence rate
- **Pituitary tumors**
  - Found in 10-60% of MEN1 patients; mean age 38
  - Initial clinical manifestation of MEN1 in 10% and 20% of familial and sporadic cases, respectively
  - MEN1 pituitary adenomas tend to be larger and more aggressive than sporadic counterparts
  - Prolactinomas (PRL) (60%), growth hormone (GH) secreting adenoma (10%), adrenocorticotrophin (ACTH) secreting (5%), and nonsecreting adenomas (15%)
    - Women with PRL adenoma: Major clinical signs are amenorrhea, infertility, galactorrhea
    - Men with PRL adenoma: Hypogonadism
    - GH adenoma: Acromegaly
    - ACTH-secreting adenoma: Cushing disease
- **Endocrine pancreatic/duodenal tumors**
  - Familial Zollinger-Ellison syndrome (ZES)
    - Most frequent clinical manifestation related to duodenal &/or pancreatic gastrinoma observed in MEN1 patients
    - Initial symptoms, such as abdominal pain or gastroesophageal reflux disease, caused by gastric acid hypersecretion
    - Severe complications include bleeding, perforation, and esophageal strictures
    - In 90% of MEN1 patients with ZES, lesions are often multiple, small, and located in duodenum
  - Insulinomas
    - 2nd most frequent pancreatic tumor in setting of MEN1
    - Hypoglycemia
  - Glucagonoma, VIPoma, and other pancreatic endocrine tumors
    - Occur in < 5% of MEN1 patients
    - ~ 80% of glucagonomas and 40% of VIPomas are malignant
    - Glucagonomas induce necrolytic migratory erythema associated with diabetes mellitus, which is secondary to abnormal glucagon secretion
    - VIPomas induce classical Verner-Morrison syndrome associated with watery diarrhea, hypokalemia, and achlorhydria
  - Nonfunctioning pancreatic endocrine tumors
    - 20-40% of MEN1 patients
    - When misdiagnosed, often discovered after local compression &/or hepatic metastases
- **Others**
  - Adrenal cortical lesions
    - Observed in 20-40% of MEN1 patients
    - Often detected about 7 years after diagnosis of MEN1
    - Most are adenomas and may produce aldosterone and cortisol
    - Often small, benign, and nonfunctional
    - Surgery for lesions < 3 cm
  - Gastric ECLomas
    - Thought to originate from proliferation of enterochromaffin-like (ECL) cells in gastric mucosa
    - Often small and multiple
    - Can be treated with endoscopic polypectomy if lesion is < 1 cm
    - Good prognosis
  - Thymic and bronchial neuroendocrine tumor
    - Observed in 5-10% of MEN1 patients
    - Thymic carcinoids are predominantly in males
    - Poor prognosis with local invasion, recurrence, and distant metastasis
  - Cutaneous proliferations
    - Present in 40-80% of MEN1 patients
    - Nodular lipomas (30%)
    - Collagenomas (5%)
    - Angiofibromas are multiple and often on face (75%)
  - Soft tissue tumors
    - Esophageal leiomyoma
    - Renal angiomyolipoma
    - Malignant gastrointestinal stromal tumors
  - Central nervous system tumors
    - Spinal ependymomas, meningioma, and astrocytoma have been described in MEN1 cases

CLINICAL DIAGNOSIS

Basis for MEN1 Diagnosis

- Diagnosis of MEN1 may be established by 1 of 3 criteria
- **Clinical**
  - Occurrence of 2 or more primary MEN1-associated endocrine tumors: Parathyroid adenoma, enteropancreatic tumor, and pituitary adenoma
- **Familial**
  - Occurrence of 1 MEN1-associated tumor in 1st-degree relative of patient with clinical diagnosis of MEN1
- **Genetic**
  - Identification of germline *MEN1* mutation in an individual who may be asymptomatic and has not yet developed serum biochemical or radiological abnormalities is indicative of tumor development

Diagnostic Criteria

- Presence of ≥ 2 of the following

MULTIPLE ENDOCRINE NEOPLASIA TYPE 1

Clinical Practice Guidelines for Multiple Endocrine Neoplasia Type 1 (MEN1): Biochemical and Imaging Screening

Tumor	Age	Biochemical Test	Imaging Test
Parathyroid	8	Calcium, PTH	
Pituitary	5	Prolactin, IGF-1	MR every 3 years
Insulinoma	5	Fasting glucose, insulin	
Gastrinoma	20	Gastrin	
Other pancreatic endocrine tumors	< 10	Chromogranin-A, pancreatic polypeptide, glucagon, VIP	MR, CT, or EUS annually
Adrenal cortical tumors	< 10		MR or CT annually
Thymic and bronchial carcinoid	15		CT or MR every 1-2 years

Adapted from Thakker RV et al: Clinical practice guidelines for multiple endocrine neoplasia type 1 (MEN1). J Clin Endocrinol Metab. 97(9):2990-3011, 2012.

- Primary hyperparathyroidism with multiglandular hyperplasia &/or adenoma or recurrent primary hyperparathyroidism
- Duodenal &/or pancreatic endocrine tumors, gastric enterochromaffin-like tumors
  - Both functioning and nonfunctioning or multisecreting tumor
- Anterior pituitary adenoma
  - Functioning (GH-secreting tumor, prolactinoma)
  - Nonfunctioning or multisecreting
- Adrenal cortical tumor
  - Both functioning and nonfunctioning
- Thymic &/or bronchial endocrine tumors (foregut carcinoids)
- 1st-degree relative with MEN1

ANCILLARY TESTS

Immunohistochemistry

- Pituitary adenoma can express 1 or several hormones
  - Prolactin, ACTH, HGH, LH, FSH, TSH
- Pancreatic endocrine tumor can express 1 or several hormones
  - Insulin, gastrin, glucagon, pancreatic polypeptide, VIP, somatostatin, or serotonin

CANCER RISK MANAGEMENT

Screening

- Optimal screening age, test, and frequencies not established, but recommend starting annual biochemical test by 5 years
  - For known carriers of *MEN1* mutations
    - Glucose, insulin, prolactin, and IGF-1 levels
- Finding of MEN1 in a patient has important implications for family members
  - 1st-degree relatives have 50% risk of developing disease and can often be identified by *MEN1* mutational analysis
- Serologic tests
  - Starting at age 8: PTH and calcium levels
  - Starting at age 20: Fasting serum gastrin, pancreatic polypeptide, VIP, and glucagon

Treatment

- **Pituitary adenoma**
  - Medical and surgical treatment for prolactin or GH-producing tumors
- **Endocrine pancreatic/duodenal tumors**
  - Surgery in most cases
- **Hyperparathyroidism**
  - Total parathyroidectomy with autotransplantation or subtotal resection

Prognosis

- MEN1 patients have decreased life expectancy, and outcomes of current treatments are not as successful due to
  - Multiple tumors
    - Tumors may be larger, more aggressive, and resistant to treatment
  - Concurrence of metastases
- Same prognosis for pituitary adenoma in MEN1 as in sporadic counterparts
- Malignancy of duodenal and pancreatic endocrine tumors
  - Gastrinomas > 40%, glucagonoma > 80%, VIPoma > 40%, nonfunctioning tumor > 70%
- Prognosis for MEN1 patients might be improved by presymptomatic tumor detection

SELECTED REFERENCES

1. Hanazaki K et al: Surgery for a gastroenteropancreatic neuroendocrine tumor (GEPNET) in multiple endocrine neoplasia type 1. Surg Today. 43(3):229-36, 2013
2. Horiuchi K et al: An analysis of genotype-phenotype correlations and survival outcomes in patients with primary hyperparathyroidism caused by multiple endocrine neoplasia type 1: the experience at a single institution. Surg Today. 43(8):894-9, 2013
3. Thakker RV et al: Clinical practice guidelines for multiple endocrine neoplasia type 1 (MEN1). J Clin Endocrinol Metab. 97(9):2990-3011, 2012
4. Zhang Y et al: Endocrine tumors as part of inherited tumor syndromes. Adv Anat Pathol. 18(3):206-18, 2011

Pituitary, Parathyroid, and Pancreatic Pathology Features

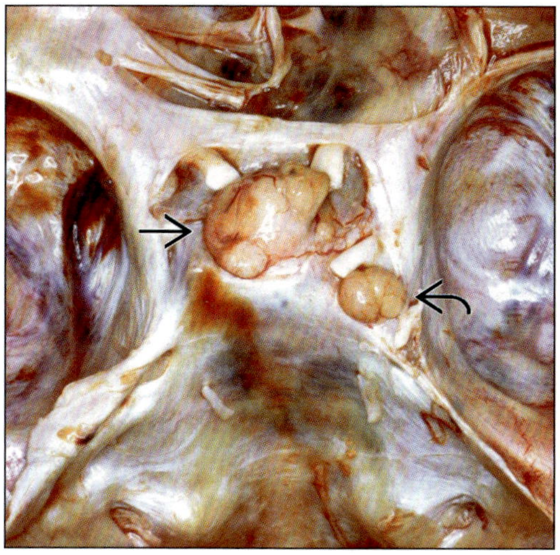
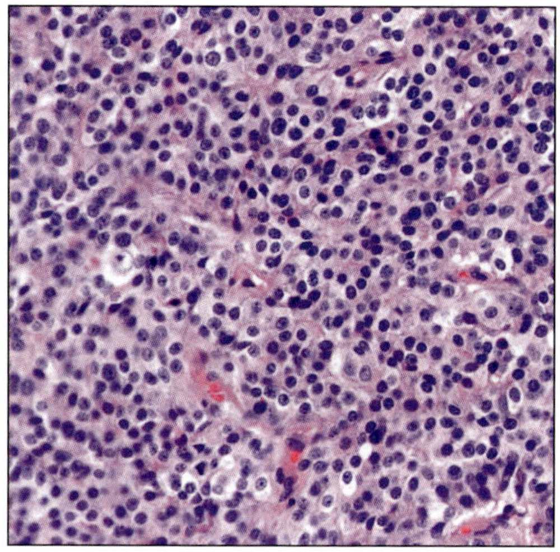

(Left) *Gross image shows a pituitary macroadenoma that extends upward into the suprasellar cistern → and laterally into the cavernous sinus ↶. Pituitary adenomas are found in 10-60% of MEN1 patients.* ***(Right)*** *Pituitary adenomas are usually arranged in a solid pattern that is formed by a homogeneous population of cells with no nuclear pleomorphism. The nuclei exhibit neuroendocrine cell features with finely dispersed chromatin and small distinct nucleoli.*

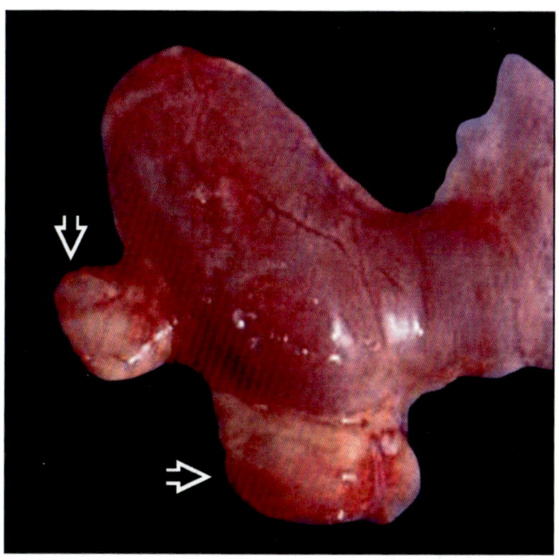
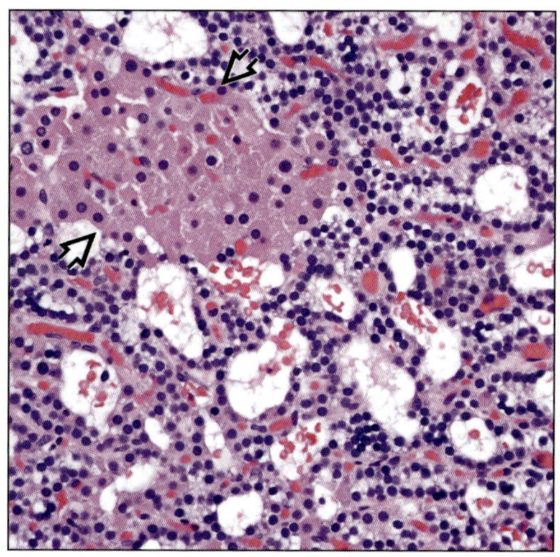

(Left) *The usual finding in specimens from patients with MEN1 and parathyroid hyperplasia is an uneven enlargement of the parathyroid glands. In this thyroid specimen, 2 attached parathyroid glands show hyperplasia ⇨. The parathyroids are markedly enlarged and of different sizes.* ***(Right)*** *Parathyroid from a patient with primary hyperparathyroidism in MEN1 setting shows nodular hyperplasia with nodules composed of chief cells and oncocytic cells ⇨.*

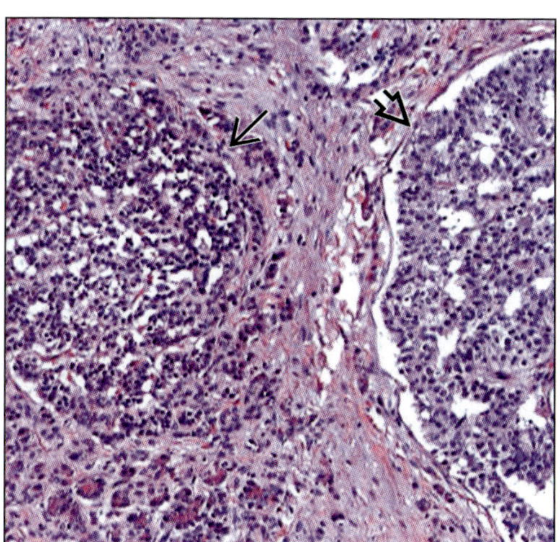
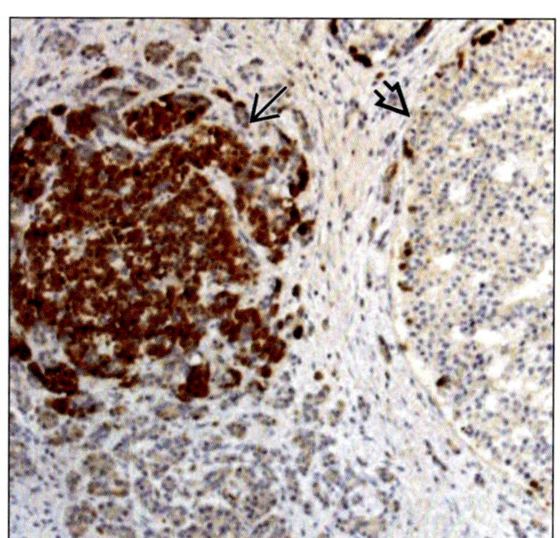

(Left) *Two distinct pancreatic endocrine cell proliferations in a patient with MEN1 are shown side by side. The lesion on the left → has irregular borders, and the lesion on the right ⇨ is well demarcated and larger.* ***(Right)*** *The smaller pancreatic endocrine lesion present in this field → is uniformly positive for glucagon (microadenoma) whereas the larger lesion ⇨ shows a pattern of immunostaining similar to that of a normal island, indicating hyperplasia.*

MULTIPLE ENDOCRINE NEOPLASIA TYPE 2/ FAMILIAL MEDULLARY THYROID CARCINOMA

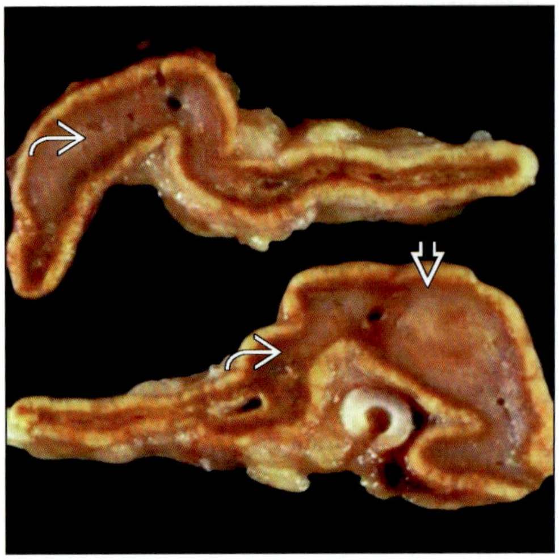

The adrenal gland from a patient with multiple endocrine neoplasia type 2A (MEN2A) shows diffuse medullary expansion ➦ as well as a well-defined nodule ⇨.

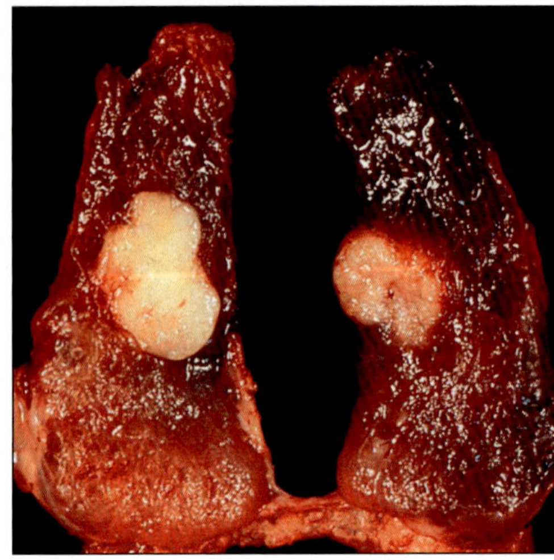

Bilateral medullary thyroid carcinoma from a patient with MEN2A shows both nodules to be well circumscribed with a pink-tan cut surface.

TERMINOLOGY

Abbreviations

- Multiple endocrine neoplasia type 2 (MEN2)
  - Multiple endocrine neoplasia type 2A (MEN2A)
  - Multiple endocrine neoplasia type 2B (MEN2B)
- Familial medullary thyroid carcinoma (FMTC)

EPIDEMIOLOGY

Incidence

- MEN2
  - Overall incidence is 1 in 30,000 live births
    - Hereditary medullary thyroid carcinoma (MTC) accounts for 25% of all MTC
- MEN2A
  - Unknown; estimated 1.25-7.5 per 10 million per year
  - Prevalence is 1 per 35,000
- MEN2B
  - Comprises about 5% of cases of MEN2
- FMTC
  - Comprises about 10-20% of cases with MEN2
- Overall incidence of MTC in patients with familial disease is 25%
  - This group represents ~ 5% of all thyroid tumors and ~ 15% of all thyroid cancer-related deaths

Age

- MEN2A
  - In late adolescence or early adulthood
  - Peak incidence of medullary carcinoma in these patients is in 4th decade
- MEN2B
  - Patients usually develop medullary carcinoma early in life, diagnosed in infancy or early childhood
- FMTC
  - Inherited medullary carcinoma without associated endocrinopathies
    - Similar to other types of thyroid cancers, peak incidence is between age 40 and 50 years

Gender

- MEN2
  - F:M = 1:1

GENETICS

RET Proto-Oncogene

- Maps to chromosome 10q11.2 and encodes a receptor tyrosine kinase called "rearranged during transfection"
  - Tyrosine kinase plays integral role in transducing signals for growth and differentiation in tissues derived from neural crest
- **MEN2A**: *RET* mutation in > 98% of cases
- **MEN2B**: *RET* mutation in 100% of cases
- **FMTC**: *RET* mutation in > 85% of cases
- MEN2 is caused by gain-of-function mutations that produce constitutively active protein or ↓ substrate specificity
- In contrast, loss-of-function mutations are associated with a subset of Hirschsprung disease (HSCR)
- Pathologic allelic variants: Major disease-causing mutations are nonconservative gain-of-function substitutions located in 1 of 6 cysteine codons in extracellular domain of encoded protein
  - Include codons 609, 611, 618, and 620 in exon 10 and codons 630 and 634 in exon 11
  - All of these variants have been identified in families with MEN2A, and some have been identified in families with FMTC
    - Mutations in these sites have been detected in 98% of families with MEN2A
  - ~ 95% of all individuals with MEN2B have single-point mutation at codon 918 in exon 16

- 2nd point mutation at codon 883 in exon 15 has been found in 3-5% of individuals with MEN2B
- For families in which MEN2A and HSCR cosegregate, models to explain how same mutation can cause gain of function and loss of function have been proposed

Genotype-Phenotype Correlations

- 1st clear genotype-phenotype associations to be found in inherited neoplasia syndromes: *RET* genotype- and MEN2-phenotype correlations
- Most striking observation: Gain-of-function mutations affected several hotspot codons, with great majority mutating cysteine residues in exons 10 and 11
- Notably, mutations of codon 634 in exon 11 are highly associated with full-blown phenotype of MEN2A, i.e., with high prevalence of pheochromocytoma and hyperparathyroidism
  - Associated fulminant course with p.C634R, which is associated with higher probability of having metastases at diagnosis of MTC than other codon 634 mutations
  - Although 25% of FMTC kindreds harbor a mutation in codon 634 (most commonly p.C634Y), p.C634R mutations are virtually absent in this subtype
  - Codon 634 mutations are also associated with development of cutaneous lichen amyloidosis (36%)
- *RET* germline p.M918T mutations are associated only with MEN2B
  - Somatic mutations at this codon are frequently observed in MTC in individuals with no known family history of MTC
    - Overrepresented in individuals with sporadic MTC who have particular germline *RET* variant, c.2439C/T
- Genotype-phenotype correlations suggest that exon 10 codon mutations, in particular at codons 609 and 611, have incidence of MTC in 77%, pheochromocytoma in 17%, and HPT in 3%
- Mutations involving cysteine codons 609, 618, and 620 in exon 10 of *RET* are associated with MEN2A or FMTC cosegregating with HSCR
- Mutations at codons 768, 804, and 891 are associated with FMTC and in rare families with MEN2A
- Mutations in codons 790 or 804 may be associated with papillary thyroid carcinoma (PTC) as well as MTC
  - 40% of family members with p.V804M mutation had concomitant medullary and PTC
- American Thyroid Association Guidelines Task Force has classified mutations based on risk for aggressive MTC
  - May be used in predicting phenotype and recommendations for age at which to perform prophylactic thyroidectomy and to begin biochemical screening for pheochromocytoma and hyperparathyroidism

CLINICAL IMPLICATIONS AND ANCILLARY TESTS

Presentation

- MEN2A, FMTC, and MEN2B can all be diagnosed based on clinical features
- With advances of *RET* testing, genotype-specific risks, and management, molecular genetic testing is virtually mandatory
  - Most often used to distinguish sporadic from hereditary MTC
- **MEN2A**
  - Diagnosed clinically by occurrence of ≥ 2 specific endocrine tumors (MTC, pheochromocytoma, or parathyroid adenoma/hyperplasia) in single individual or in close relatives
  - Makes up ~ 70-80% of cases of MEN2
  - ~ 100% of individuals with MEN2A develop MTC
  - 10-60% develop pheochromocytoma and 10-30% develop hyperparathyroidism
- **MEN2B**
  - Diagnosed clinically by presence of mucosal neuromas of lips and tongue, as well as medullated corneal nerve fibers, distinctive facies with enlarged lips, asthenic "Marfanoid" body habitus, and MTC
  - Comprises ~ 5% of cases of MEN2
  - Characterized by early development of aggressive form of MTC associated with C-cell hyperplasia (CCH)
  - 50% develop pheochromocytoma
  - 60-90% have ganglioneuromatosis
  - Presence of mucosal neuromas is identified early in life
  - ~ 100% have asthenic "Marfanoid" body habitus
- **FMTC**
  - Historically, operationally diagnosed in families with ≥ 4 cases of MTC in absence of pheochromocytoma or parathyroid adenoma/ hyperplasia
  - Because *RET* mutation accounts for all clinical subtypes of MEN2, FMTC may be viewed as MEN2A with reduced organ-specific penetrance
  - Comprises 10-20% of cases of MEN2
  - MTC is the only clinical manifestation of FMTC

Laboratory Tests

- **MTC**: In provocative testing, plasma calcitonin concentration is measured before (basal levels) as well as 2 and 5 minutes after intravenous administration of calcium (stimulated level)
  - Other calcitonin secretagogues, e.g., pentagastrin, are also used
  - Reference levels for basal calcitonin vary across laboratories: < 10 pg/mL for adult males and < 5 pg/mL for adult females are typically considered normal
  - Basal or stimulated calcitonin level of ≥ 100 pg/mL is indication for surgery
    - Caution should be used when interpreting calcitonin levels in children younger than 5 years

MULTIPLE ENDOCRINE NEOPLASIA TYPE 2/ FAMILIAL MEDULLARY THYROID CARCINOMA

- **Pheochromocytoma** is suspected when biochemical screening reveals elevated secretion of catecholamines and catecholamine metabolites
  - In MEN2, pheochromocytomas consistently produce epinephrine or both epinephrine and norepinephrine
- Diagnosis of **parathyroid abnormalities** is made when biochemical screening reveals simultaneously elevated serum concentrations of calcium and elevated or high to normal parathyroid hormone

Immunohistochemistry

- MTC: Calcitonin, calcitonin gene-related peptide (CGRP), chromogranin, and CEA
- Pheochromocytoma (PCC): Neuroendocrine markers; RET staining is not helpful to distinguish MEN2-associated PCC from sporadic counterpart

Imaging Features

- May be used in predicting phenotype and recommendations for age at which to perform prophylactic thyroidectomy and to begin biochemical screening for pheochromocytoma and hyperparathyroidism
  - MR is more sensitive than CT in detection of pheochromocytoma
- 18F-fluorodopamine positron emission tomography (PET) is best overall imaging modality in localization of pheochromocytomas
- Postoperative parathyroid localizing studies with Tc-99m sestamibi scintigraphy may be helpful if HPT recurs
- For preoperative adenoma localization, 3D single-photon emission CT may also be used

ASSOCIATED NEOPLASMS

Precursor Lesions

- Neoplastic C-cell hyperplasia (NCCH)
  - NCCH is precursor lesion in hereditary MTC
  - Clusters should have > 50 C cells
  - a.k.a. C-cell carcinoma in situ or medullary carcinoma in situ
  - These lesions harbor germline *RET* mutations
  - Postulated that CCH progresses to medullary microcarcinoma (MMC) and eventually to MTC
  - Found in vicinity of medullary carcinomas
  - Distinguishing CCH from MMC or intrathyroid spread of MTC may be difficult
- Adrenal medullary hyperplasia (AMH)
  - Common in multiple endocrine neoplasia 2A and 2B; absent or very rare in other pheochromocytoma/paraganglioma syndromes
  - Adrenals removed for pheochromocytoma should be carefully examined for additional nodules as a clue to presence of MEN2
  - AMH may present with signs of catecholamine excess or be discovered incidentally after adrenalectomy for pheochromocytoma
  - Adrenal medulla normally confined to central region ("body") of gland
    - AMH often identifiable by gross extension of gray medullary tissue into alae and tail
    - Nodules often superimposed on diffuse hyperplasia

Medullary Thyroid Carcinoma

- Often presents as painless "cold" nodule
  - Up to 50% have nodal metastases
  - Up to 20% may present with distant metastases
  - Symptoms of carcinoid and Cushing syndromes may be present
- Typically at junction of upper and middle 1/3 of lobe
  - Hereditary tumors are usually multicentric and bilateral
    - Sporadic tumors tend to present as solitary mass ± lymph node involvement
  - Always associated with C-cell hyperplasia in MEN2

Pheochromocytoma

- ≥ 30% of PCCs/paraganglioma are hereditary tumors
  - ~ 1/3 of these are MEN2 patients
  - Occult germline mutations of susceptibility genes are common in patients with apparently sporadic pheochromocytomas
- Affected by genotype
  - Multiple tumors or tumors presenting in children suggest hereditary disease
    - Sporadic tumors are solitary, usually in adults
  - Tumors with *RET* mutations are almost always intraadrenal

Parathyroid Hyperplasia and Adenoma

- 20-30% of MEN2A are associated with parathyroid hyperplasia or adenoma
- Almost never initial presentation of MEN2A
  - In contrast, hyperparathyroidism is common presentation in MEN1 (> 80%)

Ganglioneuroma of Gastrointestinal Tract

- ~ 40% of MEN2B-affected individuals have diffuse intestinal ganglioneuromatosis

Mucosal Neuroma

- May be identified in infancy and early childhood
- On palate, anterior dorsal surface of tongue, or pharynx
- Neuromas in eyelids

CANCER RISK MANAGEMENT

Genetic Testing, MEN2

- *RET* is the only gene known to be associated with MEN2
- *RET* molecular genetic testing is indicated in all individuals with diagnosis of MTC, clinical diagnosis of MEN2, or primary CCH
- Algorithm for testing is summarized in most recent American Thyroid Association MTC Practice Guidelines
  - Young age of onset, significant CCH, &/or multifocal disease suggest inherited disorder
  - All individuals with MTC, regardless of other features or family history, and those with clinical

features suspicious for MEN2 &/or with family history suspicious of MEN2 should be offered germline *RET* testing for exons 10, 11, and 13-16
- MEN2A: 98% of families have *RET* mutation in exon 10 or 11
- Families with FMTC: *RET* mutation in > 85%
- Individuals with features suggestive of MEN2B: Mutation analysis or sequencing of exons 16 and 15 to detect p.M918T and p.A883F mutations
  - If mutation negative, testing for p.V804M in exon 14 followed by sequencing of entire *RET* coding region should be performed
  - Although isolated p.V804M mutation is associated with FMTC, p.V804M co-occurring with 2nd *RET* variant seems to result in MEN2B
  - This strategy will detect > 98% of mutations in individuals with MEN2B
- *RET* molecular genetic testing may be warranted in subsets of individuals presenting with apparently isolated adrenal pheochromocytoma
  - Other differential diagnoses, such as VHL and succinate dehydrogenase-associated pheochromocytoma, should also be considered
  - Testing algorithms for genes associated with paraganglioma and pheochromocytoma have been proposed based on age of onset, location, laterality, malignancy, and family history
  - Unexpected germline *RET* mutations are rarely (if ever) found in head and neck paraganglioma in absence of other features of MEN2 or family history of MEN2 phenotype
- Other clinical presentations may prompt consideration of genetic testing
  - Exon 10 sequencing should be considered in individuals with HSCR
- Differential diagnosis in persons with intestinal ganglioneuromatosis should include MEN2B, and RET testing may be considered
- Rarely, germline *RET* mutation may not be detected in family with clinical diagnosis of MEN2A, MEN2B, or FMTC

Genetic Testing, FMTC

- Germline point mutation in *RET* gene on chromosome 10q11.2 is responsible for hereditary MTC

Testing of Relatives at Risk

- At-risk relatives should be periodically screened for
  - MTC with neck ultrasound examination and basal &/or stimulated calcitonin measurements
  - HPT with albumin-corrected calcium or ionized calcium
  - PCC with measurement of plasma or 24-hour urine metanephrine and normetanephrine
- *RET* molecular genetic testing should be offered to probands with any MEN2 subtype and to all at-risk kindreds when a germline *RET* mutation has been identified in an affected family member
- American Society of Clinical Oncologists identifies MEN2 as group 1 disorder, i.e., well-defined hereditary cancer syndrome for which genetic testing is considered part of standard management for at-risk family members
- *RET* molecular genetic testing should be performed as soon as possible after birth in all children known to be at risk for MEN2B
- In families with MEN2A or FMTC, molecular genetic testing should be offered to at-risk children by age 5 years, as MTC has been documented in childhood

SELECTED REFERENCES

1. Son EJ et al: Familial follicular cell-derived thyroid carcinoma. Front Endocrinol (Lausanne). 3:61, 2012
2. Laury AR et al: Thyroid pathology in PTEN-hamartoma tumor syndrome: characteristic findings of a distinct entity. Thyroid. 21(2):135-44, 2011
3. Nosé V: Familial thyroid cancer: a review. Mod Pathol. 24 Suppl 2:S19-33, 2011
4. Smith JR et al: Thyroid nodules and cancer in children with PTEN hamartoma tumor syndrome. J Clin Endocrinol Metab. 96(1):34-7, 2011
5. Zada G et al: Atypical pituitary adenomas: incidence, clinical characteristics, and implications. J Neurosurg. 114(2):336-44, 2011
6. Zhang Y et al: Endocrine tumors as part of inherited tumor syndromes. Adv Anat Pathol. 18(3):206-18, 2011
7. Grubbs EG et al: Do the recent American Thyroid Association (ATA) Guidelines accurately guide the timing of prophylactic thyroidectomy in MEN2A? Surgery. 148(6):1302-9; discussion 1309-10, 2010
8. Nosé V: Familial follicular cell tumors: classification and morphological characteristics. Endocr Pathol. 21(4):219-26, 2010
9. Nosé V: Thyroid cancer of follicular cell origin in inherited tumor syndromes. Adv Anat Pathol. 17(6):428-36, 2010
10. American Thyroid Association Guidelines Task Force et al: Medullary thyroid cancer: management guidelines of the American Thyroid Association. Thyroid. 19(6):565-612, 2009
11. Margraf RL et al: Multiple endocrine neoplasia type 2 RET protooncogene database: repository of MEN2-associated RET sequence variation and reference for genotype/ phenotype correlations. Hum Mutat. 30(4):548-56, 2009
12. Raue F et al: Genotype-phenotype relationship in multiple endocrine neoplasia type 2. Implications for clinical management. Hormones (Athens). 8(1):23-8, 2009
13. van Nederveen FH et al: Array-comparative genomic hybridization in sporadic benign pheochromocytomas. Endocr Relat Cancer. 16(2):505-13, 2009
14. Falchetti A et al: Multiple endocrine neoplasms. Best Pract Res Clin Rheumatol. 2008 Mar;22(1):149-63. Review. Erratum in: Best Pract Res Clin Rheumatol. 22(6):III, 2008
15. Frank-Raue K et al: Difference in development of medullary thyroid carcinoma among carriers of RET mutations in codons 790 and 791. Clin Endocrinol (Oxf). 69(2):259-63, 2008
16. Lodish MB et al: RET oncogene in MEN2, MEN2B, MTC and other forms of thyroid cancer. Expert Rev Anticancer Ther. 8(4):625-32, 2008
17. Moore SW et al: Multiple endocrine neoplasia syndromes, children, Hirschsprung's disease and RET. Pediatr Surg Int. 24(5):521-30, 2008
18. White ML et al: Multiple endocrine neoplasia. Surg Oncol Clin N Am. 17(2):439-59, x, 2008
19. Carling T: Multiple endocrine neoplasia syndrome: genetic basis for clinical management. Curr Opin Oncol. 17(1):7-12, 2005

MULTIPLE ENDOCRINE NEOPLASIA TYPE 2/ FAMILIAL MEDULLARY THYROID CARCINOMA

Components of Multiple Endocrine Neoplasia Syndromes Type 2

Pathology	FMTC	MEN2A	MEN2B
Medullary thyroid carcinoma	100%	100%	100%
C-cell hyperplasia	100%	100%	100%
Pheochromocytoma	0%	10-60%	50%
Hyperparathyroidism	0%	10-30%	0%
Lichen amyloidosis	0%	0%	< 10%
"Marfanoid" habitus	0%	0%	100%
Mucosal neuromas	0%	0%	70-100%
Intestinal ganglioneuromatosis	0%	0%	60-90%
Thick corneal nerves	0%	Rare	60-90%

Familial medullary thyroid carcinoma (FMTC), multiple endocrine neoplasia type 2A (MEN2A), multiple endocrine neoplasia type 2B MEN2B).

Differential Diagnosis of Micromedullary Thyroid Carcinoma

Characteristics	Sporadic	Familial
Multifocality	Rare (~ 10%)	Frequent (~ 90%)
Bilaterality	Rare (~ 10%)	Common (~ 70%)
Physiologic CCH	Common (~ 55%)	Rare (~10%)
Neoplastic CCH	Rare (~15%)	Frequent (90%)

ATA Recommendations for Prophylactic Thyroidectomy Depending on RET Mutation

ATA Risk Level Based on RET Mutation	Recommended Age for Prophylactic Thyroidectomy
Codons 838, 918, 922	Within 1st year of life
Codons 768, 790, 791, 804, 891	Consider surgery before age 5 years; may delay surgery up to 10 years if normal serum calcitonin, normal neck ultrasound, family history of less aggressive tumor
Codons 609, 611, 618, 620, 630	Consider surgery before age 5 years; may delay surgery up to 10 years if normal serum calcitonin, normal neck ultrasound, family history of less aggressive tumor
Codon 634	Before age 5 years

ATA: American Thyroid Association. Adapted from Grubbs EG et al: Do the recent American Thyroid Association (ATA) Guidelines accurately guide the timing of prophylactic thyroidectomy in MEN2A? Surgery. 148(6):1302-9; discussion 1309-10, 2010 and American Thyroid Association Guidelines Task Force et al: Medullary thyroid cancer: management guidelines of the American Thyroid Association. Thyroid. 19(6):565-612, 2009.

Gross and Microscopic Features in MEN2

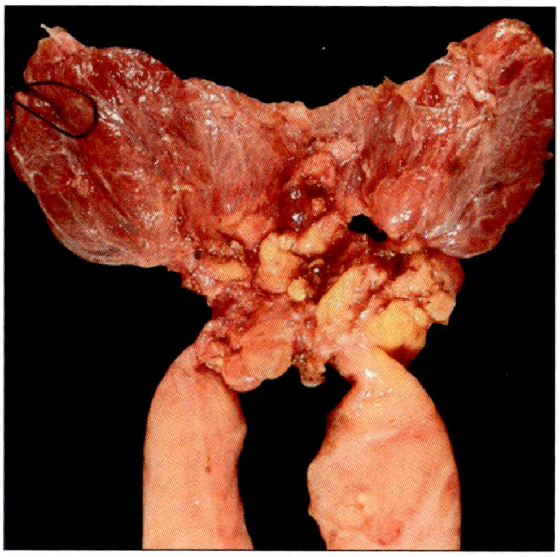

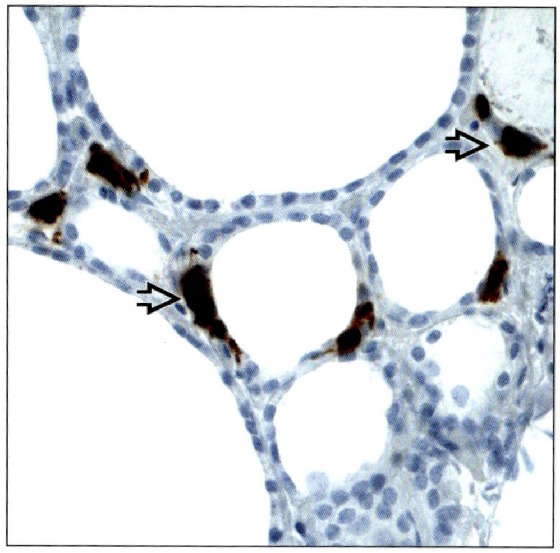

(Left) *Total prophylactic thyroidectomy plus thymectomy from a patient with a family history of MEN2 with RET mutation. The entire thyroid submitted for histological examination showed C-cell hyperplasia and 2 microscopic foci of medullary thyroid carcinoma.* ***(Right)*** *Calcitonin staining shows a normal distribution of C cells within a section of the mid portion of the thyroid lobes, indicating lack of C-cell hyperplasia.*

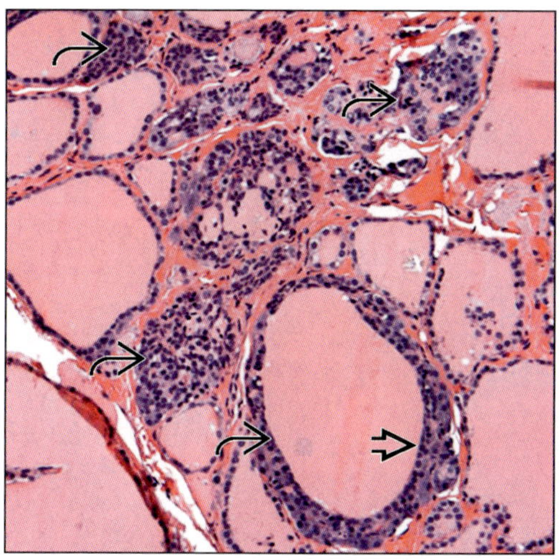

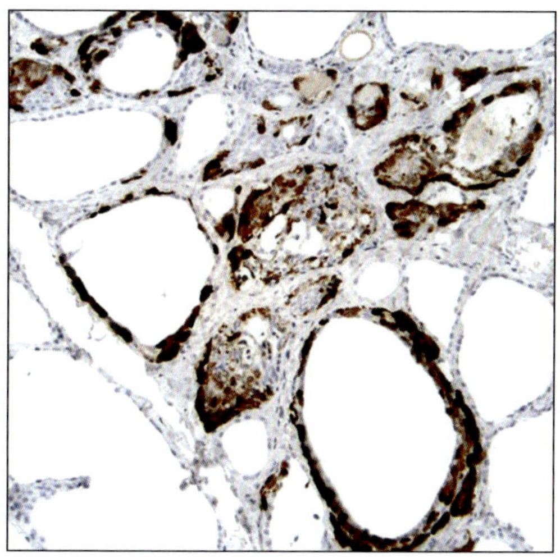

(Left) *C-cell hyperplasia is identified by H&E in a patient with MEN2 syndrome. C cells are also present surrounding an entire thyroid follicle.* ***(Right)*** *Specimen from a patient with MEN2 syndrome, who underwent prophylactic thyroidectomy, shows C-cell hyperplasia highlighted by calcitonin immunostaining. Heritable medullary thyroid carcinoma is preceded by C-cell hyperplasia (neoplastic C-cell hyperplasia).*

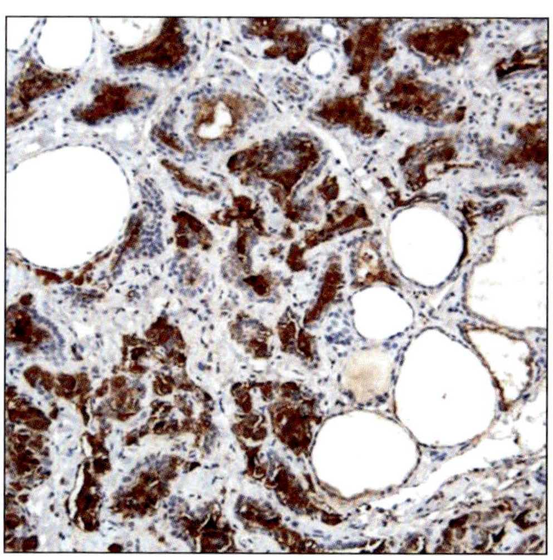

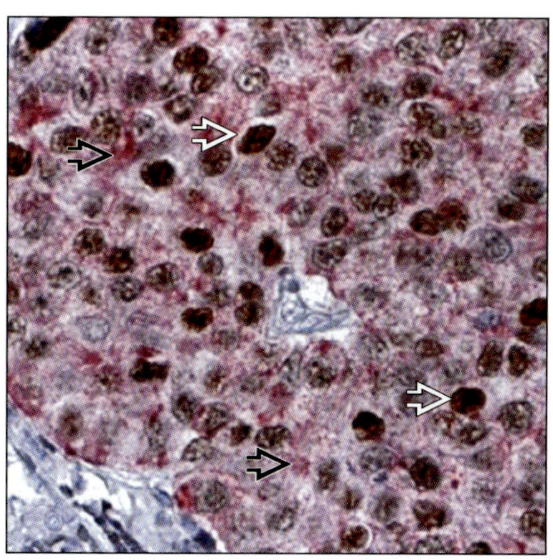

(Left) *A patient with family history of MEN2B with RET mutation had a prophylactic thyroidectomy, which showed C-cell hyperplasia and 2 foci of medullary thyroid carcinoma. Calcitonin immunostain highlights the focus of a micromedullary carcinoma.* ***(Right)*** *Double immunostaining section of a medullary thyroid carcinoma in a child with MEN2B shows cytoplasmic staining for calcitonin and nuclear staining for TTF-1.*

MULTIPLE ENDOCRINE NEOPLASIA TYPE 2/ FAMILIAL MEDULLARY THYROID CARCINOMA

Clinical, Gross, and Microscopic Features

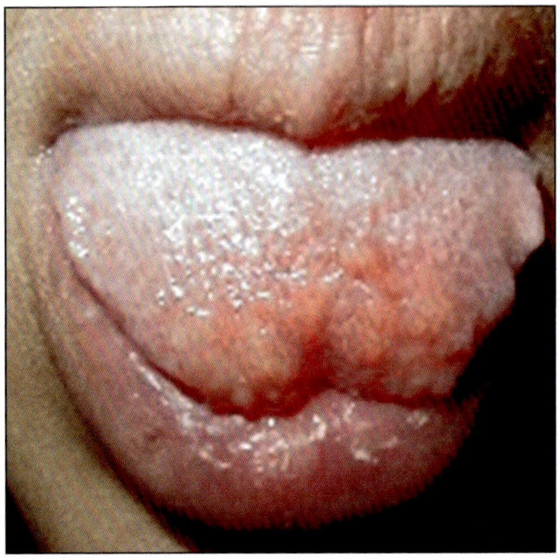
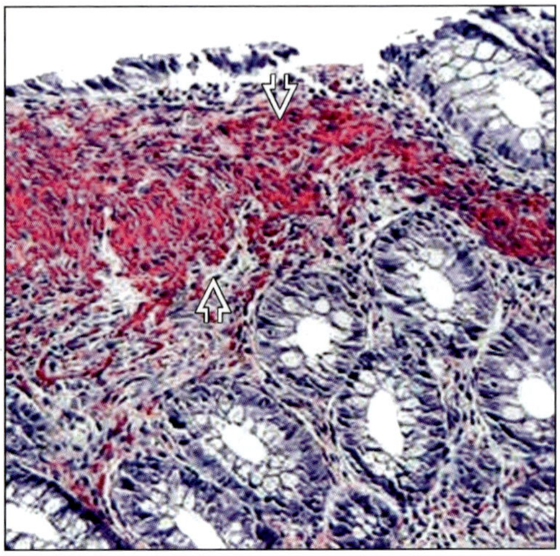

(Left) *This young patient with multiple endocrine neoplasia type 2B displays marked thickening of the lips and tongue due to ganglioneuromatosis. This patient also had a medullary thyroid carcinoma diagnosed at a young age.* ***(Right)*** *S100 immunostain from an intestinal biopsy in a patient with MEN2B shows proliferation of neuromatous fibers in MEN-associated intestinal ganglioneuromatosis.*

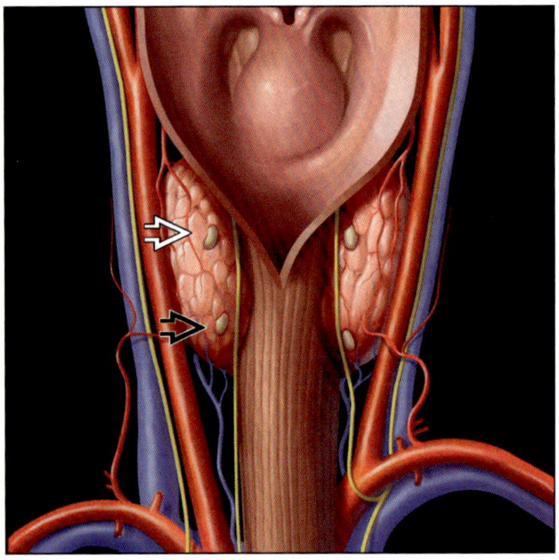
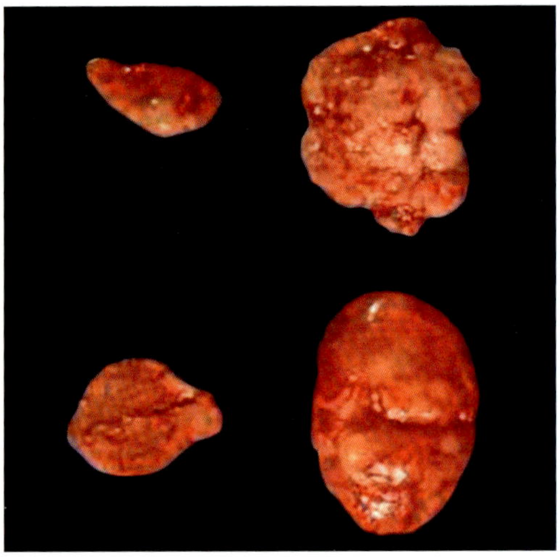

(Left) *Hyperparathyroidism in MEN2A is typically mild; it may range from a single adenoma to mild hyperplasia and rarely to severe hyperplasia. Coronal graphic displays the typical anatomic relationships of the paired superior and inferior parathyroid glands (view from behind).* ***(Right)*** *Hyperparathyroidism in MEN2A is typically mild; it may be a single adenoma or hyperplasia. This gross photograph shows mildly enlarged parathyroid glands.*

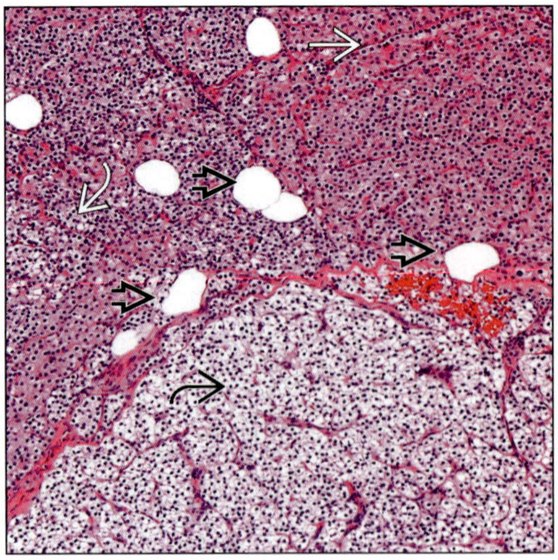
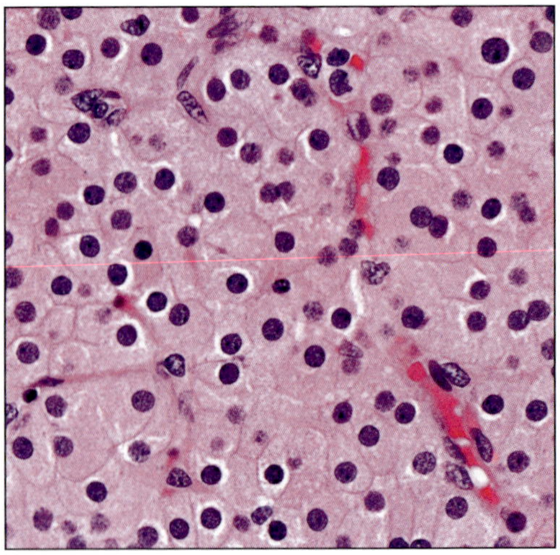

(Left) *Parathyroid glands in patients with MEN2A with primary hyperparathyroidism show nodular hyperplasia growth pattern. This photomicrograph shows clear (water-clear) cells, chief cells, and oxyphil cells intermixed with scattered fat cells.* ***(Right)*** *Parathyroid hyperplasia and neoplasia are frequently seen in patients with MEN2A. This photomicrograph of a parathyroid hyperplasia demonstrates a diffuse proliferation of mitochondrion-rich oxyphil cells (right).*

Features of Pheochromocytoma

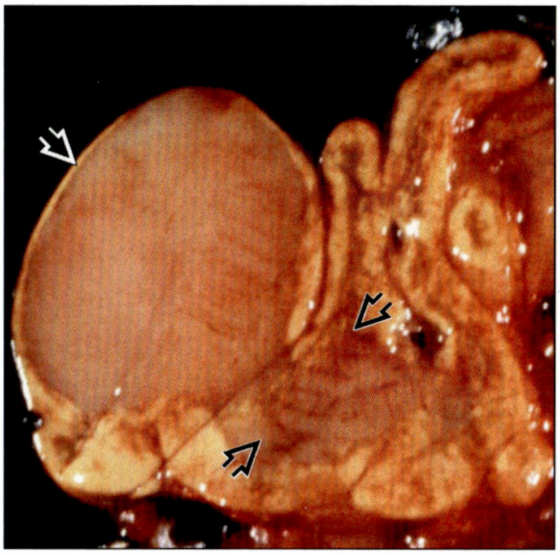

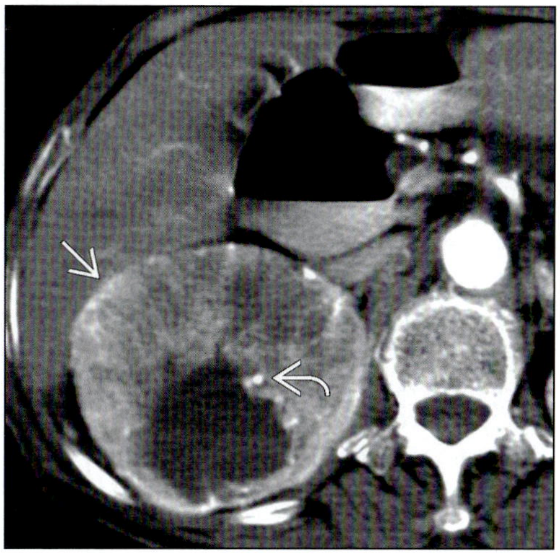

(Left) *This adrenal gland shows both MEN2-associated adrenal medullary hyperplasia ➡ and pheochromocytoma ➡. Adrenal medullary hyperplasia is characteristic of MEN2.* ***(Right)*** *Axial contrast-enhanced CT shows a large, well-circumscribed, moderately enhancing right adrenal pheochromocytoma ➡ with a hypodense area of necrosis ➡.*

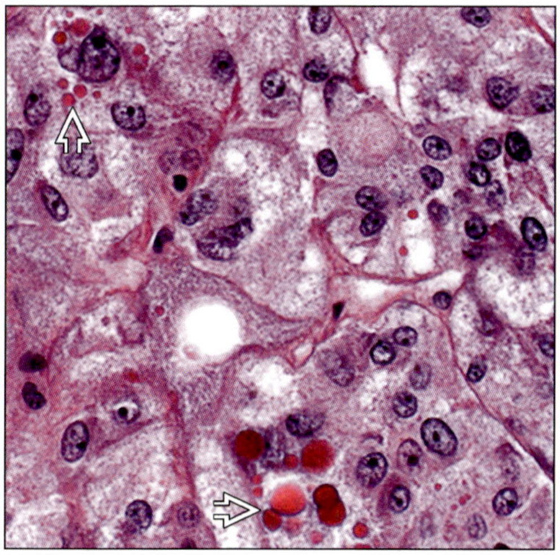

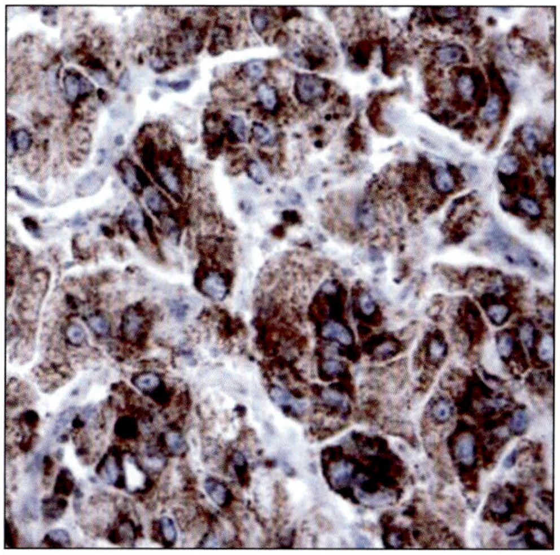

(Left) *Hyaline globules ➡ are present in some paragangliomas (PGLs) and pheochromocytomas (PCCs), especially in PCC/PGLs in patients with MEN2.* ***(Right)*** *Chromogranin-A immunostain shows granular immunoreactivity in the nests of neuroendocrine cells of a paraganglioma in a patient with MEN2A.*

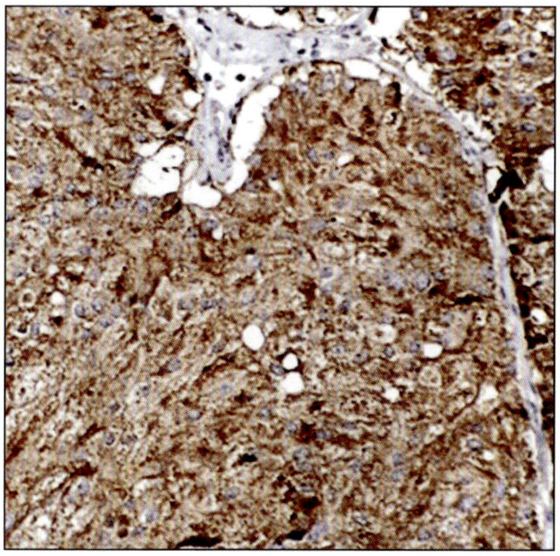

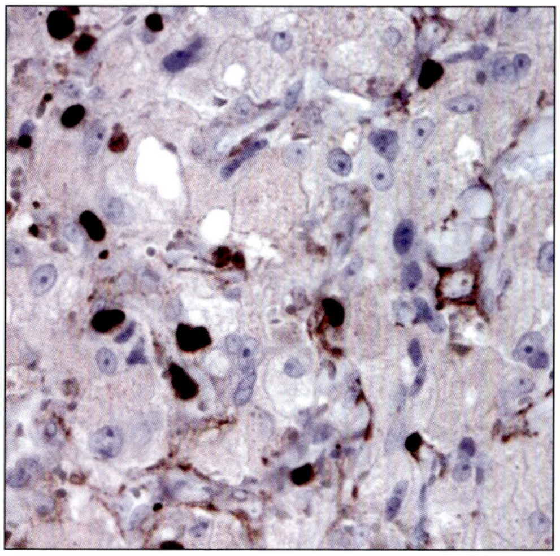

(Left) *Pheochromocytomas in MEN2 patients show granular cytoplasmic immunoreactivity for the SDHB protein. The stain is usually coarsely granular, as this protein is localized to the mitochondria.* ***(Right)*** *Immunohistochemistry for Ki-67 proliferative marker usually shows a low proliferative index in pheochromocytomas associated with MEN2. This field shows an unusually high proliferative index for a MEN2-associated pheochromocytoma.*

MYH-ASSOCIATED POLYPOSIS

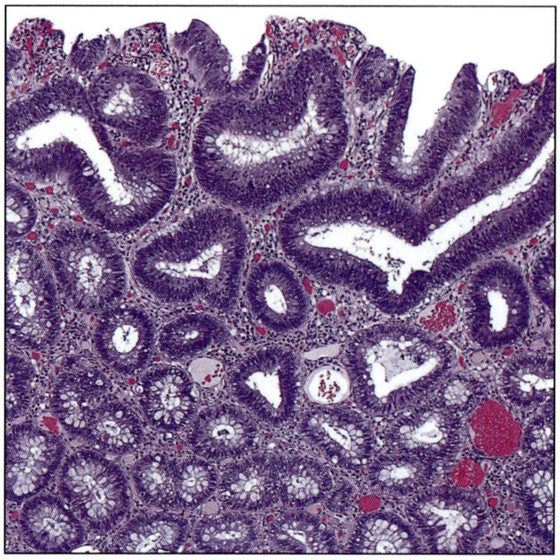

Medium-power view of a tubular adenoma from a patient with > 20 adenomas and multiple hyperplastic polyps. The adenomas in MYH polyposis are identical to sporadic adenomas.

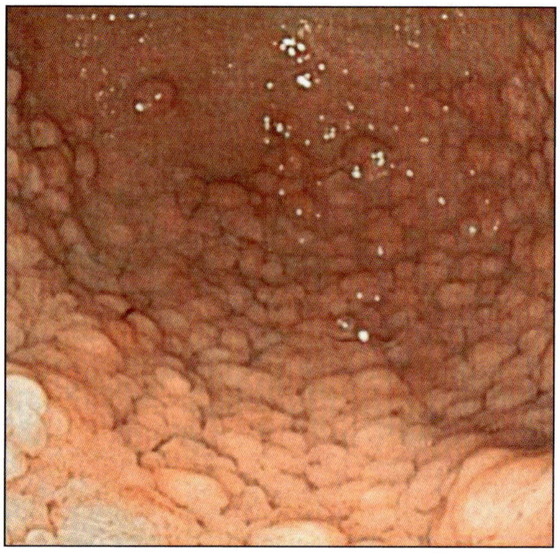

Endoscopic view shows a stomach that is carpeted with fundic gland polyps. Patients with MYH can have gastric findings similar to those of patients with familial adenomatous polyposis (FAP). (Courtesy E. Stoffel, MD.)

TERMINOLOGY

Abbreviations

- Mut Y homologue (MYH)
- MYH-associated polyposis (MAP)

EPIDEMIOLOGY

Prevalence

- < 1 in 10,000
- Mean age at diagnosis is 45, with a reported age range of 12-68 years
  - Risk of colorectal cancer (CRC) is 80% at age 70 with 50% of patients found to have CRC at time of polyposis diagnosis
  - Patients tend to be older than familial adenomatous polyposis (FAP) patients but slightly younger than typical CRC patients
    - May have right-sided CRC in younger patient suggestive of Lynch syndrome

GENETICS

MYH Gene

- Base excision repair gene
  - Biallelic germline mutations in *MYH* lead to G:C to T:A transversions in somatic genes (i.e., *APC*, *KRAS*)
    - Oxidation of guanine is normally repaired by MYH
    - Oxidated guanine binds to adenine instead of cytosine, hence the G:C to T:A transversions
    - Somatic mutations in *APC* gene leads to polyposis similar to FAP
- Autosomal recessive
  - 1-2% of population carry a single deleterious mutation
  - Parents of affected patient are both carriers
  - Unclear if carriers have an increased rate of colon cancer
    - Some reports have found slightly increased risk (1.5-2.1 relative risk) of CRC, whereas other studies have failed to show this

CLINICAL IMPLICATIONS AND ANCILLARY TESTS

Clinical Profile

- Multiple adenomas but typically not in overwhelming numbers as seen in FAP
- Easy to miss diagnosis since there is no family history and patients have fewer polyps at an older age than typical FAP patients

Genetic Testing

- In patients without a family history of polyposis, need to test for both FAP and MAP as 30% of FAP cases arise de novo
- 2 common mutations in *MYH* gene account for 80% of cases (especially in people of Northern European descent)
  - Most cost-effective method currently is to sequence *APC* gene and test for the 2 common *MYH* mutations
    - If this fails to identify mutations, then sequencing *MYH* will be necessary
  - If patients are not of Northern European descent, may be more cost effective to sequence *MYH* from the start
- Can measure G:C to T:A transversion in tumor DNA, especially in *APC* and *KRAS* genes
- MAP carcinomas are typically microsatellite stable (as opposed to Lynch cancers that are unstable)

ASSOCIATED NEOPLASMS

Identical to FAP

- Multiple adenomas and increased risk of CRC
  - Up to 42% of MAP patients have 10-100 polyps, similar to attenuated FAP
  - Up to 29% will have > 100 adenomas and resemble classic FAP
  - May have unicryptal or microadenomas
  - May also have serrated polyps (hyperplastic polyps and sessile serrated adenomas have been reported)
- Extracolonic neoplasms
  - 18-25% have duodenal adenomas
    - 4% lifetime risk of duodenal carcinoma
  - Fundic gland polyps similar to FAP
  - Congenital hypertrophy of retinal pigment epithelium, dermal cysts, osteomas, dental abnormalities, and desmoids have also been reported
    - Prevalence of these lesions may be lower than in FAP, but given rarity of syndrome, good data do not exist
  - Ovarian, bladder, and skin cancers have been reported (which can be suggestive of Lynch syndrome)

CANCER RISK MANAGEMENT

Surveillance

- Patients with known *MYH* mutations should have colonoscopic surveillance beginning between ages 20 and 30
  - If no polyps are found, may continue surveillance every 3-5 years
  - If polyps are found, may go to annual surveillance
- Upper tract endoscopic surveillance is recommended beginning at age 30-35 years
  - If no polyps are found, may continue surveillance every 3-5 years
  - If polyps are found, annual surveillance may be recommended

Surgery

- When polyps become too numerous, prophylactic colectomy with ileoanal anastomosis is treatment of choice

SELECTED REFERENCES

1. Castillejo A et al: Recurrent testicular germ cell tumors in a family with MYH-associated polyposis. J Clin Oncol. 30(23):e216-7, 2012
2. Bolocan A et al: Map syndrome (MYH Associated Polyposis) colorectal cancer, etiopathological connections. J Med Life. 4(1):109-11, 2011
3. Goodenberger M et al: Lynch syndrome and MYH-associated polyposis: review and testing strategy. J Clin Gastroenterol. 45(6):488-500, 2011
4. Lefevre JH et al: MYH biallelic mutation can inactivate the two genetic pathways of colorectal cancer by APC or MLH1 transversions. Fam Cancer. 9(4):589-94, 2010
5. de Ferro SM et al: Aggressive phenotype of MYH-associated polyposis with jejunal cancer and intra-abdominal desmoid tumor: report of a case. Dis Colon Rectum. 52(4):742-5, 2009
6. Lefevre JH et al: APC, MYH, and the correlation genotype-phenotype in colorectal polyposis. Ann Surg Oncol. 16(4):871-7, 2009
7. Lindor NM: Hereditary colorectal cancer: MYH-associated polyposis and other newly identified disorders. Best Pract Res Clin Gastroenterol. 23(1):75-87, 2009
8. Terdiman JP: MYH-associated disease: attenuated adenomatous polyposis of the colon is only part of the story. Gastroenterology. 137(6):1883-6, 2009
9. Ajith Kumar VK et al: Sebaceous adenomas in an MYH associated polyposis patient of Indian (Gujarati) origin. Fam Cancer. 7(2):187-9, 2008
10. Boparai KS et al: Hyperplastic polyps and sessile serrated adenomas as a phenotypic expression of MYH-associated polyposis. Gastroenterology. 135(6):2014-8, 2008
11. Castells A: MYH-associated polyposis: adenomas and hyperplastic polyps, partners in crime? Gastroenterology. 135(6):1857-9, 2008
12. Ellis CN: Colonic adenomatous polyposis syndromes: clinical management. Clin Colon Rectal Surg. 21(4):256-62, 2008
13. Jass JR: Colorectal polyposes: from phenotype to diagnosis. Pathol Res Pract. 204(7):431-47, 2008
14. O'Shea AM et al: Pathological features of colorectal carcinomas in MYH-associated polyposis. Histopathology. 53(2):184-94, 2008
15. Bouguen G et al: Colorectal adenomatous polyposis Associated with MYH mutations: genotype and phenotype characteristics. Dis Colon Rectum. 50(10):1612-7, 2007
16. Ponti G et al: BRAF mutations in multiple sebaceous hyperplasias of patients belonging to MYH-associated polyposis pedigrees. J Invest Dermatol. 127(6):1387-91, 2007
17. Aretz S et al: MUTYH-associated polyposis: 70 of 71 patients with biallelic mutations present with an attenuated or atypical phenotype. Int J Cancer. 119(4):807-14, 2006
18. Di Gregorio C et al: Immunohistochemical expression of MYH protein can be used to identify patients with MYH-associated polyposis. Gastroenterology. 131(2):439-44, 2006
19. Jeter JM et al: Genetics of colorectal cancer. Oncology (Williston Park). 20(3):269-76; discussion 285-6, 288-9, 2006
20. Nielsen M et al: Multiplicity in polyp count and extracolonic manifestations in 40 Dutch patients with MYH associated polyposis coli (MAP). J Med Genet. 42(9):e54, 2005
21. Ponti G et al: Attenuated familial adenomatous polyposis and Muir-Torre syndrome linked to compound biallelic constitutional MYH gene mutations. Clin Genet. 68(5):442-7, 2005
22. Al-Tassan N et al: Inherited variants of MYH associated with somatic G:C-->T:A mutations in colorectal tumors. Nat Genet. 30(2):227-32, 2002

NEUROFIBROMATOSIS TYPE 1

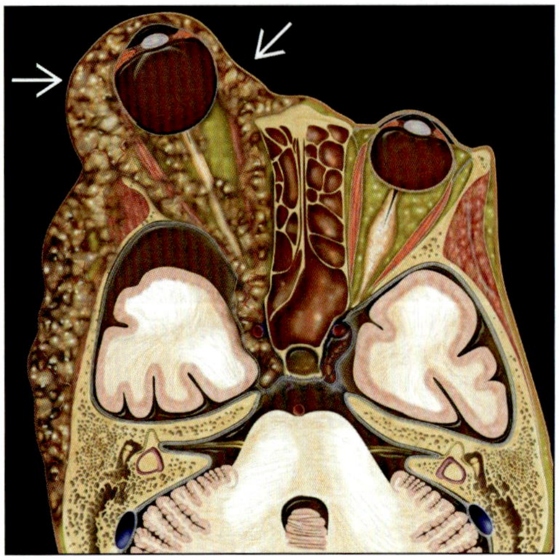

In neurofibromatosis type 1 (NF1), asymmetric deformities occur secondary to tissue overgrowth and plexiform/diffuse neurofibromas. Involvement of the orbit and ocular adnexa may be prominent ➡.

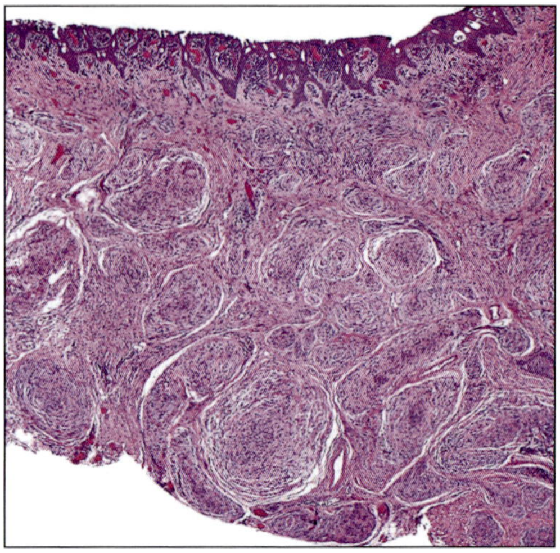

Plexiform neurofibroma is a hallmark of NF1. This eyelid example demonstrates the characteristic multinodular appearance resulting from multiple nerve fascicle involvement.

TERMINOLOGY

Abbreviations

- Neurofibromatosis type 1 (NF1)

Synonyms

- von Recklinghausen disease

Definitions

- Genetic syndrome resulting from germline mutations in *NF1* gene encoding for neurofibromin

EPIDEMIOLOGY

Incidence

- ~ 1 in 2,500-3,000 births (1 of the most common inherited syndromes)
- Occurs in all races and geographic regions

GENETICS

NF1 Gene

- Located in chromosome region 17q11.2
- Ubiquitously expressed, but levels highest in nervous system
- Encodes for neurofibromin, a tumor suppressor GTPase-activating protein that negatively regulates RAS
  - Constitutive activation of MAPK and AKT/mTOR signaling pathways
  - Also may regulate cAMP levels, which affect central nervous system manifestations
- Mosaicism or "segmental" neurofibromatosis manifests as involvement of an isolated anatomical region
- Penetrance is ~ 100% with appropriate follow-up although manifestations are variable between individuals and within families

Genetic Modifiers

- Modifier genes identified in mice and families with NF1
  - Associated with disease severity
  - Affect predisposition to peripheral nerve and central nervous system tumors

NF1-Associated Tumors

- Loss of heterozygosity in *NF1* is a feature of associated tumors
- Haploinsufficient cells in tumor microenvironment (macrophages/microglia, mast cells) also contribute to tumorigenesis

CLINICAL IMPLICATIONS AND ANCILLARY TESTS

Diagnostic Criteria (NIH 1991)

- 2 or more of the following features
  - Café au lait macules (≥ 6), with a diameter of 0.5 cm in children, or 1.5 cm after puberty
  - Cutaneous or subcutaneous neurofibromas (≥ 2) or plexiform neurofibroma
  - Freckling of the axillary or groin region
  - Glioma of the optic pathways
  - Lisch nodules identified by slit-lamp examination (≥ 2)
  - Dysplasias of skeletal system (sphenoid wing, long bone bowing, pseudoarthrosis)
  - Diagnosis of NF1 in a 1st-degree relative

NONNEOPLASTIC MANIFESTATIONS

Ophthalmic

- Lisch nodules: Nodular, hamartomatous aggregates of melanin-containing cells on surface of iris, usually asymptomatic

NEUROFIBROMATOSIS TYPE 1

Central Nervous System

- Unknown bright objects (UBOs): Asymptomatic focal areas of ↑ T2 signal on MR
  - May represent localized myelin abnormalities/ edema
- Macrocephaly, cognitive disabilities, developmental delays, and behavioral disturbances

Skin

- Café au lait spots: One of the earliest manifestations
- Axillary/inguinal (intertriginous skin) freckling

Musculoskeletal

- Sphenoid wing dysplasia/hypoplasia, scoliosis, pseudoarthrosis, bowing of long bones

Cardiovascular System

- Cerebral arteriopathy (Moyamoya disease)
- Pulmonary artery stenosis

ASSOCIATED NEOPLASMS

Central Nervous System

- Pilocytic astrocytoma
  - Most frequent central nervous system neoplasm in NF1
  - Predilection for optic pathways (15-20% of children with NF1)
  - May also occur in brainstem and anywhere along neuraxis
- Diffuse astrocytomas
  - Grades II-IV
  - Usually develop after childhood years
  - Aggressive as sporadic counterparts
- Indeterminate astrocytomas
  - Subset of low-grade astrocytomas in patients with NF1 difficult to classify
  - May demonstrate phenotypic or ultrastructural evidence of neuronal differentiation
- Glioneuronal tumors
  - Gangliogliomas and dysembryoplastic neuroepithelial tumors previously reported in NF1

Peripheral Nervous System

- Neurofibroma
  - Localized neurofibroma
    - Cutaneous, soft tissue or intraneural
    - Low cellularity
    - Variable contents of Schwann cells, perineurial cells, fibroblasts, mast cells, and axons
  - Diffuse neurofibroma
    - May develop in patients with NF1 but is not exclusive for the syndrome
    - Usually large cutaneous plaques infiltrating dermis &/or subcutis
    - May arise in internal organs
  - Cellular neurofibroma
    - Areas of increased cellularity and even limited fascicular architecture
    - Lack pronounced atypia and mitotic activity
    - Differential diagnosis with low-grade MPNST challenging, particularly when associated with plexiform neurofibroma
  - Atypical neurofibroma
    - Degenerative nuclear atypia
    - Lacks hypercellularity and mitotic activity
  - Plexiform neurofibroma
    - Complex neoplasms that by definition involve multiple peripheral nerve fascicles or a large plexus
    - Characteristic "worm-like" gross appearance
    - Deep/large plexiform neurofibromas essentially restricted to patients with NF1
    - Propensity for malignant degeneration
  - Massive soft tissue neurofibroma
    - Large neoplasm displaying prominent soft tissue infiltration, often containing hypercellular, round cell areas, and pseudo-meissnerian corpuscles
    - Usually benign, but some contain a plexiform neurofibroma component with a propensity for malignant degeneration
    - Arises only in patients with NF1
  - Rare findings in neurofibroma include presence of melanin pigment, metaplastic bone, and glandular differentiation
- Malignant peripheral nerve sheath tumor (MPNST)
  - Afflicts 8-13% of patients with NF1
  - Usually aggressive, high-grade spindle cell neoplasms
  - Differentiation is predominantly schwannian but may also be perineurial
  - Presence of heterologous elements relatively more common in NF1 setting (skeletal muscle, cartilaginous, osseous, angiosarcomatous, glandular or smooth muscle)
  - "Low-grade MPNST" applied to tumors arising in transition from neurofibroma, usually in patients with NF1
    - Hypercellularity, nuclear enlargement (~ 3x the size of a neurofibroma nucleus), and hyperchromasia
    - Mitotic activity may also be present but is not required for diagnosis

Other

- Pheochromocytoma: Usually unilateral but may be bilateral in NF1
- Glomus tumor
  - Recently recognized component of NF1
  - *NF1*-biallelic inactivation, mitotic recombination not uncommon
- Intestinal ganglioneuromatosis (involving primarily the submucosal plexus)
- Gastrointestinal stromal tumor (GIST)
  - Lacks *KIT* mutations in contrast to sporadic GIST
- Gastrointestinal schwannoma
  - More common in NF1 than NF2
  - Loss of heterozygosity in *NF1* gene
- Neuroendocrine neoplasms (carcinoid tumors)
- Juvenile myelomonocytic leukemia (JMML)
  - 100x < risk in children with NF1
- Breast carcinoma

- Increased risk and earlier age of occurrence in women with NF1
- Rhabdomyosarcoma

MOLECULAR BIOLOGY

Central Nervous System

- NF1-associated gliomas demonstrate complete *NF1* inactivation
- Haploinsufficient stromal components (e.g., microglia) also required in mouse models of NF1-associated low-grade glioma
- Development of high-grade glioma requires losses in additional tumor suppressors (e.g., *TP53*, *PTEN*)

Peripheral Nerve

- Haploinsufficient microenvironment cell components (e.g., mast cells) important for neurofibroma formation in some NF1 mouse models
- Nonmyelinating Schwann cell progenitors and Dsh(+) Schwann cell precursors are candidate cells of origin of plexiform neurofibromas in mouse models
- Neural crest-derived cutaneous neural stem cell/ progenitor candidate cell of origin for cutaneous neurofibroma
- Malignant peripheral nerve sheath tumors in addition to *NF1* loss develop oncogene amplification (e.g., *EGFR*) and tumor suppressor loss (e.g., *P16*, *TP53*)

DIFFERENTIAL DIAGNOSIS

Neurofibromatosis Type 2 (NF2)

- Mutations in the *NF2* gene encoding for merlin/ schwannomin
- Gliomas, café au lait spots, and neurofibromas may present in patients with NF2 although at a lower frequency and number than in those with NF1
- Ependymoma, meningioma, and multiple schwannomas are not a feature of NF1

Noonan Syndrome

- Results from mutations in various components of the RAS/MAPK signaling pathway
  - *PTPN11*, *KRAS*, *SOS1*, *NRAS*, and *RAF1*
- Distinctive facial features, developmental delay, short stature, congenital heart disease, café au lait spots
- Tumor predisposition lower than NF1

Legius Syndrome

- Results from loss-of-function *SPRED1* mutations leading to ↑ RAS-MAPK pathway activity
- Mild NF1-like phenotype
  - Café au lait spots, macrocephaly
  - Lack Lisch nodules, bone abnormalities, gliomas, and peripheral nerve sheath tumors

Constitutional Mismatch Repair-Deficiency Syndrome

- Homozygous or compound heterozygous mutations in mismatch repair genes
- Multiple cancers, including gliomas, colon cancer
- May be associated with clinical features of NF1 (e.g., café au lait spots)

McCune-Albright Syndrome

- Somatic mutations in *GNAS1* gene resulting in increased cAMP signaling
- May have café au lait spots (unilateral) but no axillary freckling
- Polyostotic fibrous dysplasia

Proteus Syndrome

- Somatic (mosaic) activating mutations in *AKT1* in most cases
- Localized tissue overgrowth clinically mimicking plexiform neurofibroma; scoliosis, hyperostoses, "cerebriform" connective tissue nevus, and epidermal nevi; monomorphic parotid gland adenomas, ovarian cystadenomas

Familial Café Au Lait Spots

- Rare autosomal dominant disorder
- Lack neurofibromas and noncutaneous manifestations of NF1

Multiple Endocrine Neoplasia Type 2B (MEN2B)

- Caused by genetic alterations in *RET* proto-oncogene
- Develop pheochromocytomas but also mucosal neuromas (**not** neurofibromas)
  - Diffuse and extensive involvement of all intestinal layers by ganglioneuromatosis is relatively specific to MEN2B

SELECTED REFERENCES

1. Carroll SL: Molecular mechanisms promoting the pathogenesis of Schwann cell neoplasms. Acta Neuropathol. 123(3):321-48, 2012
2. Gutmann DH et al: Neurofibromatosis type 1: modeling CNS dysfunction. J Neurosci. 32(41):14087-93, 2012
3. Patil S et al: Neoplasms associated with germline and somatic NF1 gene mutations. Oncologist. 17(1):101-16, 2012
4. Brems H et al: Glomus tumors in neurofibromatosis type 1: genetic, functional, and clinical evidence of a novel association. Cancer Res. 69(18):7393-401, 2009
5. Messiaen L et al: Clinical and mutational spectrum of neurofibromatosis type 1-like syndrome. JAMA. 302(19):2111-8, 2009
6. Rodriguez FJ et al: Gliomas in neurofibromatosis type 1: a clinicopathologic study of 100 patients. J Neuropathol Exp Neurol. 67(3):240-9, 2008
7. Hawes JJ et al: Nf1 expression is dependent on strain background: implications for tumor suppressor haploinsufficiency studies. Neurogenetics. 8(2):121-30, 2007
8. Miettinen M et al: Gastrointestinal stromal tumors in patients with neurofibromatosis 1: a clinicopathologic and molecular genetic study of 45 cases. Am J Surg Pathol. 30(1):90-6, 2006

Systemic Manifestations

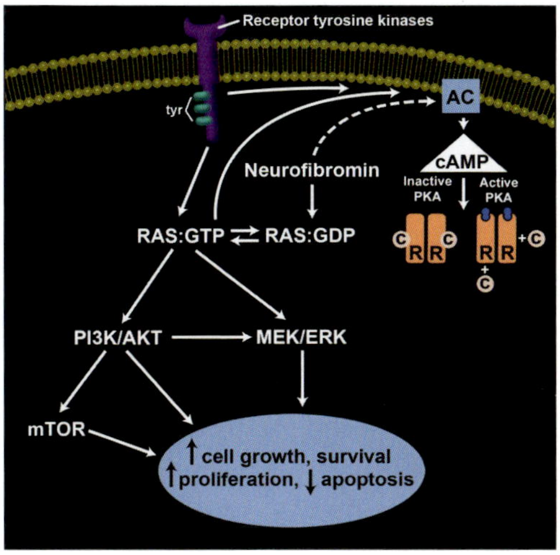

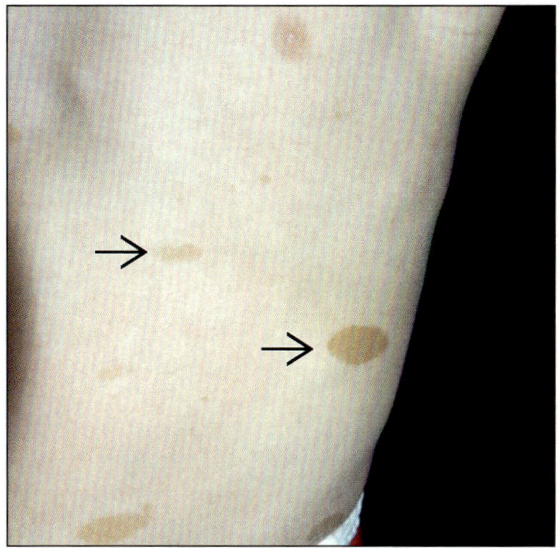

(Left) *NF1 syndrome is caused by germline mutations in the gene encoding for neurofibromin, a tumor suppressor protein that works by activating RAS GTPase function. Neurofibromin loss leads to constitutive RAS signaling and altered cAMP levels, resulting in a variety of neoplasms and other manifestations, particularly affecting the nervous system.* ***(Right)*** *Multiple café au lait spots represent an important cutaneous manifestation of NF1 →. (Courtesy K. Yohay, MD.)*

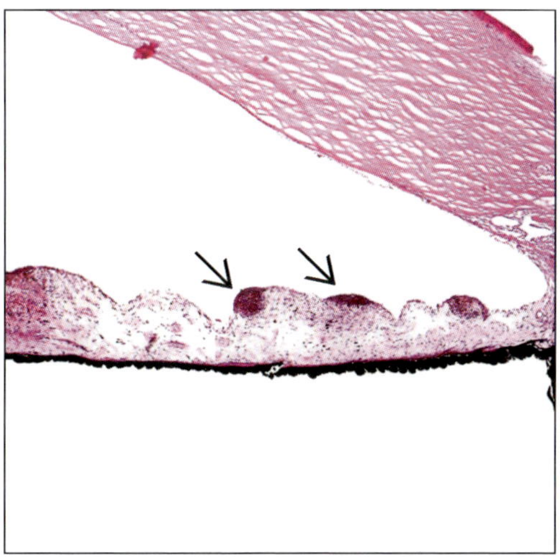

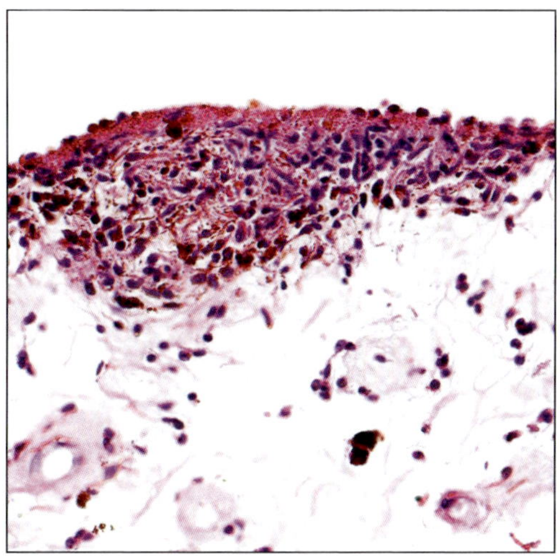

(Left) *Lisch nodules are asymptomatic nodular proliferations of pigmented cells involving the anterior surface of the iris in NF1 patients →. They represent an important diagnostic criterion that is relatively easy to identify by ophthalmologic examination.* ***(Right)*** *Lisch nodules are composed of melanin-containing cells that form superficial aggregates in the iris. They usually do not affect vision and have no malignant potential.*

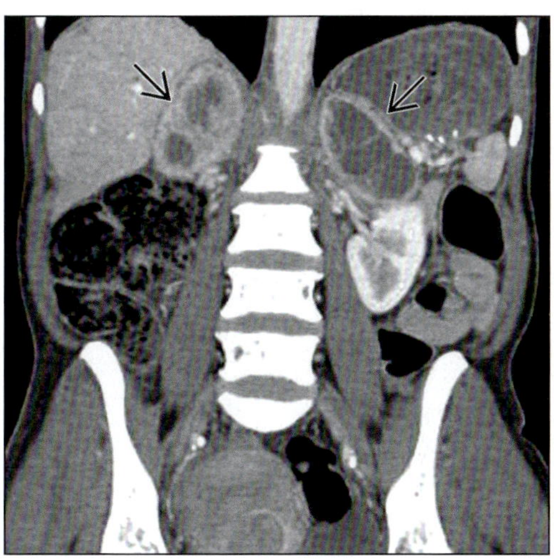

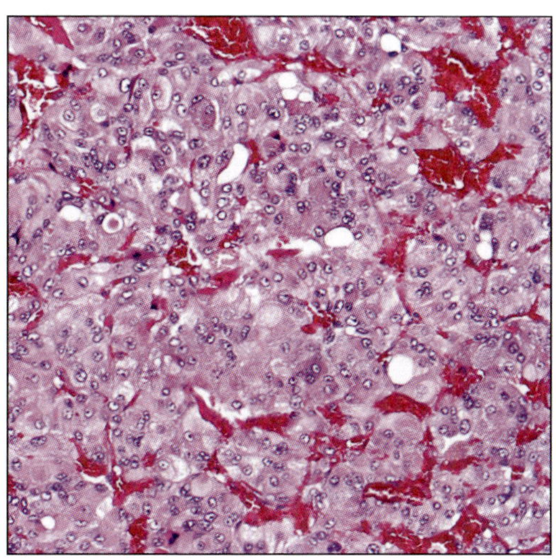

(Left) *NF1 is 1 of several syndromes characterized by the development of pheochromocytomas. Although these tumors are usually solitary/unilateral, multiple tumors may develop in a subset of patients →.* ***(Right)*** *Both sporadic and NF1-associated pheochromocytomas are characterized by variably sized nodules of large cells with ample basophilic to amphophilic cytoplasm. A rich microvascular network is a constant feature.*

Central Nervous System

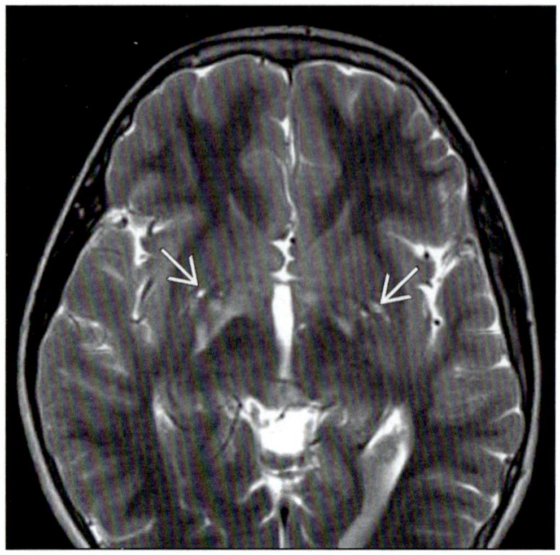

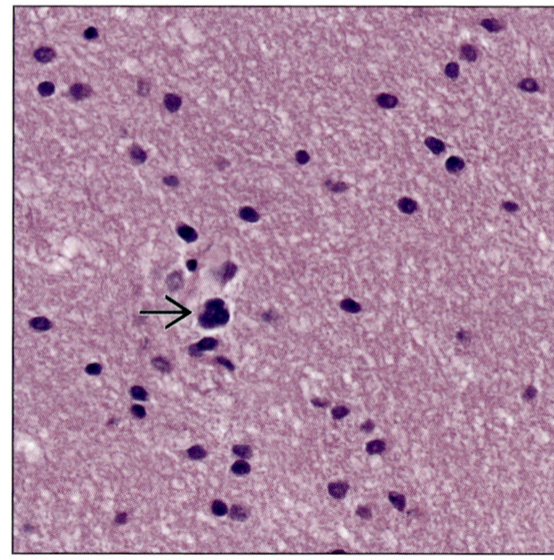

(Left) *Hyperintensities on T2-weighted MR images are a frequent finding in NF1 patients →. These are referred to as unknown bright objects and may represent focal abnormalities in myelin.* ***(Right)*** *A small increase in glial cell number and even mild atypia → are not uncommon in the setting of NF1. It is essential to identify these findings in central nervous system specimens because of the propensity of patients with NF1 to develop infiltrating gliomas of all grades.*

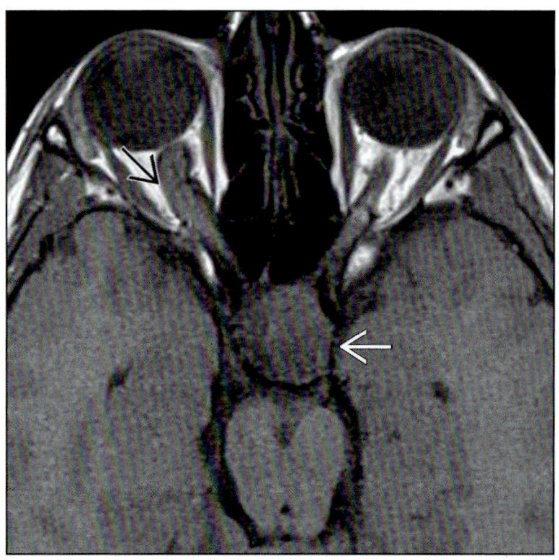

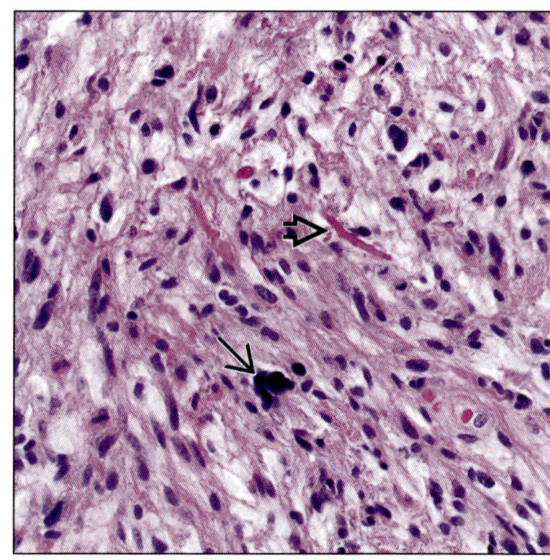

(Left) *The central nervous system hallmark of NF1 is multiple involvement of the optic pathways by low-grade gliomas. These may affect the optic nerve proper → as well as the chiasm →.* ***(Right)*** *The overwhelming majority of optic pathway gliomas are pilocytic astrocytomas. In this NF1-associated case, areas of tissue compaction, degenerative atypia →, and Rosenthal fibers → are evident. The tumors grow slowly and may even be followed without treatment in most cases.*

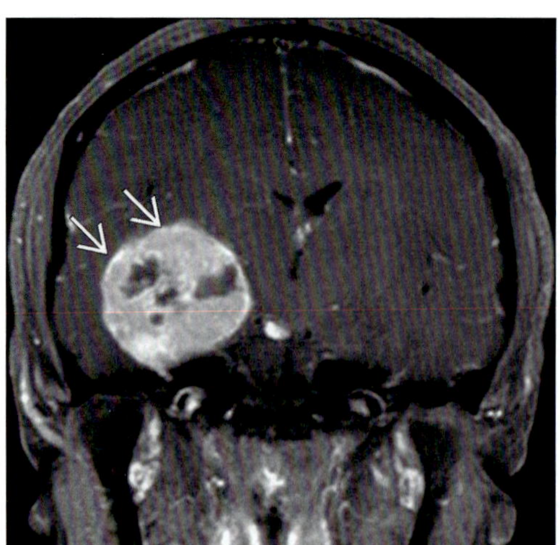

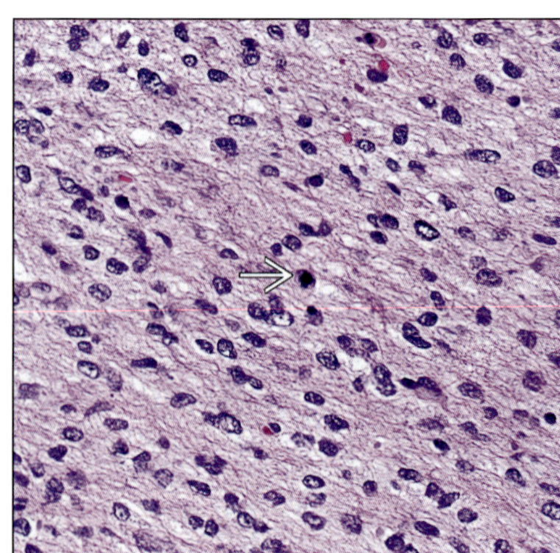

(Left) *Although pilocytic astrocytoma is the most frequent glioma in patients with NF1, all astrocytic subtypes may potentially develop, including high-grade astrocytomas as seen in this example. Heterogeneous contrast enhancement → is evident.* ***(Right)*** *High-grade astrocytomas in patients with NF1 are graded using similar criteria as in sporadic tumors. Parenchymal infiltration, atypia, and mitotic activity → are not subtle in this anaplastic (WHO grade III) astrocytoma.*

Peripheral Nervous System

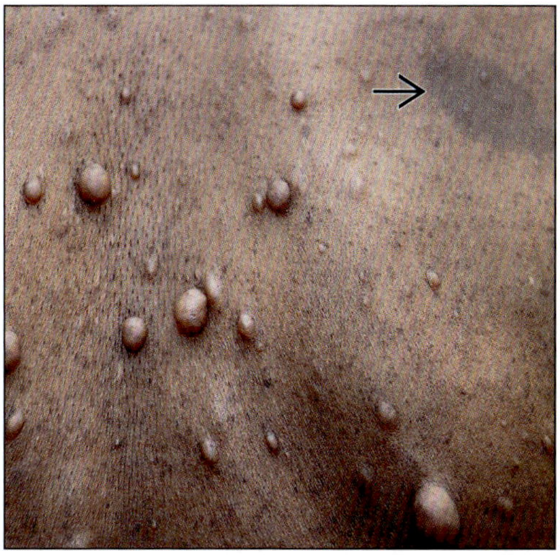

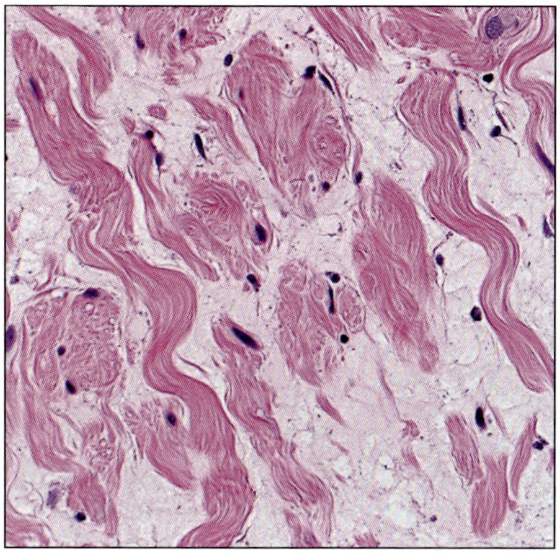

(Left) *Numerous cutaneous neurofibromas afflict a significant proportion of patients with NF1. They are characterized by sessile or pedunculated growths. An associated café au lait spot ⇒ is also present in this NF1 patient. (Courtesy K. Yohay, MD.)* ***(Right)*** *Most neurofibromas are paucicellular tumors characterized by wavy, delicate eosinophilic collagen bundles colorfully referred to as "shredded carrots." A variable myxoid stroma may be identified in almost all neurofibromas.*

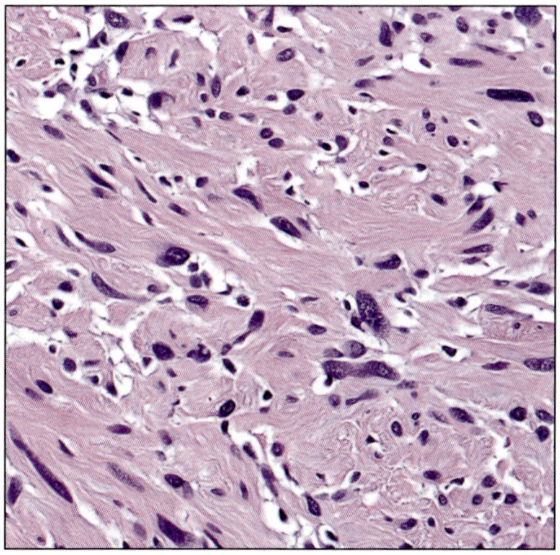

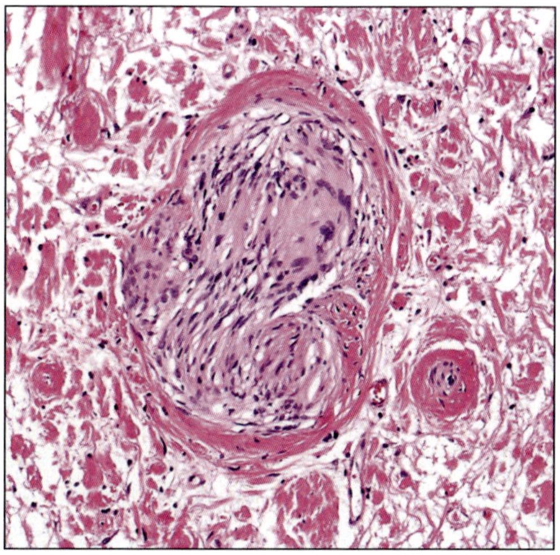

(Left) *Some neurofibromas are characterized by areas of increased cellularity and nuclear atypia. Such areas deserve particular attention when occurring in plexiform neurofibromas of NF1 patients. Distinction from a low-grade MPNST may be difficult.* ***(Right)*** *Well-circumscribed schwannian nodules may occur in neurofibromas. Although these nodules within neurofibroma are sometimes interpreted as hybrid benign nerve sheath tumors, the predominant architecture in NF1 is usually neurofibroma.*

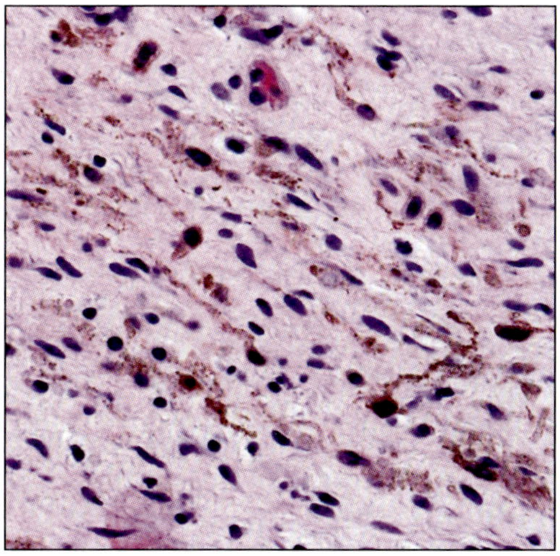

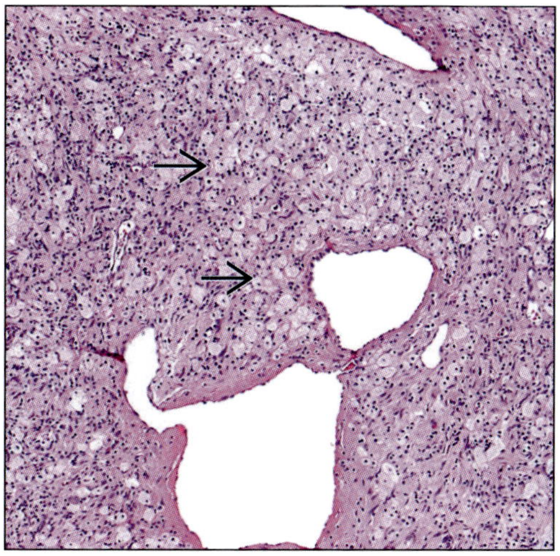

(Left) *Rarely, melanin/pigment may be observed in neurofibroma examples, particularly diffuse tumors in the setting of NF1.* ***(Right)*** *Hybrid benign nerve sheath tumors may be more frequent in syndrome settings. This section from a patient with NF1 contains large hyalinized vessels and numerous foamy macrophages ⇒, features that are more frequently encountered in schwannomas. However, more classic features of neurofibroma were present in other fields.*

NEUROFIBROMATOSIS TYPE 1

Peripheral Nervous System

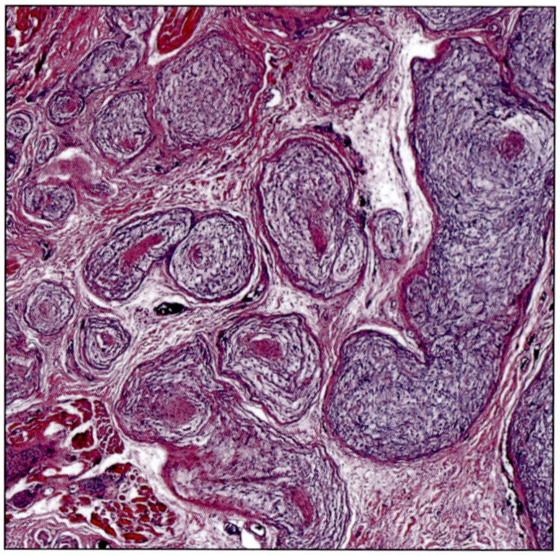

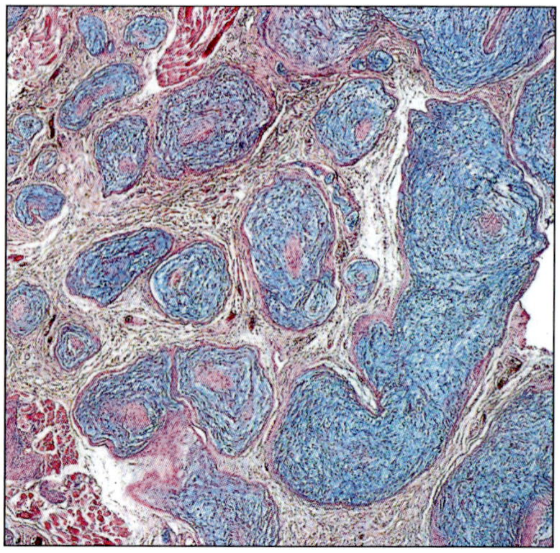

(Left) *The main diagnostic attributes of plexiform neurofibroma are evident on gross examination and low magnification, particularly a nodular or worm-like pattern of growth imparted by expansion of multiple peripheral nerve fascicles. Such tumors also demonstrate cellular complexity, including Schwann cells, perineurial cells, fibroblasts, mast cells, and peripheral nerve axons.* ***(Right)*** *Neurofibromas, including the plexiform variant, contain a myxoid stroma stained by Alcian blue.*

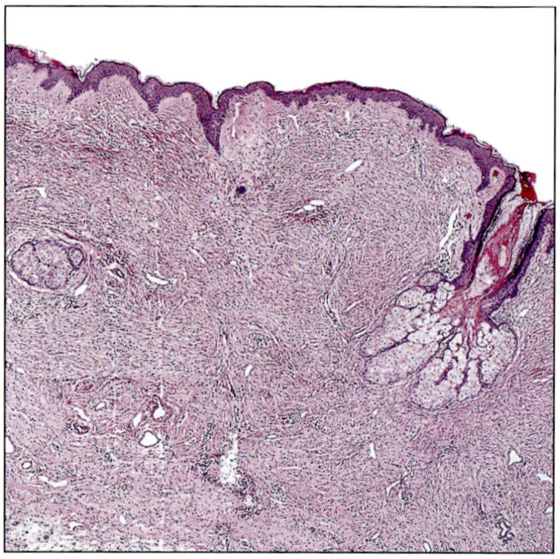

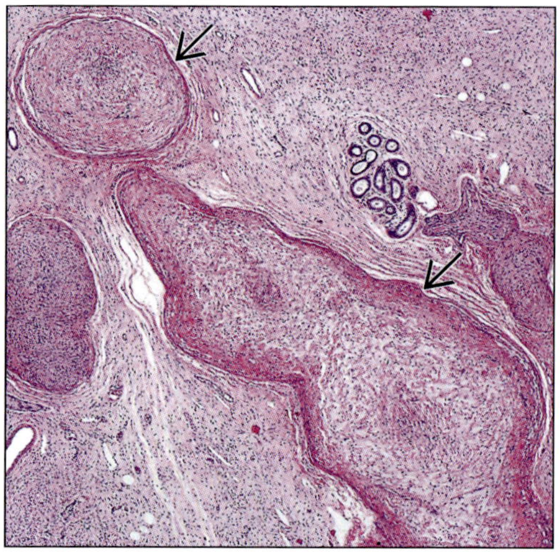

(Left) *Diffuse neurofibromas are usually characterized by large, superficial, plaque-like growths enveloping multiple cutaneous adnexa. Although relatively frequent in patients with NF1, these neurofibromas are not exclusive to the syndrome.* ***(Right)*** *Complex neurofibromas with diffuse components demonstrating dermal/subcutaneous infiltration as well as plexiform expansion of individual peripheral nerve fascicles → are not uncommon in patients with NF1.*

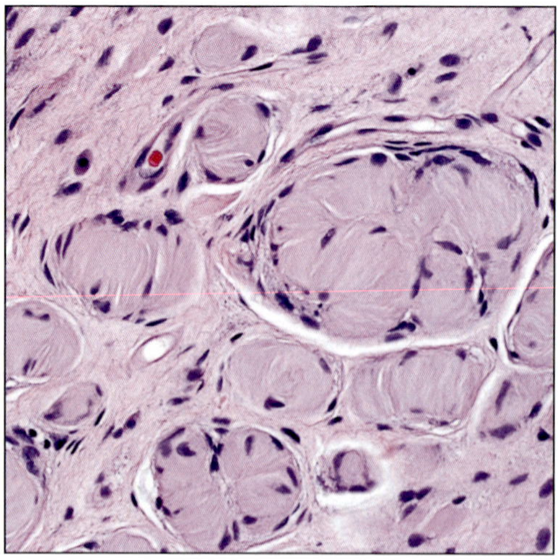

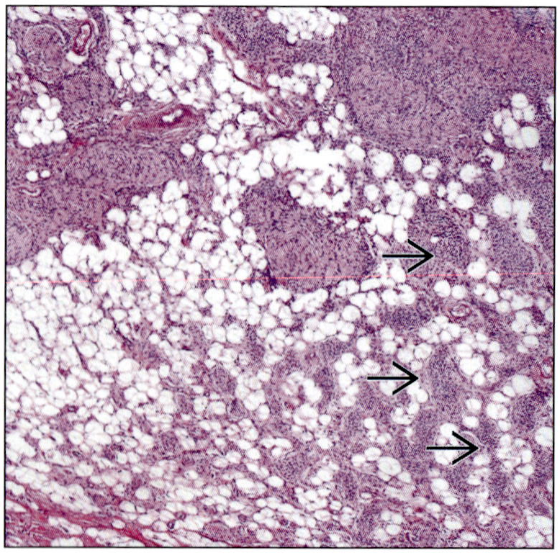

(Left) *Pseudo-meissnerian corpuscles are characteristic of diffuse neurofibromas and may be present in variable amounts. They are intensely immunoreactive with antibodies directed against S100 protein.* ***(Right)*** *The massive soft tissue neurofibroma is a particular subtype limited to patients with NF1. It is characterized by diffuse infiltration of adipose tissue and other soft tissue elements. In addition, it may have areas of closely packed round cells →.*

Malignant Peripheral Nerve Sheath Tumor

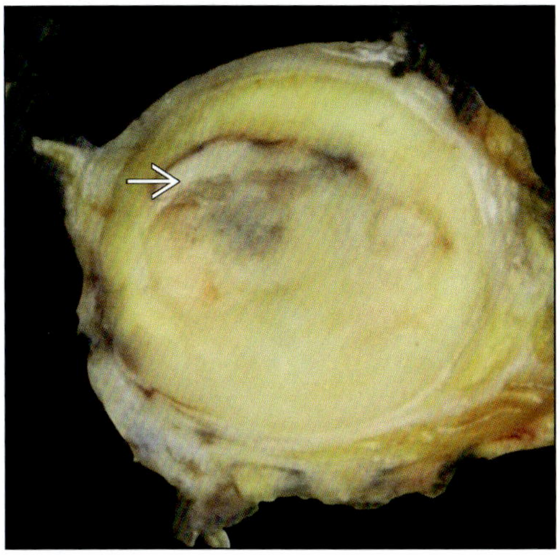
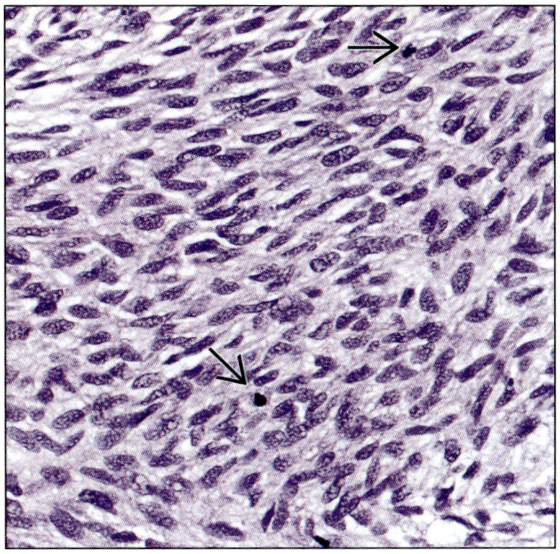

(Left) *Malignant peripheral nerve sheath tumor (MPNST) is the prototypical malignancy afflicting patients with NF1 syndrome. A suspicious finding on gross examination is the presence of necrosis* ➔. *MPNST may arise de novo or from a preexisting, usually plexiform, neurofibroma.* ***(Right)*** *MPNSTs are usually high-grade spindle cell malignancies. The neoplastic cells may be arranged in fascicles and resemble fibrosarcoma. Mitotic activity is variable but usually evident* →.

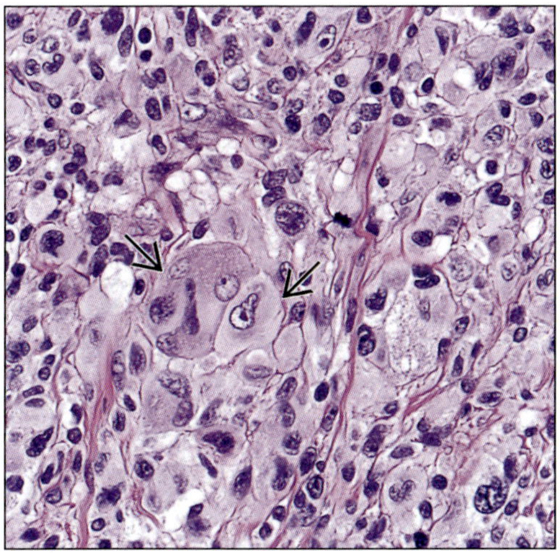
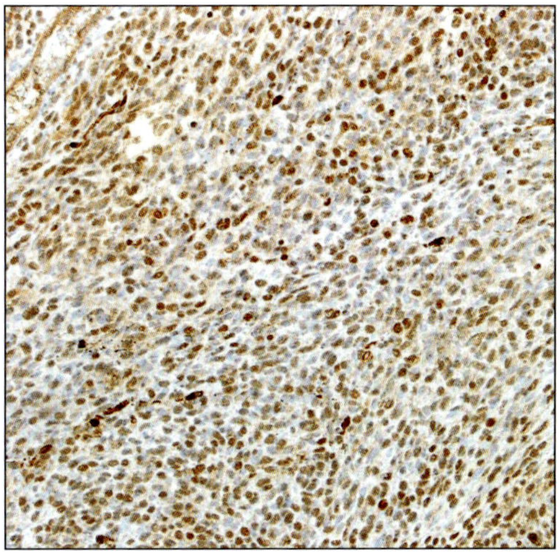

(Left) *The morphologic variability of MPNST is wide, and pleomorphism may be marked in some NF1-associated and sporadic examples. Some tumors may contain epithelioid cells with well-defined borders* →. ***(Right)*** *S100, a ubiquitous Schwann cell marker, is characteristically weaker in areas of MPNST, or altogether negative. This is a useful distinguishing feature from cellular schwannoma. However, the latter is not typically NF1 associated.*

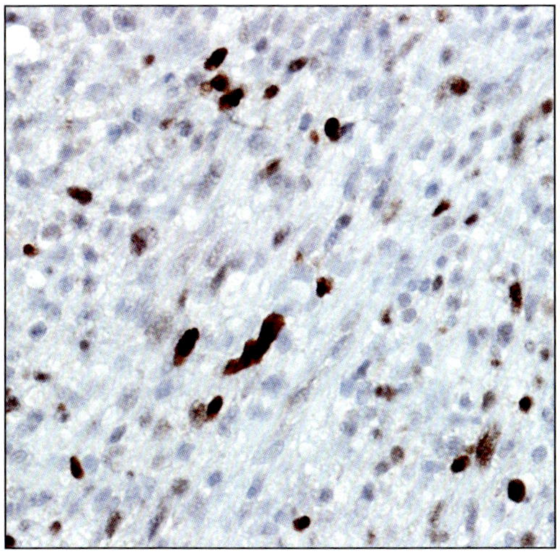
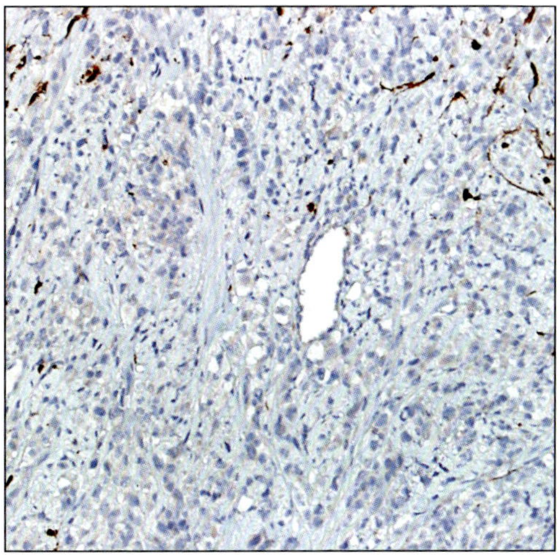

(Left) *Strong nuclear immunoreactivity for p53 in a variable number of neoplastic cell nuclei is frequent in MPNST in contrast with benign neurofibromas.* ***(Right)*** *p16 immunoreactivity is frequently lost in MPNST. p16 represents an important tumor suppressor that is frequently inactivated by gene mutations/deletions in MPNST. p16 loss at the gene or protein level may suggest malignant degeneration of neurofibromas in NF1 patients.*

NEUROFIBROMATOSIS TYPE 2

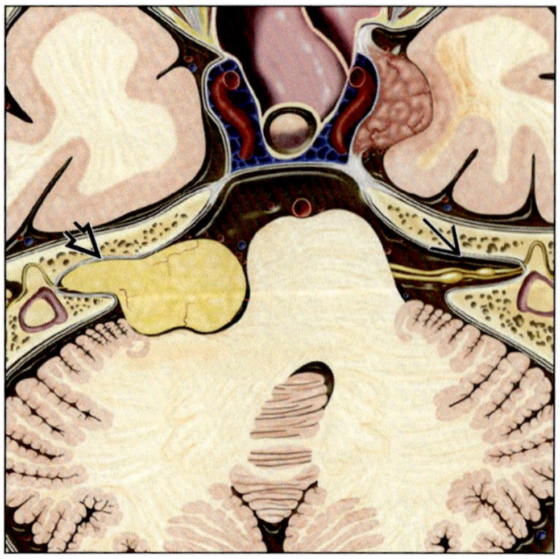

Bilateral schwannomas involving the vestibular branch of CN8 are a hallmark of neurofibromatosis type 2 (NF2). They present as a cerebellopontine angle mass ⇨ and may be multiple →.

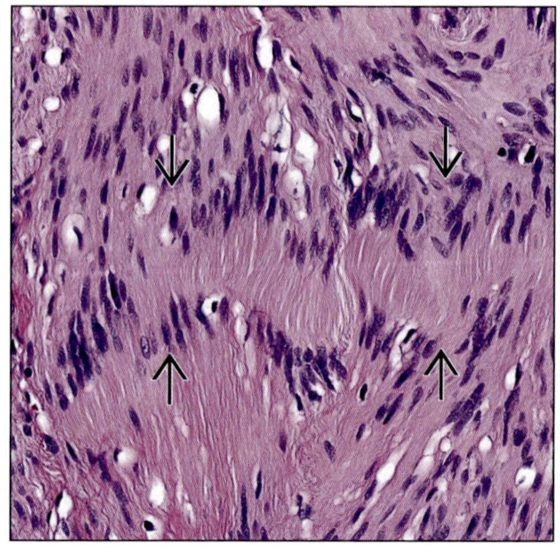

Schwannomas are the most common neoplasms affecting patients with NF2. They are composed of a solid proliferation of neoplastic Schwann cells and may contain characteristic Verocay bodies →.

TERMINOLOGY

Abbreviations

- Neurofibromatosis type 2 (NF2)

Definitions

- Inherited tumor predisposition syndrome caused by germline mutations in the *NF2* gene encoding for merlin/schwannomin

EPIDEMIOLOGY

Incidence

- 1 in 33,000 to 40,000 births
- Similar proportion of male and female patients

GENETICS AND MOLECULAR BIOLOGY

NF2 Gene Encodes for Merlin

- Inherited in 1/2 of patients and new germline mutation in remaining 1/2
- Located in chromosomal region 22q12.2
- Merlin associates with cell junctional complexes and participates in contact-dependent inhibition
- More severe phenotype in patients with frameshift or nonsense mutations
- Germline mosaicism occurs in 20-30% of patients without family history

CLINICAL IMPLICATIONS AND ANCILLARY TESTS

Nonneoplastic Manifestations

- Ophthalmic: Posterior subcapsular cataracts, retinal hamartomas, and epiretinal membranes
- Central nervous system: Glial microhamartomas
- Peripheral nervous system: Polyneuropathy
- Skin: Café au lait spots but at a lesser frequency than NF1; also hairy cutaneous plaques
- Musculoskeletal: Scoliosis

Classification Criteria

- Manchester criteria (1992)
  - Bilateral vestibular schwannoma **or**
  - NF2 in 1st-degree relative plus unilateral vestibular schwannoma or any 2 of the following: Neurofibroma, meningioma, glioma, schwannoma, posterior subcapsular lens opacity **or**
  - Unilateral vestibular schwannoma plus any 2 of the following: Neurofibroma, meningioma, glioma, schwannoma, posterior subscapular lens opacity **or**
  - ≥ 2 meningiomas plus unilateral vestibular schwannoma or any 2 of the following: Neurofibroma, glioma, schwannoma, or cataract
- Baser criteria (2011)
  - Manifests an effort to incorporate genetic information into clinical classifications

ASSOCIATED NEOPLASMS

Schwannoma

- Similar histologic features as sporadic tumors
  - Compact Antoni A areas alternating with loose Antoni B areas
  - Verocay bodies, hyalinized vessels, hemosiderin deposition
  - S100, SOX10, and pericellular collagen IV immunoreactivity; EMA limited to perineurium and neurofilament protein to rare entrapped axons
- Features occurring more frequently in NF2-associated schwannomas include whorl formation, multiple tumors involving a single nerve, and juxtaposition to meningioma

NEUROFIBROMATOSIS TYPE 2

Baser Criteria for Neurofibromatosis Type 2		
Feature	**Present Age ≤ 30 Years**	**Present Age > 30 Years**
NF2 in 1st-degree relative	2	2
Vestibular schwannoma (unilateral)	2	1
Vestibular schwannoma (2nd)	4	3
Meningioma	2	1
Meningioma (2nd)	2	1
Cutaneous schwannoma(s)	2	1
Neoplasm of cranial nerves	2	1
Mononeuropathy	2	1
Cataract(s)	2	0

Points are added: ≥ 6 = definite NF2; 4-5 = NF2 mutational analysis required for diagnosis; < 4 = NF2 unlikely.

- Mosaic pattern of INI1 immunostaining in majority of syndrome-associated schwannomas
- Bilateral vestibular schwannomas are a hallmark of NF2 (90-95% of patients)
- Plexiform schwannomas may occur in NF2 but are not specific to the syndrome
  - Nodular Schwann cell proliferation favoring cutaneous and mucosal sites
  - May be multiple

Neurofibroma

- Relatively rare in NF2 compared to NF1 but may contribute to clinical diagnosis if other criteria present

Meningioma

- Intracranial meningiomas found in ~ 1/2 of NF2 patients
- Skull base involvement is less frequent than in sporadic tumors
- "Saltatory growth": Periods of growth followed by quiescence
- Relatively high frequency of fibroblastic, transitional, and grade II meningiomas in NF2 patients but also histologic heterogeneity
- Meningioangiomatosis
  - Growth of meningothelial-like cells into superficial cortical vessels and leptomeninges
  - Associated with seizures
  - EMA(+) or EMA(-), collagen rich (Masson trichrome)

Ependymoma

- Cervical cord and cervicomedullary junction are favored sites in NF2
- Majority of NF2-associated ependymomas are low grade and asymptomatic
- Associated with a relatively high rate of truncating *NF2* mutations

Other

- Conventional MPNST and MPNST ex-schwannomas reported in NF2 but very rare
- Some malignant neoplasms may be irradiation-induced
- Nonependymal glial neoplasms may occur

SELECTED REFERENCES

1. Aboukais R et al: Intracranial meningiomas and neurofibromatosis type 2. Acta Neurochir (Wien). 155(6):997-1001, 2013
2. Dirks MS et al: Long-term natural history of neurofibromatosis Type 2-associated intracranial tumors. J Neurosurg. 117(1):109-17, 2012
3. Goutagny S et al: Long-term follow-up of 287 meningiomas in neurofibromatosis type 2 patients: clinical, radiological, and molecular features. Neuro Oncol. 14(8):1090-6, 2012
4. Baser ME et al: Empirical development of improved diagnostic criteria for neurofibromatosis 2. Genet Med. 13(6):576-81, 2011
5. Evans DG et al: Consensus recommendations to accelerate clinical trials for neurofibromatosis type 2. Clin Cancer Res. 15(16):5032-9, 2009
6. Baser ME et al: The location of constitutional neurofibromatosis 2 (NF2) splice site mutations is associated with the severity of NF2. J Med Genet. 42(7):540-6, 2005
7. Baser ME et al: Genotype-phenotype correlations for nervous system tumors in neurofibromatosis 2: a population-based study. Am J Hum Genet. 75(2):231-9, 2004
8. Kluwe L et al: Molecular study of frequency of mosaicism in neurofibromatosis 2 patients with bilateral vestibular schwannomas. J Med Genet. 40(2):109-14, 2003
9. Moyhuddin A et al: Somatic mosaicism in neurofibromatosis 2: prevalence and risk of disease transmission to offspring. J Med Genet. 40(6):459-63, 2003
10. Perry A et al: Aggressive phenotypic and genotypic features in pediatric and NF2-associated meningiomas: a clinicopathologic study of 53 cases. J Neuropathol Exp Neurol. 60(10):994-1003, 2001
11. Mérel P et al: Screening for germ-line mutations in the NF2 gene. Genes Chromosomes Cancer. 12(2):117-27, 1995
12. Rouleau GA et al: Alteration in a new gene encoding a putative membrane-organizing protein causes neuro-fibromatosis type 2. Nature. 363(6429):515-21, 1993
13. Trofatter JA et al: A novel moesin-, ezrin-, radixin-like gene is a candidate for the neurofibromatosis 2 tumor suppressor. Cell. 1993 Mar 12;72(5):791-800. Erratum in: Cell. 75(4):826, 1993
14. Wiestler OD et al: Distribution and immunoreactivity of cerebral micro-hamartomas in bilateral acoustic neurofibromatosis (neurofibromatosis 2). Acta Neuropathol. 79(2):137-43, 1989

NEUROFIBROMATOSIS TYPE 2

Molecular, Imaging, and Microscopic Features

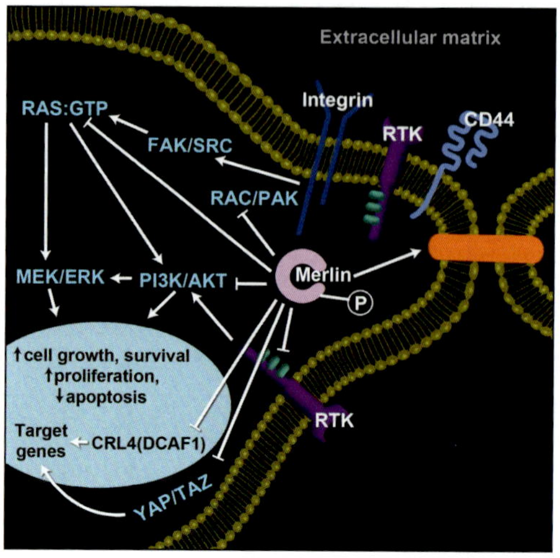

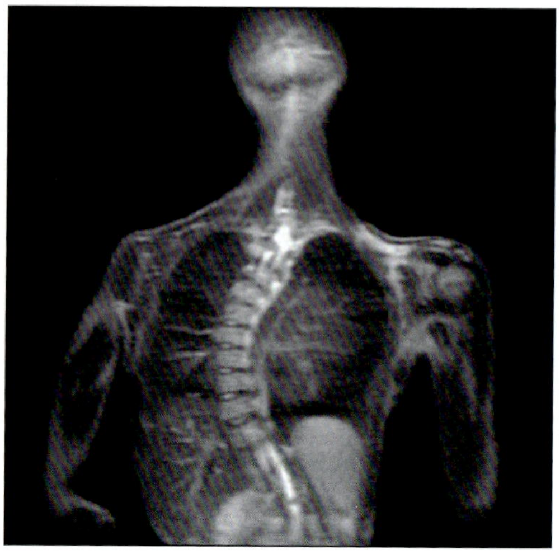

(Left) *NF2 is associated with loss of the tumor suppressor merlin. Merlin has numerous important cellular functions, including participation in intercellular junctions, contact dependent growth inhibition (through integrins, CD44), cytoskeleton dynamics, and modulation of signaling pathways, including those downstream from receptor tyrosine kinases (RTK) and YAP.* ***(Right)*** *In addition to neoplasms, patients with NF2 may develop a variety of nonneoplastic disorders, such as severe scoliosis.*

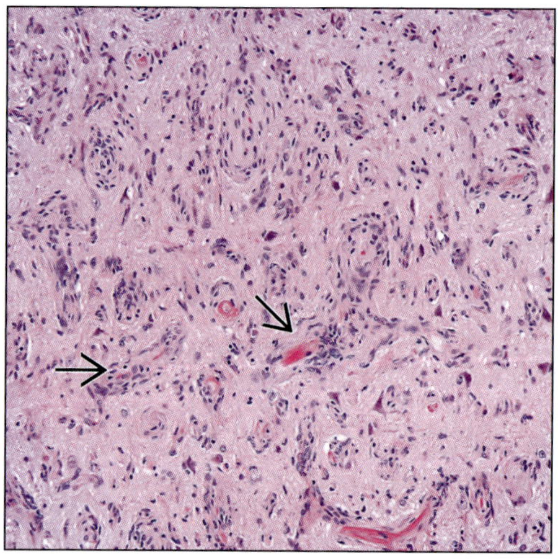

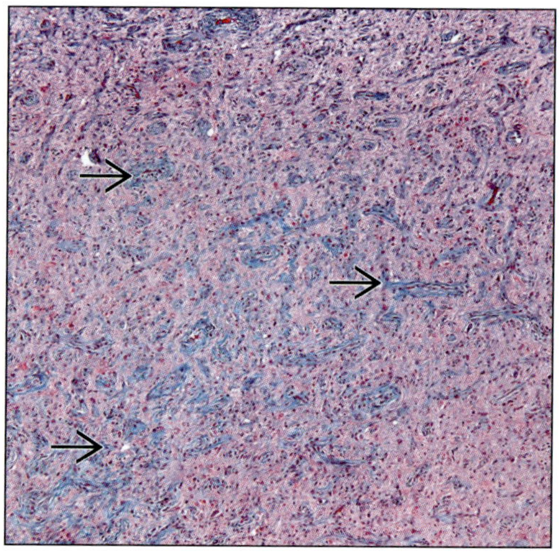

(Left) *Meningioangiomatosis afflicts some patients with NF2. It is a hamartomatous-like lesion associated with seizures and is characterized by a cortical proliferation of spindle cells, particularly surrounding small vessels* ➙*. An association with an overlying meningioma may be present in some instances.* ***(Right)*** *Perivascular collagen deposition is a diagnostically useful feature of meningioangiomatosis that may be demonstrated with histochemical stains such as Masson trichrome* ➙*.*

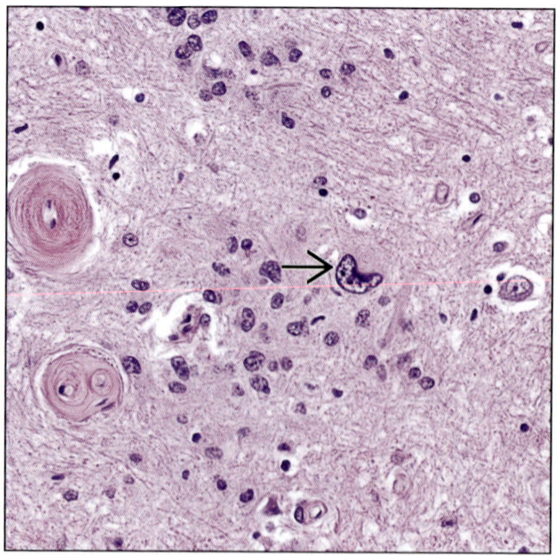

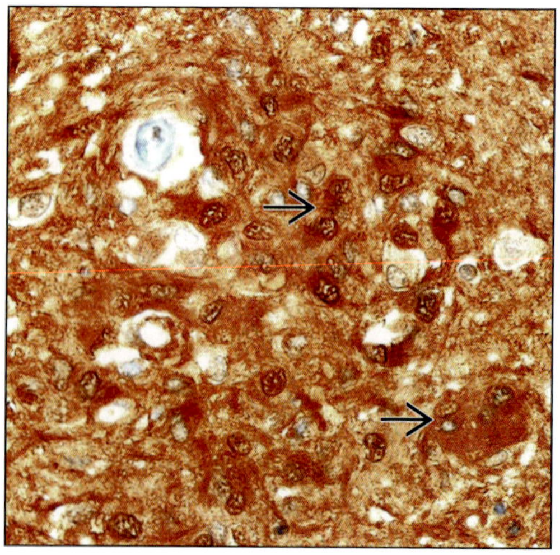

(Left) *Another nonneoplastic brain lesion afflicting patients with NF2 is the glial hamartoma, characterized by clusters of glial-like hyperchromatic cells with nuclear atypia and hyperchromasia* ➙*. Multinucleated cells may also be present. They tend to arise in cerebral cortex and basal ganglia and lack mitotic activity and potential for neoplastic change.* ***(Right)*** *Glial hamartomas in NF2 patients show strong S100 labeling* ➙ *but lack expression of other neuronal and glial markers.*

Schwannoma

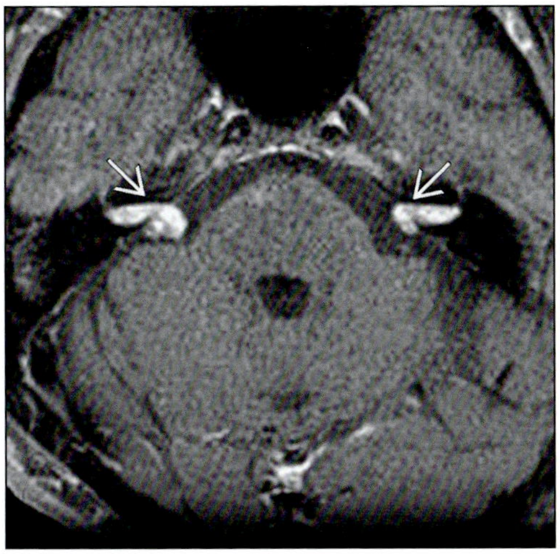
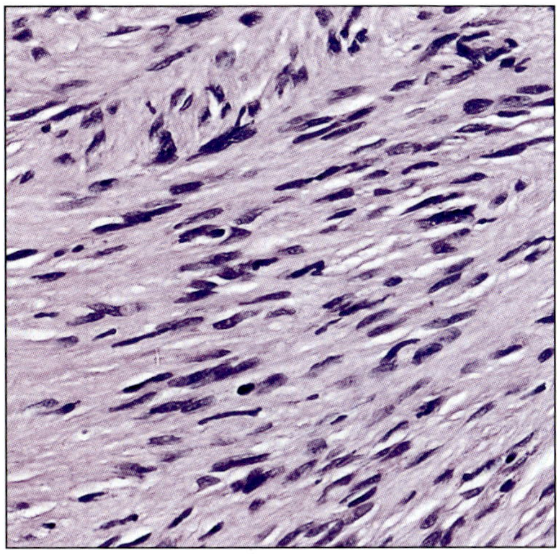

(Left) *Bilateral vestibular schwannomas are pathognomonic of NF2, presenting as enhancing masses in the cerebellopontine angle ➔. Age of presentation is variable; candidate patients may be monitored for years before this characteristic manifestation presents.* ***(Right)*** *Compact proliferations of spindle cells characterize the Antoni A pattern of schwannomas. Mitotic activity is usually low and the potential for spontaneous malignant degeneration is negligible.*

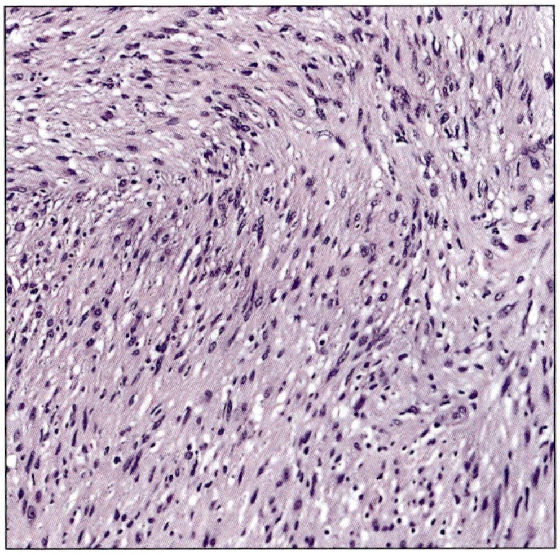
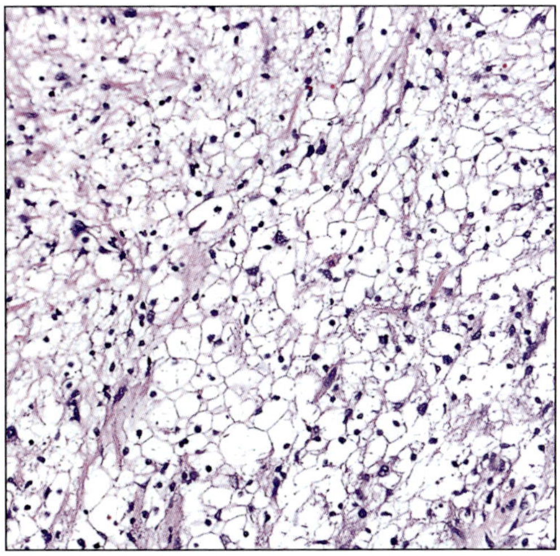

(Left) *Bland spindle cells represent the main component of sporadic and NF2-associated schwannomas. These usually aggregate in compact areas known as Antoni A. Diagnostic Verocay bodies are not always identifiable, and in such instances, immunohistochemistry may be required for confirmation.* ***(Right)*** *Antoni B patterns are relatively paucicellular in contrast to Antoni A patterns. They contain variable mixtures of Schwann cells with clear cytoplasm and foamy histiocytes.*

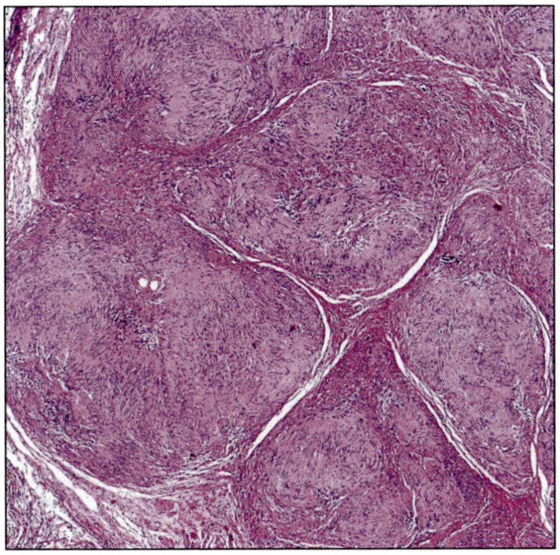
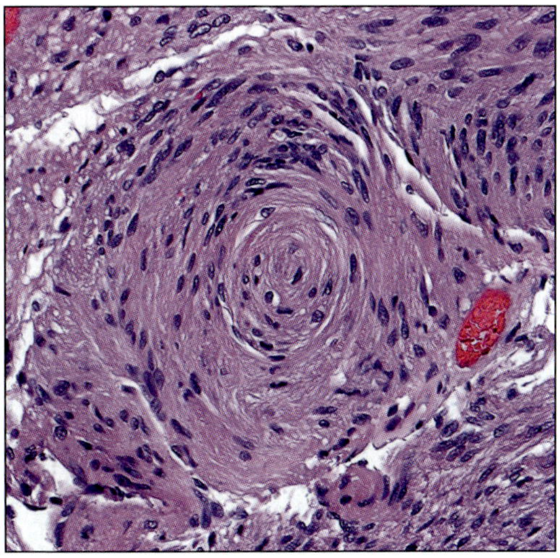

(Left) *Plexiform schwannomas form multinodular masses usually involving superficial locations. Unlike plexiform neurofibromas, which are closely associated with NF1, most plexiform schwannomas are sporadic but may affect NF2 patients, as in this example.* ***(Right)*** *Whorls resembling those encountered in meningiomas may be more frequent in NF2-associated schwannomas than in sporadic tumors. IHC may help in their distinction, particularly in small biopsies.*

Meningioma

*(**Left**) Meningiomas are the 2nd most common neoplasms in patients with NF2. They are usually dura-based and demonstrate strong, homogeneous contrast enhancement after administration of gadolinium in T1-weighted MR sequences ➔. (**Right**) The cytologic features of meningiomas are evident in intraoperative smears. They include "flat" cells with ample eosinophilic cytoplasm containing bland oval nuclei. Intercellular borders are usually indistinct.*

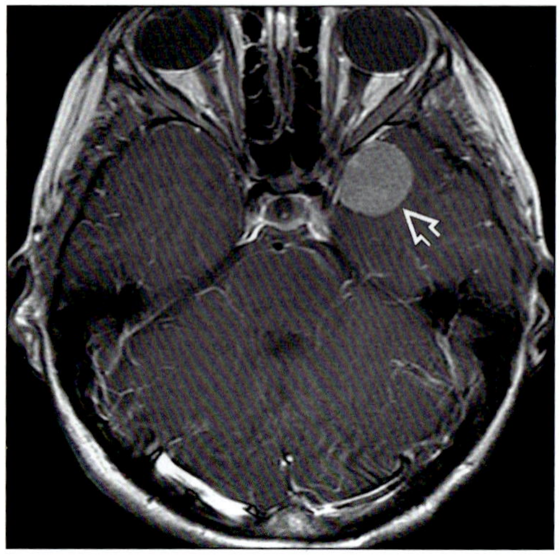

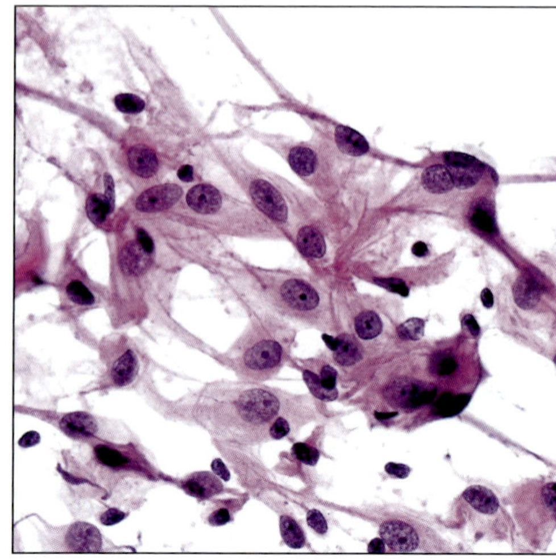

*(**Left**) The most frequent meningioma subtype is meningotheliomatous, characterized by bland cells with indistinct borders and oval nuclei. This subtype occurs at a lesser frequency in NF2 patients compared to sporadic tumors. (**Right**) One of the most useful features for grading meningiomas is the number of mitotic figures → per 10 high-power fields. Most meningiomas are low grade (WHO grade I), but the whole grading spectrum (I-III) may affect patients with NF2.*

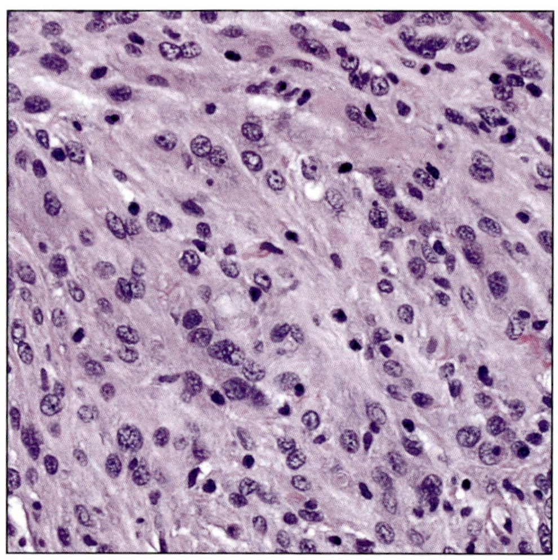

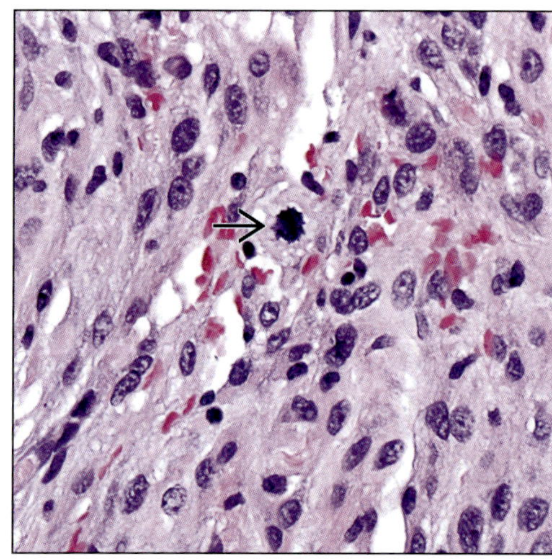

*(**Left**) The combination of multiple meningiomas → and schwannomas ➔ is characteristic of patients with NF2. (**Right**) Juxtaposition of schwannomas and meningiomas (i.e., collision tumors) represents a characteristic feature of patients with NF2. Histologically, these NF2-associated tumors may demonstrate morphologic overlap. However, the presence of wavy nuclei and Verocay bodies indicate schwannoma ➔ whereas psammoma bodies are usually limited to meningiomas →.*

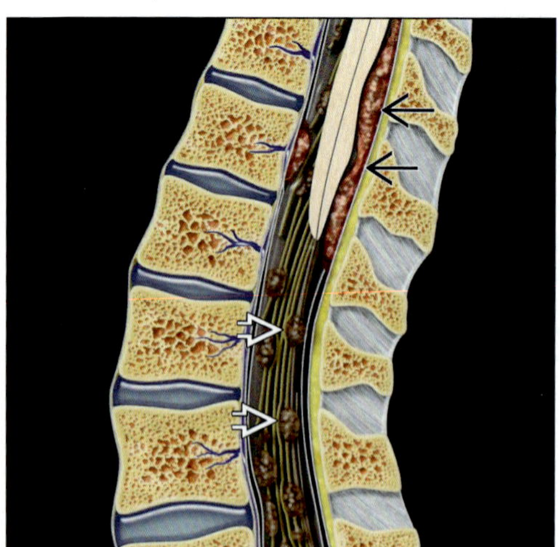

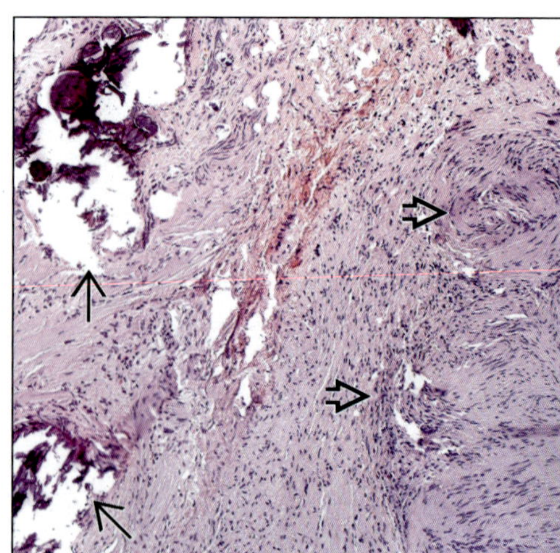

Ependymoma

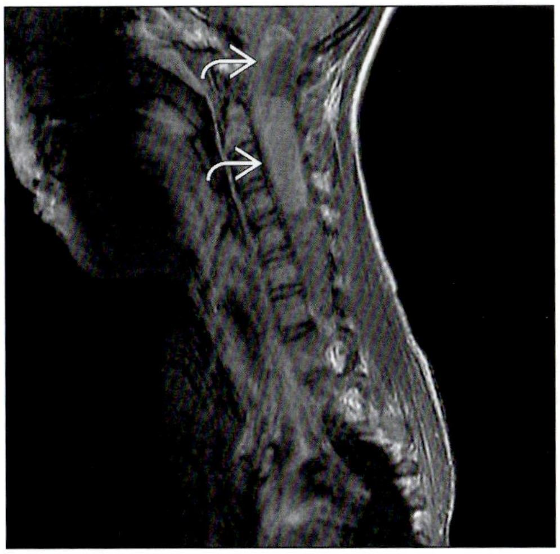

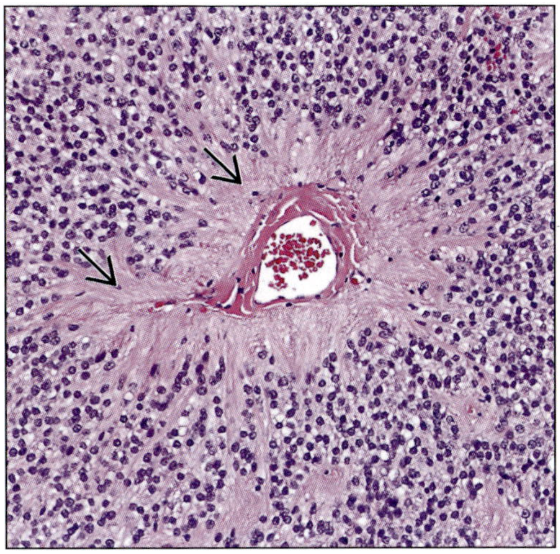

(Left) *The intraparenchymal CNS neoplasm afflicting patients with NF2 is ependymoma, which has a predilection for the cervical cord/cervicomedullary junction. These tumors are well demarcated and demonstrate contrast enhancement.* ***(Right)*** *Perivascular pseudorosettes are frequent in ependymomas. They are composed of anuclear perivascular zones containing numerous neoplastic glial cell processes.*

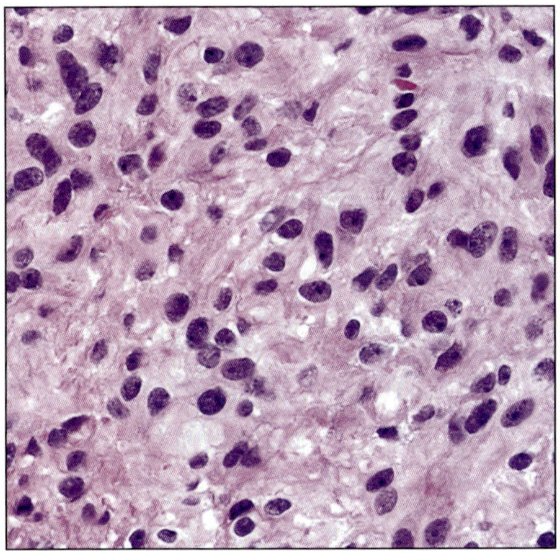

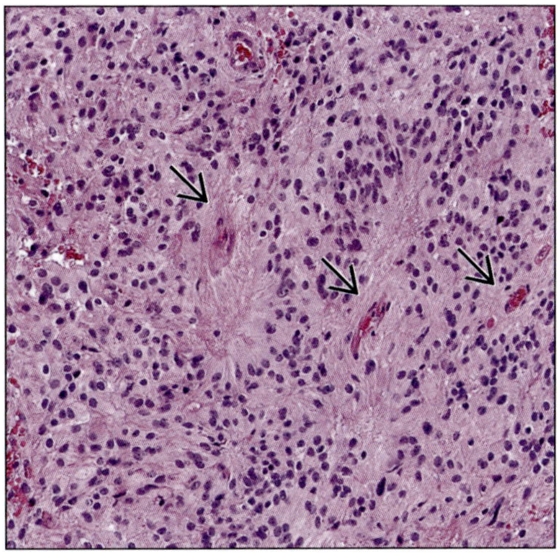

(Left) *This intramedullary neoplasm in a patient with NF2 contains bland oval nuclei, but the pseudorosettes are inconspicuous, making identification of ependymoma difficult. A high index of suspicion is required in spinal cord tumors originating in patients with NF2.* ***(Right)*** *In some ependymomas, diagnosis is straightforward and possible at low magnification. In this NF2-associated ependymoma, perivascular pseudorosettes are abundant.*

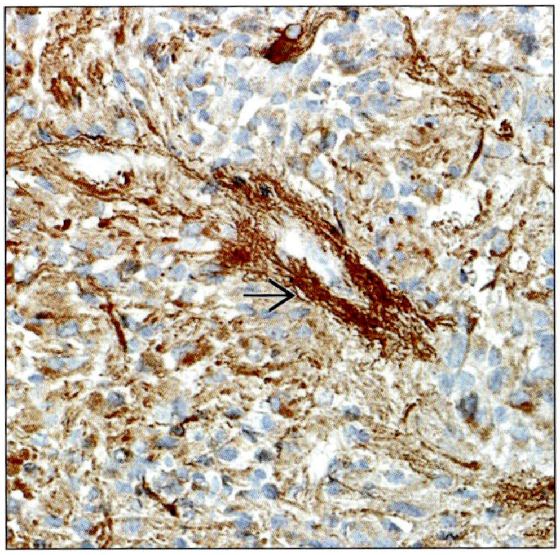

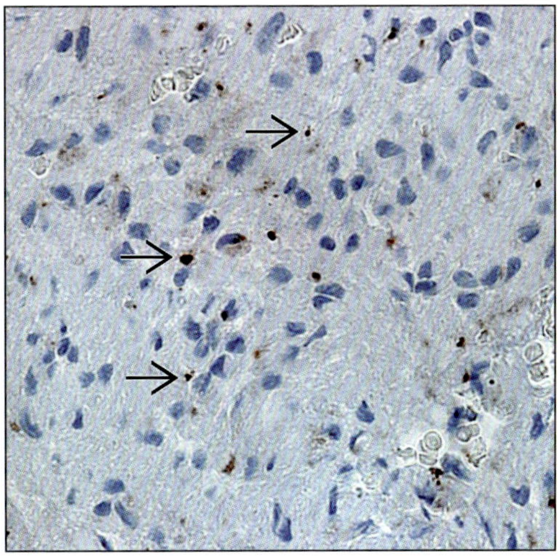

(Left) *The glial nature of ependymoma may be confirmed by immunolabeling with anti-GFAP antibodies. Although the reactivity of individual cells varies, pseudorosettes show intense immunoreactivity.* ***(Right)*** *A dot-like pattern of immunoreactivity for EMA is a diagnostically useful property of ependymoma. Although it may resemble an artifact at 1st glance, it corresponds to microlumina containing microvilli at the ultrastructural level.*

PEUTZ-JEGHERS SYNDROME

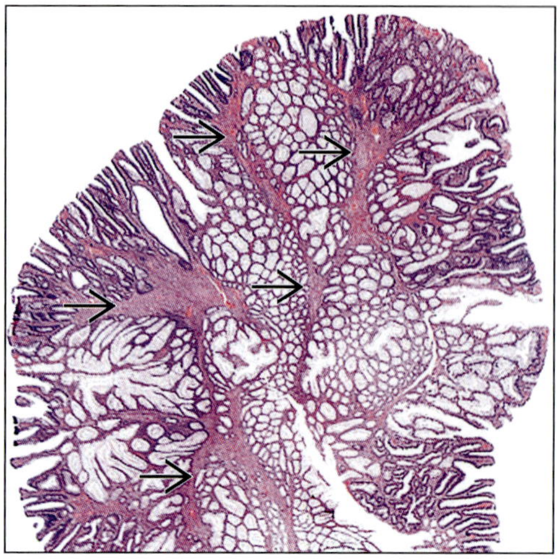

Low-power view of a Peutz-Jeghers polyp shows arborizing bands of smooth muscle ➔.

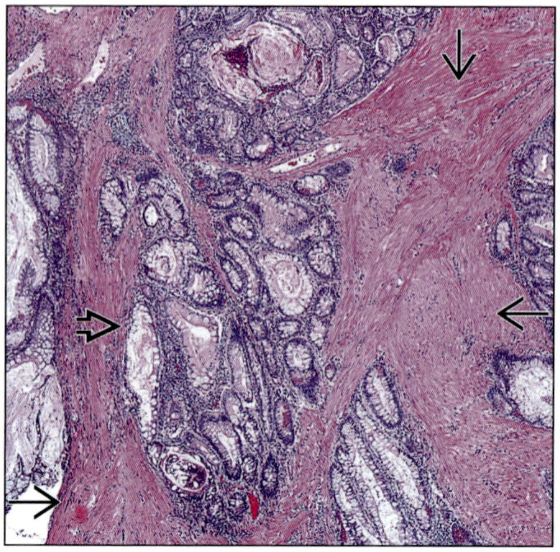

Higher power view shows benign glands ➲ trapped within muscle bundles ➔. Care must be taken not to overinterpret this as cancer.

TERMINOLOGY

Abbreviations

- Peutz-Jeghers syndrome (PJS)

Definitions

- PJS is characterized by
  - Pigmented melanotic lesions around lips, oral cavity, and genitals
  - Hamartomatous polyposis of gastrointestinal (GI) tract
  - Increased risk of cancers in the GI tract, pancreas, gynecologic tract, testis, breast, lung, and thyroid
  - Autosomal dominant inheritance
    - 25% of cases appear de novo

EPIDEMIOLOGY

Prevalence

- Exact prevalence is unknown; estimates range from 1 in 8,500 to 1 in 300,000 live births
- No gender or racial predominance

GENETICS

LKB1 Gene

- Also known as *STK11*
- Serine-threonine kinase that is thought to behave like a tumor suppressor gene
- Important in controlling cell proliferation
- Regulates mTOR pathway
  - Clinical trials using mTOR pathway inhibitors (rapamycin analogues) for chemoprevention are currently underway in PJS patients and have shown promising early results

CLINICAL IMPLICATIONS AND ANCILLARY TESTS

Clinical Presentation

- Pigmentation of lips and oral and genital mucosa seen in infancy and early childhood
  - Lips most common site (> 95%)
  - Pigmentation may fade with age
- GI tract symptoms
  - Abdominal pain due to obstruction/intussusception
    - Polyps arise in stomach (50%), small bowel (65%), and colon (50%)
  - Anemia due to occult or frank GI tract bleeding
    - Hematemesis in patients with gastric and duodenal polyposis
  - Prolapse of rectal polyps
- Associated skeletal abnormalities
  - Club foot and scoliosis

Diagnostic Criteria

- ≥ 2 histologically confirmed Peutz-Jeghers polyps (PJPs)
  - Even patients with only a single PJP seem to have an increased risk of cancer
- Any number of PJPs in a patient with a family history of PJS
- Any number of PJPs in a patient with mucocutaneous pigmentation
- Mucocutaneous pigmentation in a patient with a family history of PJS

Genetic Testing

- Sequencing the *LKB1* gene identifies a mutation in 50-70% of cases
  - Need to look for both protein-truncating mutations as well as large deletions
- Gene inactivation theorized in cases that test negative

ASSOCIATED NEOPLASMS

GI Tract Neoplasms

- Adenocarcinoma of small bowel
  - Cumulative risk: 13%
- Adenocarcinoma of colon
  - Cumulative risk: 39%
  - Mean age of diagnosis: ~ 46 years
- Adenocarcinoma of pancreas
  - Cumulative risk: 36% (100x risk in general population)
- Adenocarcinoma of stomach
  - Cumulative risk: 29%

Other Neoplasms

- Carcinoma of breast
  - Absolute risk: ~ 54%
- Ovarian sex cord tumors with annular tubules
- Adenoma malignum of cervix
- Mucinous tumors of ovaries and fallopian tubes
  - Absolute risk: 10%
- Bronchioalveolar carcinomas of lung
- Testicular sex cord and Sertoli cell tumors
  - Absolute risk: 9%
- Papillary thyroid cancer
- Overall cumulative cancer risk: 93% at age 65

MICROSCOPIC FINDINGS

Hamartomatous Polyps

- Polyps classically have arborizing bands of smooth muscle with a papillary architecture
  - Best seen in small bowel polyps; stomach and colon polyps may lack classic features and thus can be difficult to diagnose
- Epithelium is nonneoplastic and has a lobular growth pattern
  - Epithelium frequently is trapped in bands of smooth muscle; do not overinterpret this finding as carcinoma
  - Dysplasia has hardly ever been found in PJPs, suggesting that cancer may arise by a different mechanism

CANCER RISK MANAGEMENT

Endoscopic Surveillance

- Baseline upper and lower endoscopy at age 8, to be repeated every 2-3 years
- Endoscopic removal of small polyps
  - Surgery may be necessary for obstructing polyps or intussusception

Radiologic Surveillance

- Transvaginal ultrasound, serum CA-125, and Pap smears annually beginning between age 20 and 25 for gynecologic (GYN) tumors
- Endoscopic ultrasound, abdominal CT, and CA-19-9 every 1-2 years starting between age 25 and 30 for pancreas tumors
- Mammography or MR annually starting at age 25 for breast cancer

SELECTED REFERENCES

1. Korsse SE et al: Small bowel endoscopy and Peutz-Jeghers syndrome. Best Pract Res Clin Gastroenterol. 26(3):263-78, 2012
2. Arber N et al: Small bowel polyposis syndromes. Curr Gastroenterol Rep. 13(5):435-41, 2011
3. Kuwada SK et al: A rationale for mTOR inhibitors as chemoprevention agents in Peutz-Jeghers syndrome. Fam Cancer. 10(3):469-72, 2011
4. Latchford AR et al: Gastrointestinal polyps and cancer in Peutz-Jeghers syndrome: clinical aspects. Fam Cancer. 10(3):455-61, 2011
5. Latchford AR et al: Peutz-Jeghers syndrome: intriguing suggestion of gastrointestinal cancer prevention from surveillance. Dis Colon Rectum. 54(12):1547-51, 2011
6. Triggiani V et al: Papillary thyroid carcinoma in Peutz-Jeghers syndrome. Thyroid. 21(11):1273-7, 2011
7. van Lier MG et al: High cancer risk and increased mortality in patients with Peutz-Jeghers syndrome. Gut. 60(2):141-7, 2011
8. Beggs AD et al: Peutz-Jeghers syndrome: a systematic review and recommendations for management. Gut. 59(7):975-86, 2010
9. Chen HM et al: Genetics of the hamartomatous polyposis syndromes: a molecular review. Int J Colorectal Dis. 24(8):865-74, 2009

IMAGE GALLERY

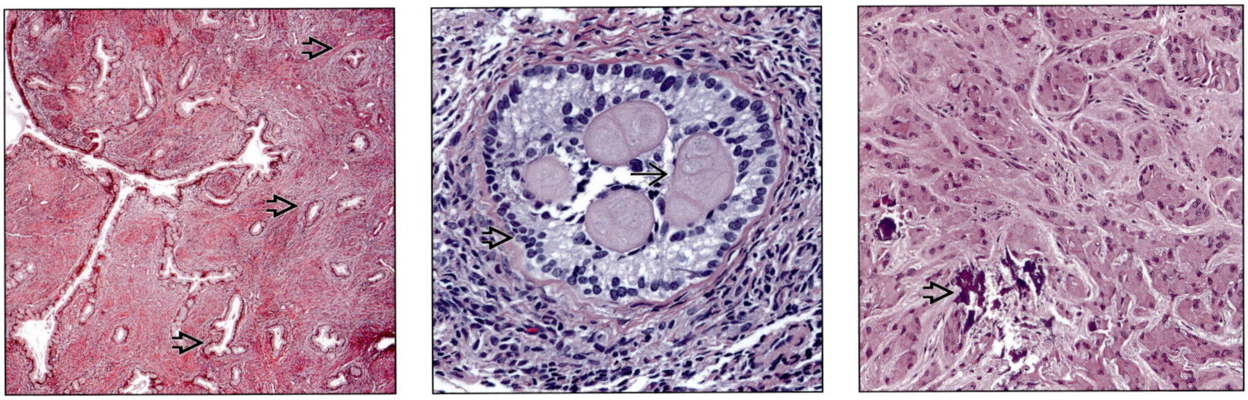

(Left) *Adenoma malignum of the cervix in Peutz-Jeghers syndrome (PJS) shows bland infiltrative glands ➾ without a desmoplastic response. (Courtesy A. Srivastava, MD.)* ***(Center)*** *Ovarian sex cord tumor with annular tubules in PJS shows circumscribed nests of tumor cells ➾ containing hyaline material ➙.* ***(Right)*** *A Sertoli cell tumor of the testis shows nests and cords of tumor cells with abundant pink cytoplasm and a hyalinized stroma with foci of calcification ➾. (Courtesy E. Oliva, MD.)*

PTEN-HAMARTOMA TUMOR SYNDROMES

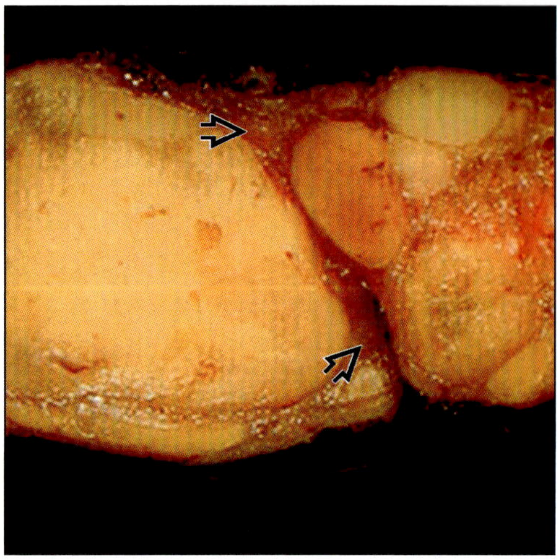

Gross photograph of thyroid adenomatous nodules shows multiple well-circumscribed and unencapsulated nodules compressing the adjacent uninvolved thyroid parenchyma ➡.

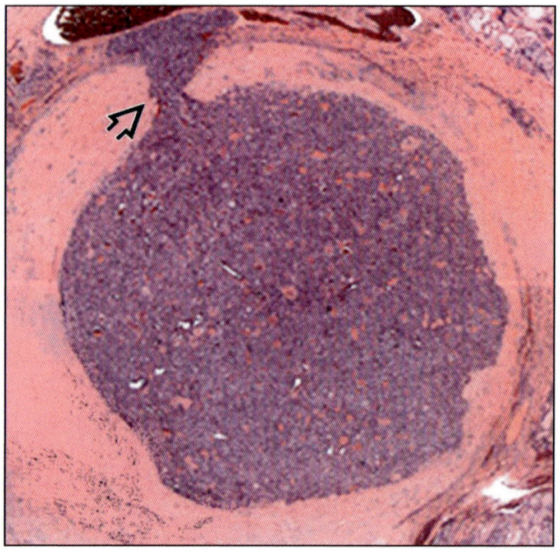

One of the major criteria for the diagnosis of PHTS is the presence of follicular carcinoma. A follicular cell proliferation present in this young patient with Cowden syndrome shows capsular invasion ➡.

TERMINOLOGY

Abbreviations

- Phosphatase and tensin homolog (*PTEN*) deleted on chromosome 10
- *PTEN*-hamartoma tumor syndrome (PHTS)
- Cowden syndrome (CS)
- Cowden disease (CD)
- Multiple hamartoma syndrome (MHAM)
- Bannayan-Riley-Ruvalcaba syndrome (BRRS)
- *PTEN*-related Proteus syndrome (PRPS)

Syndromes

- PHTS includes
  - Cowden syndrome
  - Bannayan-Riley-Ruvalcaba syndrome
  - *PTEN*-related Proteus syndrome and Proteus-like syndrome
  - Autism with macrocephaly

Definition

- PHTS is a complex disorder caused by germline inactivating mutations of *PTEN* tumor suppressor gene, which maps to 10q23.3
- PHTS is primarily composed of the Cowden and Bannayan-Riley-Ruvalcaba syndromes
  - Several other syndromes have been linked with *PTEN* mutations including *PTEN*-related Proteus syndrome, Proteus-like syndrome, and autism with macrocephaly
- **Cowden syndrome**
  - Clinical manifestations of Cowden syndrome includes hamartomatous tumors in multiple organ systems and an increased risk for malignancy
  - Affected individuals usually have macrocephaly, trichilemmomas, and papillomatous papules and present by late 20s
  - Multiple hamartoma syndrome with a high risk for benign and malignant tumors of thyroid, breast, and endometrium
  - Lifetime risk of developing breast cancer is 25-50%; reports up to 85%
    - Average age of diagnosis between 38 and 46 years
  - ~ 50% of women have benign breast conditions: Ductal hyperplasia, intraductal papillomatosis, adenosis, lobular atrophy, fibroadenomas, fibrocystic change, &/or densely fibrotic hyalinized nodules
  - Increased incidence of both multifocality and bilateral involvement has been observed for both benign and malignant breast disorders
  - ~ 2/3 of CS patients develop thyroid lesions involving follicular cells
    - Includes multinodular goiter, multiple adenomatous nodules, follicular adenoma, follicular carcinoma, and, less frequently, papillary thyroid carcinoma
    - Usually follicular, rarely papillary, but no medullary thyroid cancer has been reported
    - Risk of thyroid cancer in affected individuals ranges from 3-35% in large case series
    - ~ 70x increased incidence of nonmedullary thyroid cancer relative to the general population
  - Risk for endometrial cancer, although not well defined, may approach ~ 13-28%
- **Bannayan-Riley-Ruvalcaba syndrome**
  - Congenital disorder characterized by macrocephaly, lipomas, intestinal hamartomatous polyposis, vascular hamartomatous lesions, and pigmented macules of glans penis
  - Although diagnostic criteria for CS have been established for more than a decade, there are no agreed upon international criteria for the diagnosis of BRRS
  - Rate of occurrence and histologic types of thyroid lesions in BRRS have not been widely reported

but have appeared similar to those seen in CS, suggesting a single entity
- **PTEN-related Proteus syndrome**
  - Complex, highly variable disorder involving congenital malformations and hamartomatous overgrowth of multiple tissues as well as connective tissue nevi, epidermal nevi, and hyperostoses
  - There have been reports of *PTEN* mutations in some patients with phenotypic similarities to Proteus syndrome (PS)
    - Somatic activating mutations in *AKT1* oncogene have been delineated as the genetic cause of PS
  - Proteus-like syndrome
    - Undefined but refers to individuals with significant clinical features of PS who do not meet the diagnostic criteria for PS

EPIDEMIOLOGY

Incidence

- Estimated ~ 1 in 200,000-250,000 people

Familial

- Only 10-50% of individuals with Cowden syndrome have an affected parent
- Each child of an affected individual has a 50% chance of inheriting mutation and developing PHTS

Lifetime Risk of Developing Cancer

- Lifetime risks for a variety of cancers are increased in patients with *PTEN* mutations
  - Thyroid: 3-35%
  - Breast: 25-85%
  - Endometrium: 13-28%
  - Now extending to
    - Colorectal cancer: 9-13%
    - Kidney cancer: 13-34%%
    - Melanoma: 6%

GENETICS

PTEN

- *PTEN* is a tumor suppressor gene located on 10q23.3
- Up to ~ 80% of cases of that met criteria for Cowden syndrome and a small percentage of cases of Cowden-like syndrome result from mutations in *PTEN* gene
  - In *PTEN* sequencing-negative and clinically positive Cowden syndrome, ~ 10% have large deletions and ~ 10% have promoter mutations
- *PTEN* mutation
  - Initially reported that up to 83% of individuals meeting clinical criteria for Cowden syndrome had a detectable *PTEN* mutation
    - Overestimate attributable to the highly selected nature of earlier Cowden syndrome cohorts
  - More recent estimates are that germline *PTEN* mutations are found in ~ 20-34% of individuals who meet clinical criteria for Cowden syndrome or who meet criteria for genetic testing
- Function of *PTEN* is not entirely understood, but it is a major phosphatase for phosphoinositide-3,4,5-triphosphate
- By downregulating the levels of phosphoinositide-3,4,5-triphosphate, *PTEN* produces an inhibitory (tumor suppressor) effect on the PI3P/Akt pathway, an important carcinogenesis pathway
- Loss of *PTEN* function results in escape from programmed cell death and G1 arrest in cell cycle
- Proposed that *PTEN* has important activity both in cytoplasm and nucleus
  - Nuclear *PTEN* might be required for cell cycle arrest by downregulating cyclin-D1 and preventing phosphorylation of mitogen-activated protein kinase pathway
  - Cytoplasmic *PTEN* seems to be required for apoptosis by downregulating the phosphorylation of Akt and upregulating p27
- 75% of germline mutations result in truncated protein, lack of protein, or dysfunctional protein
- Protein produced from *PTEN* gene is a tumor suppressor, which means that it normally prevents cells from growing and dividing (proliferating) too rapidly or in an uncontrolled way

Other Loci

- In some patients who lack *PTEN* mutations, hypermethylation of the promoter of the *KLLN* (Killin) gene, leading to reduced expression of *KLLN*, has been described
  - *KLLN* gene, which is located on chromosome 10q23 and functions as a p53-regulated inhibitor of DNA synthesis, shares the same transcription site as *PTEN* gene
- Other patients have been reported with mutations in the succinate dehydrogenase *(SDH)* gene, subunits B and D
- Germline *PIK3CA* and *AKT1* mutations have also been reported in phenotypic Cowden syndrome patients without *PTEN, SDH,* or *KLLN* mutations

Diagnosis

- Up to 85% of individuals who meet the diagnostic criteria for CS and 65% of individuals with a clinical diagnosis of BRRS have a detectable *PTEN* mutation
- Preliminary data suggest that up to 50% of individuals with Proteus-like syndrome and up to 20% of individuals with *PTEN*-related Proteus syndrome have *PTEN* mutations
- *PTEN* sequence analysis, deletion/duplication testing, and FISH testing are available on a clinical basis
- **Cowden syndrome**
  - Consensus diagnostic criteria for CS have been developed and are updated each year by the National Comprehensive Cancer Network (NCCN)
  - Clinical criteria have been divided into 3 categories: Pathognomonic, major, and minor
  - **Pathognomonic criteria**
    - Adult Lhermitte-Duclos disease (LDD), defined as presence of a cerebellar dysplastic gangliocytoma
  - Mucocutaneous lesions
    - Acral keratoses

PTEN-HAMARTOMA TUMOR SYNDROMES

- Papillomatous lesions
- Mucosal lesions
- Trichilemmomas (facial)

○ **Major criteria**
- Epithelial thyroid cancer (nonmedullary), especially follicular thyroid cancer
- Macrocephaly (occipital frontal circumference ≥ 97th percentile)
- Endometrial carcinoma
- Breast cancer

○ **Minor criteria**
- Other thyroid lesions (e.g., adenoma, adenomatous nodules, multinodular goiter)
- Hamartomatous intestinal polyps
- Fibrocystic disease of the breast
- Lipomas
- Fibromas
- Genitourinary tumors (especially renal cell carcinoma)
- Genitourinary malformation
- Uterine fibroids
- Intellectual disability

○ **Operational diagnosis of CS**: Made if an individual meets any of the following criteria
- Pathognomonic mucocutaneous lesions combined with 1 of the following
- ≥ 6 facial papules, of which ≥ 3 must be trichilemmoma
- Cutaneous facial papules and oral mucosal papillomatosis
- ≥ 6 palmoplantar keratoses
- Oral mucosal papillomatosis and acral keratoses
- ≥ 4 minor criteria
- 1 major and ≥ 3 minor criteria
- ≥ 2 major criteria

- **BRRS**
  - Diagnostic criteria for BRRS have not been set
  - Based heavily on the presence of the cardinal features
    - Macrocephaly
    - Hamartomatous intestinal polyposis
    - Lipomas
    - Pigmented macules of glans penis
  - ~ 60% of patients with BRRS have detectable *PTEN* mutation
- **PTEN-related Proteus syndrome**
  - Highly variable and appears to affect individuals in a mosaic distribution
    - Somatic activating mutations in the *AKT1* oncogene have been delineated as the genetic cause of Proteus syndrome
  - It is frequently misdiagnosed despite the development of consensus diagnostic criteria
  - Mandatory general criteria for diagnosis include mosaic distribution of lesions, progressive course, and sporadic occurrence
  - Rapidly progressive, asymmetric postnatal overgrowth of tissues, with hyperostoses, vascular malformations, dysregulation of fatty tissues (both atrophy and overgrowth), and skin manifestations, such as verrucous epidermal nevi or cerebriform connective tissue nevi
  - Specific criteria for diagnosis include
  - Connective tissue nevi (pathognomonic)
  - **2 of the following**
    - Epidermal nevus
    - Disproportionate overgrowth (≥ 1)
    - Limbs: Arms/legs; hands/feet/digits
    - Skull: Hyperostoses
    - External auditory meatus: Hyperostosis
    - Vertebrae: Megaspondylodysplasia
    - Specific tumors before end of 2nd decade
    - Bilateral ovarian cystadenomas
    - Parotid monomorphic adenoma
  - **3 of the following**
    - Dysregulated adipose tissue: Lipomas or regional absence of fat
    - Vascular malformations (≥ 1): Capillary, venous, lymphatic
    - Facial phenotype: Dolichocephaly, long face, minor downslanting of palpebral fissures &/or minor ptosis, low nasal bridge, wide or anteverted nares, open mouth at rest
- **Proteus-like syndrome**
  - Exceedingly rare asymmetric overgrowth syndrome
  - Undefined but describes individuals with significant clinical features of PS yet do not meet diagnostic criteria

Genetic Counseling

- PHTS is inherited in an autosomal dominant manner
- Because CS is likely underdiagnosed, actual proportion of simplex cases (defined as individuals with no obvious family history) and familial cases (defined as ≥ 2 related affected individuals) cannot be determined
- Majority of CS cases are simplex
- Perhaps 10-50% of individuals with CS have an affected parent
- Each child of an affected individual has a 50% chance of inheriting mutation and developing PHTS
- Prenatal testing for pregnancies at increased risk is possible if disease-causing mutation in family is known

CLINICAL IMPLICATIONS AND ANCILLARY TESTS

Clinical Testing

- Sequence analysis
  - Virtually all missense mutations in *PTEN* are believed to be deleterious
  - Early studies suggest that up to 85% of individuals who meet diagnostic criteria for CS and 65% of individuals with a clinical diagnosis of BRRS have a detectable *PTEN* mutation
  - More recently, it was found that ~ 25% of individuals who meet strict diagnostic criteria for CS have a pathogenic *PTEN* mutation, including large deletions

  - Data suggest that up to 50% of individuals with a Proteus-like syndrome and up to 20% of individuals with Proteus syndrome have *PTEN* mutations
- Deletion/duplication analysis
  - Southern blotting, real-time PCR, MLPA, and other methods of detecting gene copy number variation can each be used to detect large *PTEN* deletions and rearrangements that are not detectable by PCR-based sequence analysis

Management

- Treatment of manifestations
  - Treatment for benign and malignant manifestations of PHTS is same as for their sporadic counterparts
  - Topical agents (e.g., 5-fluorouracil), curettage, cryosurgery, or laser ablation may alleviate mucocutaneous manifestations of CS
  - Cutaneous lesions should be excised only if malignancy is suspected or symptoms (e.g., pain, deformity) are significant
- Surveillance
  - To detect tumors at the earliest, most treatable stages
    - For children (< 18 years): Yearly thyroid ultrasound and skin check with physical examination
    - For adults: Yearly thyroid ultrasound and dermatologic evaluation
    - For men and women: Colonoscopy beginning at age 35-40 years with frequency dependent on degree of polyposis identified; biennial (every 2 years) renal imaging (CT or MR preferred) beginning at age 40 years
    - For women beginning at age 30 years: Monthly breast self-examination
    - Annual breast screening (at minimum mammogram; MR may also be incorporated) and transvaginal ultrasound or endometrial biopsy
    - For those with family history of a particular cancer type at an early age: Consider initiating screening 5-10 years prior to youngest age of diagnosis in family
- Testing of relatives at risk
  - When *PTEN* mutation has been identified in a proband, molecular genetic testing of asymptomatic at-risk relatives can identify those who have family-specific mutation and warrant ongoing surveillance

ASSOCIATED LESIONS AND BENIGN NEOPLASMS

Skin

- Multiple trichilemmomas, usually on face, are cutaneous hallmark of disease
  - Trichilemmomas show differentiation toward hair follicle infundibulum
- Mucocutaneous fibromas and neuromas
- Acral and palmoplantar keratoses
- Oral papillomas involving lips, gums, and tongue

Breast

- Benign lesions are often bilateral and multiple
  - Fibroadenoma
  - Adenosis
  - Apocrine cysts
  - Hamartomas

Thyroid

- Multiple adenomatous nodules are hallmark of disease
- Lymphocytic thyroiditis
- Multinodular hyperplasia
- C-cell hyperplasia

Esophagus

- Esophageal glycogen acanthosis is hallmark of CS
  - Abundant glycogen demonstrated on PAS stain ± diastase treatment
  - Pale, ballooned, and vacuolated squamous cells
  - Multiple nodular foci of squamous cell proliferation

Stomach

- Most often resemble hyperplastic polyps with prominent foveolar hyperplasia
  - Stromal smooth muscle proliferation may be prominent and mimic Peutz-Jeghers polyps
  - Distinction from gastric polyps in juvenile polyposis difficult
  - Polyps may appear virtually identical to those described in patients with Cronkhite-Canada syndrome

Colon

- Hamartomatous stroma-rich polyps with cystically dilated glands
- Ganglioneuromatous polyps with proliferation of Schwann cells and ganglion cells in lamina propria
- Inflammatory polyps that may mimic juvenile polyps
- Lymphoid polyps with prominent mucosal or submucosal reactive lymphoid aggregates
- Lipoma
- Colon adenomas may occur in patients with CS at young age
  - Isolated polyps in rectosigmoid colon may mimic mucosal prolapse

Brain

- Dysplastic gangliocytoma of the cerebellum, or adult Lhermitte-Duclos disease
  - Refers to a hamartomatous tumor of the cerebellar cortex that can occur in the setting of a *PTEN* mutation
- Cavernous hemangioma

Soft Tissue

- Characteristic disorganized overgrowth of mesenchymal elements (*PTEN* hamartoma of soft tissue)
- Vascular proliferations
- Hamartomas

PTEN-HAMARTOMA TUMOR SYNDROMES

ASSOCIATED MALIGNANT NEOPLASMS

Breast Carcinoma

- Age of diagnosis: 38-46 years
  - Occurs 10 years younger than general population
  - Male breast cancer also occurs

Follicular Thyroid Carcinoma

- Predominant thyroid tumor in PHTS

Papillary Thyroid Carcinoma

- Also reported to have greater risk than general population

Endometrial Carcinoma

- Increased risk of endometrial adenocarcinoma: 13-28% lifetime risk

Renal Cancer

- Increased risk of renal cancer

Colorectal Adenocarcinoma

- Risk of colorectal cancer was estimated at 10x higher that the general population

Other Cancers Associated With PHTS

- Glioblastoma
- Melanoma
- Merkel cell carcinoma
- Retinal glioma
- Lung cancer
- Liver cancer
- Pancreatic cancer
- Ovarian cancer
- Bladder cancer
- Liposarcoma

Other Cancers Rarely Associated With PHTS

- Ependymoma
- Medullary thyroid carcinoma
- Granulosa cell tumor
- Lipoblastoma

CANCER RISK MANAGEMENT

Breast

- Breast awareness, including prompt reporting to physicians of any changes
- Periodic breast self-exams starting at age 18 years
- Clinical breast exam every 6-12 months starting at age 25 years or individualized based on earliest known onset of breast cancer in the family
- Annual mammography and breast MR screening starting at age 30-35 years
  - Or 5-10 years before the earliest known breast cancer in the family
  - MR screening as an adjunct to mammography

Thyroid

- Baseline thyroid ultrasound at 18 years and consideration of repeating annually thereafter
- Monthly thyroid examination and palpation starting in adolescence

Uterus

- Surveillance for endometrial cancer starting at age 35-40 years
  - Or 5 years younger than the earliest familial endometrial cancer diagnosis

Kidney

- Annual urinalysis with cytology and renal ultrasound

Colon

- Consideration of baseline colonoscopy at age 35 years
  - Then every 5-10 years or more frequently if patient is symptomatic or polyps are noted

Other Tumors

- Given the high risk of malignancy, cancer surveillance is the major focus of medical management as per American Cancer Society guidelines
  - Annual comprehensive physical exam, starting at 18 years of age

SELECTED REFERENCES

1. Al-Zaid T et al: Trichilemmomas show loss of PTEN in Cowden syndrome but only rarely in sporadic tumors. J Cutan Pathol. 39(5):493-9, 2012
2. Daniels MS et al: Lifetime cancer risks of PTEN mutation carriers--letter. Clin Cancer Res. 18(15):4213; author reply 4214, 2012
3. Hobert JA et al: Elevated plasma succinate in PTEN, SDHB, and SDHD mutation-positive individuals. Genet Med. 14(6):616-9, 2012
4. Kurek KC et al: PTEN hamartoma of soft tissue: a distinctive lesion in PTEN syndromes. Am J Surg Pathol. 36(5):671-87, 2012
5. Mansoor Q et al: Proliferative retinopathy in Cowden syndrome. BMJ Case Rep. 2012, 2012
6. Mester JL et al: Papillary renal cell carcinoma is associated with PTEN hamartoma tumor syndrome. Urology. 79(5):1187, 2012
7. Milas M et al: Should patients with Cowden syndrome undergo prophylactic thyroidectomy? Surgery. 152(6):1201-10, 2012
8. Ngeow J et al: Utility of PTEN protein dosage in predicting for underlying germline PTEN mutations among patients presenting with thyroid cancer and Cowden-like phenotypes. J Clin Endocrinol Metab. 97(12):E2320-7, 2012
9. Ni Y et al: Germline SDHx variants modify breast and thyroid cancer risks in Cowden and Cowden-like syndrome via FAD/NAD-dependant destabilization of p53. Hum Mol Genet. 21(2):300-10, 2012
10. Romano C et al: PTEN gene: a model for genetic diseases in dermatology. ScientificWorldJournal. 2012:252457, 2012
11. Sawamura N et al: [A case of Cowden disease with a germline mutation in exon5 of PTEN gene diagnosed based on typical esophageal multiple polypoid lesions observed on a medical checkup.] Nihon Shokakibyo Gakkai Zasshi. 109(4):593-9, 2012
12. Son EJ et al: Familial follicular cell-derived thyroid carcinoma. Front Endocrinol (Lausanne). 3:61, 2012
13. Tan MH et al: Lifetime cancer risks in individuals with germline PTEN mutations. Clin Cancer Res. 18(2):400-7, 2012

Benign and Malignant Neoplasms Associated With PHTS

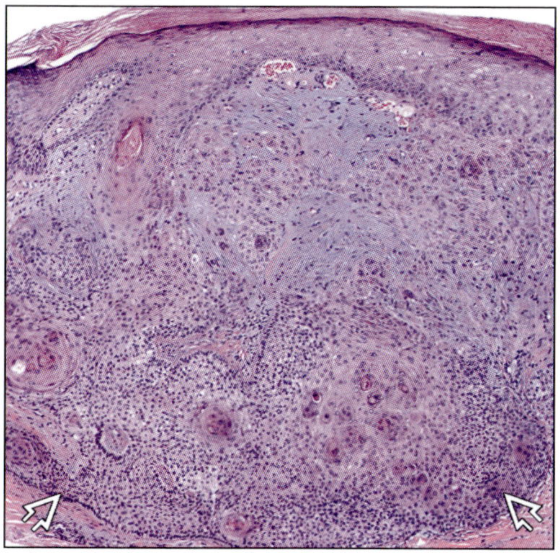

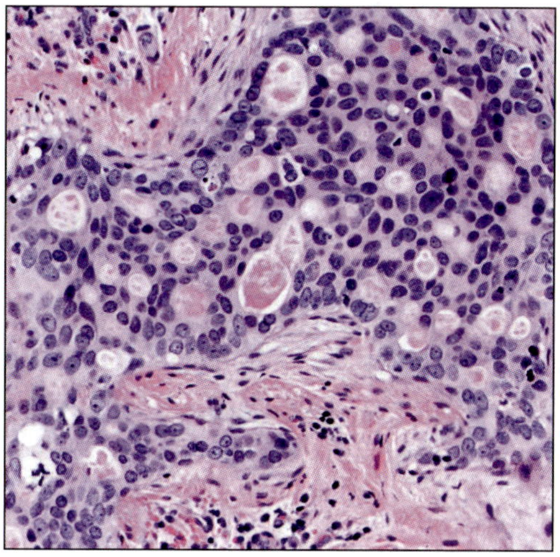

(Left) *Multiple facial trichilemmomas are common in patients with Cowden syndrome/ PHTS. Well-circumscribed epidermal proliferation ➲ with pale clear cells are reminiscent of the hair follicle infundibulum.* ***(Right)*** *Invasive ductal carcinomas present in patients with PHTS may demonstrate tubules and have intermediate- to high-grade nuclei or a prominent component of well-formed tubules, and may have rare or absent mitoses.*

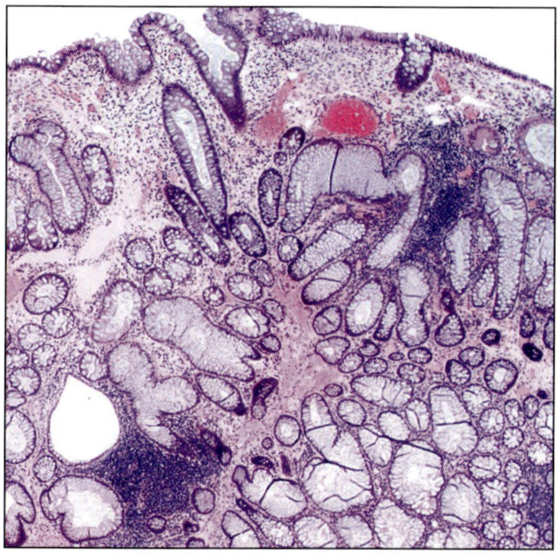

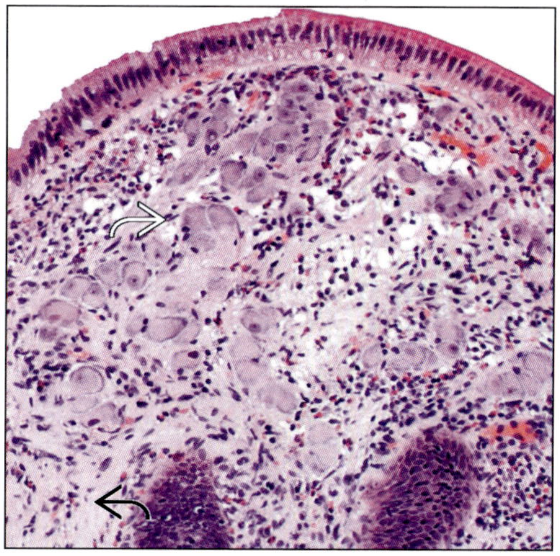

(Left) *Hematoxylin & eosin shows hamartomatous colon polyps usually present in Cowden syndrome/ PHTS. Disarray of normal crypt architecture and fibromuscular proliferation may mimic mucosal prolapse polyps.* ***(Right)*** *Hematoxylin & eosin shows ganglioneuromatous polyps, which may be seen in juvenile polyposis and Cowden syndrome. Schwann cell proliferation ➚ and numerous ganglion cells ➨ are present in the lamina propria in this polyp.*

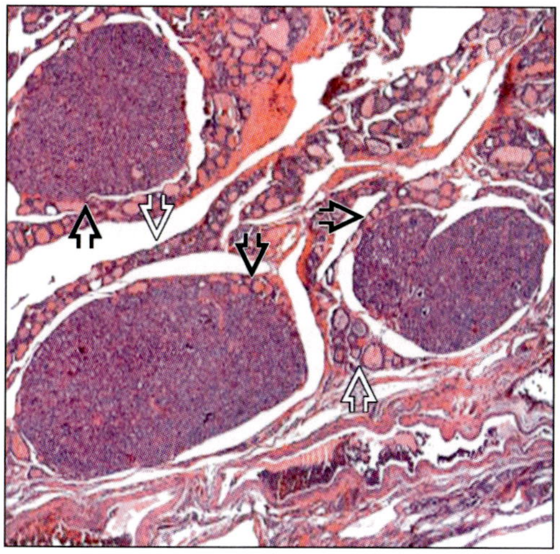

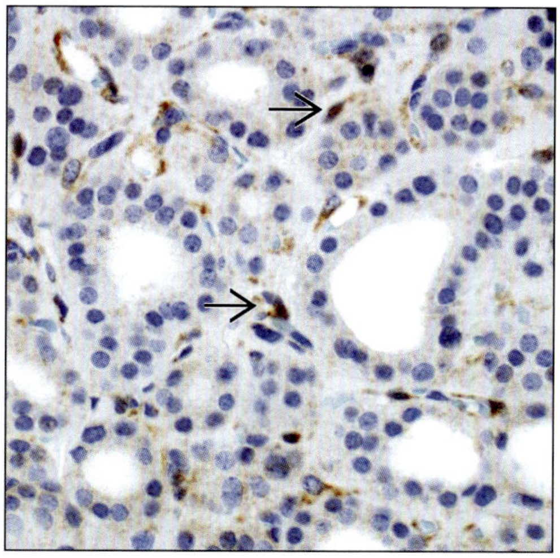

(Left) *Multiple adenomatous thyroid nodules ➲ are usually present in patients with PHTS. These adenomatous nodules may be seen in the thyroid with follicular adenoma and follicular carcinoma. Note the adjacent thyroid follicles are compressed ➲.* ***(Right)*** *Immunohistochemistry for PTEN in thyroid adenomatous nodules in patients with PHTS usually shows loss of immunoreactivity of the follicular cells. Endothelial cells maintain immunopositivity ➝.*

RHABDOID PREDISPOSITION SYNDROME

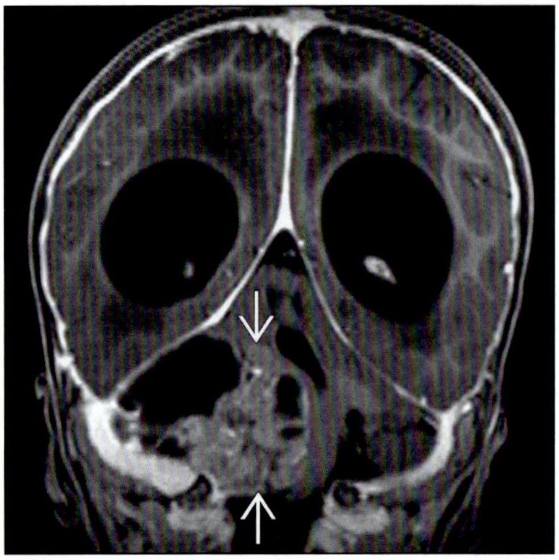

The cerebellopontine angle is a classic location for AT/RT ➡. This patient had a constitutional Chr 22 abnormality with multiple congenital anomalies in addition to AT/RT. (Courtesy C. Specht, MD.)

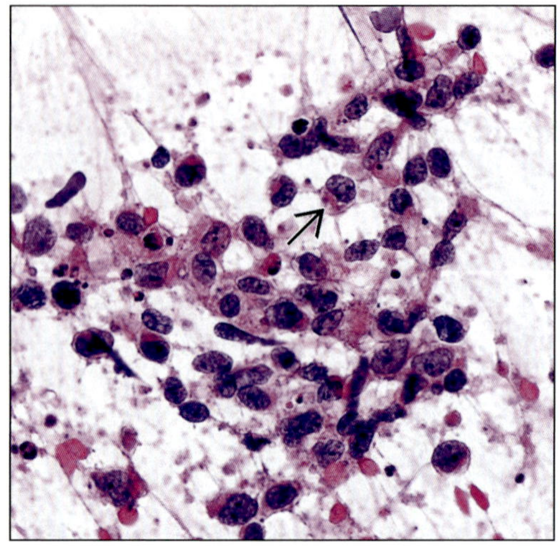

Cytologic features of rhabdoid tumors at all sites include the presence of large, variably dyscohesive cells with eosinophilic cytoplasm ➡ and eccentric nuclei with prominent nucleoli.

TERMINOLOGY

Synonyms

- Formerly called familial posterior fossa brain tumor syndrome, though not all tumors arise in the posterior fossa

Definition

- Genetic predisposition for development of rhabdoid tumors (atypical teratoid/rhabdoid tumor [AT/RT]) of the brain, renal rhabdoid tumors, and extrarenal rhabdoid tumors)

EPIDEMIOLOGY

Relatively Rare

- AT/RT represents 1-2% of pediatric brain tumors; 10% of brain tumors in infants with M:F ratio 1.6-2:1
- Rhabdoid tumors represent < 3% of pediatric renal tumors
- Median age at diagnosis of rhabdoid tumors is 6 months in patients with germline mutations vs. 18 months sporadically

GENETICS

Germline Mutations in *INI1*

- Occur in ~ 1/3 of patients with rhabdoid tumors
- Also known as *SMARCB1, hSNF5, BAF47*
- Located in chromosome region 22q11.2
- Encodes for a protein component of the ATP-dependent SWI-SNF chromatin-remodeling complex
  - Protein product interacts with HIV-1 integrase
- Classic tumor suppressor gene (i.e., inactivation through 2 hits leads to tumor formation)
- Frequency of germline mutations is highest in patients with multiple primary sites (~ 100%)
- Gonadal mosaicism in a subset
  - Multiple affected siblings, unaffected parents
- Most mutations in rhabdoid tumors are deletions, nonsense, or frameshift and lead to complete gene inactivation
- Rarely present in > 1 generation given the high penetrance and high mortality of the disease
- Few, if any, additional somatic genetic alterations in rhabdoid tumors other than *INI1* alterations

Germline Mutation in *SMARCA4/BRG1*

- Reported in a rare family with rhabdoid predisposition syndrome
- Encodes for another protein member of the SWI/SNF chromatin-remodeling complex
- Loss of heterozygosity in 2 sisters with rhabdoid tumors, INI1 protein preservation

CLINICAL IMPLICATIONS AND ANCILLARY TESTS

Genetic Testing

- Germline mutation testing and genetic counseling recommended in any patient/families with rhabdoid tumors/neoplasms associated with INI1 protein loss
- Irrespective of age: Patients with germline mutations as old as 22 years at presentation have been reported
- Prenatal DNA testing may be offered in families with documented mutation

ASSOCIATED NEOPLASMS

Atypical Teratoid/Rhabdoid Tumor

- Highly malignant neoplasm corresponding to WHO grade IV
- Composed of large cells with eccentric nuclei and macronucleoli arranged in nests or sheets
- Brisk mitotic activity and necrosis
- Variable small round blue cell component

- May predominate in younger patients
- Mesenchymal differentiation, arrangement in cords, myxoid stroma in a subset of cases
- Epithelial morphology with papillae and gland-like areas is rare
- Immunohistochemistry highlights a polyphenotypic pattern of staining
  - EMA expression is most frequent, but cytokeratin, GFAP, neurofilament protein, and smooth muscle actin may also be expressed
- Cytoplasmic aggregates of intermediate filaments by electron microscopy
- Very few genetic alterations other than *INI1* mutation
  - Loss of INI1 nuclear protein by immunohistochemistry with preservation in nonneoplastic elements is almost diagnostic
- Differential diagnosis includes choroid plexus carcinoma, CNS-PNET/medulloblastoma, epithelioid/rhabdoid glioblastoma, metastasis (melanoma, carcinoma)
  - Cribriform neuroepithelial tumor: Rare, nonrhabdoid intracranial tumor that also demonstrates INI1 protein loss but with a relatively favorable prognosis

Malignant Rhabdoid Tumors

- Renal
  - Most frequent organ affected outside of the CNS
  - Germline *INI1* mutations in almost all bilateral cases
  - Sheets of rhabdoid cells with extensive infiltration of renal parenchyma
  - Brisk mitotic activity, necrosis, vascular invasion, and extrarenal extension are common
  - Gene expression studies suggest origin from early progenitors with repression of neural development
  - Differential diagnosis includes renal medullary carcinoma, cellular mesoblastic nephroma, and clear cell sarcoma of kidney
- Extrarenal
  - May occur in deep soft tissue, skin, and viscera
  - Differential diagnosis includes melanoma, proximal variant of epithelioid sarcoma, rhabdomyosarcoma, extraskeletal myxoid chondrosarcoma, soft tissue myoepithelioma, and carcinoma

Schwannoma

- Germline mutations in *SMARCB1* are also responsible for a subset of patients with schwannomatosis
  - Mainly multiple schwannomas but also meningiomas in rare occasions
  - "Mosaic" pattern of INI1 protein loss by immunohistochemistry in syndrome-associated schwannomas suggests a milder phenotype compared to rhabdoid tumors
  - Mutations more likely to be nontruncating (e.g., splice site)
- Rare families characterized by both rhabdoid tumors and schwannomatosis in different family members

Others

- Choroid plexus carcinomas and medulloblastomas have been reported in the setting of rhabdoid predisposition syndrome, but morphologic and immunophenotypic features overlap with AT/RT
- Loss of SMARCB1 protein expression also described in epithelioid sarcoma, renal medullary carcinoma, pediatric sarcomas, hepatoblastomas, epithelioid malignant peripheral nerve sheath tumor (MPNST), and soft tissue myoepithelioma

CANCER RISK MANAGEMENT

Established Guidelines for Tumor Screening in Affected Families

- Routine imaging (CNS MR, renal ultrasound) and feasible screening approaches in the 1st few years of life for mutation carriers

SELECTED REFERENCES

1. Plotkin SR et al: Update from the 2011 International Schwannomatosis Workshop: From genetics to diagnostic criteria. Am J Med Genet A. 161(3):405-16, 2013
2. Schiffman JD et al: Update on pediatric cancer predisposition syndromes. Pediatr Blood Cancer. 60(8):1247-52, 2013
3. Lee RS et al: A remarkably simple genome underlies highly malignant pediatric rhabdoid cancers. J Clin Invest. 122(8):2983-8, 2012
4. Bourdeaut F et al: Frequent hSNF5/INI1 germline mutations in patients with rhabdoid tumor. Clin Cancer Res. 17(1):31-8, 2011
5. Eaton KW et al: Spectrum of SMARCB1/INI1 mutations in familial and sporadic rhabdoid tumors. Pediatr Blood Cancer. 56(1):7-15, 2011
6. Hasselblatt M et al: Nonsense mutation and inactivation of SMARCA4 (BRG1) in an atypical teratoid/rhabdoid tumor showing retained SMARCB1 (INI1) expression. Am J Surg Pathol. 35(6):933-5, 2011
7. Gadd S et al: Rhabdoid tumor: gene expression clues to pathogenesis and potential therapeutic targets. Lab Invest. 90(5):724-38, 2010
8. Schneppenheim R et al: Germline nonsense mutation and somatic inactivation of SMARCA4/BRG1 in a family with rhabdoid tumor predisposition syndrome. Am J Hum Genet. 86(2):279-84, 2010
9. Hasselblatt M et al: Cribriform neuroepithelial tumor (CRINET): a nonrhabdoid ventricular tumor with INI1 loss and relatively favorable prognosis. J Neuropathol Exp Neurol. 68(12):1249-55, 2009
10. Swensen JJ et al: Familial occurrence of schwannomas and malignant rhabdoid tumour associated with a duplication in SMARCB1. J Med Genet. 46(1):68-72, 2009
11. Ammerlaan AC et al: Long-term survival and transmission of INI1-mutation via nonpenetrant males in a family with rhabdoid tumour predisposition syndrome. Br J Cancer. 98(2):474-9, 2008
12. Hulsebos TJ et al: Germline mutation of INI1/SMARCB1 in familial schwannomatosis. Am J Hum Genet. 80(4):805-10, 2007
13. Judkins AR, et al. Atypical teratoid/rhabdoid tumour. In Louis DN, et al: WHO Classification of Tumours of the Central Nervous System. IARC Press. 147-149, 2007
14. Taylor MD et al: Familial posterior fossa brain tumors of infancy secondary to germline mutation of the hSNF5 gene. Am J Hum Genet. 66(4):1403-6, 2000

RHABDOID PREDISPOSITION SYNDROME

Diagrammatic and Microscopic Features

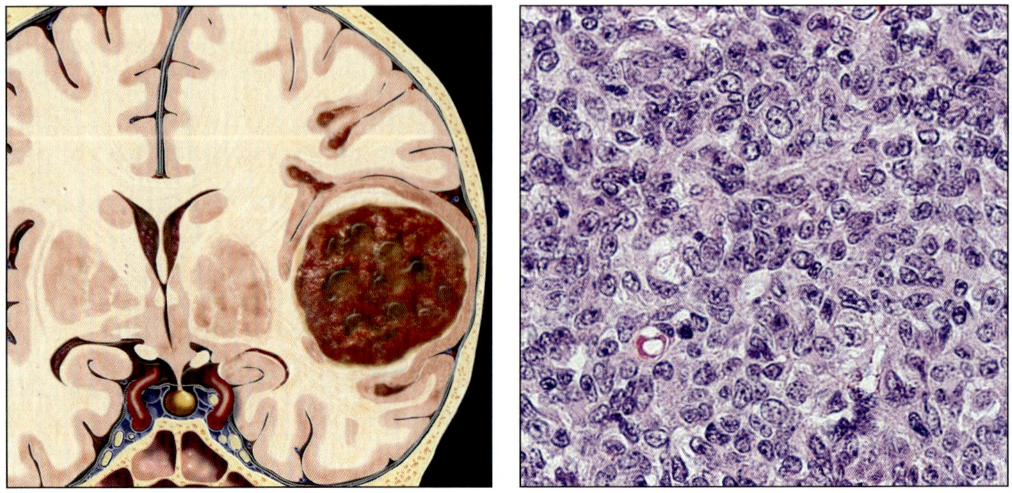

(Left) *Atypical teratoid/rhabdoid tumors (AT/RT) form variably sized masses that may appear well circumscribed. Multiple foci of necrosis are not uncommon in these high-grade, extremely aggressive pediatric tumors. Despite their genetic predisposition being ascribed to the posterior fossa in early reports, they occur throughout the neural axis, including the supratentorial compartment.* ***(Right)*** *AT/RT architecture is variable and may demonstrate sheet-like arrangements of rhabdoid cells.*

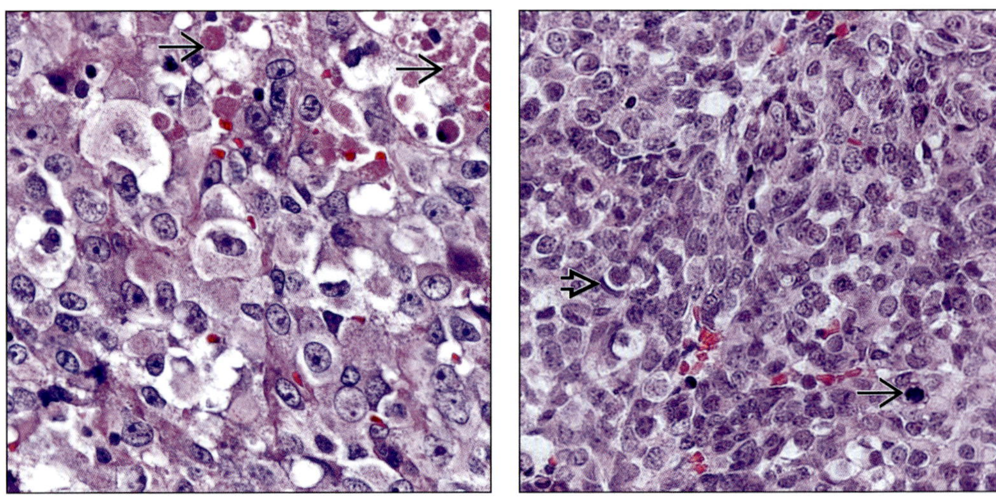

(Left) *Rhabdoid tumors in all sites contain variable numbers of large eosinophilic cells with eccentric nuclei and macronucleoli. Cell borders are usually distinct. Single cell necrosis may be a feature →.* ***(Right)*** *Mitotic activity is usually not subtle in AT/RT →. These tumors are characterized by high proliferative rates and are among the most aggressive human malignancies. Cell to cell wrapping ⇨ raises the differential with anaplastic medulloblastoma in the CNS.*

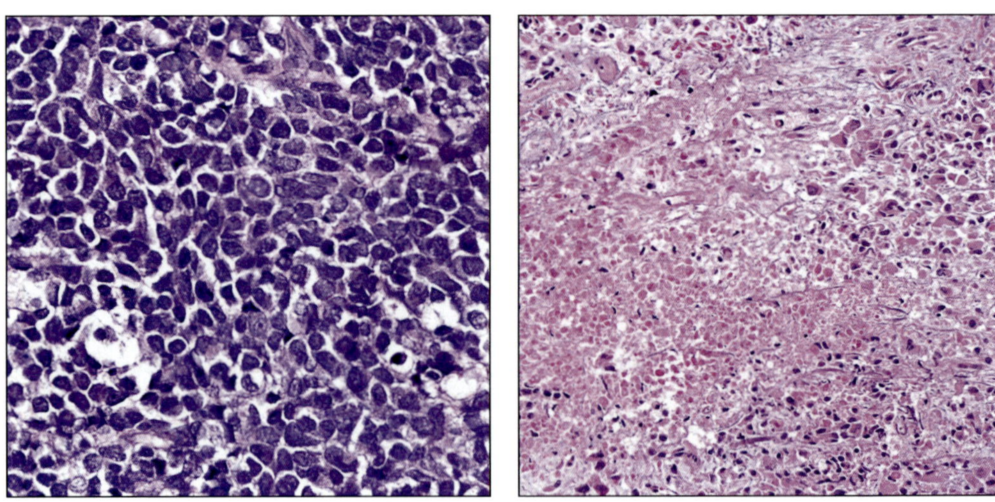

(Left) *Rhabdoid tumors may contain poorly differentiated areas of closely packed cells with high nuclear:cytoplasmic ratios lacking overt rhabdoid cytologic features, particularly when involving the CNS. A high index of suspicion is required when encountering a primitive neoplasm in a very young child. Careful search for rare rhabdoid cells and immunostaining documenting INI1 loss is helpful in the diagnosis.* ***(Right)*** *Necrosis is almost always present in rhabdoid tumors.*

Ancillary Techniques

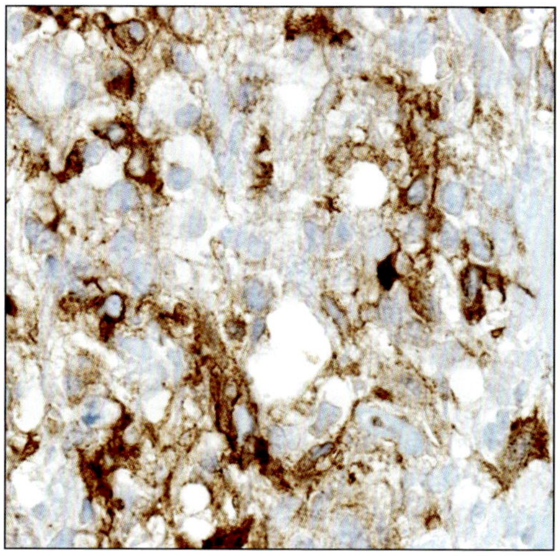
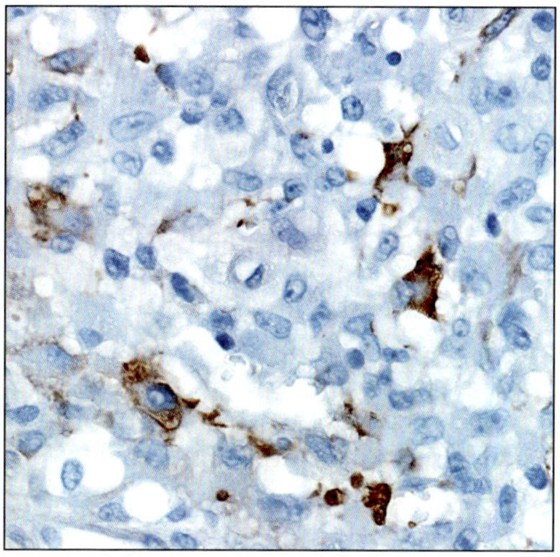

(Left) *Rhabdoid tumors typically label with numerous immunohistochemical markers. Epithelial membrane antigen (EMA) is 1 of the most frequently expressed antigens in such tumors.* ***(Right)*** *Smooth muscle actin expression occurs in a subset of cases of AT/RT and other rhabdoid tumors, although with less frequency than EMA.*

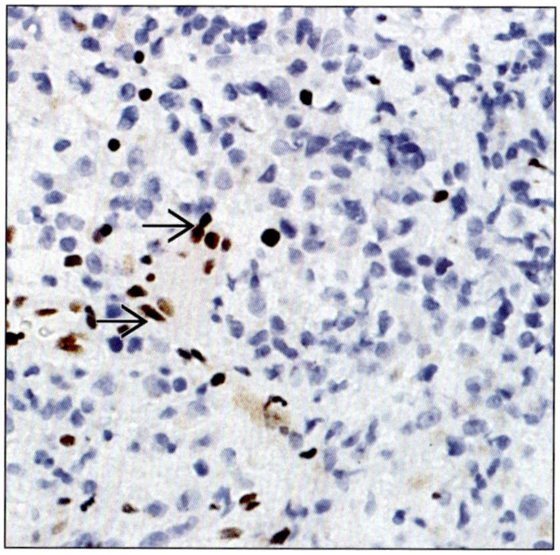
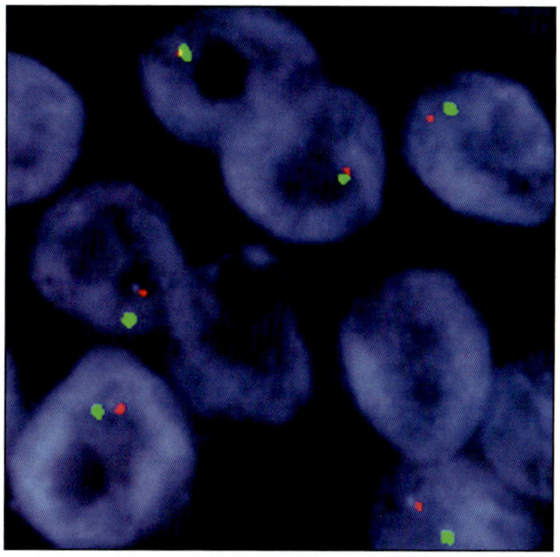

(Left) *One of the most diagnostically useful immunohistochemical findings in malignant rhabdoid tumors is the loss of INI1 expression in neoplastic cells. Preservation of reactivity in nonneoplastic elements, including stromal and endothelial cells ⇒, is essential for interpretation.* ***(Right)*** *Whole chr 22 loss/22q deletion features a variety of neoplasms, particularly rhabdoid tumors (BCR = green, NF2 = red). (Courtesy A. Perry, MD.)*

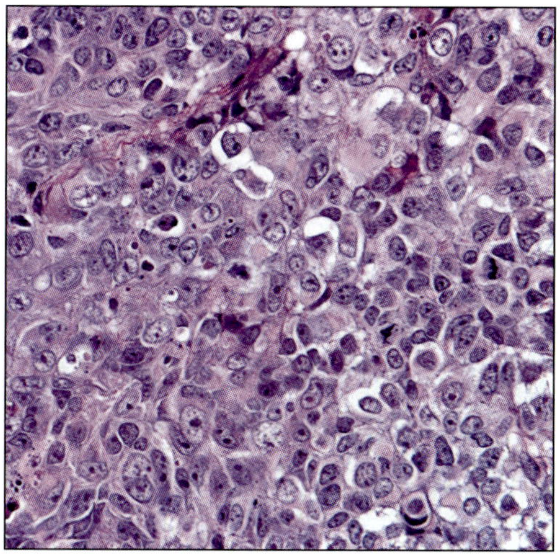
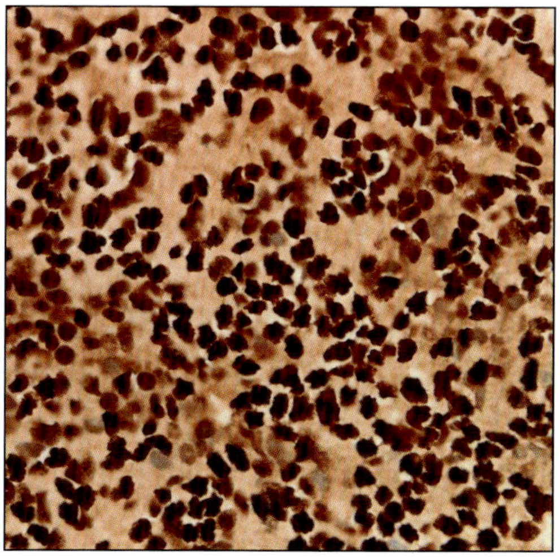

(Left) *Rarely, AT/RT may lack INI1 mutations and instead have mutations in associated proteins such as SMARCA4. As this example demonstrates, histologic and other immunophenotypic findings are identical to INI1 mutant tumors. (Courtesy C. Giannini, MD.)* ***(Right)*** *Retained INI1 (SMARCB1) in an AT/RT containing SMARCA4 mutation, although this tumor demonstrated classic histologic and immunohistochemical features of AT/RT. (Courtesy C. Giannini, MD.)*

SCHWANNOMATOSIS

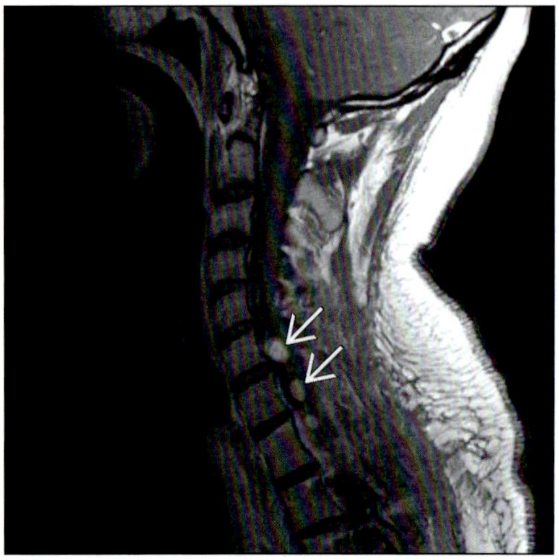

Multiple schwannomas are the hallmark of schwannomatosis ➡. The spinal nerves are frequently involved in these patients. (Courtesy J. Blakeley, MD.)

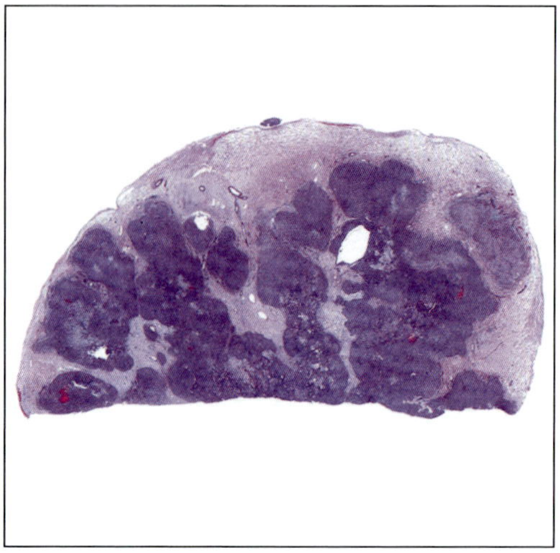

Many schwannomas in patients with schwannomatosis have features similar to sporadic tumors, including circumscription and a biphasic architecture of Antoni A and Antoni B areas.

EPIDEMIOLOGY

Incidence

- Affects ~ 1 in 40,000 individuals (similar incidence as neurofibromatosis type 2 [NF2])
- Similar incidence in males and females

ETIOLOGY/PATHOGENESIS

Inheritance Pattern

- 75-85% sporadic, 15-25% inherited

Germline Mutations in *SMARCB1* Tumor Suppressor Gene

- 40-50% of familial cases
- 8-10% of sporadic cases
- 4-hit hypothesis: (1) germline *SMARCB1* mutation → loss of Chr 22 with remaining (2) *SMARCB1* allele and (3) *NF2* gene → loss of remaining (4) *NF2* allele

CLINICAL IMPLICATIONS

Clinical Presentation

- Onset is usually in 2nd and 3rd decades
  - Wide range of ages at initial presentation (children < 10 years through senior patients)
- Multiple schwannomas, usually sparing vestibular nerve
  - Restricted to 1 anatomical region in 1/3 of patients
  - Unilateral vestibular schwannomas may occur at a low frequency and do not exclude the diagnosis
- Chronic pain is most common symptom, often debilitating
  - No clear relationship to tumor size, location, or burden
- Mood disorders, including depression and anxiety, are frequent
- Lack of family history in a majority of patients
- Meningiomas occur at a low frequency in schwannomatosis patients (~ 5%)
  - Rare families with schwannomatosis, multiple meningiomas, and germline *SMARCB1* mutation
  - Preferential location in falx cerebri
  - Usually solitary rather than multiple in schwannomatosis in contrast to NF2
- Ependymoma not a feature
- Ophthalmologic manifestations not present at a higher frequency in schwannomatosis (in contrast to NF2)

Imaging Findings

- Peripheral schwannoma location (89%)
  - Arms and legs most common
- Spinal schwannomas (74%)
- Intracranial schwannoma (nonvestibular) (9%)

Diagnostic Criteria

- Several clinical criteria proposed to distinguish schwannomatosis from NF2
  - Lack of bilateral vestibular schwannoma; lack of NF2 in 1st-degree relative; lack of germline *NF2* mutation
- Recent proposals incorporate molecular testing

Proposed Criteria for Schwannomatosis (2011 International Schwannomatosis Workshop)

- **Molecular diagnosis**
  - Schwannomas or meningiomas (≥ 2 pathologically proven) **and**
  - ≥ 2 tumors with chromosome 22 loss of heterozygosity + 2 different *NF2* mutations **or** schwannoma or meningioma + germline *SMARCB1* mutation
- **Clinical diagnosis**

- ≥ 2 schwannomas (not intradermal), 1 pathologically confirmed; no vestibular schwannomas on high-quality MR study **or**
- Schwannoma, pathologically confirmed, or intracranial meningioma and 1st-degree relative with schwannomatosis
- **Possible schwannomatosis**
  - ≥ 2 nonintradermal schwannomas **without** pathologic confirmation
- **Excludes schwannomatosis**
  - Patient with diagnostic criteria for NF2, germline *NF2* mutation, 1st-degree relative with NF2, or multiple schwannomas in a prior irradiated field only

MICROSCOPIC FINDINGS

Schwannomas

- Histologic features similar to sporadic tumors
  - Compact Antoni A areas alternating with loose Antoni B areas, Verocay bodies, hyalinized vessels, and well-formed capsule
- Myxoid changes ("myxoid schwannoma"), intraneural growth, and peritumoral edema overrepresented in schwannomatosis-associated cases
- Nerve edema
- Rare schwannoma variants reported in schwannomatosis patients include plexiform, cellular, and neuroblastoma-like
- S100 and collagen IV (pericellular) positive by immunohistochemistry; EMA(-)
- Mosaic pattern of INI1 immunostaining (i.e., loss in a subset of neoplastic cells) in most schwannomatosis-associated schwannomas

Neurofibromas

- Neurofibromas, in addition to schwannomas, are a recognized feature of neurofibromatosis type 2
- Not usually a feature of schwannomatosis patients but previously reported in at least 2 patients

Hybrid Tumors

- Tumors with hybrid neurofibroma/schwannoma features overrepresented in syndrome-associated peripheral nerve tumors, particularly in schwannomatosis
- Neurofilament (+) axons in neurofibroma-like component in 1/2 of cases
- GLUT1/EMA (+) perineurial-like cells in neurofibroma-like areas
- CD34(+) in Antoni B and neurofibroma-like areas, negative in Antoni A areas

GENETICS AND MOLECULAR BIOLOGY

SMARCB1 Function

- Tumor suppressor gene
- Other synonyms include *INI1*, *BAF47*, *hSNF5*
- Encodes for a component of the SWI/SNF protein complex
  - Chromatin-remodeling complex, ATP dependent
  - Interacts with HIV-1 integrase

Germline Mutations in *SMARCB1*

- Nontruncating, missense, or splice site in familial schwannomatosis (unlike atypical teratoid rhabdoid tumor)
- Mutations usually located at ends of *SMARCB1*
- Inherited in an autosomal dominant fashion, incomplete penetrance

SELECTED REFERENCES

1. Plotkin SR et al: Update from the 2011 International Schwannomatosis Workshop: From genetics to diagnostic criteria. Am J Med Genet A. 161(3):405-16, 2013
2. Carter JM et al: Epithelioid malignant peripheral nerve sheath tumor arising in a schwannoma, in a patient with "neuroblastoma-like" schwannomatosis and a novel germline SMARCB1 mutation. Am J Surg Pathol. 36(1):154-60, 2012
3. Harder A et al: Hybrid neurofibroma/schwannoma is overrepresented among schwannomatosis and neurofibromatosis patients. Am J Surg Pathol. 36(5):702-9, 2012
4. Merker VL et al: Clinical features of schwannomatosis: a retrospective analysis of 87 patients. Oncologist. 17(10):1317-22, 2012
5. Smith MJ et al: Frequency of SMARCB1 mutations in familial and sporadic schwannomatosis. Neurogenetics. 13(2):141-5, 2012
6. Smith MJ et al: Vestibular schwannomas occur in schwannomatosis and should not be considered an exclusion criterion for clinical diagnosis. Am J Med Genet A. 158A(1):215-9, 2012
7. Rodriguez FJ et al: Superficial neurofibromas in the setting of schwannomatosis: nosologic implications. Acta Neuropathol. 121(5):663-8, 2011
8. Boyd C et al: Alterations in the SMARCB1 (INI1) tumor suppressor gene in familial schwannomatosis. Clin Genet. 74(4):358-66, 2008
9. Patil S et al: Immunohistochemical analysis supports a role for INI1/SMARCB1 in hereditary forms of schwannomas, but not in solitary, sporadic schwannomas. Brain Pathol. 18(4):517-9, 2008
10. Sestini R et al: Evidence of a four-hit mechanism involving SMARCB1 and NF2 in schwannomatosis-associated schwannomas. Hum Mutat. 29(2):227-31, 2008
11. Baser ME et al: Increasing the specificity of diagnostic criteria for schwannomatosis. Neurology. 66(5):730-2, 2006
12. MacCollin M et al: Diagnostic criteria for schwannomatosis. Neurology. 64(11):1838-45, 2005

Microscopic Features

*(**Left**) Classic schwannoma features that may be present in tumors from patients with schwannomatosis include a circumscribed architecture, a collagenous capsule of variable thickness →, and microcysts ⇨. (**Right**) Syndrome-associated and sporadic schwannomas are characterized by the presence of compact areas rich in neoplastic Schwann cells, (Antoni A areas) →, alternating with loose, macrophage-rich regions (Antoni B areas). Microcysts may be frequent ⇨.*

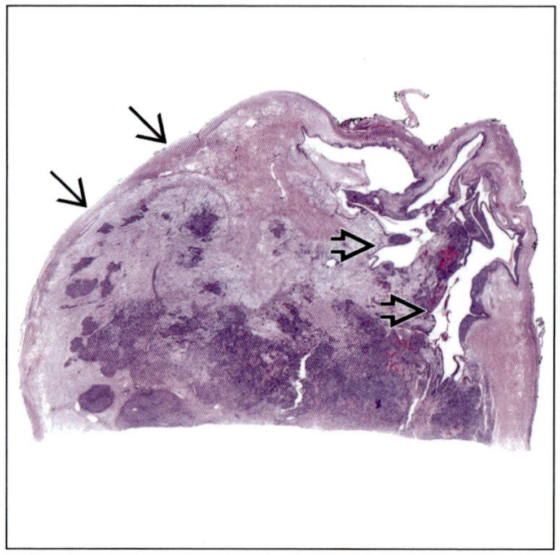

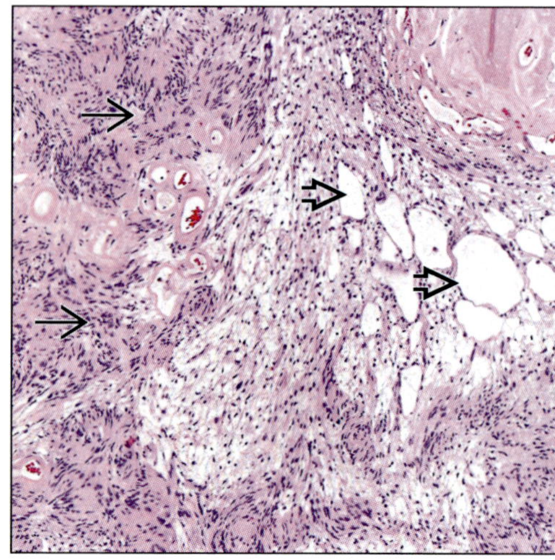

*(**Left**) One of the diagnostic hallmarks of schwannoma is the Verocay body →. This anuclear, process-rich, elongated structure is bordered by palisades of neoplastic Schwann cells. (**Right**) Antoni B areas in schwannomas are characterized by a loose stroma containing lipidized cells as well as macrophages. Delicate wisps of bland spindle cells are variably present →, suggesting the schwannian nature of the neoplasm.*

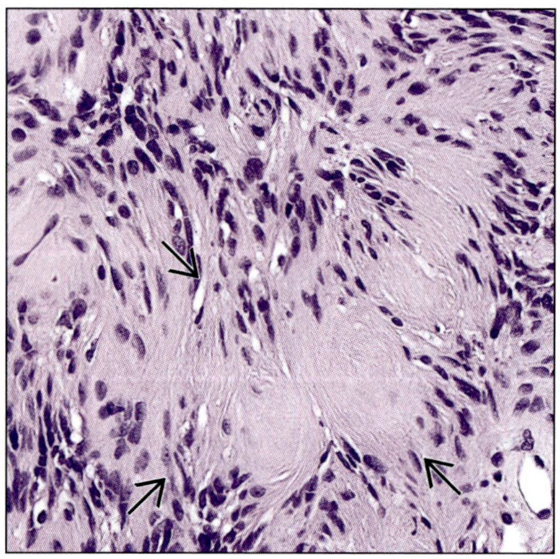

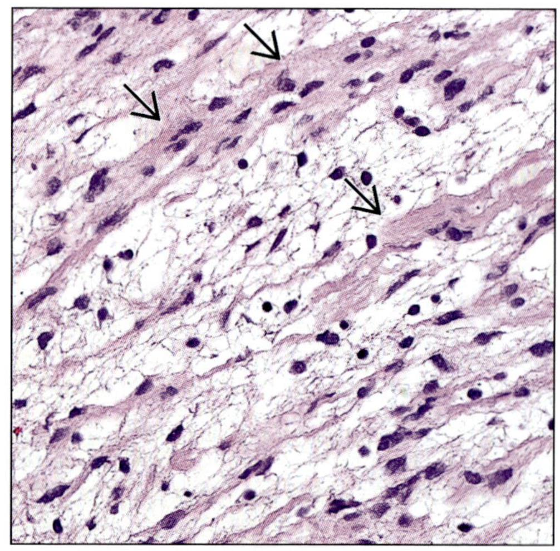

*(**Left**) A collagenous capsule is typical of most schwannomas →, including schwannomatosis-associated cases. However, capsule thickness is variable and may be altogether absent in areas. (**Right**) Cellular pleomorphism is a well-recognized feature of schwannomas → and has no prognostic significance. Classically termed "ancient change," it likely represents a degenerative phenomenon. Proliferative rates in these areas are typically low, compatible with a benign nature.*

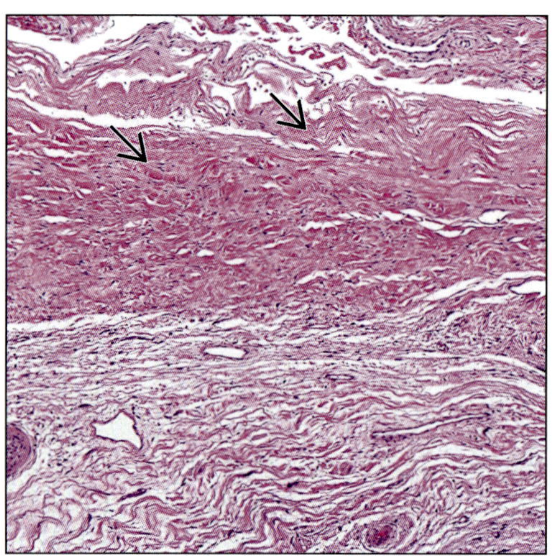

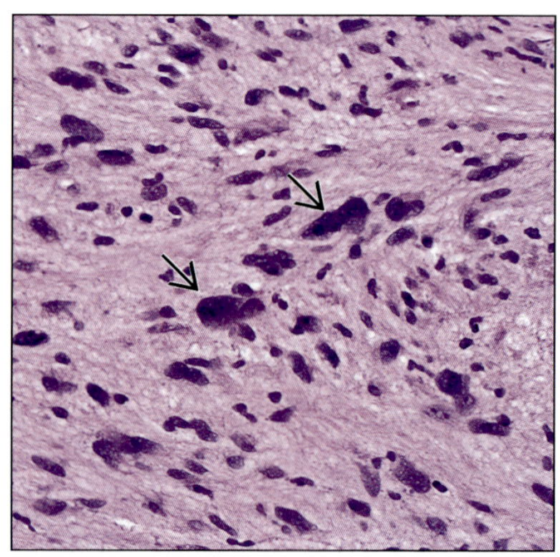

Microscopic Features

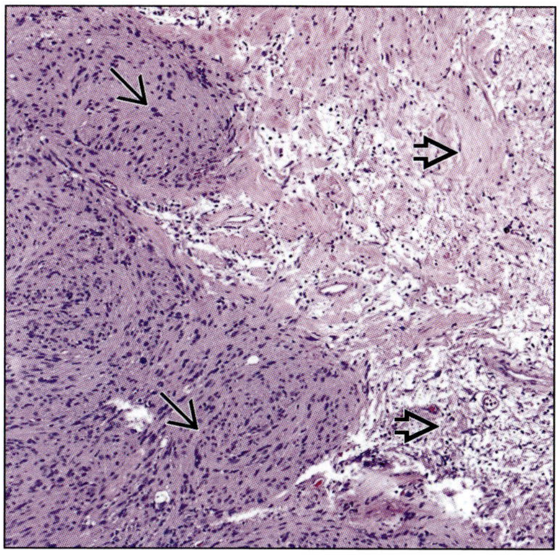

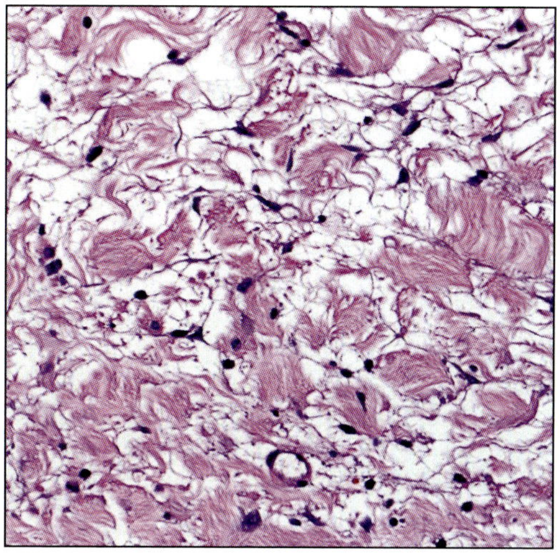

*(**Left**) Many schwannomas in schwannomatosis patients contain classic features. However, the presence of benign nerve sheath tumors with mixed features, including compact Antoni A areas typical of schwannoma → and juxtaposed to neurofibroma-like areas ⇨, occur at a relatively higher frequency in syndrome-associated tumors. (**Right**) Neurofibroma-like area in a schwannomatosis-associated benign nerve sheath tumor contains wavy nuclei in a loose stroma with associated collagen.*

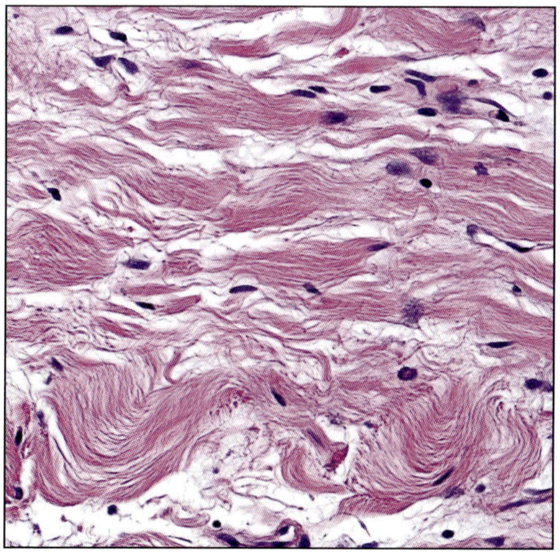

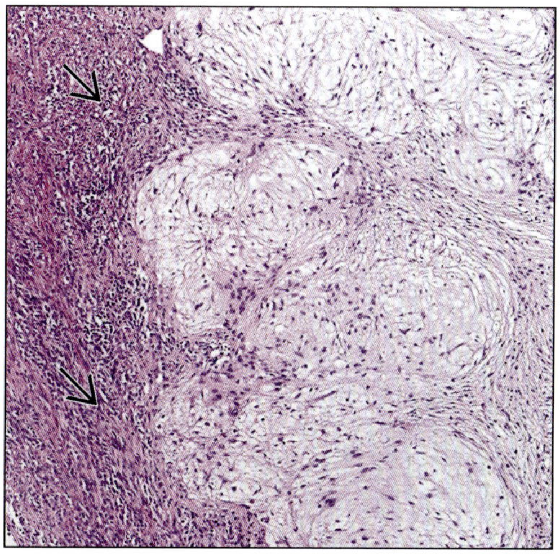

*(**Left**) The presence of delicate collagen in a loose stroma imparts a neurofibroma-like appearance to this difficult-to-classify benign nerve sheath tumor. Classic schwannoma regions were also present, which justifies its interpretation as a hybrid tumor. (**Right**) Conspicuous myxoid change (i.e., myxoid schwannoma) is seen at an increased frequency in schwannomatosis-associated tumors. Compact, Antoni A areas → may represent a minor component of these tumors.*

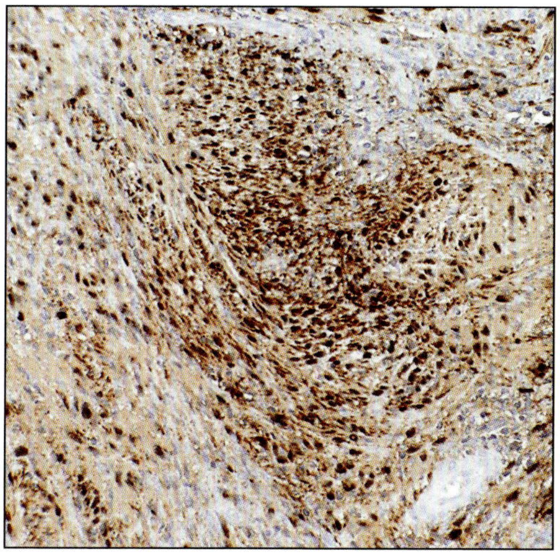

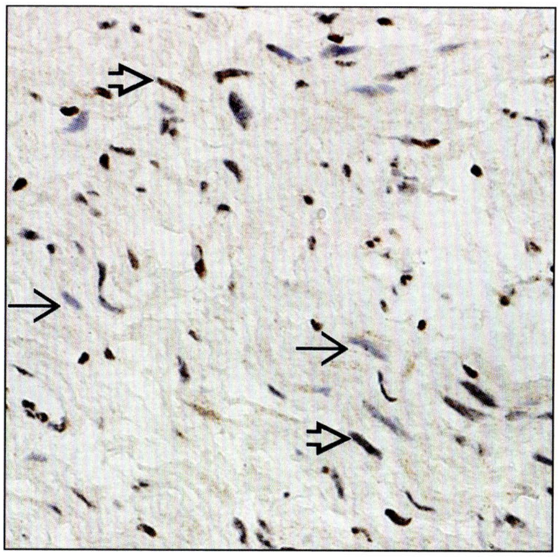

*(**Left**) The immunohistochemical hallmark of schwannoma is the expression of S100 protein in a diffuse and strong pattern. (**Right**) A mosaic pattern of INI1 immunostaining is found in most syndrome-associated schwannomas, including in schwannomatosis. Immunonegative cells → alternate with immunopositive cells ⇨. This finding suggests that INI1 protein loss is partial in these tumors, compared with the uniform INI1 loss present in rhabdoid tumors.*

TUBEROUS SCLEROSIS COMPLEX

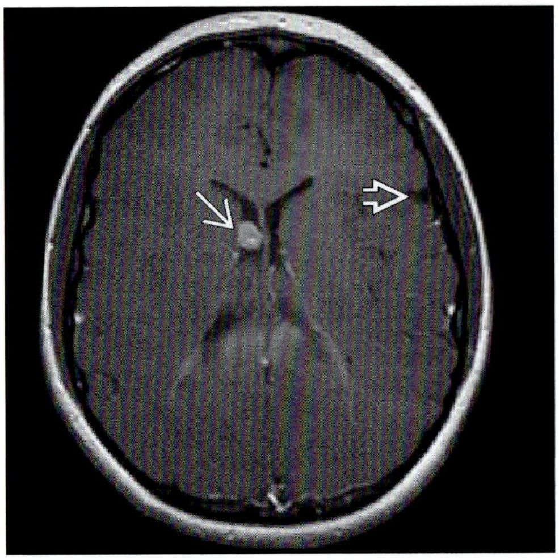

Subependymal giant cell astrocytomas (SEGAs) are characteristic of TSC, characterized by contrast-enhancing intraventricular masses ➡ near the foramen of Monro. A subtle cortical tuber ⇨ is also present.

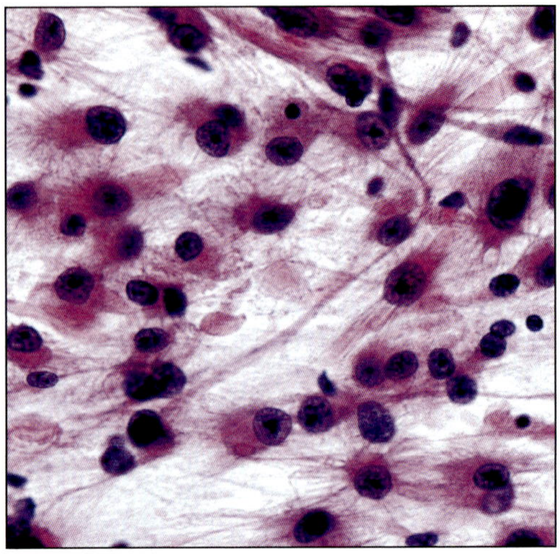

SEGAs are characterized by eosinophilic, large cells with prominent nucleoli, features particularly recognizable in smear preparations. Variable cytoplasmic processes are also present.

TERMINOLOGY

Abbreviations

- Tuberous sclerosis complex (TSC)

Definitions

- Inherited tumor predisposition syndrome resulting from mutations in *TSC1* or *TSC2* genes leading to mTOR pathway activation

EPIDEMIOLOGY

Incidence

- ~ 1:5,000-10,000
  - 2nd most common hereditary tumor syndrome involving the CNS

GENETICS

Germline Mutations in *TSC1* or *TSC2*

- Encode for tumor suppressor part of protein complex that inhibits RHEB and regulates mTOR activation
  - *TSC1* located in chromosome region 9q34 (encodes for hamartin)
  - *TSC2* located in chromosome region 16p13.3 (encodes for tuberin)
  - RHEB is a small GTPase/homolog of *RAS* and is kept in an inactive state by *TSC1*/*TSC2* complex
- mTOR is a key downstream mediator of PI3K/AKT activation
- Protein mTOR exists as part of 2 different multiprotein complexes
  - mTORC1 contains PRAS40, RAPTOR, and mLST8/GBL
    - Increases protein translation, cell growth, and survival
  - mTORC2 contains RICTOR, mSIN1, PROTOR, and mLST8
    - Functional role less understood than mTORC1 complex
    - Regulates metabolism and survival through activation of AKT
    - Plays a role in cytoskeletal organization
  - Activation leads to increased protein translation
  - Effective pharmacologic inhibition by rapamycin and analogs
- Majority of patients (70-80%) have new "spontaneous" mutations and lack a family history
  - *TSC1* and *TSC2* mutation frequency similar in familial cases
  - Mutations in *TSC2* more frequent than *TSC1* in nonfamilial cases

CLINICAL IMPLICATIONS AND ANCILLARY TESTS

Diagnostic Criteria

- Definite TSC: 2 major features or 1 major + 2 minor
- Probable TSC: 1 major + 1 minor
- Possible TSC: 1 major or > 1 minor
- **Major features**: Cortical tuber, subependymal nodule, subependymal giant cell astrocytoma (SEGA), facial angiofibroma/forehead plaque, ungual/periungual fibroma, > 3 hypomelanotic macules, Shagreen patch, multiple retinal hamartomas, cardiac rhabdomyoma, renal angiomyolipoma/lymphangioleiomyomatosis (LAM)
- **Minor features**: White matter migration lines, transmantle cortical dysplasia, retinal patch, hamartomatous rectal polyps, gingival fibroma, dental pits, hypomelanotic clustered skin lesions, bone cysts, renal cysts, nonrenal hamartomas

TUBEROUS SCLEROSIS COMPLEX

NONNEOPLASTIC MANIFESTATIONS

Skin

- Hypomelanotic macules ("ash leaf spot")
- Shagreen patch

Nervous System

- Epilepsy and mental retardation
- Cortical tubers
  - Localized cortical areas with abnormal development
    - Abnormal lamination, dysmorphic neurons, microcalcifications
  - Giant/balloon cells: Pale cytoplasm, variably immunoreactive with glial (S100, GFAP) and neuronal markers (synaptophysin, neurofilament)
- Cortical cytoarchitectural abnormalities may also be present outside tubers
- Subependymal nodules ("candle guttering lesions")
  - Giant cells arranged in clusters and fascicles with mixed glial/neuronal phenotype

Retinal Hamartoma/Astrocytoma

- Small lesions involving nerve fiber layer of retina in ~ 50% of TSC patients
- Larger lesions may grow and cause retinal detachment
- Histologically similar to SEGA

Renal Cysts

- Usually asymptomatic
- *TSC2/PKD1* contiguous gene syndrome: Coexisting TSC and autosomal dominant polycystic kidney disease (severe)

Micronodular Pneumocyte Hyperplasia

- Small nodules of bland type II pneumocytes

ASSOCIATED NEOPLASMS

Cutaneous Angiofibroma

- Previously known by misnomer "adenoma sebaceum"
- Dermal sclerosis
- Dilatation/proliferation of small vessels
- Stellate fibroblasts/multinucleated cells

Subependymal Giant Cell Astrocytoma

- Slow growth
- WHO grade I
- Mitotic activity rare to absent
- Microcalcifications in a subset, necrosis rare
- Pseudorosettes may be present and simulate ependymal neoplasms
- Composed of large cells with eosinophilic cytoplasm and macronucleoli
- Evidence of glial and neuronal differentiation by immunohistochemistry and electron microscopy
  - Consistent S100 expression, GFAP variable
  - Variable expression of synaptophysin, chromogranin, and neurofilament protein
- Excellent response to mTOR inhibitors in clinical trials

Angiomyolipoma

- Usually benign, but large tumors associated with risk for life-threatening bleeding
- Most common cause of mortality in TSC adult patients
- May be classic or epithelioid subtype
- May be a cause of LAM
- Partial response to mTOR inhibitors in some studies

Lymphangioleiomyomatosis

- Occurs in 30% of women with tuberous sclerosis
- Progressive pulmonary disorder involving lung
- Cystic changes, respiratory failure
- Lung biopsies demonstrate smooth muscle cells involving lymphatics, vessels, airways, and alveolar septa
- SMA(+), HMB-45(+)
- Majority of cases associated with tuberous sclerosis have *TSC2* mutations (rather than *TSC1*) and loss of heterozygosity
- Loss of heterozygosity in *TSC2* also frequent in sporadic LAM

Cardiac Rhabdomyoma

- ~ 50% of patients with TSC
- Most frequent initial imaging finding in TSC patients
- May cause cardiac arrhythmias but also may regress with age

Pancreatic Neuroendocrine Tumor

- Not part of diagnostic criteria, but recognized in rare TSC patients

SELECTED REFERENCES

1. Kocabaş A et al: Cardiac rhabdomyomas associated with tuberous sclerosis complex in 11 children: presentation to outcome. Pediatr Hematol Oncol. 30(2):71-9, 2013
2. Krueger DA et al: Everolimus long-term safety and efficacy in subependymal giant cell astrocytoma. Neurology. 80(6):574-80, 2013
3. Arva NC et al: Well-differentiated pancreatic neuroendocrine carcinoma in tuberous sclerosis--case report and review of the literature. Am J Surg Pathol. 36(1):149-53, 2012
4. Budde K et al: Tuberous sclerosis complex-associated angiomyolipomas: focus on mTOR inhibition. Am J Kidney Dis. 59(2):276-83, 2012
5. Henske EP et al: Lymphangioleiomyomatosis - a wolf in sheep's clothing. J Clin Invest. 122(11):3807-16, 2012
6. Marcotte L et al: Cytoarchitectural alterations are widespread in cerebral cortex in tuberous sclerosis complex. Acta Neuropathol. 123(5):685-93, 2012
7. Yates JR et al: The Tuberous Sclerosis 2000 Study: presentation, initial assessments and implications for diagnosis and management. Arch Dis Child. 96(11):1020-5, 2011
8. Kacerovska D et al: TSC2/PKD1 contiguous gene syndrome: a report of 2 cases with emphasis on dermatopathologic findings. Am J Dermatopathol. 31(6):532-41, 2009
9. Shields JA et al: Aggressive retinal astrocytomas in 4 patients with tuberous sclerosis complex. Arch Ophthalmol. 123(6):856-63, 2005
10. Lopes MB et al: Immunohistochemical characterization of subependymal giant cell astrocytomas. Acta Neuropathol. 91(4):368-75, 1996

TUBEROUS SCLEROSIS COMPLEX

Microscopic Features

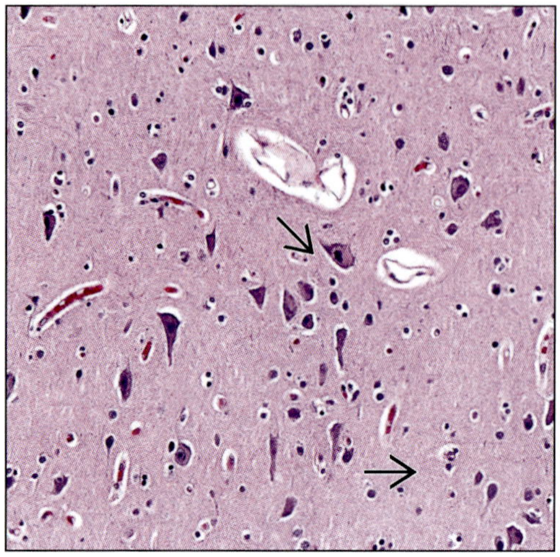

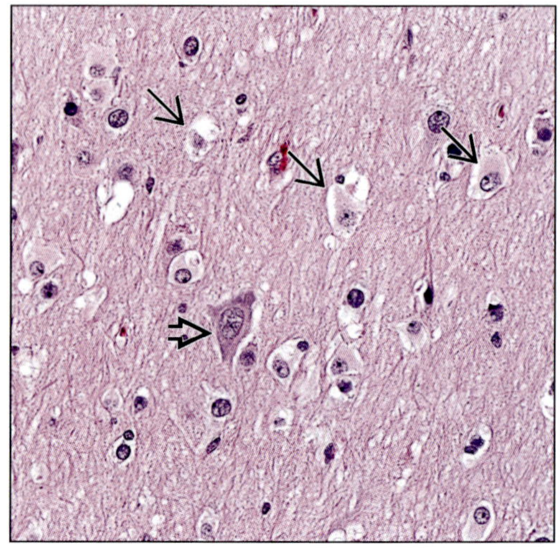

(Left) *Numerous cortical abnormalities characterize the tuberous sclerosis complex. In this example, cortical disarray → is present in a cortical tuber.* ***(Right)*** *Numerous abnormal pale cells are evident in this field →. They have an ambiguous phenotype. A distinct cortical neuron is also present in this field, which serves as a good comparison ⇨.*

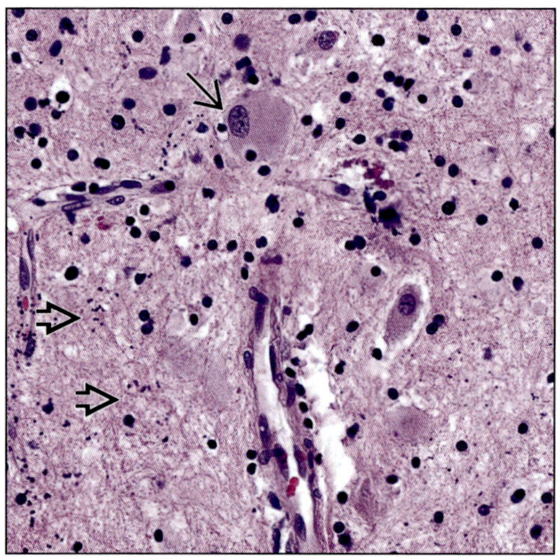

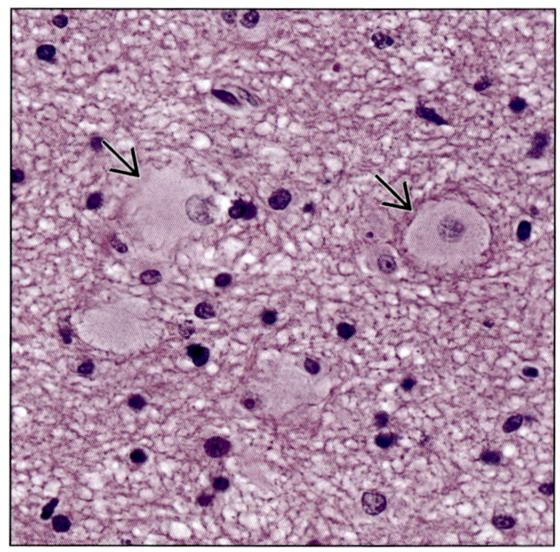

(Left) *Large, pale balloon cells → are typical of cortical tubers associated with tuberous sclerosis and are present in variable numbers. Fine, particulate calcifications are also present in this example ⇨.* ***(Right)*** *Cortical tubers are distinctive lesions associated with tuberous sclerosis complex containing enlarged pale cells (giant/balloon cells) → with an ambiguous, variable phenotype along glial and neuronal lines.*

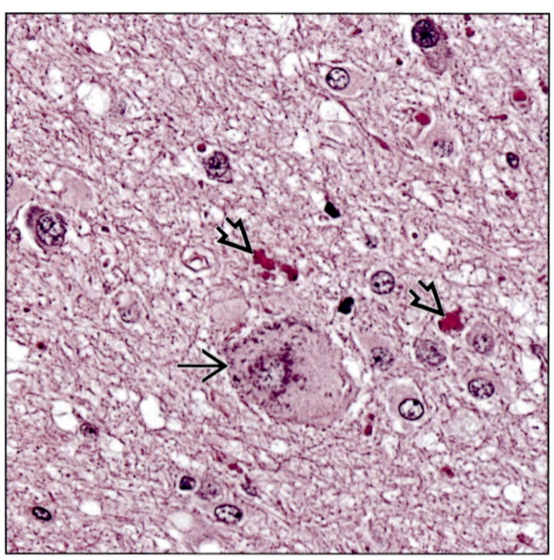

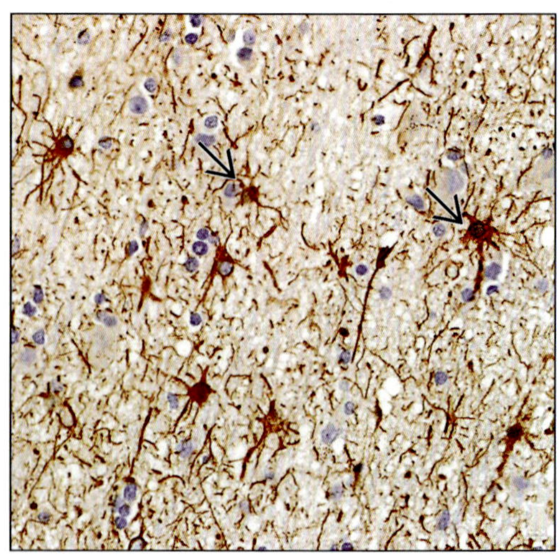

(Left) *Dysplastic neurons are also frequent in tubers →. In this example, there is abnormal pallor and uneven distribution of Nissl substance. Prominent gliosis, including Rosenthal fibers, was also present ⇨.* ***(Right)*** *In addition to abnormal neurons and pale cells, tubers are characterized by frequent gliosis. An immunohistochemical stain for GFAP is useful in highlighting reactive astrocytes and their characteristic stellate cytoplasmic processes →.*

Diagrammatic and Microscopic Features

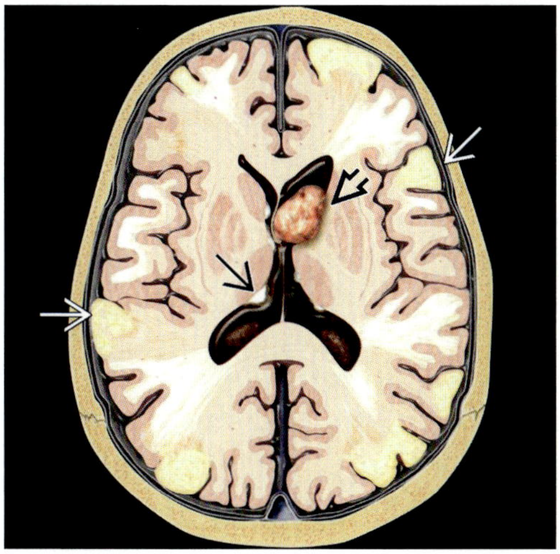

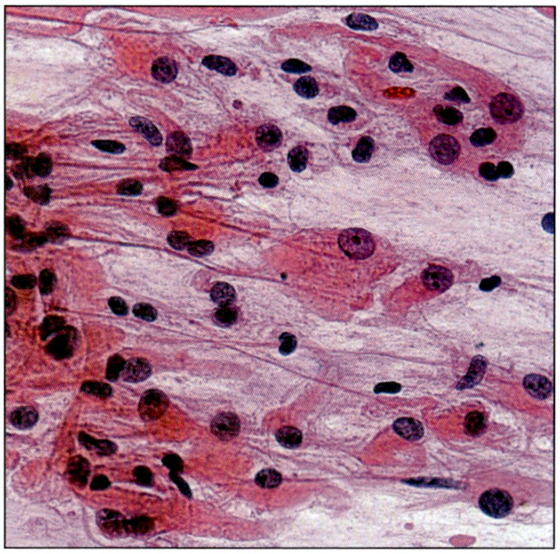

(Left) *The characteristic lesions of tuberous sclerosis in the CNS include cortical tubers →, subependymal nodules identifiable in the walls of the lateral ventricles →, and the low-grade neoplasm known as subependymal giant cell astrocytoma →.* ***(Right)*** *SEGAs may be identified on smear preparations during intraoperative evaluations. They are characterized by large eosinophilic cells with round/oval nuclei and macronucleoli.*

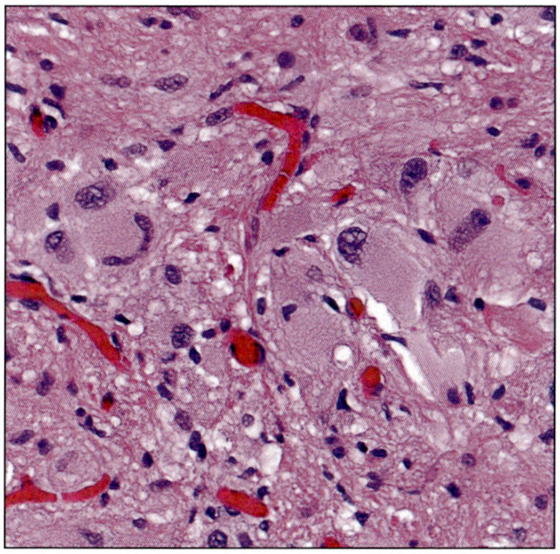

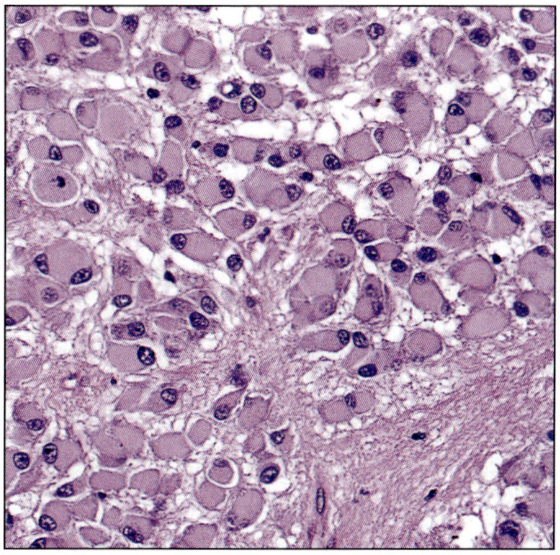

(Left) *The large cells of subependymal giant cell astrocytoma may contain voluminous eosinophilic cytoplasm with a "glassy" quality. Mitotic activity in these tumors is rare to absent, in keeping with their low-grade nature.* ***(Right)*** *Aggregates of eosinophilic cells in a fibrillar stroma characterize this SEGA.*

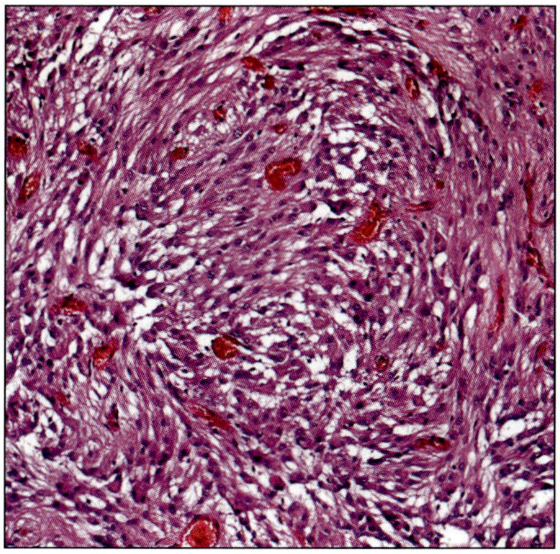

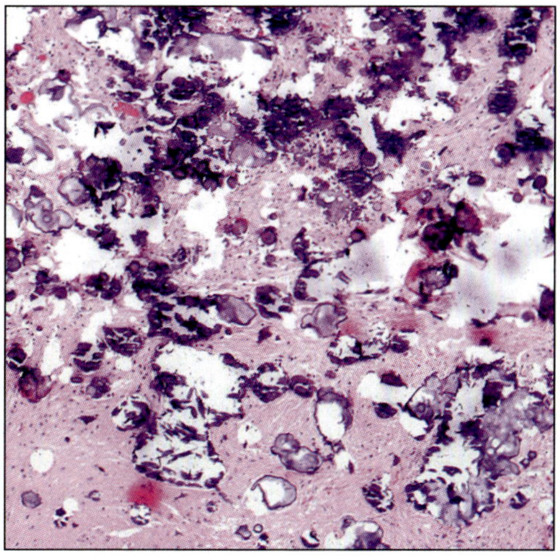

(Left) *Not infrequently, subependymal giant cell astrocytomas may contain fields of spindle cells arranged in loose fascicles. Whorling may be present in low-power magnification.* ***(Right)*** *Coarse calcifications may be a feature of some subependymal giant cell astrocytomas, as in other CNS lesions associated with tuberous sclerosis.*

Ancillary Techniques

(Left) *A glial phenotype was ascribed early on to subependymal giant cell astrocytoma, which is reflected in its name. The most consistent glial marker in these tumors is S100, which typically demonstrates diffuse staining. However, this marker is not entirely specific for glial differentiation.* ***(Right)*** *GFAP, a more specific marker of glial differentiation, is usually positive in subependymal giant cell astrocytoma, although it is more variable in frequency and intensity.*

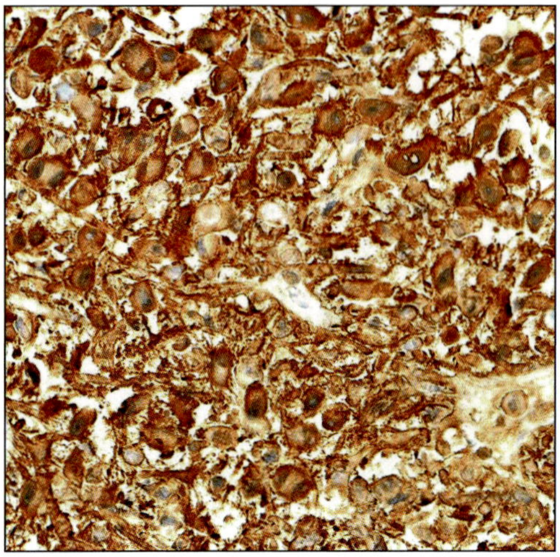
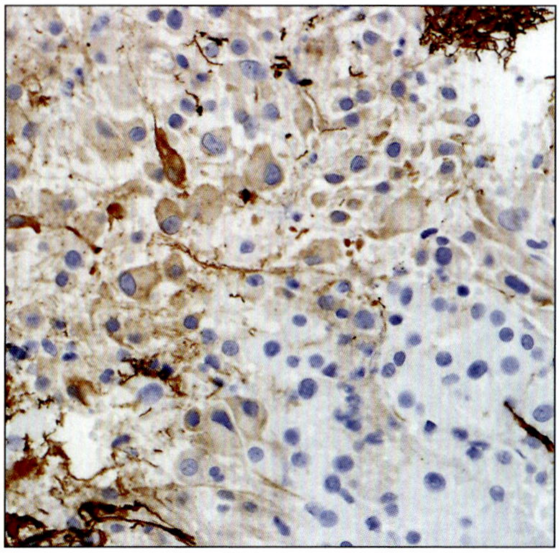

(Left) *In addition to glial markers, subependymal giant cell astrocytoma also labels with markers of neuronal differentiation, such as synaptophysin. Therefore, these tumors demonstrate differentiation along glial and neuronal lines.* ***(Right)*** *Subependymal giant cell astrocytomas usually have very low proliferative rates. In this example, the Ki-67 proliferation index is < 1%.*

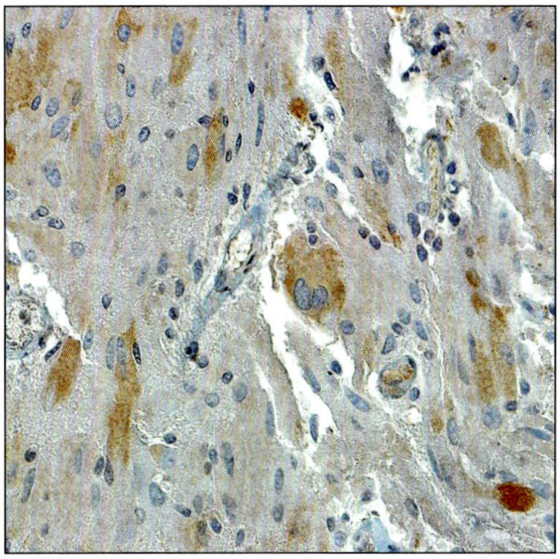
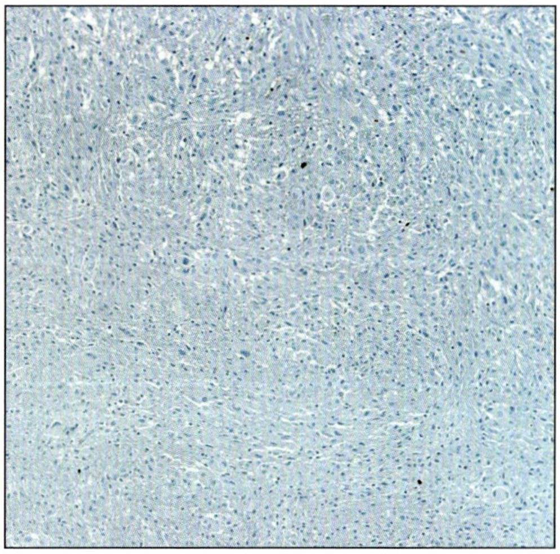

(Left) *Subependymal giant cell astrocytoma is a tumor of the nervous system that is characterized by varying numbers of mast cells* ⇒*. Other tumors with increased number of mast cells include hemangioblastoma and neurofibroma.* ***(Right)*** *Mast cells may be identified by expression of KIT on immunohistochemical preparations* ⇒*.*

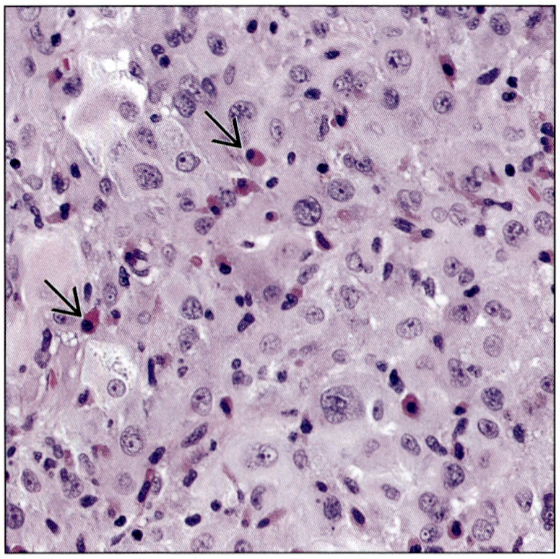
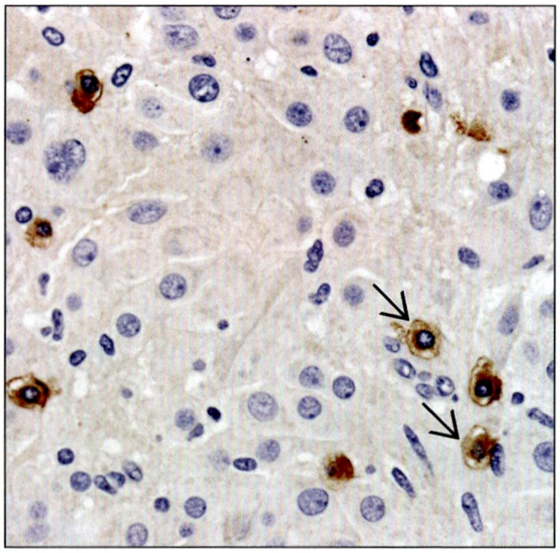

Microscopic and Imaging Features

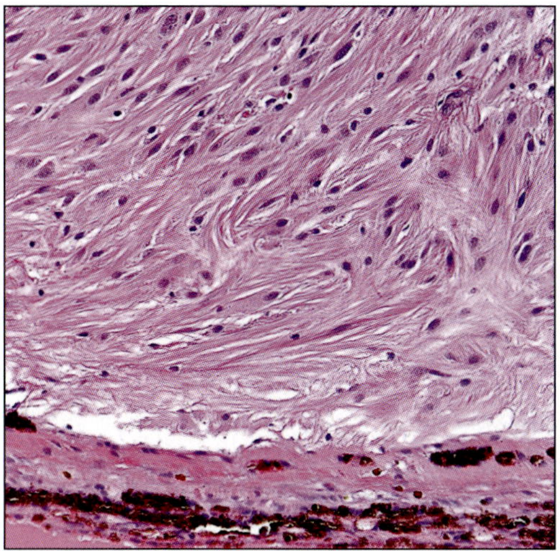
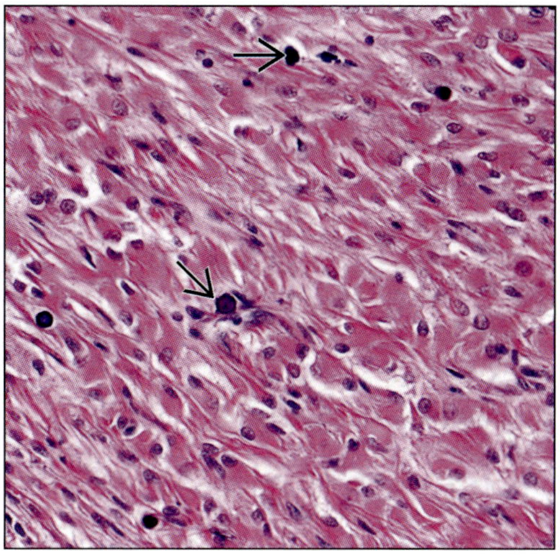

(Left) *Astrocytic hamartomas represent the typical intraocular manifestation in tuberous sclerosis patients. They are characterized by slow growth and bland spindle cell cytology. They are frequently multiple in TSC.* ***(Right)*** *Histologic similarities with subependymal nodules/ SEGA are a feature of retinal astrocytic lesions in tuberous sclerosis patients. Scattered microcalcifications ⇒ were present in this example.*

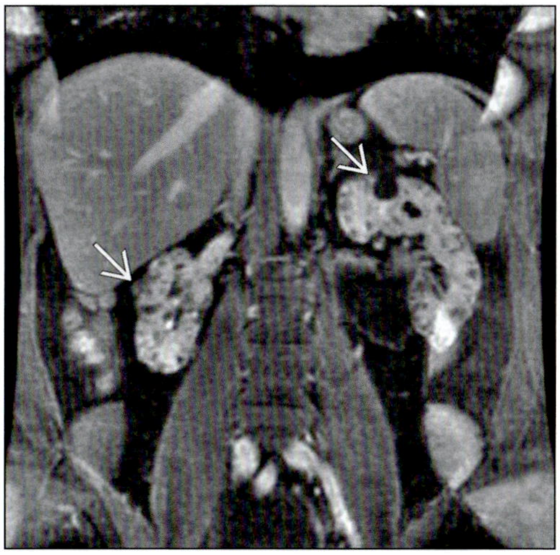
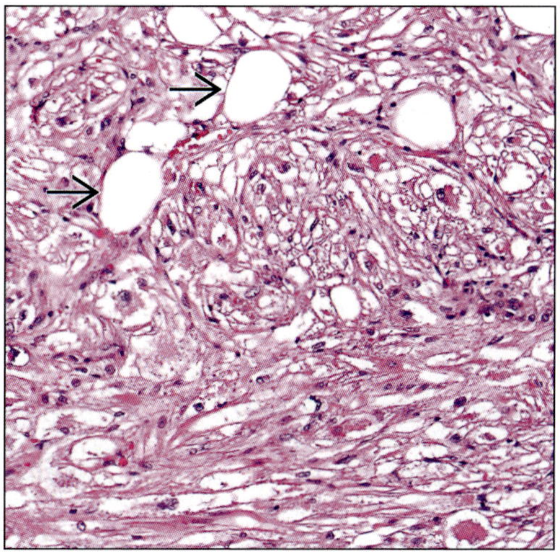

(Left) *Renal manifestations are also typical of tuberous sclerosis complex, including numerous cysts as well as bilateral neoplasms ➡ that, in this case, were interpreted radiologically as probable angiomyolipomas.* ***(Right)*** *The prototypical neoplasm involving the kidney in tuberous sclerosis patients is angiomyolipoma, which contains spindle/eosinophilic cells as well as variable amounts of adipose tissue ⇒.*

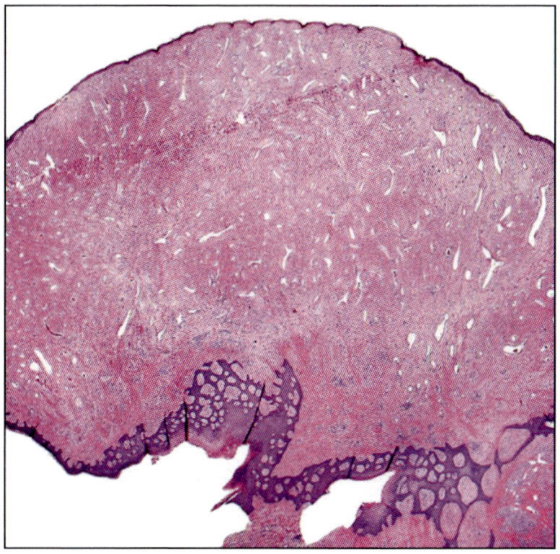
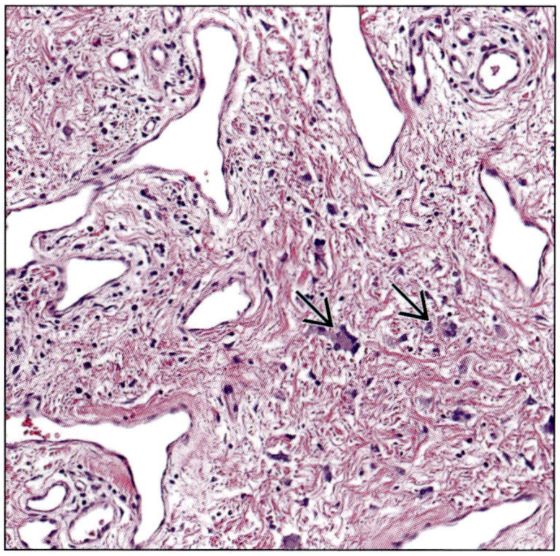

(Left) *Tuberous sclerosis patients also frequently develop cutaneous angiofibromas. As the name implies, these benign growths contain variable amounts of small vessels and collagen deposition.* ***(Right)*** *Numerous thin-walled vessels are evident in cutaneous angiofibromas. Multinucleated stromal cells ⇒ are also frequent and, despite their pleomorphic nature, should not be a cause for alarm in these benign tumors.*

VON HIPPEL-LINDAU SYNDROME

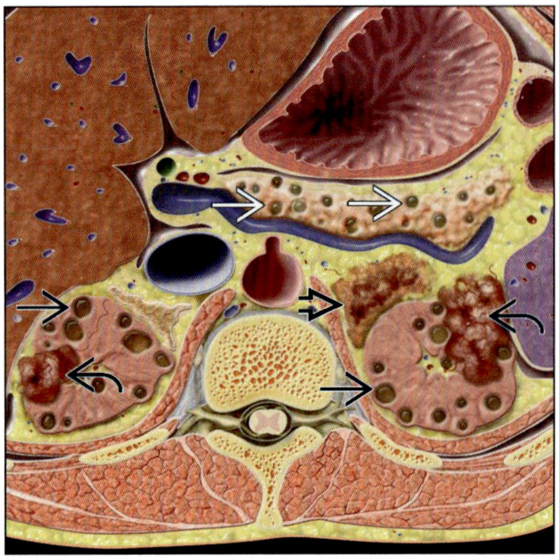

Abdominal lesions in von Hippel-Lindau (VHL) syndrome are varied and include bilateral renal cysts ➙, renal tumors, particularly renal cell carcinoma (RCC) ➙, pancreatic cysts ➙, and pheochromocytoma ➙.

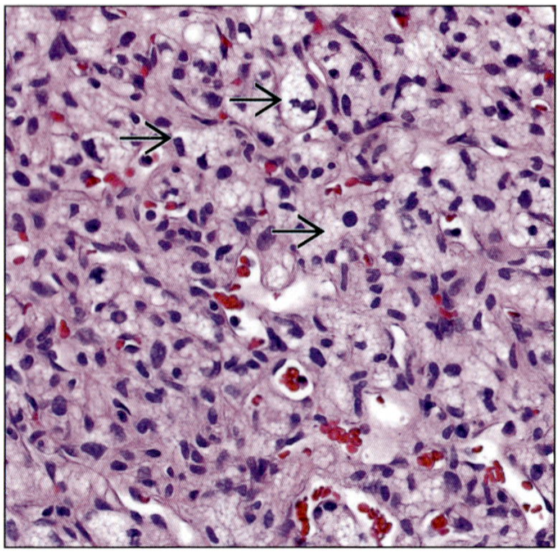

The characteristic neoplasm involving the CNS and retina in patients with VHL syndrome is hemangioblastoma, a vascularized tumor containing vacuolated stromal cells ➙.

TERMINOLOGY

Abbreviations

- von Hippel-Lindau (VHL) syndrome

Synonyms

- von Hippel-Lindau disease
- Familial cerebelloretinal angiomatosis

Definitions

- Rare autosomal dominant genetic disease resulting from mutation in *VHL* tumor suppressor gene on chromosome 3p25.3
- Characterized by retinal and CNS hemangioblastomas, pheochromocytomas, pancreatic serous cystadenoma, café au lait spots, and renal cell carcinoma
  - If no family history, diagnosis requires 2 cardinal manifestations
    - Including retinal and CNS involvement
    - Excluding cysts
  - With positive family history
    - 1 cardinal manifestation, excluding cysts
- Member of phacomatosis familial cancer syndromes

EPIDEMIOLOGY

Incidence

- 1 case per 36,000 newborns
- 6,000-7,000 patients in United States

Age

- Age at diagnosis varies from infancy to 60-70 years

Gender

- No predilection is noted

GENETICS AND MOLECULAR BIOLOGY

Tumorigenesis

- *VHL* gene encodes VHL protein, which is an E3 ubiquitin ligase
  - Major regulator of hypoxic response by targeting transcription factor hypoxia inducible factor (HIF) for degradation
- VHL disease demonstrates marked phenotypic variability and age-dependent penetrance
  - Genotype-phenotype associations in VHL disease form basis of clinical classification
- Presumed that clinical presentation reflects quantitative or qualitative altered VHL protein function

Molecular Genetics

- Autosomal dominant
- Germline mutation of *VHL* gene (3p25.3)
  - *VHL* mutation in 50% of sporadic renal cell carcinoma (RCC)
  - 2nd inactivating event predisposes to neoplasms
- VHL protein
  - Promotes destruction of hypoxia inducible factor 1 α (HIF-1-α) via ubiquitin pathway
    - Loss of function leads to increased levels of vascular endothelial growth factor (VEGF)
  - HIF-independent regulation of primary cilium and apoptosis via NF-κB pathway
    - Loss of function promotes renal cysts

Subtypes

- Classification
  - Type 1: Caused by deletions or truncation mutations of VHL gene
  - Types 2A, B, C: Caused by missense point mutations
- Genotype-phenotype correlations
  - Type 1 *VHL* (truncating and exon deletions)

- Low risk of pheochromocytoma
  - Type 2 VHL (missense mutations)
    - High risk of pheochromocytoma
    - Type 2A: Low risk of RCC
    - Type 2B: High risk of RCC
    - Type 2C: Familial pheochromocytoma without hemangioblastoma or RCC

CLINICAL IMPLICATIONS AND ANCILLARY TESTS

Surgical Approaches

- Nephron-sparing surgery
- Tumor resection when other organs affected
- Surgery for > 3 cm endocrine pancreatic tumor
- Adrenalectomy for pheochromocytoma

Prognosis

- Death due to renal cell carcinoma in 50%
  - Metastases to liver, lung, and bone
- Pheochromocytoma is cured after surgery
  - Metastatic pheochromocytoma has not been reported

ASSOCIATED NEOPLASMS

Hemangioblastoma

- Most common lesion associated with VHL disease
- Clinical, radiologic, and pathologic features similar in sporadic and VHL-associated tumors
- Cerebellum and spinal cord tumors are major central nervous system manifestations
  - Affect 60-84% of patients
- Benign vascular tumor, but may cause significant morbidity due to neurological deficits
- Clinically, patient can present with headaches, numbness, dizziness, weakness, pain in arms and legs, incontinence, or ataxia
- Retinal hemangioblastomas are typical ocular lesions of VHL disease
  - Previously referred to as hemangiomas, but histologically identical to CNS counterparts
  - Usually multifocal and bilateral
  - Clinically, patients present with painless loss of visual acuity or visual field
  - In advanced cases, can present with hemorrhage, leading to secondary glaucoma and loss of vision
- Histologic features
  - Well-circumscribed tumors
  - Piloid gliosis with Rosenthal fibers is common in adjacent CNS parenchyma
  - Highly vascular with large and small thin-walled vessels
  - Absent to rare mitotic activity
  - Reticular type
    - Composed of small nests/sheets of vacuolated cells known as stromal or interstitial
    - Reticulin abundant and highlights small lobules and individual cells
  - Cellular type
    - Architecture characterized by larger lobules
    - Increased cytoplasm, vacuolation inconspicuous
    - Glioma-like areas expressing GFAP
    - Less reticulin
  - Nuclear pleomorphism may be present
  - Extramedullary hematopoiesis
  - Cystic changes and sclerosis variable
  - Metastatic renal cell carcinoma to hemangioblastoma very rare but reported
- Histochemistry and immunohistochemistry
  - Lipid in stromal cells may be highlighted by oil red O in frozen sections
  - Reticulin helpful in highlighting small lobules and individual cells in reticular type
  - Immunophenotype typically inhibin (+), NSE(+), GFAP(+/-)
  - EMA usually negative (very rarely positive), CD10(-), CK(-)
  - Low Ki-67 labeling index
- Molecular cytogenetics
  - Different cytogenetic profiles in reticular and cellular subtypes of hemangioblastoma by comparative genomic hybridization
    - Loss of chromosome 6 associated with cellular subtype
    - Loss of 19/19p more frequent in reticular variant

Renal Cell Carcinoma

- Patients with VHL disease are at high risk of developing multiple renal cysts and RCC, affecting 2/3 of VHL patients
- RCC is clear cell type, often multicentric &/or bilateral
- Histology
  - Sporadic and VHL-associated clear cell tumors are often indistinguishable
  - Tumors are usually surrounded by a thick fibrous capsule
  - Tumors in VHL patients are usually multicystic &/or solid
  - Typically VHL tumors have microcystic growth pattern
  - Composed of cells with cleared-out cytoplasm and small nuclei
  - Early lesion: Intratubular proliferation of clear cells

Pheochromocytoma

- Catecholamine-producing neuroendocrine tumor related to chromaffin cells that arise from adrenal medulla or extraadrenal chromaffin tissue (paraganglia)
- Pheochromocytoma associated with VHL is usually asymptomatic
- Hallmark of type 2 VHL disease
- Patients with VHL disease are often very young (< 40 years)
- Tumor is usually bilateral, multiple, or extraadrenal
  - Hypertension with headache and sweating is most common presentation
- Histology
  - VHL pheochromocytoma have distinct pathological features from multiple endocrine neoplasia type 2 (MEN2) pheochromocytomas

- Presence of thick fibrous capsule
- Myxoid and hyalinized stroma
- Small to medium-sized tumor cells
- Absence of cytoplasmic hyaline globules
- Lack of nuclear atypia
- Absence of adrenomedullary hyperplasia

Pancreatic Endocrine Tumor and Pancreatic Cysts

- Tumors present in 10% of VHL patients are usually multiple and well circumscribed
- Tumors in VHL patients are usually nonsecretory
- Endocrine pancreatic tumors are characterized by solid, trabecular, &/or glandular architecture
- Stomal collagen is usually present
- Most tumors have clear cells
- Marked nuclear atypia may be present
- Mitoses are rare

Other Associated Lesions

- Papillary cystadenoma of epididymis
- Endolymphatic sac tumor
- Papillary cystadenoma of broad ligament and mesosalpinx
- Cysts of pancreas, kidney, adrenal, testis, and ovary

DIFFERENTIAL DIAGNOSIS

Cystic Renal Diseases Associated With Renal Neoplasms

- Acquired cystic kidney disease
  - Cyst frequency proportional to duration of ESRD
  - Diverse array of RCCs
- Tuberous sclerosis complex/autosomal dominant polycystic kidney disease (ADPKD) contiguous gene syndrome
  - Diffusely cystic kidneys identical to ADPKD
  - Multiple and bilateral angiomyolipomas
  - Rarely, clear cell RCC
- Autosomal dominant polycystic kidney disease
  - Risk of RCC may be increased but controversial
  - Far more numerous cysts than in VHL

Tuberous Sclerosis Complex

- Angiomyolipomas common
- Renal cancer and renal cysts rare
- Rare pancreatic lesions
- Calcified cortical lesions (i.e., tubers), subependymal nodules, and subependymal giant cell astrocytoma

Neurofibromatosis Type 1

- May develop multiple pheochromocytomas, but CNS lesions are astrocytomas rather than hemangioblastomas

CANCER RISK MANAGEMENT

Early Diagnosis

- Improves prognosis of most VHL manifestations
  - Comprehensive screening program starting in childhood
  - Lifelong routine screening for hemangioblastomas (CNS and retinal), RCCs, and pheochromocytomas

SELECTED REFERENCES

1. Maher ER et al: von Hippel-Lindau disease: a clinical and scientific review. Eur J Hum Genet. 19(6):617-23, 2011
2. Padhi S et al: A 10-year retrospective study of hemangioblastomas of the central nervous system with reference to von Hippel-Lindau (VHL) disease. J Clin Neurosci. 18(7):939-44, 2011
3. Rechsteiner MP et al: VHL gene mutations and their effects on hypoxia inducible factor HIFÎ±: identification of potential driver and passenger mutations. Cancer Res. 71(16):5500-11, 2011
4. Rohan SM et al: Clear-cell papillary renal cell carcinoma: molecular and immunohistochemical analysis with emphasis on the von Hippel-Lindau gene and hypoxia-inducible factor pathway-related proteins. Mod Pathol. 24(9):1207-20, 2011
5. Traen S et al: Central nervous system lesions in Von Hippel-Lindau syndrome. JBR-BTR. 94(3):140-1, 2011
6. Zhang Y et al: Endocrine tumors as part of inherited tumor syndromes. Adv Anat Pathol. 18(3):206-18, 2011
7. Barontini M et al: VHL disease. Best Pract Res Clin Endocrinol Metab. 24(3):401-13, 2010
8. Ellison J: Novel human pathological mutations. Gene symbol: VHL. Disease: Von Hippel-Lindau syndrome. Hum Genet. 127(4):477, 2010
9. Kaelin WG Jr: New cancer targets emerging from studies of the Von Hippel-Lindau tumor suppressor protein. Ann N Y Acad Sci. 1210:1-7, 2010
10. Safo AO et al: Pancreatic manifestations of von Hippel-Lindau disease. Arch Pathol Lab Med. 134(7):1080-3, 2010
11. Tamura K et al: Diagnosis and management of pancreatic neuroendocrine tumor in von Hippel-Lindau disease. World J Gastroenterol. 16(36):4515-8, 2010
12. Wu D et al: Observer variation in the application of the Pheochromocytoma of the Adrenal Gland Scaled Score. Am J Surg Pathol. 33(4):599-608, 2009
13. Shehata BM et al: Von Hippel-Lindau (VHL) disease: an update on the clinico-pathologic and genetic aspects. Adv Anat Pathol. 15(3):165-71, 2008
14. Nakamura E et al: Clusterin is a secreted marker for a hypoxia-inducible factor-independent function of the von Hippel-Lindau tumor suppressor protein. Am J Pathol. 168(2):574-84, 2006
15. Rickert CH et al: Cellular and reticular variants of hemangioblastoma differ in their cytogenetic profiles. Hum Pathol. 37(11):1452-7, 2006
16. Hasselblatt M et al: Cellular and reticular variants of haemangioblastoma revisited: a clinicopathologic study of 88 cases. Neuropathol Appl Neurobiol. 31(6):618-22, 2005
17. Jung SM et al: Immunoreactivity of CD10 and inhibin alpha in differentiating hemangioblastoma of central nervous system from metastatic clear cell renal cell carcinoma. Mod Pathol. 18(6):788-94, 2005

Imaging and Gross Features

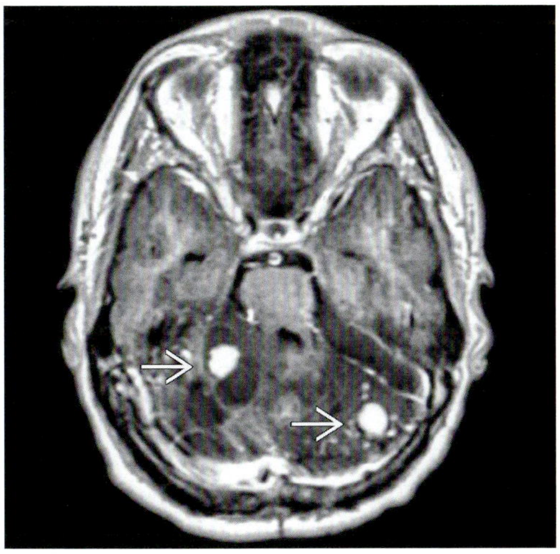

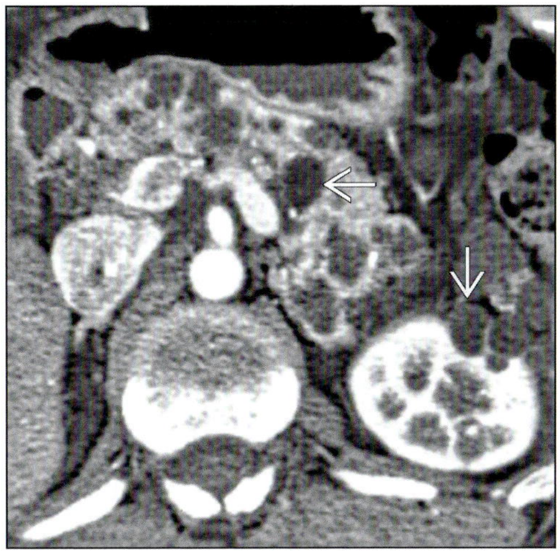

*(**Left**) Axial T1-weighted post-contrast MR shows 2 of several cerebellar hemangioblastomas →, a finding that is so characteristic as to be diagnostic of VHL syndrome by itself. The presence of multiple cysts and tumors in other organs is also characteristic of this disorder. (**Right**) Axial CT shows innumerable pancreatic and renal cysts →. Either the CNS or abdominal findings would be considered diagnostic of this disorder. A patient's family history is also useful for corroboration.*

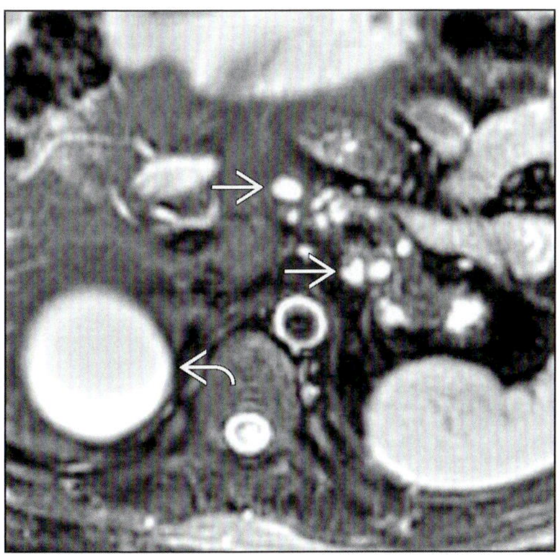

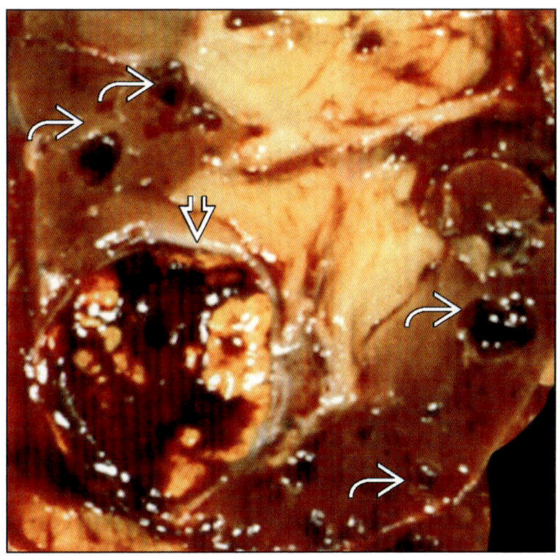

*(**Left**) Axial T2WI in a young man with multiorgan manifestations of VHL syndrome shows multiple pancreatic → and renal cysts →. (**Right**) Kidney from a patient with VHL disease shows multiple renal cysts → within the renal parenchyma. There is a yellow well-circumscribed RCC → with extensive hemorrhage.*

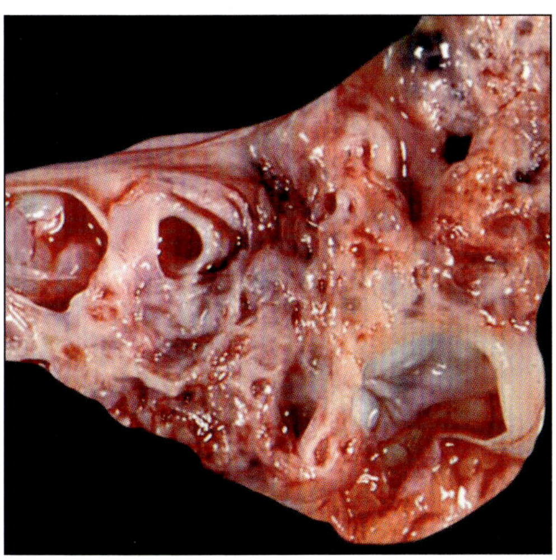

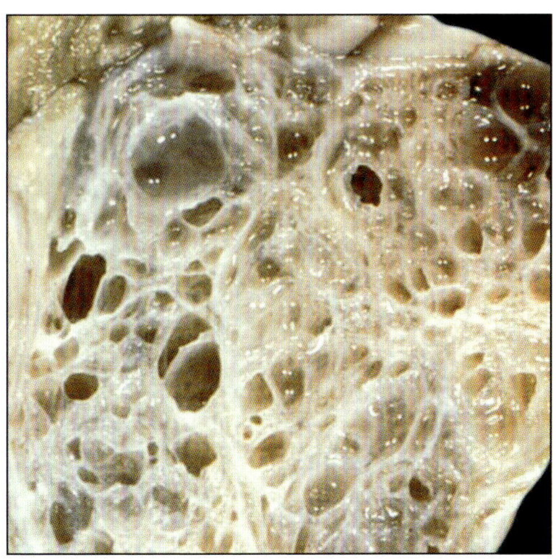

*(**Left**) This cut surface of a pancreas from a patient with VHL disease shows diffuse replacement of the normal architecture by variably sized cysts. The cysts are thin walled and have clear contents. (**Right**) Pancreas from a VHL syndrome patient shows a multicystic lesion with a cystadenoma. The cysts are derived from the pancreatic duct system, have a thin capsule, and are lined by a simple epithelium.*

Renal Cell Carcinoma

(Left) *This photomicrograph demonstrates an RCC in a patient with VHL syndrome with a predominantly solid component of the tumor. The tumor is composed of clear cells and is morphologically indistinguishable from sporadic RCC.* ***(Right)*** *RCC with a cystic component is usually present in patients with VHL syndrome. The tumor is predominantly cystic, and the cysts are lined by cells with clear cytoplasm and low-grade nuclei.*

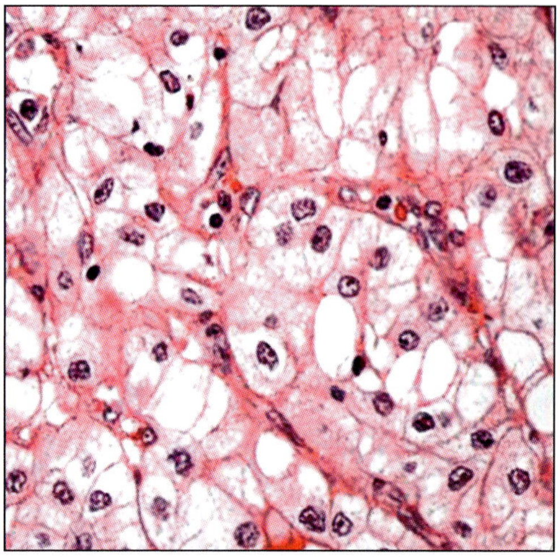

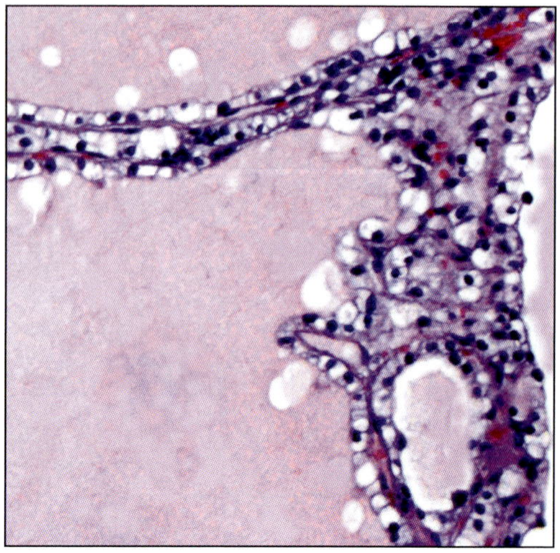

(Left) *The cyst lining from a renal cyst in a patient with VHL syndrome is composed of clear cells with ample cytoplasm and irregular grade 2 nuclei. The cyst is surrounded by a thick fibrous capsule.* ***(Right)*** *Most of the RCCs in VHL syndrome patients are solid and cystic. The solid component is composed of cells with similar appearance to the cells lining the cystic spaces.*

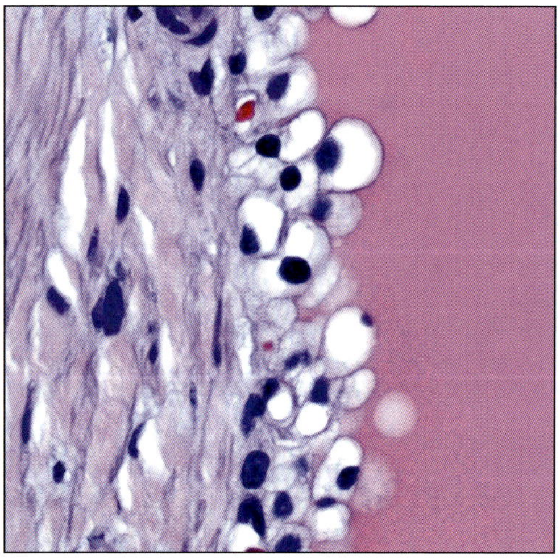

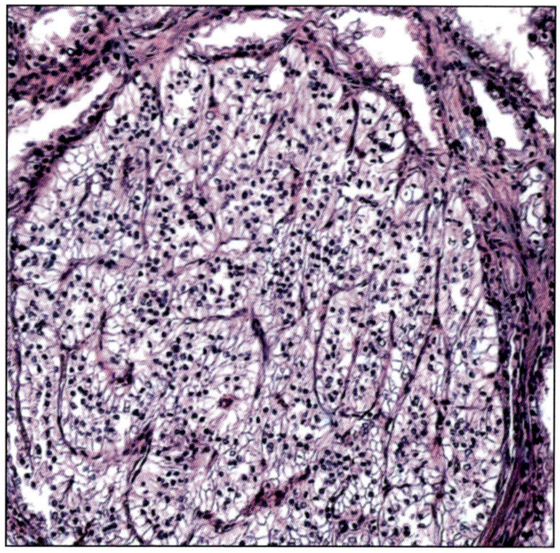

(Left) *RCC in a patient with VHL syndrome shows a solid component of the tumor. The tumor cells are arranged in cords or trabeculae and are separated by thin fibrovascular stroma. The tumor cells are round to oval with irregular nuclei.* ***(Right)*** *RCC in patients with VHL disease shows decreased clusterin staining in comparison with RCC in non-VHL disease patients.*

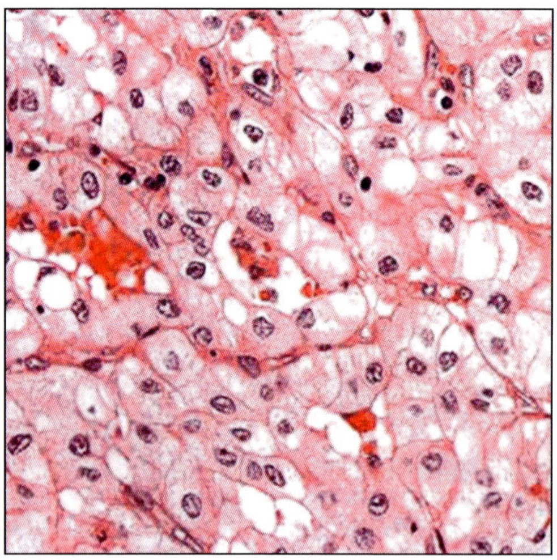

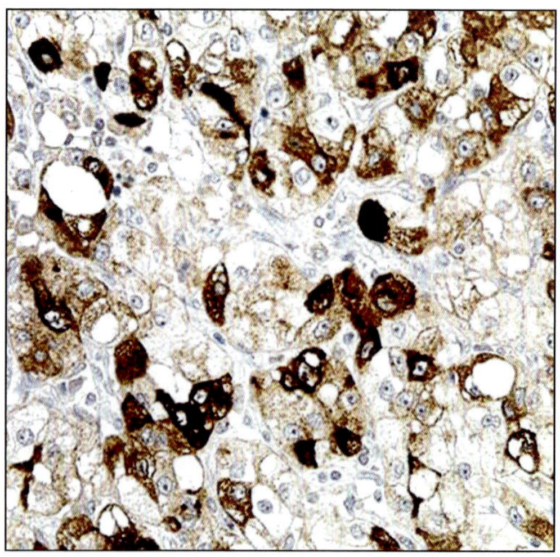

Pheochromocytoma and Pancreatic Features

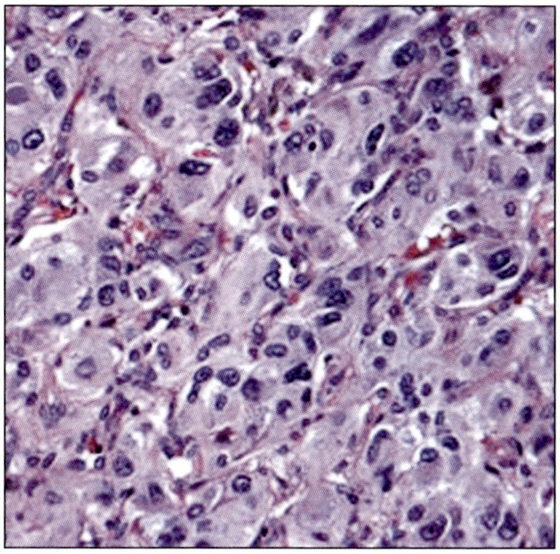
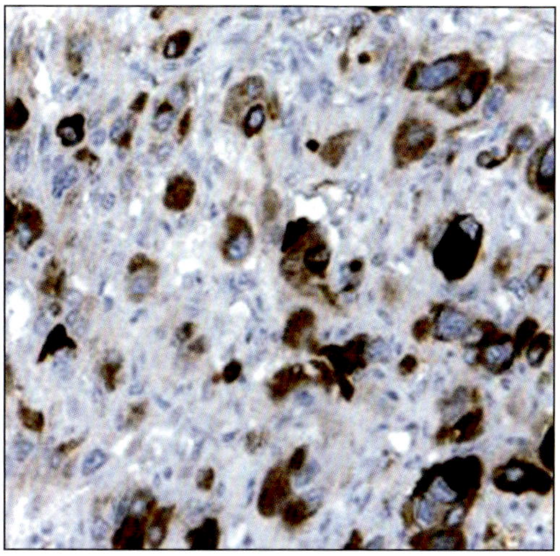

(Left) *Pheochromocytoma in association with VHL disease shows tumor cells arranged in a nested and trabecular arrangement. Tumor cells have ample cytoplasm and irregular nuclei. Note the absence of intracytoplasmic eosinophilic granules.* ***(Right)*** *Decreased clusterin staining in VHL syndrome pheochromocytoma is similar to the findings of decreased expression seen in VHL syndrome-associated RCC.*

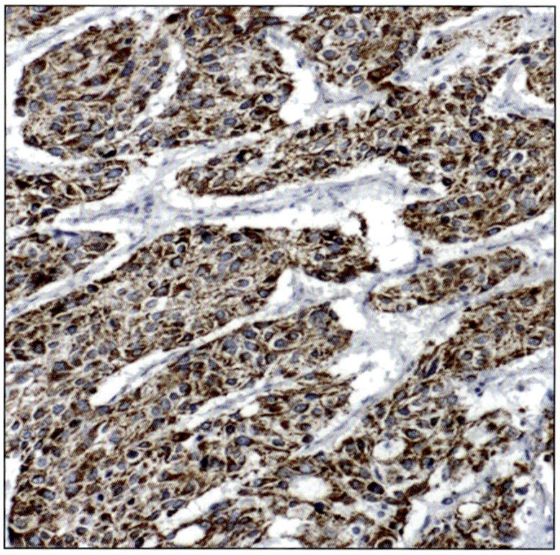
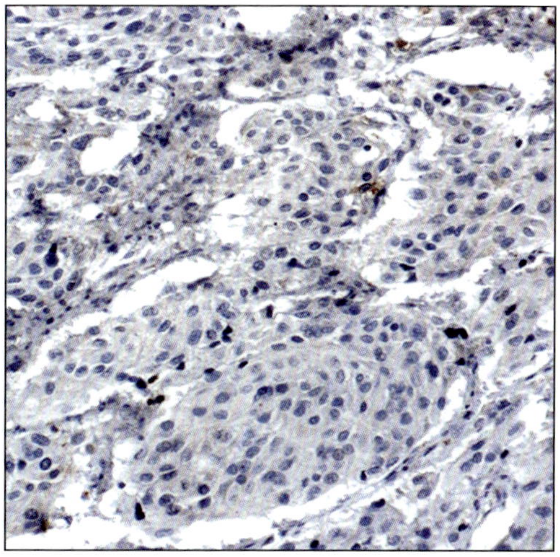

(Left) *SDHA immunostain reveals preservation of the staining of the pheochromocytoma cells in VHL syndrome-associated tumors.* ***(Right)*** *SDHB staining in VHL-associated pheochromocytoma shows loss of immunostaining, which is accompanied by preservation of SDHA. This finding is similar to the immunoexpression of these antigens in familial paraganglioma-pheochromocytoma syndromes (SDHB- and SDHD-associated pheochromocytomas).*

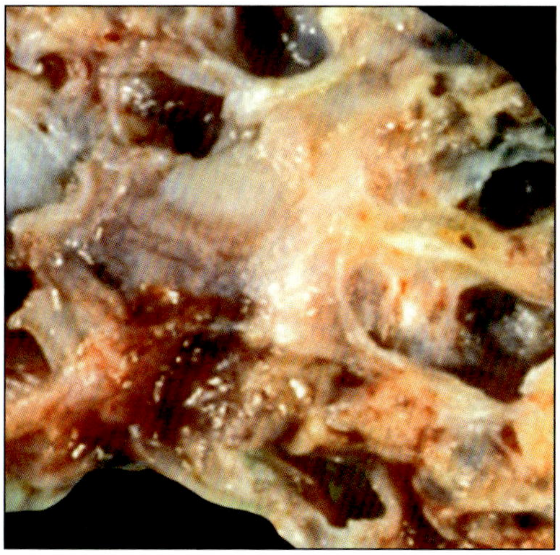
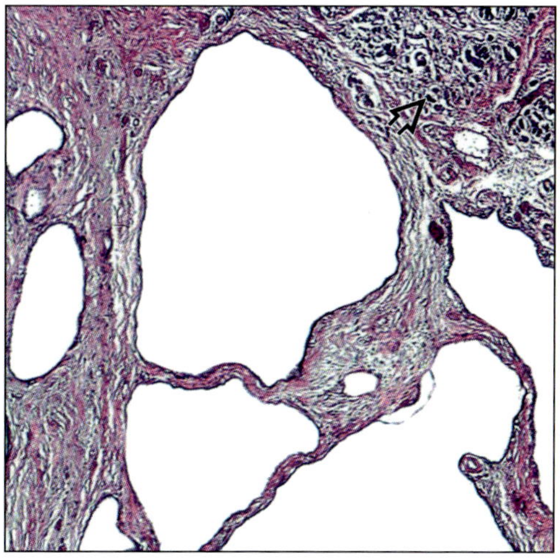

(Left) *Pancreas from a patient with VHL disease shows multiple thin-walled cysts of variable sizes. The cysts are filled with clear fluid, and there is extensive fibrosis of the pancreas.* ***(Right)*** *This photomicrograph of a pancreas from a patient with VHL disease shows multiple cysts lined by a single layer of cuboidal clear cells, surrounded by thick fibrous bands. There is residual pancreatic parenchyma ⇨.*

VON HIPPEL-LINDAU SYNDROME

Hemangioblastoma

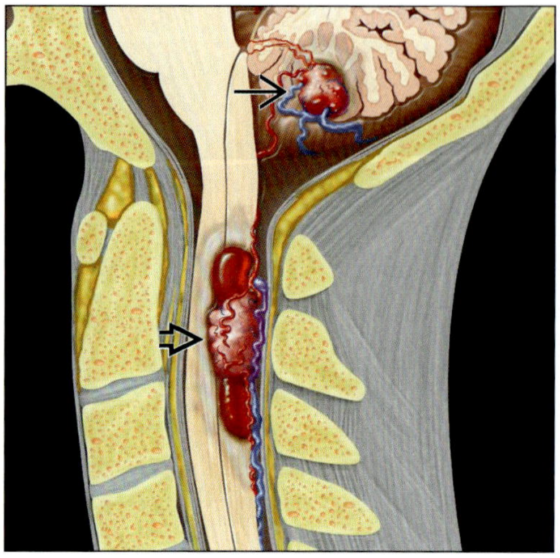

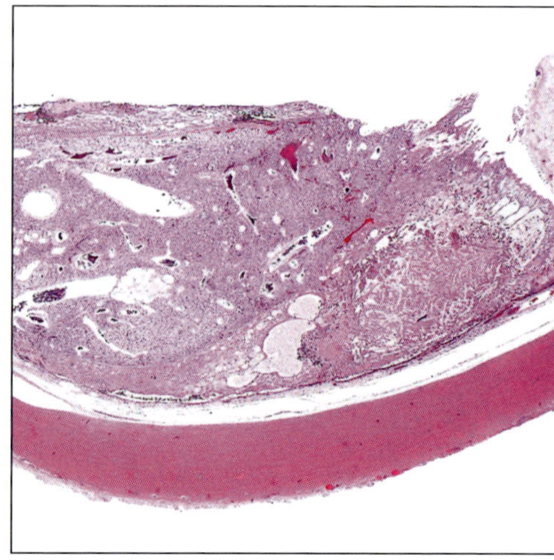

(Left) *Hemangioblastoma is the most frequently occurring tumor in VHL syndrome patients. Although they may also arise sporadically, the presence of multiple tumors is essentially pathognomonic of the disorder. The main locations involved are the cerebellum* → *and spinal cord* ⇨*.* ***(Right)*** *Although named hemangiomas in the past, given their rich vascular supply, retinal tumors afflicting VHL syndrome patients are hemangioblastomas, histologically identical to tumors involving the CNS.*

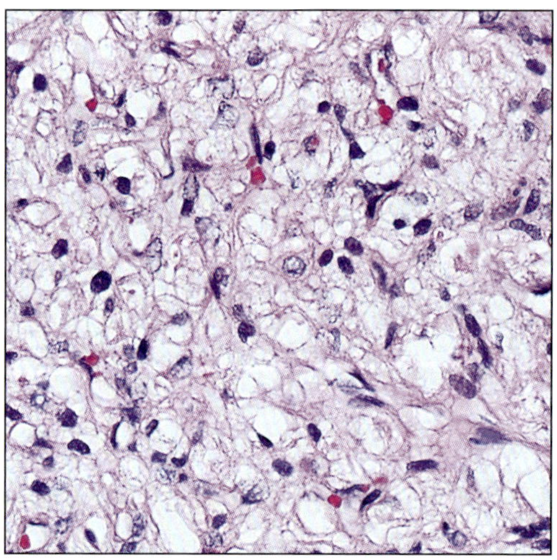

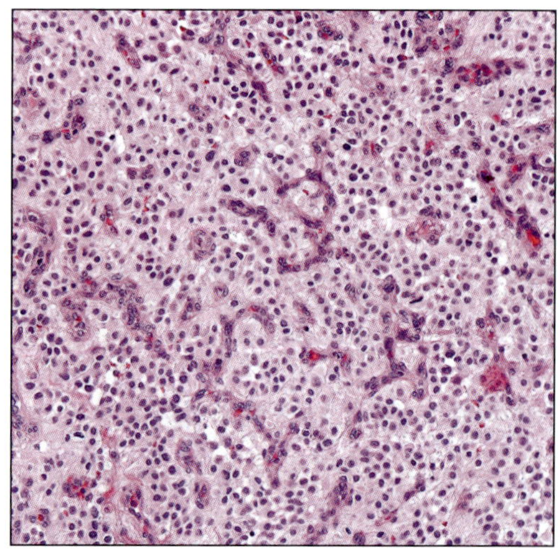

(Left) *The reticular variant of hemangioblastoma is characterized by variable numbers of stromal cells containing prominent cytoplasmic microvacuoles.* ***(Right)*** *This hemangioblastoma developed in a VHL syndrome patient and demonstrates some attributes of the cellular variant, particularly a paucity of vacuolated cells and larger lobules. There are no significant clinical or pathologic differences between VHL syndrome-associated and sporadic hemangioblastomas.*

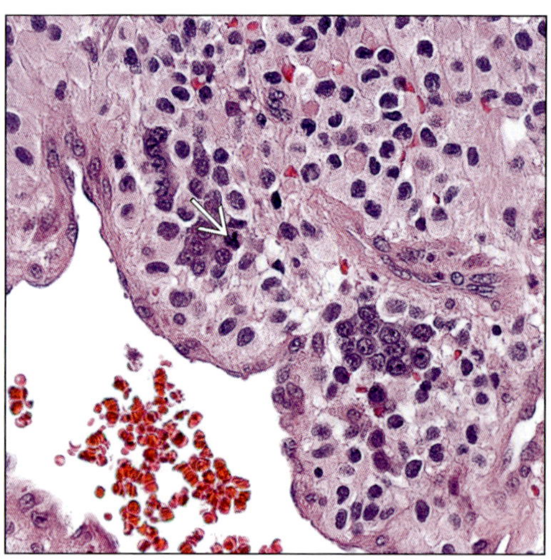

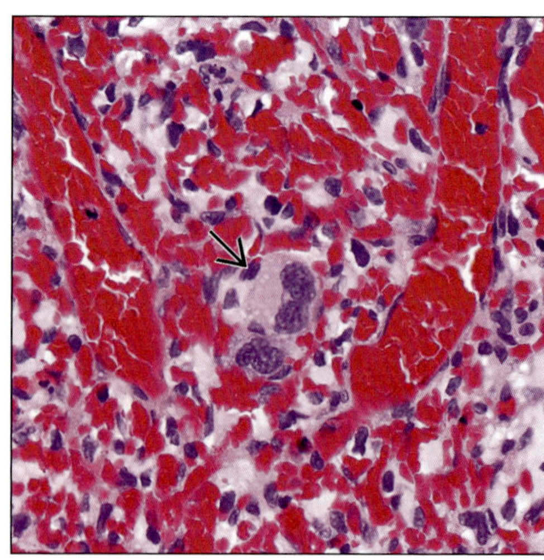

(Left) *An interesting histologic finding in a minority of hemangioblastomas is the presence of extramedullary hematopoiesis. This is characterized by variable clusters of large cells with prominent nucleoli and frequent mitotic figures* ➡*.* ***(Right)*** *Hemangioblastomas contain a rich vascular supply, and are not uncommonly grossly mistaken for blood clots or vascular malformations. This particular example demonstrates congestion as well as a multinucleated megakaryocyte* →*.*

Hemangioblastoma and Endolymphatic Sac Tumor

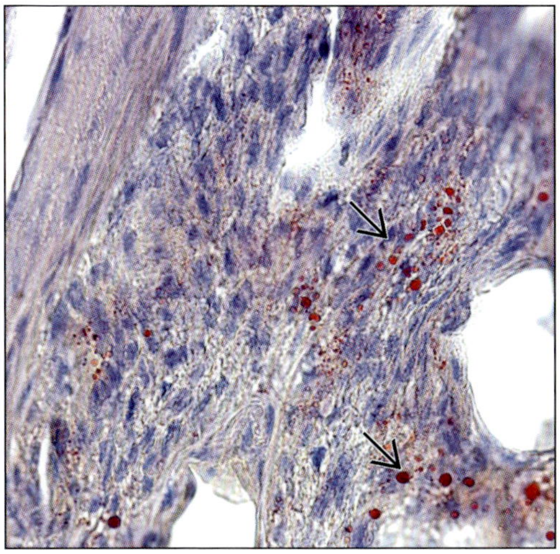
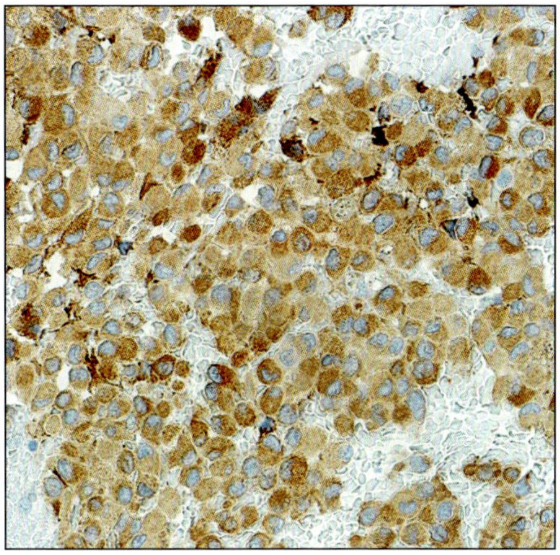

(Left) *Stromal cells contain variable amounts of intracytoplasmic lipid ⇒. In frozen section, an oil red O special stain may be particularly useful, since the characteristic microvacuolation of stromal cells may not be evident.* ***(Right)*** *A positive immunohistochemical reaction for inhibin is one of the most useful diagnostic features of hemangioblastoma, since most entities in the differential diagnosis are almost always negative.*

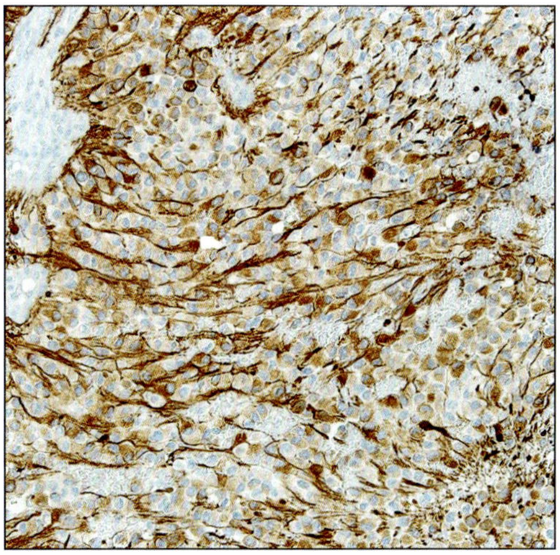
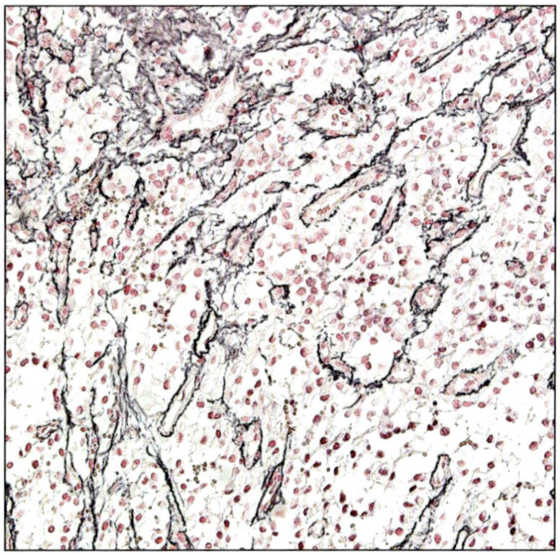

(Left) *A subset of hemangioblastomas may contain areas of glial differentiation and demonstrate overt immunoreactivity in neoplastic cells for glial markers such as GFAP.* ***(Right)*** *Reticulin stain is useful in the evaluation of hemangioblastomas, since it highlights small lobules and even individual cells. This pattern is particularly characteristic of the reticular variant.*

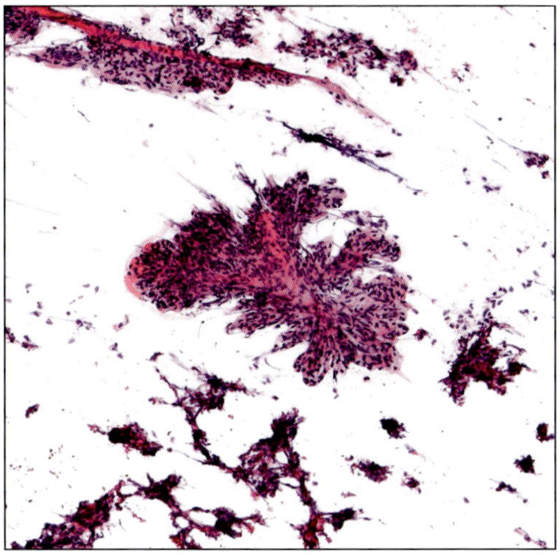
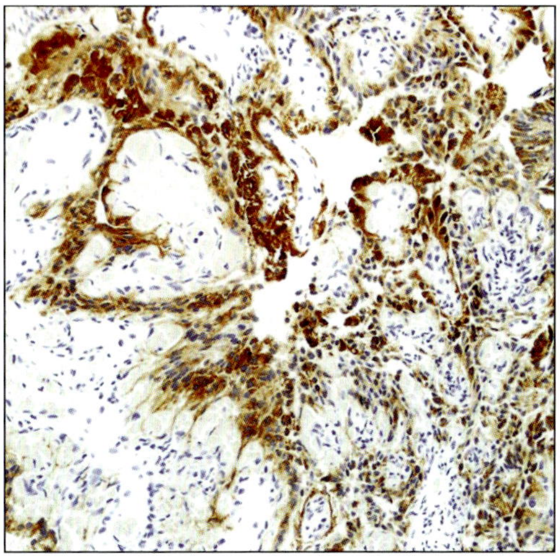

(Left) *Endolymphatic sac tumor is another rare neoplasm that may develop in patients with VHL disease. It is characterized by epithelial papillary structures, which may be easy to identify in smear preparations.* ***(Right)*** *Endolymphatic sac tumors are recognized by their epithelial cytologic and architectural features. Their epithelial phenotype may also be confirmed by immunohistochemistry. Strong EMA immunopositivity is present in this example.*

WERNER SYNDROME/PROGERIA

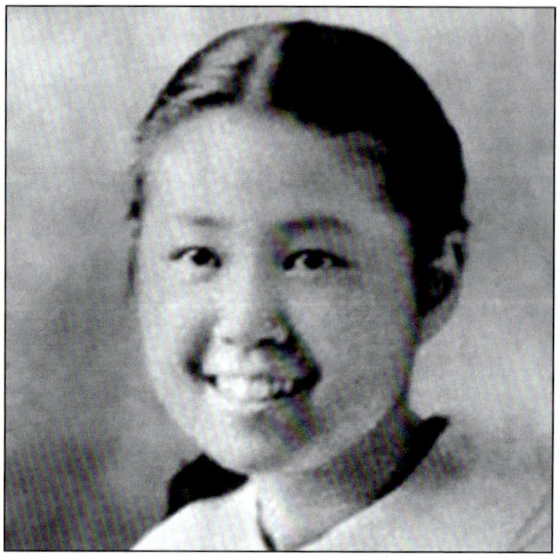

This is a patient with Werner syndrome at age 15. Her face has a normal appearance without premature aging; her hair is not yet gray. (Courtesy International Registry of Werner Syndrome.)

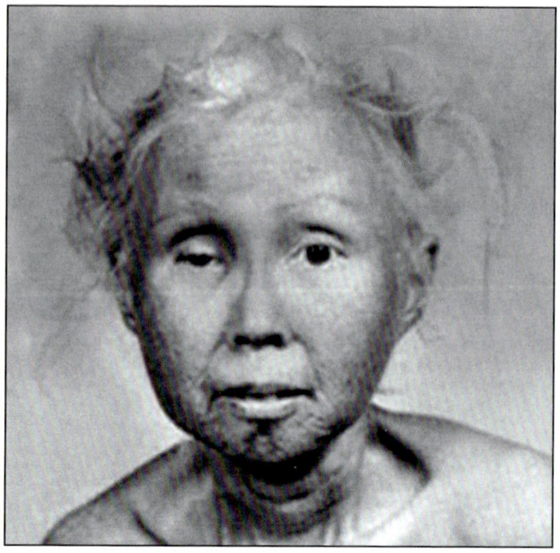

This is the same Japanese patient with Werner syndrome at age 49. Her hair is gray, and she has prematurely aged facies. (Courtesy International Registry of Werner Syndrome.)

TERMINOLOGY

Synonyms

- Adult progeria
- Progeria of the adult
- Adult premature aging syndrome

Definitions

- Premature aging after puberty
- Predisposition to cancers

EPIDEMIOLOGY

Natural History

- Normal growth until puberty
- Clinical diagnosis usually made in 30s
- Death usually in 40s to 60s
  - Often secondary to atherosclerosis or cancer

Incidence

- United States
  - ~ 1 in 200,000 to 1 million
- Japan
  - ~ 1 in 20,000 to 40,000
  - Even higher in some communities with high rates of consanguinity

Ethnicity Relationship

- More common in Japanese people
- All races affected

Age Range

- Onset of clinical findings after puberty

Gender

- M:F = 1:1

GENETICS

Mutation

- *WRN* (*RECQL2*) gene
  - Encodes Werner (RecQ DNA helicase) protein
    - Werner protein involved in DNA repair/ maintenance; has exonuclease and helicase activities
    - Most mutations lead to abnormally truncated protein that cannot translocate to nucleus
  - Mutations in *WRN* also described in age-related cataracts
  - DNA methylation of this gene may be altered in patients without mutations in *WRN*

Inheritance

- Autosomal recessive
- Heterozygote relatives of affected individuals may have very mild findings

CLINICAL IMPLICATIONS AND ANCILLARY TESTS

Clinical Presentation

- Premature graying (canities)/hair loss
  - > 98% of cases in Japanese series (Takemoto et al)
  - Mean age: 20 years
- Thin, sclerodermoid skin
  - Mean age: 25 years
  - Most prominent sites
    - Face
    - Forearms
    - Hands
    - Legs
    - Feet
- Pigmentary changes of skin
  - Diffuse or with localized freckles/lentigines
- Nails

- Dystrophic, atrophic, or hypoplastic
- Clavus/callus/hyperkeratoses
  - On soles of feet
  - Also over pressure points
    - Fingers
    - Toes
    - Ankles
    - Elbows
    - Sometimes ears
- Flat feet
- Skin ulcers
  - > 85% of cases in Japanese series (Takemoto et al)
  - Mean age: 33 years
  - May be progressive
  - Difficult to treat
  - May be complicated by osteomyelitis
- Bird-like facies
  - > 95% of of cases in Japanese series (Takemoto et al)
  - Pinched expression
  - Thin
  - Prominent eyes
  - Beaked nose
  - Circumoral radial furrows
  - Taut lips (but normal aperture)
  - Protuberant teeth
  - Micrognathia
- Short stature
  - Average height: 5 feet
- Thin extremities
- Calcification of Achilles tendon
  - > 85% of cases in Japanese series (Takemoto et al)
  - Segmental and flame-shaped pattern
- Thick trunk (central obesity)
- Abnormal voice
  - > 85% of cases in Japanese series (Takemoto et al)
  - May be hoarse
  - May be high and raspy
  - Mean age: 25 years
  - Secondary to laryngeal atrophy
- Cataracts, bilateral
  - > 75% of cases in Japanese series (Takemoto et al)
  - Mean age: 30 years
- Type 2 diabetes mellitus
  - ~ 60% in Japanese series of 185 patients
  - Mean age: 34 years
- Dyslipidemia
  - ~ 50% in Japanese series of 185 patients
- Hypogonadism
- Atherosclerosis
- Osteoporosis

Laboratory Findings

- Abnormal glucose
- Abnormal lipid panel
- Uric acid may be elevated

Imaging Findings

- Calcification of Achilles tendon

MICROSCOPIC FINDINGS

Skin

- Often epidermal, dermal, subcutaneous atrophy
- May see dermal calcifications
- Dermis may be hyalinized

ASSOCIATED NEOPLASMS

Epithelial and Nonepithelial

- Wide variety of neoplasms in Japanese series of 163 patients, but epithelial:nonepithelial ratio ~ 1:1
  - Epithelial (1 or 2 cases except where noted)
    - Thyroid cancer (4/163) most common
    - Lung cancer (3/163)
    - Pharyngeal cancer
    - Breast cancer
    - Gastric cancer
    - Hepatic cancer
    - Pancreatic cancer
    - Renal cancer
    - Bladder cancer
    - Colon cancer
    - Uterine cancer
  - Nonepithelial (1 or 2 cases except where noted)
    - Malignant fibrous histiocytoma (6/163)
    - Melanoma (6/163)
    - Meningioma (6/163)
    - Myelodysplastic syndrome (4/163)
    - Leiomyosarcoma
    - Malignant peripheral nerve sheath tumor
    - Osteosarcoma
    - Multiple myeloma

CANCER RISK MANAGEMENT

Screening

- As clinically indicated

DIFFERENTIAL DIAGNOSIS

Hutchinson-Gilford Progeria

- Premature aging from infancy
- Mutation in *LMNA*
- Severe atherosclerosis
  - Often causing death by puberty
  - Secondary to myocardial infarction, stroke
- Sclerotic skin, joint contractures, alopecia, growth impairment
- Generally lacks cataracts, hyperkeratoses, skin ulcers, diabetes mellitus

Atypical Werner Syndrome

- Heterozygous mutations in *LMNA* rather than *WRN*
- Phenotype similar to Werner syndrome
  - May be more severe
- Some suggest this could be categorized as late-onset Hutchinson-Gilford progeria

WERNER SYNDROME/PROGERIA

Acrogeria
- Onset from birth; normal lifespan
- Autosomal dominant or recessive inheritance
- Poikiloderma with marked atrophy of skin of hands/feet
- Prominent veins on trunk
- Dystrophic nails, normal scalp hair

Metageria
- Onset from birth
- Autosomal recessive
- Poikiloderma
- Atrophic extremities
- Early-onset diabetes mellitus, atherosclerosis

Rothmund-Thomson Syndrome
- Autosomal recessive, *RECQL4* mutation
- Cataracts develop in 1st 4 years of life
- Short stature
- Hypogonadism
- Telangiectasias of skin (poikiloderma)
- Increased risk of osteosarcoma, squamous cell carcinoma
- Generally lacks premature graying, sclerodermoid skin changes, osteoporosis, arteriosclerosis

Cockayne Syndrome
- Autosomal recessive, mutation in *ERCC8* or *ERCC6*
- Onset after 1st year
- Short stature, bird-like facies, canities
- Photosensitivity, poikiloderma
- No increased risk of malignancy
- Neurologic degeneration (optic atrophy, deafness, unsteady gait, demyelination of nervous system); may lead to death

DIAGNOSTIC CRITERIA

Cardinal Signs/Symptoms
- Premature graying, hair loss
- Bilateral cataracts
- Characteristic skin findings
  - Tight, atrophic skin
  - Pigmentary alteration
  - Ulceration
    - May be related to ectopic calcification
  - Atrophy
- Soft tissue calcification
- "Bird" facies
  - Pinched nasal bridge
  - Atrophy
- Abnormal voice

Further Signs/Symptoms
- Short stature
- Abnormal glucose/lipid levels
- Abnormal bones (osteoporosis)
- Malignant tumors
- Parental consanguinity or affected sibling
- Premature atherosclerosis
- Hypogonadism

Genetic Testing
- *WRN* mutation

Confirmed Diagnosis
- All cardinal signs **or** 3 cardinal signs plus *WRN* mutation

Suspected Diagnosis
- > 2 cardinal signs **or** 1-2 cardinal plus other signs

Exclusion
- Onset of signs before puberty (excluding short stature)

SELECTED REFERENCES

1. Heyn H et al: Aberrant DNA methylation profiles in the premature aging disorders Hutchinson-Gilford Progeria and Werner syndrome. Epigenetics. 8(1):28-33, 2013
2. Jiang S et al: Polymorphisms of the WRN gene and DNA damage of peripheral lymphocytes in age-related cataract in a Han Chinese population. Age (Dordr). Epub ahead of print, 2013
3. Takemoto M et al: Diagnostic criteria for Werner syndrome based on Japanese nationwide epidemiological survey. Geriatr Gerontol Int. 13(2):475-81, 2013
4. University of Washington School of Medicine, Department of Pathology: Werner Syndrome. www.wernersyndrome.org. Updated June 1 2012. Accessed July 30, 2013
5. Okabe E et al: Incidence and characteristics of metabolic disorders and vascular complications in individuals with Werner syndrome in Japan. J Am Geriatr Soc. 60(5):997-8, 2012
6. Onishi S et al: Japanese diabetic patients with Werner syndrome exhibit high incidence of cancer. Acta Diabetol. 49 Suppl 1:S259-60, 2012
7. Friedrich K et al: WRN mutations in Werner syndrome patients: genomic rearrangements, unusual intronic mutations and ethnic-specific alterations. Hum Genet. 128(1):103-11, 2010
8. Merideth MA et al: Phenotype and course of Hutchinson-Gilford progeria syndrome. N Engl J Med. 358(6):592-604, 2008
9. Muftuoglu M et al: The clinical characteristics of Werner syndrome: molecular and biochemical diagnosis. Hum Genet. 124(4):369-77, 2008
10. Hisama FM et al: WRN's tenth anniversary. Sci Aging Knowledge Environ. 2006(10):pe18, 2006
11. Huang S et al: The spectrum of WRN mutations in Werner syndrome patients. Hum Mutat. 27(6):558-67, 2006
12. Uhrhammer NA et al: Werner syndrome and mutations of the WRN and LMNA genes in France. Hum Mutat. 27(7):718-9, 2006
13. Jacob KN et al: Phenotypic heterogeneity in body fat distribution in patients with atypical Werner's syndrome due to heterozygous Arg133Leu lamin A/C mutation. J Clin Endocrinol Metab. 90(12):6699-706, 2005
14. Chen L et al: LMNA mutations in atypical Werner's syndrome. Lancet. 362(9382):440-5, 2003
15. Epstein CJ et al: Werner's syndrome a review of its symptomatology, natural history, pathologic features, genetics and relationship to the natural aging process. Medicine (Baltimore). 45(3):177-221, 1966

Clinical Photographs

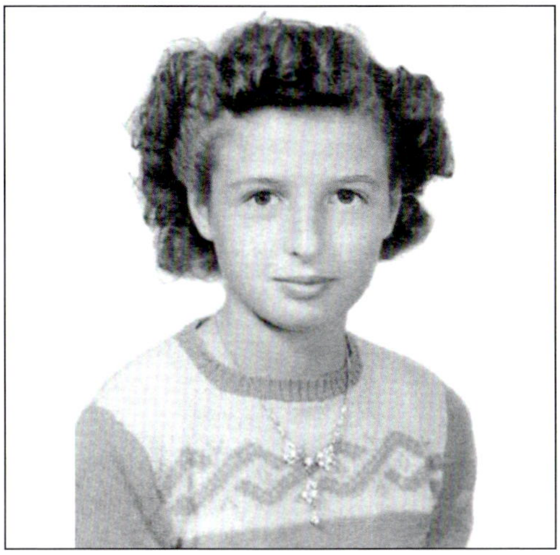

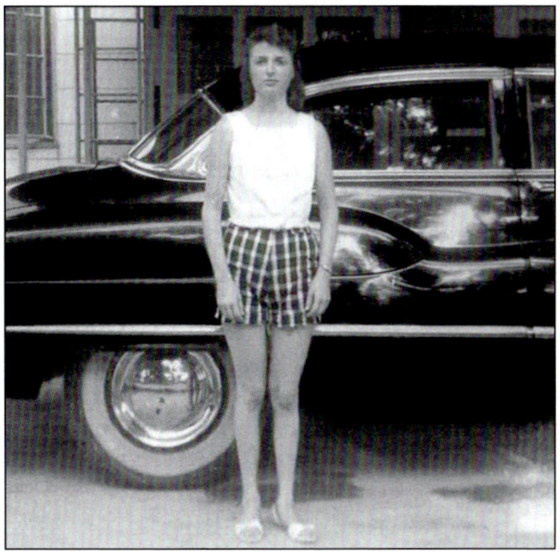

(Left) *This is a patient with Werner syndrome at age 13. Her appearance is normal. (Courtesy J. Oshima, PhD.)* ***(Right)*** *This is the same patient with Werner syndrome at age 21. She does not yet have premature gray hair but does have short stature. (Courtesy J. Oshima, PhD.)*

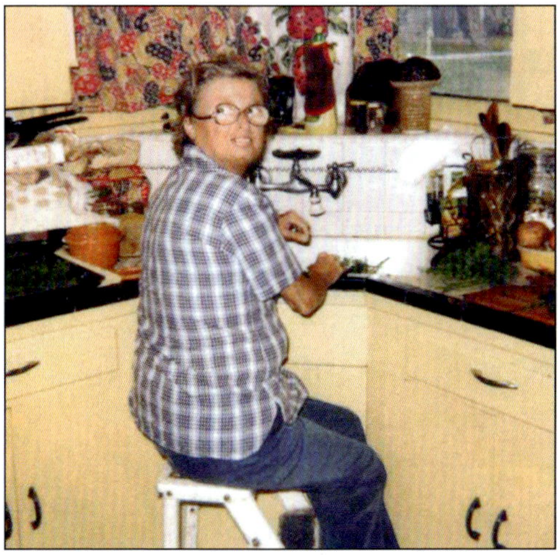

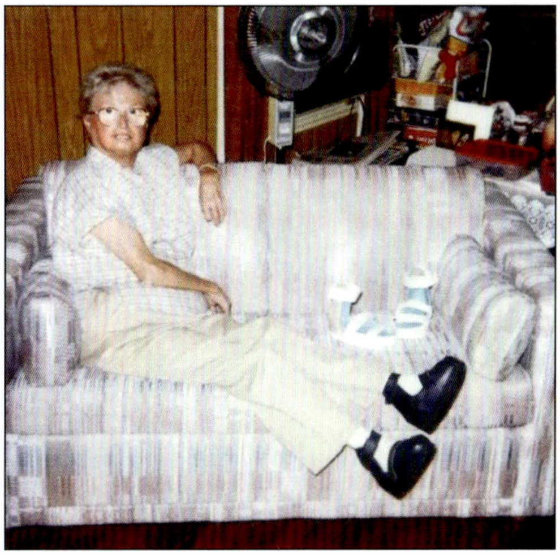

(Left) *This is the same patient with Werner syndrome at age 36. She has a prematurely aged appearance with gray hair. (Courtesy J. Oshima, PhD.)* ***(Right)*** *This is the same patient with Werner syndrome at age 40.*

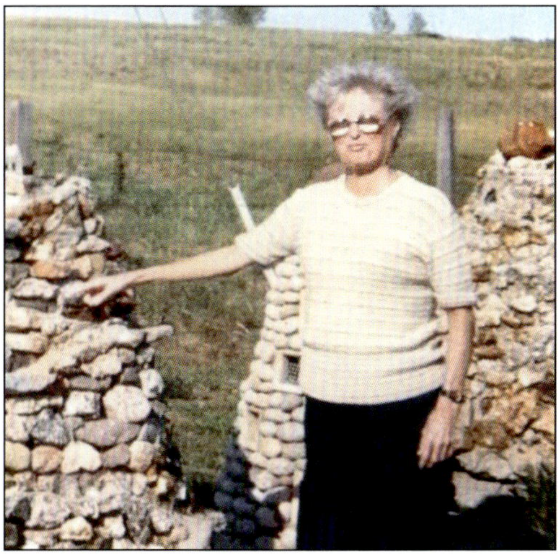

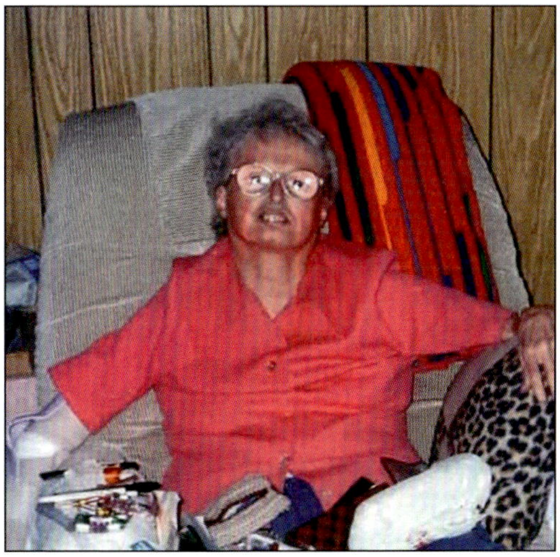

(Left) *This is the same patient with Werner syndrome at age 48.* ***(Right)*** *This is the same patient with Werner syndrome at age 54.*

WILMS TUMOR-ASSOCIATED SYNDROME

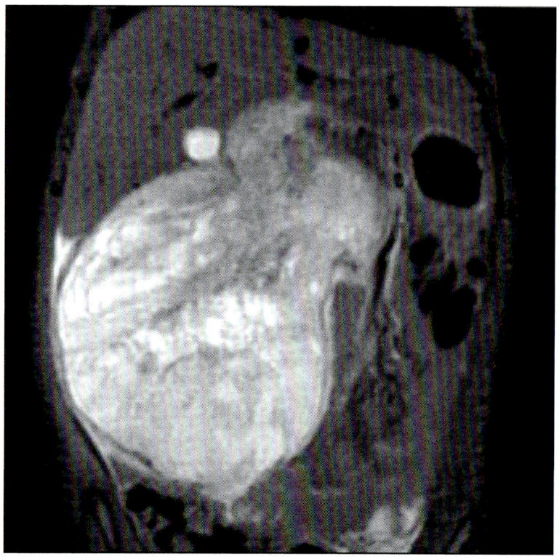

Coronal T2WI MR shows whorled high signal intensity throughout a Wilms tumor (WT). The tumor fills the right side of the abdomen and extends across the midline.

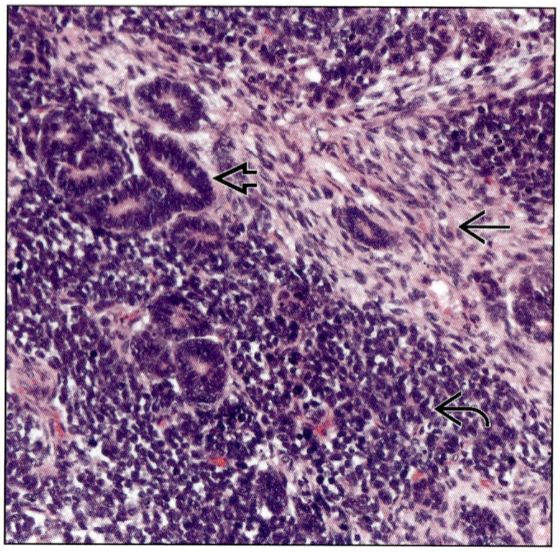

H&E shows classic triphasic histology of WT composed of an admixture of blastemal ➔, epithelial tubular ➔, and stromal spindle cells ➔. Blastemal cells are crowded small cells with abundant mitosis.

TERMINOLOGY

Abbreviations

- Wilms tumor (WT)

Definitions

- Include WT in genetic syndromes associated with *WT1* and childhood overgrowth syndromes

EPIDEMIOLOGY

Incidence

- WT diagnosed in ~ 1 in 10,000 white children
  - Vast majority of WTs are sporadic (up to 99%)
  - Familial WT comprises ~ 2% of cases
  - Congenital anomalies seen in up to 9% with syndrome diagnosis in up to 17% of WT patients
  - Childhood overgrowth syndrome seen in ~ 4% of WT patients

CLINICAL IMPLICATIONS

Prognosis of WT

- High cure rate, with estimated survival of 90% for localized disease and 70% for advanced disease
- Early screening detection for WT in individuals with syndrome is mainly to reduce complication from extensive therapy of higher stage diseases

Screening of WT

- Genetic testing and surveillance recommended for children with > 5% risk for WT
- Screening up to age 5 years expected to detect up to 95% of tumors in patients with *WT1* mutations

WT1-ASSOCIATED SYNDROMES

General Features

- Patients with WT diagnosed younger than sporadic cases (~ 1 year vs. 3-4 years)
- Higher likelihood for bilateral WT (38% vs. 5% for sporadic cases)
- Screening for WT performed by renal ultrasound ~ 3 months until 5 years of age
- WT frequently contains intralobar nephrogenic rests and often stromal predominant

WT Aniridia Genitourinary Malformations and Mental Retardation (WAGR) Syndrome

- Phenotype: Aniridia, ambiguous external genitalia (including cryptorchidism), and intellectual impairment
- High risk for renal failure, affecting ~ 40% by age 20 years
- Caused by microdeletions at Chr 11p13 that encompass *WT1* and *PAX6*
- ~ 30% risk for WT

Denys-Drash Syndrome

- Phenotype: Ambiguous genitalia, diffuse mesangial sclerosis, and genitourinary abnormalities in male
  - Nephropathy presents as hypertension and proteinuria
- Caused by point mutation in zinc finger region of *WT1* at Chr 11p13
- ~ 90% risk for WT

Frasier Syndrome

- Phenotype: Ambiguous genitalia, streak gonads, focal segmental glomerulosclerosis
- Caused by point mutation in *WT1* intron 9 donor splice site at Chr 11p13
- Low risk for WT

Conditions With Increased Risk of Wilms Tumor

Conditions	Level of Risk
WT1 deletions (including WAGR syndrome)	High
Truncating and pathogenic missense *WT1* mutations (including Denys-Drash syndrome)	High
Familial Wilms tumor	High
Perlman syndrome	High
Mosaic variegated aneuploidy	High
Fanconi anemia D1/biallelic *BRCA2* mutation	High
WT1 intron 9 splice mutations (Frasier syndrome)	Moderate
Beckwith-Wiedemann syndrome caused by 11p15 uniparental disomy, isolated *H19* hypermethylation or of unknown cause	Moderate
Simpson-Golabi-Behmel syndrome caused by *GPC3* mutations/deletions	Moderate
Isolated hemihypertrophy	Low
Bloom syndrome	Low
Li-Fraumeni syndrome/Li-Fraumeni-like syndrome	Low
Hereditary hyperparathyroidism-jaw tumor syndrome	Low
Mulibrey nanism	Low
Trisomy 18	Low
Trisomy 13	Low
2q37 deletions	Low

High risk (> 20%); moderate risk (5-20%); low risk (< 5%); screening for WT recommended for moderate- and high-risk conditions.

OVERGROWTH SYNDROMES

General Features

- Heterogeneous, poorly defined, and overlapping group of genetic conditions with manifestations of overgrowth
  - Large size at birth, large head, excessive growth or rapid increase in weight or length
- Risk for WT evaluated per syndrome rather than on collective basis
- Screening for WT in Beckwith-Wiedemann syndrome (BWS) and isolated (idiopathic) hemihypertrophy (IHH) performed by renal ultrasound ~ 3 months until age 8 years (older than in *WT1*-associated syndromes due to later age of onset)

Beckwith-Wiedemann Syndrome (BWS)

- Phenotype: Organomegaly, large birth weight, macroglossia, omphalocele, hemihypertrophy, ear anomalies, and neonatal hypoglycemia
- Renal abnormalities such as nephromegaly, renal cysts, medullary sponge kidney, medullary dysplasia, hydronephrosis, and calculi formation
- Most caused by altered expression of imprinted genes (*KCNQ1OT1*, *CDKN1C*, *LIT1*, or *H19* and *IGF2*) located at Chr 11p15.5
- < 10% results from germline *CDKN1C* mutation
- ~ 7-14% develop cancer, greatest risk at 1st decade of life
  - Most frequent is WT affecting up to 8% of cases
- Higher risk for bilateral WT (17%) and perilobar nephrogenic rest (60%) than in sporadic WT

Simpson-Golabi-Behmel Syndrome

- Phenotype: Coarse facial features, skeletal and cardiac abnormalities, accessory nipples, and possible intellectual abnormalities
- ~ 30% have renal abnormalities
- Majority (70%) caused by mutations or deletions of Glypican-3 (*GPC3*) at Chr Xq26
- ~ 9% develop WT

Isolated (Idiopathic) Hemihypertrophy (IHH)

- Phenotype: Asymmetrical growth with 1 body part larger than contralateral counterpart
- Hemihypertrophy can be associated with other syndromes such as BWS, but majority presents as isolated finding
- Abnormality in Chr 11p15 in 20-35% of cases
- ~ 3% develop WT

Perlman Syndrome

- Phenotype: Polyhydramnios, visceromegaly, facial dysmorphism, developmental delay, cryptorchidism, renal dysplasia, WT, and high infant mortality
- Unknown cause; *GPC3* mutation suggested
- ~ 33% develop WT and nephroblastomatosis

SELECTED REFERENCES

1. Huff V: Wilms' tumours: about tumour suppressor genes, an oncogene and a chameleon gene. Nat Rev Cancer. 11(2):111-21, 2011
2. Rao A et al: Genetic testing and tumor surveillance for children with cancer predisposition syndromes. Curr Opin Pediatr. 20(1):1-7, 2008
3. Scott RH et al: Syndromes and constitutional chromosomal abnormalities associated with Wilms tumour. J Med Genet. 43(9):705-15, 2006
4. Ruteshouser EC et al: Familial Wilms tumor. Am J Med Genet C Semin Med Genet. 129C(1):29-34, 2004
5. Dome JS et al: Recent advances in Wilms tumor genetics. Curr Opin Pediatr. 14(1):5-11, 2002
6. Breslow NE et al: Familial Wilms' tumor: a descriptive study. Med Pediatr Oncol. 27(5):398-403, 1996

XERODERMA PIGMENTOSUM

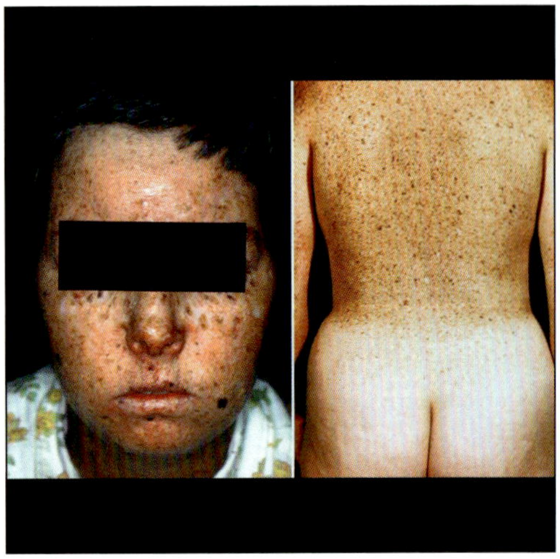

Many photo-distributed lentigines are seen in this patient with xeroderma pigmentosum. (Courtesy K. Kraemer, MD.)

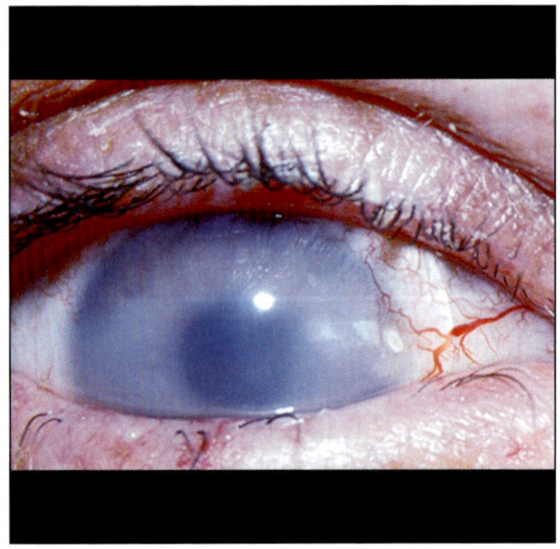

This patient with xeroderma pigmentosum has corneal clouding. (Courtesy K. Kraemer, MD.)

TERMINOLOGY

Abbreviations

- Xeroderma pigmentosum (XP)

Synonyms

- DeSanctis-Cacchione syndrome

Definitions

- Inherited disorder of nucleotide excision repair
- Characterized by photosensitivity and early onset of skin cancer and solar lentigines

EPIDEMIOLOGY

Incidence

- ~ 1 in 1 million in United States
- ~ 1 in 40,000 in Japan

Ethnicity Relationship

- More common in Japan
- More common in populations in which consanguinity is common

Age Range

- Evidence of photodamage of skin (solar lentigines)
  - As early as 1-2 years of age
- Median age of onset of nonmelanoma skin cancer: 9 years
- Mean age of presentation of hearing loss: 19 years
- Median age of onset of cutaneous melanoma: 22 years
- Often multiple primary cutaneous tumors by age 20 years
- XP variant
  - Later disease onset
    - Age 10-20 years

Natural History

- Cause of death
  - Skin cancer
    - 34% of patients
  - Neurologic degeneration
    - 31% of patients
  - Internal malignancy
    - 17% of patients
- Median age at death, if no neurologic degeneration
  - 37 years
- Median age at death, if neurologic degeneration
  - 29 years

ETIOLOGY/PATHOGENESIS

Ultraviolet (UV) Light Action Spectrum

- Inflammatory erythema of skin
  - 290-340 nm range

GENETICS

Inheritance

- Autosomal recessive

Mutations

- In genes involved in nucleotide excision repair
  - Results in high number of UV signature mutations (C to T or CC to TT)
- Complementation groups
  - Complementation is capacity of cells from 1 XP cell line to compensate for repair defects of another cell line when these 2 cell lines are fused
  - Groups A to G, defective nucleotide excision repair of UV light-induced damage
    - Group A: Mutation in *XPA*
    - Group B: Mutation in *XPB/ERCC3*
    - Group C: Mutation in *XPC*
    - Group D: Mutation in *XPD/ERCC2*
    - Group E: Mutation in *XPE/DDB2*
    - Group F: Mutation in *XPF/ERCC4*
    - Group G: Mutation in *XPG/ERCC5*

- XP variant: Mutation in *POLH* (defective DNA polymerase) causing incorrect replication of DNA
- Genotype-phenotype correlations
  - Complementation groups A, B, D, and G
    - Blistering burns with minimal sun exposure
    - More likely to have neurologic degeneration
  - Complementation groups C, E, and variant
    - Generally lack acute sunburns
    - Develop evidence of chronic sun damage, often by age 2 years, manifesting as freckling and lentigines
  - Complementation groups C, E, F, XP variant
    - Generally absent neurologic degeneration

CLINICAL IMPLICATIONS AND ANCILLARY TESTS

Clinical Presentation

- Childhood onset of photosensitivity
  - Manifests as blistering (sunburn) with minimal acute sun exposure or as early-onset lentigines
    - By age 18 months in 50% of patients
    - By age 4 years in 75% of patients
    - By age 15 years in 95% of patients
  - Chronic changes, primarily in sun-exposed areas
    - Poikiloderma (dyspigmentation with atrophy and telangiectasias), lentigines
    - Xerosis
    - Tumors
- Eye changes
  - Telangiectasias of conjunctiva
  - Photophobia
  - Cataracts
  - Keratitis
  - Corneal opacification and vascularization
- Neurologic in 25-30% of patients
  - Absent deep tendon reflexes
  - High-frequency sensorineural hearing loss
    - Especially in patients in complementation groups A and D
    - Hearing loss correlated with acute burning on minimal sun exposure
    - Mean age of presentation: 19 years
  - Cognitive impairment
  - Difficulty swallowing
  - Loss of ability to ambulate
  - Microcephaly
  - Abnormal electroencephalogram
  - Seizures

Imaging Findings

- Enlarged ventricles
- Cortical thinning

ASSOCIATED NEOPLASMS

Nonmelanoma Skin Cancer

- Carcinomas and sarcomas
  - Especially basal cell carcinoma and squamous cell carcinoma
  - Frequency compared to general population
    - 10,000x increase in XP patients < 20 years old

Cutaneous Malignant Melanoma

- 2,000x increase in XP patients < 20 years old compared to general population

Ocular Cancer

- 1,000x increase in XP patients < 20 years old compared to general population

Tongue Cancer

- 100,000x increase in XP patients < 20 years old compared to general population

Internal Malignancy

- 10-20x increase compared to general population
- Brain tumors
  - Medulloblastoma
  - Glioblastoma
- Central nervous system tumors
  - Spinal cord astrocytoma
- Carcinomas
  - Pulmonary
  - Uterine
  - Breast
  - Gastric
  - Renal cell
  - Testicular
- Leukemias

Benign Neoplasms

- Lentigines
- Conjunctival papilloma
- Actinic keratosis
- Keratoacanthoma
- Pyogenic granuloma
- Fibroma
- Multinodular thyroid
- Schwannoma

CANCER RISK MANAGEMENT

Ultraviolet Light Protection (From Sunlight and Artificial Light)

- Of skin and eyes
- From day 1 of life
- Methods include
  - Sunblock
  - Sunglasses
  - Protective clothing
  - Window tinting
  - Use of ultraviolet meters
- Oral vitamin D and calcium supplementation

Regular Examination

- Mucocutaneous
- Ocular

Avoidance of Other Carcinogens

- e.g., tobacco smoke

Possible Prophylaxis

- Oral retinoids
- T4 endonuclease V (bacterial DNA repair enzyme)

DIFFERENTIAL DIAGNOSIS

Trichothiodystrophy

- Mutations
  - *XPB* and *XPD* genes
- Autosomal recessive
- Similarities to xeroderma pigmentosum
  - Cognitive impairment
  - Photosensitivity
- Differences from xeroderma pigmentosum
  - Brittle hair
    - Hair shaft with alternating light and dark bands
  - Ichthyosis
  - Absent lentigines
  - No increased risk of internal cancer or skin cancer

Cockayne Syndrome

- Mutations
  - *XPB*, *XPD*, and *XPG* genes for combined XP/Cockayne phenotypes
  - *ERCC8* and *ERCC6* genes
  - Rarely *XPF*
- Autosomal recessive
- Clinical features
  - Cachectic dwarfism
  - Premature aged appearance
  - Microcephaly
  - Similarities to xeroderma pigmentosum
    - Photosensitivity
    - Progressive mental degeneration
  - Differences from xeroderma pigmentosum
    - Absent lentigines
    - Retinal degeneration
    - No increased risk of internal cancer or skin cancer in "pure" Cockayne phenotypes
- XP/Cockayne syndrome overlap
  - Mutations in *XPB*, *XPD*, and *XPG* genes for combined XP/Cockayne phenotypes
  - Solar lentigines
  - Increased skin cancers
  - Pigmentary retinal degeneration
  - Basal ganglion calcification

UV-Sensitive Syndrome

- Mutations
  - *CSB* and *CSA* genes
- Autosomal recessive
- Rarely reported syndrome
  - May be mild variant of Cockayne syndrome
    - Photosensitivity
    - Solar lentigines

Bloom Syndrome

- Mutations
  - *BLM* (*RECQL3*) gene
    - Results in chromosomal instability
    - Increased sister chromatid exchanges, breakage, and rearrangement
- Autosomal recessive
- Malar erythema, telangiectasias
- Café au lait macules
- Long face with prominent nose
- Short stature
- Diabetes mellitus
- Normal intelligence
- Reduced/absent fertility
- Recurrent infections
  - Respiratory
  - Gastrointestinal
- Malignancies
  - Leukemia
  - Lymphoma
  - Gastrointestinal adenocarcinoma

Rothmund-Thomson Syndrome

- Mutations
  - *RECQL4* gene
    - Encodes DNA helicase
- Autosomal recessive
- Facial erythema, edema, vesicles
  - Eventuates in poikiloderma
- Sparse hair
- Hypoplastic nails
- Acral keratoses
- Short stature
- Normal intelligence
- Malignancies
  - Osteosarcoma (10-30% of patients)
  - Squamous cell carcinoma (< 5% of patients)

SELECTED REFERENCES

1. Hadj-Rabia S et al: Unexpected extradermatological findings in 31 patients with xeroderma pigmentosum type C. Br J Dermatol. 168(5):1109-1113, 2013
2. Kashiyama K et al: Malfunction of Nuclease ERCC1-XPF Results in Diverse Clinical Manifestations and Causes Cockayne Syndrome, Xeroderma Pigmentosum, and Fanconi Anemia. Am J Hum Genet. 92(5):807-19, 2013
3. Totonchy MB et al: Auditory analysis of xeroderma pigmentosum 1971-2012: hearing function, sun sensitivity and DNA repair predict neurological degeneration. Brain. 136(Pt 1):194-208, 2013
4. DiGiovanna JJ et al: Shining a light on xeroderma pigmentosum. J Invest Dermatol. 132(3 Pt 2):785-96, 2012
5. Bradford PT et al: Cancer and neurologic degeneration in xeroderma pigmentosum: long term follow-up characterises the role of DNA repair. J Med Genet. 48(3):168-76, 2011
6. Kraemer KH et al: Xeroderma pigmentosum, trichothiodystrophy and Cockayne syndrome: a complex genotype-phenotype relationship. Neuroscience. 145(4):1388-96, 2007
7. Cleaver JE: Cancer in xeroderma pigmentosum and related disorders of DNA repair. Nat Rev Cancer. 5(7):564-73, 2005
8. Kraemer KH et al: Xeroderma pigmentosum. Cutaneous, ocular, and neurologic abnormalities in 830 published cases. Arch Dermatol. 123(2):241-50, 1987

XERODERMA PIGMENTOSUM

Associated Lesions

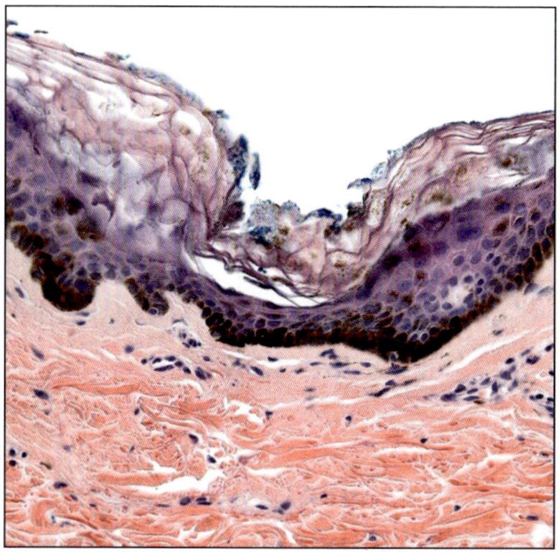

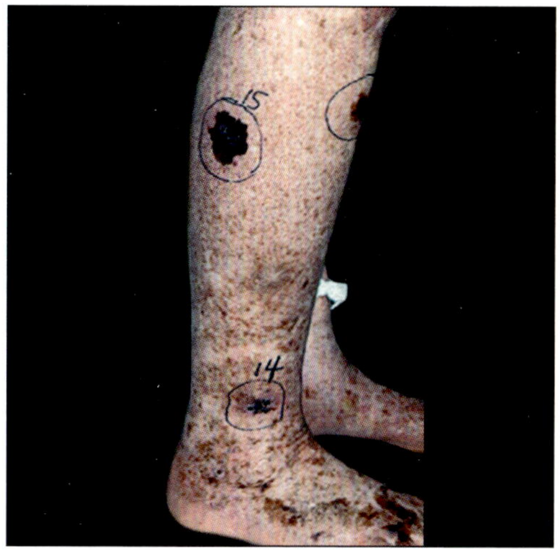

(Left) *Lentigines are common on the sun-exposed skin of patients with xeroderma pigmentosum. Histopathologically, there is an increase in basilar melanin pigment.* ***(Right)*** *The lesion labeled "15" is a malignant melanoma with a depth of 0.55 mm, on the leg of this patient with xeroderma pigmentosum. There are numerous surrounding lentigines. (Courtesy K. Kraemer, MD.)*

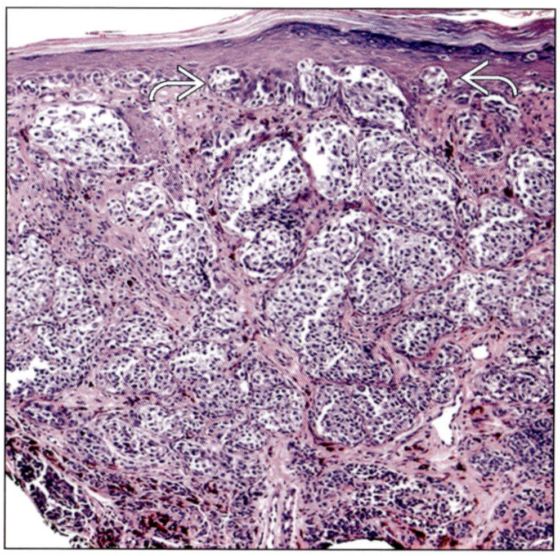

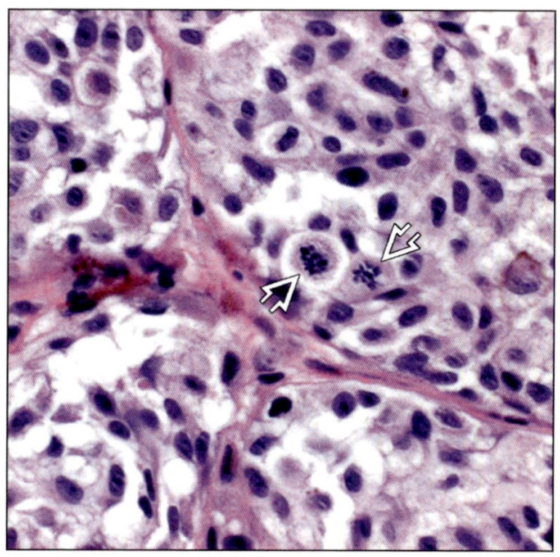

(Left) *Cutaneous melanoma can be seen in patients with xeroderma pigmentosum. Low-power examination shows pagetoid spread ➔ of a superficial spreading type of malignant melanoma. (Courtesy S. Dadras, MD.)* ***(Right)*** *High-power magnification shows prominent cytologic atypia and 2 adjacent mitoses ➔ within the dermal nests of this malignant melanoma. (Courtesy S. Dadras, MD.)*

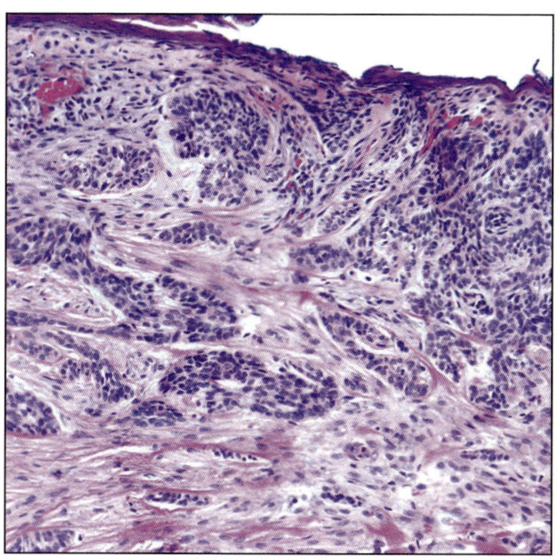

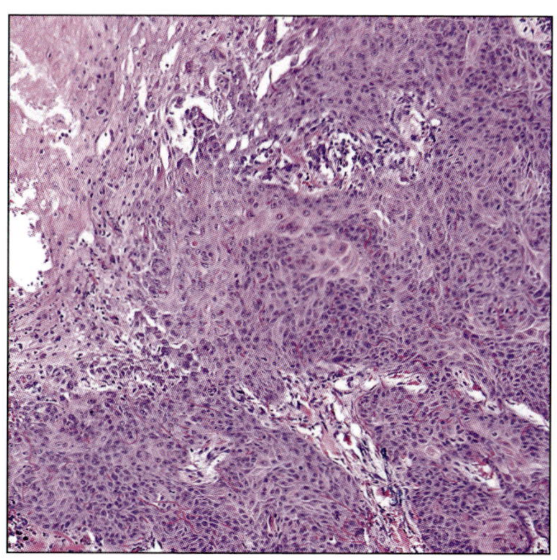

(Left) *Cutaneous basal cell carcinomas are common in patients with xeroderma pigmentosum. Histopathologically, in this example of basal cell carcinoma, there are infiltrating islands of basaloid cells with peripheral palisading.* ***(Right)*** *Cutaneous squamous cell carcinoma is also common in patients with xeroderma pigmentosum. In this example of squamous cell carcinoma of the skin, there are large islands of atypical keratinocytes in the dermis.*

Breast

BREAST CARCINOMA, FEMALE

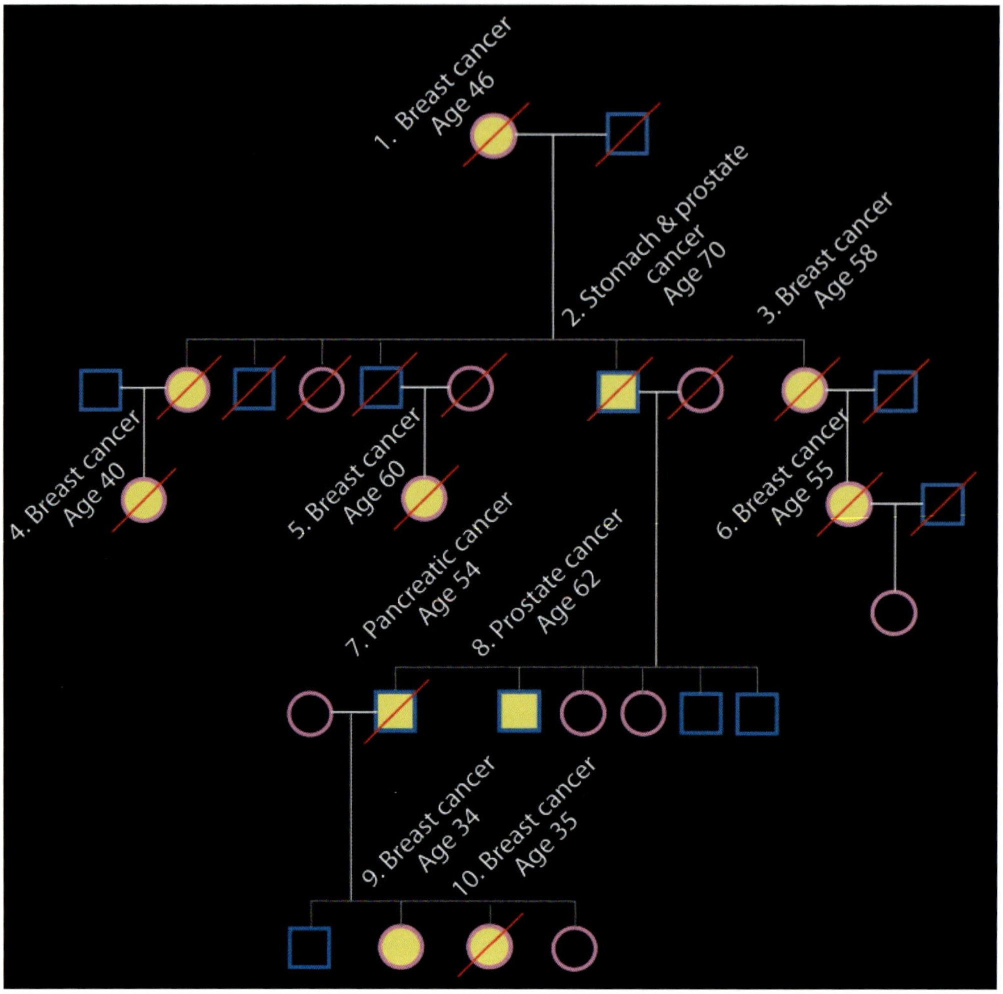

Family history is a powerful tool for detecting highly penetrant genes responsible for breast cancer susceptibility. This pedigree is very suggestive of a germline mutation due to the presence of multiple affected family members and the development of cancers at a young age. Genetic testing could determine whether any of the currently recognized mutations are present or establish the significance of a yet undescribed mutation if it consistently maps to individuals with cancer.

ETIOLOGY/PATHOGENESIS

Hereditary Breast Cancer

- Long recognized that many women with breast cancer also have affected relatives
  - ~ 27% of breast cancer is thought to be due primarily to hereditary factors
    - Only 5-10% due to highly penetrant germline mutations
    - ~ 10% of women diagnosed with breast cancer at < 45 years of age will have a germline mutation
- Familial risk not explainable by known mutations is likely due to additive effect of multiple genes
  - Multiple low penetrance genes may increase risk in families
    - These genes may also modify clinical features of high penetrance genes
  - Genome-wide association studies are searching for this group of genes
  - It is unlikely that another highly penetrant gene such as *BRCA1* or *BRCA2* will be identified
- **Features common to all major germline mutations**
  - Autosomal dominant alleles
    - Tumors occur when remaining wild-type allele is rendered nonfunctional
    - Inherited via both females and males
    - Multiple individuals in a lineage are usually affected
  - Majority of identified genes are associated with DNA repair pathways
    - Act as tumor suppressor genes in normal cells to maintain DNA integrity and control proliferation
    - Relative tissue specificity for breast cancer has not been explained
  - Breast cancers occur at earlier ages compared to sporadic cancers and are often multiple and bilateral
    - 1st mutation present at birth
    - Destabilization of genome increases likelihood of additional mutations

BREAST CARCINOMA, FEMALE

Key Facts

Etiology/Pathogenesis

- ~ 27% of breast cancer is thought to be due primarily to hereditary factors
- Only 5-10% due to highly penetrant germline mutations
- ~ 10% of women diagnosed with breast cancer at < 45 years of age will have a germline mutation
- Familial risk not explainable by known mutations is likely due to additive effect of multiple genes
- **Features in common**
- Autosomal dominant alleles
  - Inherited via females and males
- Majority of identified genes are associated with DNA repair pathways
- Breast cancers occur at earlier ages compared to sporadic cancers and are often multiple and bilateral
- Risk of nonbreast cancers increased

Diagnostic Checklist

- *BRCA1* (hereditary breast and ovarian cancer syndrome)
- *BRCA2* (hereditary breast and ovarian cancer syndrome)
- *TP53* (Li-Fraumeni syndrome)
- *CDH1* (familial gastric cancer and lobular breast cancer syndrome)
- *PTEN* (Cowden syndrome)
- *CHEK2*
- *ATM* (ataxia-telangiectasia carriers)
- *STK11/LKB1* (Peutz-Jeghers syndrome)
- *BRIP1* (*FANCJ* or *BACH1*)

- Risk of nonbreast cancers increased
- **Features specific to certain germline mutations**
  - Type of breast carcinoma
  - Risk of male breast cancer
    - Increased risk for some mutations (e.g., *BRCA1* and *BRCA2*)
    - Not reported for other mutations (e.g., *TP53*)
  - Penetrance
    - > 95% lifetime risk for some mutations
    - Other genes have lower penetrance (20% or lower lifetime risk)
  - Spectrum of nonbreast cancers
    - Types of other cancers vary according to gene and sometimes are different for specific mutations
  - Founder mutations in ethnic populations
    - Some populations have very high incidences of specific mutations
  - Homozygosity
    - Homozygosity for some mutations confers disease (e.g., *BRCA2* & *BRIP1*: Fanconi anemia; *ATM*: Ataxia-telangiectasia)
    - Homozygosity for other mutations is likely lethal (e.g., *BRCA1*)

CLINICAL ISSUES

Epidemiology

- ~ 10-25% of women with breast cancer have a 1st-degree relative (parent, sister, daughter) with breast cancer
  - Having an affected 1st-degree relative increases risk by 2-3x
- Most common family history is a mother developing breast cancer after menopause
  - This history does not increase risk of breast cancer for daughter
  - Sporadic breast cancer in this age group is very common
- **Familial patterns of breast cancer likely to be associated with germline mutations**
  - Affected 1st-degree relatives (mother, sister, daughter)
  - Multiple affected relatives
  - Carcinomas occurring at an early age (premenopausal)
  - Multiple carcinomas (bilateral or ipsilateral)
  - Relatives with nonbreast cancers associated with specific germline mutations
    - Male breast cancer for *BRCA2* and *BRCA1*
    - Ovarian, fallopian tube, or primary peritoneal cancers for *BRCA1* and *BRCA2*
    - Sarcomas for *TP53*
  - Relatives with diseases due to homozygous mutations
    - Ataxia-telangiectasia for *ATM*
    - Fanconi anemia for *BRCA2* and *BRIP1*

BRCA1 (Hereditary Breast & Ovarian Cancer Syndrome)

- **Function**
  - *BRCA1* and *BRCA2* code for large proteins
    - Proteins do not have sequence homology but do share many similar functions
  - *BRCA1* and *BRCA2* help maintain genomic stability
    - Direct role in regulation of DNA damage responses and repair and cell cycle checkpoints
    - Cells lacking *BRCA1* & *BRCA2* functional activity are prone to replication errors and genomic instability
    - Drives acquisition of mutations and chromosomal instability, contributing to tumor formation
  - *BRCA1* function is required for transactivation of the estrogen receptor (ER) gene promoter
    - May explain why 90% of *BRCA1*-associated carcinomas are negative for ER
- **Incidence: 0.1-0.3%**
  - More common in some ethnic groups: Ashkenazi Jews, Finns, French Canadians
  - Mutation can be suspected in young patients (35% risk for a patient < 30 years of age with an ER-negative poorly differentiated cancer)

BREAST CARCINOMA, FEMALE

- **High penetrance: 40-90% lifetime risk**
  - Magnitude of risk can vary for different mutations and for different types of cancers
  - Responsible for ~ 1/2 of cancers known to be due to a germline mutation (~ 2% of all breast cancers)
- **Breast cancer**
  - Mean age of onset is 44 years, but age can vary with specific mutations
  - Risk of subsequent contralateral cancer is higher
  - ~ 90% of *BRCA1* cancers share same gene expression pattern with basal-type carcinomas defined by gene expression profiling
  - Morphology of invasive carcinomas
    - Circumscribed growth pattern with pushing borders, dense lymphocytic infiltrate
    - High nuclear grade and high proliferative rate
  - Medullary carcinomas are overrepresented: 13% of cases vs. < 5% for all women
    - Majority of women with medullary carcinomas do not have *BRCA1* mutations
    - Additional *BRCA1* carcinomas have "medullary features" but not all criteria for classification as classic medullary carcinoma
  - Tumor markers
    - Lack hormone receptor positivity
    - Lack overexpression of HER2: Both *HER2* and *BRCA1* are on long arm of chromosome 17, and loss of heterozygosity may affect both
    - 10-25% of women < 50 years of age with a triple-negative carcinoma will have a *BRCA1* mutation
- **Other associated cancers**
  - Ovarian, fallopian tube, primary peritoneal (40-50% lifetime risk)
    - Usually high-grade serous carcinomas
    - ~ 80% of women with both breast and ovarian cancer will have a *BRCA* mutation
    - Average age of onset: 49-53 years (compared to 63 years in general population)
  - Male breast cancer (1-5% lifetime risk, but ~ 1/2 risk of *BRCA2*)
  - Pancreas, cervix, uterus

BRCA2 (Hereditary Breast & Ovarian Cancer Syndrome)

- **Function**
  - Although *BRCA2* is not structurally related to *BRCA1*, both genes have very similar functions and regulatory roles
- **Incidence: 0.1-0.7%**
  - More common in some ethnic groups: Ashkenazi Jews, Icelandic populations
- **High penetrance: 45-85% lifetime risk**
  - Magnitude of risk can vary for different mutations and for different types of cancers
  - Responsible for ~ 1/2 of cancers known to be due to a germline mutation (~ 2% of all breast cancers)
- **Breast cancer**
  - Mean age of onset is 47 years but can vary with specific mutations
  - Group with luminal A or B by gene expression profiling
  - Majority are high grade
    - ER positive
    - HER2 negative
- **Other associated cancers**
  - Ovary, fallopian tube, primary peritoneal (10-20% lifetime risk)
    - Usual age of onset: 55-58 years (compared to 63 years in general population)
  - Male breast cancer: 5-10% lifetime risk; ~ 5-15% of cases are associated with *BRCA2*
    - Also increased risk of early onset aggressive prostate cancer
  - Pancreas, gallbladder, stomach, bile duct, melanoma

TP53 (Li-Fraumeni Syndrome)

- **Function**
  - Central role in cell cycle control, DNA replication, DNA repair, and apoptosis
- **Incidence: 0.0025%**
  - Population in southeastern Brazil has 1/300 incidence
- **High penetrance: > 90% lifetime risk of breast cancer for women**
  - Penetrance varies for different mutations
- **Breast cancer**
  - 1/3 of malignancies in affected families
    - Early onset: Average age at diagnosis is 33 years
    - ~ 55% of women will develop breast cancer by age 45
    - ~ 2-7% of women with breast cancer were diagnosed at < 30 years of age
    - Rare for breast cancer to be diagnosed after age 50
  - Most common type is ER positive and HER2 positive (~ 55%)
  - Male breast cancer has not been reported
- **Other associated cancers**
  - Sarcomas: Most occur in children < 10 years of age
    - However, Ewing sarcoma, gastrointestinal stromal tumor (GIST), desmoid tumor, and angiosarcoma have not been reported
  - Adrenal cortical carcinoma: Most occur in children around 3 years of age
  - Brain tumors: Occur in children or in 4th-5th decades

CDH1 (Familial Gastric Cancer and Lobular Breast Cancer Syndrome)

- **Function**
  - *CDH1* encodes gene for E-cadherin
  - E-cadherin is a protein involved in cell-to-cell adhesion
  - Mutations interfere with function
    - 75-80% are truncating mutations, 20-25% are missense mutations, and 7% are large deletions
    - Loss of protein results in cells rounding up and single-cell infiltrative pattern due to lack of adhesion to adjacent cells
- **Incidence: 0.005%**
- **High penetrance: ~ 40-50% lifetime risk for women**
- **Breast cancer**
  - Women are at increased risk for lobular carcinoma

- However, majority of women with lobular carcinomas do not have *CDH1* germline mutations
  - Loss of E-cadherin prevents cell adhesion, resulting in single tumor cells with rounded contours
- **Other associated cancers**
  - 70-85% lifetime risk of developing gastric signet ring cell carcinoma in majority of families
    - Gastric carcinomas are more common than breast carcinomas in most affected families
    - Families developing only breast cancer have also been identified

PTEN (Cowden Syndrome)

- **Function**
  - Dual specificity phosphatase gene involved in control of proliferation signals and apoptosis
- **Incidence: 0.0005%**
- **High penetrance: 25-50% lifetime risk of breast cancer for women**
- **Breast cancer**
  - Early onset; most women diagnosed between 38 and 46 years of age
  - Men also at increased risk for breast cancer; magnitude of risk not yet determined
  - Other breast lesions include fibroadenomas and hamartomas
- **Other associated tumors**
  - Multiple hamartomas (including trichilemmomas)
  - Thyroid, and endometrial cancer

ATM (Ataxia-Telangiectasia Carriers)

- **Function**
  - Serine threonine kinase that phosphorylates *TP53* and *BRCA1* in response to DNA double-strand breaks
  - Homozygosity results in ataxia-telangiectasia
    - Progressive cerebellar ataxia, oculocutaneous telangiectasias, immunodeficiency, and increased risk of leukemia and lymphoma
- **Incidence: 0.5%**
- **High penetrance: 11% by age 50 and 30% by age 70**
- **Breast cancer**
  - Earlier onset than sporadic breast cancer

CHEK2

- **Function**
  - Cell cycle checkpoint gene involved in DNA repair
- **Incidence: 0.5%**
- **High penetrance: ~ 40% lifetime risk for women**
- **Breast cancer**
  - Later onset
  - Increased risk for males
  - No reported specific histologic types; 70-80% are ER positive (similar to sporadic breast cancer)

STK11/LKB1 (Peutz-Jeghers Syndrome)

- **Function**
  - Serine/threonine kinase that regulates how cells respond to proliferation signals depending on ATP availability
- **Incidence: 0.001%**
- **High penetrance: ~ 40% lifetime risk for women**
- **Breast cancer**
  - Early onset: 8% by age 40 and 32% by age 60
  - No reported specific histologic types
- **Other associated lesions**
  - Hamartomatous gastrointestinal polyps (including small intestine) and skin pigmentation (lips and buccal mucosa)
  - Skin pigmentation (lips and buccal mucosa)
  - Ovarian cancer (sex cord stromal tumors are most common): ~ 20% risk
  - Increased risk of cancer of colon, stomach, pancreas, small intestine, thyroid, lung, uterus, ovary, and cervix

Genetic Testing

- **Population to be tested**
  - American Society of Clinical Oncology recommends that patients with a > 10% mutation risk undergo testing for *BRCA1* and *BRCA2* mutations
    - This approach will detect 85% of mutation carriers
  - Patients meeting criteria for Li-Fraumeni syndrome or Li-Fraumeni-like syndrome have > 15% risk of having a mutation
  - Group of genes conferring a low increased risk for breast cancer has been identified
    - Genes functionally related to *BRCA1* and *BRCA2*: *BARD1, CHEK1, MRE11A, NBN, RAD50, RAD51D*
    - Genes in the Fanconi anemia pathway: *PALB2, RAD51C (FANCO), BRIP1, RAD51B*
    - Other genes: *MUTYH, PMS2*
    - For many of these genes, the risk of breast cancer is not yet clear
    - Limited information is available for variants of unknown significance
    - Testing for mutations in these genes may only be of value in selected cases
  - Individuals may undergo testing for rare genes in the following settings
    - Testing has excluded mutations in *BRCA1, BRCA2,* and *TP53*
    - Clinical setting is suggestive of a specific gene mutation
    - Mutation has been identified in the family
  - Counseling should occur before testing to ensure patient is aware of possible implications for individual and family
- **Predictive models**
  - National Comprehensive Cancer Network issues clinical guidelines for identifying individuals with a high risk of *BRCA1, BRCA2, TP53,* or *PTEN* mutations
    - Version 1.2013 is available at www.nccn.org/professionals/physician_gls/pdf/genetics_screening.pdf
  - *BRCA1* and *BRCA2*
    - Multiple models available
  - *TP53*
    - Classical Li-Fraumeni criteria
    - Chompret criteria
  - *PTEN*
    - Available at http://www.lerner.ccf.org/gmi/ccscore/index.php
- **Genetic testing**

BREAST CARCINOMA, FEMALE

- Full genome sequencing is required to detect all mutations
  - All testing for *BRCA1* and *BRCA2* mutations in the USA is performed by Myriad Genetics (Salt Lake City, Utah)
  - Full genome sequencing (or full exome sequencing) is commercially available and will likely decrease in cost to make testing for all genes possible in many individuals
- Limited sequence analysis can be used to detect the most likely mutation
  - Common mutations found in ethnic groups, e.g., 2 *BRCA1* and 1 *BRCA2* mutations comprise 90% of mutations found in Ashkenazi Jewish population
  - Hotspots for mutations within gene
  - Detection of a known mutation in a family
- Duplications, inversions, large deletions, and mutations in noncoding regions may not be detected by standard sequence analysis
  - 18% of genetic changes in *BRCA1* and *BRCA2* are not detected by standard testing
  - If a known mutation is not found in the initial test, additional testing may be performed
  - BRACAnalysis large rearrangement test (BART) detects some rearrangements
  - Account for 17% of deleterious mutations in individuals from the Near East/Middle East and 22% of deleterious mutations in individuals from Latin America/Caribbean
  - None of the current tests detect every deleterious change
- Variants of unknown significance (VUS)
  - Genetic polymorphism that has not yet been associated with an increased risk of cancer
  - Found in 3-7% of individuals tested for *BRCA1* and *BRCA2*
  - > 1,500 identified
  - More frequent in minority ethnic populations; however, frequency has been decreasing as more individuals are studied
  - Must be identified in multiple individuals to determine clinical significance

- **Testing families with a history of cancer**
  - Most useful, begin testing individual with cancer
    - If multiple affected individuals are present within a kindred, testing can establish linkage between cancer(s) and mutation
  - Once a mutation is detected, other family members without cancer may choose testing
  - Analysis for specific mutation in other family members is considerably less expensive

Cancer Risk Management

- **Chemoprevention**
  - Tamoxifen reduces the risk of ER-positive cancer for women with a family history of breast cancer
    - However, risk of endometrial cancer and thrombosis is increased
  - Tamoxifen reduces risk of cancers for *BRCA2* carriers but not for *BRCA1* carriers
    - However, few women have been studied
  - Tamoxifen reduces risk of subsequent ipsilateral and contralateral cancer in breast cancer patients with *BRCA1* and *BRCA2* germline mutations
  - Benefit of chemoprevention for *BRCA* carriers without breast cancer is less clear (few studies)
- **Screening**
  - Clinical breast examination 2x yearly starting at age 25
    - Patient self-breast awareness with periodic breast examinations
  - Mammography at earlier age (10 years before age at which the youngest relative with cancer was diagnosed) or more frequently
  - MR screening more sensitive than mammography in young women with dense breasts
    - However, lower specificity leads to greater numbers of biopsies for benign lesions
  - Screening, mammography, and MR may be staggered every 6 months to decrease the screening interval
- **Prophylactic surgery**
  - Women with *BRCA1* & *BRCA2* mutations are at increased risk for subsequent ipsilateral (~ 2-3% per year) and contralateral (~ 2-6%) cancer
    - Recurrence rates are higher for women with very early onset cancer (< 42 years)
    - Ipsilateral cancers are likely new primary cancers rather than true recurrences
    - Recurrence does not alter survival, as 2nd cancers are likely found at an early stage
  - Bilateral mastectomy reduces risk by 97%
    - Not all breast tissue can be removed in all patients with acceptable cosmetic results
    - Major benefit to women prior to development of breast cancer; limited or no benefit after breast cancer diagnosis with possible distant metastases
  - Bilateral salpingo-oophorectomy for mutations associated with ovarian cancer
    - Reduces risk of ovarian and fallopian tube cancer by 70-96%
    - Reduces risk of breast cancer by 50% in premenopausal women, presumably due to decrease in hormone production
    - Reduces risk of ER(-) breast cancers for *BRCA1* patients to a lesser degree; mechanism is unknown

SELECTED REFERENCES

1. Euhus DM et al: Genetic predisposition syndromes and their management. Surg Clin North Am. 93(2):341-62, 2013
2. Drohan B et al: Hereditary breast and ovarian cancer and other hereditary syndromes: using technology to identify carriers. Ann Surg Oncol. 19(6):1732-7, 2012
3. Gage M et al: Translational advances regarding hereditary breast cancer syndromes. J Surg Oncol. 105(5):444-51, 2012
4. Lynch HT et al: Hereditary breast cancer: practical pursuit for clinical translation. Ann Surg Oncol. 19(6):1723-31, 2012
5. Shannon KM et al: Genetic testing by cancer site: breast. Cancer J. 18(4):310-9, 2012

General Features

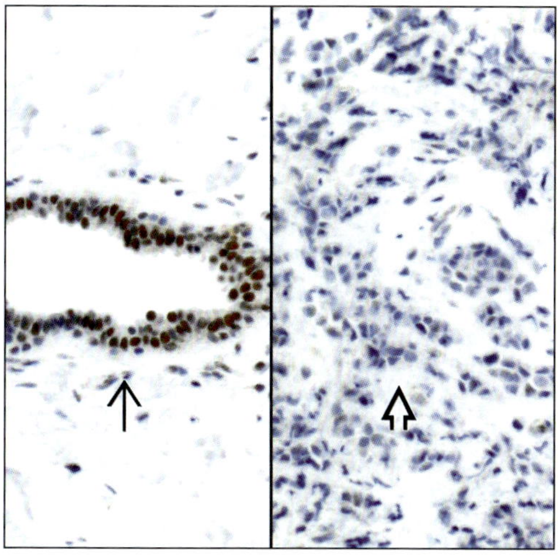

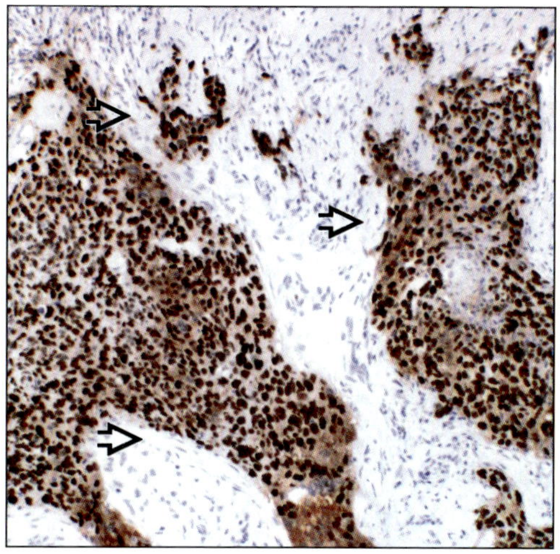

(Left) *The majority of hereditary breast cancer genes are tumor suppressors. Proteins are expressed in normal cells. BRCA2 is shown here. When the normal allele is mutated, expression is lost, resulting in genomic instability and the formation of tumors.* ***(Right)*** *TP53 is an unusual member of this group, as mutations can cause either loss of function or gain of function. Many mutated forms fail to be degraded, resulting in protein accumulation in the nucleus.*

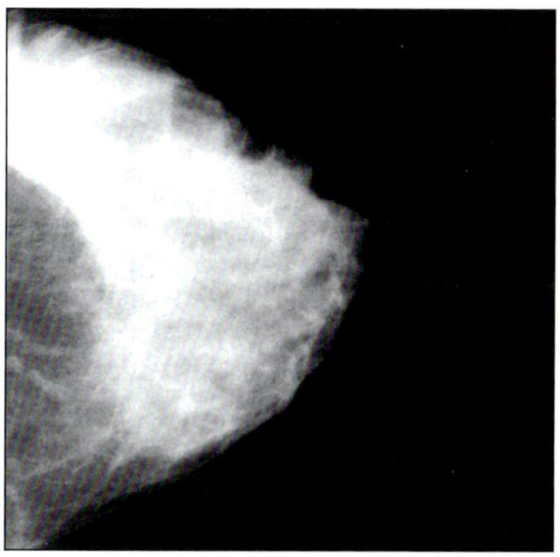

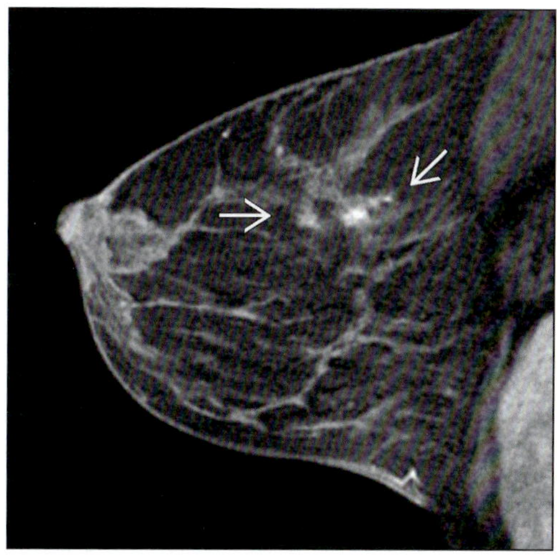

(Left) *Hereditary carcinomas arise at earlier ages as women are born with cells with the 1st alteration, leading to neoplasia. Breast tissue is often dense, making detection of tumor by mammography difficult.* ***(Right)*** *MR can be a useful technique for screening young high-risk women with dense breasts. This woman with a BRCA1 mutation has an area of clumped linear enhancement that proved to be DCIS that was not detected by screening mammography.*

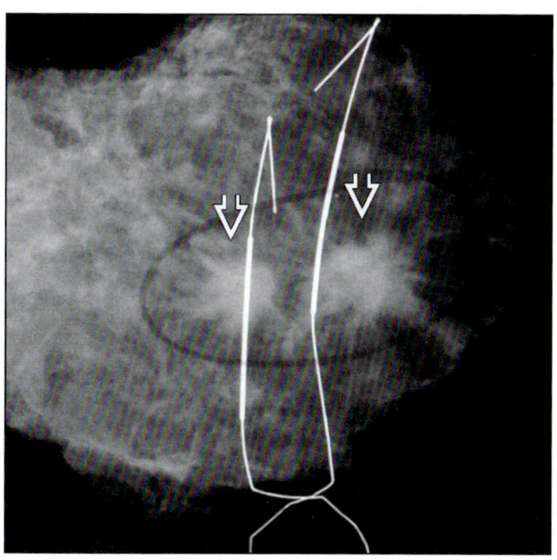

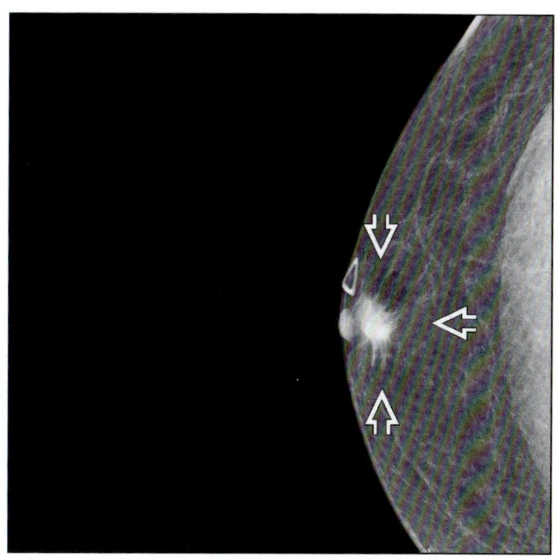

(Left) *Patients with germline mutations are more likely to develop multiple cancers, either synchronously or metachronously. Prophylactic mastectomy is an effective method to reduce the risk of cancer.* ***(Right)*** *Male breast cancer is increased by some germline mutations (including BRCA2, BRCA1, PTEN, and CHEK2), but the risk is lower than that for females. Male risk is not increased by other germline mutations (TP53). The reason for this gender specificity is unknown.*

BREAST CARCINOMA, FEMALE

BRCA1- and BRCA2-Associated Cancers

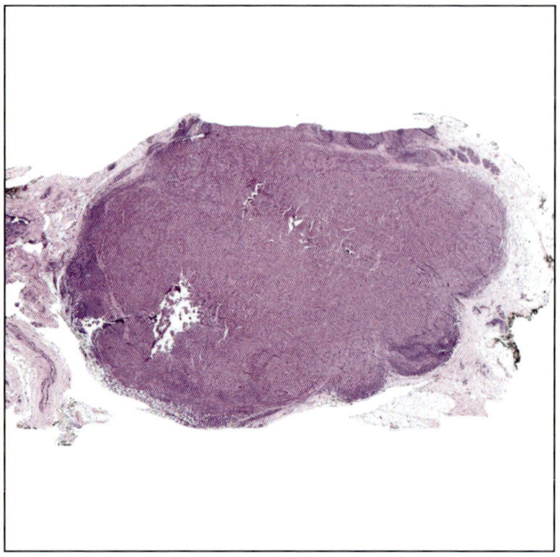

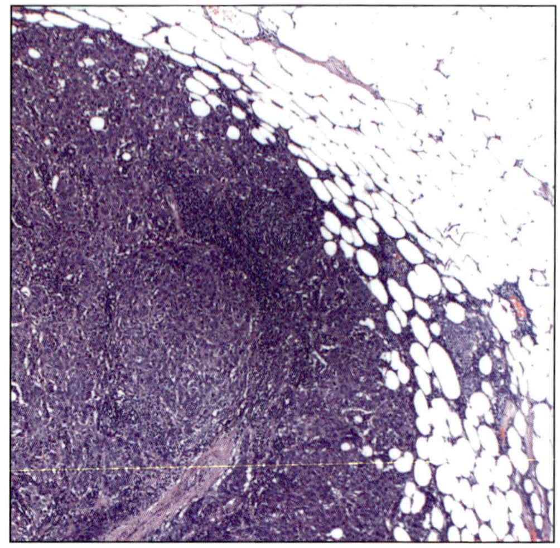

(Left) *BRCA1-associated breast cancers typically have circumscribed borders. These cancers can be mistaken for benign lesions in young women. However, growth can be quite rapid.* ***(Right)*** *BRCA1 carcinomas have high-grade nuclei, and the cells grow in a syncytial pattern. There is typically a dense lymphocytic infiltrate. Almost all carcinomas are negative for ER, PR, and HER2. 10-25% of women under the age of 50 with this type of carcinoma will have a germline mutation.*

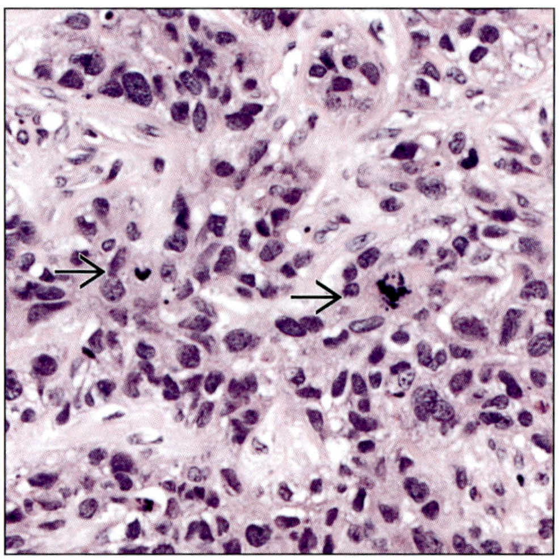

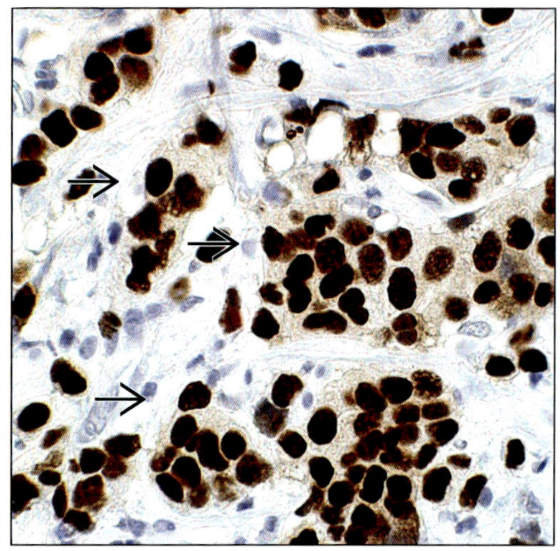

(Left) *Carcinomas associated with BRCA2 mutations are often poorly differentiated and have a high mitotic rate →. These cancers are typically classified as luminal A or B by gene expression profiling. They do not have the distinctive histologic features associated with BRCA1 mutations.* ***(Right)*** *Unlike BRCA1 cancers, BRCA2 cancers are usually positive for estrogen receptors →. Both types of carcinoma are almost always negative for HER2.*

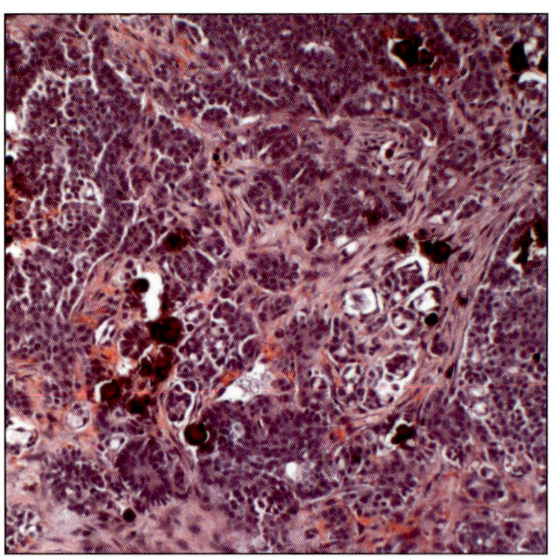

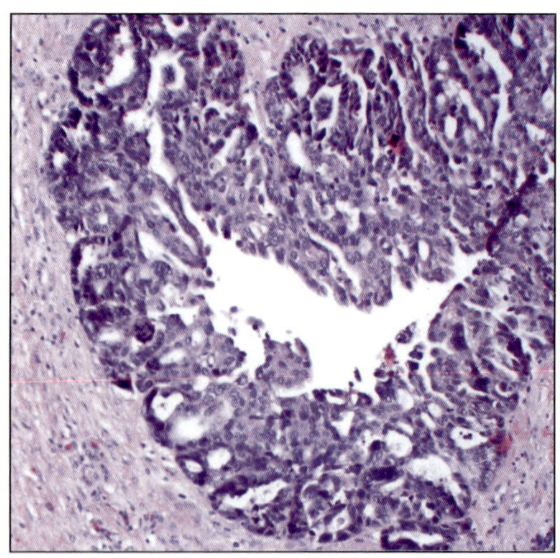

(Left) *Women with BRCA1 and BRCA2 mutations are at increased risk for ovarian carcinomas, such as this papillary serous carcinoma. Approximately 80% of women with both breast and ovarian carcinoma will have a BRCA mutation.* ***(Right)*** *Women with BRCA1 and BRCA2 mutations may choose to undergo prophylactic salpingo-oophorectomy to reduce the risk of ovarian cancer. Early tumors are frequently found in the end of the fallopian tube. Patients remain at risk for primary peritoneal carcinomas.*

TP53- and CDH1-Associated Breast Cancers

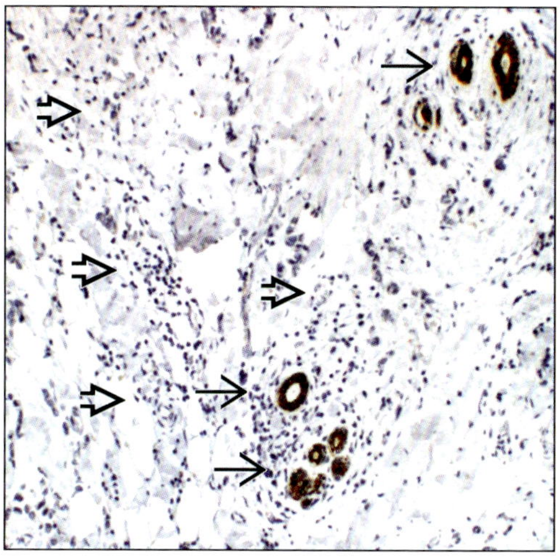

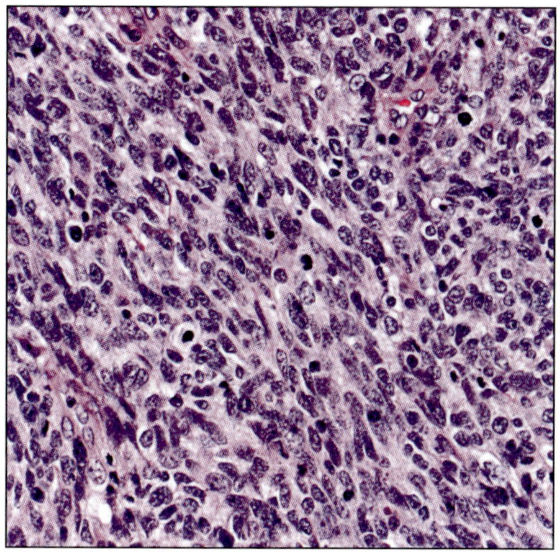

(Left) *E-cadherin is a cell adhesion molecule normally expressed by breast epithelial cells* → *. Lobular carcinomas lose expression of this protein* ⇨ *. The majority of lobular carcinomas lose E-cadherin expression due to somatic mutations.* ***(Right)*** *Individuals with Li-Fraumeni syndrome are at increased risk for a wide variety of tumors throughout their lifetimes, including adrenal carcinomas, sarcomas (alveolar rhabdomyosarcoma pictured), brain tumors, and others.*

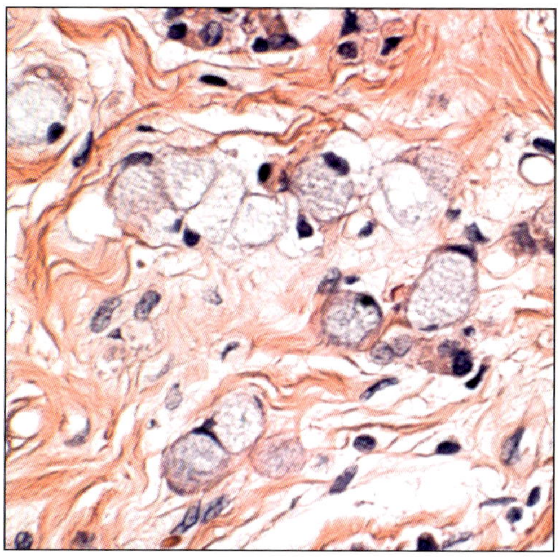

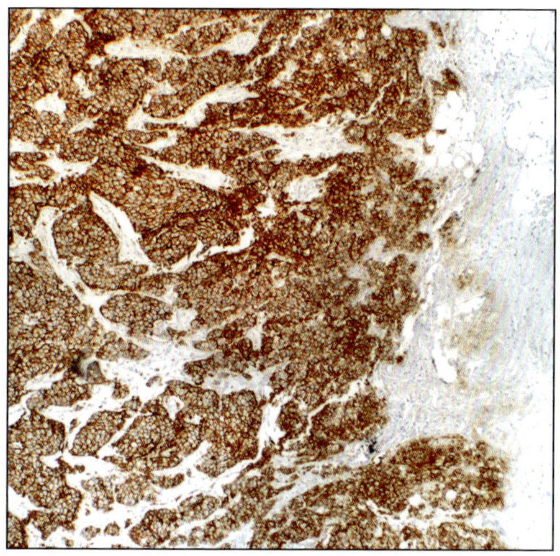

(Left) *Families with germline mutations of E-cadherin (CDH1) are at greater risk for gastric signet ring cell carcinomas rather than breast carcinomas. Both stomach and breast carcinomas have similar histologic appearances due to the loss of cell adhesion; however, the signet ring cells of gastric carcinomas typically have finely vacuolated cytoplasm.* ***(Right)*** *Over 1/2 of TP53-associated carcinomas are positive for estrogen receptor and HER2 (shown here).*

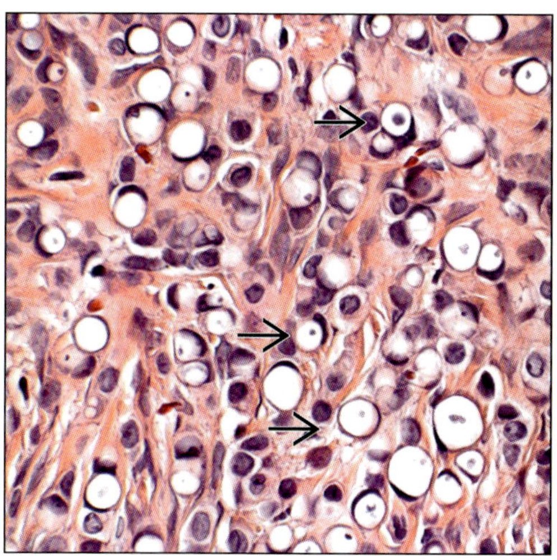

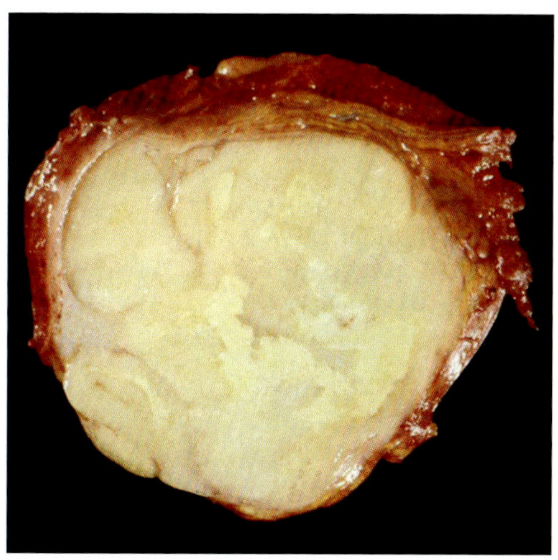

(Left) *Individuals with germline E-cadherin (CDH1) mutations develop lobular carcinomas. Due to the loss of cell adhesion, the cells are rounded and infiltrate as single cells. Many lobular carcinomas have signet ring cells that typically have a single vacuole with a mucin droplet* → *, rather than the foamy cytoplasm more typical of signet ring cell gastric carcinomas.* ***(Right)*** *80% of children with adrenal cortical carcinoma (shown here) have germline TP53 mutations. The median age of onset is 3 years.*

BREAST CARCINOMA, MALE

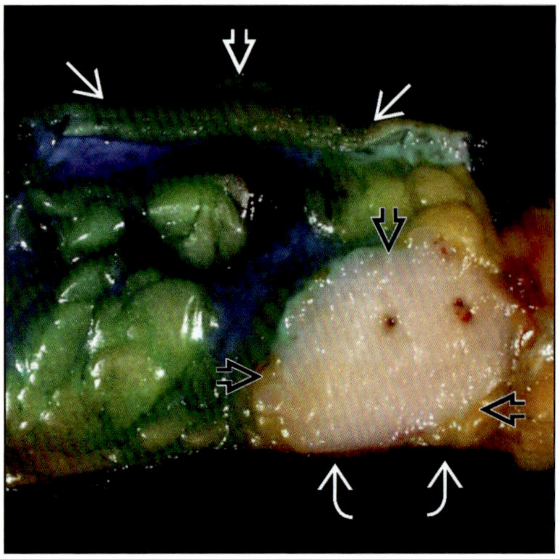

Male breast cancer (MBC) typically presents as an irregular firm mass ⊳ close to skin ➡, nipple ⊳, and chest wall ➡. Invasion of these structures can occur early in the course of the disease.

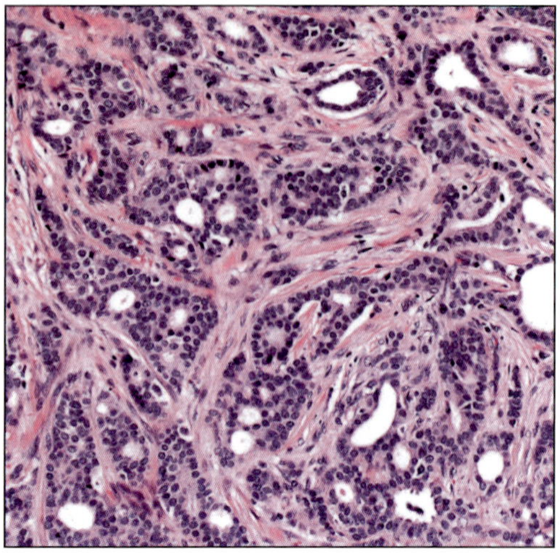

Invasive ductal carcinoma of no special type is the most common histology seen in male breast cancer and is identical in appearance to carcinomas in females. The majority express hormone receptors.

TERMINOLOGY

Abbreviations

- Male breast cancer (MBC)

ETIOLOGY/PATHOGENESIS

Environmental Exposure

- Radiation exposure
  - Occupational exposure
  - Therapeutic chest wall radiation
- Electromagnetic field exposure
- Occupational exposure to gasoline and airline fuels

Disorders Associated With Hormonal Imbalance

- Klinefelter syndrome (XXY karyotype)
- Obesity
- Testicular disorders associated with hypogonadism
  - Mumps orchitis, cryptorchidism, testicular injury
- Liver disease
- Diabetes
- Hyperthyroidism
- Alcohol abuse

Gynecomastia

- Generally not considered to be MBC risk factor
  - Some studies have suggested a slight increased risk
    - May be attributed to fact that both conditions share similar risk factors (hormonal imbalance)

Genetics (Family History)

- 5-10% of all breast cancer is attributable to mutations in high penetrance breast cancer susceptibility genes
  - ~ 15-20% of MBC patients have family history of breast or ovarian cancer
  - Risk increased in cases of an affected sister (RR 2.25) or mother and sister (RR 9.73)
- High-risk breast cancer germline mutations associated with male breast cancer
  - *BRCA1* (17q21) hereditary breast and ovarian cancer syndrome
    - For male *BRCA1* mutation carrier, estimated lifetime risk for MBC is 1.8% (< 4% of MBC is associated with *BRCA1*)
    - Lower risk than for *BRCA2* mutation carriers
  - *BRCA2* (13q12.3) hereditary breast and ovarian cancer syndrome
    - For male *BRCA2* mutation carrier, estimated lifetime risk for MBC is ~ 7% (compared with < 1% in general population)
    - There is a 60-75% chance of a *BRCA2* mutation in a family with an MBC patient
    - Also associated with increased risk for prostate cancer, pancreatic cancer, and GI tract malignancies
  - *PTEN* (10q23.3) Cowden syndrome
- Moderate/low-risk breast cancer susceptibility gene associated with male breast cancer
  - *CHEK2* (22q12.1)
- Klinefelter syndrome (47XXY karyotype)
  - Patients suffer hormonal imbalance (estrogen > testosterone)
  - Marked increased relative risk for MBC
    - Lobule formation may occur

CLINICAL ISSUES

Epidemiology

- Incidence
  - MBC accounts for < 1% of all breast cancer
    - ~ 1% of all cancers seen in men
    - 0.13% of all cancer deaths in men annually
    - Incidence has remained stable (2000-2005)
- Age
  - MBC tends to occur in slightly older age group compared to female breast cancer (FBC)

BREAST CARCINOMA, MALE

Key Facts

Terminology

- Male breast cancer (MBC)
- Accounts for ~ 1% of breast cancer cases
- In situ and invasive carcinoma occur
- Histologically identical to female breast carcinoma

Etiology/Pathogenesis

- ~ 15-20% of MBC patients report a family history of breast or ovarian cancer
- Risk associated with *BRCA1* is lower than that for *BRCA2*
  - *BRCA2* mutation carrier: Estimated lifetime risk ~ 7% for MBC (compared with < 1% in general population)
- Men with a *BRCA2* mutation are at risk for other malignancies

Clinical Issues

- Typically presents with painless firm palpable mass

Microscopic Pathology

- Similar to female breast cancer
- Same prognostic factors are used in males and females

Ancillary Tests

- ER(+) in 90%, PR(+) in 80% of MBC
- HER2 overexpression and gene amplification may be present but less frequent than incidence in FBC

Top Differential Diagnoses

- Gynecomastia
- Myofibroblastoma

    - Mean age: 67 years (MBC) vs. 61 years (FBC)
    - Younger males may also be affected
  - Compared with sporadic MBC, median age of onset for familial MBC is typically younger

Presentation

- Majority present with painless firm mass
  - Located in the subareolar region
  - Tends to be located eccentrically in relationship to nipple
  - Fixation to skin &/or pectoralis muscle is common
- Less commonly presents as nipple discharge, bloody or serous
  - May be associated with papillary ductal carcinoma in situ (DCIS)
  - Rarely presents as Paget disease of nipple
- Diagnosis may be delayed
  - MBC is rare and is often not detected early
  - Cancers usually diagnosed at higher stages as compared to FBC

Treatment

- Surgical approaches
  - Majority of males will undergo mastectomy
    - Breast conservation is not relevant for cosmesis
  - Sentinel lymph node biopsy can be performed
- Adjuvant therapy
  - Management is similar to that for postmenopausal FBC
  - Adjuvant treatment based on TNM stage, tumor grade, hormone receptors, and HER2 status

Prognosis

- Similar to that for FBC of similar stage and grade
  - Mainly determined by TNM stage, tumor grade, and receptor status
- Often more advanced at diagnosis compared with FBC
  - > 40% of MBC presents with stage III or IV disease at diagnosis, which adversely influences prognosis
  - Minimal breast tissue in males results in cancers being closer to skin and chest wall
    - Invasion of these structures occurs earlier
    - Increases likelihood of vascular invasion and nodal metastasis

IMAGE FINDINGS

General Features

- Radiographic examination can contribute to diagnosis of a mass lesion in a male patient
  - Abnormalities similar to those seen in FBC present in 80-90% of cases

Mammographic Findings

- Typically shows mass lesion that is "taller than wide"
  - Irregular spiculated margins
    - Often coarse microcalcifications
- Unlike gynecomastia, lesions tend to be eccentric in relationship to nipple
  - Gynecomastia has a flame-shaped appearance extending symmetrically from the nipple

Ultrasonographic Findings

- Distinguishes solid masses from cysts
  - Useful in identifying solid masses that are more likely to be malignant

MACROSCOPIC FEATURES

General Features

- Majority are irregular, firm, gray to white masses
  - In situ component may appear grossly as partially cystic
- Fixation to skin or pectoralis muscle is common
- Rarely, scaling exudate of nipple due to Paget disease occurs
  - Typically not seen in pathology specimens as skin is cleansed prior to surgery

Size

- 1-5 cm (usually 2-2.5 cm)

BREAST CARCINOMA, MALE

MICROSCOPIC PATHOLOGY

Histologic Features

- **Carcinoma in situ (DCIS, lobular carcinoma in situ [LCIS])**
  - DCIS accounts for ~ 10% of all MBC
    - LCIS is extremely rare in male patients
  - DCIS is microscopically similar to that seen in FBC
    - All architectural patterns have been reported
    - Greater incidence of papillary DCIS compared with FBC
    - Less likely to see comedonecrosis in DCIS in MBC compared with FBC
- **Invasive carcinoma**
  - Invasive ductal carcinoma of no special type is most common
    - Identical in appearance to that occurring in FBC
  - Special histologic types are unusual in MBC
    - Papillary carcinomas are most common special type
    - Invasive lobular carcinoma occurs rarely
    - Other special histologic types (medullary, mucinous, tubular) are also very rare
  - Graded using same system as for FBC (Elston and Ellis modification of Scarff-Bloom-Richardson histologic grading)
    - Carcinomas of grades 2 and 3 reported in 80% of cases

ANCILLARY TESTS

Immunohistochemistry

- Hormone receptors
  - Estrogen receptor (ER) positive in 90%
  - Progesterone receptor (PR) positive in 80%
- HER2
  - Overexpression occurs but less frequent than in FBC

Molecular Genetics

- Molecular analysis shows disease subtypes similar to those reported for FBC
  - Luminal subtype most common (90%)
    - Less frequent HER2 (8%) and basal (2%) subtypes in reported series

DIFFERENTIAL DIAGNOSIS

Gynecomastia

- Nonneoplastic enlargement of male breast tissue due to hyperplasia of epithelium and stroma
  - Variety of etiologies linked to an imbalance in ratio of free androgens and estrogens
  - Can be seen in infants, during puberty, or in elderly
- Often bilateral
  - If unilateral or asymmetric, can raise concern for carcinoma

Myofibroblastoma

- Clinical presentation (elderly male, palpable mass) may overlap with MBC
  - Usually discrete, well-circumscribed mass lesion
- Uniform proliferation of spindle-shaped myofibroblasts with well-circumscribed borders
  - Oval nuclei, pale cytoplasm, mitotic figures rare
  - Hyalinized bands of dense collagen separate spindle cells into groups or clusters
  - Varying degree of adipose tissue seen in some lesions
- Rarely, an epithelioid variant can be encountered
  - Can mimic invasive lobular carcinoma
    - Lesional cells express ER, PR, and AR
    - Cells are negative for cytokeratin

Metastases

- Metastatic tumors to breast can mimic primary breast carcinoma
  - Need to integrate prior history, clinical and imaging findings, and compare with prior biopsy material, if available
  - Suspect when cancer has an unusual appearance, is negative for ER and PR, &/or lacks in situ carcinoma
- Immunohistochemical markers can be helpful
  - Breast carcinoma
    - Usually CK7(+)/CK20(-), but significant overlap with other tumor immunophenotypes (e.g., lung)
    - ER(+) (70-90%), PR(+) (60-70%)
    - GCDFP-15(+) (50-75%)
    - Mammaglobin (+) (40-70%)
    - DCIS often present and can be supported by markers for myoepithelial cells
  - Lung adenocarcinoma
    - Usually CK7(+)/CK20(-)
    - TTF1(+) &/or NAPSIN-A(+) helpful
    - Very rare breast cancers are TTF1(+); often have a neuroendocrine (small cell) appearance
  - Prostate carcinoma
    - Treatment for prostate carcinoma can increase risk for breast cancer (orchiectomy, hormonal therapy)
    - Hyperplasia associated with hormonal changes can be difficult to distinguish from carcinoma in situ
    - If patient is receiving hormonal therapy, this treatment can also alter appearance of metastatic prostate cancer or breast cancer
    - Usually CK7(-), PSA(+), PAP(+)
    - Some prostate cancers are ER(+)
    - Although uncommon, some breast cancers are PSA(+)
    - PAP should be negative in breast cancer

SELECTED REFERENCES

1. Nilsson C et al: Molecular subtyping of male breast cancer using alternative definitions and its prognostic impact. Acta Oncol. 52(1):102-9, 2013
2. Deb S et al: Genotypic and phenotypic analysis of male breast cancer shows under representation of the HER2 and basal subtypes in BRCA-associated carcinomas. BMC Cancer. 12(1):510, 2012
3. Sánchez-Muñoz A et al: Male breast cancer: immunohistochemical subtypes and clinical outcome characterization. Oncology. 83(4):228-33, 2012

Imaging and Microscopic Features

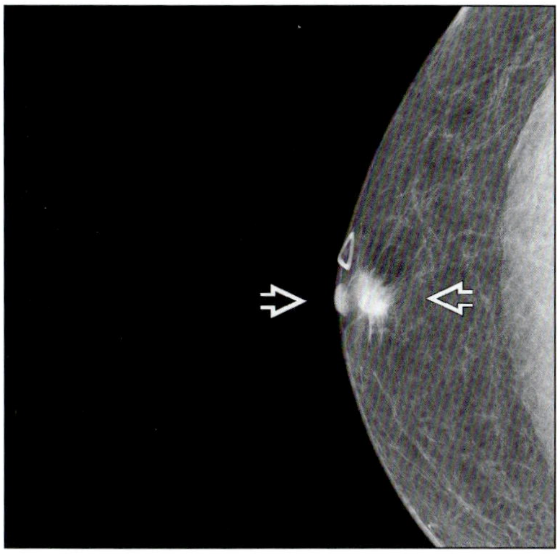

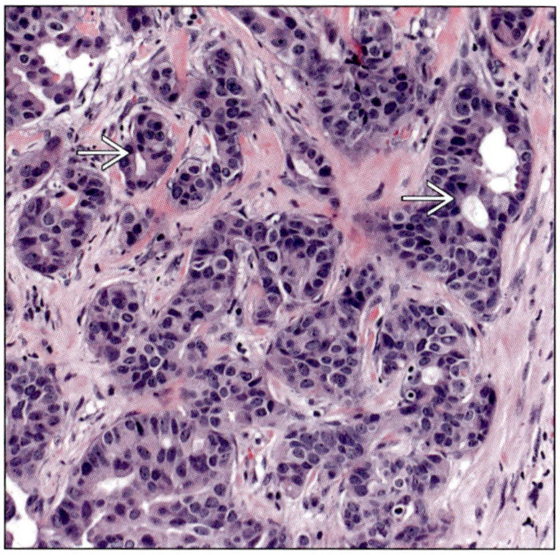

(Left) *This breast cancer was initially mistaken for gynecomastia due to the location directly behind the nipple. Most male cancers are eccentrically displaced from the nipple.* ***(Right)*** *Breast cancers arising in males and females are morphologically similar. The majority of male cancers are invasive carcinomas of no special type. These carcinomas are more likely to be higher grade compared with female breast cancer (FBC). Carcinoma in situ is rarely seen in males in isolation.*

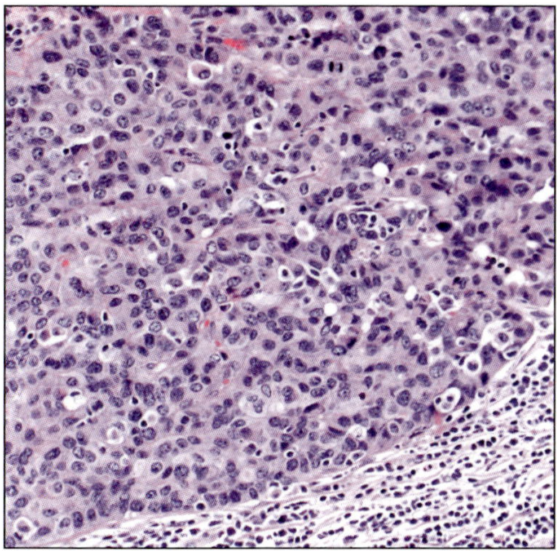

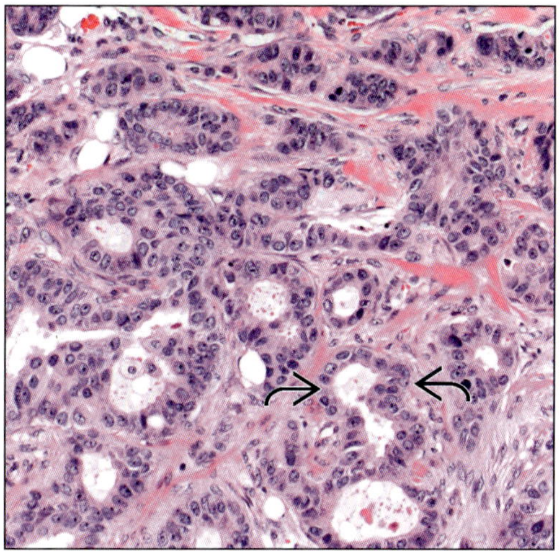

(Left) *The risk for breast cancer is lower for males with germline mutations in BRCA1 as compared to BRCA2. This male BRCA1 carrier developed a high-grade invasive ductal carcinoma.* ***(Right)*** *Breast cancer arising in male BRCA2 mutation carriers are predominantly invasive ductal carcinomas of no special type. Earlier reports suggested a higher incidence of tubulolobular and pleomorphic lobular carcinoma with BRCA2. However, this has not been seen in more recent series.*

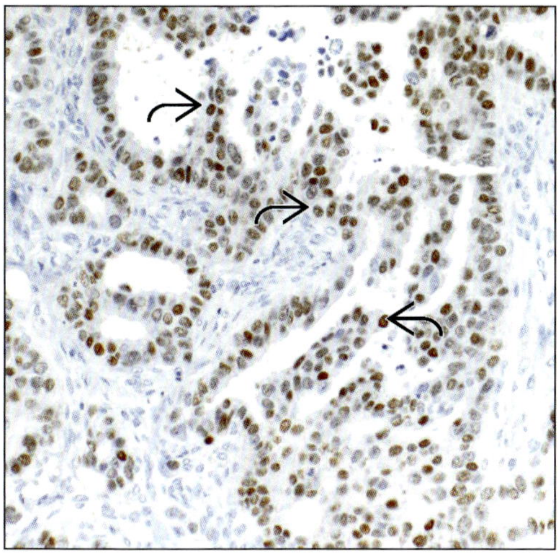

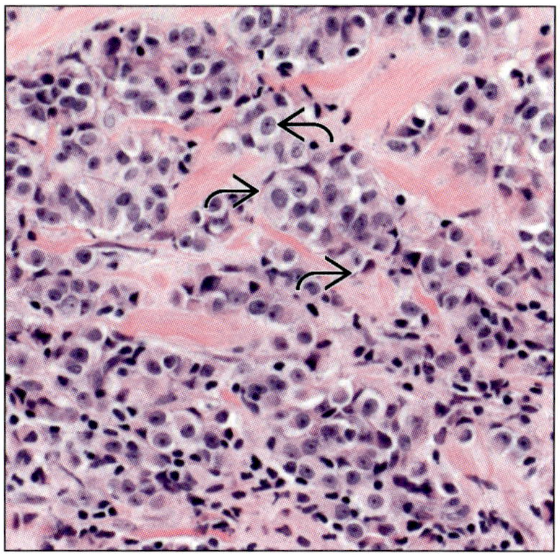

(Left) *Most MBCs express estrogen receptor and progesterone receptor. HER2 overexpression and gene amplification are less common compared with FBC.* ***(Right)*** *BRCA2 mutation carriers are at increased risk for MBC and other tumors, such as prostate and pancreatic cancer. A 70-year-old BRCA2(+) man presented with a palpable mass and was diagnosed with invasive lobular carcinoma. He was found to have an elevated serum PSA and prostate cancer.*

Blood and Bone Marrow

CHRONIC LYMPHOCYTIC LEUKEMIA/SMALL LYMPHOCYTIC LYMPHOMA

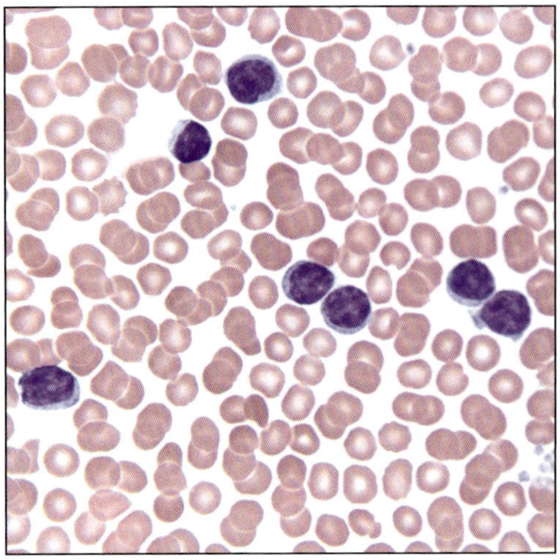

Image shows peripheral blood involved by chronic lymphocytic leukemia (CLL)/small lymphocytic leukemia (SLL). The lymphocytes have sparse cytoplasm, round to oval nuclei, and small to indistinct nucleoli.

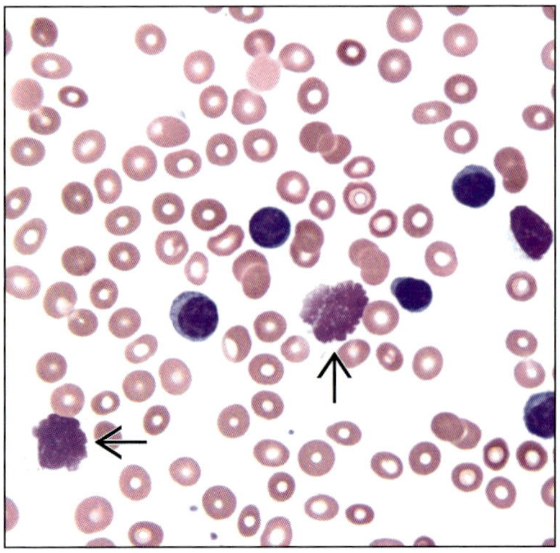

Image shows peripheral blood involved by CLL/SLL. Admixed among the neoplastic lymphocytes are "smudge cells" ⇒, an artifact of slide preparation.

TERMINOLOGY

Abbreviations

- Chronic lymphocytic leukemia (CLL)/small lymphocytic lymphoma (SLL)

Definitions

- Neoplasm of monomorphic, small round B cells in peripheral blood, bone marrow, lymph nodes, and spleen
- CLL/SLL cells usually coexpress CD5 and CD23
- SLL is used for nonleukemic cases in which tissue infiltrate has morphology and immunophenotype of CLL
- Prolymphocytes and paraimmunoblasts form proliferation centers in tissues

ETIOLOGY/PATHOGENESIS

Familial

- Relatives of patients with CLL demonstrate 8.5x increased risk of CLL

CLINICAL ISSUES

Presentation

- Lymphadenopathy, generalized
  - Occurs primarily in persons older than 50 years
  - Most patients are asymptomatic
  - Patients with SLL present with lymphadenopathy and often develop lymphocytosis
  - Patients with CLL present with lymphocytosis and fatigue and may develop lymphadenopathy
  - Organ infiltration → splenomegaly, hypersplenism, and peripheral cytopenias
  - Bone marrow becomes extensively infiltrated by neoplastic cells, resulting in severe anemia, thrombocytopenia, and neutropenia
  - Patients with CLL/SLL have significantly impaired immunologic activity
  - Autoimmunity frequently seen in CLL/SLL; up to 25% of patients develop Coombs (+) autoimmune hemolytic anemia
  - Red cell aplasia is rare occurrence
  - Serum M component present in some patients

Treatment

- CLL/SLL not considered to be curable with available therapy
- Chemoimmunotherapy combinations of fludarabine, cyclophosphamide, and rituximab (FCR) result in complete response rate of 72%

Prognosis

- Median survival: 7.5 years
  - 5-year survival (79%)
  - 10-year survival (< 30%)
  - Clinical staging systems: Rai (0-IV) and Binet (A-C) are best predictors of survival

MACROSCOPIC FEATURES

Lymph Node Features

- Lymph nodes are enlarged, and cut surface usually shows diffuse replacement
- Necrosis is rare

MICROSCOPIC PATHOLOGY

Histologic Features

- Lymph nodes
  - Vaguely nodular pattern with alternating dark zones of mature CLL cells and light zones (proliferation centers)
  - Predominant cell is small lymphocyte with clumped chromatin, usually round nucleus, and occasionally small nucleolus

CHRONIC LYMPHOCYTIC LEUKEMIA/SMALL LYMPHOCYTIC LYMPHOMA

Key Facts

Etiology/Pathogenesis

- Relatives of patients with CLL demonstrate 8.5x increased risk of CLL

Clinical Issues

- 5-year survival (79%)
- Clinical staging systems: Rai (0-IV) and Binet (A-C) are best predictors of survival

Microscopic Pathology

- Lymph nodes
  - Vaguely nodular pattern with alternating dark zones of mature CLL cells and light zones (proliferation centers)
- Peripheral blood
  - Diagnosis requires persistent (> 1 month) peripheral blood lymphocytosis (> 5 x 10^9 cells/L)
  - Mature-appearing lymphocytes with CLL immunophenotype in absence of other causes

Ancillary Tests

- Dim expression of sIg (IgM or IgM + IgD or, rarely, IgG) with κ or λ light chain restriction
- Dim CD20(+), CD19(+), CD5(+), CD23(+), FMC7(-)
- Expression of T-cell-associated antigen ZAP70 is associated with *Ig* gene mutational status
- ZAP70 on > 30% of cells by flow cytometry has worse prognosis than ZAP70(-) cases
- ~ 50% of cases have abnormal karyotypes

Top Differential Diagnoses

- Follicular lymphoma, mantle cell lymphoma
- Hairy cell leukemia, monoclonal B lymphocytosis

- Mitotic activity usually very low
- Proliferation centers contain continuum of small, medium, and large cells
- Prolymphocytes are medium-sized cells with dispersed chromatin and small nucleoli
- Paraimmunoblasts: Medium to large cells with round to oval nuclei, dispersed chromatin, central eosinophilic nucleoli
- In some cases, cells show moderate nuclear irregularity (atypical cytology), which can lead to differential diagnosis of mantle cell lymphoma
- Occasional cases show plasmacytoid differentiation
- CLL/SLL can involve lymph nodes with interfollicular pattern, surrounding reactive follicles

- Peripheral blood (PB)
  - Mature-appearing lymphocytes with scant agranular cytoplasm and homogeneously condensed chromatin without nucleoli
  - Characteristic "soccer ball" chromatin pattern and numerous smudge cells
  - Proportion of prolymphocytes (larger cells with prominent nucleoli) in blood films usually < 2%
  - ↑ numbers of prolymphocytes correlate with more aggressive disease course, *P53* abnormalities, and trisomy of chromosome 12
  - Variant CLL with ↑ prolymphocytes (CLL/PL) is defined by > 10% but < 55% prolymphocytes
  - Diagnosis requires persistent (> 1 month) PB lymphocytosis (> 5 x 10^9 cells/L) of mature-appearing lymphocytes
  - Circulating lymphocytes with CLL immunophenotype
- Bone marrow (BM)
  - Involvement may be nodular, interstitial, or diffuse
  - Proliferation centers are less common in bone marrow than in lymph nodes but can be found with extensive involvement
  - Paratrabecular aggregates are not typical
  - Advanced disease and bone marrow failure are associated with diffuse pattern of infiltration
  - Examination of bone marrow is essential for staging and helpful to monitor response to therapy

Predominant Pattern/Injury Type

- Diffuse

Predominant Cell/Compartment Type

- Hematopoietic, lymphoid

ANCILLARY TESTS

Immunohistochemistry

- B-cell antigens (CD20, CD79a, and pax-5) are positive, but CD20 expression can be very weak (dim)
- Tumor cells characteristically express CD5 and CD23
- CD23 is particularly useful in distinguishing CLL/SLL from mantle cell lymphoma
  - Should be evaluated in every case, if possible
- Some cases of CLL may express CD23 only weakly or partially; some cases of mantle cell lymphoma can be dimly CD23(+)
  - Evaluation of cyclin-D1 or t(11;14) is suggested
- p53 is expressed in ~ 10% of cases

Flow Cytometry

- Dim expression of sIg (IgM or IgM + IgD or, rarely, IgG) with κ or λ light chain restriction
- Expression of CD19, CD20 (dim), and CD79a
- CD5(+), CD23(+), CD43(+)
- CD11c(+/-), CD10(-), FMC7(-)
- Expression of CD38 on > 30% of cells is seen in ~ 1/2 of cases and reported to be associated with worse prognosis
- Expression of T-cell-associated antigen ZAP70 is associated with unmutated *Ig* variable genes
- Cases with ZAP70 on > 30% of cells by flow cytometry have worse prognosis than ZAP70(-) cases

Cytogenetics

- ~ 50% of cases have abnormal karyotypes (conventional methods); FISH is more often abnormal

- Trisomy 12 reported in 1/3 of cases with cytogenetic abnormalities
  - Correlates with atypical histology and aggressive clinical course
- Cases with trisomy 12 have predominantly unmutated *Ig* variable region genes
  - Those with 13q14 abnormalities more often have mutations
- Abnormalities of 13q reported in up to 25% of cases; associated with longer survival
- Abnormalities of 11q23 are found in small subset of cases; associated with lymphadenopathy and aggressive course
- Deletions of 6q21 or 17p13 (*TP53* locus) seen in 5% and 10% of cases, respectively
- *P53* mutations or deletions are associated with worse prognosis regardless of *IGH* mutational status

Molecular Genetics

- Mutations in *NOTCH1* and *SF3B1* predict a poor prognosis

DIFFERENTIAL DIAGNOSIS

Follicular Lymphoma

- Follicles can enlarge and coalesce to form large, grossly visible masses
- Neoplastic lymphocytes are centrocytes and centroblasts
  - Positive for CD10, CD19, CD20, and CD22; bright monoclonal sIg
  - Positive for Bcl-6 by immunohistochemistry
  - CD5(-), CD11c(-), CD43(-)

Mantle Cell Lymphoma

- Lymphocytes intermediate in size with irregular nuclear contours
  - Positive for CD5, CD19, CD20, CD22, and CD43; moderate monoclonal sIg
  - CD10(-), CD23(-/+)
- Cyclin-D1 (+) by immunohistochemistry; t(11;14)(q13;q32) positive by conventional cytogenetics or FISH

Hairy Cell Leukemia

- Patients present with splenomegaly and pancytopenia
- Indented nuclei with abundant clear cytoplasm
- Lymphocytes are positive for CD11c (bright), CD19, CD20, CD22 (bright), CD25, and CD103
- CD5(-), CD10(-), CD23(-)
- Tartrate-resistant acid phosphatase stain is strongly positive in hairy cells

Monoclonal B Lymphocytosis

- Healthy adults who have absolute increase in monoclonal B lymphocytes
- < 5 x 10^9/L B lymphocytes in peripheral blood
- Absence of lymphadenopathy or organomegaly, cytopenias, or disease-related symptoms
- May progress to frank CLL/SLL at rate of 1-2% per year

DIAGNOSTIC CHECKLIST

Pathologic Interpretation Pearls

- Dimming light during light microscopy is helpful in appreciating proliferation centers in histologic sections of lymph node
- Atypical immunophenotype occurs in ~ 10-20% of cases

SELECTED REFERENCES

1. Rossi D et al: Mutations of NOTCH1 are an independent predictor of survival in chronic lymphocytic leukemia. Blood. 119(2):521-9, 2012
2. Rossi D et al: Mutations of the SF3B1 splicing factor in chronic lymphocytic leukemia: association with progression and fludarabine-refractoriness. Blood. 118(26):6904-8, 2011
3. Lin KI et al: Relevance of the immunoglobulin VH somatic mutation status in patients with chronic lymphocytic leukemia treated with fludarabine, cyclophosphamide, and rituximab (FCR) or related chemoimmunotherapy regimens. Blood. 113(14):3168-71, 2009
4. Hallek M et al: Guidelines for the diagnosis and treatment of chronic lymphocytic leukemia: a report from the International Workshop on Chronic Lymphocytic Leukemia updating the National Cancer Institute-Working Group 1996 guidelines. Blood. 111(12):5446-56, 2008
5. Kantarjian H et al: Therapeutic advances in leukemia and myelodysplastic syndrome over the past 40 years. Cancer. 113(7 Suppl):1933-52, 2008
6. Müller-Hermelink HK et al: Chronic lymphocytic leukemia/small lymphocytic lymphoma. In: WHO Classification of Tumours of Haematopoietic and Lymphoid Tissues. Lyon, France: IARC Press. 180-182, 2008
7. Rassenti LZ et al: Relative value of ZAP-70, CD38, and immunoglobulin mutation status in predicting aggressive disease in chronic lymphocytic leukemia. Blood. 112(5):1923-30, 2008
8. Huh YO et al: The t(14;19)(q32;q13)-positive small B-cell leukaemia: a clinicopathologic and cytogenetic study of seven cases. Br J Haematol. 136(2):220-8, 2007
9. Zanotti R et al: ZAP-70 expression, as detected by immunohistochemistry on bone marrow biopsies from early-phase CLL patients, is a strong adverse prognostic factor. Leukemia. 21(1):102-9, 2007
10. Marti GE et al: Diagnostic criteria for monoclonal B-cell lymphocytosis. Br J Haematol. 130(3):325-32, 2005
11. Admirand JH et al: Immunohistochemical detection of ZAP-70 in 341 cases of non-Hodgkin and Hodgkin lymphoma. Mod Pathol. 17(8):954-61, 2004
12. Crespo M et al: ZAP-70 expression as a surrogate for immunoglobulin-variable-region mutations in chronic lymphocytic leukemia. N Engl J Med. 348(18):1764-75, 2003
13. Tobin G et al: Somatically mutated Ig V(H)3-21 genes characterize a new subset of chronic lymphocytic leukemia. Blood. 99(6):2262-4, 2002
14. Rosenwald A et al: Relation of gene expression phenotype to immunoglobulin mutation genotype in B cell chronic lymphocytic leukemia. J Exp Med. 194(11):1639-47, 2001
15. Binet JL et al: A clinical staging system for chronic lymphocytic leukemia: prognostic significance. Cancer. 40(2):855-64, 1977
16. Hernandez-Nieto L et al: Bone-marrow patterns and clinical staging in chronic lymphocytic leukaemia. Lancet. 1(8024):1269, 1977

Microscopic and Immunohistochemical Features

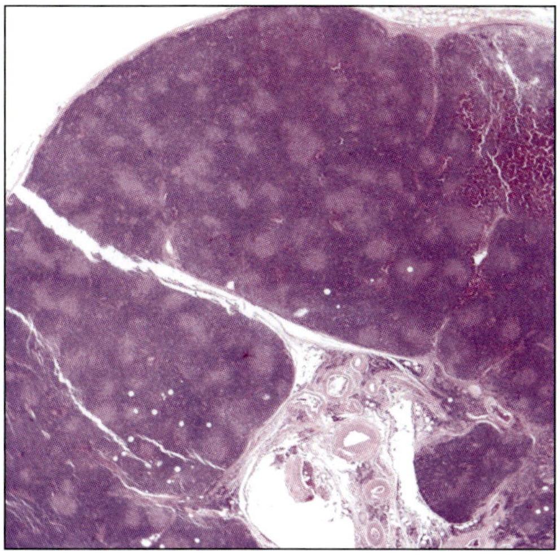

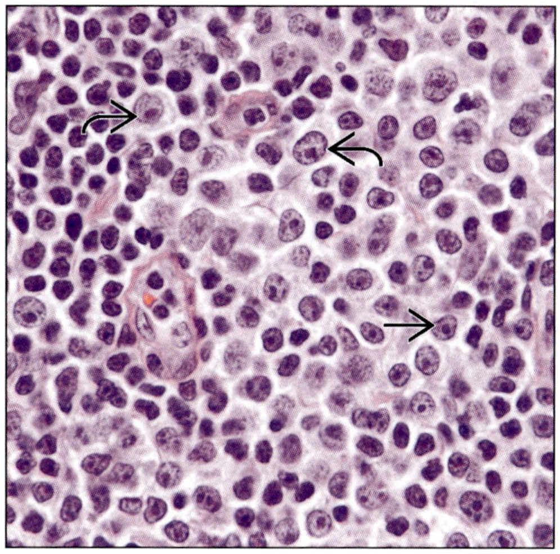

(Left) *This lymph node involved by CLL/SLL shows numerous proliferation centers (a.k.a. pseudofollicular growth centers or pseudofollicles).* ***(Right)*** *The proliferation center seen in this case of CLL/SLL is composed of small lymphocytes, prolymphocytes →, and paraimmunoblasts ↪.*

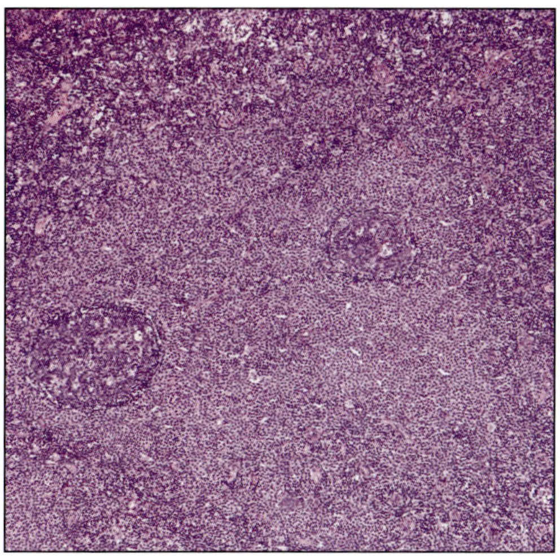

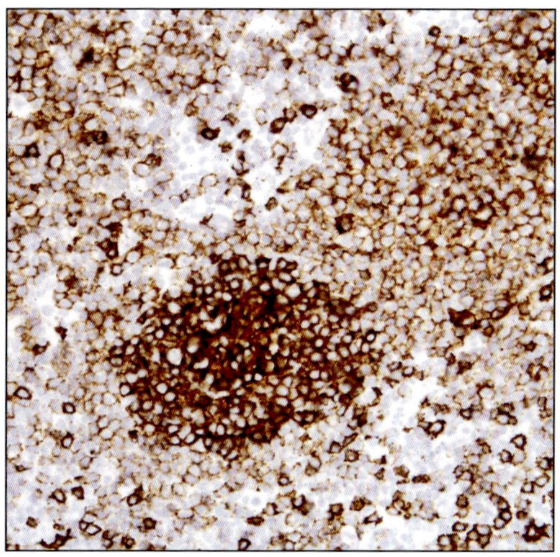

(Left) *CLL/SLL with an interfollicular pattern is characterized by darkly stained, reactive follicles surrounded by large proliferation centers. This pattern mimics marginal zone lymphoma.* ***(Right)*** *In this case of CLL/SLL (interfollicular pattern), an immunohistochemical stain demonstrates dim and variable CD20 expression in the neoplastic cells and bright CD20 expression in the central (nonneoplastic) follicle.*

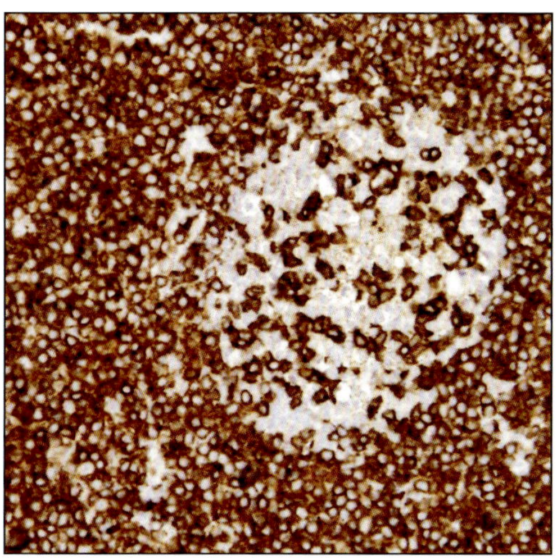

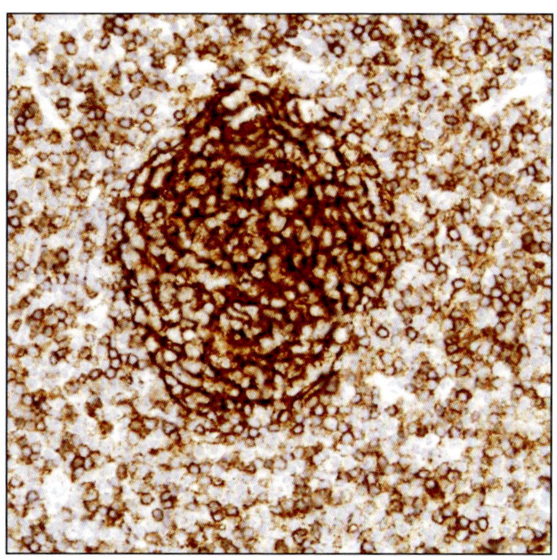

(Left) *In this case of CLL/SLL (interfollicular pattern), the neoplastic cells are highlighted by aberrant staining for the T-cell-associated marker CD5. The central benign germinal center is negative for CD5.* ***(Right)*** *In this case of CLL/SLL (interfollicular pattern), the neoplastic cells show dim CD23 expression. The central benign germinal center contains many CD23(+) follicular dendritic cells.*

Microscopic and Immunohistochemical Features

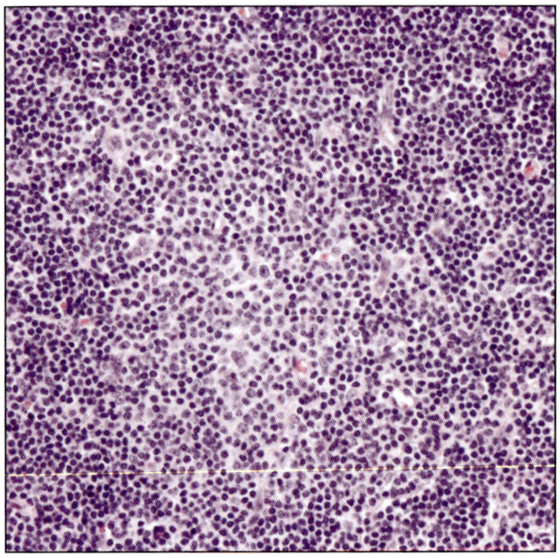
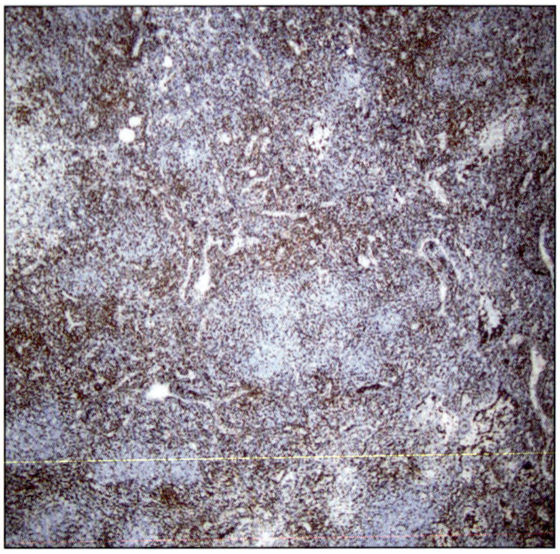

(Left) *The central proliferation center seen in this case of CLL/SLL contains a continuum of small lymphocytes, prolymphocytes, and paraimmunoblasts.* ***(Right)*** *An immunohistochemical stain for CD3 highlights background T cells. No staining is seen in the nodules of neoplastic CLL/SLL cells.*

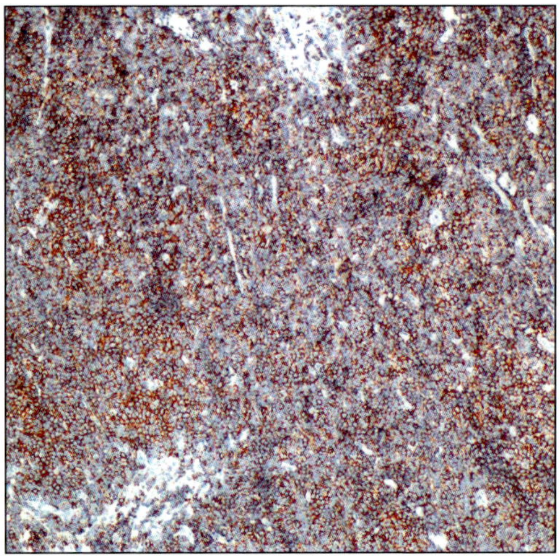
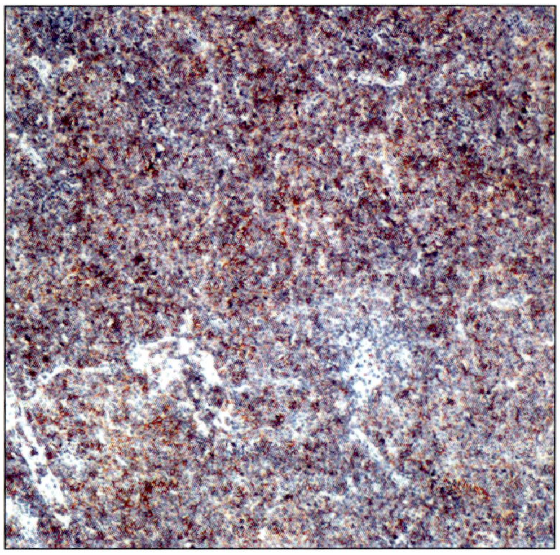

(Left) *Immunohistochemical stain for CD20 highlights CLL/SLL cells. The proliferation centers are more brightly positive than the neoplastic small lymphocytes.* ***(Right)*** *An immunohistochemical stain for CD23 highlights the vaguely nodular proliferation centers as well as the small neoplastic cells.*

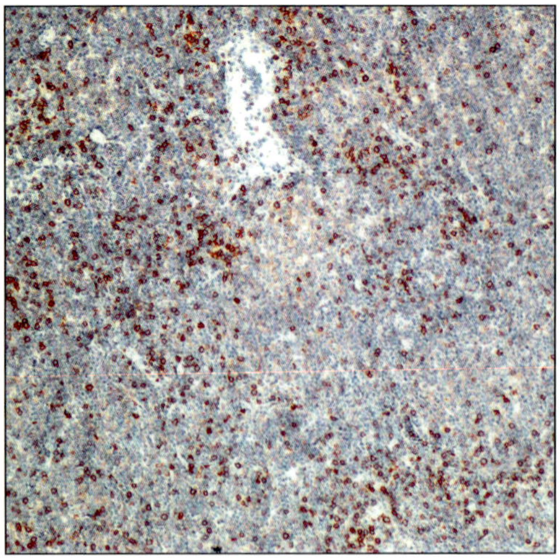
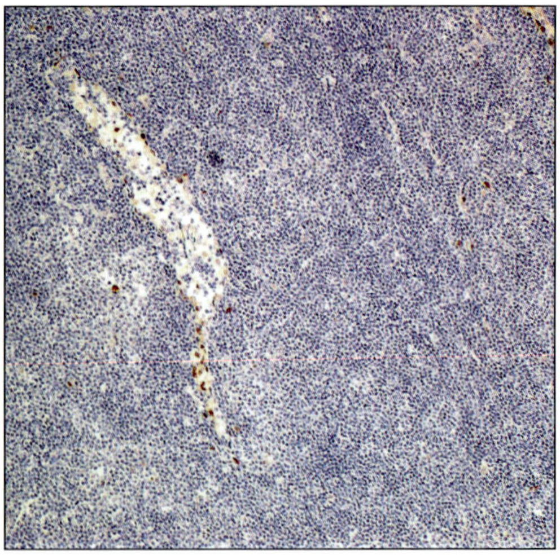

(Left) *Immunohistochemical stain for CD5 shows weakly positive expression of CD5 in the neoplastic cells. Scattered reactive T cells are darkly stained.* ***(Right)*** *An immunohistochemical stain for cyclin-D1 is negative in the neoplastic cells of CLL/SLL. Endothelial cells are positive and serve as an internal control.*

CHRONIC LYMPHOCYTIC LEUKEMIA/SMALL LYMPHOCYTIC LYMPHOMA

Microscopic and Immunophenotypic Features

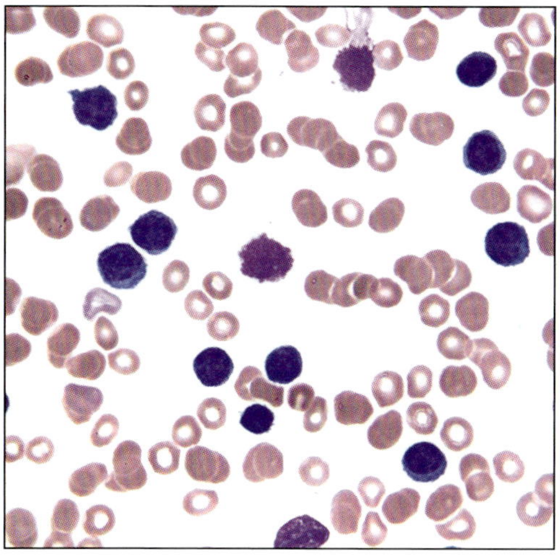

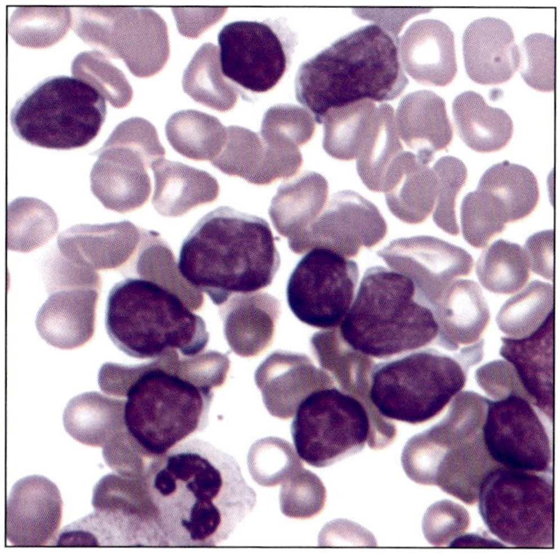

(Left) *This image shows peripheral blood involved by CLL/SLL. Characteristic features seen in this image include marked lymphocytosis and admixed smudge cells.* ***(Right)*** *Wright-Giemsa shows CLL with cytologically atypical morphology in this peripheral blood smear with a population of small and medium-sized cells, some with indented nuclei.*

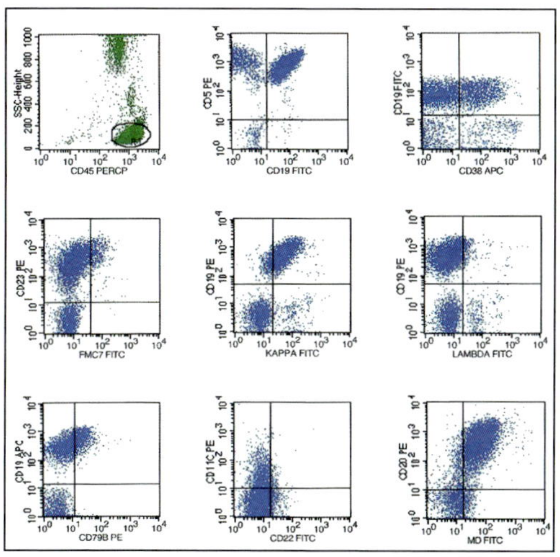

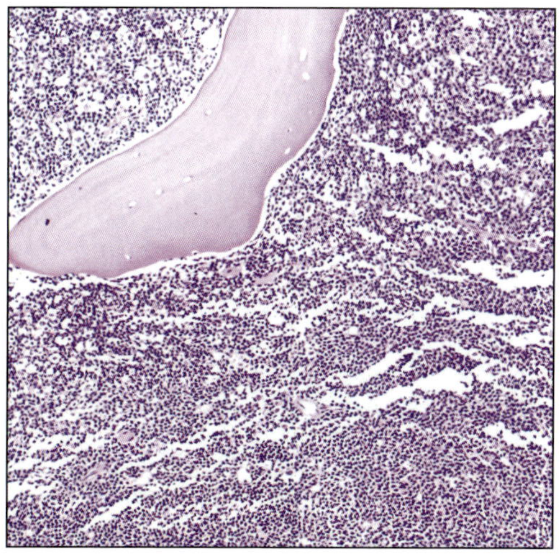

(Left) *Representative immunophenotypic analysis of CLL by flow cytometry shows that the neoplastic cells express CD5, CD11c (partial), CD19, CD20, CD23, CD38, weak surface immunoglobulin M&D, and monotypic κ light chain.* ***(Right)*** *Image shows bone marrow involvement by CLL/SLL with a diffuse pattern. The entire bone marrow space between bone trabeculae is replaced by small lymphocytes.*

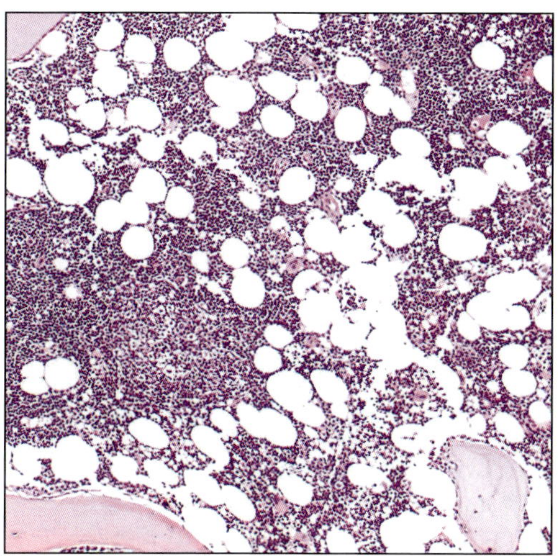

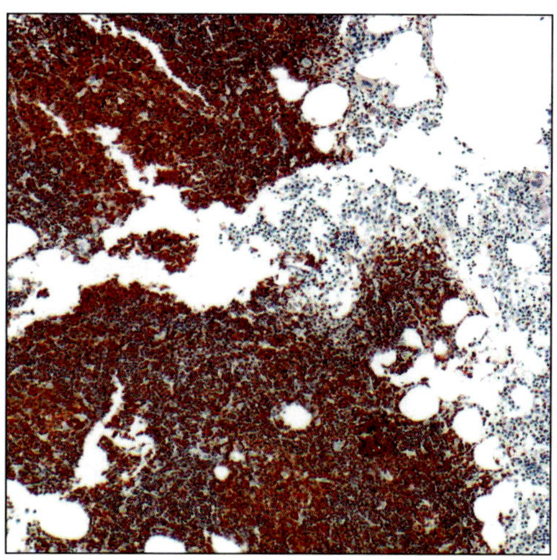

(Left) *Image shows bone marrow involvement by CLL/SLL with an interstitial pattern of lymphocytic infiltration. The mature lymphocytes infiltrate the interstitium with substantial sparing of normal hematopoietic cells.* ***(Right)*** *ZAP70 is strongly expressed in this case of CLL shown by immunohistochemistry. The expression is nuclear and cytoplasmic. ZAP70 expression in CLL is associated with a poor prognosis.*

DIFFUSE LARGE B-CELL LYMPHOMA

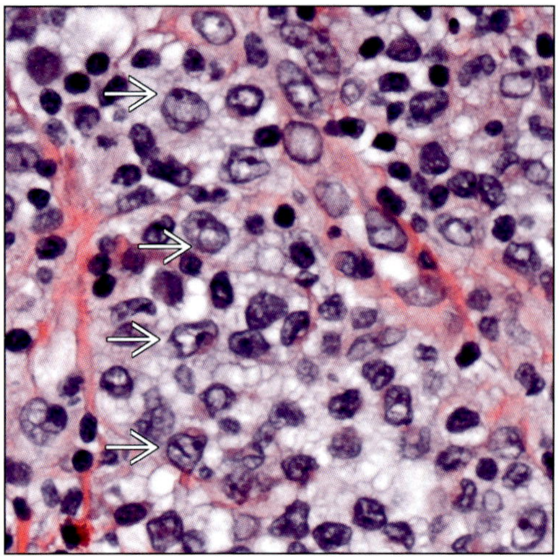

H&E stain shows a lymph node involved by diffuse large B-cell lymphoma (DLBCL). Typical centroblasts ➡ are large, noncleaved cells with vesicular chromatin and membrane-bound nucleoli.

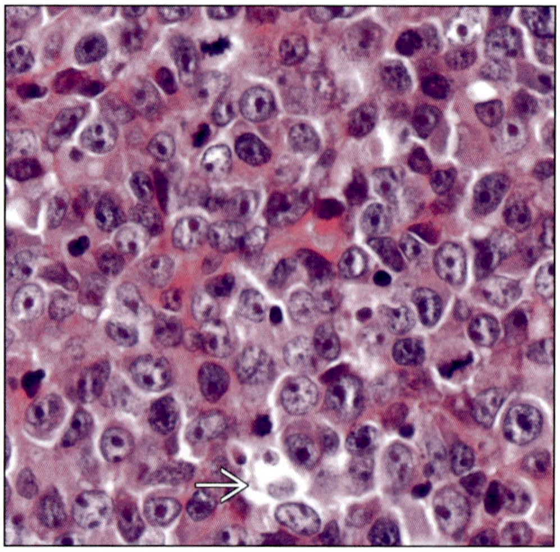

H&E stain shows a lymph node involved by DLBCL. Almost all of the cells are immunoblasts with large nuclei (compared to a histiocyte nucleus ➡) and a single, central, prominent nucleolus.

TERMINOLOGY

Abbreviations

- Diffuse large B-cell lymphoma (DLBCL)

Synonyms

- Diffuse large B-cell lymphoma, not otherwise specified (DLBCL, NOS)

Definitions

- Diffuse proliferation of large neoplastic B cells
  - Nuclei of neoplastic B cells are either equivalent to or larger than nucleus of a macrophage or are at least 2x as large as nucleus of a normal B cell
- Clinically, immunophenotypically, and genetically heterogeneous
- Multiple variants and subgroups are recognized by 2008 WHO classification system
  - Common morphologic variants (centroblastic, immunoblastic, anaplastic)
  - Rare morphologic variants
  - Molecular subgroups
    - Germinal center B-cell-like (GCB)
    - Activated B-cell-like (ABC)
  - Immunohistochemical subgroups
    - CD5(+) DLBCL
    - GCB
    - Non-GCB

ETIOLOGY/PATHOGENESIS

Sporadic

- Largely unknown
- May arise de novo (without a preceding disorder) or from an underlying, lower grade malignancy, such as follicular lymphoma (i.e., transformation)
- Patients with an underlying immunodeficiency at increased risk of developing DLBCL (often in association with Epstein-Barr virus [EBV] infection)

Familial

- Relatives of patients with DLBCL demonstrate 10x increased risk of DLBCL

CLINICAL ISSUES

Epidemiology

- Incidence
  - Predominantly disease of adults and elderly, but also occurs in children and young adults

Presentation

- Enlarging mass at nodal or extranodal sites
  - Gastrointestinal tract is a frequent extranodal site
  - Presenting symptoms may be related to mass effect
- ~ 50% of patients are at stage I or II at presentation; up to 1/3 present at stage IV
  - Bone marrow involvement occurs less frequently than in patients with low-grade B-cell lymphomas

Prognosis

- 5-year overall survival for patients with DLBCL ranges from 25-75%, depending on prognostic factors present at diagnosis

MICROSCOPIC PATHOLOGY

Histologic Features

- Diffuse growth pattern
  - Neoplasm replaces normal architecture with diffuse and usually dense lymphoid infiltrate
  - Sometimes present as vague nodules
  - Sclerosis is frequent in extranodal sites
- Centroblastic morphology
  - Typical: Medium to large cells (10-14 μm) with fine chromatin, 2-3 small nucleoli often closely apposed to nuclear membrane, and scant basophilic cytoplasm

DIFFUSE LARGE B-CELL LYMPHOMA

Key Facts

Terminology
- Diffuse proliferation of large neoplastic B cells
- Often involves nodal or extranodal sites
- Bone marrow involvement less common than in lower grade B-cell lymphomas
- Clinically, immunophenotypically and genetically heterogeneous

Etiology/Pathogenesis
- Most commonly sporadic; may be familial
  - Relatives of patients with diffuse large B-cell lymphoma (DLBCL) demonstrate a 10x increased risk of DLBCL

Microscopic Pathology
- Diffuse growth of large cells
- Usually express pan-B markers: CD20, CD22, CD79-a, pax-5
- GCB subgroup: > 30% CD10(+) or CD10(-), Bcl-6(+), MUM1(-)
- Proliferation fraction (Ki-67) usually high (> 30-40%)

Ancillary Tests
- Concurrent rearrangements of *MYC* and *BCL2* &/or *BCL6* (so-called double-hit or triple-hit lymphomas) indicate a poorer prognosis

Top Differential Diagnoses
- DLBCL subtypes
- Other lymphomas of large B cells
- Burkitt lymphoma
- Plasmablastic lymphoma
- Follicular lymphoma (grade 3B)

  - Multilobated: Medium to large cells with lobated nuclei (> 3 lobes)
- Immunoblast morphology
  - Large lymphocyte with centrally located nucleolus and moderate basophilic cytoplasm
- Anaplastic morphology
  - Large to very large bizarre, pleomorphic cells, some resembling Reed-Sternberg cells or hallmark cells of anaplastic large cell lymphoma; may grow in cohesive pattern
- Polymorphic variant: Mixture of centroblasts, immunoblasts, multilobated cells, and cells with overlapping cytologic features
- Rare morphologic variants: Myxoid stroma or fibrillary matrix, pseudorosette formation, spindle-shaped, signet ring, cytoplasmic granules, cytoplasmic projections, intercellular junctions

ANCILLARY TESTS

Immunohistochemistry
- Pan B-cell antigens (+)
- GCB subgroup: > 30% CD10(+) or CD10(-), Bcl-6(+), MUM1(-)
- Bcl-2(+/-), CD30(-/+), CD5(-/+)
- Proliferation fraction (Ki-67) usually high (> 30-40%)

Cytogenetics
- t(14;18): 1 of the most frequent translocations; detected in 20-30% of cases
- Abnormalities involving chromosome 3q27 region (*BCL6* gene) are seen in up to 30% of cases
- *MYC* translocations are identified in up to 10% of cases
- Concurrent rearrangements of *MYC* and *BCL2* &/or *BCL6* (so-called double-hit or triple-hit lymphomas) indicate a poorer prognosis

Gene Expression Profiling
- Expression microarray studies have identified molecular subgroups of DLBCL
  - GCB type: Gene expression profile similar to germinal center B cells
  - ABC type: Gene expression profile similar to activated peripheral B cells

DIFFERENTIAL DIAGNOSIS

DLBCL Subtypes
- Primary DLBCL of central nervous system
  - Recognized as distinct subtype in 2008 WHO classification
  - All primary or intraocular lymphomas are considered in this category
  - Bcl-6 and MUM1(+) in most cases
  - CD10(+) in up to 20% of cases
  - EBV(-) in immunocompetent patients
  - Patients may have sporadic systemic relapses, particularly in testes and breasts
- Primary cutaneous DLBCL, leg type
  - Not limited to lower extremities
  - Multiple tumors frequent, sometimes ulcerated
  - Large monotonous lymphoid cells (immunoblastic morphology)
  - No epidermotropism
  - Positive for CD20, Bcl-2, Bcl-6, MUM1, and FOXP1
  - CD10 usually negative
- EBV(+) DLBCL in patients > 50 years old
  - No history of chronic inflammation, immunodeficiency, or previous lymphoma
  - Believed to be related to senescence of immune system
  - Frequent extranodal involvement
  - EBV always positive (EBER and LMP1)
  - MUM1(+) in most cases
  - CD10 and Bcl-6 usually negative

Other Lymphomas of Large B Cells
- Primary mediastinal (thymic) large B-cell lymphoma
  - Young females
  - Anterosuperior mediastinal mass
  - Locally aggressive with local compressive effects

DIFFUSE LARGE B-CELL LYMPHOMA

- Large cells with pale cytoplasm (often is retraction artifact) and sclerosis (compartmentalization)
- Thymic components, such as Hassall corpuscles, may be identified
- Positive for pan-B-cell markers
- CD30 often (+) but usually weak &/or focal (~ 75%)
- CD23 (70%), Bcl-6, and MUM1 (most cases)

- DLBCL associated with chronic inflammation
  - History of longstanding chronic inflammation
  - Associated with EBV (EBER and LMP1 [-])
  - Pleural cavity, bone (especially femur), and periarticular joint tissues
  - CD30 may be positive
- Lymphomatoid granulomatosis
  - Patients may have underlying immunodeficiency disorder
  - Lung is most common site of involvement (almost essential for diagnosis)
    - Other extranodal sites: Skin, kidney, liver, and central nervous system
  - Angiocentric and angiodestructive polymorphic lymphoid infiltrate with necrosis
  - Positive for CD20, CD30 (variable), and EBV (LMP1 and EBER)
- Anaplastic kinase (ALK)-positive large B-cell lymphoma
  - Rare (~ 100 reported cases)
  - Immunoblastic/plasmablastic morphology
  - Intrasinusoidal growth pattern
  - Positive for ALK, EMA, CD138, Vs38c, and monotypic cytoplasmic light chain
  - Negative for CD20, CD30, EBV, and T-cell antigens (except for CD4)
  - *ALK* gene at 2p23 can be involved in translocations with
    - Clathrin (*CTCL*) gene on 17p23, resulting in CTCL-ALK fusion protein
    - Nucleophosmin (*NPM*) gene on 5q35, resulting in NPM-ALK fusion protein
    - Complex *SEC31A-ALK* fusion also reported
- Plasmablastic lymphoma
  - Large neoplastic cells, most of which resemble immunoblasts or plasmablasts
  - Plasma cell-associated markers expressed (CD138, CD38, Vs38c, and EMA)
  - CD56 frequently positive
    - CD56 expression is rare in DLBCL
  - Almost always negative for CD20 and pax-5
  - CD45 (LCA) weak or negative
  - Some cases positive for some T-cell markers, including CD4 and CD7
  - EBV frequently positive (~ 75%)
- Primary effusion lymphoma
  - Serous effusions (pleural, pericardial, and peritoneal cavities) without tumor masses
  - Usually in context of HIV infection
  - Positive for CD45 (LCA) and plasma cell markers
  - Negative for B-cell markers
  - EBV infection common (EBER[+], LMP1[-])
  - Usually associated with human herpesvirus 8 (HHV8)

Burkitt Lymphoma

- Monomorphic medium-sized cells with multiple small nucleoli
- Numerous mitoses and "starry sky" pattern
- Characteristic immunophenotype: Positive for CD10, Bcl-6 (strong), and CD20; negative for Bcl-2
- Ki-67 positive in virtually 100% of tumor cells (uniformly strong)
- Chromosomal translocations involving *MYC* gene at 8q24 are characteristic

Follicular Lymphoma (Grade 3B)

- CD21, CD23, and CD35 highlights follicular dendritic cells in follicular areas

SELECTED REFERENCES

1. Menon MP et al: The histological and biological spectrum of diffuse large B-cell lymphoma in the World Health Organization classification. Cancer J. 18(5):411-20, 2012
2. Jaffe ES et al: Aggressive B-cell lymphomas: a review of new and old entities in the WHO classification. Hematology Am Soc Hematol Educ Program. 2011:506-14, 2011
3. Meyer PN et al: Immunohistochemical methods for predicting cell of origin and survival in patients with diffuse large B-cell lymphoma treated with rituximab. J Clin Oncol. 29(2):200-7, 2011
4. Snuderl M et al: B-cell lymphomas with concurrent IGH-BCL2 and MYC rearrangements are aggressive neoplasms with clinical and pathologic features distinct from Burkitt lymphoma and diffuse large B-cell lymphoma. Am J Surg Pathol. 34(3):327-40, 2010
5. Choi WW et al: A new immunostain algorithm classifies diffuse large B-cell lymphoma into molecular subtypes with high accuracy. Clin Cancer Res. 15(17):5494-502, 2009
6. Johnson NA et al: Lymphomas with concurrent BCL2 and MYC translocations: the critical factors associated with survival. Blood. 114(11):2273-9, 2009
7. Niitsu N et al: Clinical features and prognosis of de novo diffuse large B-cell lymphoma with t(14;18) and 8q24/c-MYC translocations. Leukemia. 23(4):777-83, 2009
8. Tilly H et al: Diffuse large B-cell non-Hodgkin's lymphoma: ESMO clinical recommendations for diagnosis, treatment and follow-up. Ann Oncol. 20 Suppl 4:110-2, 2009
9. Fu K et al: Addition of rituximab to standard chemotherapy improves the survival of both the germinal center B-cell-like and non-germinal center B-cell-like subtypes of diffuse large B-cell lymphoma. J Clin Oncol. 26(28):4587-94, 2008
10. Le Gouill S et al: The clinical presentation and prognosis of diffuse large B-cell lymphoma with t(14;18) and 8q24/c-MYC rearrangement. Haematologica. 92(10):1335-42, 2007
11. Lin P et al: High-grade B-cell lymphoma/leukemia associated with t(14;18) and 8q24/MYC rearrangement: a neoplasm of germinal center immunophenotype with poor prognosis. Haematologica. 92(10):1297-301, 2007
12. Lossos IS et al: Prognostic biomarkers in diffuse large B-cell lymphoma. J Clin Oncol. 24(6):995-1007, 2006

Morphologic Features

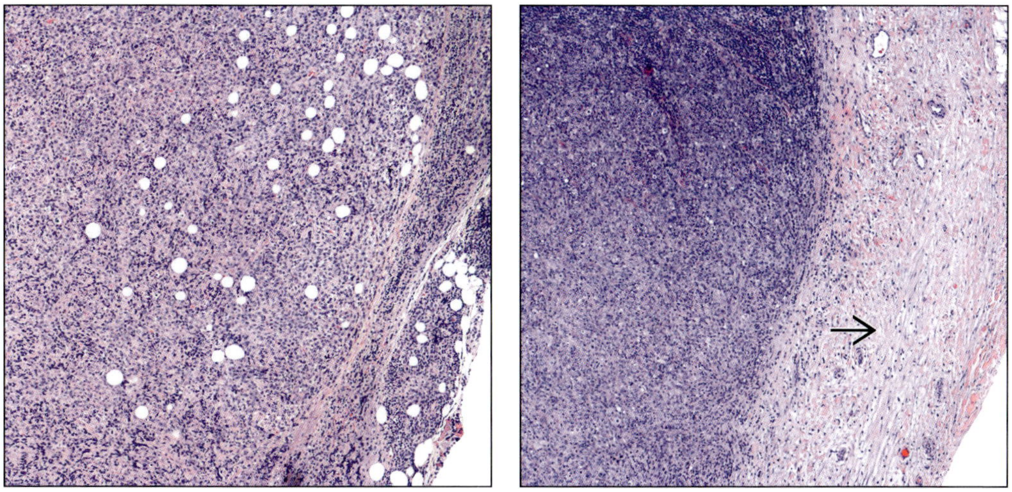

(Left) *H&E stain shows DLBCL involving a lymph node with a diffuse growth pattern and loss of normal nodal architecture. The neoplasm extends into the fibroadipose tissue.* ***(Right)*** *H&E stain shows DLBCL involving a lymph node with prominent, reactive capsular fibrosis ⇒.*

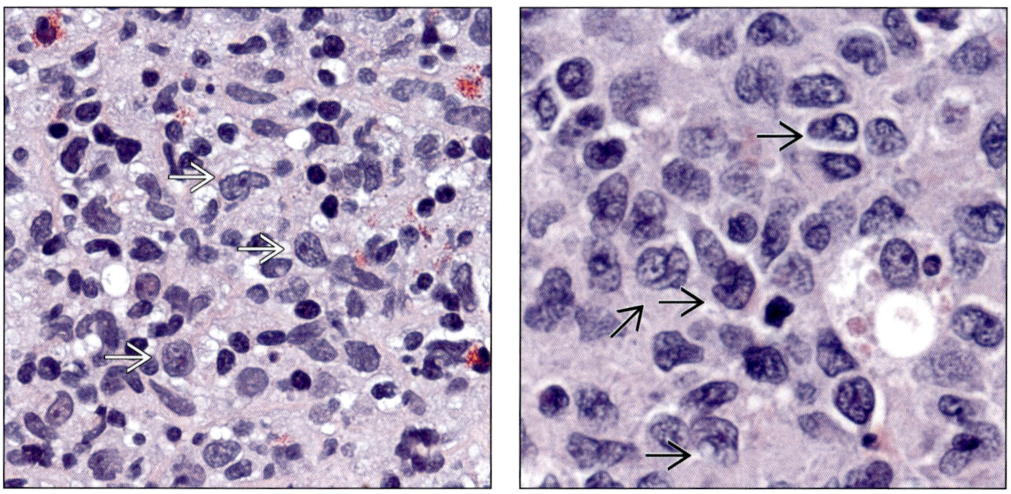

(Left) *H&E stain shows DLBCL composed of centroblasts ➡ and admixed small reactive lymphocytes and occasional eosinophils.* ***(Right)*** *This high-magnification view of DLBCL reveals an infiltrate composed of multilobated centroblasts ⇒. The tumor cells are large, and some have deeply lobated nuclei.*

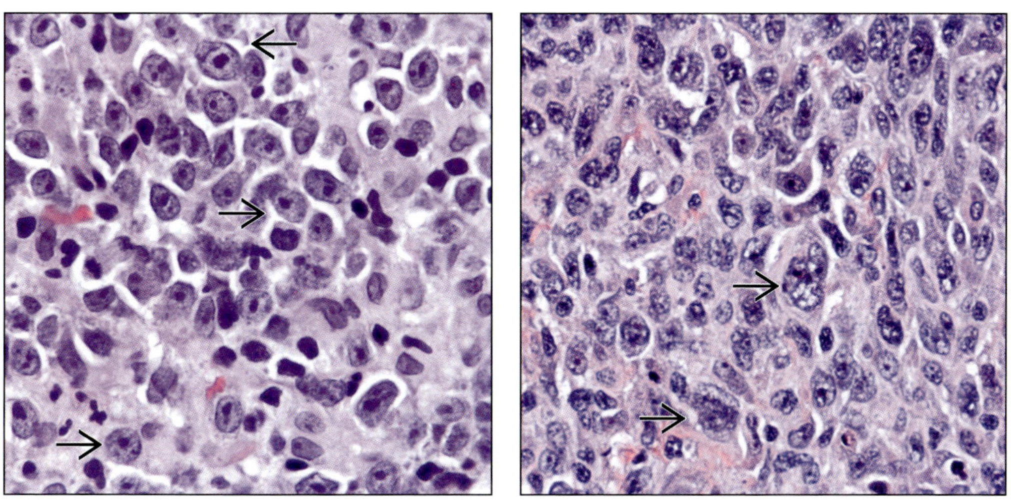

(Left) *The immunoblastic variant of DLBCL is composed of a monotonous population of large cells with central prominent nucleoli ⇒.* ***(Right)*** *The anaplastic variant of DLBCL demonstrates markedly pleomorphic cells ⇒ that are mostly large in size with irregular nuclei, vesicular chromatin, and distinct nucleoli. These tumor cells were positive for CD20 and CD30 and negative for CD10, CD5, and CD3.*

DIFFUSE LARGE B-CELL LYMPHOMA

Morphologic and Immunophenotypic Features

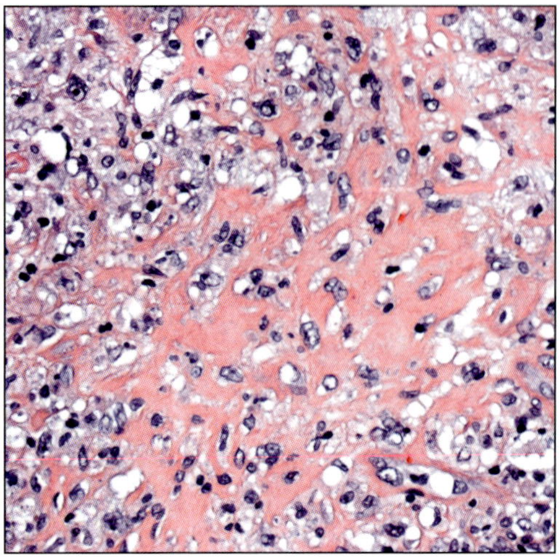
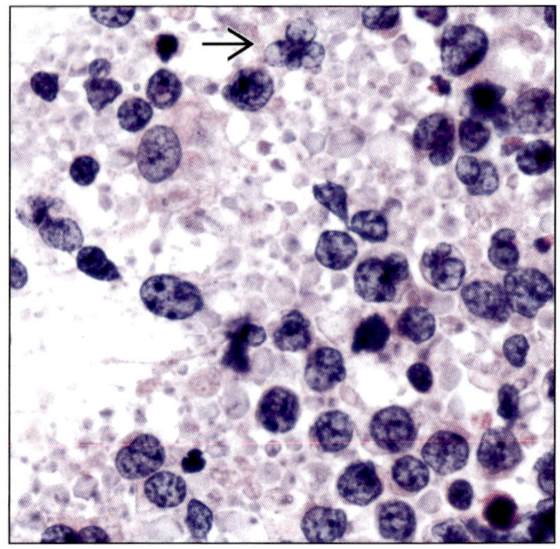

(Left) *Image shows DLBCL (centroblastic variant) with marked sclerosis. The centroblasts are large with vesicular nuclear chromatin and cleaved nuclei. Sclerosis is frequently seen in cases of DLBCL involving extranodal sites and retroperitoneum.* ***(Right)*** *H&E stain of a touch imprint of DLBCL shows medium to large lymphoid cells, some with small nucleoli apposed to the nuclear membrane. Few multilobated cells are also seen →.*

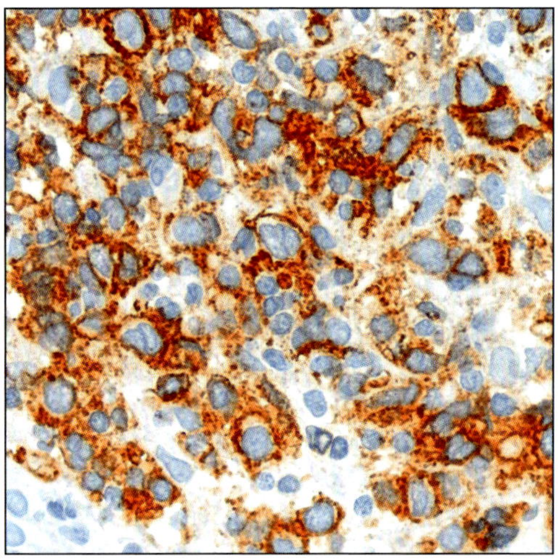
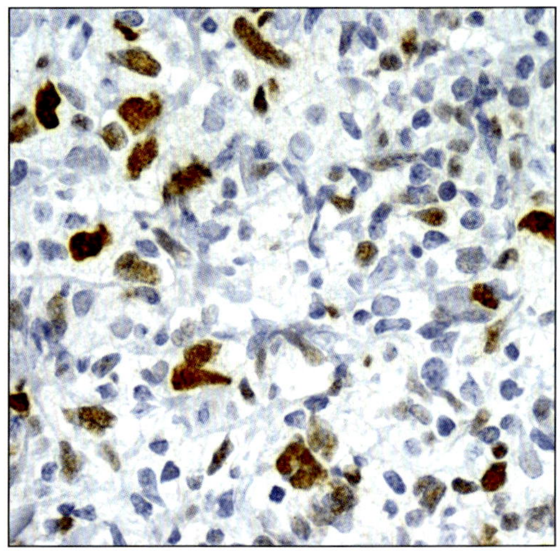

(Left) *Image shows a CD10(+) DLBCL. Almost all of the cells are immunoblasts with large nuclei and show cytoplasmic immunopositivity for CD10.* ***(Right)*** *A Bcl-6 stain shows subset positivity in this case of DLBCL. The expression of both CD10 and Bcl-6 is consistent with a germinal center cell phenotype. DLBCL cells, when positive for Bcl-6, usually show variable degrees of nuclear positivity. In contrast, Burkitt lymphoma cells are usually strongly and uniformly positive for Bcl-6.*

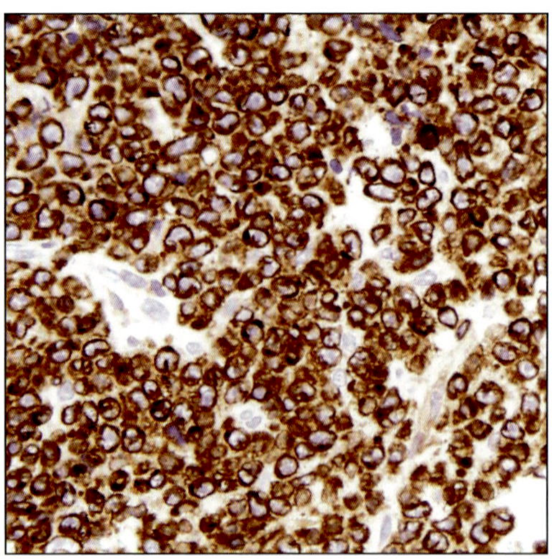
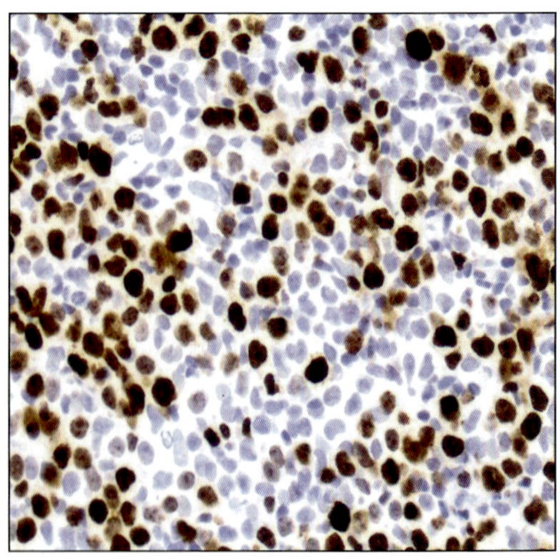

(Left) *Image shows a Bcl-2(+) DLBCL. Neoplasm replaces normal architecture with diffuse and usually dense lymphoid neoplastic cells that are strongly positive for Bcl-2.* ***(Right)*** *Nuclei of neoplastic B cells of DLBCL are equivalent to or larger than nucleus of a macrophage, or are at least 2x as large as nucleus of a normal B cell with high proliferative rate. The proliferation rate of this DLBCL is ~ 40-50% as measured by MIB-1 (Ki-67).*

Differential Diagnosis

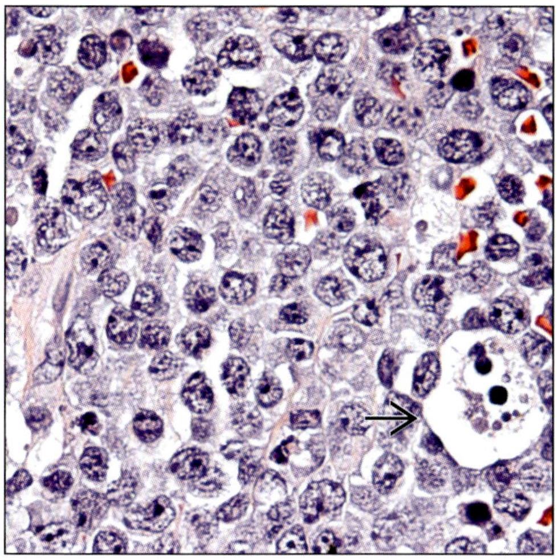
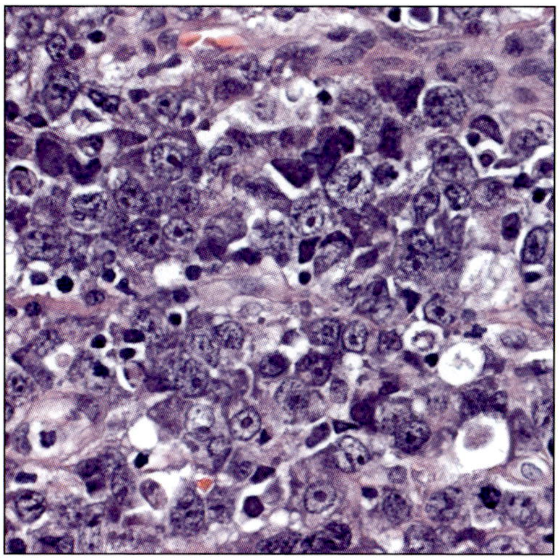

(Left) *H&E stain shows the characteristic morphologic features of Burkitt lymphoma. The tumor cells are fairly monotonous with multiple small nucleoli. Admixed tingible-body macrophages ⇨ impart a "starry sky" pattern at low magnification.* ***(Right)*** *Plasmablastic lymphoma is composed of large, pleomorphic tumor cells, some with features of immunoblasts. These tumor cells were positive for CD38, CD138, and CD10, and were negative for CD20 and pax-5.*

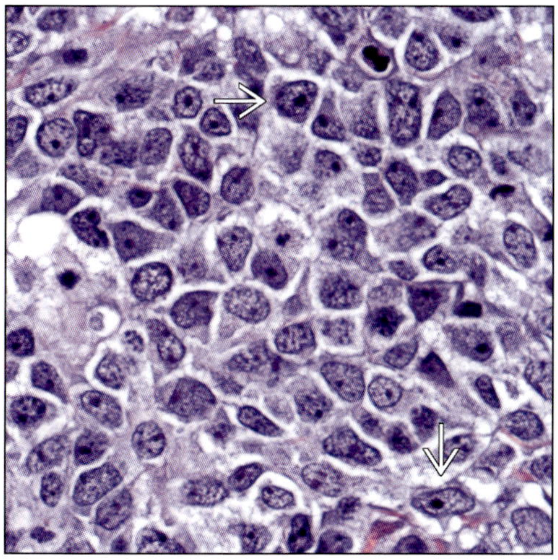
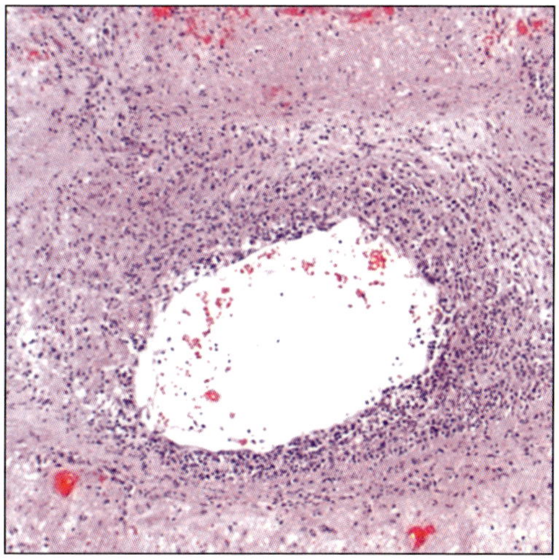

(Left) *Primary cutaneous DLBCL (leg type) is composed of large cells, some with immunoblastic features ➡. This tumor extensively involved the dermis and subcutaneous tissue.* ***(Right)*** *H&E stain shows lymphomatoid granulomatosis involving the lung with characteristic features, including extensive necrosis and an angiocentric pattern of infiltration.*

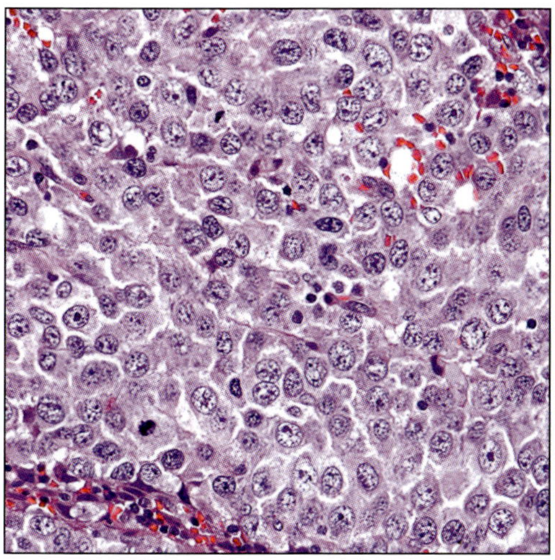
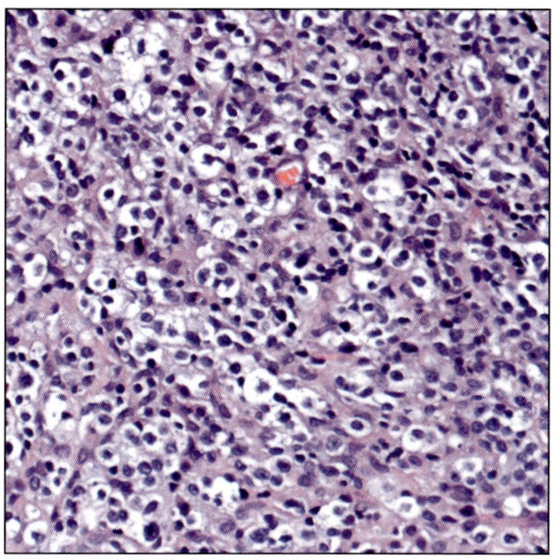

(Left) *ALK(+) large B-cell lymphoma is composed of immunoblasts with a plasmacytic appearance. These tumor cells were focally positive for CD79a and ALK (cytoplasmic and coarsely granular) and negative for CD30.* ***(Right)*** *This tumor, which presented in the anterior mediastinum, is composed of large cells with pale cytoplasm and sclerosis (features of primary mediastinal large B-cell lymphoma). These cells were positive for CD20, CD30 (focal), and MUM1, and were negative for CD10.*

FOLLICULAR LYMPHOMA

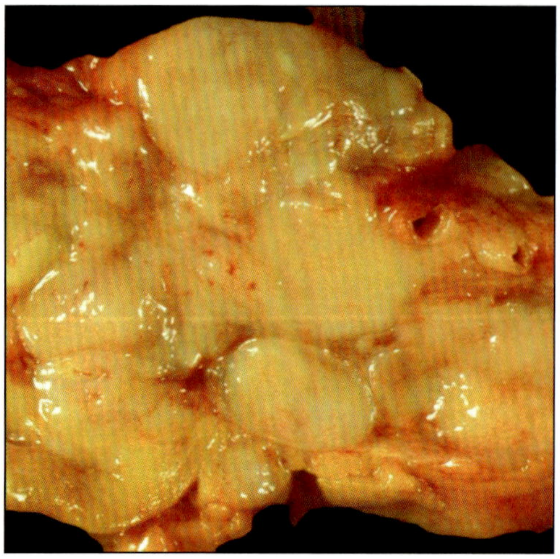

Gross photograph shows matted mesenteric lymph nodes involved by low-grade follicular lymphoma (FL). This specimen was obtained at time of autopsy.

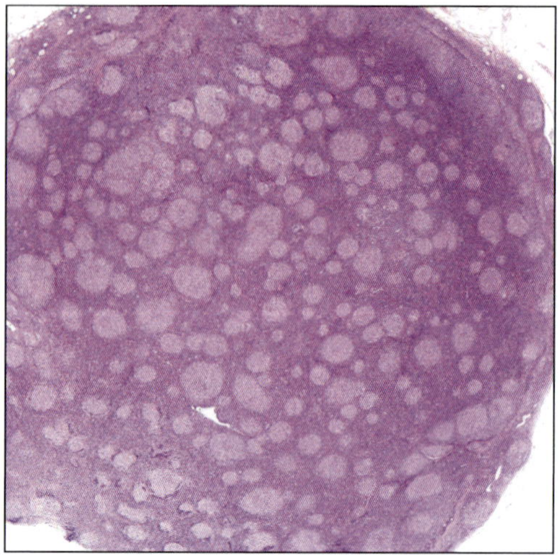

FL involving the lymph node shows follicles throughout the cortex and medulla. The large number and random distribution of follicles supports the diagnosis of lymphoma.

TERMINOLOGY

Abbreviations

- Follicular lymphoma (FL)

Synonyms

- Follicle (germinal) center cell lymphoma
- Centroblastic/centrocytic lymphoma

Definitions

- B-cell neoplasm composed of germinal center B cells (centrocytes and centroblasts)
  - Follicular, follicular and diffuse, and diffuse growth patterns

ETIOLOGY/PATHOGENESIS

t(14;18)(q32;q21) Resulting in Overexpression of Bcl-2

- Bcl-2 is antiapoptotic and confers survival advantage
- t(14;18) is considered initiating molecular event of FL
  - Insufficient to induce lymphomagenesis by itself
  - Other molecular changes necessary for development of lymphoma

Germline Susceptibility Factors

- Genotypic analysis has identified novel susceptibility locus at 6p21.3
  - Contains single gene, chromosome 6 open reading frame 15 (C6orf15)
- 4x increased lymphoma risk in 1st-degree relatives of patients with FL
- Association of single nucleotide polymorphisms of estrogen receptor gene with reduced risk of FL

Imbalance of Other Proteins Involved in Apoptosis

- Overexpression of cell death suppressor proteins Bcl-xL and Mcl-1
- Decreased expression of cell death promoting proteins BAX and BAD
- Overexpression of inhibitors of apoptosis proteins (IAP)

Immunologic Microenvironment

- CD40L(+) T cells in secondary follicles inhibit FL cell death
- Follicular dendritic cells contribute to preventing apoptosis of FL cells

CLINICAL ISSUES

Epidemiology

- Incidence
  - ~ 20% of non-Hodgkin lymphoma (NHL); 2nd most common NHL in USA and Western Europe
  - Uncommon in Asia and underdeveloped countries
- Age
  - Median = 59 years
- Gender
  - M:F = 1:1.7

Site

- Cervical and inguinal lymph nodes are more frequently affected
- Commonly affected extranodal sites
  - Bone marrow, spleen, liver, and peripheral blood
- FL uncommonly arises at extranodal sites
  - Skin, gastrointestinal tract, thyroid gland, testis

Presentation

- Insidious onset
- Often asymptomatic at time of initial diagnosis
- Almost always disseminated (stages III-IV)

Natural History

- Indolent clinical course but frequent relapses
- Some cases progress to diffuse large B-cell lymphoma (DLBCL)

FOLLICULAR LYMPHOMA

Key Facts

Terminology

- B-cell neoplasm composed of germinal center B cells (centrocytes and centroblasts)

Etiology/Pathogenesis

- Overexpression of antiapoptotic Bcl-2 due to t(14;18)(q32;q21)
- Susceptibility locus at 6p21.3 and higher risk in 1st-degree relatives of patients with follicular lymphoma (FL)

Clinical Issues

- ~ 20% of non-Hodgkin lymphoma (NHL), 2nd overall, in USA and Western Europe
- Usually asymptomatic although disseminated at presentation
- Overall 10-year survival is up to ~ 80%

Microscopic Pathology

- Closely packed neoplastic follicles, fairly uniform in size and shape
- Neoplastic follicles composed of variable amounts of centrocytes and large centroblasts
- Grading has prognostic and therapeutic significance

Ancillary Tests

- B cells positive for Bcl-2, Bcl-6, and CD10
- Bcl-2(+) in 85-90% of FL grade 1 and grade 2; 50% in FL grade 3

Top Differential Diagnoses

- Reactive follicular hyperplasia
- Nodular lymphocyte predominant HL
- Mantle cell lymphoma
- Nodal marginal zone lymphoma

Treatment

- In the past, "watch and wait" strategy was usually employed for asymptomatic patients
- Chemotherapy is currently used upfront more often for patients with stages III-IV disease
  - Rituximab, cyclophosphamide, Adriamycin (doxorubicin), vincristine, and prednisone (R-CHOP)
  - Bulky disease or signs of progression necessitate chemotherapy
- Radiation has value for subset of patients with stages I and II disease

Prognosis

- Overall 10-year survival is up to ~ 80%
- Adverse prognostic factors summarized in FL International Prognostic Index 2 (FLIPI 2)
  - High serum β2-microglobulin
  - Bulky lymph nodes > 6 cm
  - Bone marrow involvement
  - Hemoglobin < 12 g/dL
  - Age > 60 years
- FLIPI 2 prognostic model stratifies patients into different prognostic risk groups
  - Model developed in post-rituximab era using prospective analysis
- Pathologic adverse prognostic factors include
  - High histologic grade and diffuse areas > 25% with predominance of large cells
    - These areas are designated as DLBCL
  - High proliferation index
  - Complex karyotype
  - del6q23-26; del17p and mutation of *TP53*

IMAGE FINDINGS

General Features

- Widespread lymphadenopathy; often small lymph nodes

MACROSCOPIC FEATURES

General Features

- Replacement of nodal parenchyma by "fish-flesh" tumor; ± nodularity

MICROSCOPIC PATHOLOGY

Histologic Features

- Lymph node
  - Partial or complete effacement of architecture
  - Closely packed neoplastic follicles, fairly uniform in size and shape
  - Follicles usually poorly circumscribed with faint or absent mantle zones
  - "Cracking" artifact may surround neoplastic follicles
  - Neoplastic follicles are composed of centrocytes and centroblasts
    - Cells randomly distributed throughout individual follicles, without polarity
    - Infrequent mitoses and absent or scanty tingible body macrophages
    - Centrocytes: Small to large with angulated, elongated, or twisted nuclei, with dark chromatin and scant cytoplasm
    - Centroblasts: Large cells with oval or multilobated nuclei, vesicular chromatin, 1-3 nucleoli, and moderate cytoplasm
  - Diffuse areas with or without sclerosis
    - More frequent in mesenteric and retroperitoneal lymph nodes
    - Scattered interfollicular neoplastic lymphocytes are not considered diffuse growth pattern
    - Follicular dendritic cell meshworks are absent in diffuse areas
- Bone marrow
  - Paratrabecular aggregates of centrocytes and, less frequently, centroblasts in bone marrow
    - Aspirate smears may have scant lymphoma cells or are negative

FOLLICULAR LYMPHOMA

- Interstitial &/or diffuse patterns in advanced disease
- Peripheral blood
  - Marked leukemic involvement in 5-10% of patients
  - Neoplastic cells have highly cleaved nuclei and are known as "buttock cells"
  - Low-level involvement is detected by molecular methods in ~ 90% of patients
- Liver
  - Portal tracts are preferentially involved
  - Large mass lesions usually indicate transformation to DLBCL
- Spleen
  - Preferential involvement of white pulp
- Unusual morphologic variants of FL
  - Floral variant
    - Mantle zone lymphocytes penetrate into neoplastic follicles, imparting irregular shapes
    - Better highlighted with follicular dendritic cell markers, e.g., CD21
    - Often grade 3
  - Plasmacytic differentiation
    - Focal plasmacytic differentiation can occur rarely in FL, intrafollicular or interfollicular
    - Extreme degrees with intracytoplasmic inclusions appear as "signet ring cells"
  - Marginal zone differentiation
    - Monocytoid cells with clear cytoplasm at periphery of neoplastic follicles
    - Has been correlated with poorer prognosis

Cytologic Features

- Diagnosis of FL can be established by FNA with ancillary support
  - In smears, aggregates of cells bound by follicular dendritic cells
  - Variable mixture of centrocytes and centroblasts
  - Usually, absence of tingible body macrophages

Grading of FL

- Grading has prognostic and therapeutic significance
- Most reliably performed on lymph node biopsy specimen
- System is based on mean number of centroblasts per high power field (HPF)
  - Count 10 HPFs and divide by 10
- Grade 1: 0-5 centroblasts/HPF
- Grade 2: 6-15 centroblasts/HPF
- Grade 3: > 15 centroblasts/HPF
  - Grade 3A: Centrocytes admixed with centroblasts
  - Grade 3B: Sheets of centroblasts with rare or no centrocytes
- Remember: Cutoff values are based on 40x objective and 18 mm field-of-view ocular
  - Many microscopes have larger field-of-view ocular
    - 20 mm field-of-view ocular: Divide 10 HPF count by 12
    - 22 mm field-of-view ocular: Divide 10 HPF count by 15
- 2008 WHO classification recommends lumping cases of FL grades 1-2 together as low grade
  - Minimal differences in outcome between patients with FL grade 1 vs. grade 2
  - Diffuse areas > 25% of grade 3 FL should be diagnosed as DLBCL

Histologic Discordance (Discrepant Histology) in Patients With FL

- FL involving different lymph node groups may show different grades
  - Occurs in up to 1/3 of patients who undergo staging laparotomy
- Lymph node can be involved by grade 3 FL or DLBCL with bone marrow showing grade 1 FL
  - Occurs in ~ 10-20% of patients with grade 3 FL or DLBCL
  - Low-grade bone marrow involvement does not affect prognosis

Reporting Pattern in FL

- Most reliably performed on lymph node biopsy specimen
- Follicular: > 75% follicular
- Follicular and diffuse: 25-75% follicular
- Focally follicular: 1-25% follicular
- Diffuse: 0% follicular

Diffuse Follicular Lymphoma

- Diffuse growth of small centrocytes with few or absent centroblasts
  - Immunophenotype: CD10(+), Bcl-6(+), Bcl-2(+)
  - *IGH-BCL2* fusion gene or t(14;18)(q32;q21) present
- Rare diagnosis; more common in core needle biopsy specimens
  - Extensive sampling may reveal focal follicular pattern

Intrafollicular Neoplasia/In Situ Follicular Lymphoma

- Lymph node with widely spaced follicles of which a subset have Bcl-2(+) germinal centers
  - Bcl-2 expression by germinal centers is characteristically bright
  - Bcl-2(+) follicles have immunophenotype of FL and t(14;18)
  - Using histologic criteria alone, diagnosis of FL can be difficult or not possible
- Patients with intrafollicular neoplasia may
  - Have FL elsewhere simultaneously or develop FL subsequently
  - Have other types of non-Hodgkin lymphoma or Hodgkin lymphoma simultaneously or subsequently
  - Not develop lymphoma on clinical follow-up

Clinically Aggressive B-Cell Lymphoma

- FL transformation to more clinically aggressive B-cell lymphomas occurs in ~ 30% of FL patients
- Usually transforms into DLBCL
  - Accounts for most disease-related deaths
- Transformed tumor less often resembles Burkitt lymphoma (BL) or tumor with features intermediate between BL and DLBCL
- Transformation is commonly associated with
  - Resistance to therapy and median survival ~ 1 year
  - Inactivation of *TP53* or *P16*; activation of *MYC*

Pediatric FL

- Localized disease, usually involves neck lymph nodes
- Extranodal sites also affected: Testes, Waldeyer ring
- High histological grade; usually with large follicles
- Usually Bcl-2(-) and lacks t(14;18)(q32;q21) or *IGH-BCL2*
- Most patients have good prognosis without disease progression

ANCILLARY TESTS

Immunohistochemistry

- Monotypic surface Ig(+); pan-B-cell markers (+)
- CD10(+), Bcl-6(+)
    - CD10 and Bcl-6 more brightly expressed within follicles than in interfollicular regions
- HGAL(+), LMO2(+)
- Bcl-2(+) in 85-90% of FL grade 1 and grade 2; 50% in FL grade 3
    - Bcl-2(+) is useful to distinguish FL from reactive follicles that are Bcl-2(-)
- Follicular dendritic cell meshworks are present in follicles
    - Variable expression of CD21, CD23, or CD35
- CD23(+/-), IRF-4/MUM1(-)
- FLs are usually CD5(-), CD43(-)
    - Small subset (< 5%) can be CD5(+) or CD43(+)
- CD2(-), CD3(-), CD4(-), CD7(-), CD8(-)
- Proliferation rate of FLs assessed by Ki-67
    - Percentage of Ki-67(+) cells correlates with grade
        - Most low-grade FLs show low proliferation rate (< 20%)
        - High-grade FLs show moderate to high proliferation rate (> 40%)
    - Approximately 20% of low-grade FLs have moderate/high proliferation rate
        - These FLs appear to behave more aggressively, similar to grade 3A FL
- Grade 3 FLs
    - Can be CD10(-), Bcl-2(-), IRF-4/MUM1(+)

Cytogenetics

- 80-90% of cases have t(14;18)(q32;q21)
    - Juxtaposes *BCL2* at 18q21 adjacent to *IGH* on derivative chromosome 14
    - Is rarely (10%) the only karyotypic abnormality
- Other common chromosomal aberrations in FL include
    - Deletions of 1p, 6q, 10q, 17p
    - Gains of 1, 6p, 7, 8, 12q, 18q, X
- Complex karyotype correlates with poorer prognosis

In Situ Hybridization

- FISH can detect t(14;18)(q32;q21) in up to 90% of FL cases
    - Large probes can detect multiple breakpoints

PCR

- Monoclonal *IGH* and Ig light chain gene rearrangements
    - Variable regions of Ig genes undergo extensive and ongoing mutations
    - Mutations can cause false-negative result when using PCR to assess for Ig gene rearrangements
        - Multiple primer sets are therefore required for analysis
- There are multiple breakpoints in *BCL2* that must be individually assessed by PCR
    - Major breakpoint cluster region (MBR): ~ 50-60% of FLs with t(14;18)
    - Minor breakpoint cluster region (MCR): ~ 5-10% of FLs
    - Intermediate cluster region (ICR): ~ 10-15% of FLs
    - 5' breakpoint region: ~ 5% of FLs

Array CGH

- ~ 90% of FLs have abnormalities detected by CGH or array CGH
    - Gains: 2p15, 7p, 7q, 8q, 12q, 18p, 18q
    - Losses: 1p36, 3q, 6q, 9p, 11q, 13q, 17p
- Abnormalities associated with worse prognosis
    - Loss of 6q or 9p21
    - Gain of chromosome X
- Abnormalities associated with transformation to DLBCL
    - Gains of 2, 3q, and 5

Molecular Genetics

- *IGH-BCL2*/t(14;18)(q32;q21) is insufficient to induce lymphomagenesis
    - *IGH-BCL2* fusion gene can be detected in blood of 50% of healthy individuals by using sensitive nested PCR methods
- *BCL6/3q27* rearrangement occurs in ~ 15% of FLs
    - More common in grade 3B tumors
- Inactivation of tumor suppressor genes *TP53, P15, P16*
    - Occurs in FLs but is more common at time of transformation to DLBCL
- *MYC* rearrangement is associated with transformation to DLBCL

Gene Expression Profiling

- Initial study from Leukemia/Lymphoma Molecular Profiling Project showed
    - Host response in FLs has prognostic importance
    - 2 gene expression profiles: Immune response (IR) 1 and IR2
        - IR1: Good prognosis: Genes related to T cells and macrophages
        - IR2: Poor prognosis: Genes related to monocytes and dendritic cells
    - These studies included FLs ± t(14;18)(q32;q21)
- Other groups have shown importance of host response but emphasize different gene signatures
- Recent studies have analyzed t(14;18)(+) FL and t(14;18)(-) FL separately
    - FL with t(14;18)(q32;q21)
        - Enriched germinal center B-cell genes
    - FL without t(14;18)(q32;q21)
        - Enriched activated B-cell-like, NF-κB, and proliferation genes

FOLLICULAR LYMPHOMA

DIFFERENTIAL DIAGNOSIS

Reactive Follicular Hyperplasia (RFH)

- Children and young adults; patients with autoimmune disease
- Features that distinguish RFH from FL
  - Lymph node architecture preserved with follicles located mostly in cortex
  - Follicles vary in size and shape; widely spaced
  - Polarization of germinal centers into light and dark zones
  - Frequent mitoses and tingible body macrophages in germinal centers
  - Sharply demarcated mantle zones surround germinal centers
  - Immunophenotype: Polytypic B cells; Bcl-2(-)
  - No evidence of monoclonal Ig gene rearrangements

Progressive Transformation of Germinal Centers

- Partial lymph node replacement
- Nodules are 3-4x larger than background reactive follicles
- Small lymphocytes with mantle cell immunophenotype infiltrate and eventually replace germinal centers
- Immunophenotype: Polytypic B cells; Bcl-2(-)
- No evidence of monoclonal Ig gene rearrangements

Nodular Lymphocyte-Predominant Hodgkin Lymphoma

- Large, vague nodules
- Most cells in nodules are small round lymphocytes
  - Admixed with fewer LP ("popcorn") cells
- LP cells are CD20(+), CD45(+), CD10(-), Bcl-2(-)
- Small cells in tumor nodules are mostly reactive B cells
- CD4(+) and CD57(+) T cells commonly form rosettes around LP cells

Lymphocyte-Rich Classical Hodgkin Lymphoma

- Large vague nodules
- Most cells in nodules are small round lymphocytes
  - Admixed with Hodgkin and Reed-Sternberg (HRS) cells
  - HRS cells are CD15(+), CD30(+), CD45/LCA(-)
- No evidence of monotypic B cells or monoclonal *Ig* gene rearrangements

Mantle Cell Lymphoma (MCL)

- Usually MCL completely effaces lymph node architecture
  - Nodular pattern can resemble FL
- MCL cells are small with irregular nuclear contours; no centroblasts
- Hyalinized blood vessels and histiocytes with eosinophilic cytoplasm are common
- Immunophenotype
  - Monotypic B-cell population
  - CD5(+), CD43(+), cyclin-D1 (+)
- Detection of t(11;14)(q13;q32) by cytogenetics, FISH, or PCR

Nodal Marginal Zone Lymphoma

- Partial effacement of lymph node architecture with marginal zone expansion
- Neoplastic lymphocytes include small lymphocytes, lymphocytes with monocytoid nuclei, and large cells
  - Frequent plasmacytic differentiation
  - Neoplastic lymphocytes colonize and may replace germinal centers
- Bcl-2(-) in residual centrocytes of germinal centers
- Bcl-2(+) in marginal zone lymphocytes
- Immunophenotype
  - Monotypic B-cell population; Bcl-2(+)
  - CD5(-), CD10(-), cyclin-D1 (-), Bcl-6(-)
  - No evidence of t(14;18)(q32;q21)

SELECTED REFERENCES

1. Freedman A: Follicular lymphoma: 2012 update on diagnosis and management. Am J Hematol. 87(10):988-95, 2012
2. Kridel R et al: Pathogenesis of follicular lymphoma. J Clin Invest. 122(10):3424-31, 2012
3. Cheung KJ et al: High resolution analysis of follicular lymphoma genomes reveals somatic recurrent sites of copy-neutral loss of heterozygosity and copy number alterations that target single genes. Genes Chromosomes Cancer. 49(8):669-81, 2010
4. Eide MB et al: Genomic alterations reveal potential for higher grade transformation in follicular lymphoma and confirm parallel evolution of tumor cell clones. Blood. 116(9):1489-97, 2010
5. Gradowski JF et al: Follicular lymphomas with plasmacytic differentiation include two subtypes. Mod Pathol. 23(1):71-9, 2010
6. Montes-Moreno S et al: Intrafollicular neoplasia/in situ follicular lymphoma: review of a series of 13 cases. Histopathology. 56(5):658-62, 2010
7. Wrench D et al: Molecular signatures in the diagnosis and management of follicular lymphoma. Curr Opin Hematol. 17(4):333-40, 2010
8. Carlotti E et al: Transformation of follicular lymphoma to diffuse large B-cell lymphoma may occur by divergent evolution from a common progenitor cell or by direct evolution from the follicular lymphoma clone. Blood. 113(15):3553-7, 2009
9. Cheung KJ et al: Genome-wide profiling of follicular lymphoma by array comparative genomic hybridization reveals prognostically significant DNA copy number imbalances. Blood. 113(1):137-48, 2009
10. Federico M et al: Follicular lymphoma international prognostic index 2: a new prognostic index for follicular lymphoma developed by the international follicular lymphoma prognostic factor project. J Clin Oncol. 27(27):4555-62, 2009
11. Leich E et al: Follicular lymphomas with and without translocation t(14;18) differ in gene expression profiles and genetic alterations. Blood. 114(4):826-34, 2009
12. Schwaenen C et al: Microarray-based genomic profiling reveals novel genomic aberrations in follicular lymphoma which associate with patient survival and gene expression status. Genes Chromosomes Cancer. 48(1):39-54, 2009

FOLLICULAR LYMPHOMA

Microscopic Features

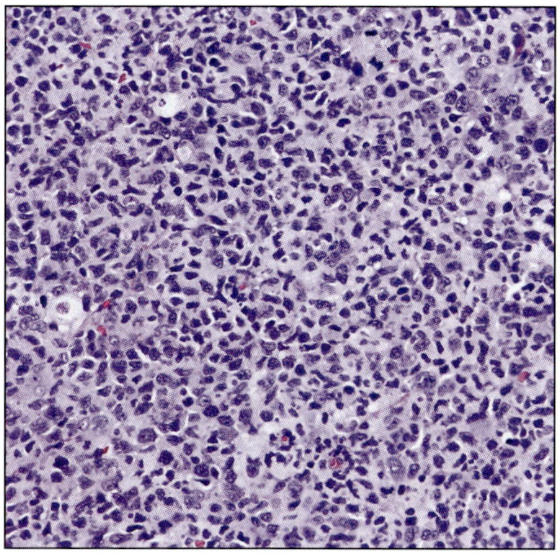

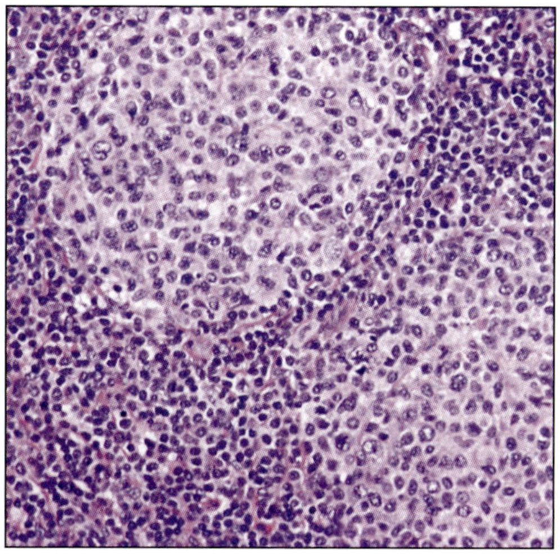

(Left) *Image shows follicular lymphoma (FL) involving lymph node. The follicles are composed of numerous centrocytes and fewer centroblasts, supporting grade 2.* ***(Right)*** *FL, grade 3A, follicular pattern is shown. The follicles are composed of many centroblasts, but centrocytes are also present.*

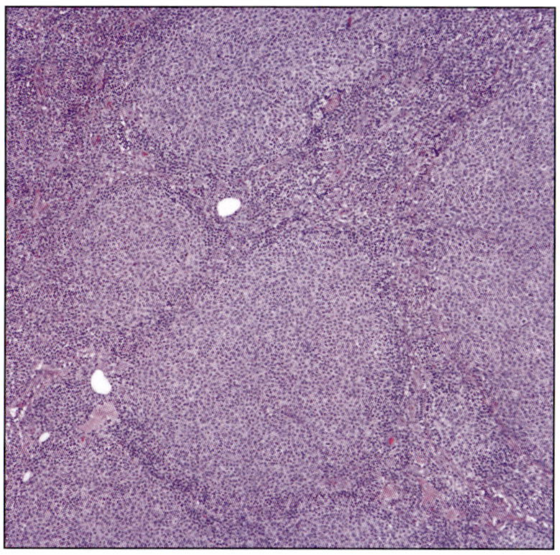

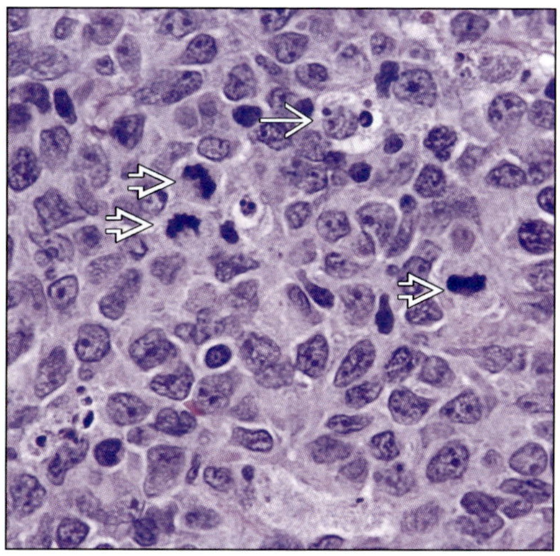

(Left) *H&E shows FL, grade 3B, replacing a lymph node. The neoplastic follicles are composed of numerous large cells, many of which are consistent with centroblasts.* ***(Right)*** *FL, grade 3B is shown, replacing a lymph node. The architecture is replaced by neoplastic follicles composed of numerous centroblasts. In this neoplastic follicle, mitotic figures ⇨ and tingible body macrophages ➔ are seen. No small centrocytes are noted.*

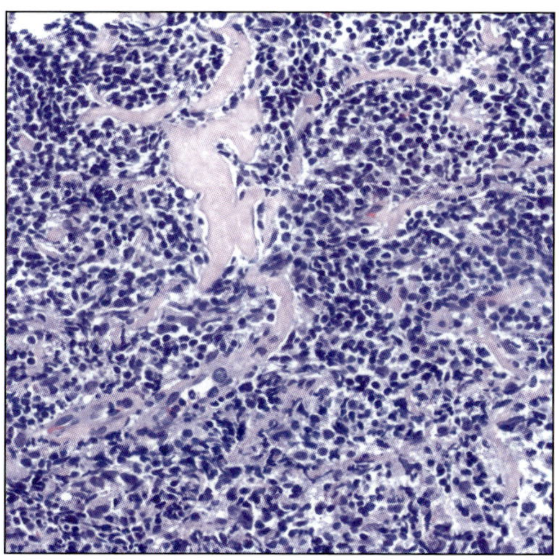

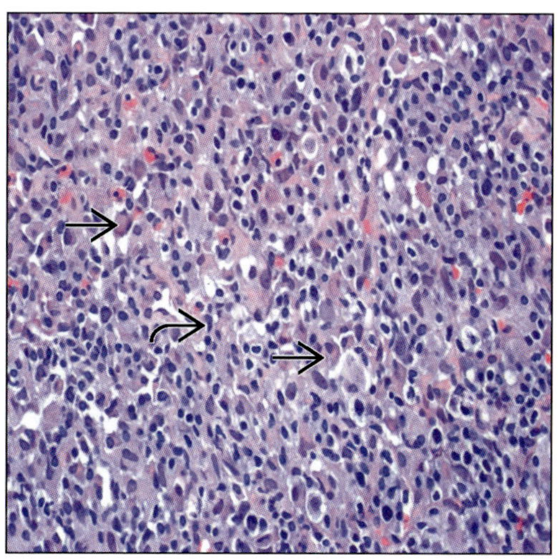

(Left) *FL, low grade, involves a retroperitoneal lymph node. This field shows sclerosis that is associated with the neoplastic lymphoid infiltrate.* ***(Right)*** *FL with plasmacytic differentiation involves a lymph node. Scattered plasma cells → admixed with centrocytes ↪ are noted. Flow cytometric immunophenotyping demonstrated a population of CD10(+) B cells, and FISH revealed the IgH/BCL2 fusion gene.*

Microscopic and Immunohistochemical Features

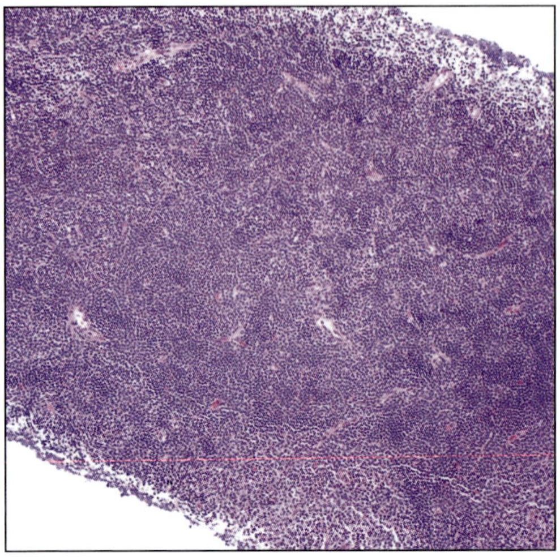

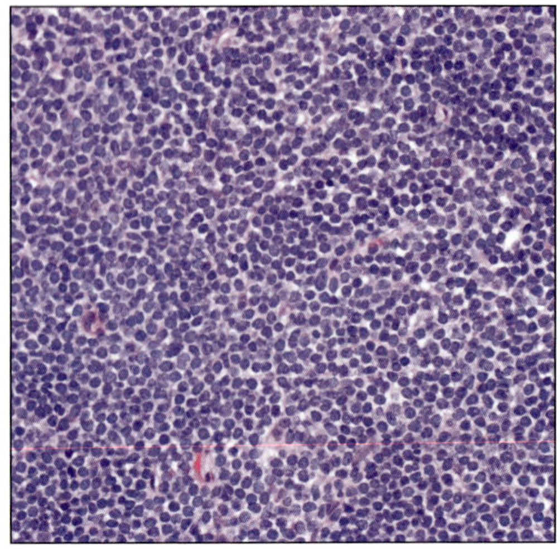

(Left) *Initial sections of this core needle biopsy revealed FL with a diffuse growth pattern. Subsequent deeper levels of the block showed rare follicles. The diagnosis of FL was further confirmed by reactivity of the neoplastic cells with CD10, Bcl-6, and Bcl-2.* ***(Right)*** *Image shows diffuse FL involving lymph node. The neoplasm had a diffuse growth pattern and was composed predominantly of centrocytes, supporting grade 1. The proliferation rate was less than 5%.*

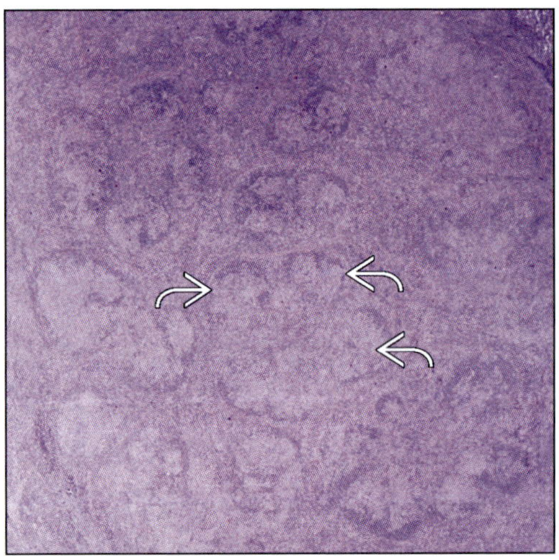

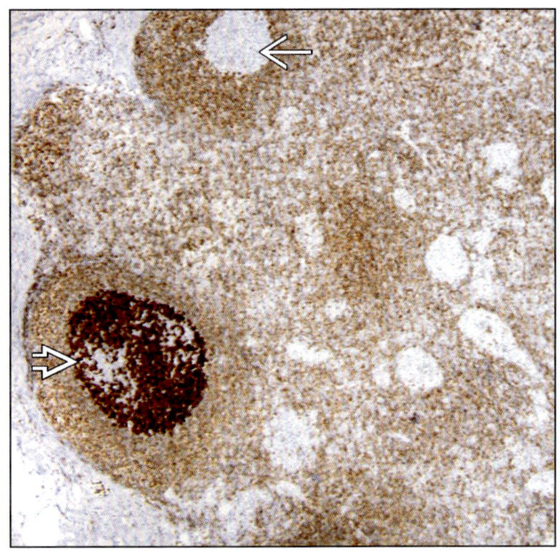

(Left) *The floral variant of FL involving lymph node is depicted. The fused or fragmented follicles have the appearance of flower petals.* ***(Right)*** *Immunohistochemical stain for Bcl-2 reveals a single positive germinal center showing intrafollicular neoplasia. A nearby hyperplastic germinal center is Bcl-2(-). Routine histologic examination revealed a benign-appearing germinal center with a predominance of small centrocytes.*

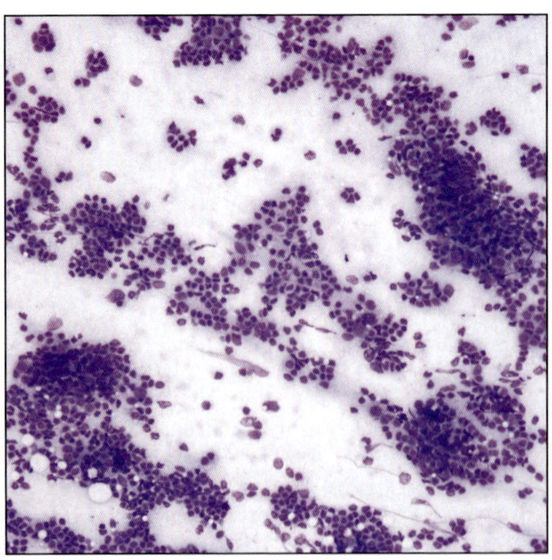

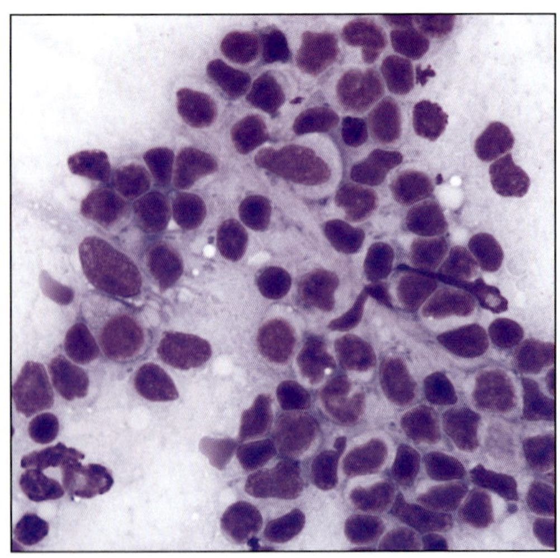

(Left) *Fine needle aspiration of a lymph node from a patient with FL, grade 2, shows aggregates of monotonous lymphoid cells bound by follicular dendritic cells.* ***(Right)*** *Fine needle aspiration of a lymph node from a patient with FL, grade 2, demonstrates a mixture of centrocytes and centroblasts.*

Immunohistochemical Features

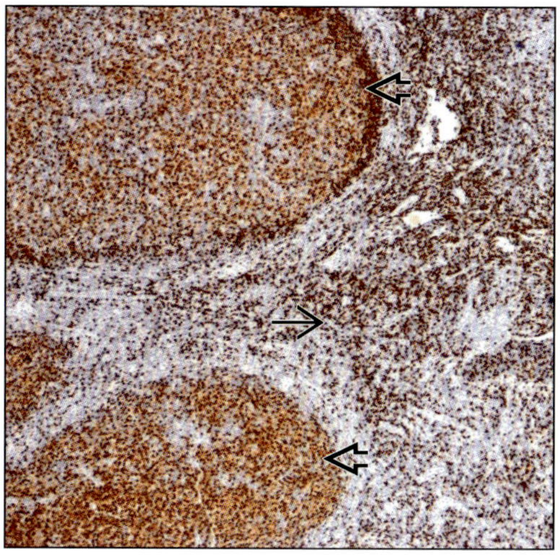
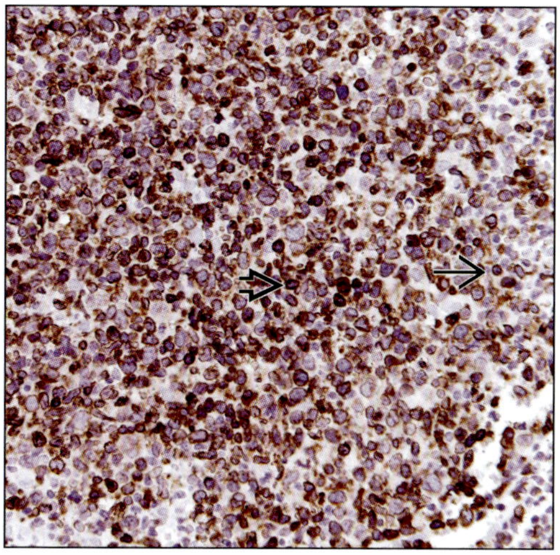

(Left) *pax-5 immunohistochemistry highlights B lymphocytes in neoplastic follicles as well as in interfollicular areas in this FL involving a lymph node.* ***(Right)*** *Immunohistochemical stain for Bcl-2 from a lymph node involved by FL shows that the neoplastic cells are positive. In this case, the neoplastic cells stained more strongly than small reactive T cells, which are also Bcl-2(+).*

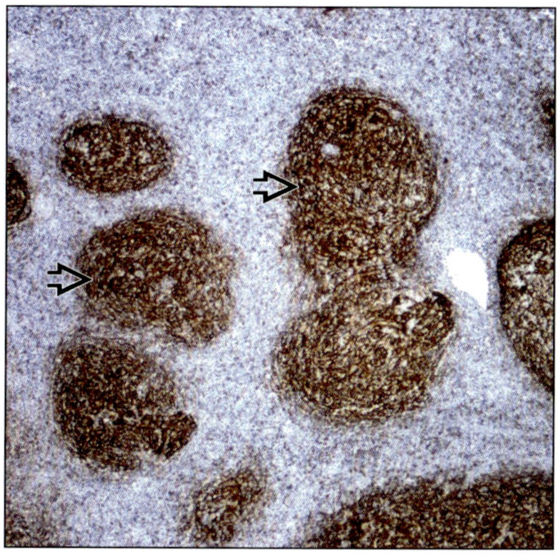
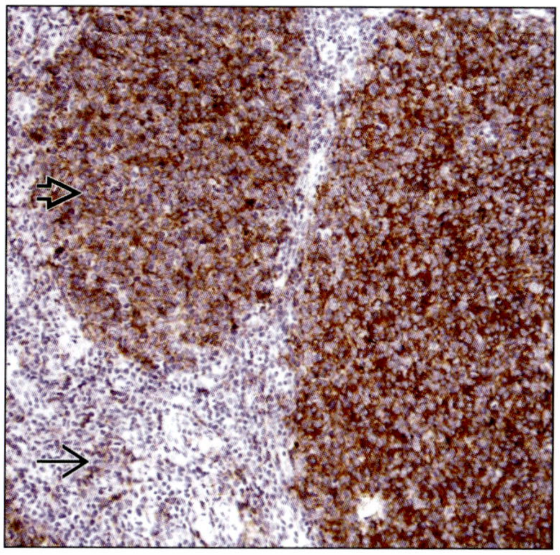

(Left) *FL involves a lymph node. Immunostain for CD21 highlights follicular dendritic cells within follicles. CD21 is very useful in establishing the presence of follicles.* ***(Right)*** *Immunohistochemical stain for CD10 in a case of FL shows that the neoplastic cells are strongly positive within neoplastic follicles and faintly positive in interfollicular areas.*

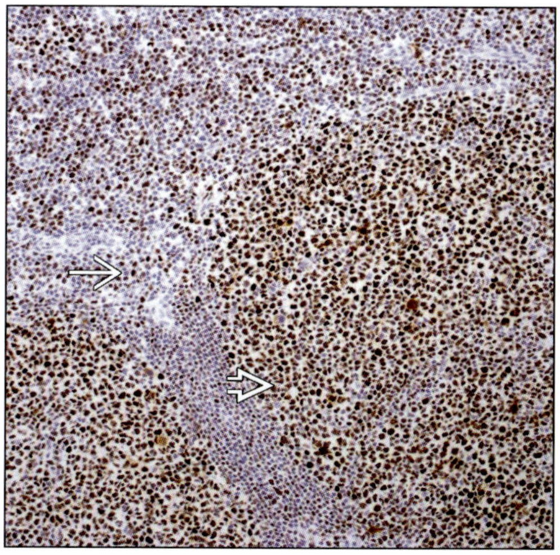
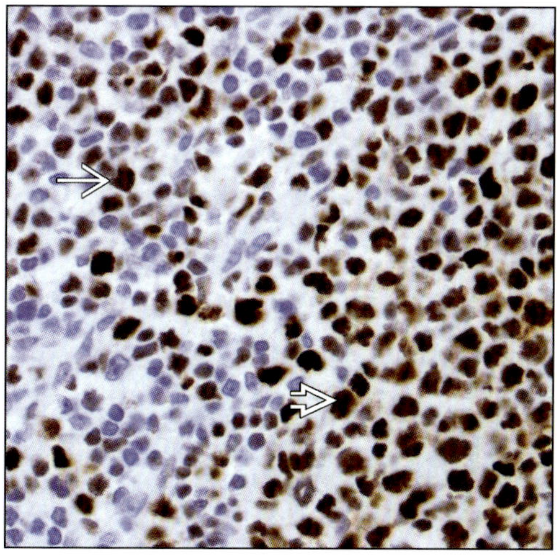

(Left) *Immunostain for Bcl-6 highlights germinal center B cells within follicles as well as within interfollicular B cells in a case of FL. The reactivity is stronger in germinal centers than in interfollicular regions.* ***(Right)*** *FL assessed for Bcl-6 by immunohistochemistry highlights germinal center B cells within follicles as well as within interfollicular B cells. The difference in intensity of expression is attributable to the microenvironment.*

FOLLICULAR LYMPHOMA

Immunohistochemical Features and Ancillary Techniques

(Left) Immunohistochemical stain for Ki-67 in a case of FL, grade 3A, shows a germinal center with a proliferation rate of 40-50%. There is usually a good correlation between the grade of FL and the proliferation rate. ***(Right)*** *Paradoxically high proliferation rate (~ 60%) is seen in a neoplastic follicle in a case of FL grade 2. Histological cases of low-grade FL associated with high Ki-67 appear to behave more aggressively than those with a low proliferation rate.*

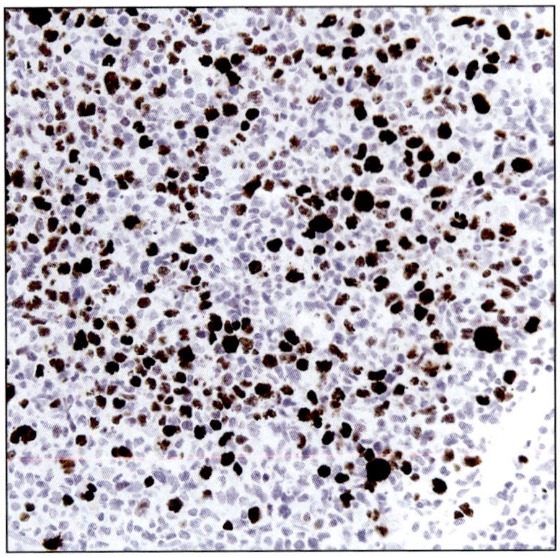

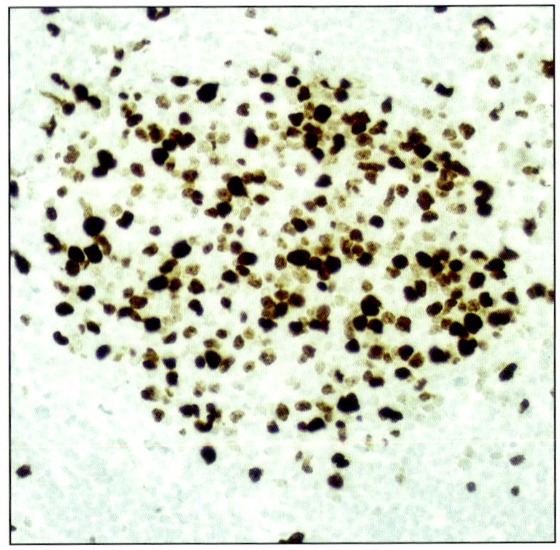

(Left) *Flow cytometric immunophenotyping of a lymph node fine aspirate specimen from a patient with FL reveals that the lymphoma cells express CD19 and CD10.* ***(Right)*** *Flow cytometric immunophenotyping of a lymph node fine aspirate specimen from a patient with FL reveals that the lymphoma cells express monotypic immunoglobulin κ light chain. In this example, the lymphocytes expressing κ outnumber the few lymphocytes expressing λ.*

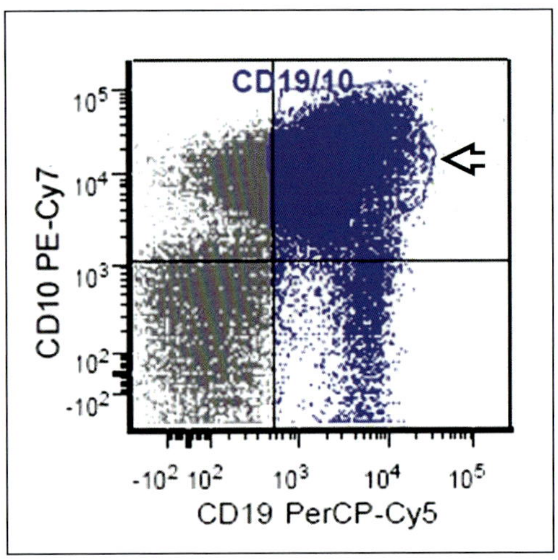

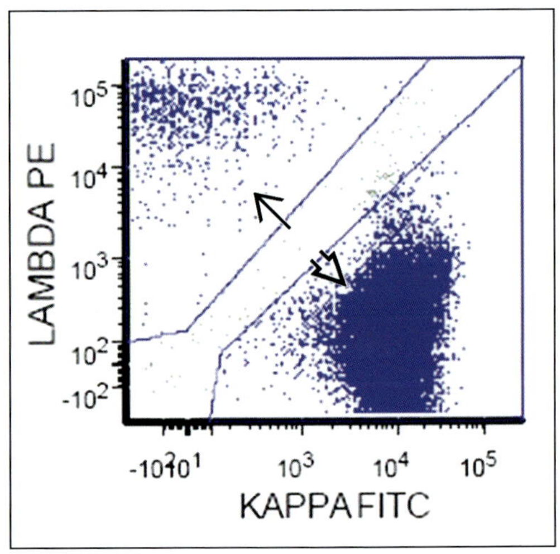

(Left) *Real-time PCR assesses for the IgH/BCL2 fusion gene involving the major breakpoint cluster region. Threshold, negative control, high positive control, and low positive amplification are highlighted. (Courtesy S. Chen, MD.)* ***(Right)*** *FISH was performed on a fixed, paraffin-embedded tissue section of FL using dual-fusion probes for Bcl-2 (red) and IgH (green). The t(14;18)(q32;q21)/IgH-BCL2 fusion gene is a yellow signal.*

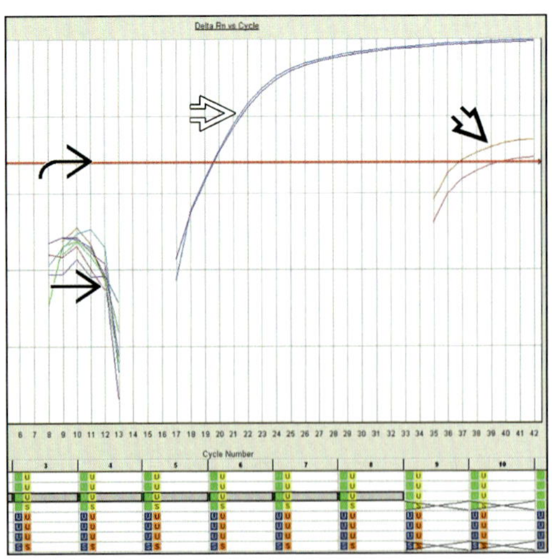

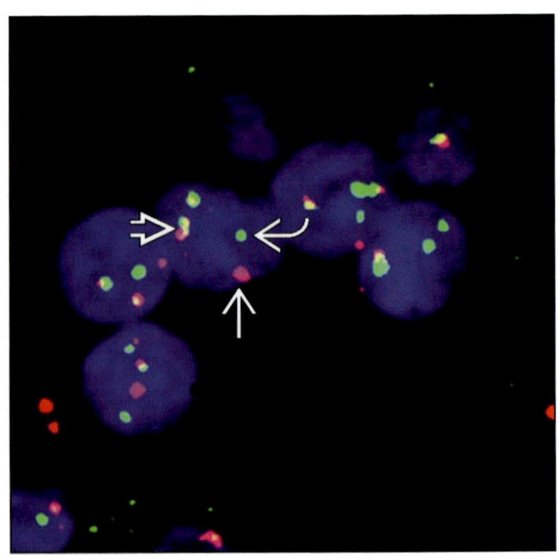

Follicular Lymphoma Involving Extranodal Sites

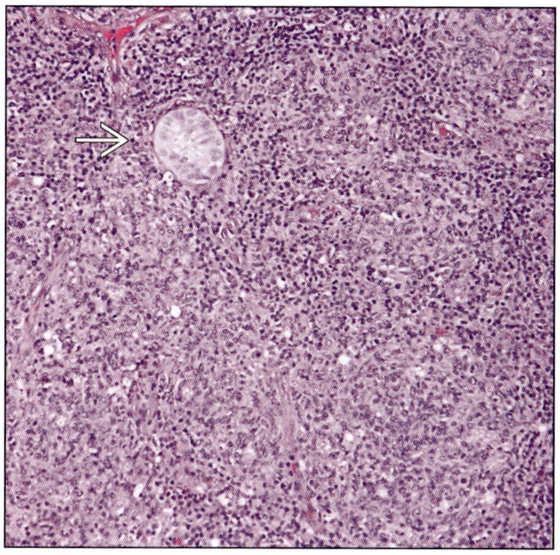

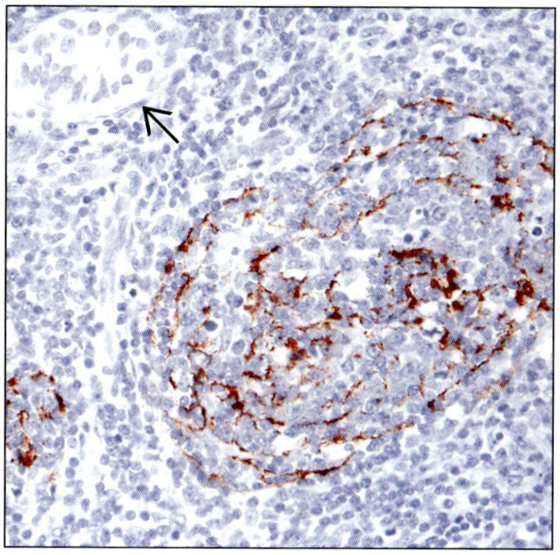

(Left) *Image shows FL involving the testis in a 6-year-old boy. Most of the testis is replaced by tumor nodules, but a seminiferous tubule ➡ can be seen in the field. Most children with FL have a clinically indolent course even when the lymphoma is grade 3.* ***(Right)*** *The anti-CD21 antibody highlights follicular dendritic cells within a neoplastic follicle in FL involving the testis in a 6-year-old boy. A seminiferous tubule ➡ is present and can be seen at the upper right corner of this image.*

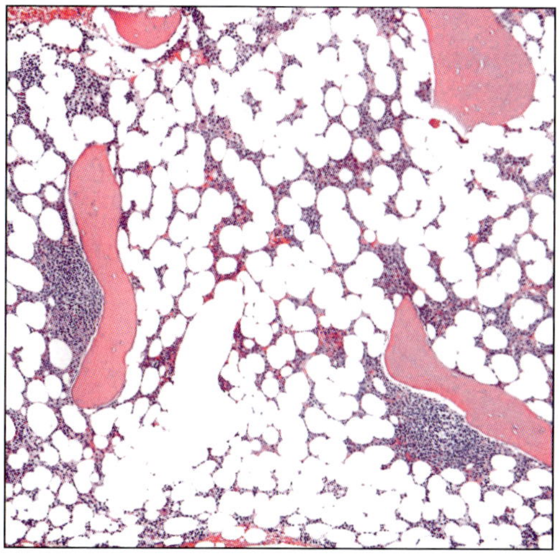

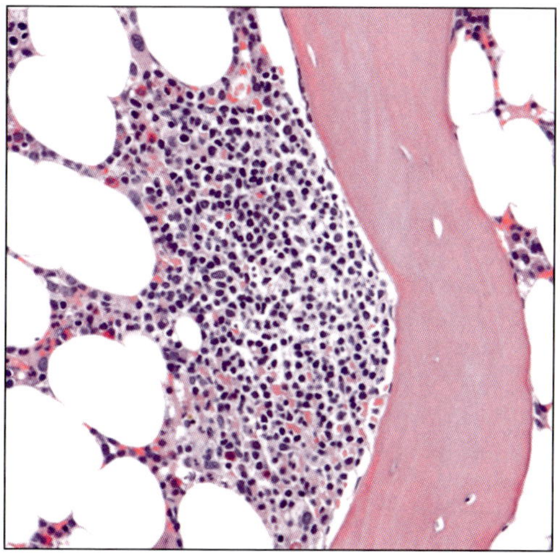

(Left) *Bone marrow core biopsy specimen is involved by FL. The neoplasm has a purely paratrabecular pattern, which is highly suggestive of FL.* ***(Right)*** *Bone marrow core biopsy specimen involved by FL is shown. In many patients with this pattern of involvement, flow cytometry or molecular studies are negative for a monotypic B-cell population or t(14;18)(q32;q21) because the lymphoma cells are not aspirated.*

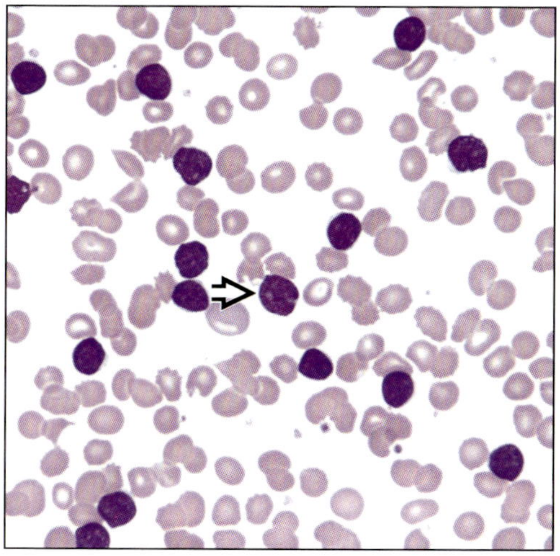

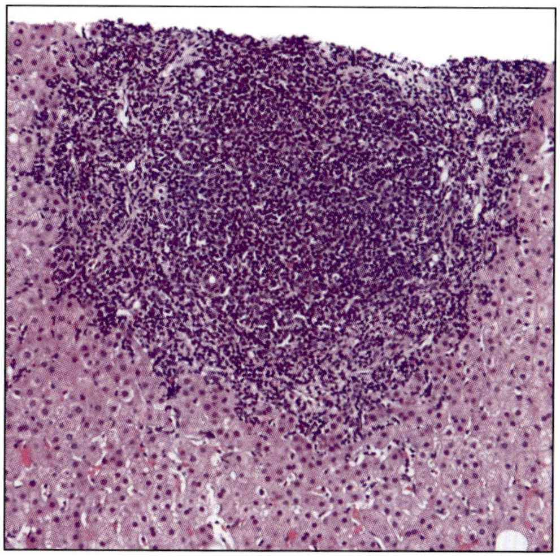

(Left) *A peripheral blood smear from a patient with FL demonstrates leukemic involvement by centrocytes with deeply cleaved nuclei, so-called buttock cells ⇨.* ***(Right)*** *A core needle biopsy of liver involved by FL shows expansion of a portal tract. The lymphoid infiltrate is composed mostly of centrocytes.*

HODGKIN LYMPHOMA

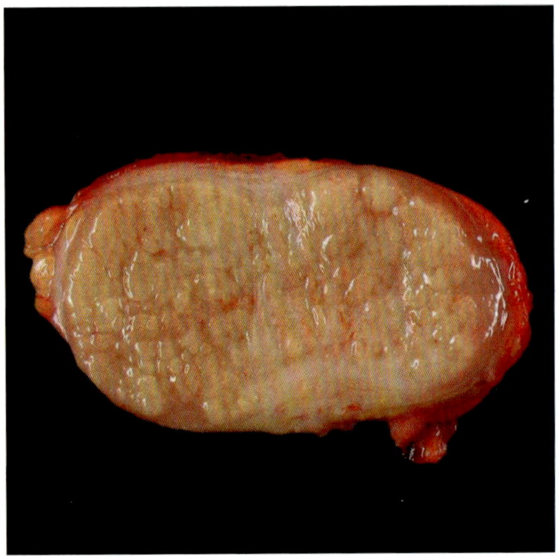

Image shows the cut surface of a lymph node from a patient with NSCHL. Note the nodular appearance and the intervening bands of fibrosis. The texture upon bisecting such lymph nodes is often described as gritty.

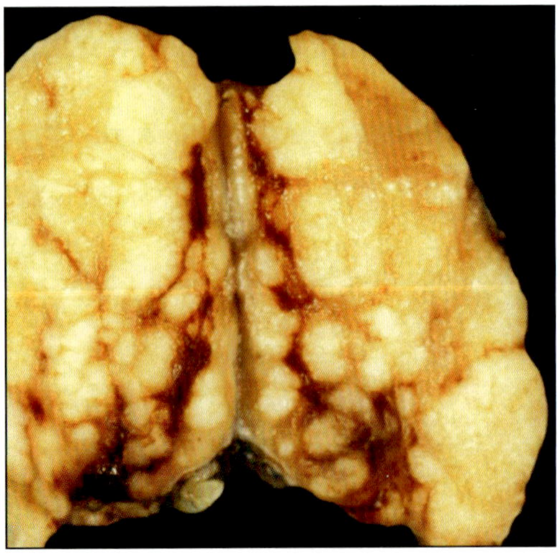

Image shows a bisected lymph node from a patient with nodular lymphocyte-predominant HL (NLPHL). There are multiple nodules of variable size throughout the lymph node parenchyma. (Courtesy P. Lin, MD.)

TERMINOLOGY

Abbreviations

- Hodgkin lymphoma (HL)
- Classical Hodgkin lymphoma (CHL)

Definitions

- CHL (95% of HL) is a lymphoid neoplasm composed of neoplastic Hodgkin and Reed-Sternberg (HRS) cells in a reactive inflammatory background
  - Composed of 4 subtypes that demonstrate distinct features
    - CHL, nodular sclerosis subtype (NSCHL) (70% CHL): Neoplastic HRS cells and reactive inflammatory cells form nodules surrounded by fibrous bands
    - CHL, mixed cellularity subtype (MCCHL) (20-25% CHL): Neoplastic HRS cells and reactive inflammatory cells form diffuse or interfollicular pattern
    - CHL, lymphocyte-rich subtype (LRCHL) (4-5% CHL): Neoplastic HRS cells are surrounded by small, reactive lymphocytes in a nodular or diffuse pattern
    - CHL, lymphocyte-depleted subtype (LDCHL) (< 1% CHL): Neoplastic HRS cells may be scant, frequent or pleomorphic in a variably fibrotic background depleted of small lymphocytes
- Nodular lymphocyte-predominant HL (NLPHL) (5% of HL) is a lymphoid neoplasm composed of neoplastic lymphocyte-predominant (LP) cells in a reactive inflammatory background

ETIOLOGY/PATHOGENESIS

CHL

- HRS cells
  - Arise from late germinal center or early post-germinal center B cells
  - Have undergone immunoglobulin (Ig) gene rearrangements with somatic mutations
  - In some cases, crippling (e.g., nonsense) Ig mutations occur but cells do not undergo apoptosis
  - Lack B-cell antigen receptors
- HRS cells lose much of the normal B-cell phenotype
  - Severe impairment of transcription factor networks regulating B-cell gene expression
    - Low or undetectable levels of transcription factors: *OCT2*, *BOB1*, *PU.1*, and early B-cell factor-1 (*EBF1*)
    - Because *EBF1* also suppresses expression of myeloid and T-cell genes, low level of *EBF1* expression in HRS may contribute to aberrant expression of T-cell markers or myeloid markers
    - Numerous B-cell genes are inactivated by epigenetic silencing (e.g., promoter hypermethylation) including *CD19*
    - Deregulated expression of *NOTCH1*, activated B-cell factor 1 (*ABF1*), and inhibitor of differentiation and DNA binding 2 (*ID2*) inhibit overall B-cell development
- HRS cells utilize antiapoptotic mechanisms to achieve survival
- Microenvironment plays a critical role
  - Reactive cellular infiltrate is induced, in part, by HRS cells, which produce a variety of cytokines, chemokines, and growth factors
    - Protects HRS cells from apoptosis
    - Suppresses T-cell and NK-cell immune response against HRS cells
- Notes about subtypes
  - NSCHL: HRS cells have increased production of IL-13, which may be responsible for broad bands of birefringent collagen
  - LDCHL: May represent progression from other types of CHL
- Infectious agents

HODGKIN LYMPHOMA

Key Facts

Terminology

- CHL (95% of HL) is a lymphoid neoplasm composed of neoplastic Hodgkin and Reed-Sternberg (HRS) cells in a reactive inflammatory background
  - Composed of 4 subtypes: NSCHL, MCCHL, LRCHL, and LDCHL
- NLPHL (5% of HL) is a lymphoid neoplasm composed of neoplastic lymphocyte-predominant (LP) cells in a reactive inflammatory background

Etiology/Pathogenesis

- HRS cells arise from late germinal center B cells
  - Demonstrate many defects in B-cell differentiation
  - Utilize antiapoptotic mechanisms to survive
- LP cells arise from centroblastic-stage germinal center B cells and demonstrate frequent *BCL6* abnormalities
- Familial factors
  - Familial HL accounts for ~ 4.5% of all HL
  - Specific HLA haplotypes have been associated with HL risk
  - Genome-wide association studies have also identified several susceptibility loci

Microscopic Pathology

- Both CHL and NLPHL are characterized by the presence of (typically) few, scattered neoplastic cells in a background of numerous reactive inflammatory cells
- Neoplastic HRS cells include bilobed or multilobated Reed-Sternberg forms and mononuclear Hodgkin cells, which display large eosinophilic nucleoli and abundant slightly basophilic cytoplasm

---

- Epstein-Barr virus (EBV) likely plays a role in pathogenesis of HL but is only found in a proportion of cases
  - NSCHL: EBV expression detected in HRS cells in ~ 20% of cases
  - MCCHL: EBV expression detected in HRS cells in ~ 75% of cases
  - LRCHL: EBV expression intermediate between NSCHL and MCCHL
  - LDCHL: EBV expression common, particularly in patients with HIV infection
  - No other associated viruses have been identified
- Primary immunodeficiencies
  - CHL has been reported in patients with ataxia-telangiectasia and Wiskott-Aldrich syndrome
- Secondary immunodeficiencies
  - Patients with HIV infection have an increased risk of HL
  - CHL may develop in the post-transplant setting (particularly after renal transplant) and is almost always EBV associated
- Familial factors
  - Familial HL accounts for ~ 4.5% of all HL
  - Specific HLA haplotypes have been associated with HL risk
  - Genome-wide association studies have also identified several susceptibility loci

NLPHL

- LP cells are clonal with rearranged, somatically mutated Ig variable region genes that are functional, indicating that normal counterpart is likely antigen-selected germinal center B lymphocytes
- No association with latent EBV infection
- *IGH-BCL6* translocations have been found in a subset of NLPHL cases
- *BCL6* rearrangements are frequent in NLPHL
- Aberrant somatic hypermutations in several genes including *PAX5*, *PIM1*, *RHOH/TTF*, and *MYC* have been identified
- NLPHL is associated with progressive transformation of germinal centers (PTGC), which may precede or occur concurrently with NLPHL, although diagnosis of PTGC alone does not increase risk of subsequent development of NLPHL
- Several NLPHL families have been identified
  - Whole exome sequencing and linkage studies revealed truncating germline mutation in *NPAT* gene in a family of 4 cousins with NLPHL

CLINICAL ISSUES

Epidemiology

- Incidence
  - HL accounts for ~ 20-30% of all lymphomas in USA and Europe
  - CHL accounts for 95% of HL (NSCHL > MCCHL > LRCHL > LDCHL)
    - NSCHL is more frequent in developed countries compared to developing countries
  - NLPHL accounts for 5% of HL
- Age
  - NSCHL: Peak incidence at 15-34 years of age
  - MCCHL, LRCHL, LDCHL, NLPHL: Older age group than peak of NSCHL (≥ 30-50 years)
- Gender
  - NSCHL: Slightly more prevalent in women
  - MCCHL, LRCHL, LDCHL, NLPHL: M:F ≥ 2:1

Site

- NSCHL: Mediastinal or cervical lymph nodes
- MCCHL: Cervical or supraclavicular lymph nodes (mediastinal involvement uncommon); spleen
- LRCHL: Peripheral lymph nodes, especially supradiaphragmatic; may involve Waldeyer ring, unlike other forms of CHL
- LDCHL: Retroperitoneal or abdominal lymph node involvement more frequent than peripheral lymph node involvement
- CHL generally spreads to contiguous structures
  - Involvement of lymphoid structures on both sides of diaphragm or at extranodal sites beyond site of

contiguous spread (including bone marrow) is an indication of advanced stage disease
- NLPHL: Cervical, axillary, or inguinal lymph nodes most common
  - Bone marrow involvement often indicates more aggressive behavior/transformation

Presentation
- B symptoms common in NSCHL, MCCHL, and LDCHL
- LDCHL often presents at advanced stage
- NLPHL often presents with asymptomatic lymphadenopathy

Treatment
- Chemotherapy ± radiation
- Autologous stem cell transplantation following high-dose chemotherapy may be considered in relapsed/refractory disease

Prognosis
- CHL
  - With modern therapy, all subtypes at similar stages have a similar prognosis
    - > 90% survival at 5 years in patients with early stage disease
    - Adverse prognostic factors: Advanced stage, massive mediastinal involvement, older age (> 45 years), male gender
- NLPHL
  - > 80% 10-year survival
  - Indolent course but frequent relapses that are responsive to therapy
  - Large cell lymphoma may coexist with or follow NLPHL
    - Diffuse large B-cell lymphoma (DLBCL): Good prognosis if localized
    - T-cell/histiocyte-rich large B-cell lymphoma (THRLBCL): Poorer prognosis

MICROSCOPIC PATHOLOGY

Histologic Features
- Both CHL and NLPHL are characterized by the presence of (typically) few, scattered neoplastic cells in a background of numerous reactive inflammatory cells
- CHL
  - Neoplastic HRS cells include bilobed or multilobated Reed-Sternberg forms and mononuclear Hodgkin cells, which display large eosinophilic nucleoli and abundant slightly basophilic cytoplasm
    - Presence of a classic Reed-Sternberg cell (≥ 2 nuclear lobes/nuclei with ≥ 1 nucleolus in each lobe/nucleus) is required at initial diagnosis
    - Once a diagnosis of CHL has been rendered, diagnostic Reed-Sternberg cells do not have to be present to make diagnosis at a secondary site or on subsequent biopsy
  - Some HRS cells are pyknotic, so-called mummified forms
  - NSCHL
    - Lymph node architecture effaced by neoplastic nodules surrounded by broad, birefringent collagen bands
    - Nodules are composed of inflammatory cells (eosinophils, histiocytes, neutrophils, and plasma cells) and admixed HRS cells
    - HRS cells may show retraction artifact in formalin-fixed tissue sections, so-called lacunar cells
    - Neutrophilic or eosinophilic abscesses may occur
    - Syncytial variant: Confluent aggregates of HRS cells and fewer collagen bands (may mimic large cell lymphoma or metastatic carcinoma)
  - MCCHL
    - Complete or partial effacement of lymph node architecture; interfollicular pattern can occur
    - Thick fibrous bands not present; otherwise similar to NSCHL
    - Histiocytes can be singly scattered or present as ill-defined or epithelioid granulomas
  - LRCHL
    - Commonly nodular pattern in lymph node but may rarely show diffuse architecture
    - Nodules are composed of expanded mantle zones (small lymphocytes) with underlying loose follicular dendritic cell (FDC) meshworks; nodules may contain eccentrically located germinal centers
    - HRS cells are located within nodules (outside of germinal centers, if present)
    - Few histiocytes, plasma cells uncommon, rare to no eosinophils or neutrophils
  - LDCHL
    - Lymph node architecture is usually diffusely effaced
    - Generalized depletion of small lymphocytes
    - Eosinophils, neutrophils, and plasma cells are usually scant or absent
    - 3 morphologic patterns: (1) **diffuse fibrosis** with scant HRS cells admixed with few or abundant fibroblasts, fibrillary stroma, and scant lymphocytes; (2) **reticular or sarcoma-like** with abundant HRS cells, including pleomorphic, bizarre (sarcomatous) cells; (3) **mixed cellularity-like** with numerous HRS cells
    - ± coagulative necrosis, sinusoidal invasion, or disordered nonbirefringent fibrillary fibrosis
    - If nodular sclerosing fibrosis is present, process is classified as NSCHL
  - Bone marrow involvement
    - Often patchy with discrete focal lesions composed of a polymorphous infiltrate of lymphocytes, histiocytes, plasma cells, and eosinophils with few HRS cells
    - Commonly associated with fibrosis
    - Multiple levels (step sections) should be performed when evaluating for marrow involvement of CHL if lesions not apparent on initial sections
    - Clinically often manifests as cytopenias
- NLPHL

- Neoplastic LP cells are large with a variety of morphologic appearances, and are typically confined within expanded, intact FDC meshworks
  - Multilobated "popcorn" cells with vesicular chromatin, multiple small nucleoli, and scant cytoplasm
  - Multinucleated or mummified cells
  - Round cells without multilobation
  - Some forms may be morphologically indistinguishable from HRS cells
- Background is composed predominantly of small lymphocytes as well as histiocytes (eosinophils and neutrophils rare)
- Low-magnification view shows complete or partial effacement of lymph node architecture
  - Classical nodular pattern is most common (expansile nodules composed mostly of small lymphocytes and fewer histiocytes; usually no reactive follicles)
  - Serpiginous nodular pattern demonstrates confluent irregular nodules
  - Nodular pattern with extranodular LP cells (most commonly seen at recurrence)
  - Nodular pattern with T-cell-rich background
  - THRLBCL-like (i.e., with diffuse areas indistinguishable from THRLBCL), but with at least 1 typical nodule
- Adjacent reactive follicular hyperplasia with PTGC may precede or be adjacent to NLPHL
- Large cell lymphoma may coexist with or follow NLPHL
  - Sheets of large cells outside of the NLPHL nodules indicates transformation to DLBCL
  - Scattered large cells in a diffuse architecture may indicate transformation to THRLBCL, although there is no consensus on pathologic criteria to distinguish between NLPHL with diffuse (THRLBCL-like) areas vs. evolving transformation to THRLBCL
  - Incorporation of clinical criteria (such as marrow or liver involvement or elevated LDH) may be needed to diagnose transformation to THRLBCL
- Bone marrow involvement
  - Uncommon
  - If present, consider progression to THRLBCL
- Fibrosis in up to 40% of cases with recurrence

Cytologic Features

- CHL
  - HRS cells in inflammatory background can be appreciated in fine needle aspiration smears
  - Must confirm morphologic impression with immunohistochemical stains performed on cell block
  - Difficult to subtype
- Features of NLPHL on fine needle aspiration are not well documented
  - Would be difficult to distinguish from THRLBCL given absence of architectural information

ANCILLARY TESTS

Immunohistochemistry

- CHL: HRS cells
  - Express CD30 (> 95% of cases) and CD15 (70-80%) with characteristic membranous pattern with accentuation in Golgi area
  - Express pax-5 (dim); variably express CD20 (often heterogeneous) and CD79a (~ 10-20%)
  - Express Ki-67, p53, MUM1, CCL17, fascin (+/1), Bcl-2 (+/-)
  - Variable expression of T-cell antigens in up to 15% of cases
  - No expression of CD45/LCA, EMA, immunoglobulin, clusterin
  - Rare expression of OCT2, BOB1; no expression of PU.1
  - Background CD4(+) T cells form rosettes around HRS cells
- NLPHL: LP cells
  - Express CD20, CD22, CD79a, OCT2, BOB1, PU.1
  - Express CD45/LCA, Ki-67, BCL6, EMA (50% of cases), MUM1 (50% of cases)
  - Express IgD in 25% of cases (typically younger patients)
  - Negative for CD30, CD15, Bcl-2, T-cell antigens
  - Small population of follicular T-helper cells (positive for CD3, CD4, CD57, PD.1) form rosettes around LP cells
  - Nodules demonstrate intact FDC meshworks as highlighted by immunohistochemical studies for CD21, CD23, or CD35

Flow Cytometry

- Will not detect HRS or LP cells
- Polytypic B cells (useful to exclude involvement by B-cell non-Hodgkin lymphoma)
- T cells with normal immunophenotype; possibly increased CD4:CD8 ratio in CHL

Cytogenetics

- NLPHL: Abnormalities of chromosome 3q27 (*BCL6* locus) involved in up to 60% of cases

In Situ Hybridization

- Expression of EBV-encoded mRNA (*EBER*) can be detected by in situ hybridization in CHL (not present in NLPHL)

Molecular Genetics

- Monoclonal Ig gene rearrangements shown by single-cell PCR of HRS cells; difficult to isolate single HRS in routine practice; therefore, PCR often polyclonal (reflecting background B cells) unless abundant HRS cells present (i.e., syncytial variant)

DIFFERENTIAL DIAGNOSIS

NSCHL

- Other types of CHL
- NLPHL
- Primary mediastinal large B-cell lymphoma

HODGKIN LYMPHOMA

Characteristics of Classical Hodgkin Lymphoma Subtypes

	NSCHL	MCCHL	LDCHL	LRCHL
Frequency of subtype	70%	20-25%	< 1%	4-5%
Clinical Features				
M:F	1:1	2:1	4:1	2:1
Median age	15-34 years	38 years	57 years	30-50 years
Preferential sites	Mediastinal and cervical nodes	Peripheral nodes, spleen	Retroperitoneal and abdominal nodes, spleen, and bone marrow	Peripheral nodes
B symptoms	~ 40%	Common	Common	Rare
Histopathologic Features				
Architecture	Broad collagen bands surround cellular nodules	Diffuse or interfollicular growth patterns	Diffuse fibrosis, reticular and mixed cellularity-like variants	Nodular growth pattern; rarely diffuse
Cytologic features	Lacunar cells and mummified cells	Frequent HRS cells admixed with cellular inflammatory background	Many HRS cells in background depleted of lymphocytes	Few HRS cells in mantle zones surrounding small germinal centers
Special Markers				
EBER association	20%	70%	75%	40%

- B-cell lymphoma, unclassifiable, with features intermediate between DLBCL and CHL
- Anaplastic large cell lymphoma (ALCL), ALK(+), or ALK(-)
- Peripheral T-cell lymphoma, not otherwise specified (PTCL, NOS)
- Metastatic carcinoma
- Primary myelofibrosis

MCCHL
- Other types of CHL
- PTCL, NOS
- THRLBCL
- Infectious mononucleosis lymphadenopathy

LRCHL
- Other types of CHL
- NLPHL
- THRLBCL
- Small B-cell lymphomas
- Reactive paracortical immunoblastic hyperplasia

LDCHL
- Other types of CHL, particularly post therapy
- ALCL, ALK(+), or ALK(-)
- PTCL, NOS
- Metastatic carcinoma
- Metastatic melanoma
- Sarcoma

NLPHL
- NSCHL, nodular LRCHL
- THRLBCL
- Follicular lymphoma
- PTGC
- Reactive lymphoid hyperplasia

SELECTED REFERENCES

1. Kuppers R: New insights in the biology of Hodgkin lymphoma. Hematology Am Soc Hematol Educ Program. 2012:328-34, 2012
2. Saarinen S et al: Exome sequencing reveals germline NPAT mutation as a candidate risk factor for Hodgkin lymphoma. Blood. 118(3):493-8, 2011
3. Biasoli I et al: Nodular, lymphocyte-predominant Hodgkin lymphoma: a long-term study and analysis of transformation to diffuse large B-cell lymphoma in a cohort of 164 patients from the Adult Lymphoma Study Group. Cancer. 116(3):631-9, 2010
4. Churchill HR et al: Programmed death 1 expression in variant immunoarchitectural patterns of nodular lymphocyte predominant Hodgkin lymphoma: comparison with CD57 and lymphomas in the differential diagnosis. Hum Pathol. 41(12):1726-34, 2010
5. Eberle FC et al: Histopathology of Hodgkin's lymphoma. Cancer J. 15(2):129-37, 2009
6. Kuppers R: The biology of Hodgkin's lymphoma. Nat Rev Cancer. 9(1):15-27, 2009
7. Nam-Cha SH et al: Lymphocyte-rich classical Hodgkin's lymphoma: distinctive tumor and microenvironment markers. Mod Pathol. 22(8):1006-15, 2009
8. Schmitz R et al: Pathogenesis of classical and lymphocyte-predominant Hodgkin lymphoma. Annu Rev Pathol. 4:151-74, 2009
9. Mourad WA et al: Morphologic, immunphenotypic and clinical discriminators between T-cell/histiocyte-rich large B-cell lymphoma and lymphocyte-predominant Hodgkin lymphoma. Hematol Oncol Stem Cell Ther. 1(1):22-7, 2008
10. Fraga M et al: Diagnosis of Hodgkin's disease: an update on histopathological and immunophenotypical features. Histol Histopathol. 22(8):923-35, 2007
11. Stamatoullas A et al: Conventional cytogenetics of nodular lymphocyte-predominant Hodgkin's lymphoma. Leukemia. 21(9):2064-7, 2007
12. de Jong D et al: Lymphocyte-rich classical Hodgkin lymphoma (LRCHL): clinico-pathological characteristics and outcome of a rare entity. Ann Oncol. 17(1):141-5, 2006

Microscopic Features of NSCHL

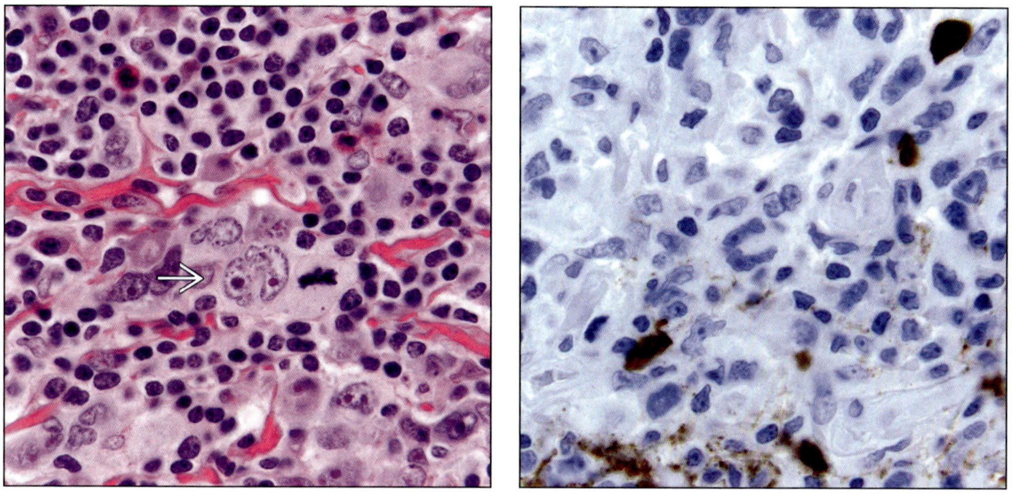

(Left) *A diagnostic Reed-Sternberg cell ➔ is at the center of the image in a background of small lymphocytes, eosinophils, and few plasma cells.* ***(Right)*** *Hodgkin and Reed-Sternberg (HRS) cells have a dysregulated B-cell program and do not express CD20 in this example. In some cases, CD20 expression is present in HRS cells, but in a heterogeneous (weak, variable) pattern. A few small B cells in this field do express the B-cell marker CD20 (internal positive control).*

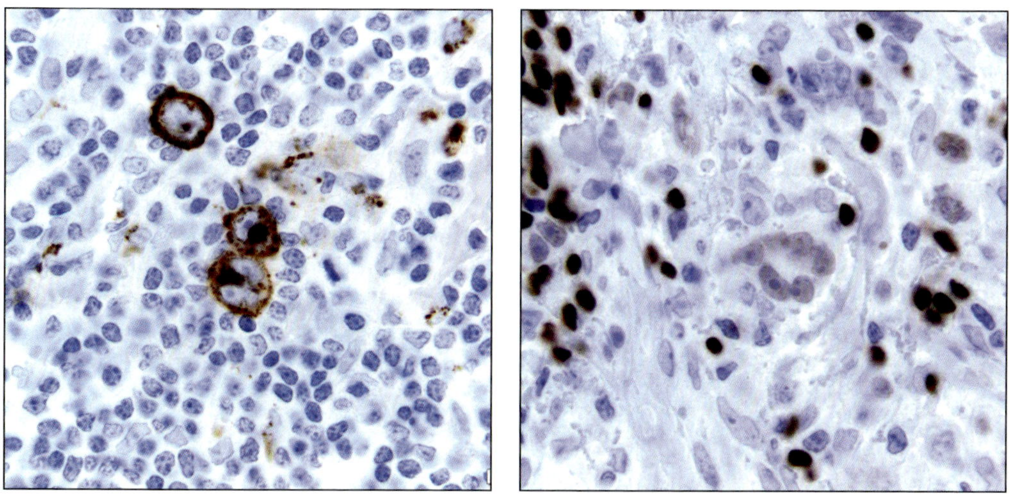

(Left) *CD15 is expressed in HRS cells. There is a strong staining pattern in the Golgi region.* ***(Right)*** *The small B cells in the background are strongly positive for pax-5. The HRS cells (in this case, a multinucleated Reed-Sternberg cell) weakly express pax-5.*

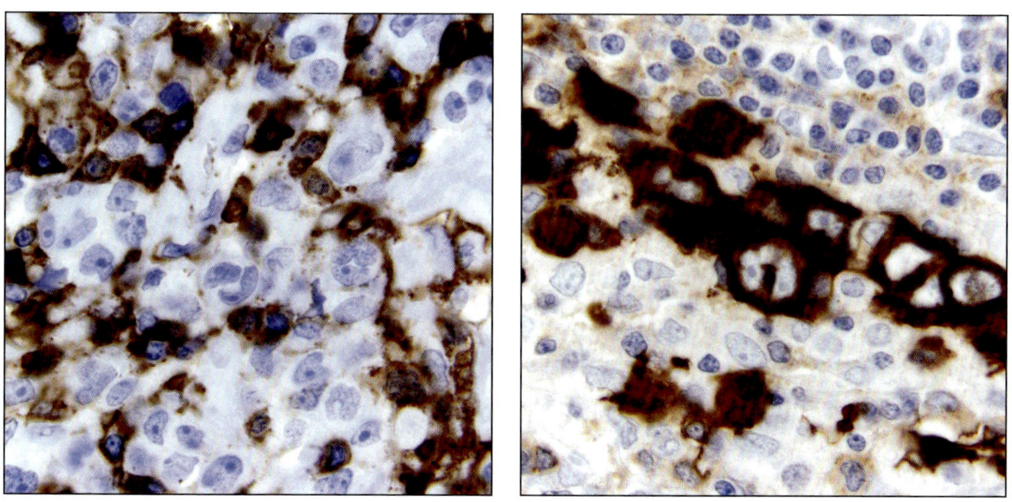

(Left) *The HRS cells do not express the leukocyte common antigen (CD45), but the small lymphocytes in the background do express CD45.* ***(Right)*** *The HRS cells strongly express CD30.*

HODGKIN LYMPHOMA

Microscopic Features

(Left) *Low magnification view of a lymph node from a patient with NLPHL demonstrates an expanded nodule with a moth-eaten appearance due to the presence of large neoplastic LP cells in a background of small lymphocytes.* ***(Right)*** *Staining with CD21 demonstrates that the nodules in NLPHL are enmeshed in expanded, intact follicular dendritic cell (FDC) meshworks.*

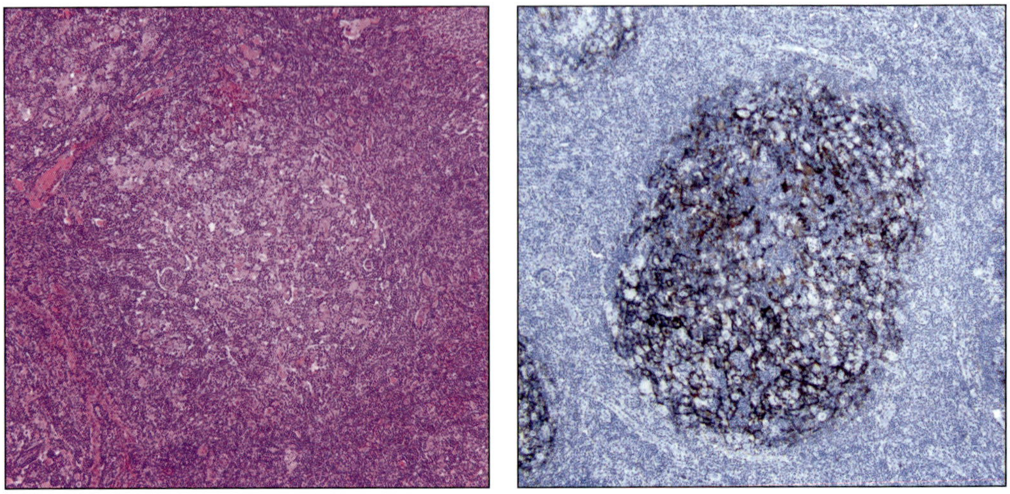

(Left) *Several lymphocyte predominant (LP) cells with multilobulated nuclei and multiple small, basophilic nucleoli are present in a background of small lymphocytes.* ***(Right)*** *CD45 expression is present in a membranous pattern in the multiple LP cells seen in the center of the field, as well as in the small lymphocytes in the background.*

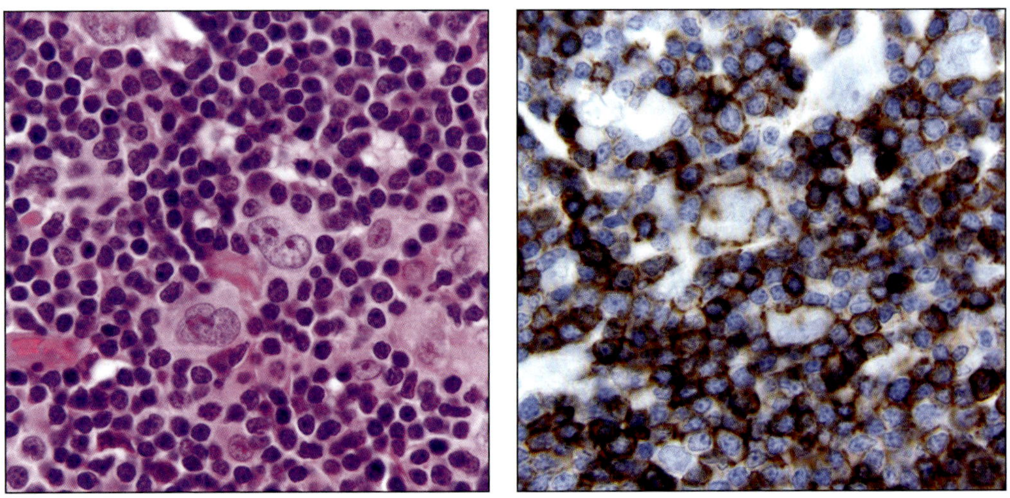

(Left) *CD20 highlights frequent small B cells in the background. The large LP cells are also CD20 positive. Note that the cells encircling the central LP cell do not express CD20 ➔ because they are follicular T-helper cells.* ***(Right)*** *The large, irregular LP cells show nuclear staining for pax-5. In this field, there are only a few reactive B cells, which are also strongly positive for pax-5.*

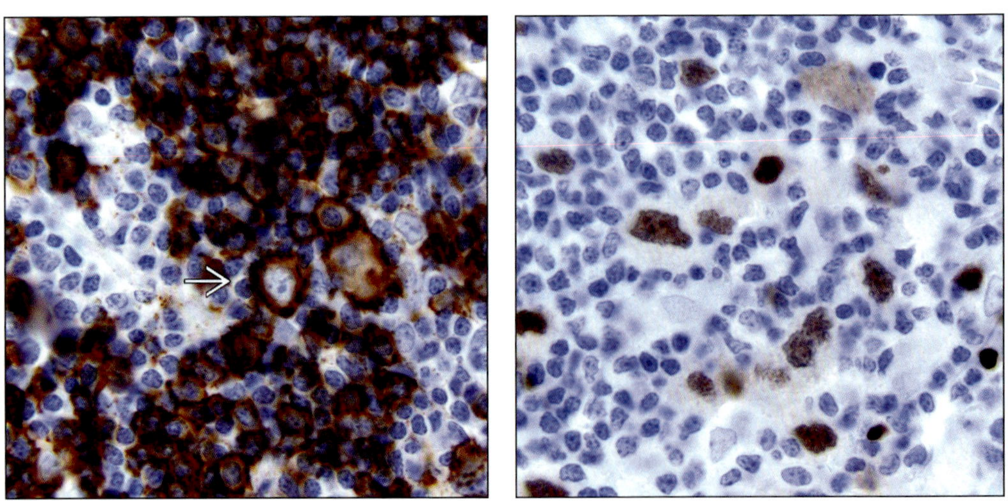

Microscopic Features

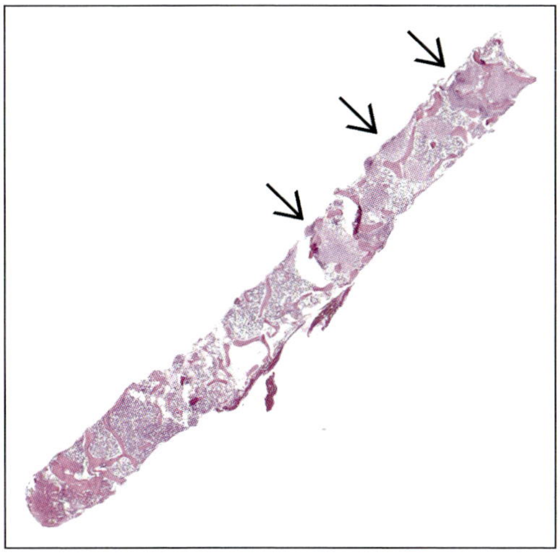

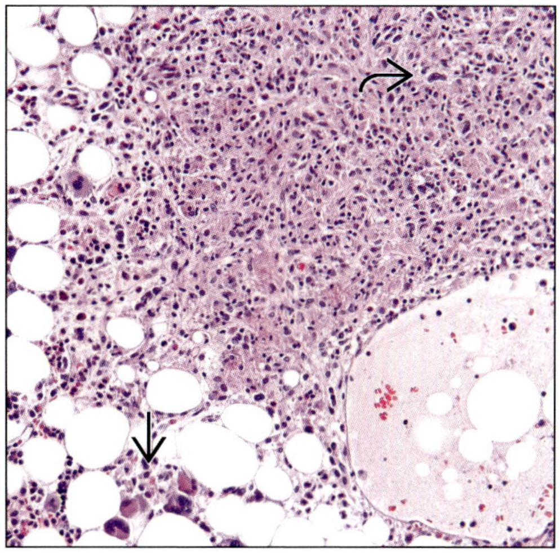

(Left) *H&E stain shows bone marrow involvement by CHL. Note the focal, patchy pattern of involvement ⇒. In cases of suspected marrow involvement by CHL, multiple levels (step sections) should be performed to ensure adequate evaluation.* ***(Right)*** *High magnification of the marrow biopsy demonstrates a large aggregate of histiocytes, lymphocytes, eosinophils, plasma cells, and rare HRS cells ↪. Normal marrow is at the periphery ⇒.*

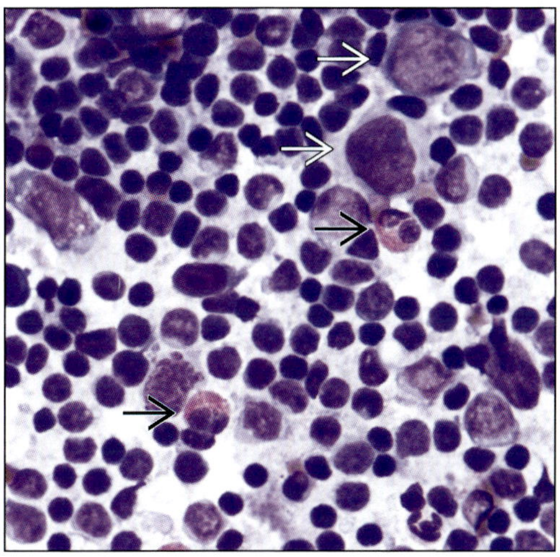

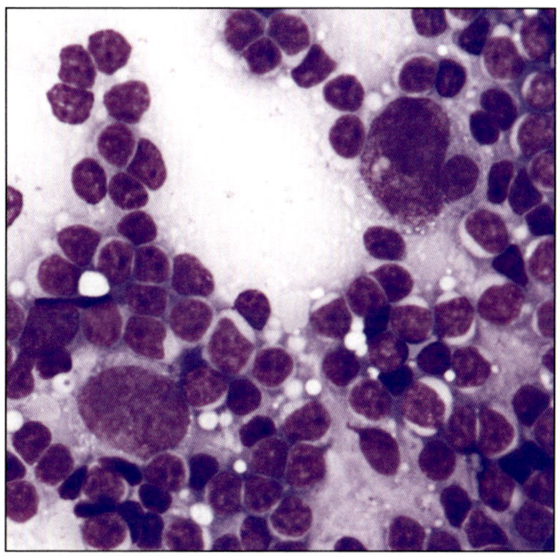

(Left) *Image shows a touch imprint of a lymph node involved by MCCHL. Scattered HRS cells ➡ are present in a mixed background of small lymphocytes, eosinophils ⇒, and neutrophils. (Courtesy C. Yin, MD, PhD.)* ***(Right)*** *Image shows a touch imprint of a lymph node involved by LRCHL. Large HRS cells are present in a background of numerous small lymphocytes. (Courtesy S. Wang, MD.)*

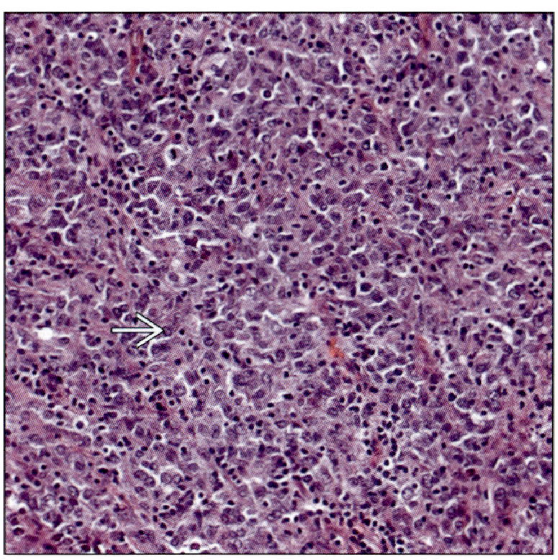

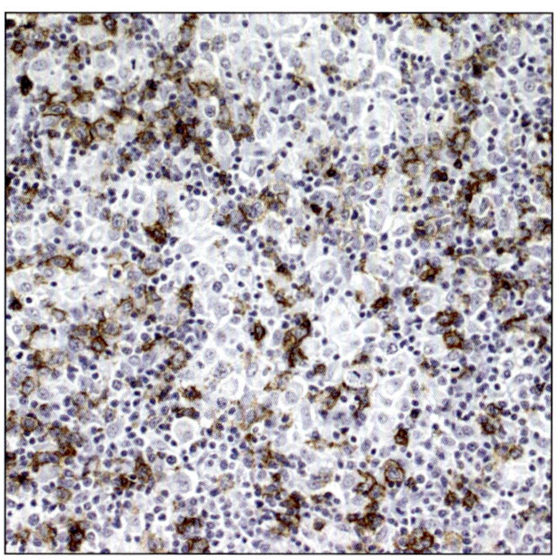

(Left) *Image shows DLBCL arising from NLPHL. The sheets of large cells ➡ are diagnostic of transformation. NLPHL was identified in other parts of the lymph node. (Courtesy P. Lin, MD.)* ***(Right)*** *This image shows THRLBCL arising from NLPHL. CD20 highlights the neoplastic large cells and rare small reactive B lymphocytes. Note that the B cells are markedly depleted in comparison with typical NLPHL. Many small T cells and histiocytes are also present. (Courtesy P. Lin, MD.)*

LYMPHOPLASMACYTIC LYMPHOMA/WALDENSTRÖM MACROGLOBULINEMIA

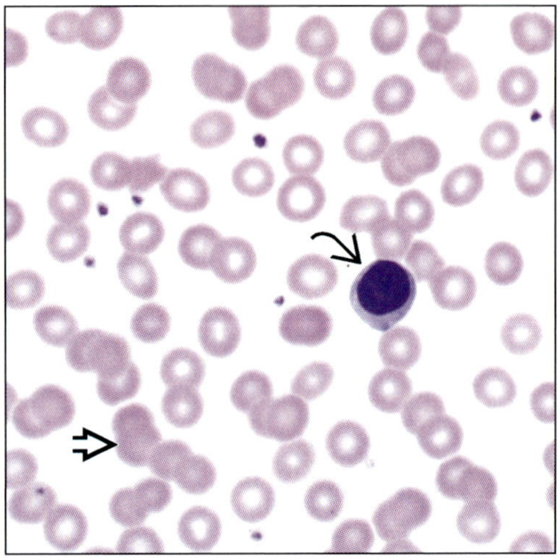

Rouleaux ⇨ and a plasmacytoid lymphocyte ⇨ are evident on this peripheral blood smear from a patient with Waldenström macroglobulinemia.

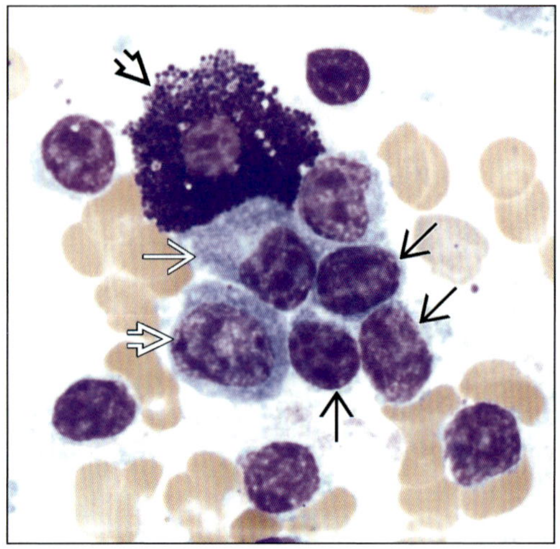

Spectrum of small lymphocytes ⇨, a plasmacytoid lymphocyte ⇨, and a plasma cell ⇨ (1 with a mast cell ⇨), in this bone marrow aspirate are characteristic of lymphoplasmacytic lymphoma.

TERMINOLOGY

Abbreviations

- Lymphoplasmacytic lymphoma (LPL)
- Waldenström macroglobulinemia (WM)

Definitions

- LPL/WM is characterized by clonal expansion of small mature B lymphocytes with variable plasmacytoid differentiation
- WM is found in significant subset of patients with LPL and is defined as LPL with bone marrow (BM) involvement and IgM monoclonal protein

ETIOLOGY/PATHOGENESIS

Etiology

- Mature B cell; evidence indicates memory B cell is likely cell of origin

Pathogenesis

- Genetic factors
  - Up to 20% of WM patients have 1st-degree relatives with WM or closely related B-cell disorder
  - Patients with familial history of WM or plasma cell disorder are diagnosed at younger age and with greater bone marrow involvement
  - Recent data demonstrate somatic mutation of *MYD88*, predicting an amino acid change L265P in ~ 90% of WM
    - *MYD88* mutation triggers IRAK-mediated NF-*k*B signaling, thus driving NF-*k*B-dependent prosurvival signaling
- Chronic immune stimulation
  - WM risk is elevated among individuals with autoimmune disorders and those with hepatitis, human immunodeficiency virus infection, and rickettsiosis
- Predisposition
  - Monoclonal gammopathy of unknown significance (MGUS) of IgM type is associated with significantly increased risk to
    - WM
    - Non-Hodgkin lymphomas
    - Chronic lymphocytic leukemia
    - Light chain amyloidosis

CLINICAL ISSUES

Epidemiology

- Incidence: 3 per 1 million people each year
- Mean age at diagnosis: 65 years
- Male predominance

Site

- Bone marrow is primary site
- Blood, lymph nodes, and extranodal sites are often involved

Presentation

- 20-30% of patients are asymptomatic at diagnosis
- Anemia-related symptoms: Fatigue, shortness of breath, and chest pain
- Thrombocytopenia-related bleeding tendency
- Constitutional symptoms including weight loss and night sweats
- Splenomegaly and adenopathy
- Hyperviscosity occurs in up to 20% of patients

Laboratory Tests

- CBC
  - Anemia and thrombocytopenia
  - Lymphocytosis
- Cryoglobulin test is positive in subset of cases
- Serum/urine protein electrophoresis (SPEP/UPEP)
  - Typically IgM monoclonal paraprotein
  - Rarely IgG or IgA

LYMPHOPLASMACYTIC LYMPHOMA/WALDENSTRÖM MACROGLOBULINEMIA

Key Facts

Terminology
- LPL/WM is characterized by clonal expansion of small mature B lymphocytes with variable plasmacytoid differentiation
- WM is found in significant subset of patients with LPL and is defined as LPL with bone marrow involvement and IgM monoclonal protein

Etiology/Pathogenesis
- Up to 20% of WM patients have 1st-degree relatives with WM or closely related B-cell disorder
- Somatic mutation of *MYD88*, predicting an amino acid change L265P is seen in ~ 90% of WM

Clinical Issues
- Bone marrow is primary site
- Typically IgM monoclonal paraprotein

Microscopic Pathology
- Blood and bone marrow show spectrum of lymphocytes, plasmacytoid lymphocytes, and plasma cells
- Bone marrow reveals combination of paratrabecular, nonparatrabecular lymphoid nodules, and diffuse &/or interstitial infiltrate
- Mast cells often increased; most prominent within particles on aspirate smears

Ancillary Tests
- Usually express IgM, CD19, CD20, CD22, CD79a
- Negative for CD5, CD10, CD23, CD43, and CD103
- Deletion 6q is reported in 40-50% of patients
- *MYD88* mutation status helpful in differential diagnosis

Treatment
- Not standardized; many options have been used in different practices
- Radiation for localized disease
- "Watch and wait" policy for asymptomatic patients
- Initiation of therapy is considered in patients with
  - Constitutional symptoms such as fever, fatigue, night sweats, weight loss
  - Hyperviscosity
  - Severe neuropathy
  - Amyloidosis
  - Symptomatic cryoglobulinemia
  - Cold agglutinin disease
  - Evidence of disease transformation
- Various combinations of chemotherapy for symptomatic patients
  - Rituximab in combination with purine analogue &/or alkylating agent
  - Cyclophosphamide/doxorubicin/vincristine/prednisone plus rituximab (R-CHOP)
  - Newer agents such as thalidomide or bortezomib are being investigated in clinical trials
- Plasmapheresis to reduce amount of circulating IgM
- Splenectomy for chemotherapy-resistant patients
- Stem cell transplantation
  - Autologous stem cell transplantation (ASCT) is feasible, safe, and associated with significant cytoreduction in relapsed or refractory patients
  - Allogeneic stem cell transplantation is used only in patients with advanced and refractory disease for whom no other options are available

Prognosis
- Median survival: 50-60 months
- Transformation to large cell lymphoma can occur
- 6q deletion does not appear to affect clinical outcome
- Adverse prognostic factors
  - Age > 65 years
  - Presence of constitutional symptoms
  - Anemia &/or thrombocytopenia
  - Decreased albumin level
  - Increased β-2-microglobulin level

MICROSCOPIC PATHOLOGY

Histologic Features
- Blood
  - May show lymphocytosis with spectrum of lymphocytes, plasmacytoid lymphocytes, and plasma cells
  - Rouleaux formation of red blood cells
  - Cold agglutinin and cryoglobulin may be present
- Bone marrow
  - Involved in almost all cases
  - Often, combination of paratrabecular, nonparatrabecular lymphoid nodules, and diffuse &/or interstitial infiltrate
  - Infiltrate composed predominantly of small lymphocytes with variable number of plasmacytoid lymphocytes and plasma cells
  - Pseudointranuclear (Dutcher bodies) and intracytoplasmic inclusions (Russell bodies) are most prominent on core biopsy section
  - Mast cells often increased; most prominent within particles on aspirate smears
  - May have amyloid
- Lymph node
  - Neoplastic cells infiltrate paracortex and hilum with patent or dilated sinuses
  - May have preserved architecture or attenuated germinal centers
  - Infiltrate consists of monotonous small lymphocytes with variable number of plasmacytoid lymphocytes and plasma cells
  - Increased mast cells and hemosiderin

ANCILLARY TESTS

Immunohistochemistry
- Helpful in assessing architecture or when flow is not available

LYMPHOPLASMACYTIC LYMPHOMA/WALDENSTRÖM MACROGLOBULINEMIA

- CD20 helpful to identify subtle infiltrate
- Congo red stain identifies amyloid deposits
- κ and λ in situ hybridizations reveal monoclonal plasma cells

Flow Cytometry
- Identify monoclonal B- and plasma cell populations
- Characteristics of lymphoma cells
  - Usually express IgM, CD19, CD20, CD22, CD79a
  - Presence of cytoplasmic immunoglobulin
  - Typically negative for CD5, CD10, CD23, CD43, and CD103
  - Variable CD25, CD11c, and CD38

Cytogenetics
- No specific abnormalities
- Most frequent finding of deletion 6q is reported in 40-50% of patients
- t(9;14)(p13;q32) is occasionally seen in LPL

PCR
- *IGH* gene rearranged
- Biased VH3 and VH3-23 usage
- *MYD88* mutation identified in > 90% of WM

DIFFERENTIAL DIAGNOSIS

Marginal Zone Lymphoma (MZL)
- Mucosa-associated lymphoid tissue (MALT) lymphoma
  - LPL/WM can rarely involves extranodal sites, creating difficulty in differential diagnosis
  - IgM paraprotein is rare
  - Often exhibits characteristic monocytoid B cells, lymphoepithelial lesions, reactive follicles
  - Translocations of t(11;18)(q21;q21) *API2-MALT1*, t(14;18)(q32;q21) *IGH-MALT1*, t(1;14)(p22;q32) *BCL10-IGH* are seen
  - *MYD88* mutation uncommon
- Nodal MZL
  - Can involve bone marrow, and LPL/WM can rarely involve lymph node, raising differential diagnosis between the 2 diseases
  - Primarily a nodal-based disease
  - Monocytoid lymphoid B cells prominent
  - IgM paraprotein only seen in minority of patients
  - *MYD88* mutation uncommon
- Splenic marginal zone lymphoma (SMZL)
  - Splenomegaly prominent
  - May have villous lymphocytes in peripheral blood
  - Sinusoidal infiltration pattern on bone marrow core biopsy
  - Deletion 7q usually associated with SMZL
  - Minor subset exhibits *MYD88* mutation
  - Spleen histology is diagnostic

IgM Monoclonal Gammopathy of Undetermined Significance (IgM MGUS)
- Serum M protein < 30 g/L
- Bone marrow clonal plasma cells < 10%
- No end-organ damage
- No evidence of B-cell lymphoma or other M-protein producing disease
- Subset exhibits *MYD88* mutation; positive rate varies depends on study

Other B-Cell Chronic Lymphoproliferative Disorders
- Expression of CD5, CD23 helpful to exclude chronic lymphocytic leukemia/small lymphocytic lymphoma
- Expression of CD5, cyclin-D1, and cytogenetic finding of t(11;14) helpful to exclude mantle cell lymphoma
- Expression of CD10 and cytogenetic findings of t(14;18) helpful to exclude follicular lymphoma
- Histology features also helpful in differential diagnosis

DIAGNOSTIC CHECKLIST

Clinically Relevant Pathologic Features
- Based on combination of following findings
  - Presence of spectrum lymphocytes, plasmacytoid lymphocytes, and plasma cells
  - Flow cytometric study demonstrates monoclonal B cells with typical immunophenotype and monoclonal plasma cells
  - Monoclonal paraprotein by SPEP/UPEP

SELECTED REFERENCES

1. Jiménez C et al: MYD88 L265P is a marker highly characteristic of, but not restricted to, Waldenström's macroglobulinemia. Leukemia. 27(8):1722-8, 2013
2. Varettoni M et al: Prevalence and clinical significance of the MYD88 (L265P) somatic mutation in Waldenstrom's macroglobulinemia and related lymphoid neoplasms. Blood. 121(13):2522-8, 2013
3. Kyle RA et al: Progression in smoldering Waldenstrom macroglobulinemia: long-term results. Blood. 119(19):4462-6, 2012
4. Treon SP et al: MYD88 L265P somatic mutation in Waldenström's macroglobulinemia. N Engl J Med. 367(9):826-33, 2012
5. Adamia S et al: Genetic abnormalities in Waldenström's macroglobulinemia. Clin Lymphoma Myeloma. 9(1):30-2, 2009
6. Federico M et al: Prognostic factors in low-grade non-Hodgkin lymphomas. Curr Hematol Malig Rep. 4(4):202-10, 2009
7. Sahota SS et al: CD27 in defining memory B-cell origins in Waldenström's macroglobulinemia. Clin Lymphoma Myeloma. 9(1):33-5, 2009
8. Treon SP et al: Advances in the biology and treatment of Waldenström's macroglobulinemia: a report from the 5th International Workshop on Waldenström's Macroglobulinemia, Stockholm, Sweden. Clin Lymphoma Myeloma. 9(1):10-5, 2009
9. Koshiol J et al: Chronic immune stimulation and subsequent Waldenström macroglobulinemia. Arch Intern Med. 168(17):1903-9, 2008
10. Treon SP et al: Characterization of familial Waldenstrom's macroglobulinemia. Ann Oncol. 17(3):488-94, 2006
11. Walsh SH et al: Lymphoplasmacytic lymphoma/ Waldenström's macroglobulinemia derives from an extensively hypermutated B cell that lacks ongoing somatic hypermutation. Leuk Res. 29(7):729-34, 2005

Microscopic Features and Differential Diagnosis

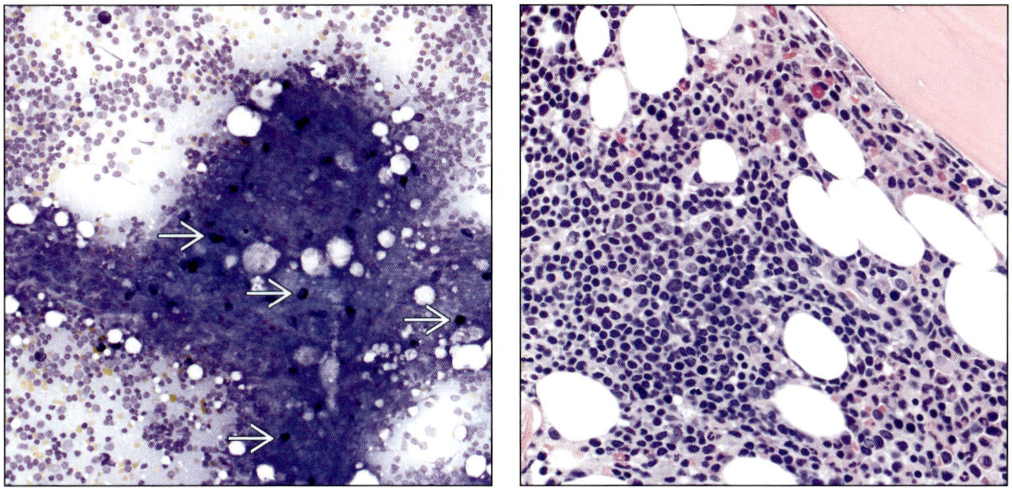

(Left) *Increased mast cells (darkly stained cells →) within bone marrow aspirate particles, although not specific, are highly characteristic of lymphoplasmacytic lymphoma.* ***(Right)*** *Nonparatrabecular lymphoid aggregate on bone marrow core biopsy is depicted here. Bone marrow involvement by lymphoplasmacytic lymphoma usually exhibits mixed diffuse, paratrabecular, nonparatrabecular nodular, and interstitial patterns.*

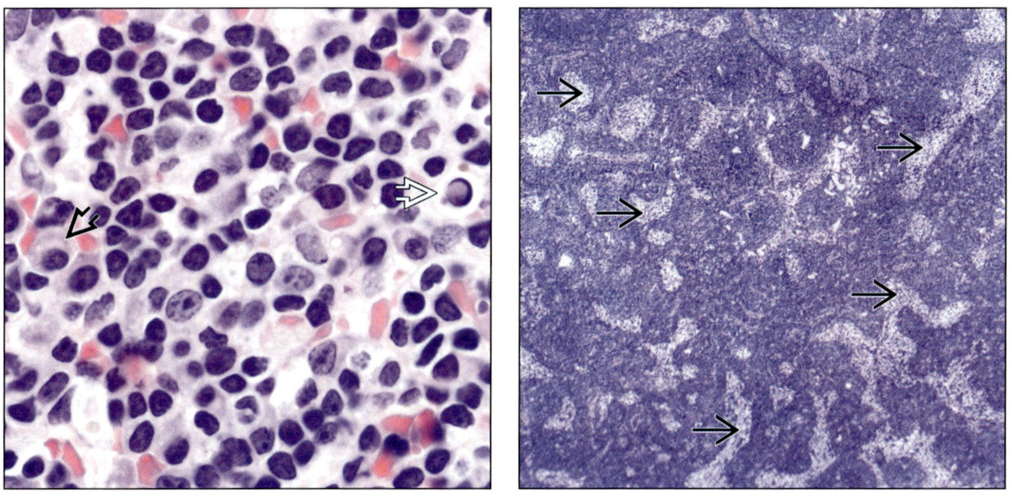

(Left) *At high power, lymphoplasmacytic lymphoma is shown to be composed of small mature lymphocytes, plasma cells ⇨, and rare scattered large cells. Note the Dutcher body →.* ***(Right)*** *Low-power view of lymphoplasmacytic lymphoma and Waldenström macroglobulinemia involving lymph node shows a diffuse pattern of growth with patent sinuses → that contain histiocytes. (Courtesy P. Lin, MD.)*

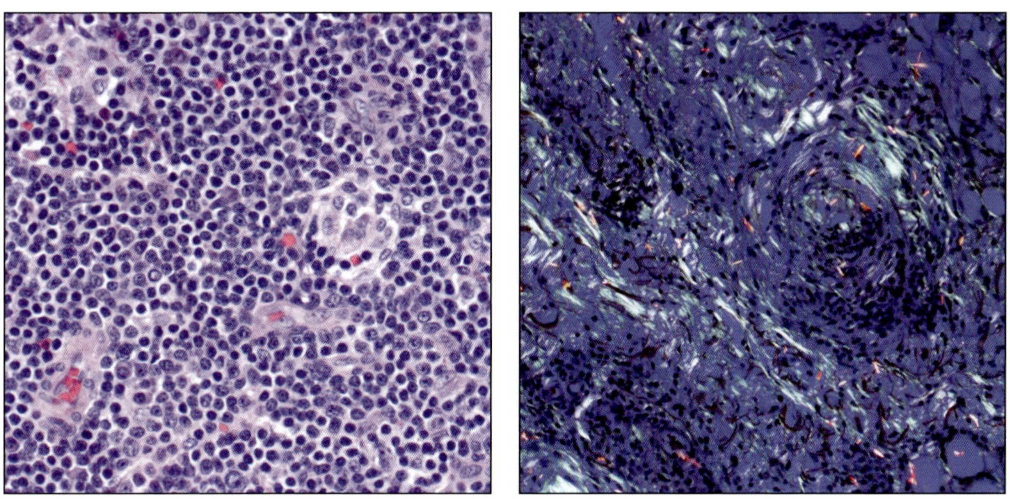

(Left) *This image shows LPL/WM involving a lymph node. The proliferating cells are small lymphocytes, and a subset of cells has plasmacytoid features. (Courtesy P. Lin, MD.)* ***(Right)*** *Congo red stain reveals an amyloid deposit in this soft tissue biopsy from a patient with marginal zone lymphoma. A previous history of marginal zone lymphoma helped in establishing the diagnosis.*

MANTLE CELL LYMPHOMA

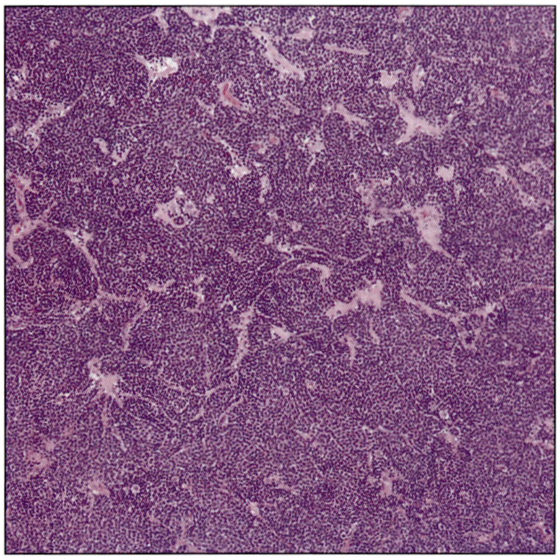

Image shows mantle cell lymphoma (MCL) with a nodular and diffuse pattern associated with hyalinized blood vessels. Hyalinized blood vessels are a common feature in MCL.

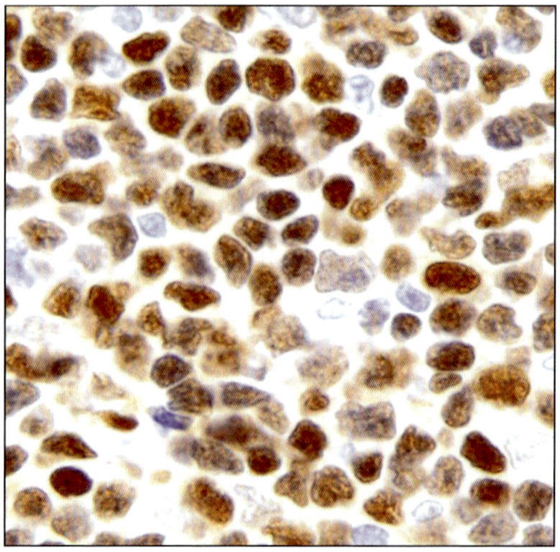

Cyclin-D1 immunostain shows nuclear expression in the cells of MCL. As demonstrated here, the nuclei often show cell-to-cell variation in the intensity of cyclin-D1 expression.

TERMINOLOGY

Abbreviations

- Mantle cell lymphoma (MCL)

Synonyms

- Centrocytic lymphoma
- Lymphocytic lymphoma, intermediate grade of differentiation
- Intermediate lymphocytic lymphoma

Definitions

- Clinically aggressive B-cell lymphoma usually composed of monomorphic small to medium-sized cells and associated with t(11;14)/*CCND1-IGH*

ETIOLOGY/PATHOGENESIS

t(11;14)(q13;q32)

- Juxtaposes *CCND1* at 11q13 with *IGH* at 14q32 and results in cyclin-D1 overexpression, Rb phosphorylation, and release of E2F
- Facilitates cell cycle progression from G1 to S phase

Familial

- Reports of familial MCL are rare

CLINICAL ISSUES

Presentation

- Median age: 6th-7th decades; male predominance
- Most patients present with Ann Arbor clinical stage III/IV; B symptoms in 40-50%
- Lymphadenopathy, generalized
- Extranodal sites are common, particularly GI tract, bone marrow, spleen, peripheral blood

Treatment

- Aggressive chemotherapy ± stem cell transplantation
- HyperCVAD chemotherapy regimen used at many medical centers

Prognosis

- Currently considered incurable; median survival: 2-5 years

MICROSCOPIC PATHOLOGY

Histologic Features

- Architectural effacement by monomorphic lymphoid proliferation with vaguely nodular, diffuse, or mantle zone growth pattern
- Monotonous population of small to medium-sized lymphoid cells with variably irregular nuclear contours, condensed chromatin, and scant cytoplasm
  - Rare variant has relatively abundant "monocytoid" cytoplasm
- Hyalinized blood vessels, "naked" germinal centers, and benign histiocytes with eosinophilic cytoplasm frequently seen
- 2 aggressive variants of MCL are recognized by 2008 WHO classification
  - Blastoid: Cells resemble lymphoblasts, small to intermediate in size, with immature chromatin and high mitotic rate (≥ 10/10 high-power field [HPF], x 400)
  - Pleomorphic: Heterogeneous population of cells, including large cells, often with prominent nucleoli and high mitotic rate
- Liver: MCL preferentially involves portal tracts
- Spleen: MCL preferentially replaces white pulp
- Bone marrow: MCL has nonparatrabecular and paratrabecular pattern
- Peripheral blood: Overt leukemia in ~ 10% of patients, but occasional MCL cells are common (in ~ 75% of patients)

MANTLE CELL LYMPHOMA

Key Facts

Terminology
- Clinically aggressive B-cell lymphoma associated with t(11;14)(q13;q32) and cyclin-D1 overexpression

Etiology/Pathogenesis
- Reports of familial MCL are rare

Clinical Issues
- Elderly people; male predominance
- Most patients present with clinical stage III/IV disease
- B symptoms, lymphadenopathy, extranodal involvement
- Currently considered incurable with median survival of 2-5 years

Microscopic Pathology
- Architectural effacement by lymphoma with nodular, diffuse, or mantle zone growth pattern
- Monotonous population of small to medium-sized cells with variably irregular nuclear contours

Ancillary Tests
- Immunohistochemistry: Cyclin-D1(+)
- Flow cytometry: CD5(+), CD19(+), CD20(+), CD43(+/-), FMC-7(+), CD10(-), CD23(-)
- Cytogenetics: t(11;14)(q13;q32) or *CCND1-IGH* (FISH)
- Gene expression profiling
  - Unique profile
  - Proliferation predicts prognosis

Top Differential Diagnoses
- Chronic lymphocytic leukemia/small lymphocytic lymphoma
- Follicular lymphoma
- Nodal marginal zone B-cell lymphoma

ANCILLARY TESTS

Immunohistochemistry
- Cyclin-D1 overexpression is almost constant feature
- Rare cyclin-D1(-) variants described, but this entity is controversial

Flow Cytometry
- CD5(+), CD19(+), CD20(+), CD22(+), CD79b(+), FMC-7(+), SOX11(+/-), and monotypic Ig
- Bcl-2(+), CD11c(+/-)
- CD3(-), CD10(-), CD23(-), CD43(+/-)
- Rare cases have atypical immunophenotype: CD5(-) or CD10(+) or CD23(+) (dim ~ 10%)

Cytogenetics
- Numerous methods can be used for demonstrating t(11;14)(q13;q32)
  - FISH is convenient because it can be performed on fixed tissue sections
  - Conventional cytogenetics if fresh material available

Molecular Genetics
- PCR detects 1 major breakpoint (MTC) in 30-50% of cases

Gene Expression Profiling
- MCL has proliferation signature that can be used to divide patients into prognostic subgroups

DIFFERENTIAL DIAGNOSIS

Chronic Lymphocytic Leukemia/Small Lymphocytic Lymphoma
- Proliferation centers; mixture of small lymphocytes, prolymphocytes, and paraimmunoblasts
- Cells express dim surface Ig, CD5, and CD23, but not cyclin-D1

Follicular Lymphoma
- Sharply circumscribed nodules composed of centrocytes and centroblasts
- Cells express CD10 but not CD5, CD43, or cyclin-D1

Nodal Marginal Zone B-Cell Lymphoma
- Neoplastic B cells ± monocytoid cytoplasm; reactive germinal centers are common; CD5(-) and cyclin-D1(-)

Lymphoblastic Lymphoma
- Mimics classic blastoid variant of MCL
- Younger patients; TdT(+) and cyclin-D1(-)

Diffuse Large B-Cell Lymphoma
- Mimics pleomorphic blastoid variant of MCL
- CD5(-) and cyclin-D1(-)

Reactive Follicular Hyperplasia
- Thinner mantle zones composed of small, round, mature lymphocytes surrounding prominent germinal centers
- No evidence of monoclonality

Castleman Disease, Hyaline Vascular Type
- Large localized mass in young person
- Architecture not entirely effaced
- Hyaline-vascular follicles, "onion skin" lymphocytes concentrically layered around germinal centers

SELECTED REFERENCES

1. Jares P et al: Molecular pathogenesis of mantle cell lymphoma. J Clin Invest. 122(10):3416-23, 2012
2. Jares P et al: Genetic and molecular pathogenesis of mantle cell lymphoma: perspectives for new targeted therapeutics. Nat Rev Cancer. 7(10):750-62, 2007
3. Rosenwald A et al: The proliferation gene expression signature is a quantitative integrator of oncogenic events that predicts survival in mantle cell lymphoma. Cancer Cell. 3(2):185-97, 2003

MANTLE CELL LYMPHOMA

Microscopic and Immunohistochemical Features

*(**Left**) The case of mantle cell lymphoma (MCL) shown in this image demonstrates a completely diffuse pattern of growth. (**Right**) H&E shows MCL with a nodular pattern. This pattern, in part, resembles follicular lymphoma at low-power magnification, but the neoplastic nodules lack centroblasts.*

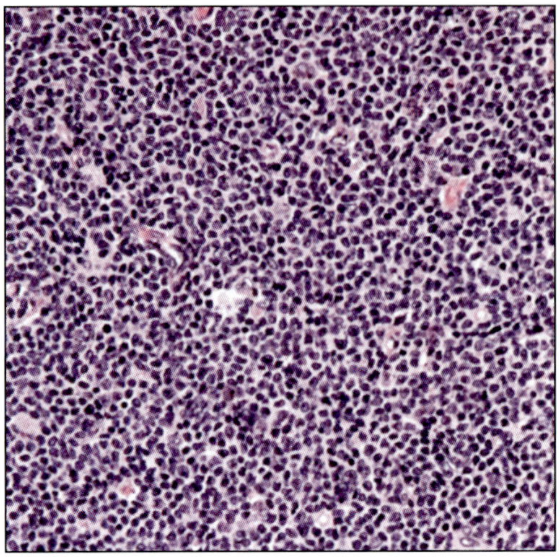

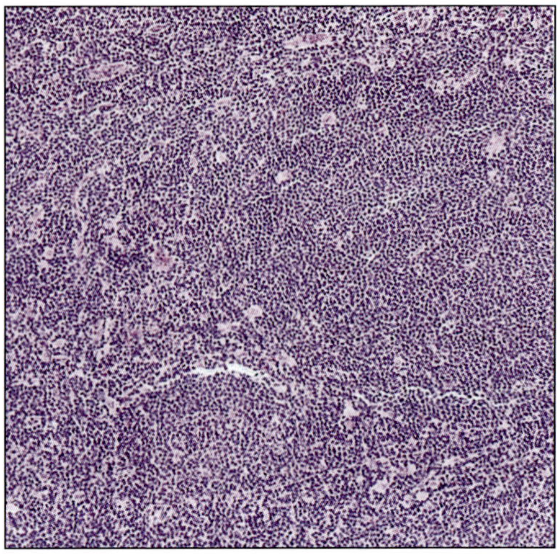

*(**Left**) Image shows MCL with a mantle zone pattern. In this pattern, the neoplasm surrounds reactive germinal centers. (**Right**) A case of MCL shows "naked" reactive germinal centers and many benign histiocytes with eosinophilic cytoplasm (so-called pink histiocytes). Pink histiocytes are a helpful clue for the diagnosis of MCL but are not specific.*

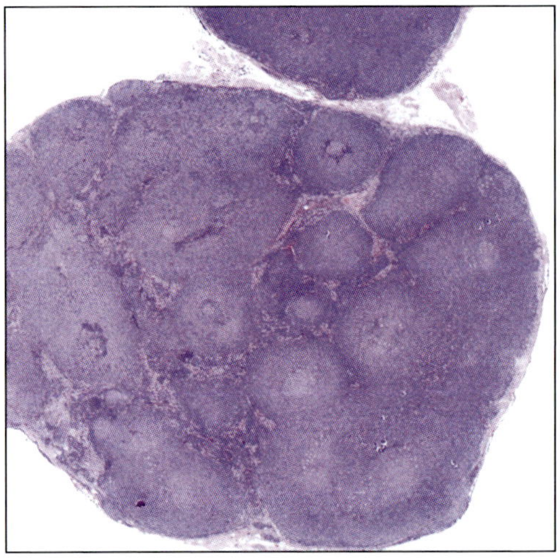

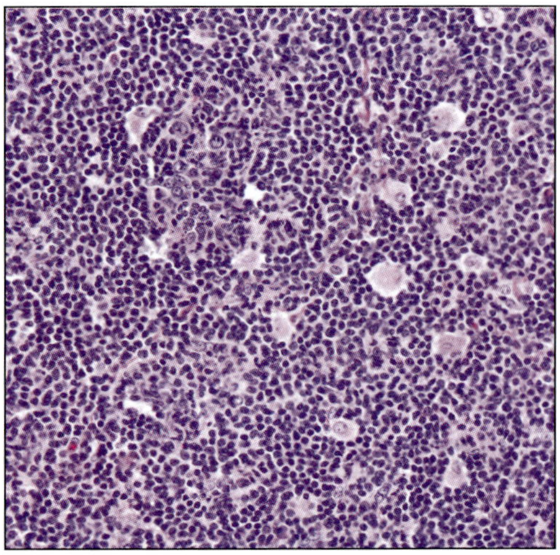

*(**Left**) Smear of a lymph node prepared at the time of a frozen section shows MCL. In addition to the neoplastic lymphoid cells, a benign pink histiocyte is shown in this field. (**Right**) Cyclin-D1 immunostain shows nuclear expression in the cells of MCL. This immunostain is helpful for recognizing MCL at extranodal sites, especially in small biopsy specimens.*

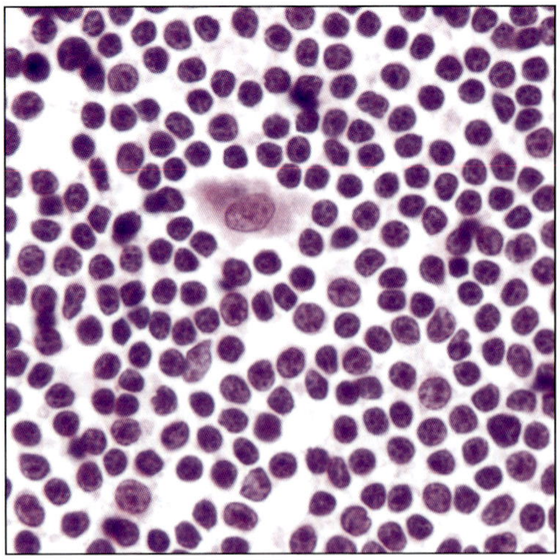

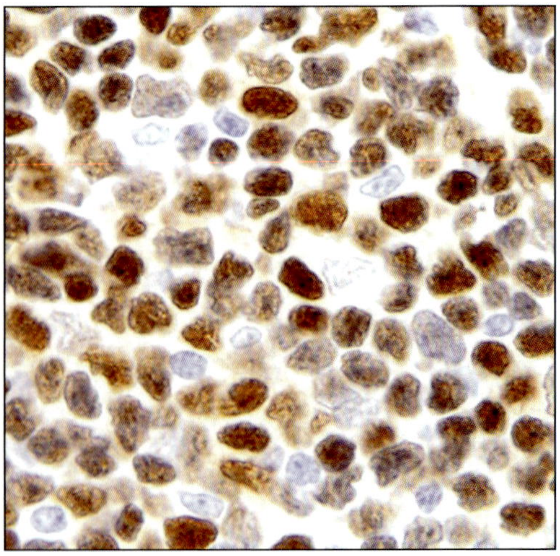

MANTLE CELL LYMPHOMA

Microscopic and Immunohistochemical Features

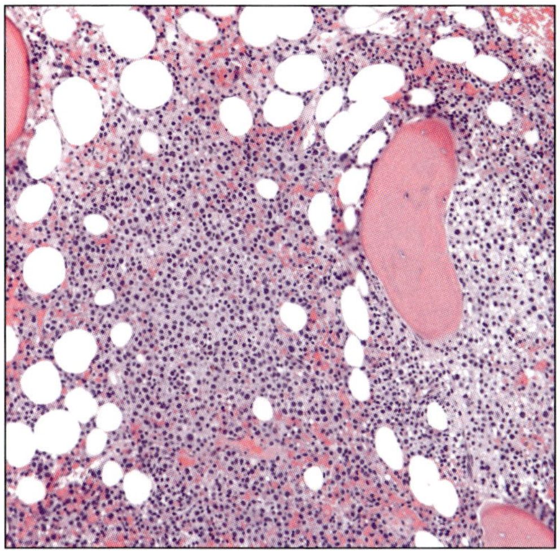

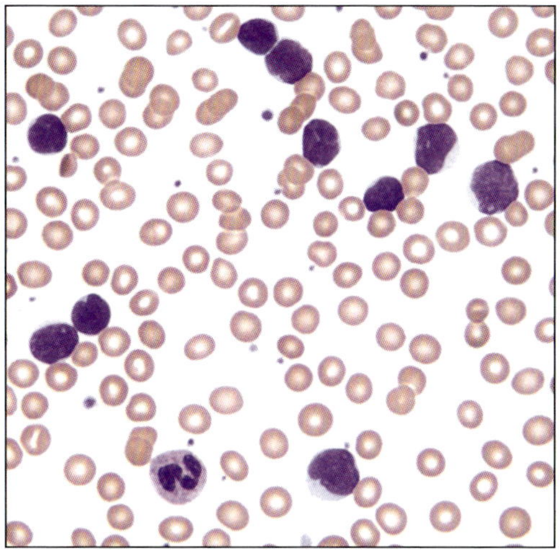

(Left) *MCL involving bone marrow is illustrated. In this case, the neoplastic cells had relatively abundant "monocytoid" cytoplasm mimicking marginal zone lymphoma. However, the neoplastic cells expressed cyclin-D1, and conventional cytogenetics showed the t(11;14)(q13;q32).* ***(Right)*** *Wright-Giemsa stain shows a case of MCL in the leukemic phase. The neoplastic lymphocytes of MCL often show variation in size and shape in a blood smear, as seen in this case.*

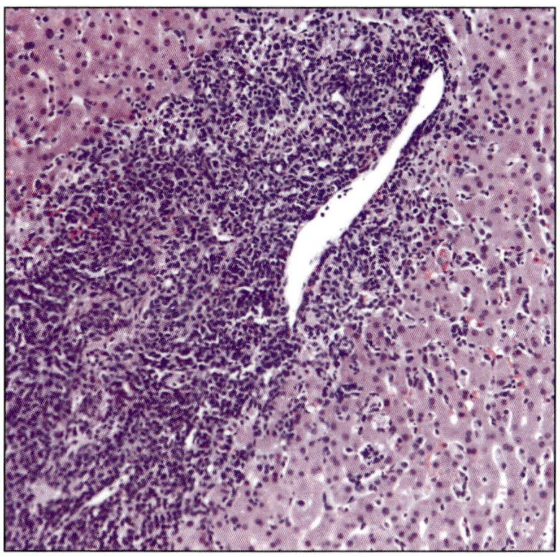

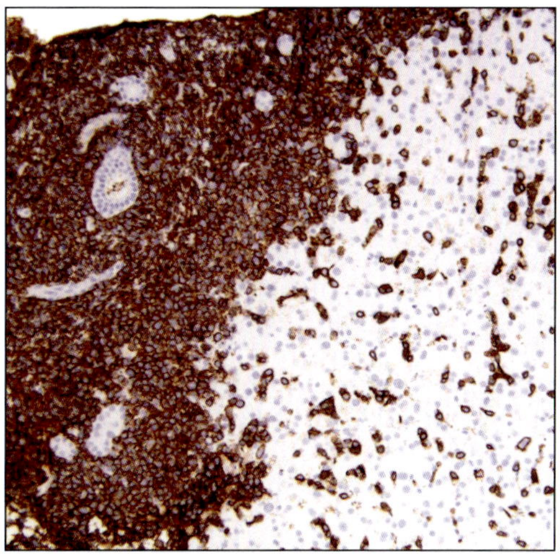

(Left) *Image shows MCL involving the liver. The neoplasm fills a portal tract and infiltrates sinusoids.* ***(Right)*** *CD20 immunostain highlights MCL cells within a portal tract and sinusoids of this liver biopsy.*

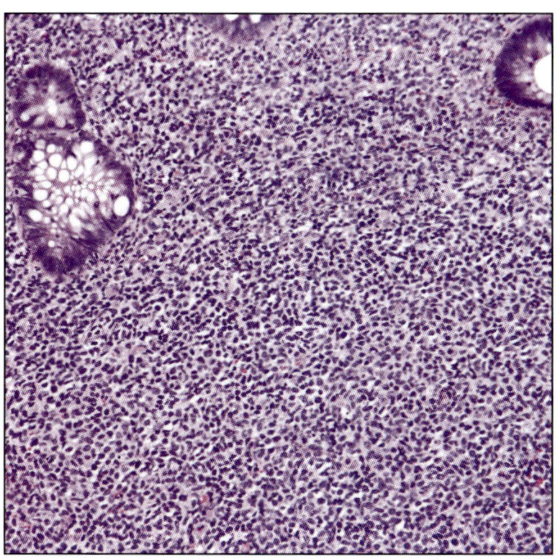

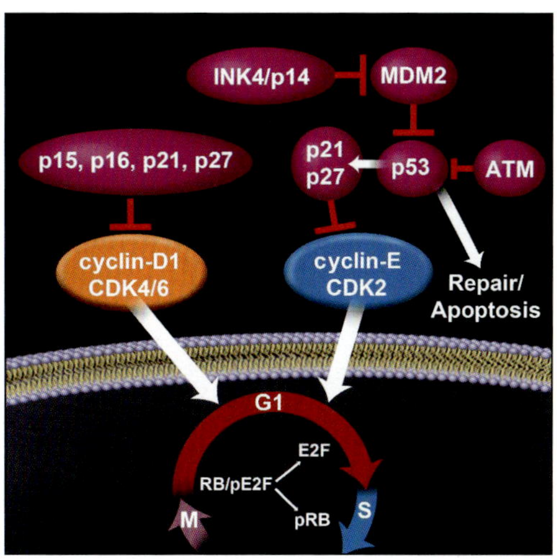

(Left) *MCL involving the colonic mucosa is shown. MCL has a tropism for the gastrointestinal tract and commonly involves this site at the time of diagnosis. However, GI symptoms occur in only 10-20% of patients.* ***(Right)*** *Schematic of the cell cycle shows the G1 to S transition and the role of cyclin-D1-cyclin-dependent kinase complexes. Some of the genes of interest in the pathogenesis of MCL are also shown.*

MYELOID NEOPLASMS

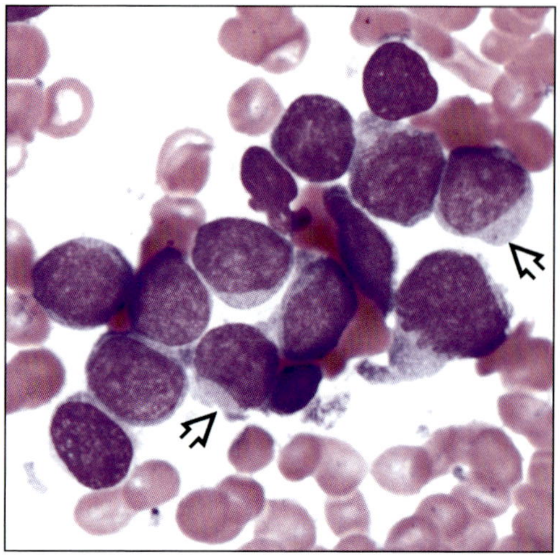

Bone marrow aspirate smear is from a patient with acute myeloid leukemia without maturation. A subset of blasts contains cytoplasmic granules ⮚, indicative of myeloid differentiation.

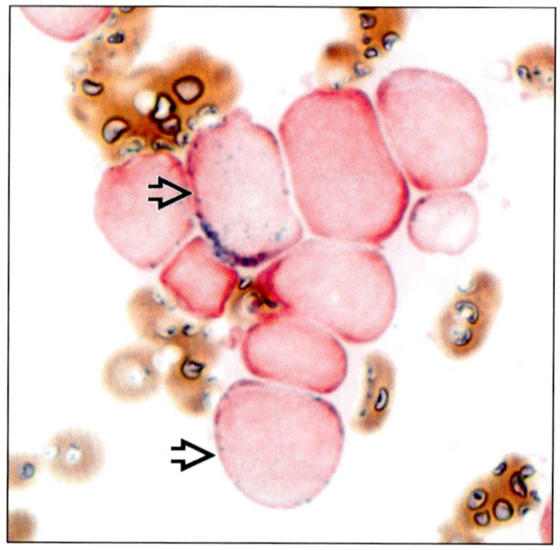

Cytochemical myeloperoxidase stain is positive in a subset of blasts ⮚ in this bone marrow aspirate smear from a patient with acute myeloid leukemia without maturation.

TERMINOLOGY

Synonyms

- Acute myeloid leukemia
- Acute myelogenous leukemia

Definitions

- Clonal hematopoietic neoplasms
- Acute myeloid leukemia (AML)
  - Blasts/blast equivalents comprise > 20% of nucleated peripheral blood (PB) &/or bone marrow (BM) cells
- Myelodysplastic syndrome (MDS)
  - Heterogeneous group of molecularly distinct entities
  - Variable degree of ineffective hematopoiesis due to simultaneous proliferation and apoptosis
  - < 20% blasts in PB and BM
  - Cytopenia of PB, hypercellular BM
  - Dysplasia in 1 or more lineages
  - Increased risk for AML
- Juvenile myelomonocytic leukemia (JMML)
  - Clonal hematopoietic disorder of childhood
  - Characterized by proliferation of myelomonocytic cells

ETIOLOGY/PATHOGENESIS

Constitutional Disorders Predispose to Hematologic Malignancy

- Down syndrome (DS)
  - 10-20x increased risk for AML
  - > 500x increased risk for acute megakaryoblastic leukemia
- Fanconi anemia (FA)
  - 10% of patients develop leukemia; majority are AML with a median age of 11-14 years at diagnosis
  - 600x increased risk for AML
  - 5,000x increased risk for MDS
  - Up to 80% of patients develop BM failure
  - Mutations in at least 15 FA genes located on various chromosomes
  - DNA cross-link repair defect
- Bloom syndrome (BS)
  - ~ 15% of patients develop MDS and leukemia, particularly AML and acute lymphoblastic leukemia (ALL)
  - *BLM* gene encodes DNA helicase that allows unwinding of DNA for repair
  - Mutations in *BLM* gene result in DNA repair defect
- Diamond-Blackfan anemia (DBA)
  - 3-4% of patients develop hematologic malignancy, particularly AML
  - Mutations in genes coding for ribosomal subunits, most frequently *RPS19*, preventing subunit from being incorporated into ribosome
  - Free subunits bind MDM2, a ubiquitin ligase that otherwise targets p52 for degradation, leading to increase in p53, thus favoring apoptosis
- Neurofibromatosis type 1 (NF1)
  - Increased risk for leukemia, particularly JMML
  - Increased risk for AML with monosomy 7
  - Increased risk for monosomy 7 syndrome
  - Neurofibromin 1 (NF1) is a negative regulator of RAS signaling pathway
  - Mutations in *NF1* result in activated RAS pathway, thus enhanced cell proliferation, survival, and suppressed apoptosis
- Noonan, Noonan-like syndrome (NS)
  - Predisposes to JMML
  - Mutations in *PTPN11* and *CBL* genes
  - *PTPN11* encodes SHP-2 protein, which controls phosphorylation of specific RAS pathway inhibitors
    - Mutations in *PTPN11* lead to sustained activation of RAS pathway
  - CBL plays a role in internalization and degradation of tyrosine kinase receptor dimers once the growth factor signal terminates

MYELOID NEOPLASMS

Key Facts

Terminology
- AML, MDS, and JMML are clonal hematopoietic neoplasms
- Blasts/blast equivalents comprise > 20% of nucleated PB &/or BM cells in AML
- MDS exhibits dysplasia in 1 or more lineages
- JMML is characterized by proliferation of myelomonocytic cells

Etiology/Pathogenesis
- AML develops with accumulation of multiple genetic hits
  - Class I and class II mutations
  - RAS signaling pathway mutations
- Initiating mutation or transforming event is unknown in MDS
- In JMML, mutations lead to constitutive activation of RAS pathway and cell proliferation
- Increased incidence of JMML is seen in many constitutional syndromes; underscores the needs to rule out the syndromes in any JMML patient

Clinical Issues
- Symptoms related to bone marrow failure
- AML may have extramedullary involvement
- Liver and spleen are almost always involved in JMML

Microscopic Pathology
- Assess circulating leukemic cells
- Assess dysplasia in all 3 lineages in MDS
- Predominantly neutrophils and monocytes with immature forms and minimal dysplasia in JMML

    - Mutations in *CBL* result in failure of degradation, thus sustained activation of receptors
- Severe congenital neutropenia (SCN)
  - Increased risk for AML, particularly patients on chronic recombinant human granulocyte colony stimulating factor therapy
  - Mutation of granulocyte colony stimulating factor (G-CSF) receptor gene strongly associated with AML development
- Familial platelet disorder with propensity to develop myeloid malignancy (FPD/AML)
  - Increased risk for acute leukemia, particularly AML
  - RUNX family of proteins binds to core-binding factor beta to form core-binding factor complex
    - Plays major role in myeloid and lymphoid development and maturation
    - Mutations of *RUNX1* gene lead to aberrant hematopoiesis and ultimately leukemia
- CCAAT/enhancer binding protein alpha (CEBPA)-dependent familial AML
  - Increased risk for AML with the following features
    - Particularly AML M1, M2 morphology subtypes
    - Auer rods
    - CD7 expression
    - Normal karyotype
  - Onset age varies from 4-46 years old
  - Complete penetrance
  - CEBPA is a member of leucine zipper transcription factors
    - Regulates myeloid differentiation by inducing granulocytic development
  - *CEBPA* encodes 2 transcription products: 42 kDa long form and 30 kDa short form
    - Short form has inhibitory function
    - Mutations lead to preferential production of 30 kDa short form; result in suppressed CEBPA function and increased risk for AML
  - CEBPA-dependent AML should be suspected in any family with autosomal dominant pattern of AML, particularly M1 and M2 morphology subtype
- Familial monosomy 7
  - Increased risk of MDS (most often) and AML (often with preceding MDS)
  - Median age at onset is 8 years
  - Equal incidence between males and females
  - Exact mechanism unknown
  - Results in deregulated growth in hematopoietic cells at various levels of differentiation, including multilineage progenitors
- Childhood monosomy 7
  - Increased risk for JMML, followed by MDS
  - Median age at onset is 3 years
  - M:F = 3-10:1

Familial Leukemia
- Multiple reports of acute leukemia in family members
- Mutations in genes responsible for maintaining telomere length are proposed
- May result from additive interactions of complex genetic and environmental factors, as well as common variants in metabolic enzymes

Environmental Exposures
- Radiation
- Chemotherapy
- Benzene

Molecular Bases of Leukemogenesis in AML
- Accumulation of multiple genetic hits
- Class I and class II mutations
  - Class I: Pro-proliferation signals
    - e.g., *FLT3, KIT;* encode receptor tyrosine kinase upstream of RAS pathway
    - e.g., *JAK2;* encodes component of JAK/STAT pathway
  - Class II: Impairment of cellular maturation
    - e.g., *PML-RARA, CEBPA, RUNX1-RUNX1T1*
- RAS signaling pathway mutations
  - *NRAS* mutations are more common than *KRAS* mutations in hematologic malignancies
  - *NF1* mutations are present in rare hematologic malignancies

- *RAS* and *NF1* mutations are overrepresented in AML with monocytic differentiation

Molecular Bases of Pathogenesis of MDS

- Initiating mutation or transforming event is unknown
- Clonal hematopoietic stem cell disease leads to ineffective hematopoiesis and apoptosis
- Clonal evolution with additional mutations leads to transformation to high-grade MDS and AML

Molecular Bases of Pathogenesis of JMML

- Mutations in various genes of RAS/MAPK signaling pathway are characteristic and lead to constitutive activation of RAS pathway and cell proliferation
  - Inactivating mutation in *NF1* gene in 10-15% of cases
  - Inactivating mutation in *CBL* gene
  - Activating mutations in *NRAS, KRAS* in 25-30% of cases
  - Activating mutations in *PTPN11* in ~ 35% of cases
  - *CBL* and *RAS/PTPN11* mutations are mutually exclusive
- Increased incidence of JMML is seen in the following syndromes; underscores the needs to rule out the syndromes in any JMML patient
  - Noonan syndrome
    - 50% of patients with Noonan syndrome have *PTPN11* mutation
  - Neurofibromatosis type 1
    - Patients with NF1 have 200-500x increased risk for JMML
  - Childhood monosomy 7
    - 6-24% of children with JMML have monosomy 7 at diagnosis
- May evolve to AML, most frequently AML with monocytic differentiation

CLINICAL ISSUES

Epidemiology

- Incidence
  - AML
    - Age-adjusted incidence: 3.4 cases per 100,000 individuals
    - ~ 10,000 new cases in USA each year
  - MDS
    - Annual incidence of > 30/100,000 among those aged > 70 years
    - Precedes or is related to majority of AML in elderly
    - Overall slight male predominance: M:F = 1.8:1
    - Exception is MDS del(5q), which has a female predominance
  - JMML
    - 1.3 per million children 0-14 years of age per year
    - M:F = 2:1
- Age
  - AML
    - All ages affected; median age: 63 years
    - 80% of adult acute leukemias are AML; incidence increases with age
    - AML with myelodysplasia-related changes is more prevalent in older adults
    - AML with recurrent genetic abnormalities (e.g., t[15;17], t[8;21], inv[16]/t[16;16], t[9;11]) are more prevalent in younger age groups
    - AML with t(1;22) occurs in infants and children < 3 years of age
  - MDS
    - Primarily a disease of elderly patients
    - Median age: 70 years in Western countries
    - Median age: ~ 10 years younger in Asian countries
    - Only ~ 10% of MDS patients are < 50 years old
    - Rare in children
  - JMML
    - 75% of cases occur in children < 3 years of age
    - Median age at diagnosis: 2 years

Presentation

- Symptoms related to bone marrow failure
  - Anemia: Fatigue, pallor, weakness
  - Thrombocytopenia: Bleeding, petechiae
  - Neutropenia: Recurrent infections
- Extramedullary involvement
  - Skin lesions
  - Gingival hyperplasia
  - Myeloid sarcomas
- JMML
  - May present with hepatosplenomegaly; liver and spleen are almost always involved
  - Skin, lymph nodes, and respiratory tract are common sites of involvement
  - Café au lait spots, tumor of CNS, and malignant tumor of peripheral nerve sheath raise suspicion of NF1
  - Abnormal face, short statue, webbed neck, cardiac defects, thoracic skeletal abnormalities, and bleeding diatheses raise suspicion of NS

Treatment

- AML
  - Chemotherapy is the mainstay of treatment
  - Radiation may be used for local control of disease
  - Bone marrow transplantation
- MDS
  - WHO prognostic scoring system (WPSS)-based risk-adapted treatment strategy
  - Low-risk patients may be monitored
  - Intermediate- or high-risk patients may choose
    - Azacytidine and its derivative decitabine to reverse effects of hypermethylation
    - Lenalidomide as immunomodulation and antiangiogenesis to induce apoptosis, particularly for MDS with 5q-
- JMML
  - Resistant to essentially all chemotherapy
  - Stem cell transplantation (SCT) is curative
  - RAS pathway inhibitors are in development or clinical trials

Prognosis

- AML
  - Highly dependent on genetic profile
    - Cytogenetics
    - Molecular genetics
  - Other factors affect prognosis

        - Prior chemotherapy &/or radiation history
        - Underlying hematopoietic neoplasm (e.g., MDS)
        - Increasing age (> 60 years old)
        - Elevated LDH
        - Performance status
    - Overall aggressive disease with high mortality and high relapse rate
- MDS
    - International prognostic scoring system (IPSS)
        - Based on number of cytopenia(s), % BM blasts, and cytogenetic abnormalities
        - Useful for predicting survival and risk of transformation to AML
    - WHO prognostic scoring system (WPSS)
        - Categorizes patients based on uni- or multilineage cytopenia, dysplasia, % BM blasts, cytogenetic findings, and transfusion dependency
        - Useful at diagnosis and during the course of disease evaluation in adult patients
        - Particularly helpful for identification of very low-risk group
        - Better prediction for survival and probability of leukemic evolution than IPSS
    - Age at diagnosis is a major risk factor for survival
    - Bone marrow fibrosis shifts patient to more advanced risk group
- JMML
    - 5-year event-free survival after SCT is ~ 50%
        - Leading cause of death is leukemic relapse
    - Median survival without SCT is 1 year
    - Age > 2 years at diagnosis, high fetal hemoglobin (HbF), and low platelet count correlate with worse prognosis
    - JMML developing in patients with Noonan syndrome may regress spontaneously

MACROSCOPIC FEATURES

General Features

- Myeloid sarcomas
    - Soft fleshy whitish or yellowish mass with variable foci of necrosis

MICROSCOPIC PATHOLOGY

Peripheral Blood

- Cytopenia
    - Anemia
    - Thrombocytopenia
    - Neutropenia
- Circulating leukemic cells
- Assess for dysplasia in neutrophils and platelets
- JMML often present with leukocytosis with median WBC count of 25,000-30,000/μL
    - Predominantly neutrophils and monocytes with immature forms and minimal dysplasia
    - Blasts < 20%, typically < 5%
- Assess red blood cell morphology for evidence of disseminated intravascular coagulation

Bone Marrow Aspirate

- Enumeration of blasts or leukemic cells; % blasts based on morphology, not by flow cytometry
- Assess for dysplasia in all 3 lineages, require ≥ 10% of cell lineage
- JMML
    - Hypercellular with myeloid hyperplasia
    - Minimal dysplasia
    - Monocytic lineage accounts for 5-10% of all cells
    - Blasts < 20%

Bone Marrow Core Biopsy

- Assess hematopoietic architecture
- Assess relative proportion of each lineage
- Assess overall number and distribution of immature cells or leukemic cells
- Assess megakaryocytic dysplasia
- Evaluate any concurrent malignancy

Diagnostic Criteria

- JMML
    - Absolute monocytes in PB > 1,000/μL
    - < 20% blasts in PB and BM
    - Absence of *BCR-ABL1* fusion
    - Plus 2 of the 5 following criteria
        - Circulating myeloid precursors
        - WBC > 10,000/μL
        - Increased HbF for age
        - In vitro granulocyte monocyte colony stimulating factor (GM-CSF) hypersensitivity of myeloid progenitors
        - Clonal cytogenetic abnormality: Mutation in *RAS, PTPN11, NF1*, or *CBL* gene, or monosomy 7

ANCILLARY TESTS

Cytology

- Myeloperoxidase (MPO)
    - Positive MPO: Confirms myeloid lineage
    - Negative MPO: Does not exclude myeloid lineage
    - ~ 5% of acute monoblastic leukemias may be MPO positive
- Nonspecific esterase (NSE)
    - Positive NSE: Confirms monocytic lineage

Immunohistochemistry

- Useful if flow cytometry is inadequate or not performed
- Fewer antibodies available than flow cytometry
    - CD34 for blasts; use CD117 if blasts are negative for CD34
    - MPO or CD33 for myeloid lineage quantification and distribution, i.e., abnormal localization of immature precursors (ALIP)
    - CD71, glycophorin A, or hemoglobin A for erythroid lineage quantification and colony formation assessment
    - CD61 or CD42b for megakaryocytic lineage quantification, abnormal clustering or localization, and morphology
    - CD68: Myeloid and monocytic
    - Lysozyme: Monocytic

MYELOID NEOPLASMS

Flow Cytometry
- Should be performed in all new cases
- Establish leukemic cell lineage
- Determine % blasts in PB &/or BM
- Establish immunophenotype, particularly aberrant marker expression as "fingerprint" for future monitoring or for maturation pattern
- Blast markers
  - CD34: Not all blasts express CD34
  - CD117: Also stains promonocytes and mast cells
  - TdT: Stains a subset of AML
- Myeloid markers
  - MPO, CD33, CD13
- Monocytic markers
  - CD14, CD36/CD64 coexpression, CD163, CD4 (weak), CD33 (bright)
- Gain of abnormal antigens such as CD56, CD19, CD7, CD5 on myeloid or monocytic cells
- Megakaryocytic markers
  - CD31, CD41, CD42b, CD61
- Erythroid markers
  - Glycophorin A, hemoglobin A, CD71 (not specific)

Cytogenetics
- Essential for new cases
- Diagnostic: AML and MDS with recurrent clonal cytogenetic abnormalities
- Prognostic: Favorable, intermediate, and unfavorable risk groups for AML and MDS
- JMML
  - Normal karyotype in 65% of cases
  - Monosomy 7 in ~ 25% of cases

Molecular Genetics
- Perform as per institution, protocol requirements, anticipated minimal residual disease monitoring
- Karyotypically normal AML should be evaluated for *FLT3, NPM1*, and *CEBPA* mutations
- JMML should be evaluated for *RAS, NF1, PTPN11*, or *CBL* mutations

FISH
- Cryptic cytogenetic abnormalities
- Prognostic: Favorable, intermediate, and unfavorable risk groups for MDS

DIFFERENTIAL DIAGNOSIS

Acute Lymphoblastic Leukemia (ALL)
- Typically has smaller blasts with scant cytoplasm
- Immunophenotype reveals lymphoid lineage

Therapy-Related Myeloid Neoplasm
- Exhibits dysplasia
- History of chemotherapy for other malignancy

Chronic Myelomonocytic Leukemia (CMML)
- Has monocytosis and should be differentiated from JMML
- Typically diagnosed in older patient population

Chronic Myeloid Leukemia (CML)
- Rarely CML arises in young patients and should be differentiated from JMML
- Exhibits predominantly granulocytic lineage proliferation
- Translocation 9;22 is diagnostic of CML

Atypical Chronic Myeloid Leukemia (aCML)
- May exhibit slightly increased monocytes and should be differentiated from JMML
- Typically seen in elderly patients
- Reveals predominantly granulocytic proliferation with significant dysplasia

DIAGNOSTIC CHECKLIST

Clinically Relevant Pathologic Features
- CEBPA-dependent AML should be suspected in any family with autosomal dominant pattern of AML, particularly M1 and M2 morphology subtype
- Rule out related syndromes in any JMML patient

SELECTED REFERENCES

1. Grimwade D: The changing paradigm of prognostic factors in acute myeloid leukaemia. Best Pract Res Clin Haematol. 25(4):419-25, 2012
2. Kühnl A et al: Molecular markers in acute myeloid leukaemia. Int J Hematol. 96(2):153-63, 2012
3. Ward AF et al: Targeting oncogenic Ras signaling in hematologic malignancies. Blood. 120(17):3397-406, 2012
4. Grimwade D et al: Diagnostic and prognostic value of cytogenetics in acute myeloid leukemia. Hematol Oncol Clin North Am. 25(6):1135-61, vii, 2011
5. Seif AE: Pediatric leukemia predisposition syndromes: clues to understanding leukemogenesis. Cancer Genet. 204(5):227-44, 2011
6. Komrokji RS et al: Myelodysplastic syndromes classification and risk stratification. Hematol Oncol Clin North Am. 24(2):443-57, 2010
7. Motyckova G et al: The role of molecular tests in acute myelogenous leukemia treatment decisions. Curr Hematol Malig Rep. 5(2):109-17, 2010
8. Vardiman JW et al: The 2008 revision of the World Health Organization (WHO) classification of myeloid neoplasms and acute leukemia: rationale and important changes. Blood. 114(5):937-51, 2009
9. Wang S et al: Noonan syndrome/leukemia-associated gain-of-function mutations in SHP-2 phosphatase (PTPN11) enhance cell migration and angiogenesis. J Biol Chem. 284(2):913-20, 2009
10. Benson KF et al: Familial leukemia. Best Pract Res Clin Haematol. 19(2):269-79, 2006
11. Michaud J et al: In vitro analyses of known and novel RUNX1/AML1 mutations in dominant familial platelet disorder with predisposition to acute myelogenous leukemia: implications for mechanisms of pathogenesis. Blood. 99(4):1364-72, 2002
12. Luna-Fineman S et al: Childhood monosomy 7: epidemiology, biology, and mechanistic implications. Blood. 85(8):1985-99, 1995
13. Fong CT et al: Down's syndrome and leukemia: epidemiology, genetics, cytogenetics and mechanisms of leukemogenesis. Cancer Genet Cytogenet. 28(1):55-76, 1987

Microscopic Features and Immunophenotype

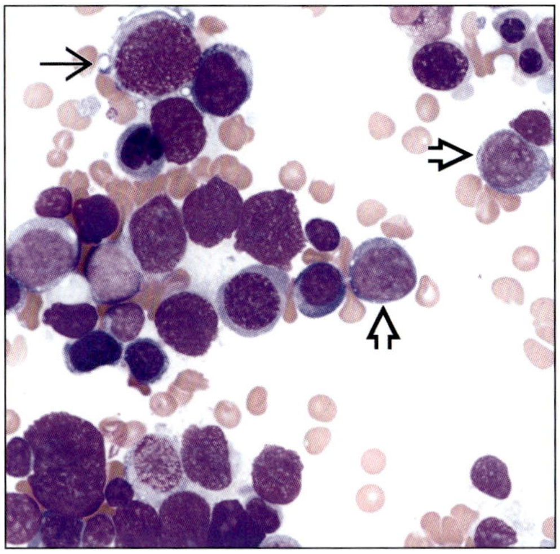

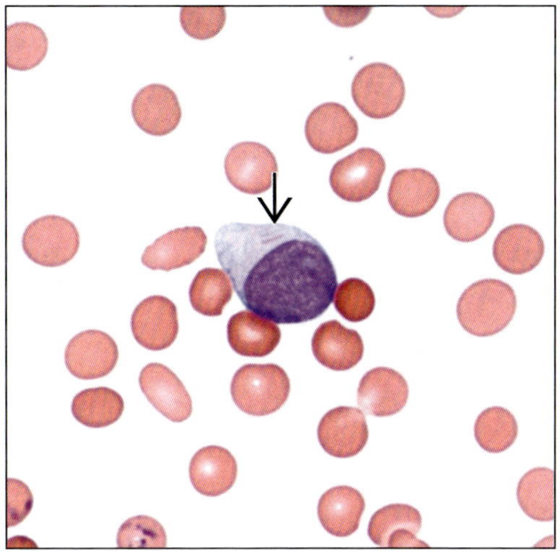

(Left) *Bone marrow aspirate smear shows a case of AML that is tricky/difficult to diagnose because of the markedly increased erythroid precursors* → *admixed with myeloid blasts* ⇨. *Such cases raise the possibility of acute erythroid leukemia vs. MDS. (Courtesy K. Reichard, MD.)* ***(Right)*** *Auer rods are a hallmark feature of a myeloid neoplasm* →, *representing compact linear aggregation of MPO granules. This patient was diagnosed with AML by other studies. (Courtesy K. Reichard, MD.)*

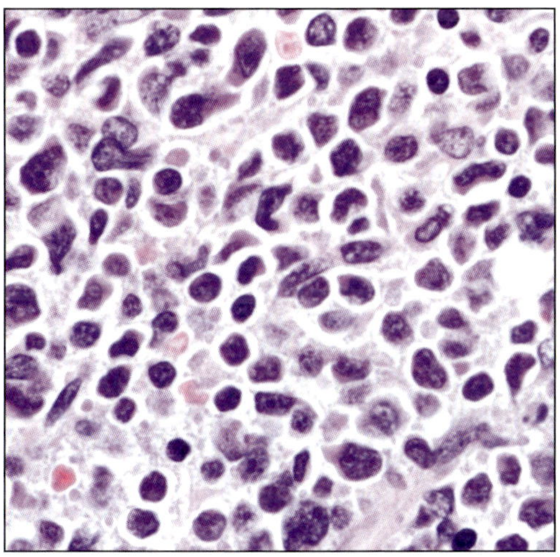

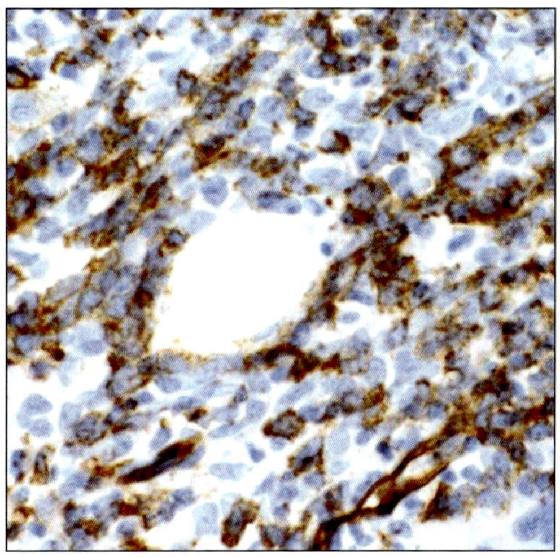

(Left) *Bone marrow core biopsy of AML without maturation exhibits hypercellular marrow with predominant blasts.* ***(Right)*** *On occasion, flow cytometry is suboptimal or unavailable. Immunohistochemical (IHC) stains can verify an acute leukemia using lineage-specific and blast markers. CD34 reveals > 20% blasts in this acute leukemia. (Courtesy K. Reichard, MD.)*

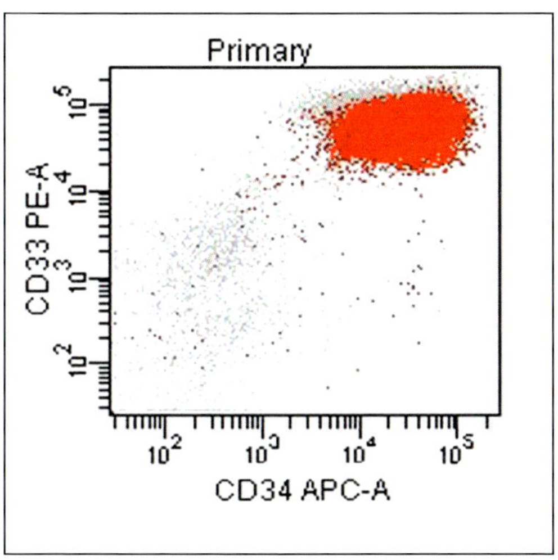

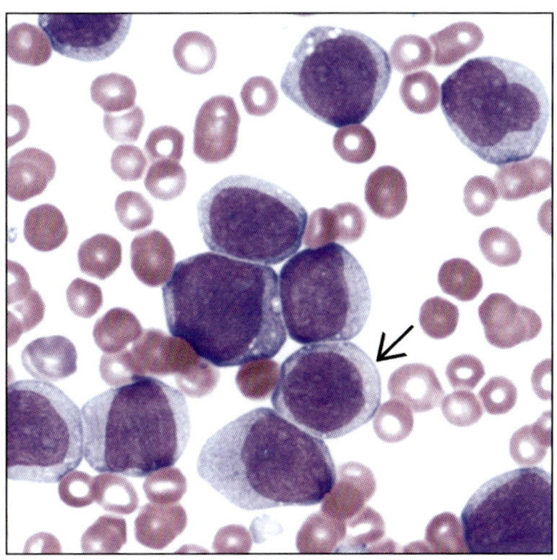

(Left) *Flow cytometric analysis of AML without maturation demonstrates coexpression of CD34 and CD33, indicative of both immaturity and myeloid differentiation.* ***(Right)*** *Peripheral blood smear demonstrates the typical cytology of monoblasts. They are large with round nuclei, variably prominent nucleoli, and abundant cytoplasm, which may contain fine azurophilic granules* →. *(Courtesy K. Reichard, MD.)*

Ancillary Techniques and Microscopic Features

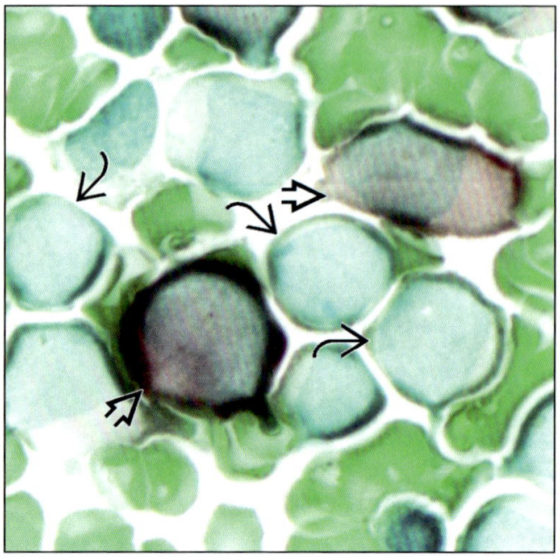
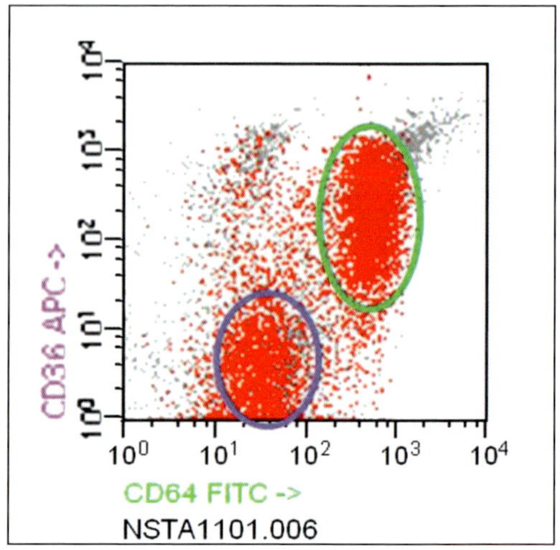

(Left) *Nonspecific esterase (NSE) stain reveals NSE(+) monoblasts ⇨. The myeloblasts ↪ are negative.* ***(Right)*** *Flow cytometric analysis of acute myelomonocytic leukemia (AMML) demonstrates 2 blast populations. The blasts in the green circle demonstrate expression of both CD36 & CD64, consistent with monocytic differentiation. The myeloblasts in the blue circle are negative for both monocytic markers; they are identified as myeloblasts by myeloid markers.*

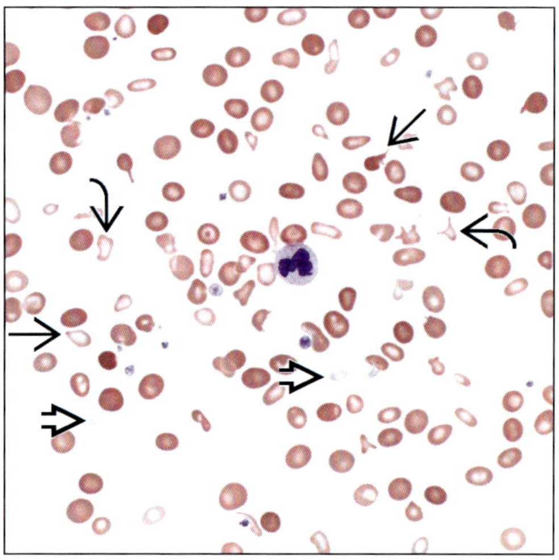
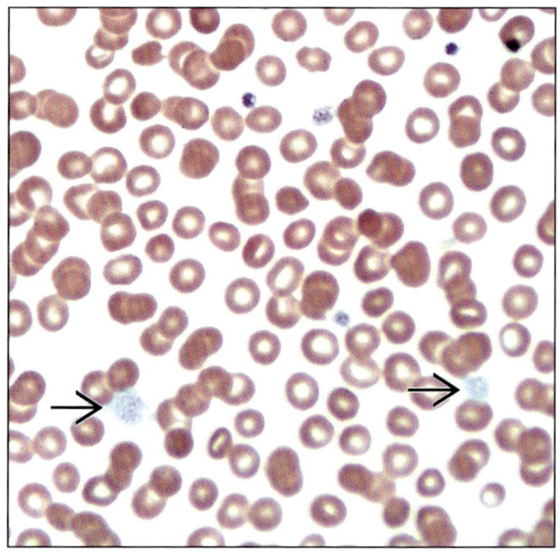

(Left) *This peripheral blood smear is from a 56-year-old man with pancytopenia. The red cells show prominent anisopoikilocytosis with teardrop cells → and small hypochromatic irregularly shaped poikilocytes ↪. The platelets are mildly decreased in number and include hypogranular forms ⇨.* ***(Right)*** *Large and hypogranular platelets → are another dysplastic finding in MDS blood films.*

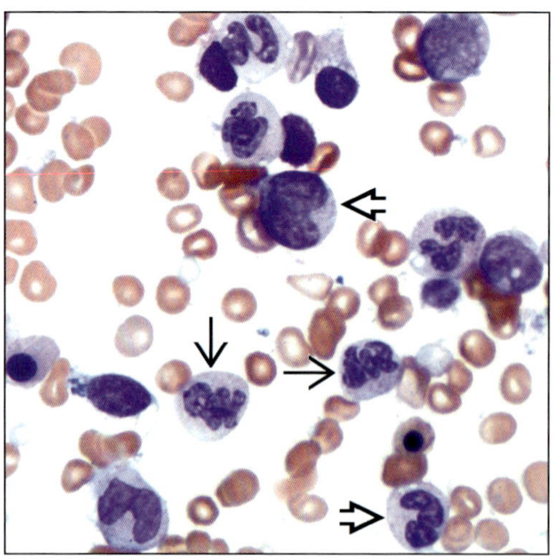
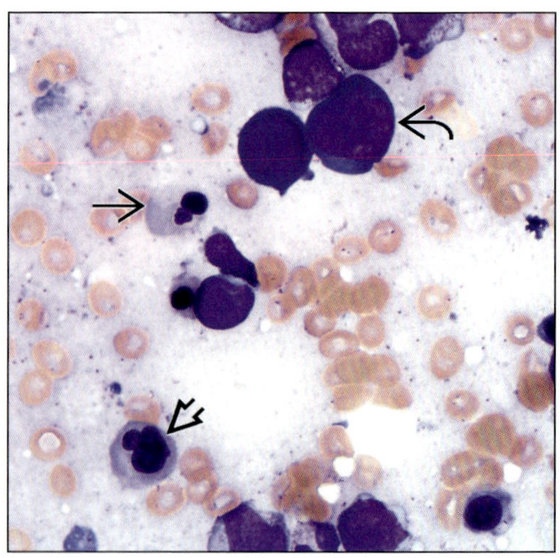

(Left) *Dysgranulopoiesis in ≥ 10% of the myeloid lineage is the predominant finding in this bone marrow aspirate from a patient with MDS. Dysplastic features include irregular and abnormal nuclear segmentation → and cytoplasmic hypogranulation ⇨.* ***(Right)*** *Dysplastic features in erythroid precursors in MDS include nuclear budding →, hyperlobation ⇨, and megaloblastic changes ↪.*

Microscopic Features and Immunohistochemical Stains

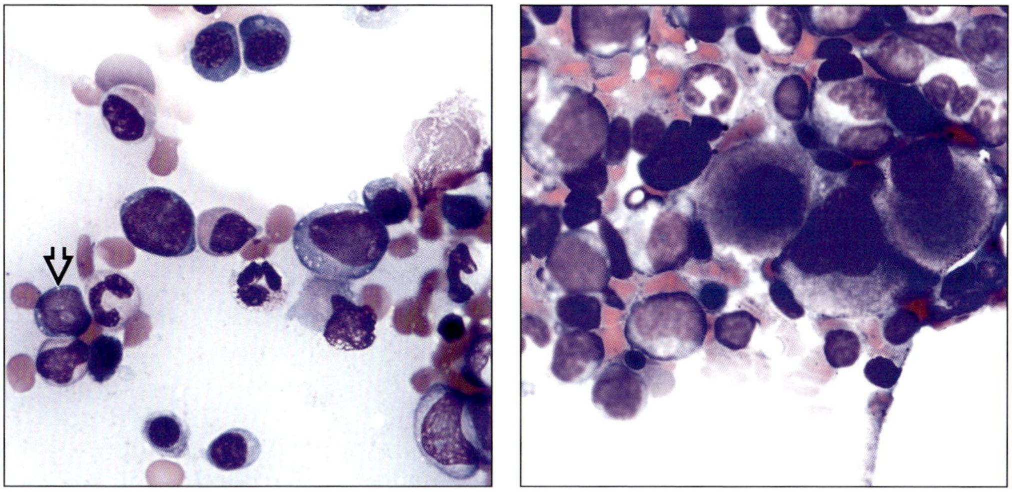

(Left) *Blasts in MDS may be small ⇨ and are particularly difficult to identify in poorly prepared or suboptimally stained smears. Some cases of refractory anemia with excess blasts may not have prominent dysplastic features.* ***(Right)*** *Small dysplastic megakaryocytes with hypolobated and hyperchromatic nuclei are clustered together in this aspirate smear from the same patient.*

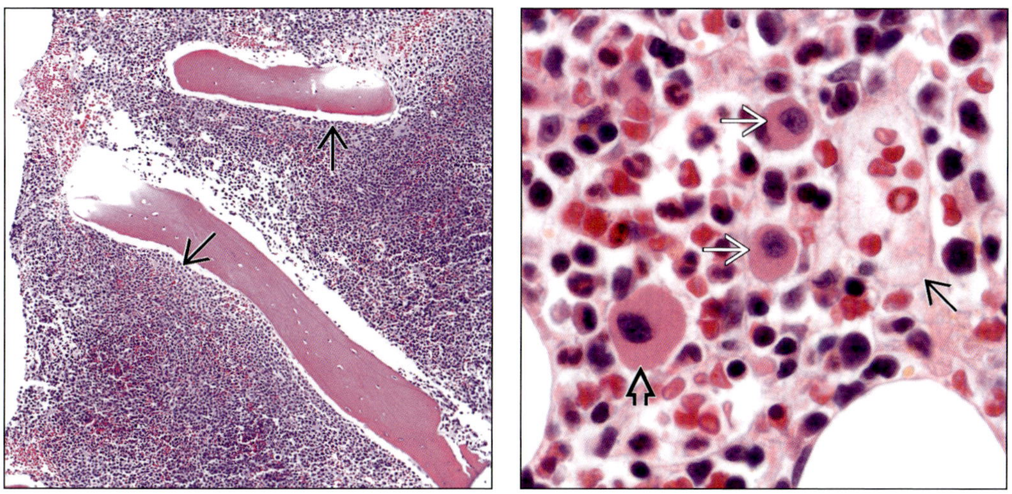

(Left) *MDS bone marrows are typically hypercellular with intact hematopoiesis. Immature myeloid precursors normally line the trabecular bone → but are also clustered in intratrabecular areas termed abnormal localization of immature precursors (ALIP).* ***(Right)*** *Higher power examination shows dysmegakaryopoiesis with monolobated ⇨ and small ➡ megakaryocytes. The erythroid and myeloid lineages show complete maturation, and sinuses are patent →.*

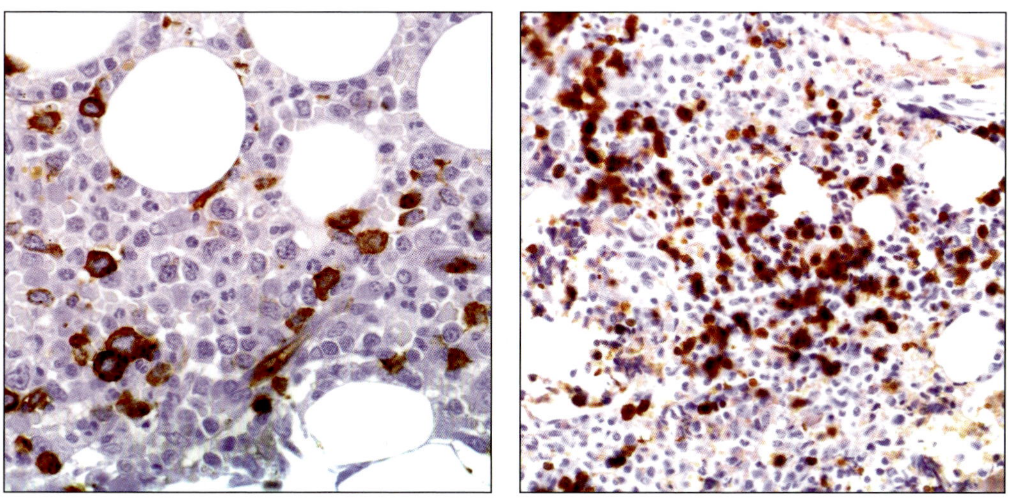

(Left) *The same biopsy has an uneven distribution of CD34(+) blasts that are slightly increased (~ 5%) and fulfill minimum criteria for a diagnosis of refractory anemia with excess blasts.* ***(Right)*** *Disruption of the normal bone marrow architecture is illustrated with the hemoglobin A stain. The erythroid precursors are scattered without good colony formation.*

MYELOID NEOPLASMS

Microscopic Features and Ancillary Techniques

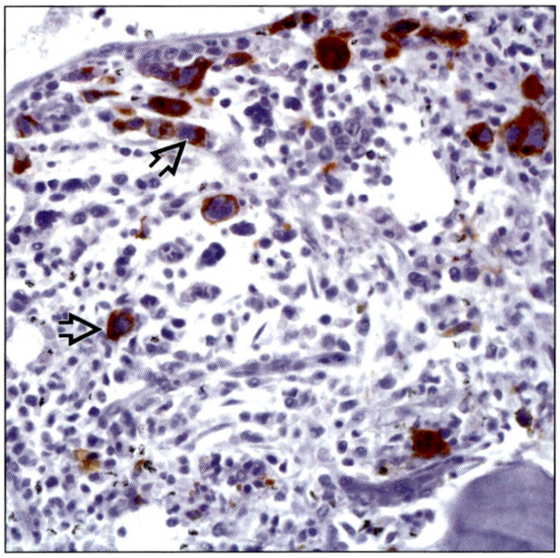

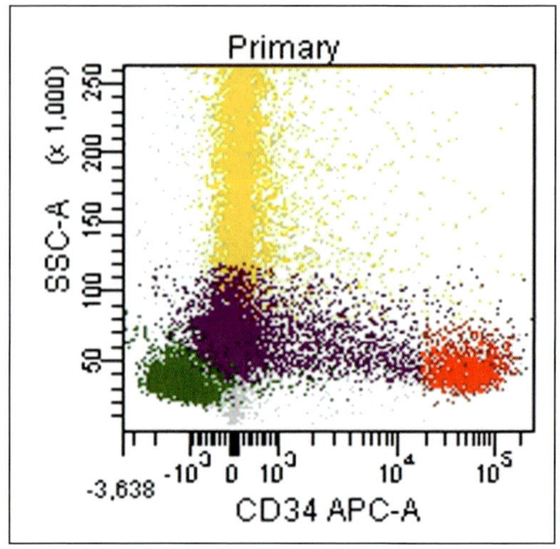

(Left) *Megakaryocytes are increased despite thrombocytopenia. The megakaryocytes are visualized by CD42b staining and include small cells ⇨.* ***(Right)*** *A CD34(+) blast population (red) was detected in the MDS marrow aspirate by flow cytometric (FCM) analysis. The blasts have abnormally bright CD34 expression. Blast percentages should be based on visual inspection of the bone marrow rather than FCM analysis because of hemodilution and erythroid cell lysis of FCM specimens.*

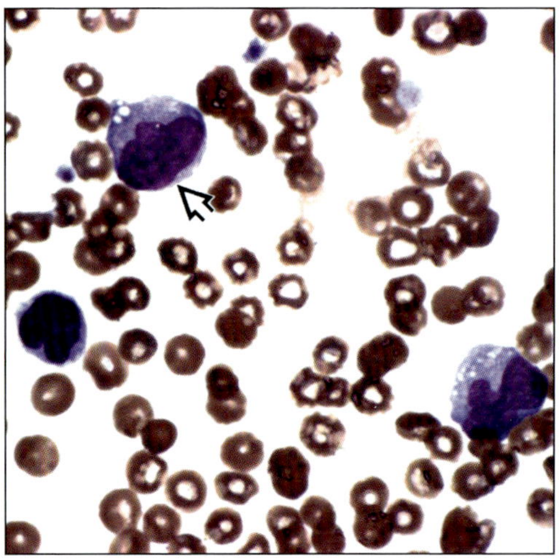

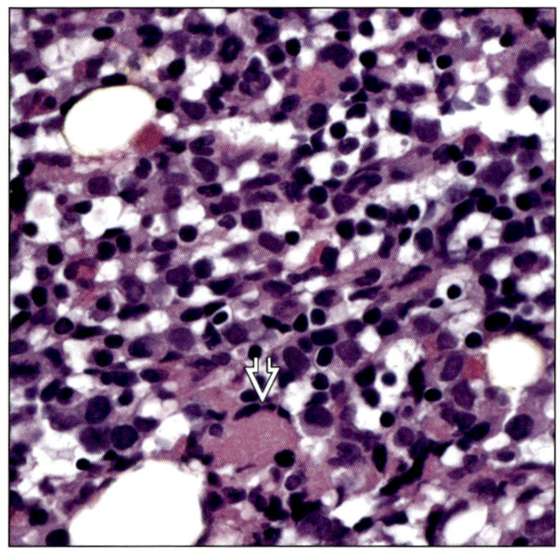

(Left) *Peripheral blood from an 11-month-old boy with hepatosplenomegaly, leukocytosis, and monocytosis shows an immature monocyte ⇨. Cytogenetic study revealed monosomy 7, supporting the diagnosis of juvenile myelomonocytic leukemia (JMML).* ***(Right)*** *Bone marrow core biopsy from the same patient shows trilineage hematopoiesis, occasional hypolobulated megakaryocytes ➡, and left-shifted myeloid and erythroid precursors.*

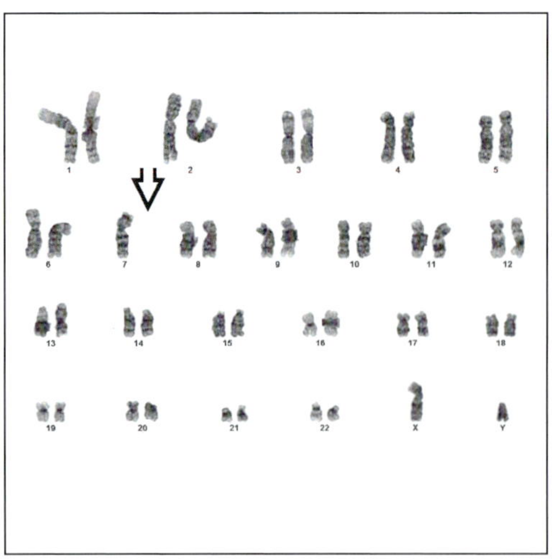

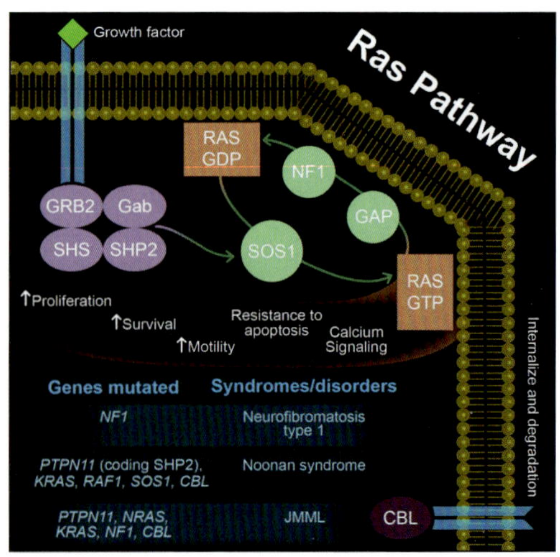

(Left) *Monosomy 7 ⇨ can be seen in JMML, childhood monosomy 7 syndrome, familial monosomy 7, MDS/AML ± associated syndromes or prior therapy history, and familial MDS/AML, among others. Monosomy 7 may occur as an isolated abnormality or concurrently with other abnormalities.* ***(Right)*** *Mutations of RAS pathway are frequently found and may play important roles in the pathogenesis of neurofibromatosis type 1, Noonan syndrome, and JMML.*

Differential Diagnosis

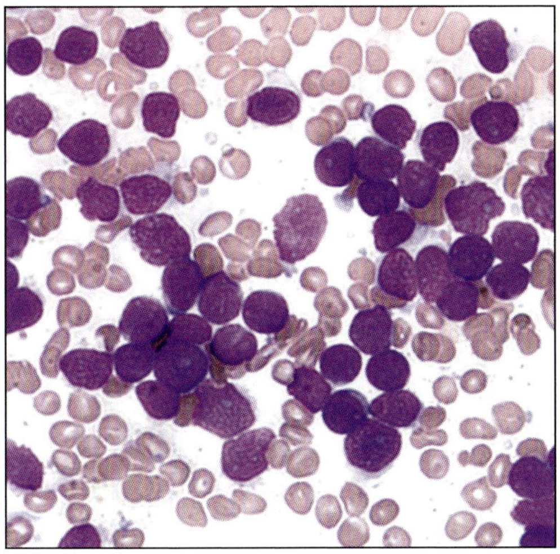

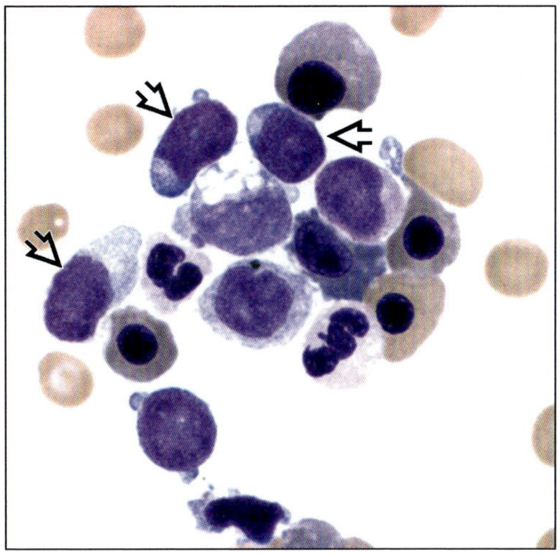

(Left) *Typical small uniform lymphoblasts (L1 blasts) are seen in this bone marrow smear from a 3-year-old boy with a new diagnosis of ALL. The blasts have scant cytoplasm.* ***(Right)*** *Bone marrow aspirate smear shows therapy-related myeloid neoplasm that developed after topoisomerase II inhibitor treatment for acute lymphoblastic leukemia. Note the myeloblasts ➪. (Courtesy K. Foucar, MD.)*

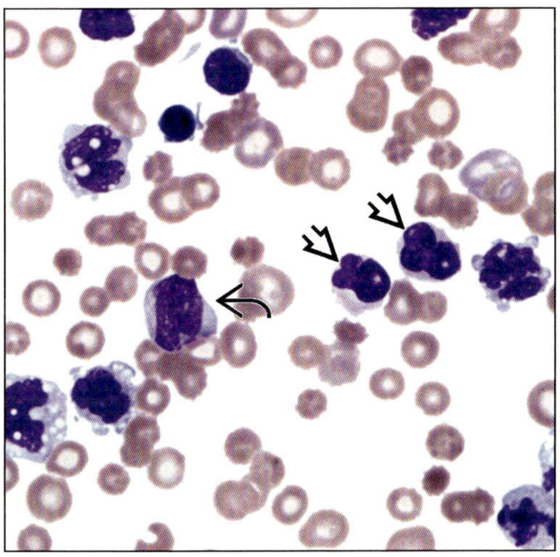

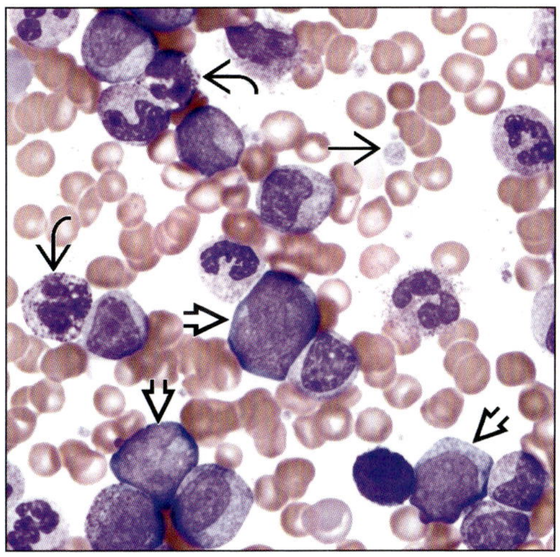

(Left) *Peripheral blood from a 5-month-old girl with 11q23-associated AML is shown. Dysplastic neutrophils ➪ and immature cell ⮫ are prominent.* ***(Right)*** *Wright stain of peripheral blood from a patient with CML shows leukocytosis, left shift, presence of blasts ➪, basophilia ⮫, and frequent large platelets →. There is no significant dysplasia. t(9;22) is diagnostic of chronic myeloid leukemia (CML).*

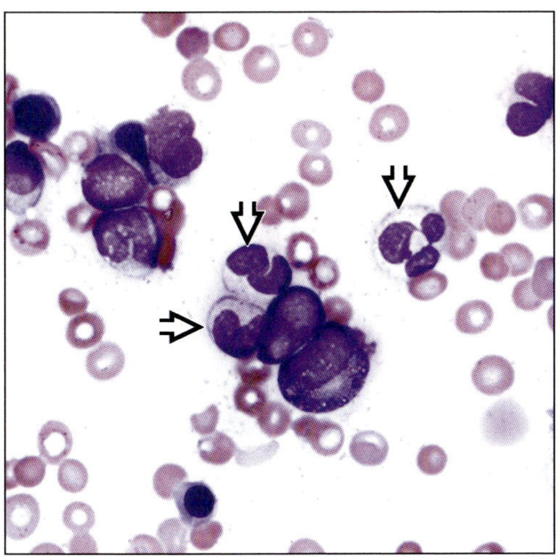

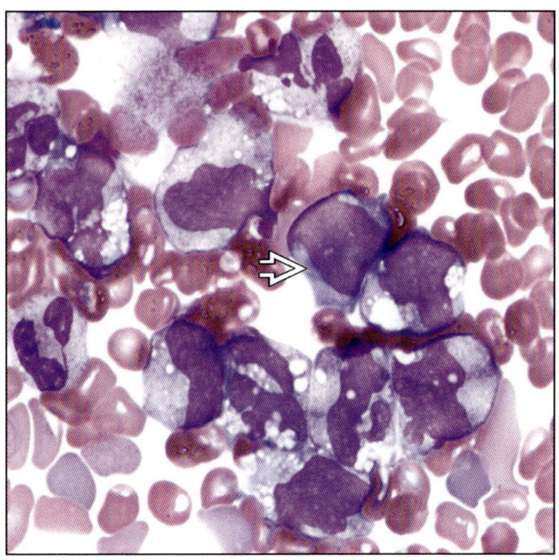

(Left) *Wright stain of bone marrow aspirate smear from a patient with atypical CML (aCML) shows abundant granulocytes and precursors. aCML typically exhibits significant dysplasia. Neutrophils demonstrated here show abnormal nuclear hypolobation and hypogranulation ➪.* ***(Right)*** *Blood smear from a patient diagnosed with chronic myelomonocytic leukemia, type 2 (CMML-2) shows monocytosis with an occasional immature cell ➪. CMML is usually seen in older patients.*

PLASMA CELL MYELOMA

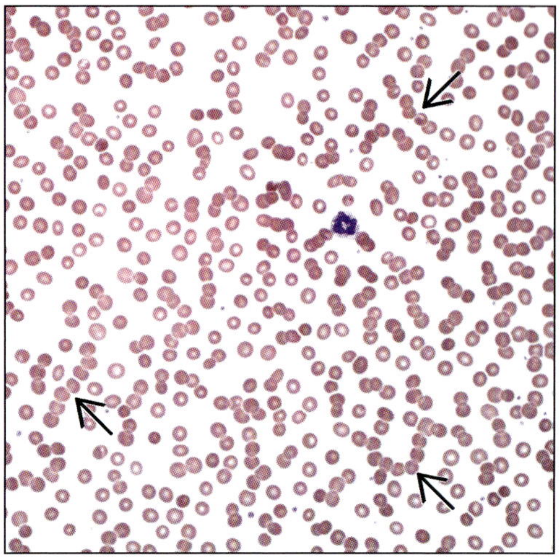

Rouleaux formation ➔ is the linear arrangement of ≥ 4 red cells that resemble a stack of coins. It indicates increased protein (i.e., globulins, fibrinogen) when seen in thin areas of the smear.

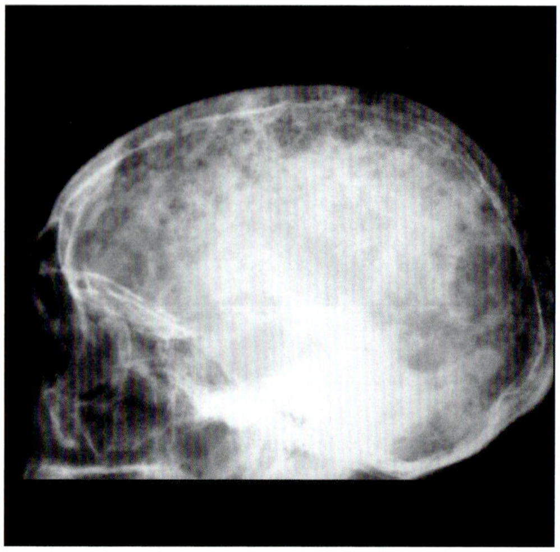

A lateral radiograph of the calvarium shows multiple lytic bone lesions. Lytic bone lesions or a combination of osteoporosis, osteolysis, or pathologic fractures are found in ~ 75% of plasma cell myeloma (PCM) patients.

TERMINOLOGY

Abbreviations

- Plasma cell myeloma (PCM)

Synonyms

- Multiple myeloma

Definitions

- Accumulation of clonal plasma cells (PCs) in bone marrow
  - Associated monoclonal (M) protein in serum &/or urine in majority of cases
- 2008 WHO Classification of Tumors of Plasma Cell Neoplasms
  - PCM diagnosis requires > 30 g/L serum M component **or**
  - > 10% clonal PCs in bone marrow **or**
  - Evidence of myeloma-related symptoms
- Multifocal bone marrow involvement in most cases
  - Asymptomatic (smoldering) PCM: No related organ or tissue impairment
  - Symptomatic PCM: End-organ damage or bone lesions
- Preceded by monoclonal gammopathy of undetermined significance (MGUS) in all patients

ETIOLOGY/PATHOGENESIS

Environmental Exposure

- Increased susceptibility as people age (declining immune system)
- Linked to chemical, toxin, or radiation exposure
  - Herbicides, insecticides, asbestosis
  - Rubber, plastic, wood, or petroleum products
- Associated with some autoimmune, inflammatory, or infectious disorders

Proposed Pathogenesis

- Immature B cells, after VDJ recombination, migrate from bone marrow to lymphoid tissue
  - B cells that survive antigen selection in germinal centers have marked intrinsic genetic instability
    - Develop genetic abnormalities from IgH switch recombination errors or somatic hypermutation
  - Genetically abnormal PCs/plasmablasts home to bone marrow
    - PCs have primarily hyperdiploid or immunoglobulin heavy (IgH) chain abnormalities
    - Induce stromal cells to produce cytokines
    - PCs undergo additional genetic alterations
    - Ultimate immortalization of PC clone
  - MGUS precedes PCM
    - 100x more common than PCM
    - 1% MGUS converts to PCM per year indefinitely
  - PCM
    - Random secondary genetic hit is associated with MGUS progression to PCM
    - Role for miRNAs, i.e., miRNA-15a, miRNA-16
  - Extramedullary PCM
    - Additional genetic hits allow for PC growth independent of marrow microenvironment

CLINICAL ISSUES

Epidemiology

- Incidence
  - ~ 20,000 cases diagnosed in USA in 2008
    - Incidence is increasing as population ages
  - Genetic predisposition
    - Familial clustering
- Age
  - Peak incidence is 8th decade of life
    - Rarely observed in people < 35 years old
- Gender
  - Slight male predominance

PLASMA CELL MYELOMA

Key Facts

Terminology
- Plasma cell myeloma (PCM) diagnosis requires
  - > 30 g/L serum M component **or**
  - > 10% clonal PCs in bone marrow **or**
  - Evidence of myeloma-related symptoms
- Preceded by MGUS in all patients
- Asymptomatic PCM: No related organ or tissue impairment

Clinical Issues
- Unique triad of clinical features: Bone marrow plasmacytosis, osteolytic bone lesions, monoclonal gammopathy
  - Accounts for 10-15% of hematopoietic malignancies
- Median overall survival
  - > 8 years for standard-risk PCM after tandem stem cell transplantation
  - 3 years for high-risk disease after therapy

Microscopic Pathology
- Peripheral blood: Rouleaux formation
- Bone marrow: Clonal PC infiltrate, osteoclastic bone lesions, possible amyloid

Ancillary Tests
- Cytogenetic/FISH studies
  - Have prognostic and therapeutic implications
- Intermediate-risk disease (mSMART)
  - Cytogenetics: Deletion 13 or hypodiploidy
  - FISH: t(4;14)
- High-risk disease
  - FISH: t(14;16), t(14;20), del17p

    - M:F = 3:2
- Ethnicity
  - High incidence in African Americans: 9.5/100,000
  - Caucasian American incidence is 4.1/100,000

Presentation
- Unique triad: Bone marrow plasmacytosis, osteolytic bone lesions, monoclonal gammopathy
  - Clinical and laboratory findings reflect or are secondary to these abnormalities
    - Most common presenting symptoms are bone pain, fatigue, weight loss
    - Anemia of chronic disease
    - Renal failure if excess light chain
    - Recurrent bacterial infections from hypogammopathy and immunodeficiency
- Asymptomatic myeloma
  - Distinguish from symptomatic PCM by absence of end-organ damage
    - Develop symptomatic PCM at 10% per year in 1st 5 years, 3% per year in next 5 years, 1% per year for last 10 years
    - 50x increased risk for amyloidosis
  - Higher risk of progression than MGUS
- Plasma cell leukemia (PCL)
  - Primary PCL comprises 2-5% of PCM
    - Peripheral blood plasmacytosis (> 20% of WBCs or > 2 x 10^9/L)
    - Present with renal failure, lymphadenopathy, &/or organomegaly
    - Decreased incidence of bone lesions
  - Secondary PCL
    - Circulating plasmacytosis late in course of PCM

Laboratory Tests
- Serum protein electrophoresis (SPEP)
  - Identifies and quantifies monoclonal protein (M component)
  - Immunofixation electrophoresis to determine immunoglobulin type
  - Decrease in uninvolved immunoglobulins (~ 90% of cases)
- Urine protein electrophoresis (UPEP) or serum free light chain (FLC) assay
  - FLC is best for screening
    - If abnormal, perform UPEP; requires 24-hour urine collection
- Nephelometric quantitation of immunoglobulins
- Chemistry panel
  - Increased β2 microglobulin (75% at diagnosis)
    - Surrogate marker for tumor burden
  - Subset of PCM patients have
    - Increased uric acid, creatinine, or calcium
    - Decreased albumin

Treatment
- Evolving rapidly so clinical trials are recommended
  - Multiple trials utilizing novel drugs, specific subsets of patients
    - Elderly, relapsed/refractory disease, severe renal failure
    - High-risk myeloma
- Standard-risk disease
  - High-dose chemotherapy with autologous stem cell transplantation (ASCT)
  - Alternative therapy if elderly, renal insufficiency, comorbid condition
- Intermediate-risk disease (Mayo Stratification of Myeloma and Risk Adapted Therapy [mSMART])
  - Bortexomib-based regimen
- High-risk disease
  - Induction includes novel agents, followed by ASCT
- Anti-PCM drugs: Usually 2-3 drug regimens initially
  - Alkylating agents, anthracyclines, corticosteroids
  - Immunomodulatory drugs (IMiDS): Thalidomide, lenalidomide, pomalidomide
  - Protease inhibitors: Bortezomib, carfilzomib
  - Other novel agents
    - Multikinase inhibitors, farnesyl transferase inhibitors, histone deacetylase inhibitors, heat shock protein 90 inhibitors, MLN9708
    - Various monoclonal proteins: IL-6, CS1
- Bisphosphonates for bone disease

PLASMA CELL MYELOMA

Prognosis

- Features associated with worse prognosis
  - Increased proliferative rate
    - High plasma cell labeling index or Ki-67 rate
    - Abnormal karyotype on conventional cytogenetics
    - High proliferative gene expression signature
  - Increased tumor burden
    - International staging system: Utilizes β2 microglobulin and albumin levels
    - Circulating PCs
  - High-risk genetic features
    - Based on karyotype, fluorescent in situ hybridization (FISH) studies, or gene expression profile
    - Plasmablastic morphology is associated with high-risk cytogenetics
- International Myeloma Working Group proposed molecular classification
  - More favorable prognosis if
    - Hyperdiploid (45%)
    - Cyclin-D translocations (18%): t(11;14)(q13;q32), t(6;14)(p21;q32), t(12;14)(p13;q32)
  - More aggressive disease if
    - Nonhyperdiploid (40%), especially hypodiploid
    - *MMSET* translocation (15%): t(4;14)(p16;q32)
    - *MAF* translocation (~ 8%): t(14;16)(q32;q23), t(14;20)(q32;q11), t(8;14)(q24;q32)
    - Other (15%): Includes *TP53* deletion
- Asymptomatic PCM with > 10% clonal PCs
  - FLC ratio (involved/uninvolved) > 100
    - 70-80% risk of progression in next 2 years
- Median overall survival with contemporary therapy using mSMART
  - > 8 years for standard risk PCM
  - 4-5 years for intermediate-risk disease
  - 3 years for high-risk disease

IMAGE FINDINGS

Radiographic Findings

- Bone survey to evaluate for osteolytic lesions
  - If no lesions identified, may require MR, CT, or PET scans to detect

MICROSCOPIC PATHOLOGY

Cytologic Features

- Peripheral blood
  - Rouleaux formation
  - Normochromic normocytic anemia
    - Anemia of chronic disease
    - Decreased erythropoietin due to renal failure
    - Replacement of marrow by PCs
  - Plasma cells
    - Worse prognosis, need to exclude PCL
  - Leukopenia or thrombocytopenia
    - < 20% of cases at diagnosis
  - Neutrophilia (rare)
- Bone marrow
  - PC infiltrate
    - Assess PC volume (PC % x cellularity %)
    - Infiltration pattern, associated fibrosis
  - Amyloid, osteoclastic bone lesions

ANCILLARY TESTS

Immunohistochemistry

- CD138 (syndecan-1), kappa and lambda light chains
  - Quantify clonal PC population in tissue sections
  - Expression of CD56 (~ 70%) or cyclin-D1 (~ 33%)

Flow Cytometry

- Routinely underestimates PC % by 60-70%
  - Technical difficulties in evaluating PCs
    - PCs stick to things that alter expression patterns
    - PCs autofluoresce and get false-positive results
- PCM is CD138(+), CD38(+), CD19(-), CD45(+/-), CD56(+/-)
  - Often weaker CD38, brighter CD138 than normal
  - Aberrant expression of other lineage antigens, i.e., CD20 (15-20%), CD28 (40%), CD33 (15%), CD52 (30%), CD117 (27%)
- Primary PCL has increased frequency of CD20(+), CD56(-), CD117(-)

Cytogenetics

- Perform on all newly diagnosed patients
  - PCs require IL-4 stimulation to proliferate
  - Informative in 30-40% of PCM
- Abnormal karyotype indicates increased proliferation
  - Worse prognosis than normal karyotype
    - Intermediate risk disease (mSMART) if deletion 13 or hypodiploidy
    - 1q amplification associated with shorter survival
  - Most prevalent findings
    - Gains in chromosomes 1q, 3, 5, 7, 8, 11,15,19, 21
    - Losses in chromosomes 1p, 6q, 8, 13q, 14q, 16q
    - Translocations involving 14q32 (*IGH@*)
- Interphase FISH
  - Detects abnormalities in > 90% PCM
  - Use for risk stratification and therapy (mSMART)
    - Standard risk: t(11;14), t(6;14)
    - Intermediate risk: t(4;14)
    - High risk: del17p, t(14;16), t(14;20)
  - Trisomies may ameliorate impact of adverse FISH
  - Monosomy or del13q found in ~ 50% PCM
- PCL often has complex or hypodiploid karyotype
  - Increased del17p, t(11;14), chromosome 1q+

Molecular Genetics

- Multiple genetic lesions associated with progression
  - Activating mutations
    - MAPK/STAT3 pathway: *NRAS, KRAS, FGFR3*
    - NF-κB pathway
  - Inactivating mutations
    - RB pathway (*RB1*), P53 pathway (*TP53*)
  - Myc dysregulation

Gene Expression Profiling

- Most informative test but not available for routine clinical use
- 7 distinct gene expression profiles described

PLASMA CELL MYELOMA

2008 WHO Classification of Plasma Cell Neoplasms**			
	Monoclonal Gammopathy of Undetermined Significance	Asymptomatic Plasma Cell Myeloma†	Symptomatic Plasma Cell Myeloma
M protein in serum	< 30 g/L	≥ 30 g/L &/or ≥ 10% plasma cells	Yes (M protein often ≥ 30 g/L IgG, ≥ 25 g/L IgA, or > 1g/24 hr urine LC)
BM clonal plasma cells	< 10%	≥ 10%	Yes, or plasmacytoma
CRAB*	No	No	Yes

*†Diagnose if ≥ 30 g/L M protein &/or ≥ 10% PCs. *International Myeloma Working Group Diagnostic Criteria: Calcium ↑ > 1 mg/dL above upper limit of normal; renal dysfunction: Creatinine > 2 g/dL; anemia: Hemoglobin 2 g/dL below lower limit of normal; bone lesions: Lytic lesions or osteoporosis with fracture. **No B-cell disorder present. LC = light chain.*

- 2 high-risk disease signatures
  - High proliferation (1q abnormalities)
  - *MMSET* gene associated
- 2 moderate-risk disease signatures
  - Hyperdiploid; *MAF/MAFB* gene signature
- 3 low-risk gene signatures
  - Low bone disease associated
  - *CCND1* or *CCND3* gene associated

DIFFERENTIAL DIAGNOSIS

Reactive Polyclonal Plasmacytosis

- Systemic infections
  - HIV, other bacterial or viral infections
- Autoimmune disorders
  - Systemic lupus erythematosus, rheumatoid arthritis
- Drug-induced agranulocytosis, hypersensitivity
  - Levamisole (in cocaine), others
- Carcinomas, lymphomas, rare leukemias
  - Classical Hodgkin lymphoma

MGUS

- Small clonal PC population (< 10%), small paraprotein
  - No signs of disease-related end-organ damage or bone lesions

Solitary Plasmacytoma of Bone or Extraosseous Plasmacytoma

- Clonal PCs in lesion
  - No clonal population in random bone biopsy
  - No evidence of lymphoma with plasmacytic differentiation
- Negative skeletal survey
  - MR useful to exclude occult lesions
- No anemia, hypercalcemia, or renal involvement

Osteosclerotic Myeloma (POEMS Syndrome)

- Osteosclerotic bone lesions associated with
  - **P**olyneuropathy, **o**rganomegaly, **e**ndocrine abnormalities, **M** protein (~ 1.1 g/dL), **s**kin changes
  - Possible Castleman disease

Monoclonal Immunoglobulin Deposition Diseases

- Primary amyloidosis
- Monoclonal light and heavy chain deposition diseases

Lymphoplasmacytic Lymphoma

- Monoclonal B-cell and monoclonal PC populations
  - Usually intact IgM monoclonal protein
  - Hyperviscosity, often associated with Waldenström macroglobulinemia

DIAGNOSTIC CHECKLIST

Clinically Relevant Pathologic Features

- Genomic aberrations
  - Have prognostic and therapeutic implications
  - Many novel anti-PCM agents will allow for personalized therapy

Pathologic Interpretation Pearls

- Consider PCM in differential diagnosis of unusual bone marrow infiltrate

SELECTED REFERENCES

1. Baker A et al: Uncovering the biology of multiple myeloma among African Americans: a comprehensive genomics approach. Blood. 121(16):3147-52, 2013
2. Fernández de Larrea C et al: Plasma cell leukemia: consensus statement on diagnostic requirements, response criteria and treatment recommendations by the International Myeloma Working Group. Leukemia. 27(4):780-91, 2013
3. Kastritis E et al: Extensive bone marrow infiltration and abnormal free light chain ratio identifies patients with asymptomatic myeloma at high risk for progression to symptomatic disease. Leukemia. 27(4):947-53, 2013
4. Larsen JT et al: Serum free light chain ratio as a biomarker for high-risk smoldering multiple myeloma. Leukemia. 27(4):941-6, 2013
5. Mikhael JR et al: Management of Newly Diagnosed Symptomatic Multiple Myeloma: Updated Mayo Stratification of Myeloma and Risk-Adapted Therapy (mSMART) Consensus Guidelines 2013. Mayo Clin Proc. 88(4):360-76, 2013
6. Kumar S et al: Trisomies in multiple myeloma: impact on survival in patients with high-risk cytogenetics. Blood. 119(9):2100-5, 2012
7. Dimopoulos M et al: Consensus recommendations for standard investigative workup: report of the International Myeloma Workshop Consensus Panel 3. Blood. 117(18):4701-5, 2011
8. Paiva B et al: Utility of flow cytometry immunophenotyping in multiple myeloma and other clonal plasma cell-related disorders. Cytometry B Clin Cytom. 78(4):239-52, 2010
9. Bartl R et al: Histologic classification and staging of multiple myeloma. A retrospective and prospective study of 674 cases. Am J Clin Pathol. 87(3):342-55, 1987

PLASMA CELL MYELOMA

Laboratory Tests and Microscopic Features

*(**Left**) This SPEP from an older man with lytic bone lesions has an M component in the β2 region. The M component measures 35 g/L. An M component is found in ~ 97% of PCM cases by SPEP or UPEP analysis. (**Right**) Immunofixation electrophoresis identifies the M component to be IgAκ with slight free κ light chain. Distribution of M components in PCM includes IgG (~ 50%), IgA (~ 20%), light chain (~ 20%), IgD (~ 2%), biclonal (~ 2%), IgE/IgM (< 1%), and nonsecretory (~ 3%).*

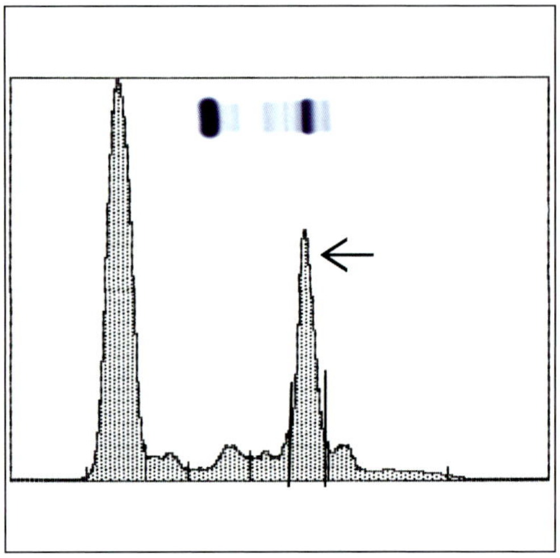

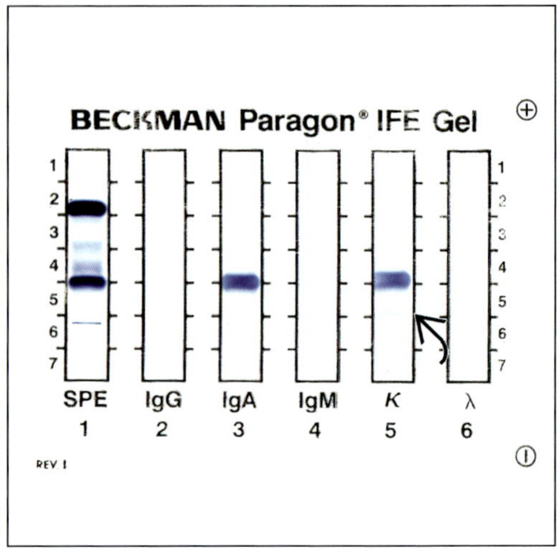

*(**Left**) Features of plasma cell (PC) atypia include cellular and nuclear enlargement, nuclear pleomorphism, multinucleation, dispersed nuclear chromatin, prominent nucleoli, and cytoplasmic fraying or shedding. (**Right**) Classification schemes for PCM are based on the degree of PC differentiation. Genetic abnormalities are associated with some morphologies. This low-risk PCM morphology looks like reactive PCs. The PCs have eccentric cartwheel nuclei with few nucleoli.*

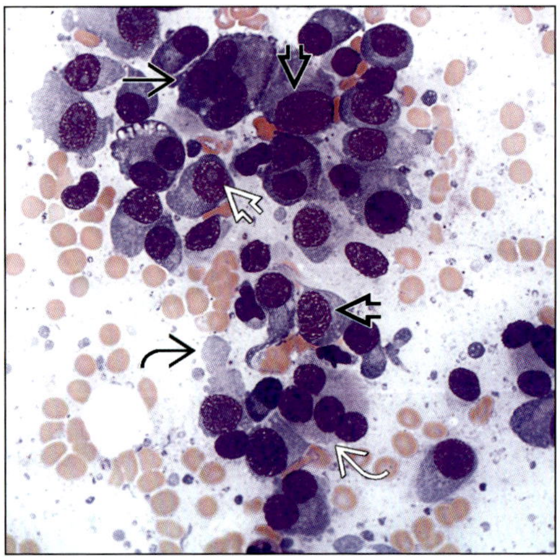

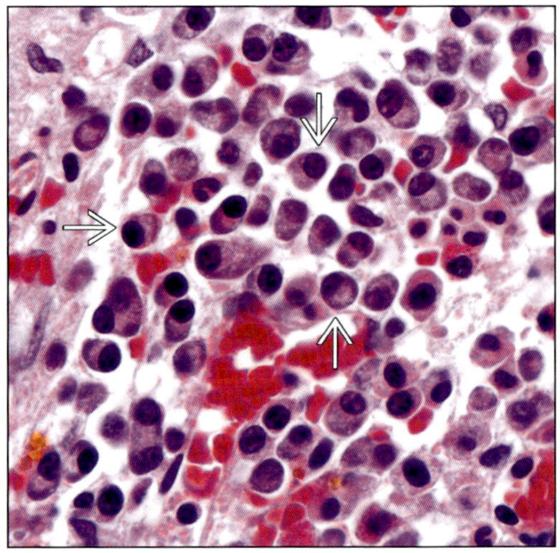

*(**Left**) The lymphoid or small cell type of PCM has round, lymphocyte-like nuclei and is associated with a better prognosis. A t(11;14) is identified in ~ 10% of cases and CD20(+) in ~ 20% of cases. (**Right**) Plasmablastic PCM is considered an aggressive disease, although the definition of plasmablasts differs. Plasmablasts in aspirates are described as having large concentric nuclei (> 10 μm) or large nucleoli (> 2 μm), fine reticular chromatin, and cytoplasm that is < 1/2 of the nuclear area.*

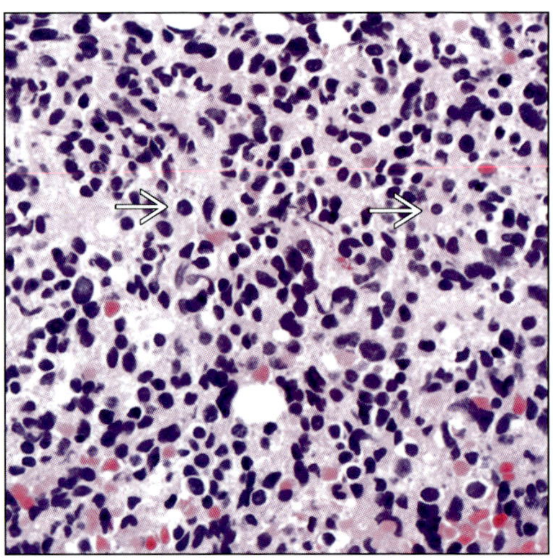

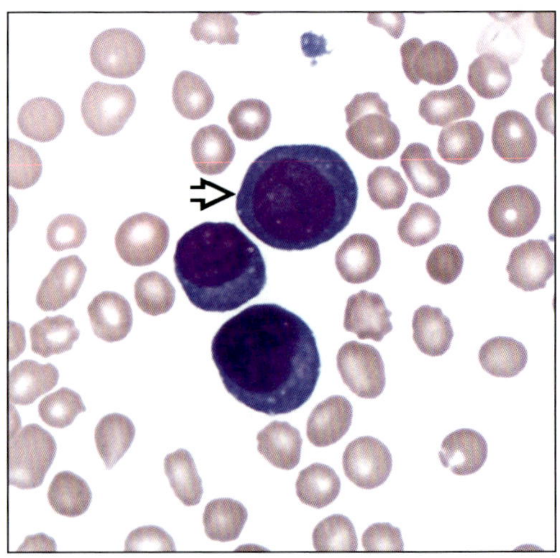

PLASMA CELL MYELOMA

Microscopic Features

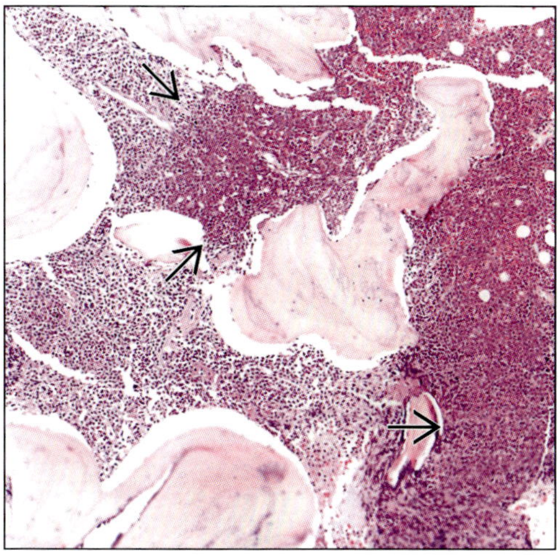
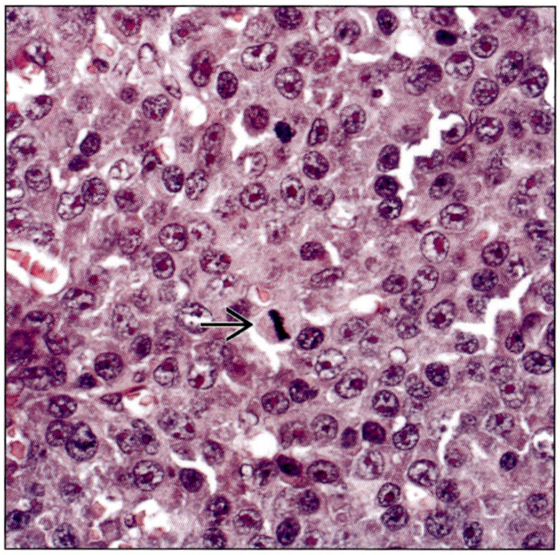

(Left) *Areas with sheets of plasmablasts → are distinct in this bone biopsy with PCM. Plasmablastic areas are often packed and fibrotic, and thus plasmablasts are typically poorly represented in aspirate smears. Plasmablastic PCM is associated with high-risk cytogenetic abnormalities, IgAλ disease, and poor patient responses to standard therapy.* ***(Right)*** *Plasmablastic myeloma resembles immunoblastic lymphoma in biopsy sections and is always associated with increased mitoses →.*

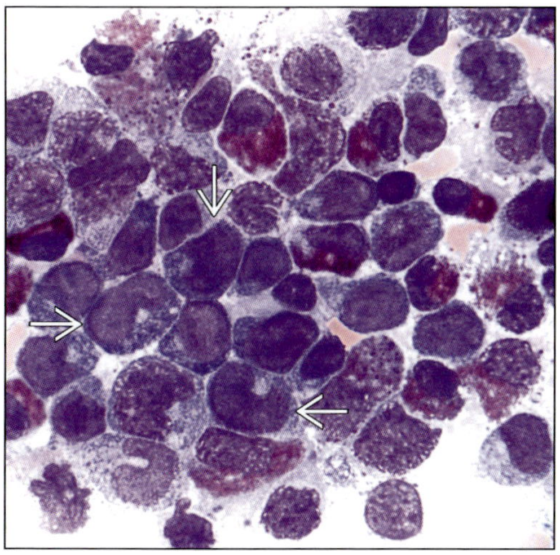
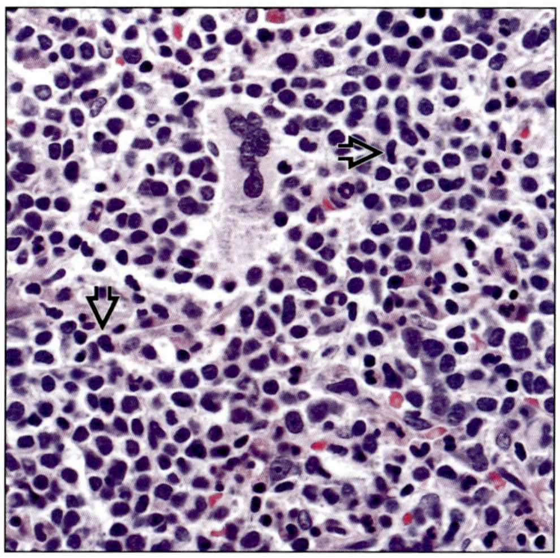

(Left) *As PCM is a heterogeneous disease with complex genetic abnormalities, it is not surprising that neoplastic PCs have a variety of appearances. The variant types are usually considered to be of intermediate-grade morphology unless high-risk genetic aberrations are identified with ancillary testing. This PCM → has cleaved nuclei with a high nuclear to cytoplasmic ratio.* ***(Right)*** *Sheets of the "cleaved" myeloma cells ⇨ surround a megakaryocyte in the bone marrow biopsy.*

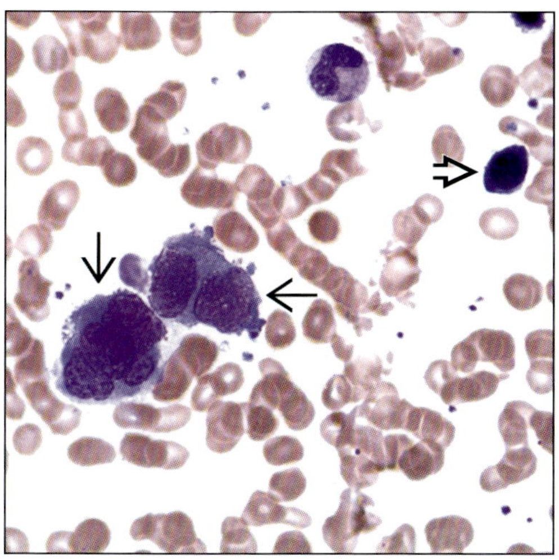
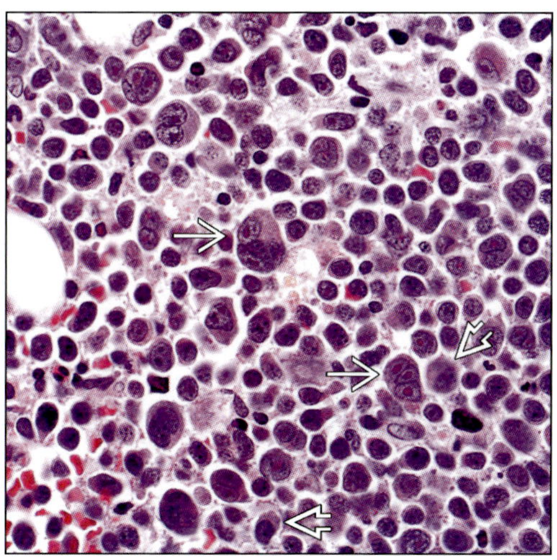

(Left) *This bone marrow aspirate smear has large, polymorphous PCs → and a small lymphocyte ⇨ in the background for comparison.* ***(Right)*** *The polymorphous type of PCM has marked cellular pleomorphism and multinucleated cells with prominent nucleoli →. Some of the large cells may resemble Reed-Sternberg cells or anaplastic large cell lymphoma. One clue to the diagnosis of PCM is the presence of recognizable PCs ⇨ in the background infiltrate.*

PLASMA CELL MYELOMA

Microscopic Features

(Left) *PCM must be considered in the differential diagnosis of any morphologically unusual bone marrow infiltrate. This bone marrow is extensively involved by large cells with abundant pale to clear cytoplasm that is worrisome for metastatic carcinoma.* ***(Right)*** *The cells appear to be forming nests, further supporting the impression of carcinoma. Immunohistochemical stains show that the cells are cytokeratin negative and express CD138, CD56, and kappa light chain, diagnostic of PCM.*

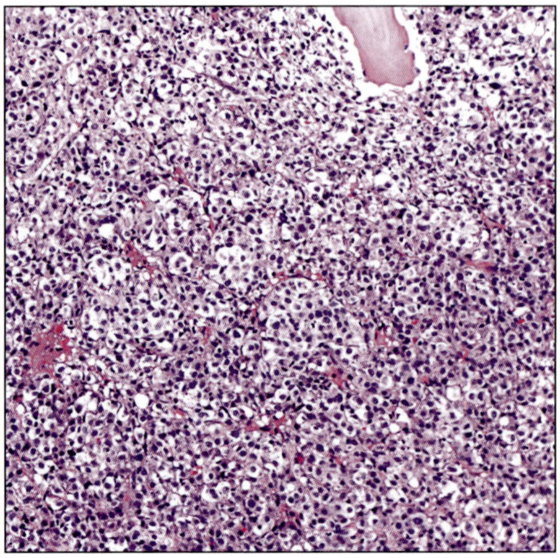

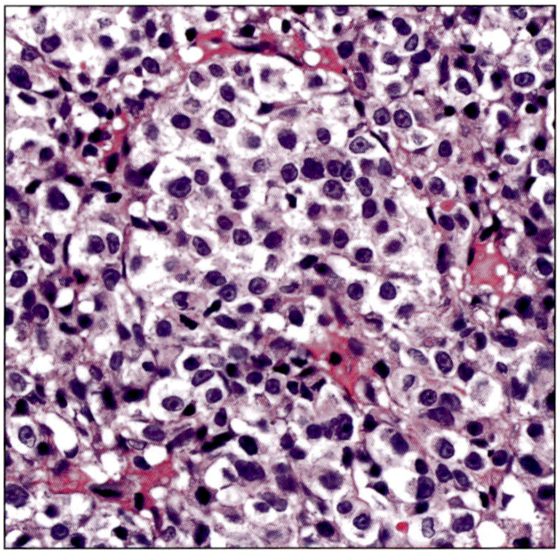

(Left) *PCM infiltrates → may be widely spaced and irregularly distributed with large areas of bone marrow sparing ⇒.* ***(Right)*** *A higher power view of a paratrabecular nodule shows myeloma cells with intranuclear inclusions called "Dutcher bodies" →. Dutcher bodies are caused by increased or blocked immunoglobulin secretions. These secretory globules are actually in the cytoplasm of the cells, although they appear to invaginate into the nucleus. The nuclear membrane is intact.*

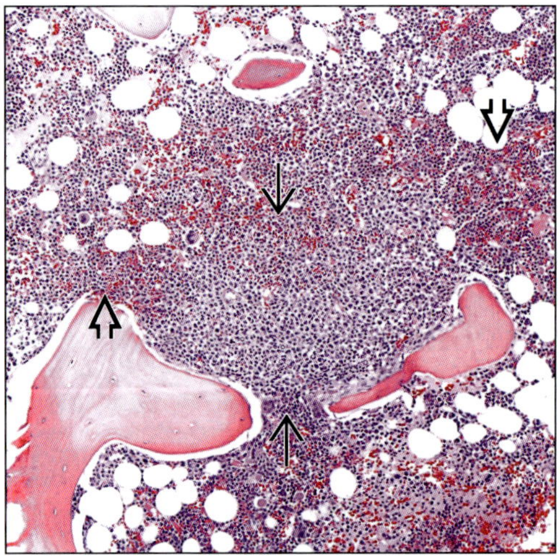

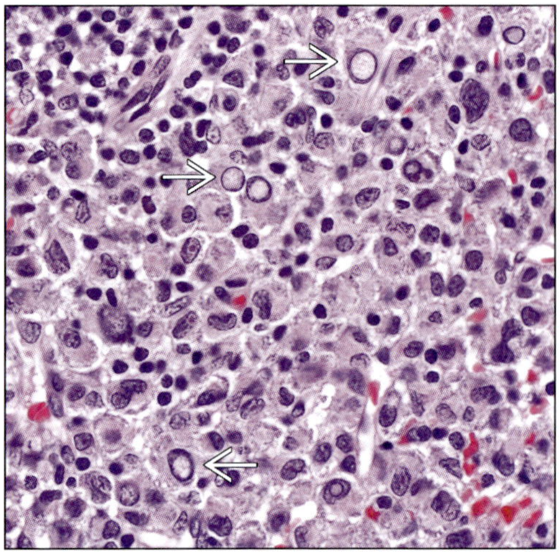

(Left) *Immunoglobulin accumulations may appear as uniform, round, colorless globules called "Russell bodies" →. When multiple Russell bodies are in the cytoplasm of myeloma cells, they are called Mott cells →. Additional terms for when the entire cytoplasm is replaced by Russell bodies is a morula cell or a grape cell.* ***(Right)*** *This PCM has a signet ring appearance due to abundant cytoplasmic secretions that mimic the appearance of a signet ring cell carcinoma.*

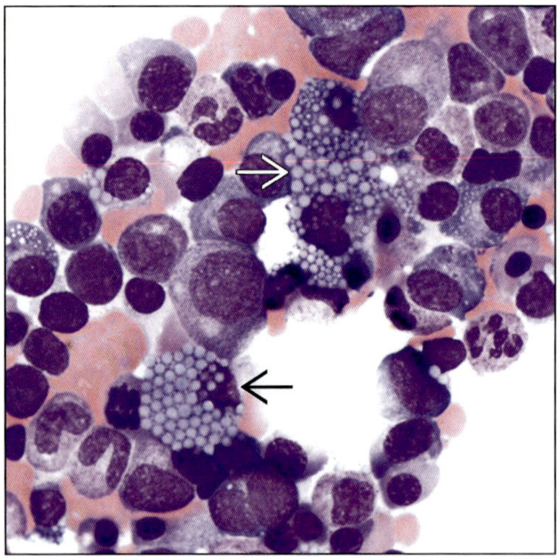

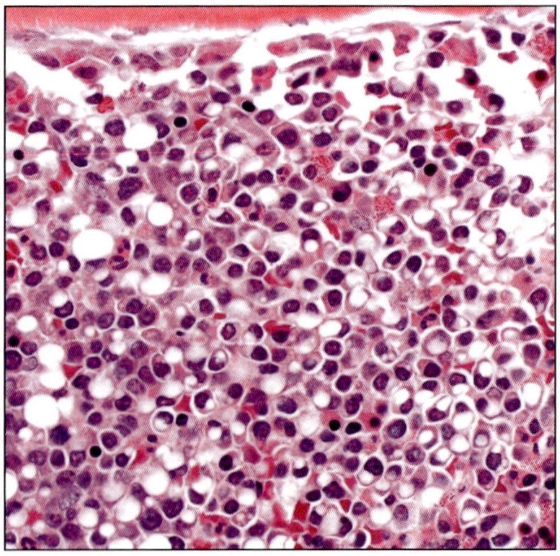

Microscopic Features and Immunohistochemical Stains

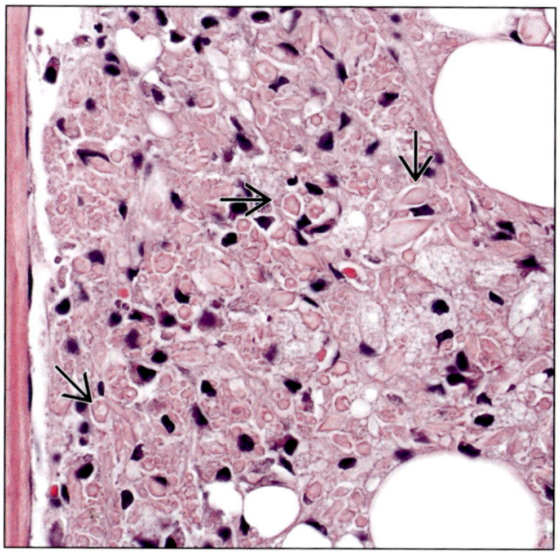
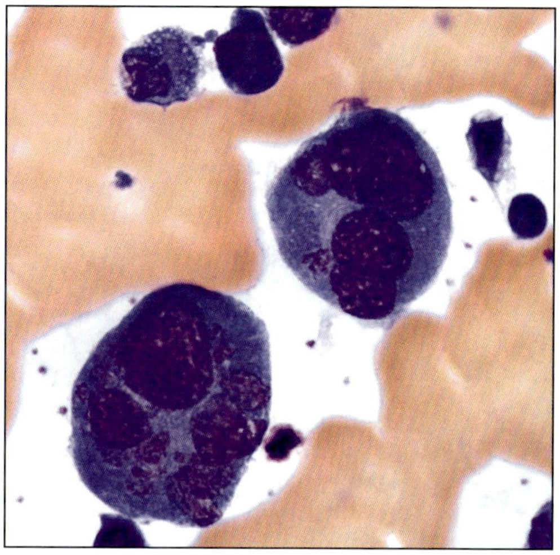

(Left) Myeloma cells that resemble histiocytes fill this bone marrow. These cells contain pink crystals with diamond or more elongated shapes ➡. Crystals form when immunoglobulins crystallize or combine with other compounds. They may resemble Auer rods, or stain blue or purple. **(Right)** These large, pleomorphic PCs in a bone marrow aspirate smear resemble abnormal megakaryocytes. Immunophenotyping is essential for the correct identification of myeloma with variant morphologies.

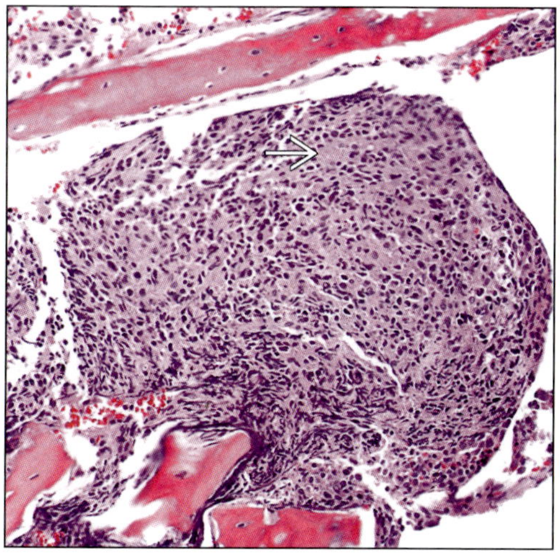
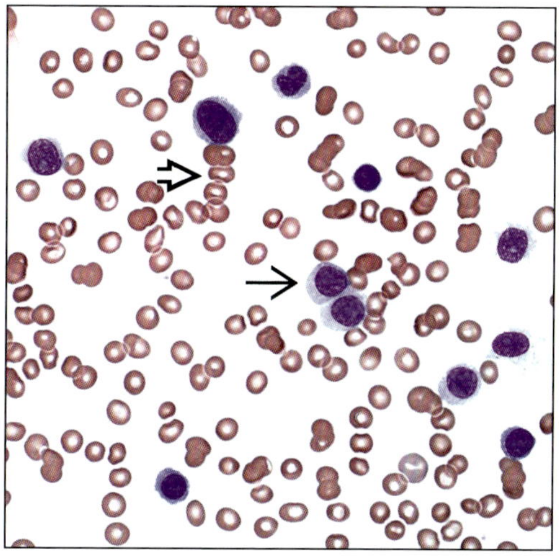

(Left) Approximately 9% of PCM at diagnosis are associated with fibrosis (pink background stroma) ➡ and a worse prognosis. **(Right)** This 57 year old presented with leukocytosis, anemia, thrombocytopenia, and new onset renal failure. The majority of leukocytes (70%) are kappa light chain-restricted PCs ➡, diagnostic of PCL. The PCs are intermediate in size and have round nuclei, variably prominent nucleoli, and moderately abundant cytoplasm. Rouleaux formation is present ➡.

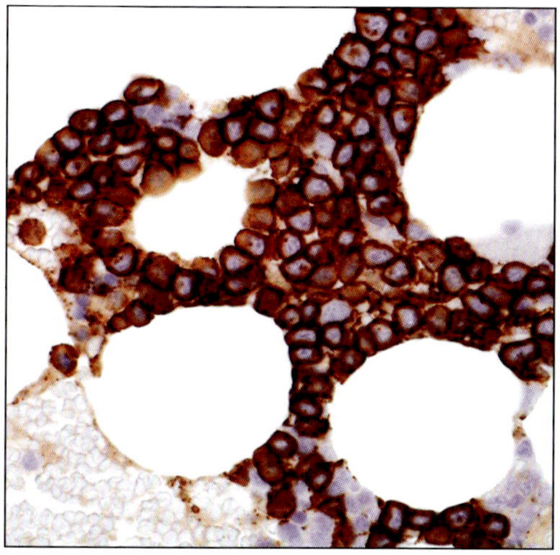
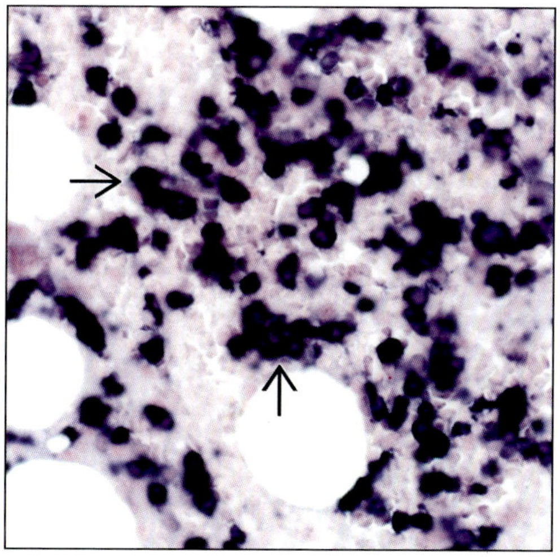

(Left) CD138 is the most specific marker for PCs in marrow and helps to evaluate for percentage of PC involvement, particularly when PCs are unevenly distributed in biopsy sections. **(Right)** Although CD138 highlights PCs in bone marrow, it does not distinguish between reactive and clonal populations. Clonality is best assessed by light chain evaluation; in situ hybridization is often more reliable than immunohistochemistry. PCs are kappa light chain positive ➡ in this biopsy.

PLASMA CELL MYELOMA

Immunohistochemical Stains and Flow Cytometry

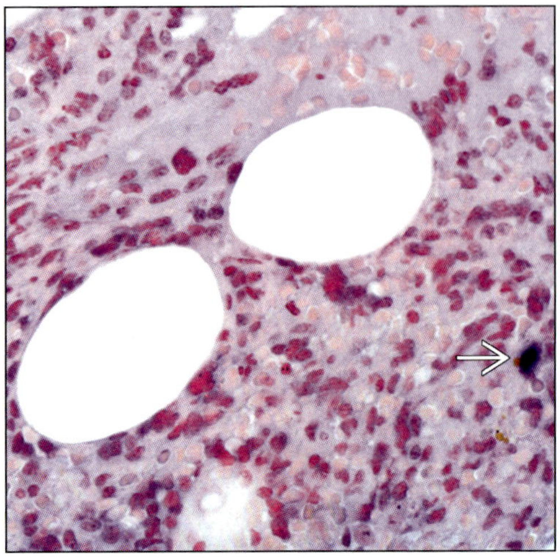

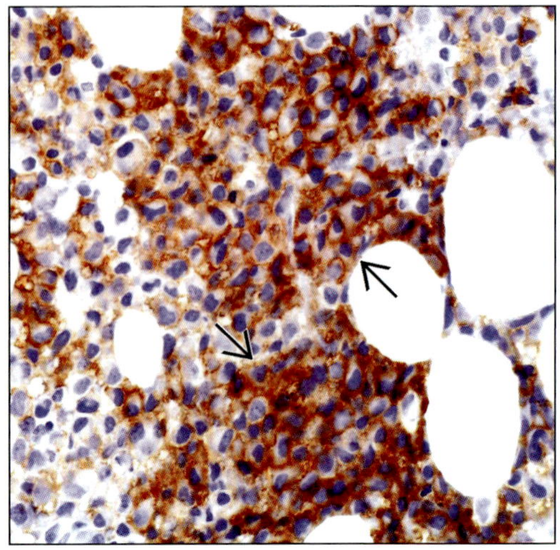

(Left) *This biopsy has only rare lambda-positive PCs ➡, confirming a clonal kappa-positive PC infiltrate in the background. As CD138 stains a variety of undifferentiated epithelial and mesenchymal neoplasms, light chain expression also confirms a plasmacytic process.* ***(Right)*** *Aberrant immunophenotypes are seen in > 80% of PCM cases at diagnosis, including CD56(+) ➡ in a majority of cases (~ 70%). Lineage infidelity is a feature of PCM with myeloid, T-cell, and B-cell marker expression possible.*

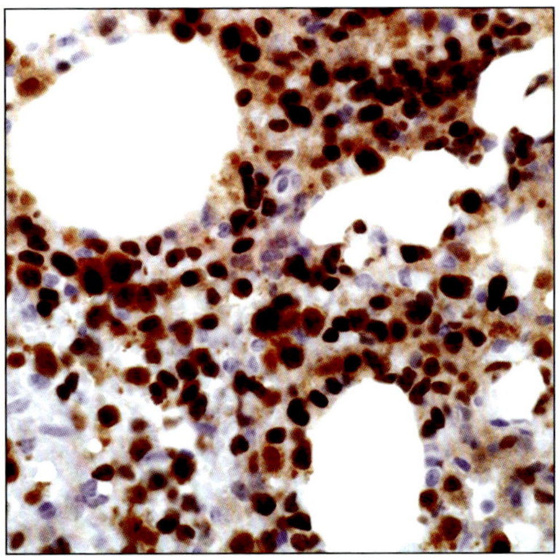

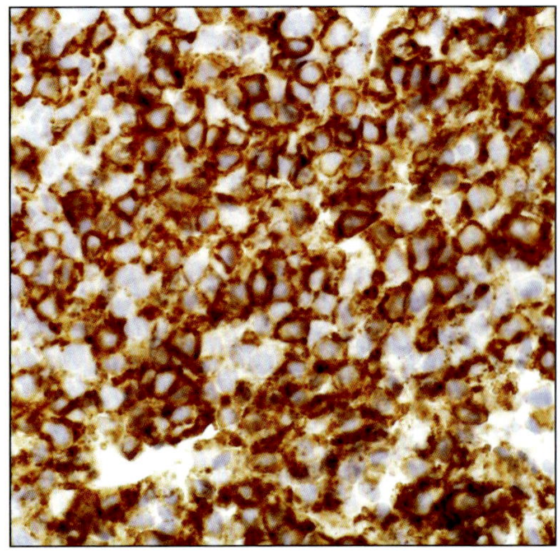

(Left) *Cyclin-D1 expression is seen in ~ 1/3 of PCM with only ~ 10% of these having an associated t(11;14)(q13q32) karyotypic abnormality.* ***(Right)*** *Bright CD20 expression is found in 15-20% of PCM. CD20 expression is not specific, but when it is associated with cyclin-D1(+), t(11;14), and small cell type of PCM, it confers a better prognosis. CD20(+) PCM needs to be distinguished from B-cell lymphoma, particularly lymphoplasmacytic lymphoma.*

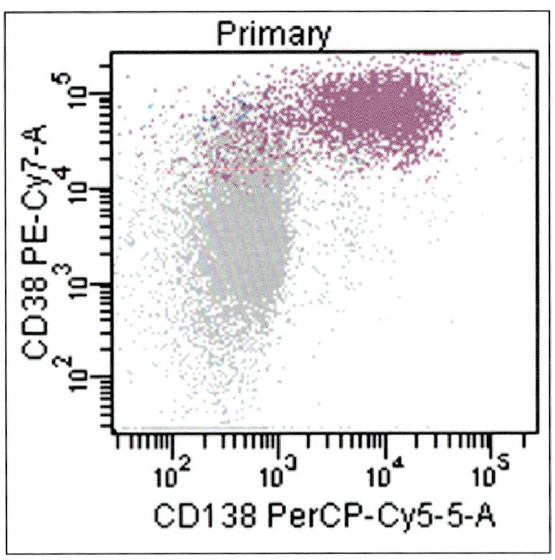

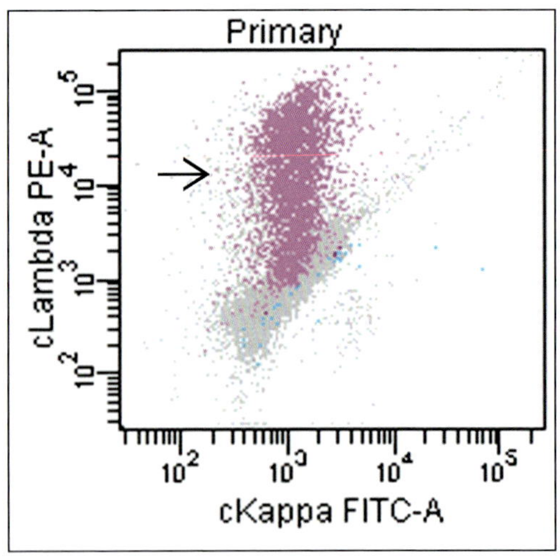

(Left) *FCM identifies the PCs (pink) in this bone marrow by their bright CD138 and CD38 coexpression. Gating on CD38 alone is problematic, as neoplastic PCs often have dimmer CD38 than normal, and activated/immature T cells, hematogones, and monocytes may be brightly CD38 positive.* ***(Right)*** *Evaluation for PC immunoglobulin requires permeabilization of the cell membrane to allow antibodies to enter the cytoplasm. PC clonality is identified by finding light chain restriction ➡.*

Ancillary Techniques and Differential Diagnosis

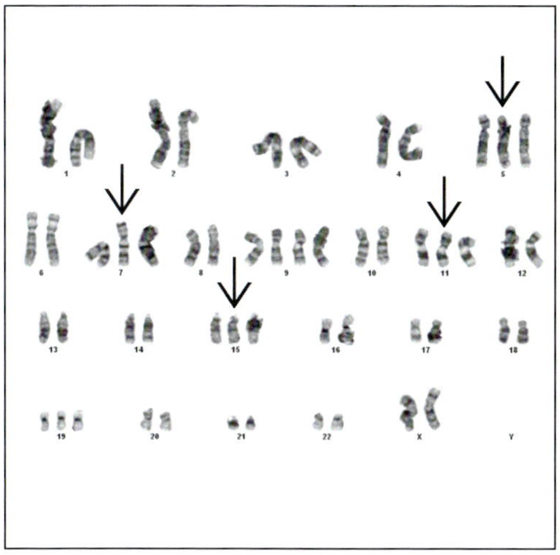

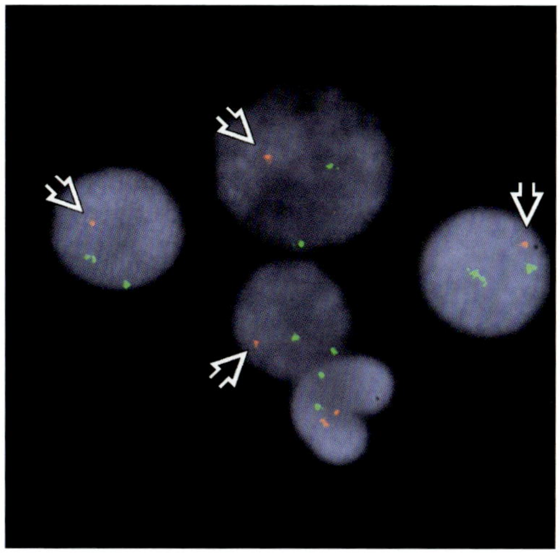

(Left) *Karyotype: 52~53,XX, +5,+7,+9,+9,+11,+15, +19[cp11]/46,XX[9]. Hyperdiploid karyotypes with multiple trisomies* → *of the odd-numbered chromosomes are common in PCM. Hyperdiploid PCM has a better prognosis than other abnormal karyotypes, unless there are concurrent chromosome 1q gains.* ***(Right)*** *Interphase FISH analysis shows 2 normal copies of 11q22.3 region (ATM; green) in all MM cells and evidence for deletion of 17p13.1 region (TP53; red)* ⇨ *in a subset.*

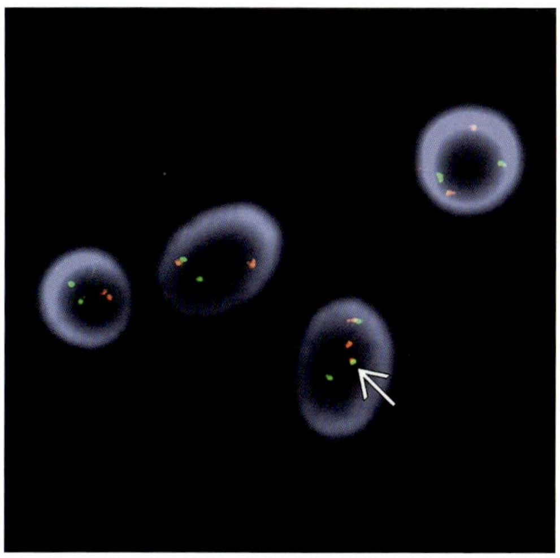

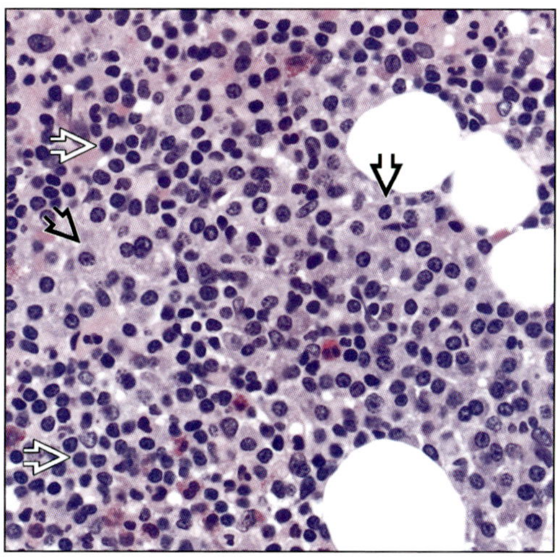

(Left) *Interphase FISH shows an FGFR3/IgH@ fusion* ➡ *associated with t(4;14)(p16.3;q32.3) (IgH: Green; MMSET/FGFR3: Red). Patients with the t(4;14) tend to be more responsive to bortezomib-based therapy. The findings of del17p, t(14.16), or t(14;20) indicate high-risk disease.* ***(Right)*** *Lymphoplasmacytic lymphoma is differentiated from PCM by small monoclonal B cells* ⇨*, clonal PCs* ⇨*, and increased mast cells, usually accompanied by an IgM paraprotein.*

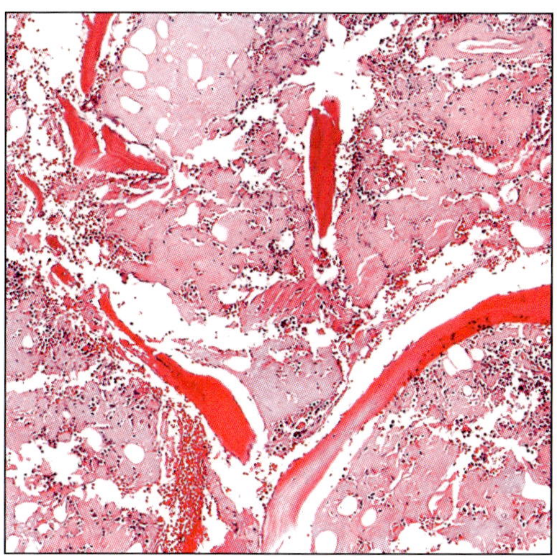

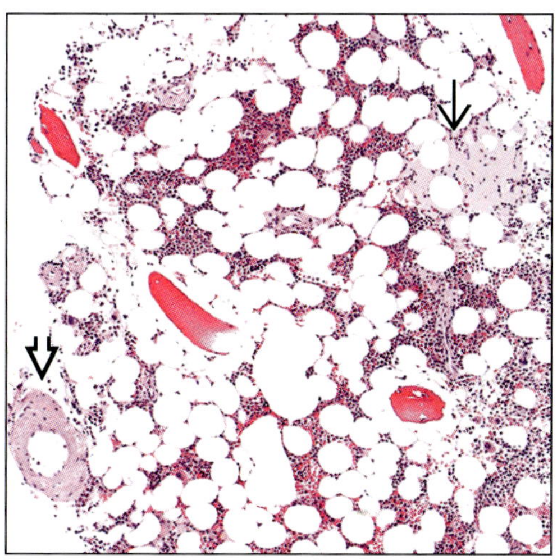

(Left) *This marrow with primary amyloidosis is filled with dense, waxy, amorphous material. Apple-green birefringence is present under polarized light when Congo red staining is performed. Most patients with primary amyloidosis have MGUS; ~ 20% are associated with PCM. The t(11;14) is relatively common.* ***(Right)*** *Amyloid is a manifestation of end-organ damage (i.e., symptomatic) in PCM and is seen in ~ 10% of patients. Focal involvement of stroma* → *&/or vessel walls* ⇨ *is typical.*

Bone and Soft Tissue

CHONDROSARCOMA

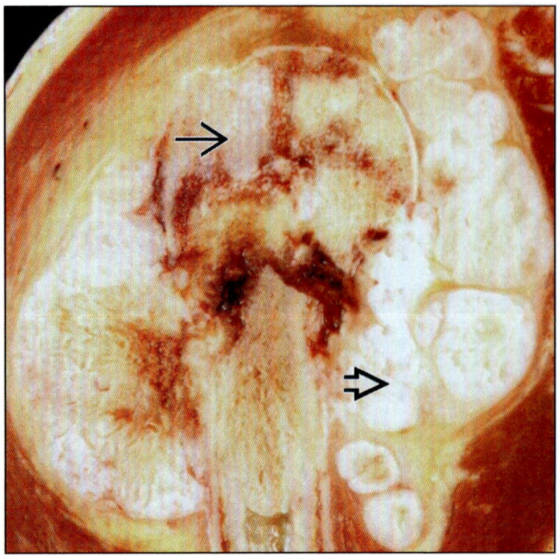

The gross appearance of chondrosarcoma varies with the grade and constitution of the tumor. Most cases show a glassy cut surface that is blue-gray → to tan-white ⇨. (Courtesy A. Hough, MD.)

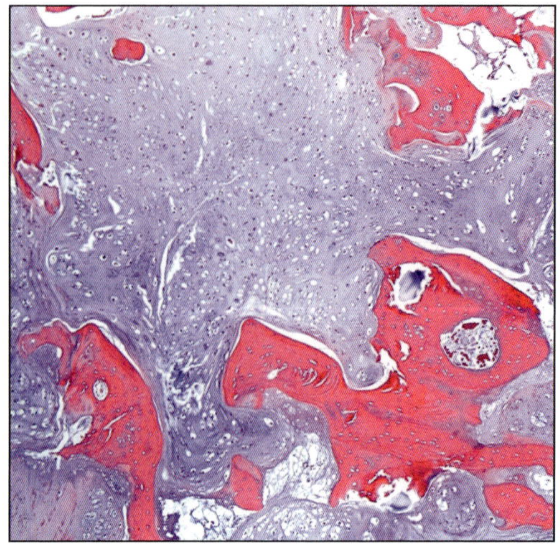

This image shows the classic low-power appearance of a conventional chondrosarcoma: Sheets and lobules of atypical cartilage demonstrating extensive intertrabecular bone infiltration and destruction.

TERMINOLOGY

Definitions

- Malignant cartilaginous matrix-producing tumor of bone
  - Primary chondrosarcoma arises in medullary cavity (i.e., conventional type) or on surface (i.e., periosteal/juxtacortical type) of bone
  - Secondary chondrosarcoma arises in association with preexisting benign tumor (e.g., enchondroma, osteochondroma) or diseased bone (e.g., radiation, Paget disease)
  - Chondrosarcoma with dedifferentiation contains areas of high-grade noncartilaginous sarcoma adjacent to traditional areas of conventional chondrosarcoma

ETIOLOGY/PATHOGENESIS

Sporadic

- > 90% of cases
- Can also arise in the setting of a solitary nonsyndromic osteochondroma (rare)

Enchondromatosis

- May be sporadic (Ollier disease) or familial
  - Familial cases occur predominantly in men and appear to show autosomal dominant transmission
- Asymmetric distribution of multiple enchondromas
  - Marked variability in size, location, number, and age at onset of lesions
- Maffucci syndrome
  - Enchondromatosis associated with soft tissue hemangiomas
- Risk of malignant transformation in these benign lesions is 35-40%

Hereditary Multiple Exostosis/Osteochondromas (HME/HMO)

- Autosomal dominant
- Asymmetric distribution of multiple exostoses or osteochondromas
  - Localization of lesions to surface of bone distinguishes this condition from enchondromatosis
- Risk of malignant transformation is 5-25%

Wilms Tumor

- Rare cases documented of Wilms tumor of the kidney and chondrosarcoma occurring in the same patient

CLINICAL ISSUES

Site

- Sporadic
  - Can arise in any bone derived from endochondral ossification
  - Most originate in pelvis, especially ilium, followed by proximal femur, proximal humerus, distal femur, and ribs
    - In long bones, chondrosarcoma usually involves metaphysis or diaphysis
  - Infrequently develops in small bones of hands and feet (1% of chondrosarcoma)
  - Chondrosarcomas of cranium usually involve skull base
- Hereditary
  - Arise in a preexisting enchondroma or osteochondroma in syndromic patients

Presentation

- Sporadic
  - Patients present with pain, enlarging mass, and, infrequently, fracture
  - Symptoms often present for a long time

CHONDROSARCOMA

Key Facts

Terminology

- Malignant cartilaginous matrix-producing tumor
- Secondary chondrosarcoma arises in association with a preexisting benign tumor or diseased bone
- Periosteal chondrosarcoma arises on bone surface

Etiology/Pathogenesis

- > 90% of cases are sporadic
  - Can also arise in the setting of a solitary nonsyndromic osteochondroma (rare)
- Enchondromatosis
  - May be sporadic (Ollier disease) or familial
  - Maffucci syndrome
- Hereditary multiple exostosis/osteochondromas
  - Asymmetric distribution of multiple exostoses or osteochondromas
- Wilms tumor
  - Rare cases documented of Wilms tumor of the kidney and chondrosarcoma occurring in the same patient

Clinical Issues

- Conventional intramedullary chondrosarcoma accounts for > 90% of all chondrosarcomas
- Chondrosarcomas arising in osteochondroma and periosteal chondrosarcoma are rare

Macroscopic Features

- Neoplastic hyaline cartilage is blue or gray-tan and glistening

Microscopic Pathology

- Infiltration of preexisting bone is important histologic finding and distinguishes chondrosarcoma from a benign cartilaginous tumor

  - Skull base tumors frequently cause headache, diplopia, and cranial nerve palsies
- Hereditary
  - Worsening of clinical symptoms related to preexisting growths/lesions
  - Sudden, increased rate of growth in preexisting enchondroma or osteochondroma after puberty

Treatment

- Aggressive curettage for low-grade (grade 1/3) chondrosarcomas
  - Especially if tumor is located in appendicular skeleton
- High-grade chondrosarcomas (grades 2/3 and 3/3) require wide surgical resection
  - Include dedifferentiated tumors
- Radiation has been used to treat unresectable tumors
  - Frequently used for tumors arising in spine or skull base
- Chondrosarcomas arising in pelvis are treated with resection regardless of grade because local recurrence in this region is very difficult to treat
- Prophylactic removal of osteochondromas if possibility of morbidity is low

Prognosis

- Histologic grade is the single most important prognostic factor
  - Applies to both sporadic type and those arising in the setting of enchondromatosis
  - Prognosis of chondrosarcoma arising in osteochondroma(tosis) is excellent unless there is dedifferentiation (i.e., component of high-grade noncartilaginous sarcoma)
- Grade 1 chondrosarcomas behave in a locally aggressive manner
  - Deaths usually result from local recurrence
  - Metastases are rare
  - 5-year survival for grade 1 chondrosarcoma is ~ 85%
- Grade 2 and grade 3 chondrosarcomas have much worse prognosis
  - 5-year survival rate is ~ 50%
- Dedifferentiated chondrosarcoma has dismal prognosis
  - Most patients die within 2 years of diagnosis
- Recurrent tumors may have increase in histologic grade
- Periosteal chondrosarcomas tend to recur locally, and metastases are rare

IMAGE FINDINGS

Radiographic Findings

- Lytic with scattered radiodensities
- Densities often take the form of rings and arcs and irregular spiculations
  - Rings and arcs represent peripheral enchondral ossification and reactive bone formation
  - Spiculations caused by irregular calcification of matrix
- Low-grade tumors may contain significant areas of mineralization, bone expansion, endosteal scalloping, and thickening of cortex
- High-grade tumors have large radiolucent areas and cortical destruction, frequently with a significant soft tissue mass
  - Includes dedifferentiated tumors
- Permeation of cortex is rarely seen, except in most aggressive lesions
- Periosteal chondrosarcoma shows irregular mineralization on surface of bone

MR Findings

- MR is helpful in identifying extent of tumor
- Dark on T1-weighted images
- Bright on T2-weighted images
- In osteochondroma, a cartilage cap with a thickness of > 1.5-2 cm should raise suspicion of possible malignant transformation
  - Thickened cap is not diagnostic for malignancy
- In periosteal chondrosarcoma, there is a T2 bright mass arising on surface of bone with areas of mineralization

CHONDROSARCOMA

CT Findings

- Unmineralized and mineralized components of tumor are clearly delineated in intramedullary and surface lesions

Bone Scan

- Avid technetium uptake on bone scan

MACROSCOPIC FEATURES

General Features

- Low-grade tumors fill medullary cavity, expand bone, scallop endosteal surface, and produce cortical thickening
- High-grade tumors destroy cortex and form a soft tissue mass that is frequently well delineated by raised periosteum
- Neoplastic hyaline cartilage is gray-tan and glistening
  - Has lobulated architecture that may be accentuated by thin, fibrous septa
- Mineralized portions of matrix appear as scattered, punctate, chalk-like deposits
- Regions of prominent endochondral ossification are seen as hard, ivory areas of bone formation
- Myxoid matrix is translucent, gray, and mucinous or watery
- In chondrosarcoma arising in osteochondroma, cartilage cap is thick and frequently shows cystic changes
- In sporadic periosteal chondrosarcoma, a large (usually > 5 cm) gray, glistening mass is attached to surface of bone
  - May contain gritty areas corresponding to calcification and ossification
  - Tumor scallops the underlying cortex and can invade into medullary cavity
- Areas of dedifferentiation may appear tan-white and firm or fleshy

Size

- Usually large (≥ 10 cm)

MICROSCOPIC PATHOLOGY

Histologic Features

- Infiltrative growth pattern encasing preexisting trabecular bone
- Neoplastic matrix is either hyaline or myxoid
  - Fibrocartilage is rare, and elastic cartilage is not found
- Hyaline matrix is homogeneous and usually basophilic
  - Occasionally, it may be pink
- Myxoid matrix is frothy or bubbly
  - Almost always basophilic
- Cartilage may mineralize or undergo endochondral ossification
- Neoplastic chondrocytes vary in size
  - Have moderate amounts of eosinophilic cytoplasm, occasionally vacuolated
- Tumor cells in hyaline cartilage are round to oval and confined to lacunar spaces
- Tumor cells in myxoid areas are bipolar or stellate and arranged singly or in cords and strands
  - Cytoplasmic processes of neighboring cells come in close or direct contact with one another and form a complex cellular network
  - Tumor cells do not form tight cohesive nests or clusters
- Neoplastic cells demonstrate varying degrees of cytologic atypia
- May contain foci of enchondroma
- Chondrosarcoma arising in osteochondroma is usually low grade
  - Diagnosis of chondrosarcoma in osteochondroma is somewhat subjective
    - Cartilage cap has nodular appearance with fibrous septae delineating lobules
    - Infiltration into stalk is unequivocal evidence of malignant transformation
- In periosteal chondrosarcoma, hyaline-type cartilaginous tumor is seen on surface of bone
  - Usually low to intermediate grade with areas of calcification and ossification
  - Distinguishing periosteal chondroma from periosteal chondrosarcoma is also often subjective
    - Chondrosarcoma shows more cellularity, atypia, invasion of underlying cortex, and, sometimes, infiltration into underlying medullary cavity
- Dedifferentiated chondrosarcoma shows abrupt transition from (most commonly) low-grade chondrosarcoma to high-grade pleomorphic sarcoma

ANCILLARY TESTS

Molecular Genetics

- Isocitrate dehydrogenase genes *IDH1* and *IDH2* are mutated in many chondrosarcomas
  - Primary chondrosarcoma: 38-70%
  - Secondary chondrosarcoma: 86%
  - Periosteal chondrosarcoma: 100%

DIFFERENTIAL DIAGNOSIS

Enchondroma

- Does not grow with infiltrative pattern
- Does not show soft tissue extension
- Relatively less cellular and lacks significant atypia

Chondromyxoid Fibroma

- Has well-delineated margins
- Contains fibromyxoid tissue and abundant blood vessels
- Radiographically, chondromyxoid fibroma shows nonaggressive features and is well circumscribed
- Frequently contains osteoclast-type giant cells

Clear Cell Chondrosarcoma

- Arises in epiphysis of long tubular bone, usually proximal femur and proximal humerus
- Contains clear cells, metaplastic bone formation, and osteoclast-type giant cells, features that are not present in conventional chondrosarcoma

CHONDROSARCOMA

Grading of Chondrosarcoma

Grade	Cellularity	Cytologic Features
1	Hypocellular	Nuclei are small and dark or slightly enlarged with fine chromatin
2	More cellular	Nuclei are larger, irregular, and have coarse chromatin; mitoses infrequent
3	Hypercellular	Severe pleomorphism and mitoses

Enchondroma vs. Low-Grade Chondrosarcoma

	Enchondroma	Low-Grade Chondrosarcoma	Notes
Pain	Not attributed directly to neoplastic cartilage (more often related to pathologic fracture)	Pain attributed to neoplastic cartilage	May be difficult to assess due to proximity of enchondromas to joints
Histologic features	In long bones, generally low cellularity and absence of chondrocyte atypia; lacks myxoid change and chondrocyte necrosis	Increased cellularity, double-nucleated chondrocytes, myxoid change, and chondrocyte necrosis	Cytologic and histologic features may overlap; degree of overlap is even more apparent in patients with multiple enchondromas (endochondromatosis)
Mitotic activity	Absence	Low level	Mitotic activity is extremely rare in enchondromas
Growth pattern	Lacks infiltration	Infiltrative	This feature is diagnostic of low-grade chondrosarcoma

Chondroid Chordoma

- Can be difficult to differentiate from low-grade chondrosarcoma
- Usually arises in skull base
- Expresses both keratin and brachyury (not expressed by chondrosarcoma)
  - Both chondrosarcoma and chondroid chordoma are S100 protein positive

Fracture Callus

- On histologic features alone, a fracture callus can easily be misdiagnosed as chondrosarcoma
- Nodules of cartilage are small
- Cartilage undergoes endochondral ossification
- Should be easy to distinguish radiographically

DIAGNOSTIC CHECKLIST

Pathologic Interpretation Pearls

- On core biopsy, it can be impossible to differentiate between enchondroma and low-grade chondrosarcoma
  - In these instances, radiographic features of tumors should be correlated with histology
- In difficult cases, open biopsy should target interface between tumor and normal bone
  - Best area to identify infiltrative growth pattern that is diagnostic of chondrosarcoma
- In tubular bones, this distinction is not crucial as both enchondroma and low-grade chondrosarcoma can be treated with thorough curettage

SELECTED REFERENCES

1. Schoenfeld AJ et al: Chondrosarcoma of the mobile spine: a review of 21 cases treated at a single center. Spine (Phila Pa 1976). 37(2):119-26, 2012
2. Streitbuerger A et al: The treatment of locally recurrent chondrosarcoma: Is extensive further surgery justified? J Bone Joint Surg Br. 94(1):122-7, 2012
3. Vanel D et al: Enchondroma vs. chondrosarcoma: A simple, easy-to-use, new magnetic resonance sign. Eur J Radiol. Epub ahead of print, 2012
4. Amary MF et al: IDH1 and IDH2 mutations are frequent events in central chondrosarcoma and central and periosteal chondromas but not in other mesenchymal tumours. J Pathol. 224(3):334-43, 2011
5. Verdegaal SH et al: Incidence, predictive factors, and prognosis of chondrosarcoma in patients with Ollier disease and Maffucci syndrome: an international multicenter study of 161 patients. Oncologist. 16(12):1771-9, 2011
6. Lin PP et al: Secondary chondrosarcoma. J Am Acad Orthop Surg. 18(10):608-15, 2010
7. Eefting D et al: Assessment of interobserver variability and histologic parameters to improve reliability in classification and grading of central cartilaginous tumors. Am J Surg Pathol. 33(1):50-7, 2009
8. Porter DE et al: Severity of disease and risk of malignant change in hereditary multiple exostoses. A genotype-phenotype study. J Bone Joint Surg Br. 86(7):1041-6, 2004
9. Ahmed AR et al: Secondary chondrosarcoma in osteochondroma: report of 107 patients. Clin Orthop Relat Res. (411):193-206, 2003
10. Papagelopoulos PJ et al: Periosteal chondrosarcoma. Orthopedics. 25(8):839-42, 2002
11. Bovée JV et al: Chondrosarcoma of the phalanx: a locally aggressive lesion with minimal metastatic potential: a report of 35 cases and a review of the literature. Cancer. 86(9):1724-32, 1999
12. Evans HL et al: Prognostic factors in chondrosarcoma of bone: a clinicopathologic analysis with emphasis on histologic grading. Cancer. 40(2):818-31, 1977

CHONDROSARCOMA

Gross, Imaging, and Microscopic Features

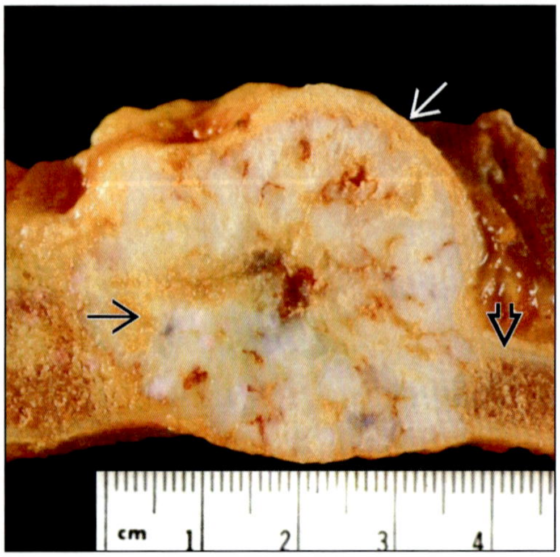

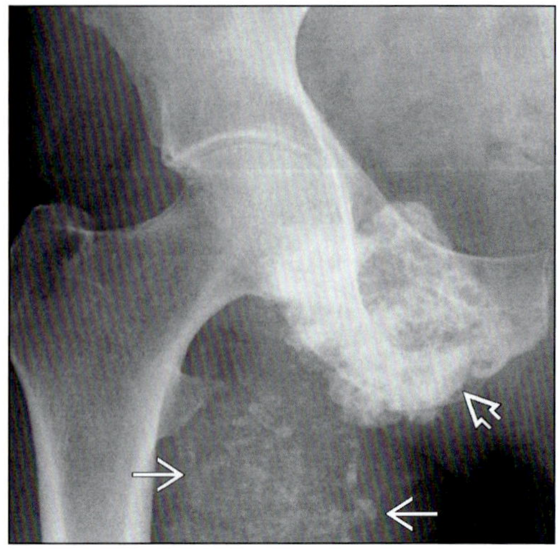

(Left) *Conventional chondrosarcoma shows a nodular intramedullary proliferation of cartilage → that often breaches the cortex ⇨ and extends into the adjacent soft tissue ➡. (Courtesy A. Hough, MD.)* ***(Right)*** *This image of a large exophytic chondrosarcoma arising in an osteochondroma of the pelvis reveals the production of chondroid matrix ➡, which characteristically shows a "snowstorm" appearance on radiograph. The base portion of the tumor is seen proximally ➡.*

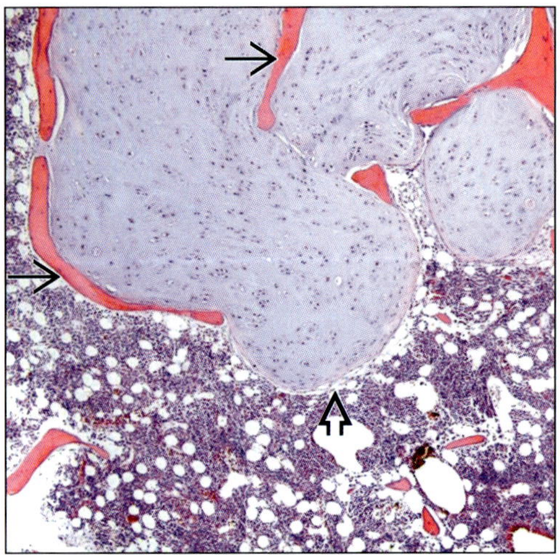

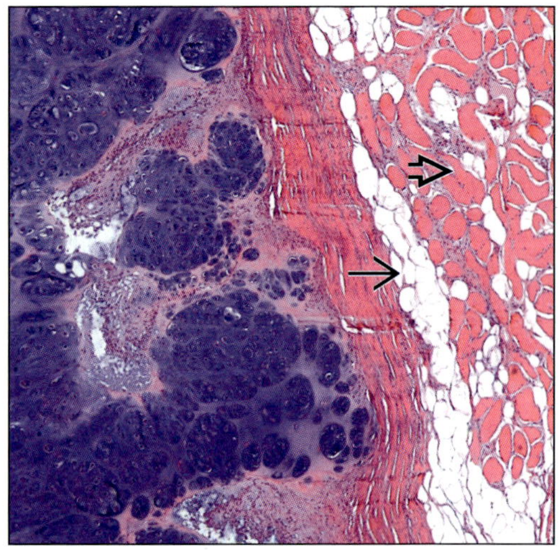

(Left) *A cartilaginous neoplasm demonstrating infiltration of normal trabecular → or cortical bone &/or invasion of the marrow cavity is diagnostic of chondrosarcoma. Note the rounded pushing border ⇨ present at the leading edge of the tumor.* ***(Right)*** *Infiltrative soft tissue extension by a cartilaginous neoplasm is also diagnostic of a chondrosarcoma. Note the involvement of fibroadipose tissue → and skeletal muscle ⇨.*

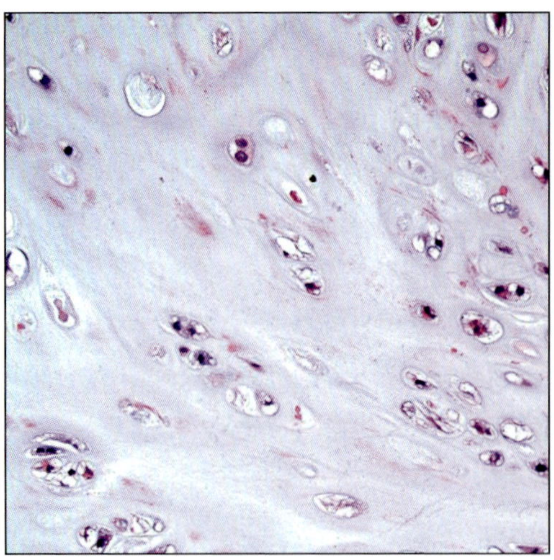

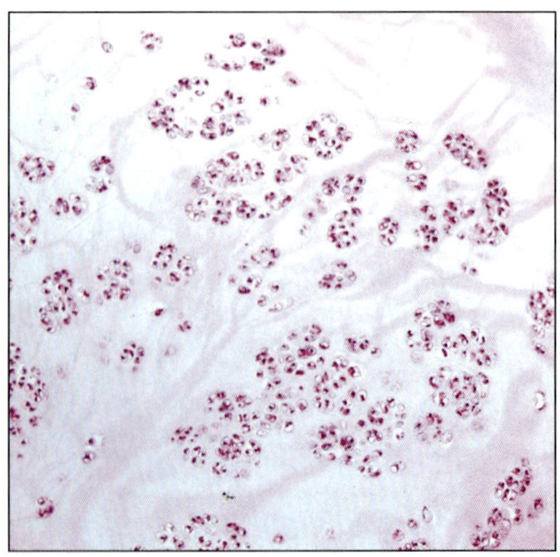

(Left) *Low-grade (grade 1) chondrosarcoma often demonstrates very low cellularity and an absence of pleomorphism, thereby making histologic distinction from a benign enchondroma challenging. However, atypical cytologic changes such as chondrocyte binucleation, formation of small nucleoli, and myxoid degeneration of the matrix may be seen.* ***(Right)*** *Clustering of chondrocytes may be identified in chondrosarcoma. However, this finding can be seen in benign cartilaginous tumors as well.*

Microscopic Features

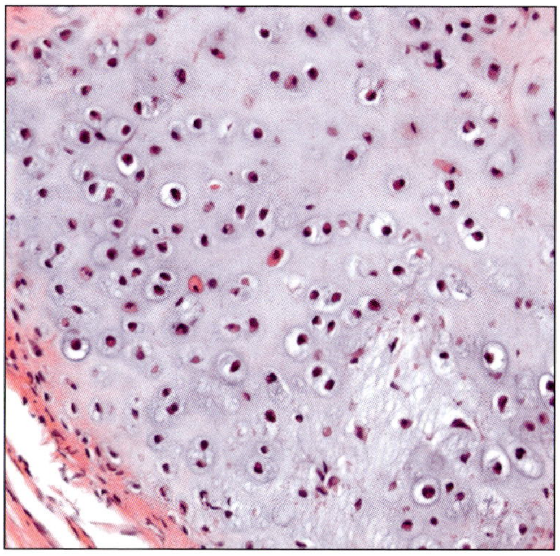
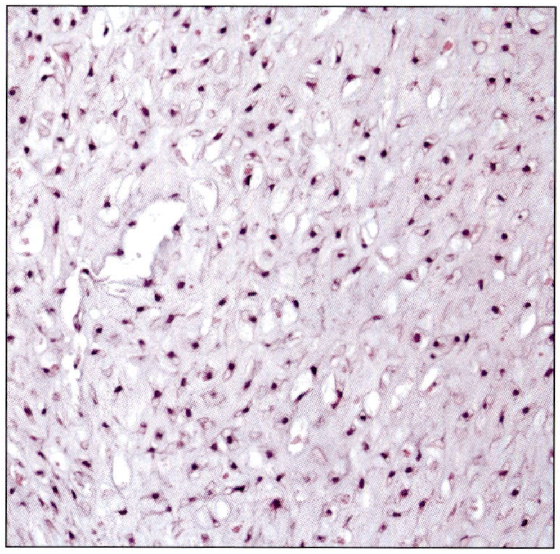

(Left) *Intermediate-grade (grade 2) chondrosarcoma displays a greater degree of cellularity than low-grade examples but lacks significant nuclear pleomorphism. With the exception of cartilaginous tumors in the small bones of the hands and feet, this increase in cellularity usually favors a chondrosarcoma over enchondroma.* ***(Right)*** *Intermediate-grade chondrosarcoma may show prominent myxoid degeneration of the matrix, leading to potential difficulty in identification.*

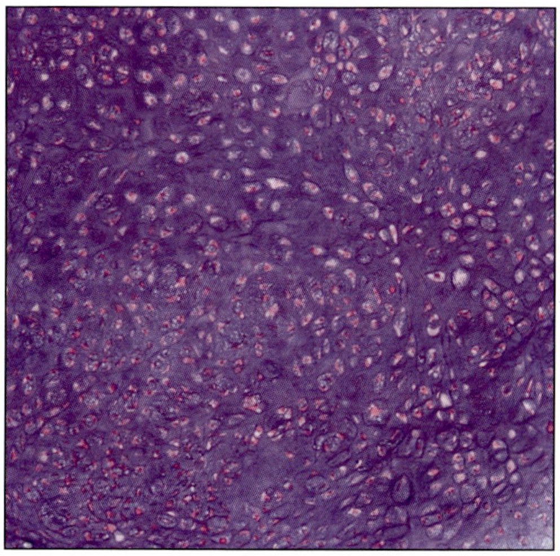
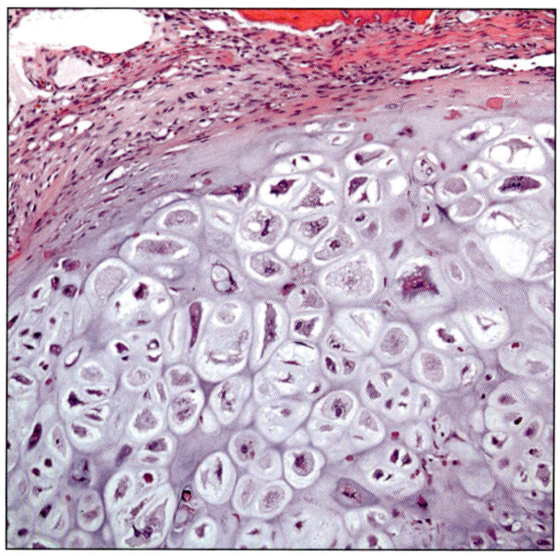

(Left) *In some chondrosarcomas, the cartilaginous matrix is prominently dark blue-purple rather than light blue-gray. This change in color is often seen in more cellular (grade 2) chondrosarcomas.* ***(Right)*** *High-grade (grade 3) chondrosarcoma demonstrates not only an increase in cellularity but also an increase in nuclear pleomorphism. Mitotic figures are often readily seen in higher grade tumors as well.*

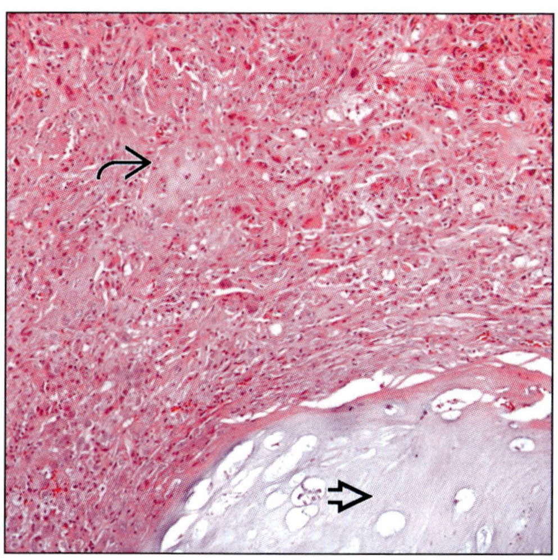
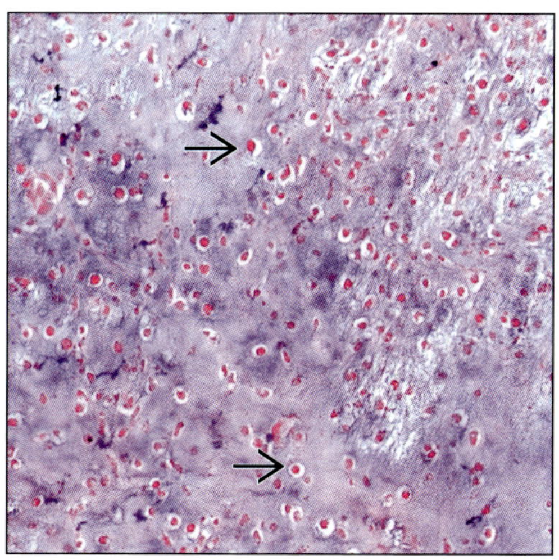

(Left) *Dedifferentiation in a chondrosarcoma is marked by the presence of a generally high-grade noncartilaginous sarcoma* ↷ *immediately adjacent to a more conventional hyaline-type chondrosarcoma component* ⇨*. In most cases, the conventional chondrosarcoma component is histologically low grade.* ***(Right)*** *Chondrocyte necrosis is a common finding in chondrosarcoma and is represented by loss of nuclear staining, leading to the appearance of purely pink cells* → *within lacunae.*

CHORDOMA

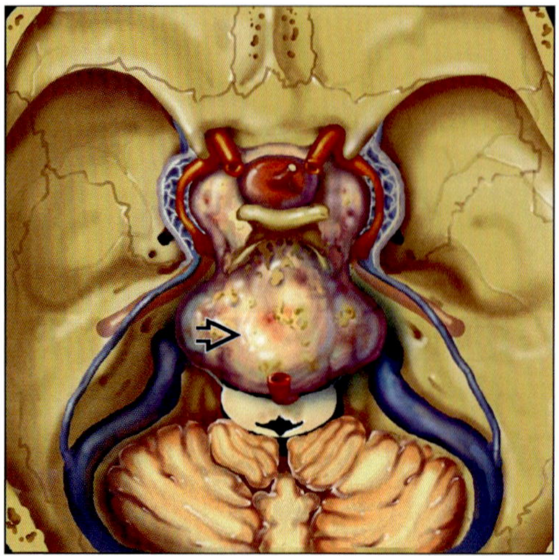

Chordomas ⇨ classically occur in the midline of the body, and one of the more common locations (~ 35% of cases) is at the base of the skull in the region of the clivus.

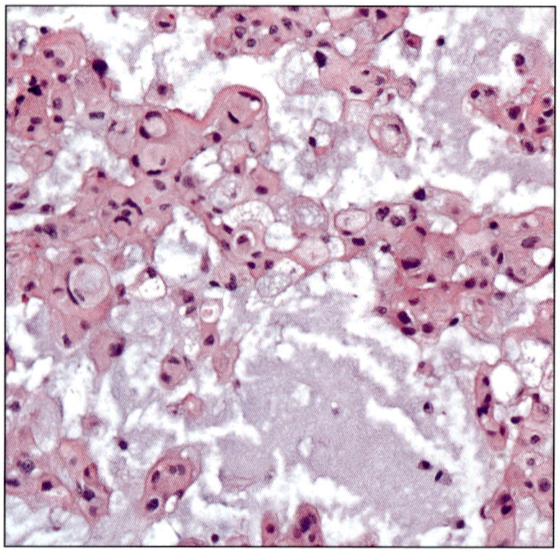

This image shows the classic histologic appearance of a conventional chordoma: Nests and cords of plump eosinophilic cells, clear cells, and physaliferous cells within a myxoid stroma.

TERMINOLOGY

Definitions

- Primary malignant tumor of bone with a phenotype that recapitulates notochord and usually arises within bones of axial skeleton
- Chondroid chordoma: Tumor with areas of conventional chordoma and regions resembling low-grade hyaline-type chondrosarcoma
- Dedifferentiated chordoma: Tumor with areas of conventional chordoma juxtaposed to high-grade sarcoma

ETIOLOGY/PATHOGENESIS

Sporadic and Familial

- Thought to arise from notochordal remnants
- Benign notochordal cell tumor (BNCT) may be a precursor lesion to chordoma
- Variety of genetic abnormalities can be identified in sporadic and familial tumors
  - Familial tumors (familial chordoma) have been associated with upregulation of T-brachyury, a nuclear transcription factor
  - Appears to be increased incidence of chordoma in patients with tuberous sclerosis

CLINICAL ISSUES

Epidemiology

- Incidence
  - Accounts for ~ 5% of primary malignant bone tumors
- Age
  - Wide range: 30-70 years
    - Generally earlier in familial chordoma (30-50 years)
  - Only 5% of tumors develop in patients < 20 years
    - Tumors in children usually arise in skull base and are often a part of tuberous sclerosis complex (TSC)
- Gender
  - Men affected more frequently than women

Site

- Virtually restricted to axial skeleton
  - Rare cases reported to arise outside axial skeleton
- Most (~ 50%) arise in sacrococcygeal region
- ~ 35% arise in skull base
- ~ 15% arise in mobile spine
- Chondroid chordoma usually arises in skull base
- Dedifferentiated chordoma usually arises in sacrococcygeal region
  - Dedifferentiation is most often seen in recurrences

Presentation

- Depends on site of origin
  - Skull base: Diplopia, headaches, cranial nerve palsies
  - Mobile spine: Pain, neurologic symptoms
  - Sacrum: Pain, constipation, incontinence, bladder dysfunction, erectile dysfunction

Treatment

- Standard of care is surgery ± radiation therapy
  - No effective chemotherapy is currently available

Prognosis

- Affected by tumor location, size, and resectability
- Sacral chordomas have best prognosis and longest overall survival because they are most likely to be resected with negative margins
  - Local recurrences for sacrococcygeal tumors are common after incomplete excision
  - 5- and 10-year survival rates range from 60-95% and 40-60%, respectively
- In mobile spine, 5-year survival rate is ~ 55%, with local recurrence rate ranging from 62-75%

CHORDOMA

Key Facts

Terminology
- Primary malignant tumor of bone with a phenotype that recapitulates notochord and usually arises within bones of axial skeleton

Etiology/Pathogenesis
- Benign notochordal cell tumor (BNCT) thought to be a precursor lesion to chordoma

Clinical Issues
- Accounts for ~ 5% of primary malignant bone tumors
- Usually diagnosed between 4th and 8th decades
- Virtually restricted to axial skeleton

Image Findings
- Destructive
- Lytic
- Invariably extends into soft tissues, forming a sizable, well-defined mass; may show calcifications

Macroscopic Features
- Gelatinous and lobulated
- Well delineated from surrounding tissues
- Dedifferentiated component is solid and fish flesh-like in appearance

Microscopic Pathology
- Histologically, chordoma is classified into 3 groups: Conventional chordoma, chondroid chordoma, and dedifferentiated chordoma
  - Chondroid chordoma can mimic chondrosarcoma
  - Dedifferentiated chordomas contain high-grade sarcomatous areas and have worst prognosis

---

  - Primarily due to difficulty in achieving complete resection
- In skull base, factors such as large size, female gender, and age > 40 years are associated with a worse outcome
  - In a series in which patients were treated with surgery and radiation, 46% developed local progression with median follow-up of 69 months
  - Others have reported a 5-year local control rate of 59%
- No apparent difference in overall survival for patients with chondroid chordomas (controversial)
- Dedifferentiated chordoma has worst prognosis of all chordomas
  - Usually rapidly fatal with systemic spread occurring in ~ 90% of cases
- Rate of metastatic spread of chordoma varies widely
  - Range: < 5-43% (highest for dedifferentiated chordoma)
- Common sites of dissemination include lung, skin, and bone

IMAGE FINDINGS

Radiographic Findings
- Lytic and destructive
- Invariably extends into soft tissues, forming a sizable, well-defined mass; may show calcifications
- In sacrum, soft tissue component is characteristically anterior
  - May displace the rectum and extend along sacral nerve roots into sciatic notch
- Sacral tumors are notoriously difficult to see on conventional radiographs

MR Findings
- Extremely bright on T2-weighted images; may show lobulated pattern
- Foci of calcification are frequently seen
- Soft tissue extent is better seen

CT Findings
- Has water content and appears radiolucent
- Bone destruction
- Calcifications may be seen

MACROSCOPIC FEATURES

General Features
- Soft, tan-gray, gelatinous, and lobulated
- Well delineated from surrounding tissues
- Dedifferentiated component is solid and fish flesh-like in appearance

Size
- Tumors in skull base are smallest, usually 2-5 cm in diameter
- Sacral tumors can be very large, usually > 10 cm

MICROSCOPIC PATHOLOGY

Histologic Features
- Histologically, chordoma is classified into 3 groups: Conventional chordoma, chondroid chordoma, and dedifferentiated chordoma
  - Familial and sporadic cases have similar findings
- Conventional chordoma has lobular growth pattern, infiltrates marrow space, encases preexisting bony trabeculae, and usually breaches the cortex, forming a well-demarcated soft tissue mass
  - Composed of large epithelioid cells arranged in cohesive nests and cords
  - One tumor cell may wrap or "hug" another
  - Nuclei are of moderate size, darkly staining, and may contain a small nucleolus or pseudoinclusions
  - Most cells have eosinophilic or clear cytoplasm (the latter due to ≥ 1 large intracytoplasmic vacuoles)
  - Physaliferous cells contain numerous small intracytoplasmic vacuoles that impart a "bubbly" appearance to cytoplasm

- Physaliphorous cells are not pathognomonic of chordoma, as other types of tumors may have similar-appearing cells and some chordomas may lack them
- In some tumors, physaliphorous cells have a large single cytoplasmic vacuole that causes them to mimic adipocytes
  - Pleomorphism and spindling of tumor cells may be present
  - Mitotic activity is usually limited
    - Foci of necrosis are common, especially in larger tumors
  - Extracellular stroma is myxoid, frothy, basophilic
- Chondroid chordoma contains areas of conventional chordoma as well as chondroid regions
  - Chondroid regions merge with or abruptly abut conventional component
  - Chondroid areas are composed of neoplastic cells distributed individually in lacunar-like spaces
    - Neoplastic cells are surrounded by solid-appearing hyalinized matrix similar in appearance to hyaline cartilage
  - Quantity of chondroid component is variable
    - In some tumors, chondroid areas may be so abundant as to make it difficult to distinguish chordoma from chondrosarcoma
- Dedifferentiated chordoma is composed of a high-grade sarcoma juxtaposed with conventional chordoma
  - Sarcoma is usually a high-grade, undifferentiated pleomorphic sarcoma
  - Dedifferentiation results from ongoing cumulative mutations in conventional chordoma cells
- In some tumors, areas of benign notochordal cell tumor may be seen adjacent to chordoma, suggesting malignant transformation

ANCILLARY TESTS

Immunohistochemistry

- Conventional chordoma typically expresses epithelial markers, including keratins and epithelial membrane antigen (EMA)
- Vast majority show nuclear expression of brachyury
- Most tumors show variable expression of S100
- Variable numbers also stain with antibodies to carcinoembryonic antigen (CEA) and glial fibrillary acidic protein (GFAP)
- Immunohistochemical stain can be very helpful in distinguishing chondrosarcoma from chordoma, especially on a small biopsy
  - Chondrosarcomas are negative for epithelial markers (particularly keratin) and brachyury

Molecular Genetics

- Some familial cases may show similar genetic alterations as sporadic cases

Electron Microscopy

- Neoplastic cells in conventional chordoma have villous-like surface projections, abundant cytoplasmic glycogen, and mitochondria-rough endoplasmic reticulum complexes
- Contain cytoplasmic processes that wrap around adjacent cells
- Cells have well-developed desmosomes, intracytoplasmic lumina, and tonofilaments

DIFFERENTIAL DIAGNOSIS

Metastatic Adenocarcinoma

- Mucinous adenocarcinoma can mimic chordoma on small biopsy sample
  - Immunohistochemical stains are helpful as adenocarcinomas are S100 protein positive and brachyury negative

Chondrosarcoma

- On small biopsies, especially from skull base, it can be difficult to distinguish chordoma from myxoid chondrosarcoma
  - Immunohistochemical stains for keratins and brachyury are helpful as chondrosarcoma is negative for those markers
  - Both tumors stain for S100 protein

Benign Notochordal Cell Tumor

- Contains cells with abundant clear cytoplasm (adipocyte-like) or eosinophilic cytoplasm
- Has same immunohistochemical profile as chordoma
- Unlike chordoma, BNCTs are usually confined to bone and lack extracellular myxoid matrix histologically
- Radiographically, chordoma is lytic whereas BNCT is sclerotic and does not show contrast enhancement

SELECTED REFERENCES

1. Walcott BP et al: Chordoma: current concepts, management, and future directions. Lancet Oncol. 13(2):e69-76, 2012
2. Le LP et al: Recurrent chromosomal copy number alterations in sporadic chordomas. PLoS One. 6(5):e18846, 2011
3. Yang XR et al: T (brachyury) gene duplication confers major susceptibility to familial chordoma. Nat Genet. 41(11):1176-8, 2009
4. Tirabosco R et al: Brachyury expression in extra-axial skeletal and soft tissue chordomas: a marker that distinguishes chordoma from mixed tumor/myoepithelioma/parachordoma in soft tissue. Am J Surg Pathol. 32(4):572-80, 2008
5. Deshpande V et al: Intraosseous benign notochord cell tumors (BNCT): further evidence supporting a relationship to chordoma. Am J Surg Pathol. 31(10):1573-7, 2007
6. O'Connell JX et al: Base of skull chordoma. A correlative study of histologic and clinical features of 62 cases. Cancer. 74(8):2261-7, 1994
7. Coffin CM et al: Chordoma in childhood and adolescence. A clinicopathologic analysis of 12 cases. Arch Pathol Lab Med. 117(9):927-33, 1993

CHORDOMA

Imaging, Gross, and Microscopic Features

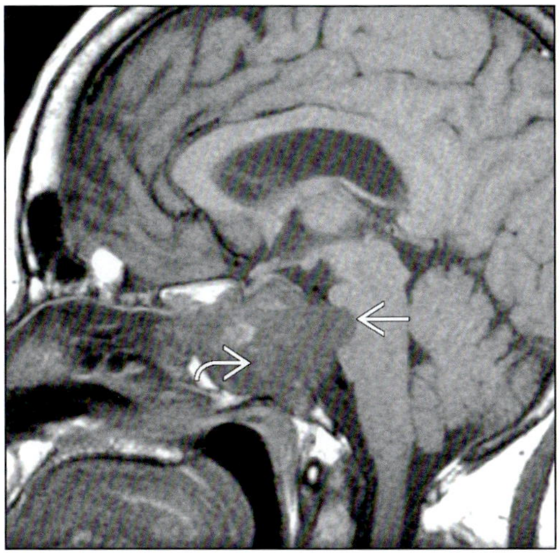

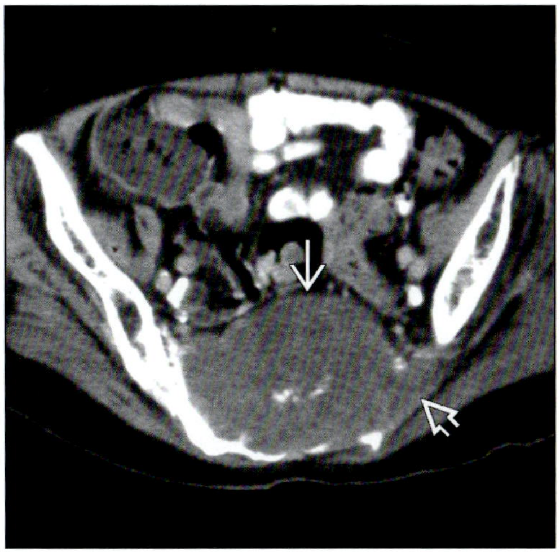

(Left) *Sagittal T1 MR image shows near-complete involvement of the clivus with expansile low-signal tumor ➡ and the classic "thumb" ➡ of chordoma focally compressing the pons.* ***(Right)*** *Axial CECT shows a large lytic lesion ➡ destroying the majority of the sacrum and extending into the adjacent soft tissues ⇨. Sacral tumors can be large at presentation, as this one was.*

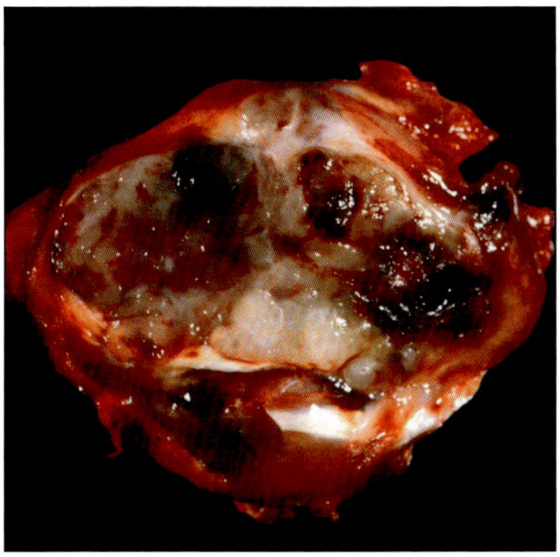

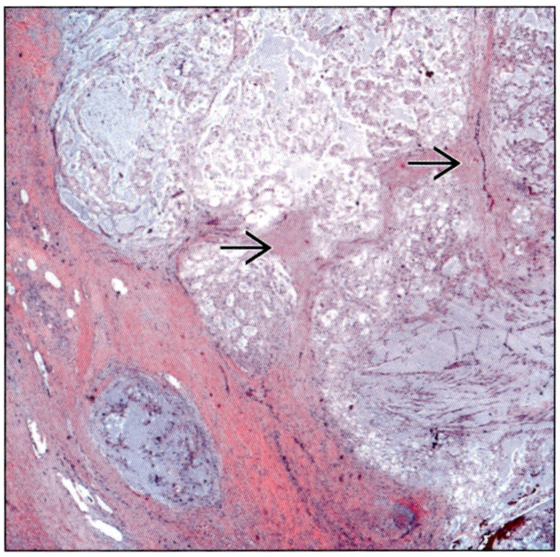

(Left) *This gross photograph shows the standard macroscopic features of a conventional chordoma. Most tumors are generally well circumscribed, tan-gray, focally hemorrhagic &/or myxoid, and demonstrate a nodular architecture. (Courtesy A. Hough, MD.)* ***(Right)*** *At low magnification, most chordomas demonstrate prominent lobularity with large nodules of tumor divided by thick fibrous septae →.*

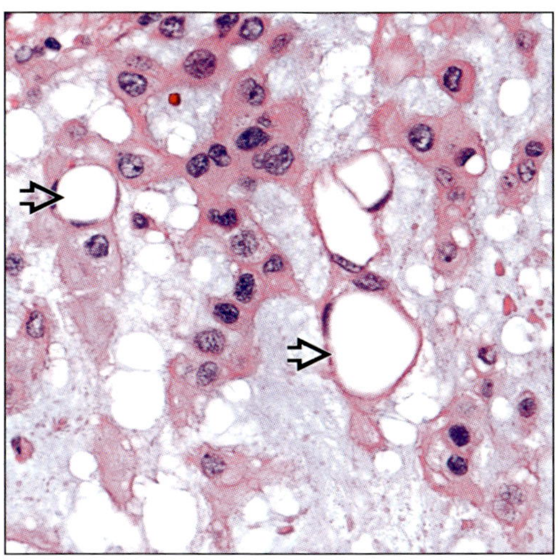

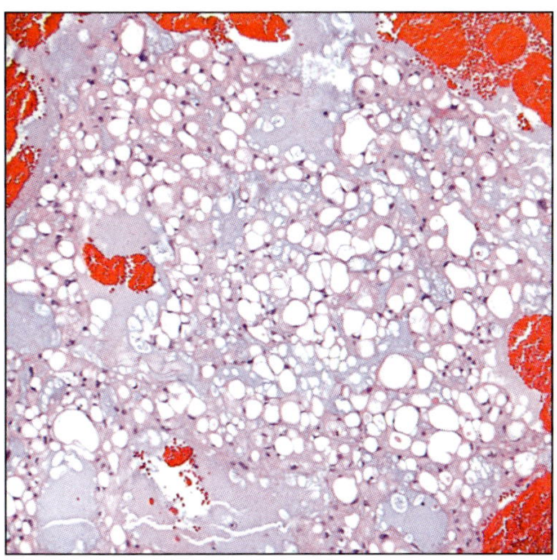

(Left) *Chordoma cells that contain a single large cytoplasmic vacuole ⇨ often resemble mature adipocytes and, when extensive, may potentially lead to confusion with an adipocytic neoplasm.* ***(Right)*** *This microscopic field demonstrates numerous clear chordoma cells and somewhat resembles adipose tissue. Note, however, that there is also a large number of conventional eosinophilic tumor cells to help support a diagnosis of chordoma.*

CHORDOMA

Microscopic Features

(Left) *Some chordoma cells contain numerous tiny intracytoplasmic vacuoles that give the cell a "bubbly" appearance. These cells are known as physaliferous cells ⇨. The number of physaliferous cells varies widely from tumor to tumor and even from 1 microscopic field to another.* ***(Right)*** *This image shows a dramatic and abrupt demarcation between conventional chordoma ⇨ and a sheet of physaliferous cells. In general, however, physaliferous cells are not usually numerous.*

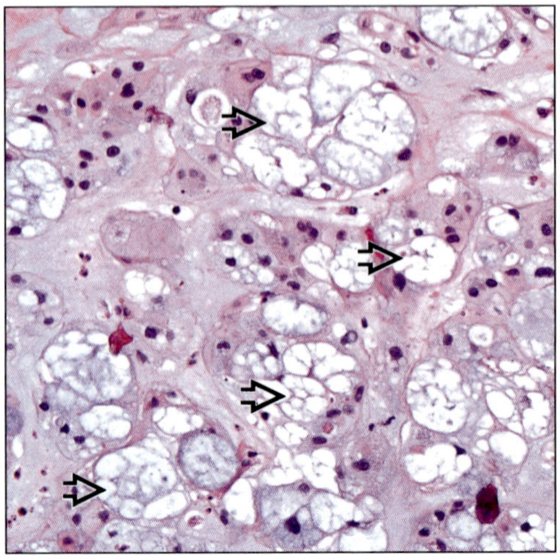

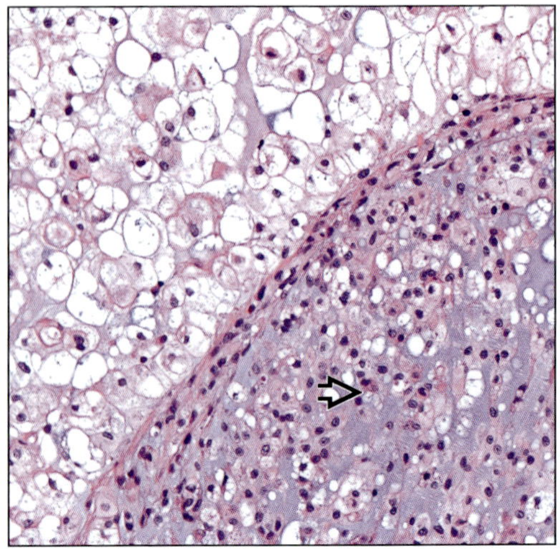

(Left) *It is not uncommon for occasional chordoma cells to display nuclear hyperchromasia, enlargement, &/or pleomorphism →. Within the context of otherwise conventional morphology, this finding is not prognostically significant. Similarly, mitotic figures are usually not prominent in chordomas.* ***(Right)*** *Tumor necrosis ↷ is a common finding in chordomas. Most often, it is localized and patchy; however, in larger tumors, it can be extensive.*

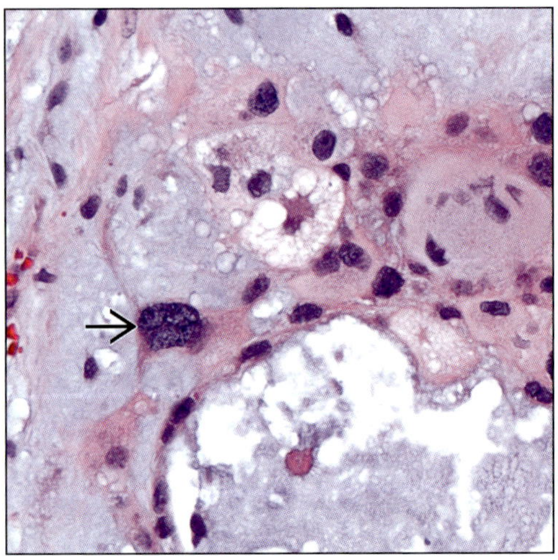

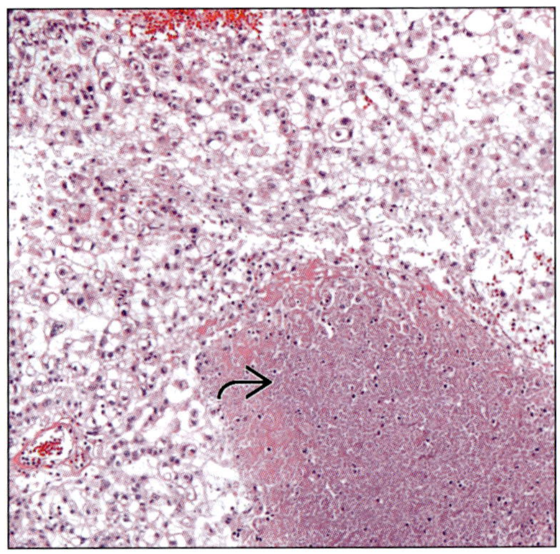

(Left) *Although most chordoma tumor cells are epithelioid, a spindled morphology may be seen occasionally. In a limited biopsy sample, this finding may raise the possibility of a myxoid chondrosarcoma of bone.* ***(Right)*** *Some chordomas demonstrate foci in which the tumor cells form a solid sheet of cells without the characteristic myxoid stroma. This morphology is usually not diffuse, however, and more conventional areas are often present elsewhere.*

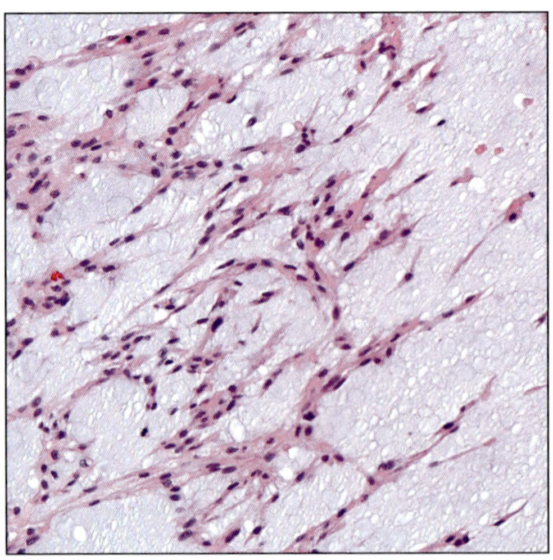

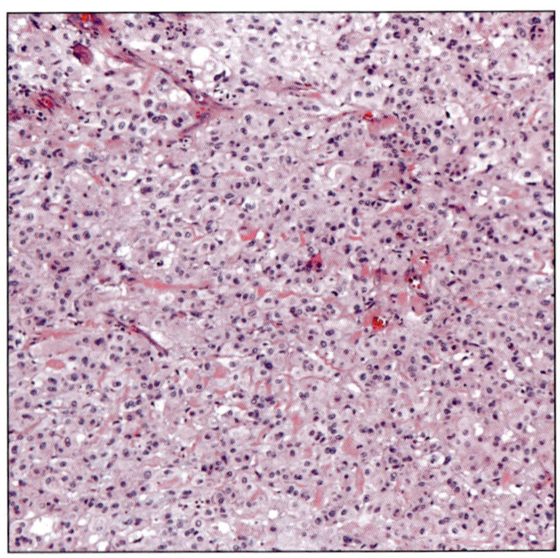

Microscopic and Immunohistological Features

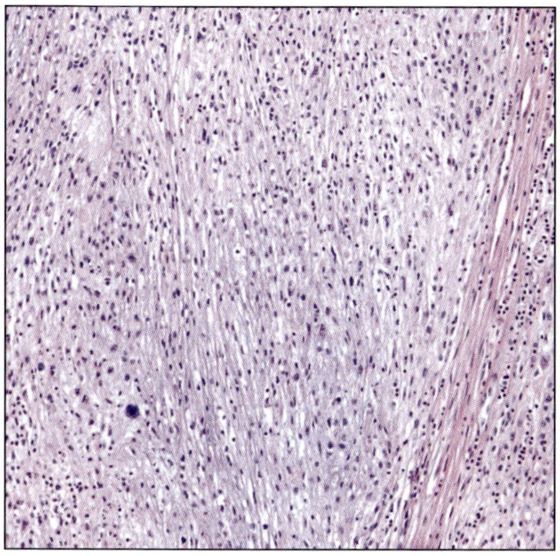

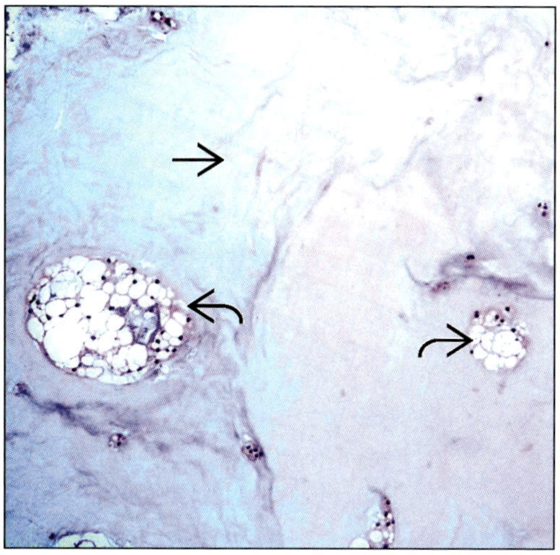

(Left) *This chordoma contained a few cellular areas composed of spindled tumor cells without well-developed myxoid stroma. Importantly, these areas did not show features of frank sarcoma that would suggest dedifferentiation.* ***(Right)*** *Chondroid chordomas show areas of conventional chordoma* → *associated with a hyaline-type chondroid matrix* →*. Depending on the extent of the chondroid portion, this variant may be difficult to distinguish from a chondrosarcoma.*

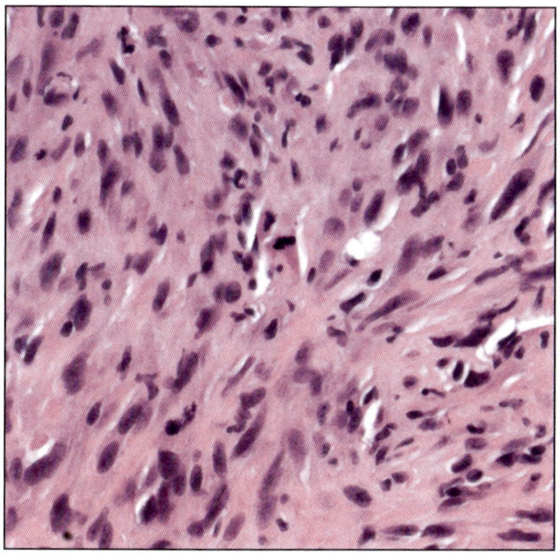

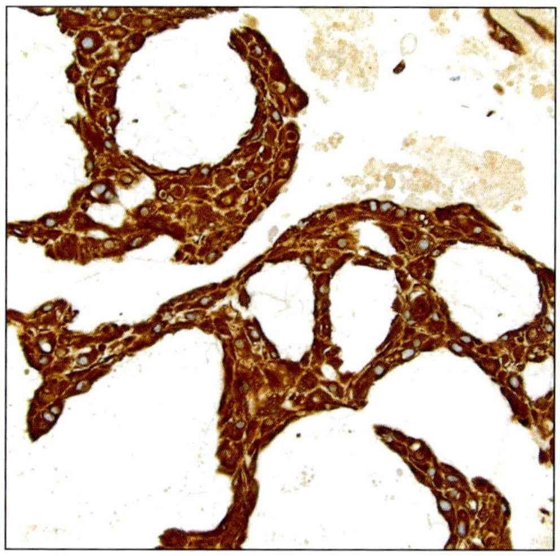

(Left) *A dedifferentiated chordoma contains areas of conventional chordoma (not shown in this image) juxtaposed to areas that have the appearance of a cellular &/or pleomorphic spindle cell sarcoma. (Courtesy M. Gokden, MD.)* ***(Right)*** *Most chordomas demonstrate strong diffuse expression of epithelial antigens, particularly keratins. Epithelial membrane antigen (EMA) is also commonly expressed but may show a more patchy staining pattern.*

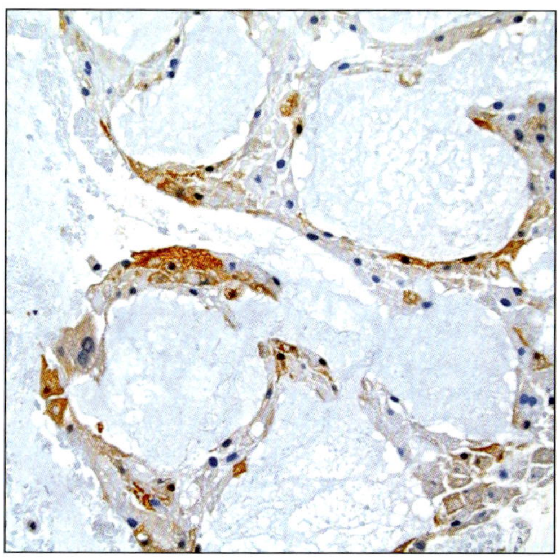

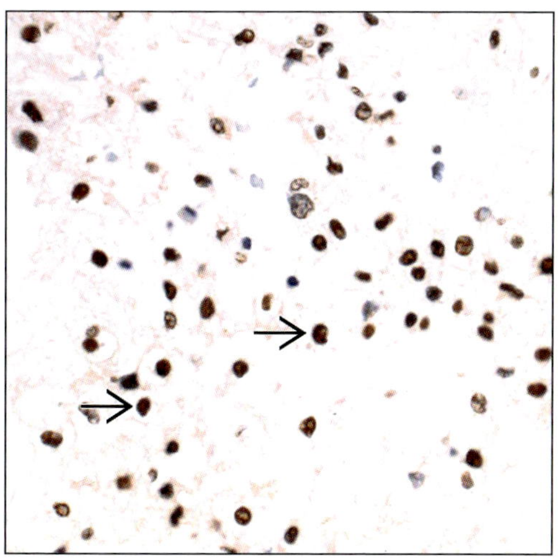

(Left) *The expression of S100 protein in chordomas is often less strong and diffuse than that seen for keratins. Importantly, care must be taken as chondrosarcomas can also show expression of this marker.* ***(Right)*** *Chordoma is 1 of very few tumors that express T-brachyury, a nuclear transcription factor found in notochordal cells and tumors that have a notochordal phenotype. Only nuclear staining* → *is considered positive. (Courtesy M. Gokden, MD.)*

MALIGNANT PERIPHERAL NERVE SHEATH TUMOR

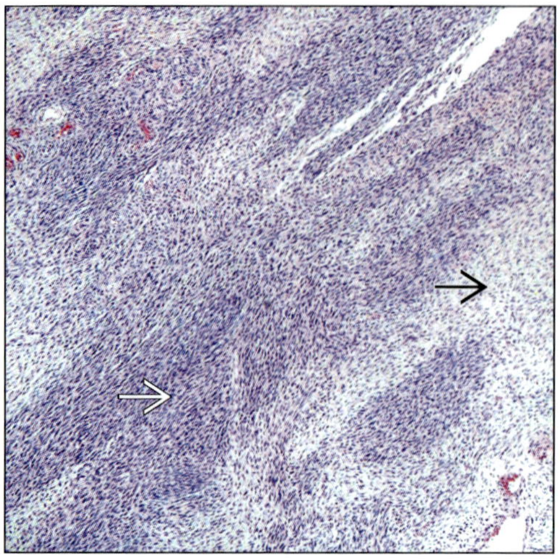

At low magnification, malignant peripheral nerve sheath tumor (MPNST) classically shows a marbled or tapestry pattern of alternating regions of high ➔ and low ➔ cellularity.

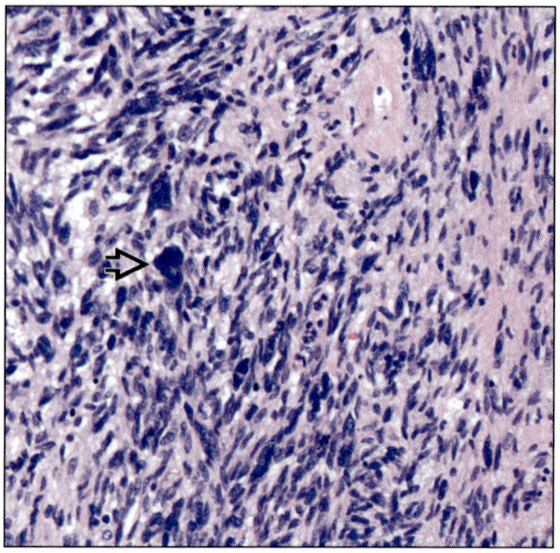

Although some cases of MPNST can show monomorphic nuclear cytology, most examples show at least focal nuclear hyperchromasia and pleomorphism ➔, as well as a brisk mitotic rate.

TERMINOLOGY

Abbreviations

- Malignant peripheral nerve sheath tumor (MPNST)

Synonyms

- Neurofibrosarcoma, malignant schwannoma, neurogenic sarcoma

Definitions

- Sarcoma arising from a nerve or benign nerve sheath tumor or showing nerve sheath differentiation
  - Diagnostic criteria
    - Arises from a nerve or benign nerve sheath tumor, or
    - Shows histological evidence of nerve sheath differentiation in patient with neurofibromatosis type 1 (NF1), or
    - Shows histological plus immunohistochemical or ultrastructural evidence of nerve sheath differentiation in patient without NF1

ETIOLOGY/PATHOGENESIS

Genetic Predisposition

- 50% of cases are associated with NF1
  - Lifetime incidence: 2-16%
- 40% of cases are sporadic

Environmental Exposure

- 10% of cases are associated with radiation

Molecular Pathogenesis

- NF1 caused by germline mutation of *NF1* tumor suppressor gene
  - Somatic loss of 2nd *NF1* allele required for tumorigenesis
- Malignant transformation in both NF1-associated and sporadic MPNST often involves *INK4A* and *TP53* and their downstream pathways

CLINICAL ISSUES

Epidemiology

- Incidence
  - Rare: 5-10% of soft tissue sarcomas
- Age
  - Mostly adults (20-50 years)
    - Wide age range: 10-70 years
    - Average age in NF1: 30 years
    - Average age in sporadic MPNST: 40 years
- Gender
  - M ~ F

Site

- Common sites: Thigh, buttock, trunk, upper arm, retroperitoneum, head and neck
  - Mostly deep seated
  - Central body axis more common in NF1
- Most (70%) arise in major nerve trunks
  - Sciatic nerve most common
  - Brachial plexus, sacral plexus, paraspinal nerves

Presentation

- Painful mass
- Neurological deficit in some

Treatment

- Surgical approaches
  - Wide excision/resection
  - Amputation
- Adjuvant therapy
  - Radiation
- Drugs
  - Generally poor response to chemotherapy

MALIGNANT PERIPHERAL NERVE SHEATH TUMOR

Key Facts

Terminology
- Sarcoma arising from a nerve or benign nerve sheath tumor or showing nerve sheath cellular differentiation

Etiology/Pathogenesis
- 50% of cases are associated with NF1
- 10% of cases are associated with radiation

Clinical Issues
- Mostly adults (20-50 years)
- Most (70%) arise in major nerve trunks
- Local recurrence: > 40%
- Metastasis: 30-60%
- 5-year survival: 15-34%

Microscopic Pathology
- Mostly high-grade sarcomas
- Spindle cell MPNST (80%)
  - Long fascicles of closely spaced hyperchromatic spindle cells
  - Small round blue cells
  - Pleomorphic cells
  - Extensive necrosis with perivascular preservation
- Epithelioid MPNST (5%)
- Heterologous differentiation (15%)

Ancillary Tests
- S100: 50-60% (usually focal)

Top Differential Diagnoses
- Synovial sarcoma
- Cellular schwannoma
- Atypical neurofibroma
- Malignant melanoma

Prognosis
- Poor
  - Local recurrence: > 40%
  - Metastasis: 30-60%
    - Lungs, bone, pleura most common
  - > 60% die of disease
  - 5-year survival: 15-34%
  - NF1 patients have worse overall prognosis
    - Probably due to higher incidence of large central axis tumors

IMAGE FINDINGS

General Features
- Morphology
  - Large heterogeneous mass
  - Fusiform mass within major nerve trunk

MACROSCOPIC FEATURES

General Features
- Similar to other soft tissue sarcomas
  - Pseudoencapsulated
  - Gray-tan
  - Firm to fleshy
  - Necrosis and hemorrhage common
- Fusiform or eccentric mass when arising in major nerve trunk
- Coexisting neurofibroma in some
  - Solitary or plexiform

Size
- Most > 5 cm
- Sometimes very massive

MICROSCOPIC PATHOLOGY

Histologic Features
- Wide spectrum of cytoarchitectural patterns
  - Mostly high-grade sarcomas
    - High mitotic rate and necrosis
    - Only ~ 15% are low grade
  - Nerve sheath differentiation
    - Nuclear palisading is uncommon (15%), usually focal
    - Tactoid differentiation with whorling or Wagner-Meissner-like features
  - Intraneural tumors
    - Plexiform architecture
    - Microscopic extension within nerve fascicle
  - Tumors arising from preexisting benign nerve sheath tumor
    - Neurofibroma most common, transitional areas, usually in NF1 patients
    - Schwannoma, ganglioneuroma, ganglioneuroblastoma, or pheochromocytoma; very rare
  - Diffuse sarcomatous proliferation with no evidence of nerve or nerve sheath origin
- Spindle cell MPNST (80%)
  - Long fascicles of uniform, closely spaced, hyperchromatic spindle cells
  - Alternating cellular fascicles and hypocellular areas ("tapestry" or "marbled" pattern)
  - Storiform arrays
  - Small round blue cells
  - Pleomorphic cells
    - Multinucleated giant cells
  - Extensive necrosis with perivascular preservation
  - Hemangiopericytoma-like vascular pattern in some
- Epithelioid MPNST (5%)
  - Multinodular architecture
  - Cords and clusters in some
  - Large epithelioid cells
    - Abundant eosinophilic cytoplasm
    - Large vesicular nuclei with macronucleoli
    - Clear cytoplasm in some
  - Often mixed with spindle cells
- Heterologous differentiation (15%)
  - Osseous and osteosarcomatous

- Chondroid and chondrosarcomatous
- Rhabdomyosarcomatous (malignant triton tumor)
- Angiosarcomatous
- Glandular
- Neuroepithelial (rosettes)

Cytologic Features

- Spindle cells
  - Hyperchromatic nucleus with dispersed coarse chromatin
  - Tapered and wavy nuclei in well-differentiated tumors
  - Very brisk mitotic activity in high-grade tumors
- Epithelioid cells
  - Abundant eosinophilic or clear cytoplasm
  - Vesicular nucleus with prominent inclusion-like nucleolus

ANCILLARY TESTS

Immunohistochemistry

- S100 protein (+) in about 60%, usually focal
- Nestin (+) in 50-80%
- SOX10(+) in ~ 30%, usually focal

Cytogenetics

- Complex structural and numeric chromosomal abnormalities
  - Frequent loss of *NF1* at 17q11
  - Frequent loss of *TP53* at 17q13

DIFFERENTIAL DIAGNOSIS

Monophasic or Poorly Differentiated Synovial Sarcoma

- Nuclei have softer, less coarse chromatin
- Usually has lower mitotic rate
- TLE1(+)
  - MPNST rarely (2%) positive
- Usually cytokeratin (+) and EMA(+)
  - MPNST usually negative
- Usually S100(-)
- t(X:18) identified ~ 90% of cases
  - *SSX* gene on chromosome X fuses to *SS18* gene (formerly termed *SYT*) on chromosome 18

Cellular Schwannoma

- Usually located in retroperitoneum, pelvis, posterior mediastinum, gastrointestinal tract
- Exclusively Antoni A areas; often lacks Verocay bodies
- Focal necrosis and mitotic figures may be present
- Lacks malignant cytological atypia
- Strong, diffuse S100 staining
  - MPNST usually has only focal staining

Atypical Neurofibroma

- Large, hyperchromatic spindle cells
- Degenerated (smudged) chromatin
- Low mitotic rate and generally low cellularity
- Usually retains cytoarchitectural features of neurofibroma
  - Edematous fibrillary or myxoid matrix with collagen bundles ("shredded carrots" pattern)

Malignant Melanoma

- Spindle cell/sarcomatoid melanoma
  - May have clustered or thèque-like areas
  - Diffusely S100(+)
    - MPNST often focally S100(+) (60% of cases)
  - Usually HMB-45(-) and Melan-A (-)
- Epithelioid melanoma
  - Amelanotic melanoma may be indistinguishable from epithelioid MPNST
  - Usually HMB-45(+) and Melan-A (+)
    - MPNST is negative for these markers

Clear Cell Sarcoma (CCS)

- Predilection for acral extremities
- Multinodular, vaguely nested architecture
- Uniform epithelioid and spindle cells
- Diffuse S100, HMB-45, and Melan-A staining in most
- t(12:22) (~90% of cases)
  - *EWSR1* gene on chromosome 22 fuses to *ATF1* gene on chromosome 12
  - Variant t(2;22) (*CREB1-EWSR1*) identified in gastrointestinal forms of CCS

Ewing Sarcoma

- Usually a primary bone tumor but may present as soft tissue primary
  - MPNST is exceedingly rare as primary bone tumor
- Small round blue cell tumor
  - Often with glycogenated (clear) cytoplasm
  - Diffusely CD99(+), usually S100(-)
    - MPNST sometimes CD99(+) but usually weak/focal and nonmembranous
  - Several balanced translocations and fusions involving *EWSR1* gene (on chromosome 22) identified in Ewing sarcoma
    - t(11;22), *EWSR1-FLI1* (90% of cases)
    - t(21;22), *EWSR1-ERG* (5-10% of cases)
    - Others including t(2;22), t(7;22), t(17;22)

Embryonal Rhabdomyosarcoma

- Small round blue cells and spindle cells
- Scattered rhabdomyoblasts
- S100(-), desmin (+), and myogenin (+)

SELECTED REFERENCES

1. Masliah-Planchon J et al: MicroRNAome profiling in benign and malignant neurofibromatosis type 1-associated nerve sheath tumors: evidences of PTEN pathway alterations in early NF1 tumorigenesis. BMC Genomics. 14:473, 2013
2. Rahrmann EP et al: Forward genetic screen for malignant peripheral nerve sheath tumor formation identifies new genes and pathways driving tumorigenesis. Nat Genet. 45(7):756-66, 2013
3. Gottfried ON et al: Neurofibromatosis Type 1 and tumorigenesis: molecular mechanisms and therapeutic implications. Neurosurg Focus. 28(1):E8, 2010
4. Jagdis A et al: Prospective evaluation of TLE1 as a diagnostic immunohistochemical marker in synovial sarcoma. Am J Surg Pathol. 33(12):1743-51, 2009

Microscopic Features

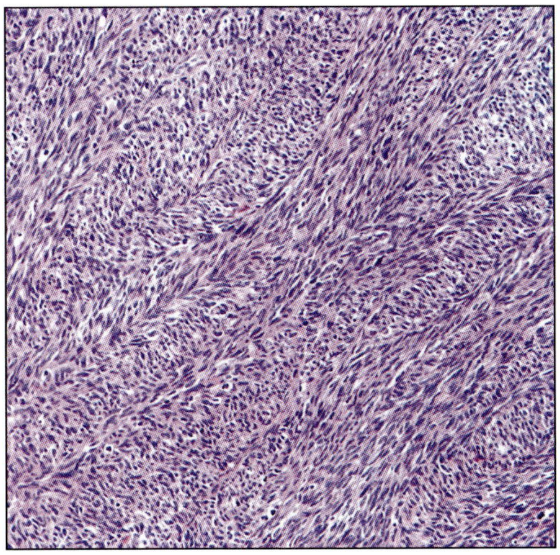

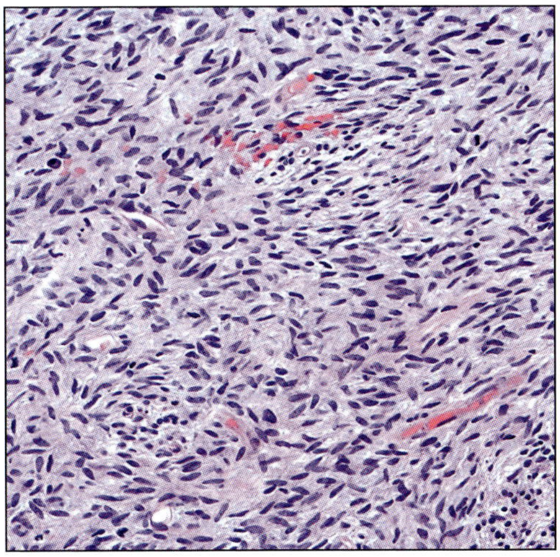

(Left) *Some cases of MPNST demonstrate a marked fascicular growth pattern with a herringbone architecture, similar to what is often seen in adult-type fibrosarcoma, fibrosarcomatous dermatofibrosarcoma protuberans, and other morphologically similar cellular spindle cell sarcomas.* ***(Right)*** *In the less cellular regions of an MPNST, the tumor cells exhibit typical features of neural derivation, including thin, elongated, and buckled nuclei with tapered ends.*

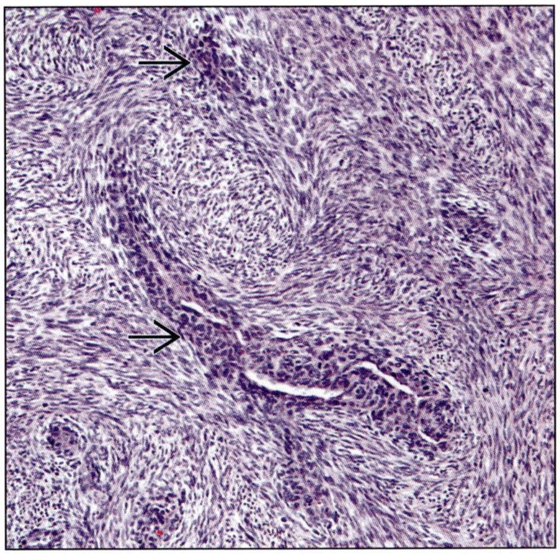

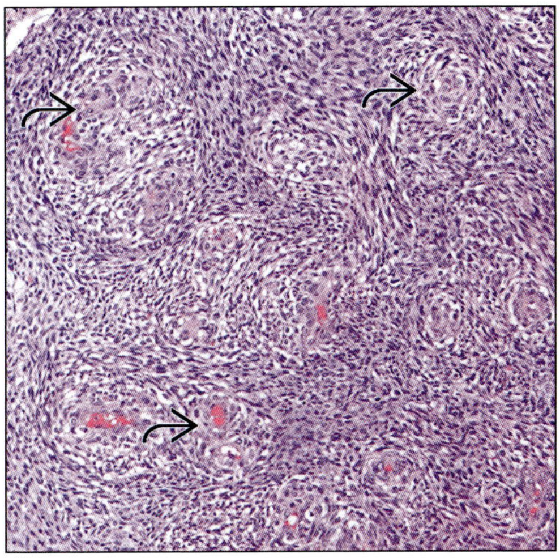

(Left) *A characteristic but underappreciated feature of many MPNSTs is an accentuation* → *of tumor cells around the stromal blood vessels. Sometimes, the tumor cells will proliferate and appear to "herniate" into the lumen of the vessel.* ***(Right)*** *In some cases of MPNST, the perivascular tumor cells* ⤻ *are so prominent that they may resemble true glands or epithelial islands, leading to potential confusion with biphasic synovial sarcoma.*

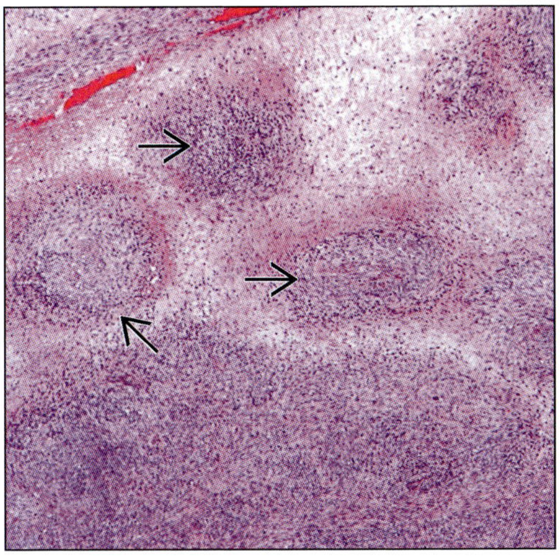

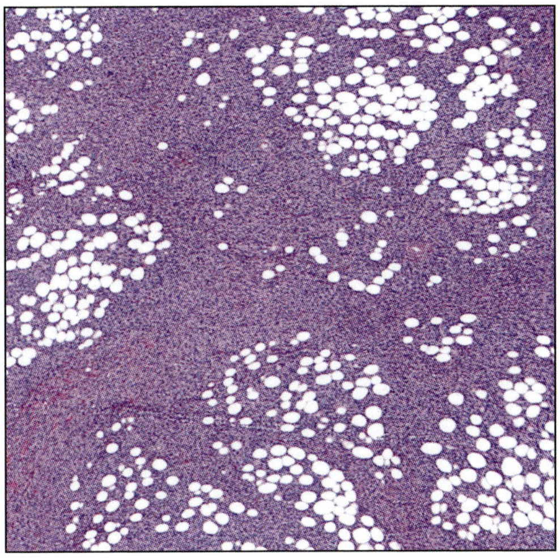

(Left) *Coagulative necrosis is a common finding in MPNST and may range from scattered foci to extensive zones. Within geographic zones of necrosis, it is common to see viable tumor cells around stromal blood vessels (peritheliomatous pattern* →*), resembling "islands in an ocean."* ***(Right)*** *Although not a typical finding in most cases, MPNST may show diffuse infiltration of peritumoral fat in a honeycomb fashion, mimicking the growth of dermatofibrosarcoma protuberans.*

MALIGNANT PERIPHERAL NERVE SHEATH TUMOR

Microscopic Features

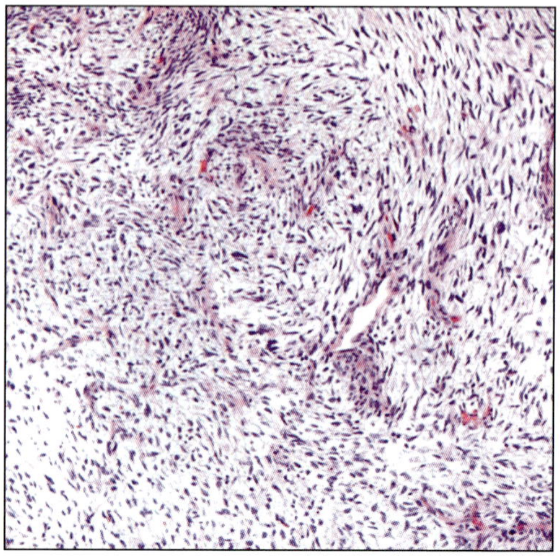

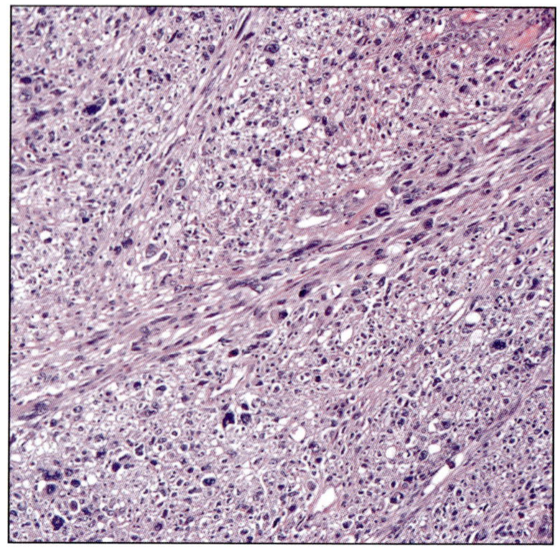

(Left) *Myxoid stromal change is common in MPNST. In some cases, this change is extensive, and it can be difficult to distinguish this tumor from myxofibrosarcoma, myxoid dermatofibrosarcoma protuberans, and others. Areas of more conventional morphology are helpful in these cases.* ***(Right)*** *Diffuse nuclear pleomorphism and anaplasia are not common findings in MPNST and can make the diagnosis very difficult. Demonstration of origin from a nerve or a benign nerve sheath tumor is helpful.*

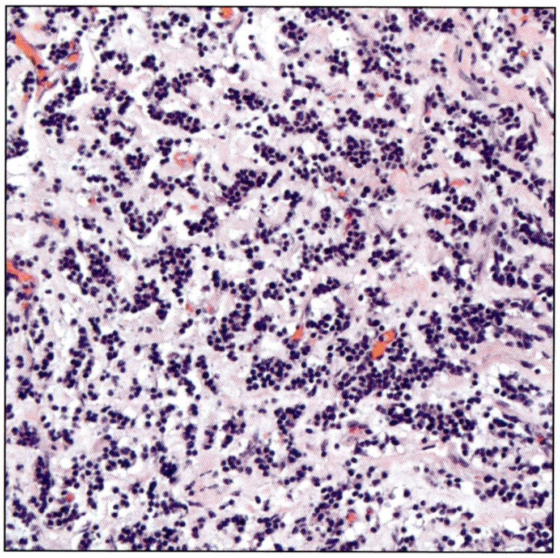

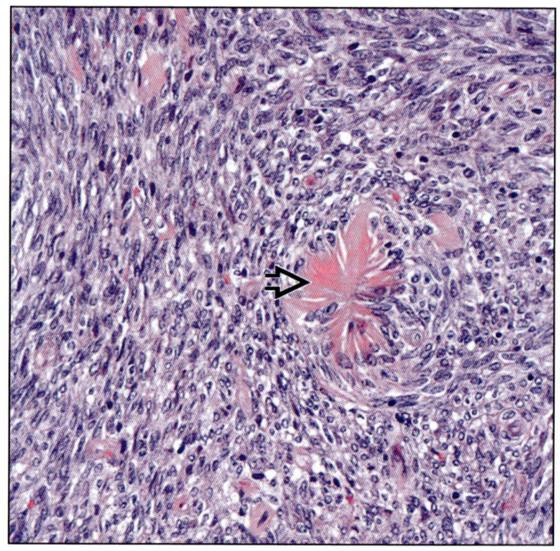

(Left) *Rare cases of MPNST contain a small round blue cell morphology that mimics a variety of round cell sarcomas or even a hematolymphoid process. The diagnosis usually requires demonstration of areas of more conventional MPNST morphology.* ***(Right)*** *Occasionally, MPNST will contain structures suggestive of neural origin such as cellular whorls; Verocay-like palisading, tactoid bodies; and fibrillar rosettes ⇨.*

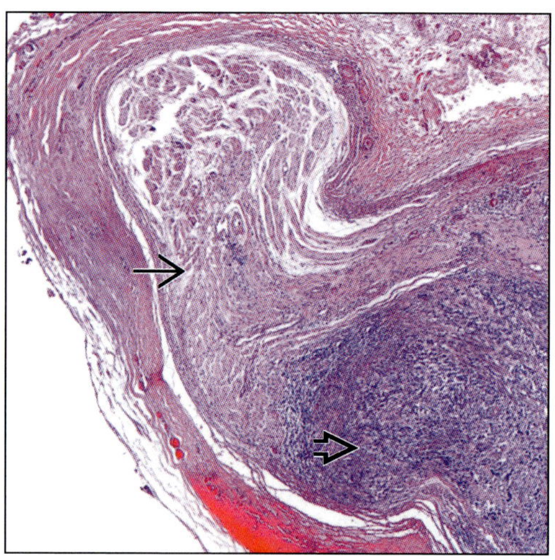

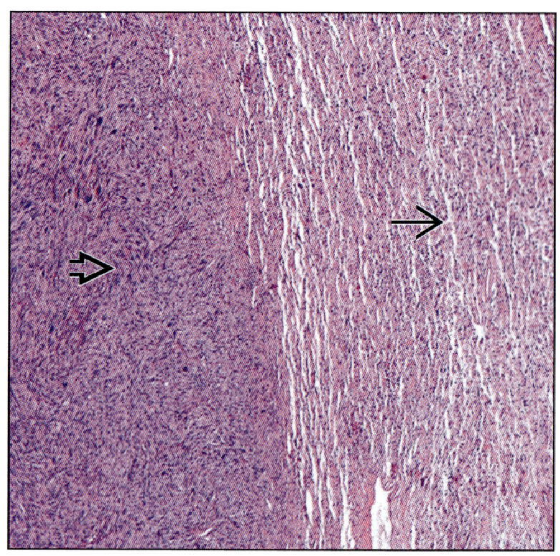

(Left) *Demonstration of origin from a nerve (either microscopically → or grossly/intraoperatively) by a spindle cell sarcoma ⇨ is diagnostic of MPNST. Importantly, origin from a nerve seen histologically must be distinguished from simple neural/perineural invasion, which is seen in a variety of malignancies.* ***(Right)*** *Demonstration of a spindle cell sarcoma ⇨ arising in association with a benign nerve sheath tumor (usually a neurofibroma →) is also diagnostic of MPNST.*

Variant Microscopic Features

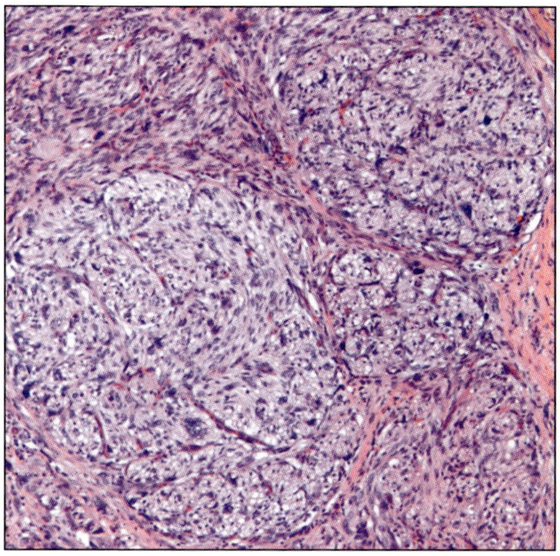
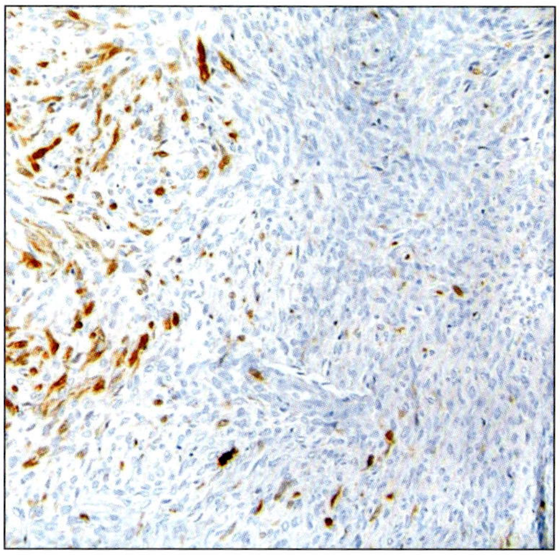

(Left) *In some cases of MPNST, residual nerve trunks/fibers can be identified that are almost completely replaced by tumor yet are still recognizable enough to clinch the diagnosis.* ***(Right)*** *Expression of S100 protein in MPNST is characteristically focal and patchy and is seen only in up to 60% of cases. Strong, diffuse expression of this antigen is very uncommon in conventional spindle cell MPNST and should raise the possibility of a cellular schwannoma.*

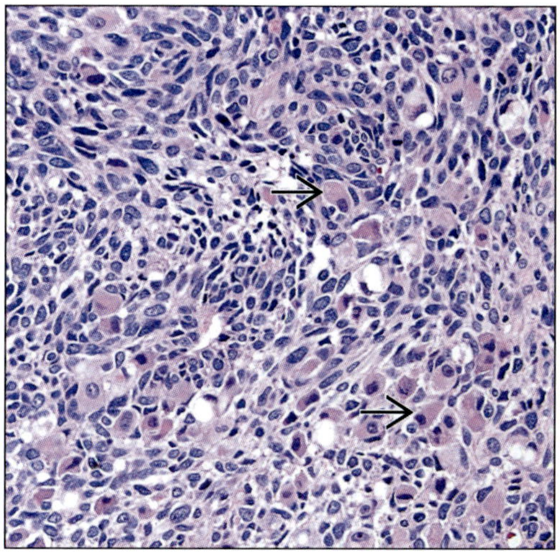
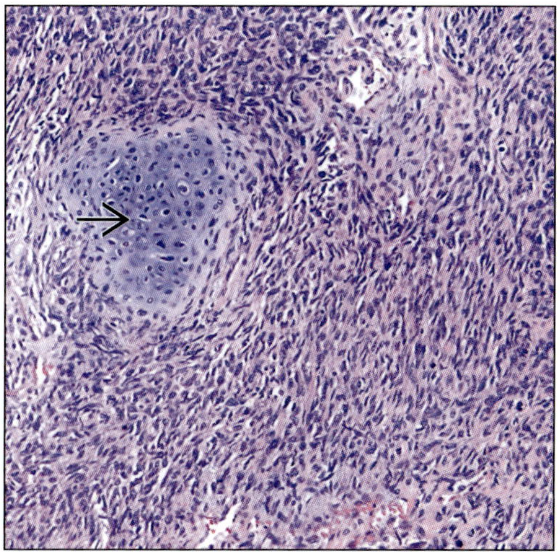

(Left) *A small subset of MPNST cases contain heterologous elements such as rhabdomyoblasts* ➙*. (Such cases are also known as a malignant triton tumor.) These elements are morphologically distinct but do not appear to affect the prognosis.* ***(Right)*** *Other heterologous elements that can be identified in MPNST include histologically benign or malignant cartilage* ➙*, bone, and vascular structures. Glands and squamous islands are exceptional findings.*

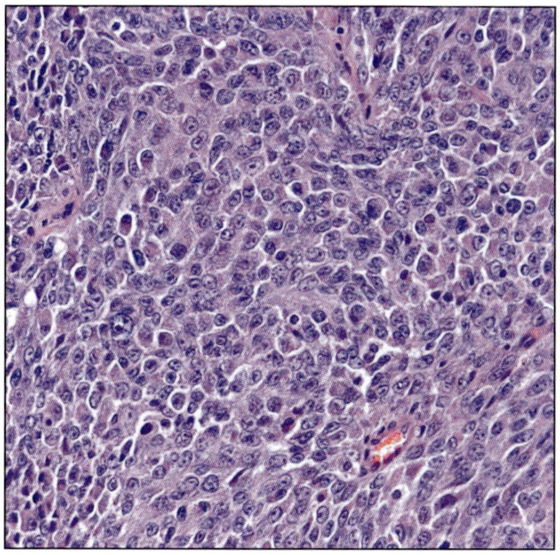
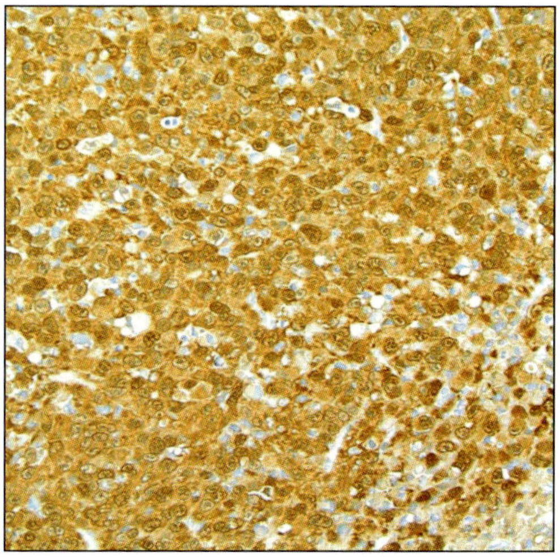

(Left) *Epithelioid MPNST is a less common variant of MPNST; it is generally composed of large nodules of epithelioid cells divided by fibrous septae. Large nucleoli and a variably prominent myxoid stroma are common features. A rhabdoid morphology may also be seen.* ***(Right)*** *Characteristically, epithelioid MPNST is diffusely positive for S100 protein, unlike conventional MPNST in which S100 staining is focal or negative. Melanocytic markers (e.g., HMB-45) are negative.*

MELANOTIC NEUROECTODERMAL TUMOR OF INFANCY

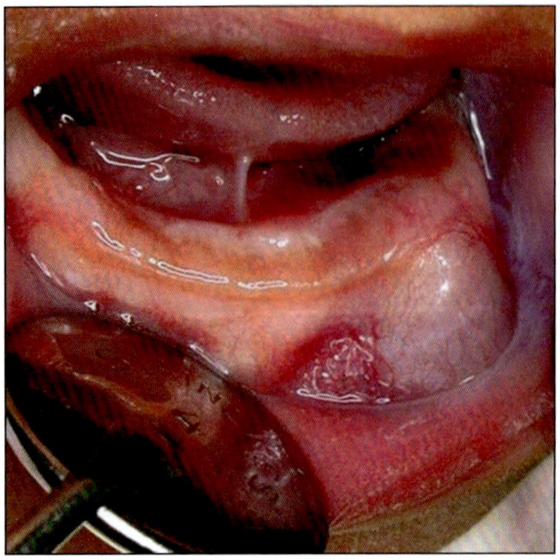

Clinical photo shows a maxillary expansion with an intact overlying mucosa in a child. The clinical features of the melanotic neuroectodermal tumor may mimic an eruption cyst. (Courtesy J. Hille, MDS, DDS.)

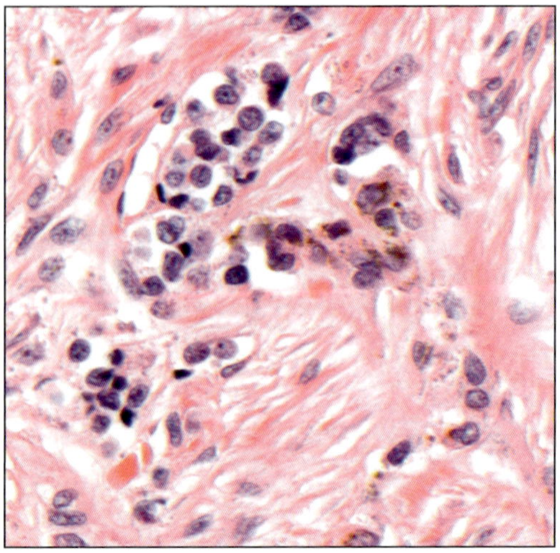

The neuroblastic small cells separated by a fibrocollagenous stroma demonstrate an alveolar pattern of growth. Epithelial cells with abundant eosinophilic cytoplasm and melanin pigment are scattered.

TERMINOLOGY

Abbreviations

- Melanotic neuroectodermal tumor of infancy (MNTI)

Synonyms

- Retinal anlage tumor
- Melanotic progonoma

Definitions

- Rare, fast-growing, pigmented neoplasm of likely neural crest origin

ETIOLOGY/PATHOGENESIS

Disputed Histogenesis

- Neural crest (neuroectodermal) origin

Familial Setting

- Reports of familial cases: Unknown gene

CLINICAL ISSUES

Epidemiology

- Age
  - Most present in 1st year of life (> 90%)

Site

- Most MNTI cases arise in maxilla, although occurrence in other intraosseous and extraosseous anatomic locations has been described, including the skull, brain, epididymis, testis, skin, and mediastinum
- Most involve craniofacial sites
  - Upper and lower jaw
    - Maxilla: 69%
    - Mandible: 6%
  - Skull: 11%

Presentation

- Rapidly enlarging, firm, expansile mass
- Intact overlying mucosa
- Erosion into adjacent bone
- Nontender
- Bluish discoloration

Laboratory Tests

- Elevated urinary vanillylmandelic acid may be present

Treatment

- Complete local excision
  - Local recurrence rate: 10-15%
  - Usually recurs in 1st postoperative year

Prognosis

- Benign to intermediate clinical course
  - Recurrence rate: 10-15%
  - Metastatic spread in < 5%

MACROSCOPIC FEATURES

Gross Features

- Firm
- Well circumscribed
- Gray to blue-black cut surface

MICROSCOPIC PATHOLOGY

Predominant Pattern/Injury Type

- Glandular/alveolar
  - Spaces lined by cuboidal pigmented epithelial cells
  - Small neuroblastic cells found within spaces
- Solid
  - Background of fibrocollagenous stroma

Predominant Cell/Compartment Type

- Dual population of cells
  - Flat to cuboidal pigmented epithelial cells

MELANOTIC NEUROECTODERMAL TUMOR OF INFANCY

Key Facts

Terminology
- Rare, fast-growing, pigmented neoplasm of likely neural crest origin

Clinical Issues
- Most present in 1st year of life
- Commonly involve craniofacial sites
  - Maxilla: 69%
- Rapidly enlarging expansile mass
- Elevated urinary vanillylmandelic acid may be present

Microscopic Pathology
- 3 distinct components
  - Clusters of small round neuroblastic cells
  - Primitive gland-like structures
  - Fibrocollagenous stroma

Top Differential Diagnoses
- Primitive neuroectodermal tumor
  - Sheets of small to medium round blue cells
  - Characteristic t(11;22)
- Neuroblastoma
  - Sheets and lobules of small round hyperchromatic cells
- Congenital epulis
  - Characteristic location in labial aspect of dental ridge
  - Protruding round or ovoid nodule
- Alveolar rhabdomyosarcoma
  - Aggregates and nests of poorly differentiated small hyperchromatic cells
  - Characteristic immunohistochemical and cytogenetic findings

Immunohistochemistry

Antibody	Reactivity	Staining Pattern	Comment
AE1/AE3	Positive	Cell membrane & cytoplasm	Epithelial cells
HMB-45	Positive	Cytoplasmic	Epithelial cells
Mart-1	Positive		Neuroblastic and epithelial cells
NSE	Positive	Cytoplasmic	Frequently expressed by neuroblastic cells and epithelial cells
Synaptophysin	Positive	Cytoplasmic	Neuroblastic cells and variably expressed in epithelial cells
CD57	Positive	Cell membrane & cytoplasm	Neuroblastic cells and epithelial cells

- Small neuroblastic cells
- Fibrocollagenous stroma

Microscopic Features
- Biphasic cell population of large epithelioid cells with intracellular melanin granules and smaller, round, neuroblast-like cells in a variably vascularized fibrous stroma
- 3 distinct components
  - Clusters of small round neuroblastic cells
    - Small round hyperchromatic nuclei
    - Scant cytoplasm
    - Arranged in small islands and cords
    - Crush artifact frequently encountered
  - Primitive gland-like structures
    - Larger cells with round vesicular nuclei
    - Abundant cytoplasm with melanin granules
    - Alveolar or glandular arrangements
  - Fibrocollagenous stroma

DIFFERENTIAL DIAGNOSIS

Primitive Neuroectodermal Tumor
- Sheets of small to medium round blue cells
- Frequent mitoses and foci of necrosis
- Characteristic t(11;22)

Neuroblastoma
- Predominantly located in retroperitoneum
- Sheets and lobules of small round hyperchromatic cells
- Homer Wright rosettes

Congenital Epulis
- Characteristic location in labial aspect of dental ridge
- Protruding round or ovoid nodule
- Microscopically resembles adult granular cell tumor
  - Polygonal cells with abundant eosinophilic cytoplasm
  - Lack pseudoepitheliomatous hyperplasia

Alveolar Rhabdomyosarcoma
- More commonly located in extremities
- Aggregates and nests of poorly differentiated small hyperchromatic cells
- Separated by fibrous septae
- Characteristic immunohistochemical and cytogenetic findings

SELECTED REFERENCES

1. Mendis BR et al: Melanotic neuroectodermal tumor of infancy: a histopathological and immunohistochemical study. J Investig Clin Dent. 3(1):68-71, 2012
2. Singh C et al: Cigar-shaped melanin granules in melanotic neuroectodermal tumor of infancy. Diagn Cytopathol. 40(8):716-8, 2012

MELANOTIC NEUROECTODERMAL TUMOR OF INFANCY

Clinical, Imaging, and Microscopic Features

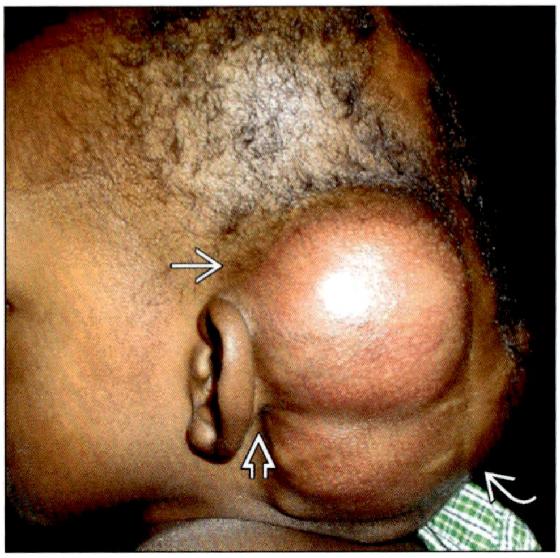
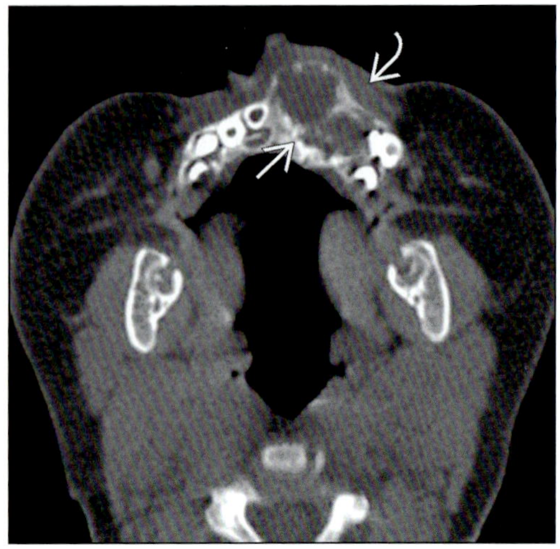

(Left) *Clinical photograph shows a huge mass extending toward parietal squama superiorly and in the upper neck inferiorly behind the displaced left ear. The overlying skin looks normal.* ***(Right)*** *Axial bone CT shows the most common appearance, location, and age for melanotic neuroectodermal tumor: Maxillary expansion with osteolysis and adjacent soft tissue changes in an infant.*

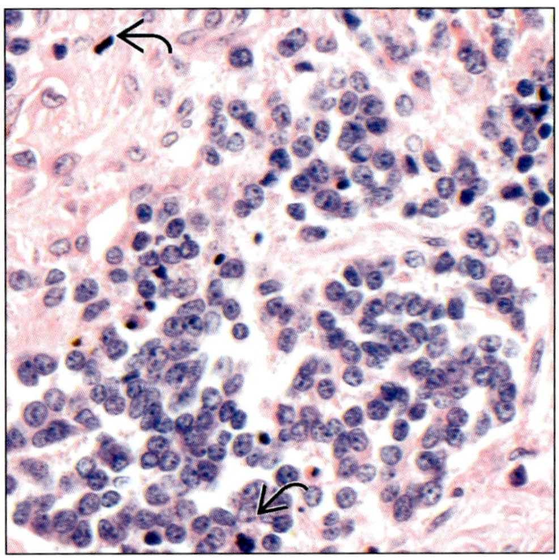
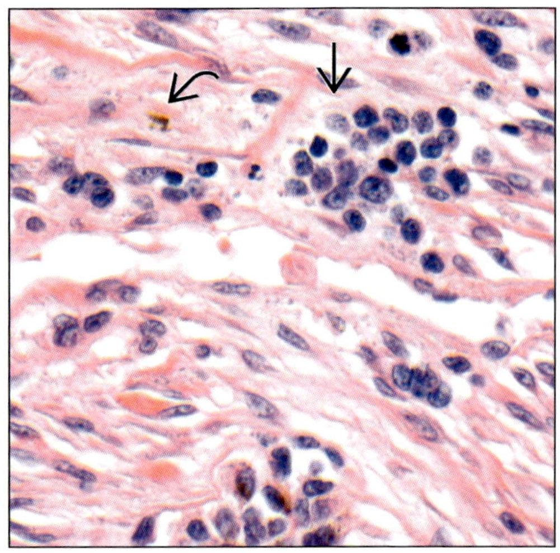

(Left) *High-power view of this nest of small neuroblastic round cells highlights the scant amount of cytoplasm and the small nucleoli with dispersed salt-and-pepper chromatin. Mitotic figures are rarely observed.* ***(Right)*** *Dense fibrous stroma is shown with scattered small neuroblastic cells arranged individually and in nests in this melanotic neuroectodermal tumor of infancy (MNTI). Note that the pigment deposition is minimal.*

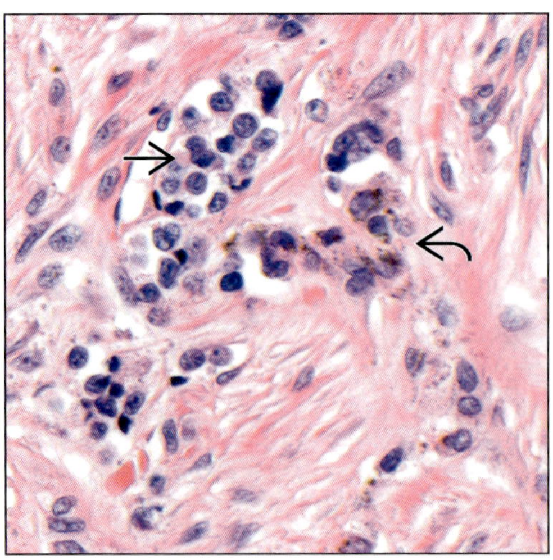
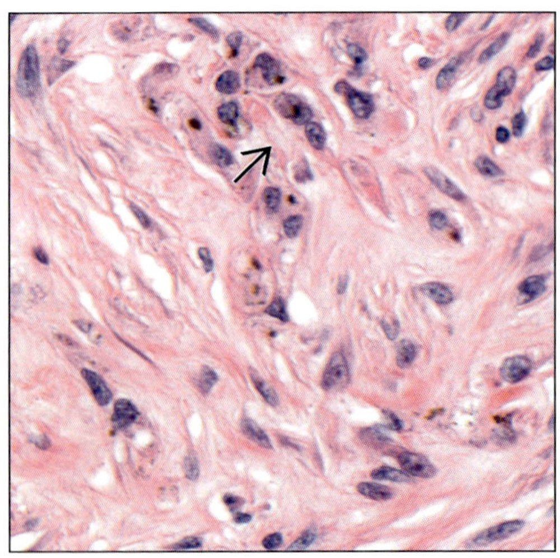

(Left) *A mixture of pigmented epithelial cells and small neuroblastic cells separated by dense fibrocollagenous stroma show an alveolar pattern of growth in this MNTI. Note the crush artifact in the small hyperchromatic small cells.* ***(Right)*** *Dense fibrous stroma is shown with scattered small neuroblastic cells arranged individually and in cords with pigment deposition in this MNTI. Note the lack of a prominent epithelial component in this field.*

Imaging, Gross, and Microscopic Features

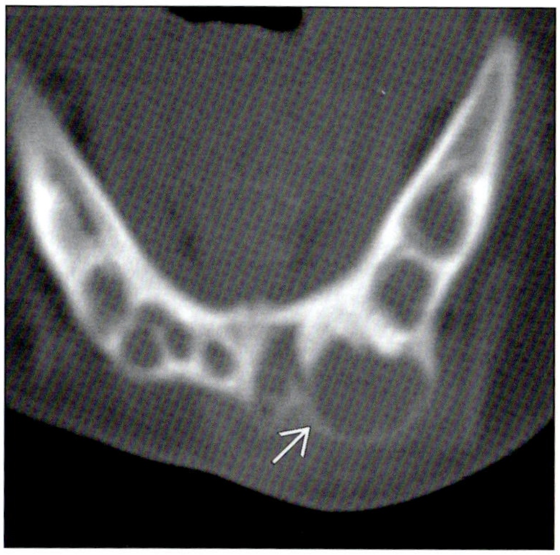

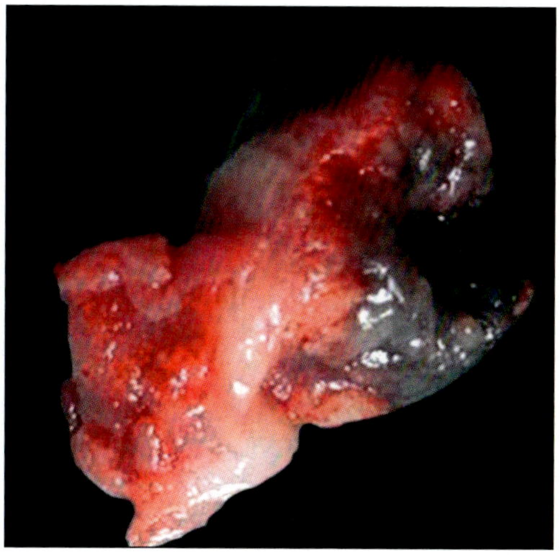

(Left) *CT shows a maxillary expansion with osteolysis* → *and adjacent soft tissue changes in an infant. These are the most common appearance, location, and age for melanotic neuroectodermal tumor. (Courtesy J. Hille, MDS, DDS.)* ***(Right)*** *Gross specimen of a melanotic neuroectodermal tumor of infancy in the maxilla of a young child shows a dark pigmented area in 1 side of the specimen corresponding to an area of heavy pigment deposition.*

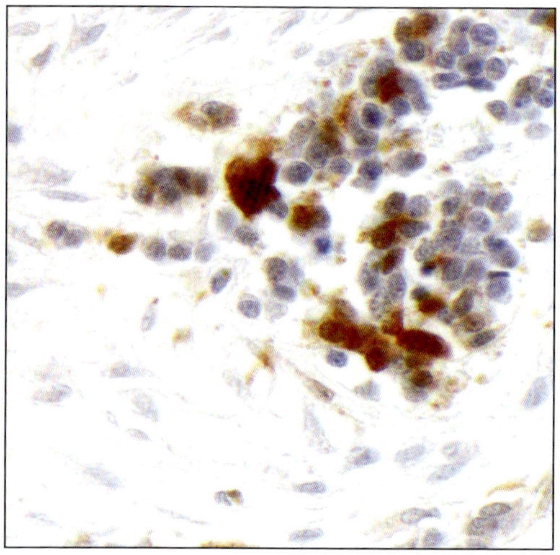

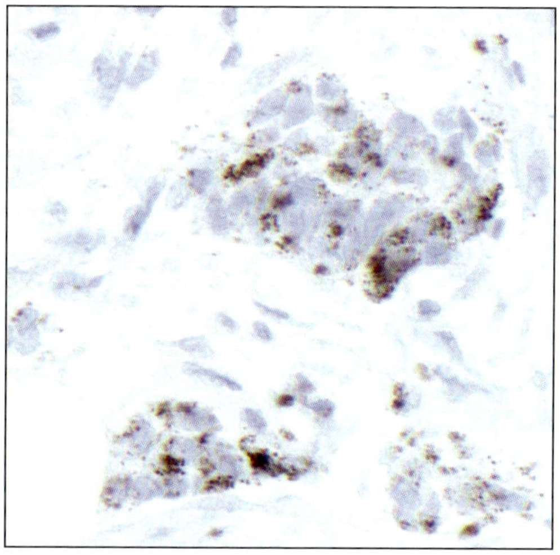

(Left) *Immunohistochemical staining for NSE shows strong cytoplasmic reactivity in both the epithelial and small neuroblastic cellular components.* ***(Right)*** *Immunohistochemical staining for Melan-A shows a finely granular cytoplasmic reactivity predominantly in the small neuroblastic cellular component. This figure also shows rare immunopositivity in the epithelial cells.*

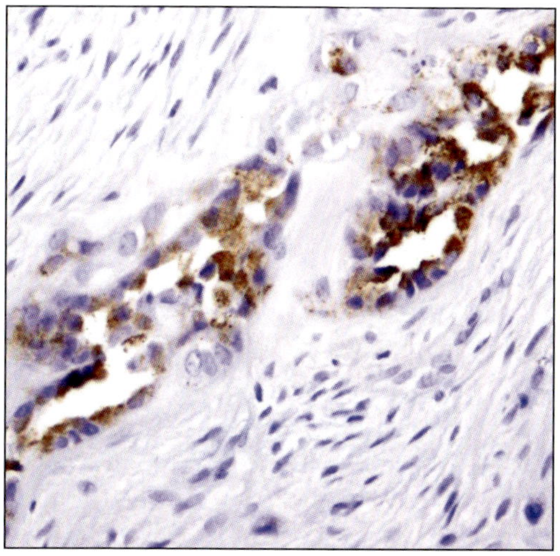

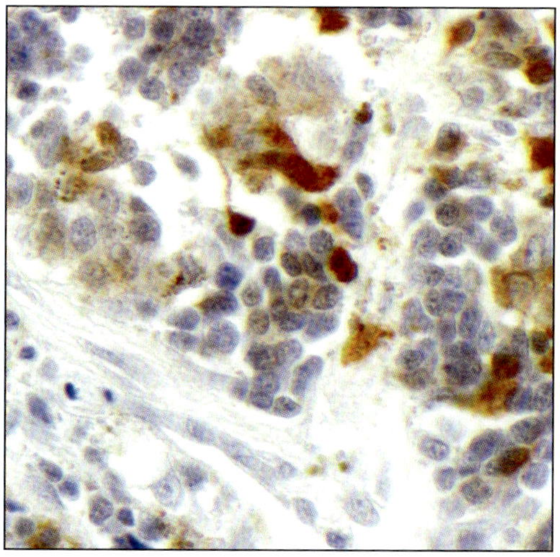

(Left) *Immunohistochemical reactivity for HMB-45 is observed in the cytoplasm of the epithelial cells. The other makers for these cells are keratins, vimentin, NSE, and epithelial membrane antigen.* ***(Right)*** *Immunohistochemical staining for synaptophysin shows strong cytoplasmic reactivity in both the epithelial and small neuroblastic cellular components.*

OSTEOSARCOMA

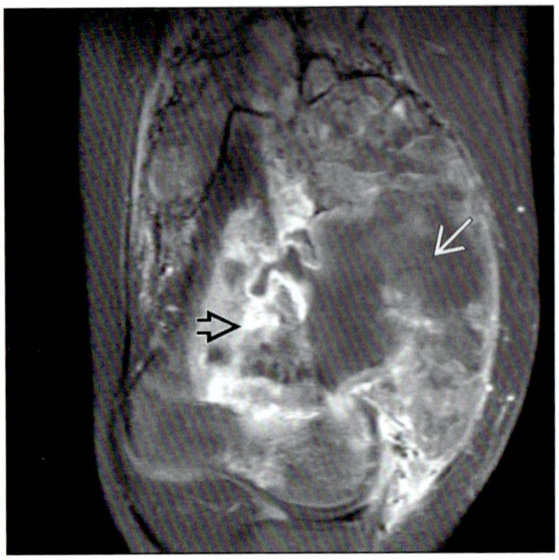

Coronal T1WI C+ MR of an osteosarcoma of the distal femur shows a very destructive bone lesion ➢ with a large soft tissue mass ➔.

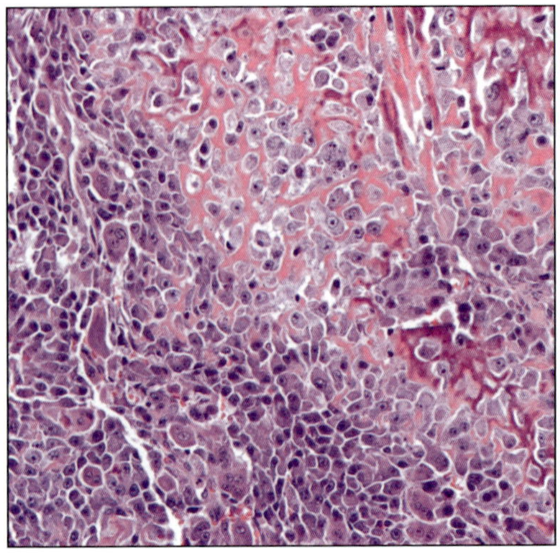

Conventional osteosarcoma demonstrates sheets of malignant osteoblasts intimately associated with the production of pink, lace-like osteoid and neoplastic bone.

TERMINOLOGY

Synonyms

- Osteogenic sarcoma

Definitions

- High-grade malignant tumor in which neoplastic cells directly produce bone

ETIOLOGY/PATHOGENESIS

Neoplastic Process

- Primary osteosarcomas arise de novo without a known predisposing condition
- Secondary osteosarcomas arise within a diseased bone
  - Paget disease of bone
  - Radiation exposure
  - Chemotherapy
  - Trauma
  - Foreign body (e.g., orthopedic implants)
  - Certain genetic abnormalities

Genetic Susceptibility

- Hereditary retinoblastoma: Germline mutation in *RB1* gene
- Li-Fraumeni syndrome: Germline mutation in *TP53*
- Rothmund-Thomson syndrome
  - Skin lesions, photosensitivity, hypogonadism, psychomotor retardation, and various skeletal abnormalities

CLINICAL ISSUES

Epidemiology

- Incidence
  - Most common primary malignant tumor of bone; exclusive of hematopoietic malignancies
    - Accounts for ~ 20% of primary bone sarcomas
- Age
  - Most patients are young, between 10 and 20 years
    - Females usually younger than males, probably due to earlier skeletal development
  - 2nd peak occurs in patients > 50 years (usually secondary osteosarcoma)
- Gender
  - More common in males than females (1.3:1)

Site

- Most commonly arises in long tubular bones
  - Distal femur > proximal tibia > proximal humerus
    - 50% of cases located in knee region
- In older individuals, pelvis and axial skeleton are most common locations
- < 10% occur in mandible and craniofacial bones

Presentation

- Progressively enlarging painful mass
  - Pain is deep seated and frequently noted months prior to diagnosis
  - Intensity of pain increases over time, eventually producing unremitting discomfort
- May appear as visible and palpable mass
- Overlying skin may be warm, erythematous, edematous, and cartographed by prominent engorged veins
  - Ulceration of skin secondary to pressure ischemia can occur
- Large tumors may restrict range of motion
- May cause joint effusions when tumor involves epiphysis or periarticular structures
- Patients with advanced cases may have weight loss and cachexia
- In 5-10% of cases, heralding event is pathologic fracture through tumor

Laboratory Tests

- Elevated serum alkaline phosphatase

OSTEOSARCOMA

Key Facts

Terminology
- High-grade malignant tumor in which neoplastic cells produce bone

Etiology/Pathogenesis
- Primary osteosarcomas arise de novo without a known predisposing condition
- Secondary osteosarcomas arise within a diseased bone
  - Paget disease of bone
  - Radiation exposure
  - Chemotherapy
  - Trauma
  - Foreign body
  - Certain genetic abnormalities
- Hereditary retinoblastoma: Germline mutation in *RB1* gene
- Li-Fraumeni syndrome: Germline mutation in *TP53*
- Rothmund-Thomson syndrome
  - Skin lesions, photosensitivity, hypogonadism, psychomotor retardation, and various skeletal abnormalities

Clinical Issues
- Most patients are young, between 10 and 20 years
- Distal femur > proximal tibia > proximal humerus

Microscopic Pathology
- Admixture of 2 elements in varying proportions
  - High-grade sarcoma with epithelioid, plasmacytoid, fusiform, ovoid, small round cells, clear cells, mono- or multinucleated giant cells, or spindle cells
  - Bone matrix produced directly by tumor

Treatment
- Surgical approaches
  - Limb salvage; complete excision with wide negative margins is optimal
    - Biopsy tract is often removed with tumor
  - Amputation necessary if major vessels and nerves compromised, if tumor involves region that cannot be reconstructed, or if pathologic fracture or surgical intervention has contaminated large volumes of tissue
- Adjuvant therapy
  - Preoperative chemotherapy often administered
    - May diminish tumor in size
    - Tumor often undergoes more extensive mineralization and develops a more developed pseudocapsule facilitating excision
    - Chemotherapeutic efficacy can be determined by histologic assessment of amount of necrosis induced in tumor
    - Tumor-induced necrosis of ≥ 90% considered good response and important prognostic indicator
- Drugs
  - Cisplatin, high-dose methotrexate, ifosfamide
- Radiation
  - Definitive treatment used for unresectable tumors because of size &/or site
  - Definitive radiation may be used to treat tumors in patients with widely metastatic disease who are considered incurable
  - Adjuvant radiation may be used if surgical excision is associated with positive margins

Prognosis
- Relapse-free survival rates reported to vary from 50-80% (median: ~ 70%)
- Of conventional osteosarcoma subtypes, chondroblastic variant has been shown to be associated with a poor preoperative chemotherapy response

IMAGE FINDINGS

Radiographic Findings
- Permeative and destructive lesion
- Centered around metaphysis of long bones (very rarely epiphysis)
- Poorly defined with a lack of sclerotic rim
- Mixed lytic and blastic mass transgressing cortex and forming large soft tissue components
  - 90% extend into soft issue
- Visible matrix present in 90% of cases
  - Periphery of lesion usually less mineralized than central area
- Soft tissue components may have fine "cloud-like" pattern of radiodensity
- In some instances, tumor is entirely lytic or sclerotic
  - Entirely lytic appearance is characteristic of telangiectatic variant
- Lower grade lesions tend to be more mineralized
- Periosteal reaction
  - Reactive woven bone is deposited between cortex and periosteum elevated by tumor
  - Appears either as multiple layers (onion skin) or radiating (sunburst) appearance
  - Codman triangle: Term used to describe periosteal reaction at diaphyseal end of tumor at angle created by cortex and elevated periosteum
- Rarely, imaging appears deceptively benign
- < 10% of lesions are diaphyseal

MR Findings
- Heterogeneous metaphyseal mass
- MR helpful in detecting skip lesions in same or adjacent bone
- Osteoid shows low signal on all sequences
- T1WI: Nonosteoid portions of tumor are near isointense to skeletal muscle
- Fluid sensitive sequences: Tumor appears heterogeneous

OSTEOSARCOMA

CT Findings
- Useful in defining bone matrix
- Useful when planning surgery and delineating extent of tumor

Bone Scan
- Increased activity in primary tumor and metastasis

MACROSCOPIC FEATURES

General Features
- Intramedullary
- Usually centered in metaphysis, but can involve any portion of bone
- Tumors containing abundant mineralized bone are tan-white and hard
- Nonmineralized cartilaginous components are glistening and gray
  - May be mucinous if matrix is myxoid, or more rubbery if hyaline in nature
- Areas of hemorrhage and cystic change
  - When extensive, produce a friable, bloody, and spongy mass (telangiectatic osteosarcoma)
- Tumor usually destroys overlying cortex and forms eccentric or circumferential soft tissue component displacing periosteum peripherally
- Dislodged periosteum becomes sharp interface between mass and bordering skeletal muscle and fat
- Layer of reactive bone at proximal and distal regions where periosteum 1st lifted from cortex
- Growth into joint space may occur
  - Growth may occur through synovium, via extension along cortical surface, or through tendoligamentous and joint capsule insertion sites
- Open growth plates often function as effective barriers to advancing tumors
  - Penetration of physis and invasion through epiphysis to base of articular surface occurs in some cases
- Skip metastases appear as intramedullary firm, ovoid, tan-white nodules located adjacent to or far from main mass
- Variants of osteosarcoma confined to surface of bone occur but are uncommon

MICROSCOPIC PATHOLOGY

Histologic Features
- Admixture of 2 elements in varying proportions
  - High-grade sarcoma with epithelioid, plasmacytoid, fusiform, ovoid, small round cells, clear cells, mono- or multinucleated giant cells, or spindle cells
  - Bone matrix produced directly by tumor
    - Mineralized (bone) and unmineralized (osteoid)
- Nuclei are hyperchromatic, and central or eccentric in position
  - Brisk mitotic activity and prominent nucleoli are common
  - Degree of atypia variable but frequently severe
  - Numerous mitoses, commonly including atypical forms
- Cytoplasm is eosinophilic and variable in volume
- Tumor cells intimately related to surface of neoplastic bone
  - Tumor cells diminish in size and appear less atypical as they are surrounded and imprisoned by matrix
    - In heavily mineralized portions of tumor, neoplastic cells lack atypia
    - This phenomenon is referred to as normalization
- Neoplastic bone is woven in architecture and varies in quantity
  - Deposited as primitive, disorganized trabeculae producing coarse, lace-like pattern or broad, large sheets formed by coalescing trabeculae
  - Bone is frequently mineralized
  - In some instances, neoplastic bone uses preexisting trabeculae as a scaffold
  - Neoplastic lamellar bone is very rare
- Bone is eosinophilic or basophilic and may have pagetoid appearance caused by haphazardly deposited cement lines
- Neoplastic cartilage, when present, is usually hyaline, but may be predominately myxoid, particularly in tumors arising in jaw bones
- Malignant chondrocytes demonstrate severe cytologic atypia
- Fibroblastic foci manifest as cytologically malignant spindle cells arranged in a herringbone or storiform pattern without direct bone formation

ANCILLARY TESTS

Immunohistochemistry
- Immunoprofile is nonspecific and of minimal help in diagnosis
- May be positive for keratin and epithelial membrane antigen
- Cartilaginous areas are positive for S100
- CD99 is frequently positive

Molecular Genetics
- Virtually all osteosarcomas contain clonal chromosomal aberrations
- Aberrations are complex, comprising abundance of numerical and structural alterations
- No specific translocation has been identified in conventional osteosarcoma

DIFFERENTIAL DIAGNOSIS

Fibrosarcoma (Malignant Fibrous Histiocytoma)
- Fibrosarcoma lacks tumor bone directly abutted by neoplastic cells
- Distinction between intraosseous fibrosarcoma and osteosarcoma is frequently an academic one
  - Chemotherapeutic regimens are similar

Fracture Callus
- Bone is rimmed by osteoblasts

- Fracture site shows fibrocartilage, a finding not seen in either osteosarcoma or chondrosarcoma
- Atypical mitotic figures are not seen
- Radiographic features frequently assist in making this distinction

Osteoblastoma

- Distinction between osteoblastoma-like osteosarcoma and aggressive osteoblastoma is often challenging
- Features supporting diagnosis of osteosarcoma include
  - Infiltration of preexisting bony trabeculae
  - Large size (> 5 cm)
  - Atypical mitotic figures
  - Prominent and abundant lace-like tumor bone deposition
- Osteoblastoma typically shows interconnecting trabeculae of tumor bone lined by plump osteoblasts

Chondrosarcoma

- In chondroblastic osteosarcomas and some gnathic osteosarcomas, bone may be scarce
- Extensive sampling will generally reveal foci of bone
- Cartilaginous tumor with marked atypia, particularly in 2nd and 3rd decades of life, is highly suspicious for osteosarcoma
- Presence of *IDH1* or *IDH2* mutations supports diagnosis of chondrosarcoma

Dedifferentiated Chondrosarcoma

- Characterized by presence of low-grade cartilage juxtaposed to high-grade sarcoma (dedifferentiated component)
- Rarely, dedifferentiated component may be osteosarcoma

Myositis Ossificans

- Both soft tissue and parosteal myositis ossificans may be mistaken for osteosarcoma
- Distinct zonal pattern is characteristic of myositis ossificans and is not seen in osteosarcoma
  - Grossly and on imaging, periphery of lesion is mineralized whereas center lacks mineralization
  - Microscopically, central portion of lesion shows granulation tissue/nodular fasciitis-like appearance whereas periphery shows woven bone lined by osteoblasts, with outermost layer of lamellar bone in mature lesions

Giant Cell Tumor

- May show reactive woven bone formation around periphery
- Unlike osteosarcoma, bone in giant cell tumor is lined by osteoblasts and not atypical tumor cells

Metastatic Carcinoma

- Metastatic breast and prostate carcinoma may evoke robust osteoblastic reaction
- Appropriate immunohistochemical studies assist in making this distinction

Ewing Sarcoma

- Small cell variant of osteosarcoma may mimic Ewing sarcoma
- In > 95% of cases, FISH will demonstrate rearrangement of *EWSR1* gene

Aneurysmal Bone Cyst

- May mimic telangiectatic osteosarcoma
- Cells in cyst wall not severely atypical

DIAGNOSTIC CHECKLIST

Pathologic Interpretation Pearls

- At least focal bone production by malignant cells is necessary to render diagnosis of osteosarcoma
- Ancillary tests do not help in identifying bone
- Distinction between bone and nonosseous collagen may be difficult, and at times arbitrary
- Delicate lace-like deposition of mineralized eosinophilic matrix is highly suggestive of neoplastic bone

Assessment of Chemotherapy Effect

- Complete (grade 4) or near complete (grade 3) > 90% necrosis of tumor is associated with survival advantage
- Assessment of necrosis should be performed by histologically evaluating a central slice of tumor and sampling remaining halves
- Extent of necrosis on preoperative chemotherapy may be used to alter postoperative regimen

SELECTED REFERENCES

1. Deyrup AT et al: Sarcomas arising in Paget disease of bone: a clinicopathologic analysis of 70 cases. Arch Pathol Lab Med. 131(6):942-6, 2007
2. Mankin HJ et al: Survival data for 648 patients with osteosarcoma treated at one institution. Clin Orthop Relat Res. (429):286-91, 2004
3. Ozaki T et al: Genetic imbalances revealed by comparative genomic hybridization in osteosarcomas. Int J Cancer. 102(4):355-65, 2002
4. Bridge JA et al: Cytogenetic findings in 73 osteosarcoma specimens and a review of the literature. Cancer Genet Cytogenet. 95(1):74-87, 1997
5. Nishida J et al: Malignant fibrous histiocytoma of bone. A clinicopathologic study of 81 patients. Cancer. 79(3):482-93, 1997
6. Raymond AK et al: Osteosarcoma. Specimen management following primary chemotherapy. Hematol Oncol Clin North Am. 9(4):841-67, 1995
7. Glasser DB et al: Survival, prognosis, and therapeutic response in osteogenic sarcoma. The Memorial Hospital experience. Cancer. 69(3):698-708, 1992
8. Unni KK et al: Osteosarcoma: pathology and classification. Semin Roentgenol. 24(3):143-52, 1989
9. Rosen G et al: Primary osteogenic sarcoma: eight-year experience with adjuvant chemotherapy. J Cancer Res Clin Oncol. 106 Suppl:55-67, 1983
10. Dahlin DC et al: Osteosarcoma of bone and its important recognizable varieties. Am J Surg Pathol. 1(1):61-72, 1977

OSTEOSARCOMA

Gross, Imaging, and Microscopic Features

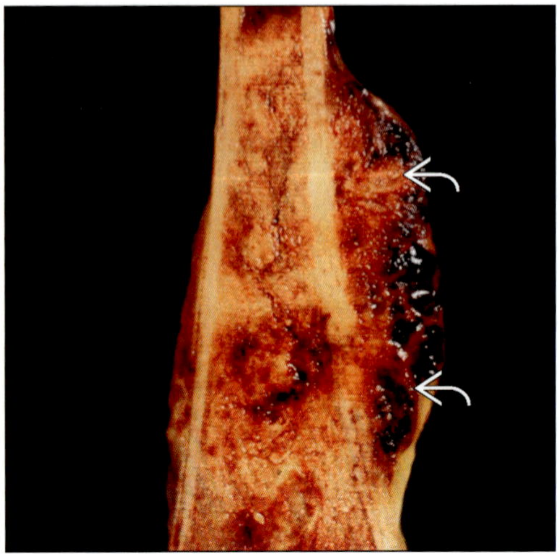

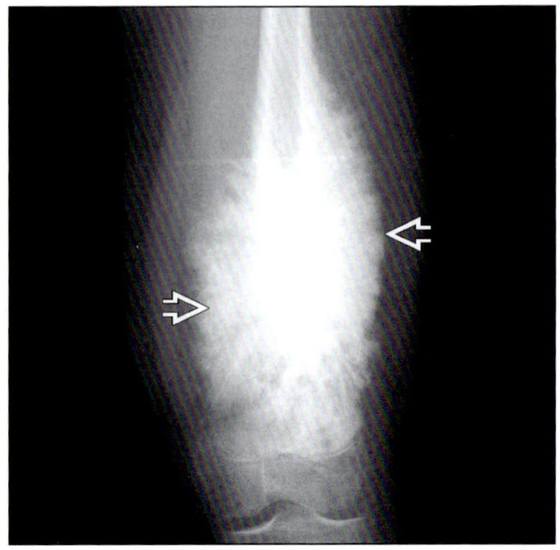

(Left) *Osteosarcoma most commonly arises in the region of the knee (distal femur shown here). This gross photograph shows the characteristic metadiaphyseal origin of this destructive tumor as well as foci of soft tissue extension ➔. (Courtesy A. Hough, MD.)* ***(Right)*** *This anteroposterior radiograph of an osteosarcoma of the left femur shows an extensive and impressive periosteal reaction ➔. This particular pattern is described as a sunburst pattern.*

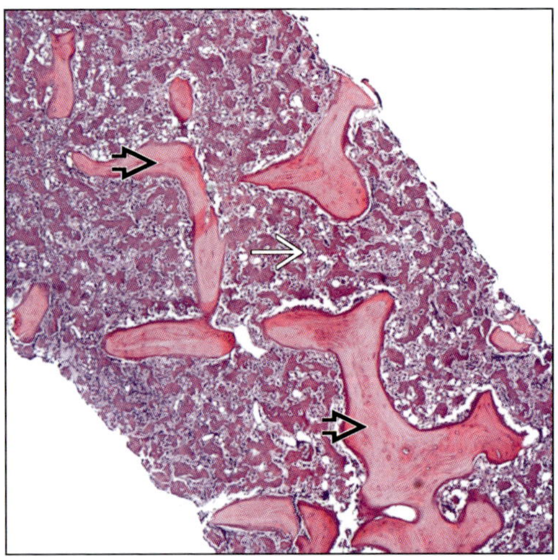

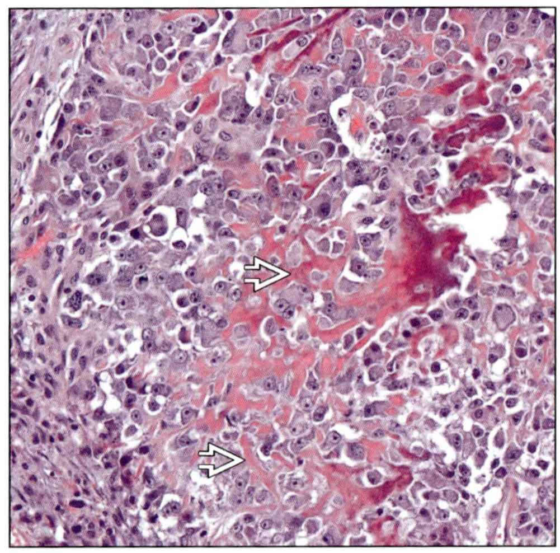

(Left) *Osteosarcoma is a highly permeative neoplasm. This image shows the malignant cells ➔ and neoplastic woven bone growing between and around normal host mature trabecular bone ⇨.* ***(Right)*** *Malignant osteoblasts directly associated with the production of osteoid or woven (immature) bone is characteristic of osteosarcoma. Osteoid ➔ is classically depicted as very thin seams of glassy pink material that insinuate between individual neoplastic cells ("filigree pattern").*

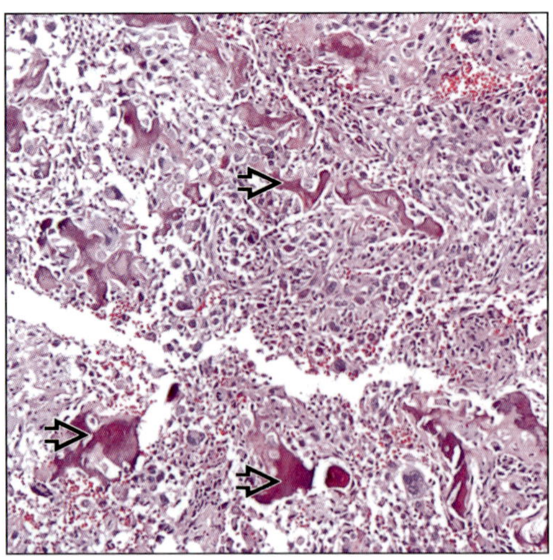

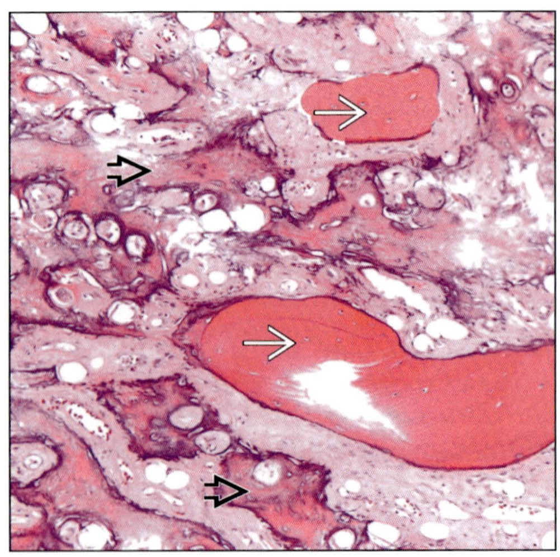

(Left) *Foci of neoplastic bone production vary widely in size, shape, and distribution from 1 tumor to the next. Mineralized foci demonstrate a purple or blue glassy appearance ⇨.* ***(Right)*** *Osteosarcomas treated by specific chemotherapy regimens often show areas in which the infiltrating malignant cells are eliminated, leaving behind the neoplastic bone ⇨ they had produced. Note that the overall permeative relationship with the host trabecular bone ➔ is retained.*

Microscopic Features

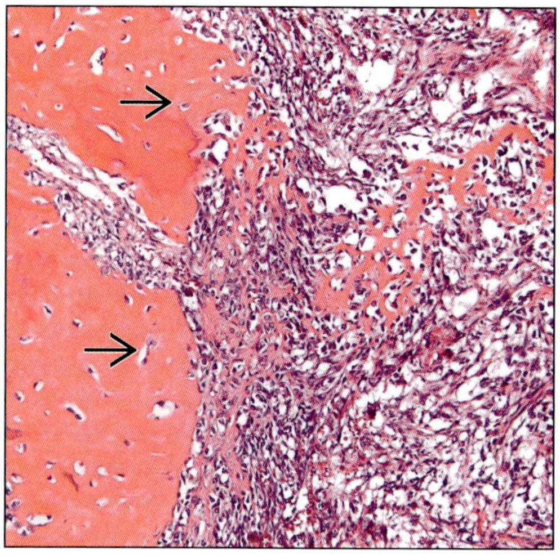

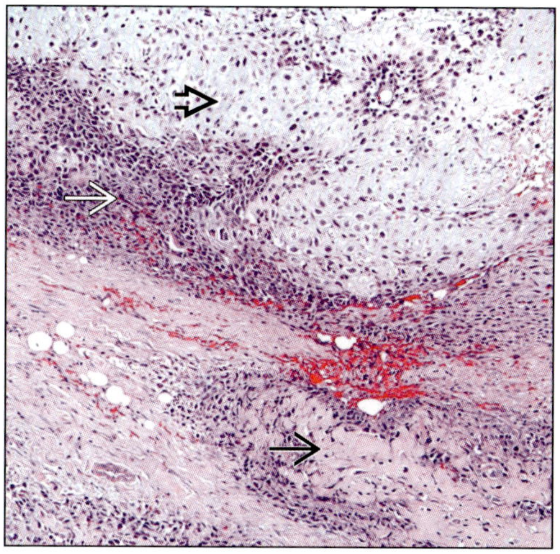

(Left) As bone is produced, the neoplastic cells → may become entrapped within it and will show a reduction in size and loss or decrease in cytologic atypia. This phenomenon has been described as normalization. **(Right)** Although the majority of osteosarcomas are osteoblastic (bone forming), some tumors demonstrate areas of malignant cartilage ⇨ (chondroblastic osteosarcoma). Note the increased peripheral cellularity ➡ and presence of osteoid →.

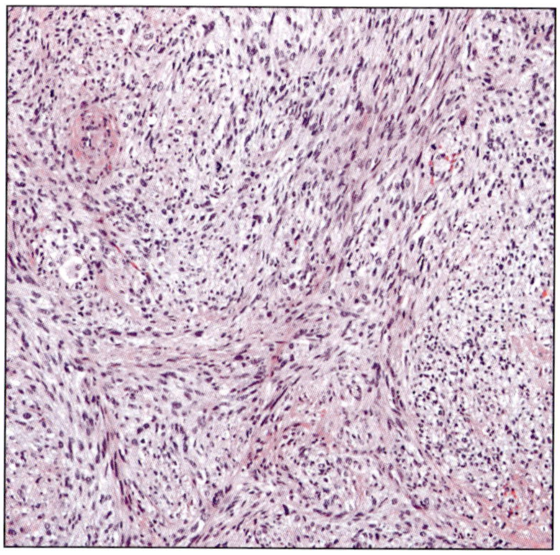

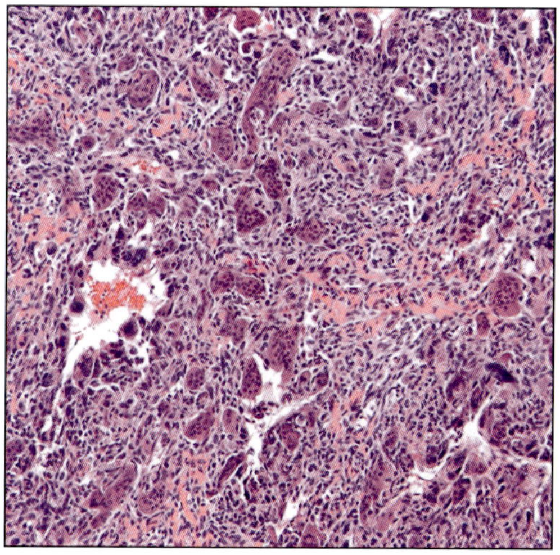

(Left) Some areas within an osteosarcoma may demonstrate a spindled and fascicular morphology (fibroblastic osteosarcoma). Neoplastic bone formation in these areas may be very focal or absent. **(Right)** This image shows a giant-cell-rich osteosarcoma. In these tumors, the osteoclast-like giant cells are often numerous and can lead to diagnostic confusion with other entities, such as malignant giant cell tumor and metastatic carcinoma containing giant cells.

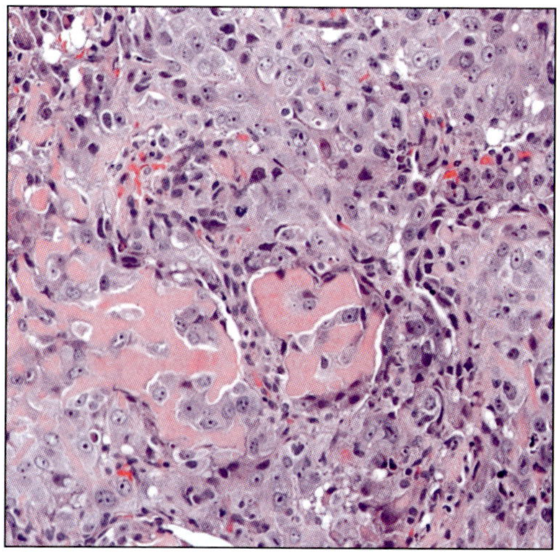

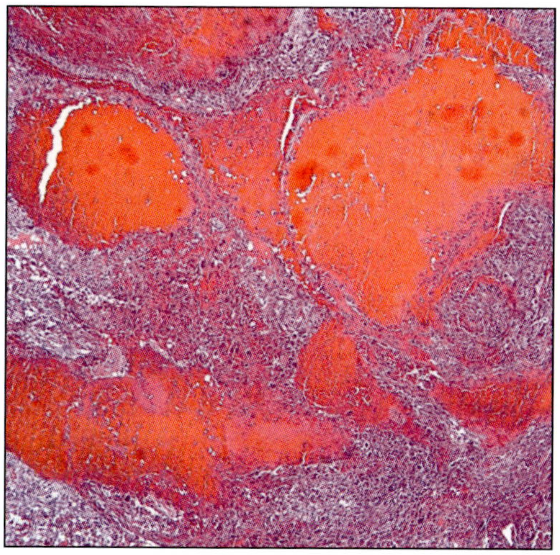

(Left) This image shows an osteosarcoma with a prominent population of plump epithelioid malignant osteoblasts. This cellular morphology may mimic a metastatic osteoblastic carcinoma. Note the osteoid production. **(Right)** Most osteosarcomas contain hemorrhagic foci; however, in some cases these hemorrhagic and cystic changes are extensive (telangiectatic osteosarcoma). This variant resembles an aneurysmal bone cyst.

RHABDOMYOSARCOMA

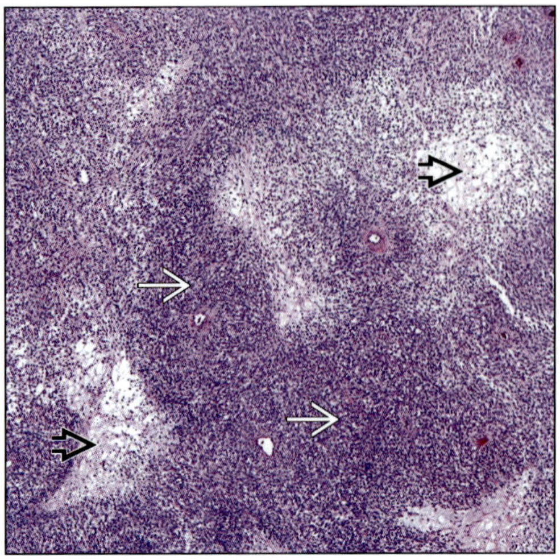

At low magnification, embryonal rhabdomyosarcoma (ERMS) characteristically shows a mixture of both hypercellular ➡ and hypocellular ⇨ areas.

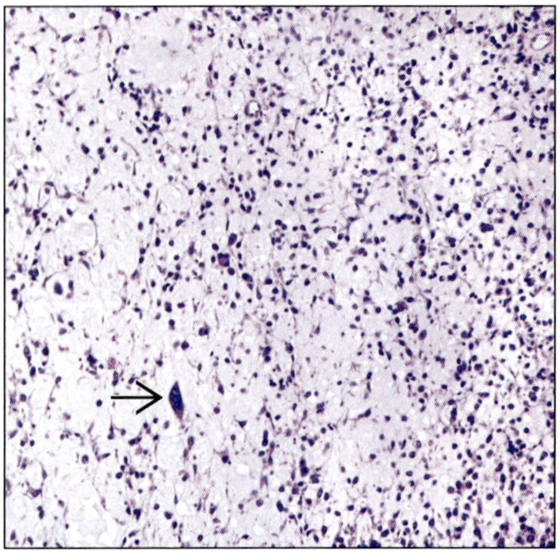

ERMS is generally composed of primitive spindled to ovoid cells with eosinophilic cytoplasm. Nuclear pleomorphism ⇨ &/or anaplasia may be focal or diffuse.

TERMINOLOGY

Abbreviations

- Rhabdomyosarcoma (RMS)

Definitions

- Malignant mesenchymal neoplasm that shows variable differentiation toward skeletal muscle
- Most common subtypes include embryonal, alveolar, spindle cell, sclerosing, and pleomorphic

ETIOLOGY/PATHOGENESIS

Genetic Events

- Alveolar rhabdomyosarcoma (ARMS) has characteristic balanced translocations
  - t(2;13)(q35;q14), *PAX3-FOXO1*
    - Most common (60% of cases)
  - t(1;13)(p36;q14), *PAX1-FOXO1*
    - Approximately 15% of cases
- Embryonal and other subtypes of RMS do not show reproducible translocations

Genetic Associations

- Certain inherited diseases increase the risk of developing RMS
  - Li-Fraumeni syndrome
  - Neurofibromatosis type 1 (NF1)
  - Beckwith-Wiedemann syndrome
  - Costello syndrome
  - Noonan syndrome

CLINICAL ISSUES

Epidemiology

- Incidence
  - RMS is most frequent soft tissue sarcoma in children and young adults
    - Embryonal rhabdomyosarcoma (ERMS) is most common subtype (60-70% of RMS)
    - ARMS is 2nd most common subtype (30% of RMS)
    - Spindle cell, sclerosing, and pleomorphic subtypes are much less common
- Age
  - Mostly children and adolescents
    - ERMS generally affects younger population than ARMS
  - Most cases of RMS in adults are pleomorphic, spindle cell, and sclerosing subtypes
  - Very rare cases of RMS are congenital
- Gender
  - M = F
    - Pleomorphic subtype more common in men

Site

- Embryonal subtype
  - Head and neck (particularly orbital and parameningeal sites)
  - Genitourinary region (bladder, prostate, paratesticular soft tissue)
  - Other sites including vagina, retroperitoneum, pelvis, biliary tract
  - Much less frequent involvement of trunk and limbs than ARMS
- Alveolar subtype
  - Most common in deep soft tissue of the extremities
  - Also head and neck, trunk, pelvis, retroperitoneum, perineum
- Pleomorphic subtype
  - Deep soft tissues of the extremities (particularly thigh)
  - Also abdomen, retroperitoneum, other sites
- Spindle cell subtype
  - Most common in head and neck region (50% of cases)
  - Paratesticular region
  - Retroperitoneum, extremities, vulva, other sites

RHABDOMYOSARCOMA

Key Facts

Terminology

- Malignant mesenchymal neoplasm that shows variable differentiation toward skeletal muscle
- Most common subtypes include embryonal (including botryoides), alveolar, spindle cell, sclerosing, and pleomorphic

Clinical Issues

- Rhabdomyosarcomas (RMS) are most frequent soft tissue sarcomas in children and young adults
  - Embryonal RMS (ERMS) subtype is most common
- Site varies depending on subtype; however, head and neck and extremities are common
- Multimodality approach to therapy (surgery, chemo, and radiation)
- Main prognostic parameters are histologic type, disease stage, and site
  - Pleomorphic and sclerosing subtypes are most aggressive

Macroscopic Features

- Tan-white fleshy to firm fibrous cut surface with hemorrhage, necrosis
- Botryoid variant of ERMS grows exophytically from mucosal surface

Microscopic Pathology

- Varies widely by subtype
- Rhabdomyoblasts most common in embryonal and spindle cell subtypes
- Wreath-like giant cells seen in ARMS

Ancillary Tests

- Desmin diffusely positive in most cases of RMS
- Myogenin and MYOD1 focally to diffusely positive

- Sclerosing subtype
  - Extremities and head and neck sites are most common

Presentation

- Suddenly enlarging mass
  - Local symptoms pertaining to site of origin (e.g., deafness, proptosis in head and neck, or urinary retention in genitourinary sites)
- Most are painful, but may be painless

Treatment

- Multimodality approach
- Childhood RMS is generally sensitive to both chemotherapy and radiation therapy
- Complete resection is recommended, if possible

Prognosis

- Main prognostic parameters are histologic type, disease stage, and site
- Favorable sites are head and neck (nonparameningeal), genitourinary (nonbladder, nonprostate), and bile duct
- Botryoid and spindle cell variants in children and adolescents have better prognosis
  - Spindle cell subtype in adults is more clinically aggressive
- ERMS has significantly better prognosis than ARMS
- Pleomorphic subtype shows an aggressive clinical course with frequent metastases
- Sclerosing subtype also has a poor prognosis (often unresectable)

MACROSCOPIC FEATURES

General Features

- Varies in size (usually large)
- Tan-white fleshy to firm fibrous cut surface
- Margins usually infiltrative
- May contain hemorrhage, cystic degeneration, necrosis
- Botryoid RMS (variant of ERMS)
  - Exophytic, polypoid tumor arising from underneath a mucosal surface
  - More circumscribed margins
  - Gelatinous cut surface

MICROSCOPIC PATHOLOGY

Histologic Features

- Embryonal subtype
  - Wide variety of patterns
    - Often loose fascicles and sheets of spindled, stellate, &/or ovoid cells with hyperchromatic or vesicular nuclei
  - Variable cellularity and myxoid stroma
  - Rhabdomyoblasts variable in number
    - Cells with eccentric nuclei and variable amounts of eosinophilic cytoplasm
    - Cytoplasmic cross-striations may be visible
    - Varying shapes (strap cells, tadpole cells, spider cells)
  - Mitoses usually easily discernible
  - Necrosis
  - Botryoid RMS characteristically shows a tightly packed cellular layer of tumor cells (cambium layer) closely abutting the overlying epithelial surface
    - Often contains loose myxoid stroma and may be of relatively low cellularity
  - Anaplastic variant of ERMS shows marked nuclear anaplasia
    - Tumors with sheets of anaplastic cells rather than focal or scattered anaplasia associated with worse prognosis
    - Atypical mitotic figures
    - More conventional areas of ERMS are often present
- Alveolar subtype
  - Poorly differentiated round cells with hyperchromatic, relatively monomorphic nuclei and scanty cytoplasm
    - Nuclear anaplasia is very rare

RHABDOMYOSARCOMA

- Sheets and nests of tumors cells separated by variably thick fibrous septae
  - Central necrosis and loss of cellular cohesion in tumor nests gives the tumor an alveolar appearance
- Rare clear cell appearance
- Rhabdomyoblasts can be present, but are less frequent than in ERMS
- Multinucleated giant cells are characteristic, when present
  - Nuclei are arranged at periphery of giant cell (wreath cell)
- Solid variant of ARMS lacks alveolar growth pattern but has similar cytomorphology to conventional ARMS
  - Solid sheets of neoplastic cells
  - Foci of more conventional ARMS may be present
  - More likely to be translocation negative

- Pleomorphic subtype
  - Densely cellular
  - Morphology is that of an undifferentiated pleomorphic sarcoma
    - Marked nuclear pleomorphism and anaplasia
    - Sheet-like, fascicular, or storiform growth patterns
    - Tumor cells have eosinophilic cytoplasm
    - Atypical mitotic figures and necrosis are common
  - Pleomorphic rhabdomyoblasts may be present
- Spindle cell RMS
  - Elongated spindled cells growing in a predominantly fascicular pattern
    - May have storiform foci
  - Nuclei can be vesicular or hyperchromatic
  - Mitoses common
    - Atypical figures more common in adult cases
  - Variable number of rhabdomyoblasts (spindled or polygonal)
  - Variable amounts of intervening collagen
  - No round cell or pleomorphic areas
  - Necrosis may be seen
- Sclerosing subtype
  - Hyalinized or sclerotic stroma
    - Can mimic osteoid or chondroid matrix (if myxoid)
  - Pseudovascular, microalveolar, cord-like, single cell strand patterns
  - Some areas are solid or fascicular
  - Composed of small round blue cells and spindle cells with scant eosinophilic or clear cytoplasm
  - Rhabdomyoblasts are rare
- Mixed embryonal and alveolar RMS
  - Presence of focal alveolar pattern is associated with reduced survival
  - Tumors with any evidence of alveolar features (morphologic or molecular) behave like and should be classified as ARMS
- Post-chemotherapy RMS
  - Cells often appear more differentiated
    - Larger, more mature rhabdomyoblasts are often evident
    - Possibly residual, better differentiated component is left after selective destruction of undifferentiated tumor cells
  - Fibrosis, myxoid changes, and necrosis are common

ANCILLARY TESTS

Immunohistochemistry

- Desmin diffusely positive in most cases of RMS
  - Expression is more likely to be less diffuse or focal in embryonal and pleomorphic RMS
  - Perinuclear dot-like expression pattern in sclerosing RMS
- Myogenin and MYOD1 variably positive
  - Nuclear expression is specific for RMS
    - Cytoplasmic staining is nonspecific and should be disregarded
  - Expression in ARMS is characteristically strong and diffuse
    - Expression is usually more focal in other subtypes
  - MYOD1 is more likely to be expressed in sclerosing RMS than myogenin
- Variable positivity for smooth muscle actin
- H-caldesmon (-), S100(-)

Molecular Genetics

- Almost all RMS show regions of loss of heterozygosity (LOH)
- Most frequent LOH at chromosome 11
  - 80% of ERMS
  - Both long and short arms
  - LOH at 11p15.5 considered hallmark of ERMS
  - Genes located in 11p15.5 region include those encoding proteins involved in growth regulation
    - Subject to genomic imprinting (parent of origin-specific gene expression)
    - e.g., *IGF2* (paternally expressed) and *CDKN1C* (maternally expressed)
  - Genetic alterations can lead to disruption of imprinted gene expression and cause disease
- ERMS lack *PAX3/7-FOXO1* fusions characteristic of ARMS

DIFFERENTIAL DIAGNOSIS

Embryonal RMS

- Fetal rhabdomyoma
  - Lacks mitoses, nuclear pleomorphism, necrosis
- MPNST and malignant triton tumor
  - Occur more commonly in adults
  - Desmin and myogenin expression limited to rhabdomyosarcomatous component, if present
- Infantile fibrosarcoma
  - Most occur congenitally or in first 2 years of life
  - Characteristic t(12;15) with *NTRK3-ETV6* fusion
  - Does not express myogenic markers

Alveolar RMS

- Ewing sarcoma
  - Soft tissue examples typically occur in older age group than ARMS
  - Strong, diffuse membranous expression of CD99
  - Presence of t(11;22) (*FLI1-EWSR1*) or variants
- Desmoplastic small round cell tumor

RHABDOMYOSARCOMA

Immunohistochemistry

Antibody	Reactivity	Staining Pattern	Comment
Desmin	Positive	Cytoplasmic	
CD56	Positive	Cytoplasmic	
Actin-sm	Positive	Cytoplasmic	Variable positivity
WT1	Positive	Cytoplasmic	Some tumors display cytoplasmic rather than nuclear staining
Myogenin	Positive	Nuclear	Cytoplasmic staining not diagnostic
MYOD1	Positive	Nuclear	Cytoplasmic staining not diagnostic
CD99	Positive	Cell membrane	Some tumors
AE1/AE3	Negative		
Caldesmon	Negative		
CD34	Negative		
S100	Negative		

  - Keratin (+), desmin (+), myogenin (-)
  - Presence of t(11;22) (*WT1-EWSR1*)
- Leukemia/lymphoma
  - Absence of wreath cells
  - Expression of hematopoietic markers (e.g., CD45, CD3, CD20, TdT)
- Malignant extrarenal rhabdoid tumor
  - Predominantly infants
  - Prominent nucleoli are common
  - Loss of nuclear INI-1 by immunohistochemistry
  - Cytokeratin (+), desmin (-), myogenin (-)
- Neuroblastoma
  - NB84 (+), desmin (-), myogenin (-)
  - Infants and young children, often in characteristic locations (follows distribution of sympathetic ganglia)

Pleomorphic RMS

- Pleomorphic leiomyosarcoma
  - Smooth muscle actin (+), desmin (+), H-caldesmon (+), myogenin (-)
  - Often shows better differentiated areas with typical cytoarchitectural features of leiomyosarcoma (fascicular bundles, cigar-shaped nuclei)
- Undifferentiated pleomorphic sarcoma
  - Lacks expression of myogenic markers
  - Distinction is largely academic prognostically
- Malignant triton tumor
  - Contains areas of conventional MPNST
  - Helpful to demonstrate origin from nerve, benign nerve sheath tumor, or within the setting of NF1

Spindle Cell RMS

- Low-grade myofibroblastic sarcoma
  - No rhabdomyoblasts
  - Myogenin (-)
- Leiomyosarcoma
  - Intersecting fascicular architecture with cytologic features of smooth muscle differentiation (cigar-shaped nuclei)
  - Strong smooth muscle actin (+) and H-caldesmon (+); myogenin (-)
- Inflammatory myofibroblastic tumor
  - Prominent stromal inflammatory component, particularly plasma cells
  - ALK1 expression in most cases

Sclerosing RMS

- Extraskeletal osteosarcoma
  - Usually highly pleomorphic
  - Negative for myogenic markers
- Angiosarcoma
  - Expresses vascular markers (CD31, CD34, ERG, etc.)
- Sclerosing epithelioid fibrosarcoma
  - Very similar histologically
  - Younger age group
  - May express MUC4; negative for myogenic markers

SELECTED REFERENCES

1. Williamson D et al: Fusion gene-negative alveolar rhabdomyosarcoma is clinically and molecularly indistinguishable from embryonal rhabdomyosarcoma. J Clin Oncol. 28(13):2151-8, 2010
2. Davicioni E et al: Molecular classification of rhabdomyosarcoma--genotypic and phenotypic determinants of diagnosis: a report from the Children's Oncology Group. Am J Pathol. 174(2):550-64, 2009
3. De Giovanni C et al: Molecular and cellular biology of rhabdomyosarcoma. Future Oncol. 5(9):1449-75, 2009
4. Ognjanovic S et al: Trends in childhood rhabdomyosarcoma incidence and survival in the United States, 1975-2005. Cancer. 115(18):4218-26, 2009
5. Smith AC et al: Growth regulation, imprinted genes, and chromosome 11p15.5. Pediatr Res. 61(5 Pt 2):43R-47R, 2007
6. Gordon T et al: Cytogenetic abnormalities in 42 rhabdomyosarcoma: a United Kingdom Cancer Cytogenetics Group Study. Med Pediatr Oncol. 36(2):259-67, 2001

RHABDOMYOSARCOMA

Microscopic Features

__(Left)__ Some cases of embryonal RMS (ERMS) are very cytologically bland and may be confused with a benign lesion, such as fetal rhabdomyoma. Detection of mitotic activity, nuclear pleomorphism, &/ or necrosis is helpful. __(Right)__ Rhabdomyoblasts → are commonly seen in embryonal and most other subtypes of RMS and are helpful in making the diagnosis. Depending on the morphology, they may be referred to as "strap cells" or "tadpole cells," among other terms.

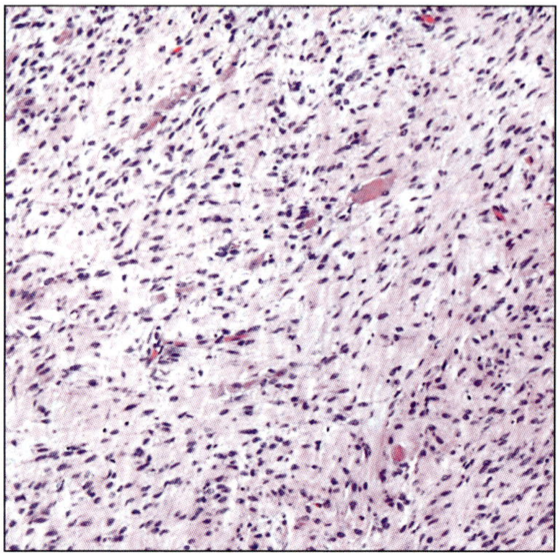

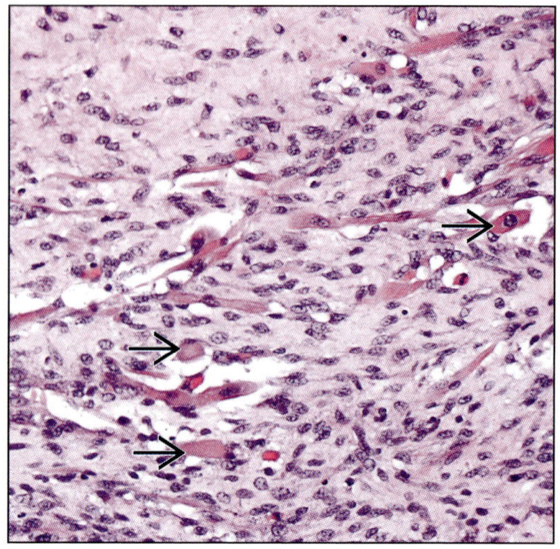

__(Left)__ The botryoid variant of ERMS occurs in a mucosal location and often gives the macroscopic impression of a polyp or "bunch of grapes." Another typical finding is a cambium layer →, which is an increase in tumor cell density directly beneath the epithelium. __(Right)__ Alveolar RMS is composed of relatively monomorphic small round cells with minimal cytoplasm arranged in nests divided by fibrous septae. Many nests typically show a central loss of cellular cohesion →.

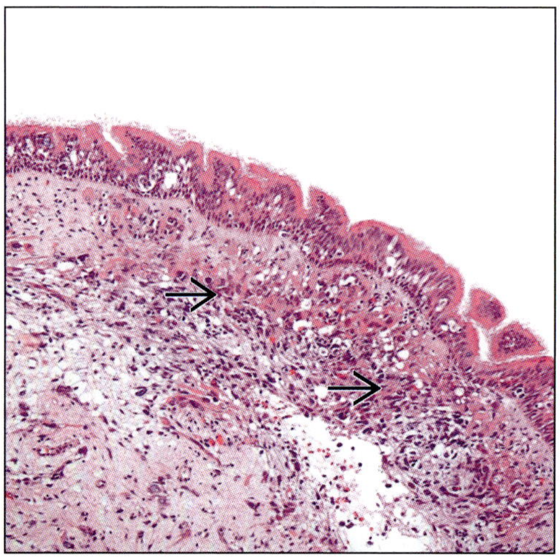

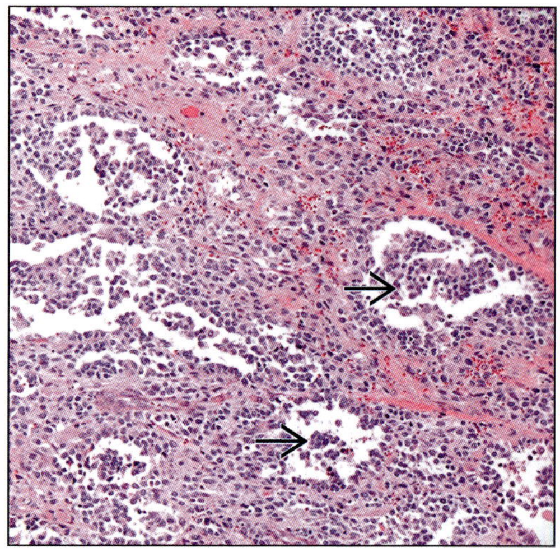

__(Left)__ Another characteristic finding in alveolar RMS is the multinucleated giant cell with peripherally arranged nuclei (wreath cells) →. Although diagnostically useful when present, this cell type is usually very focal or completely absent. __(Right)__ A small subset of cases of alveolar RMS are composed predominantly or exclusively of sheets of neoplastic cells without the usual nested and "pseudoalveolar" growth pattern. This is known as the solid variant of alveolar RMS.

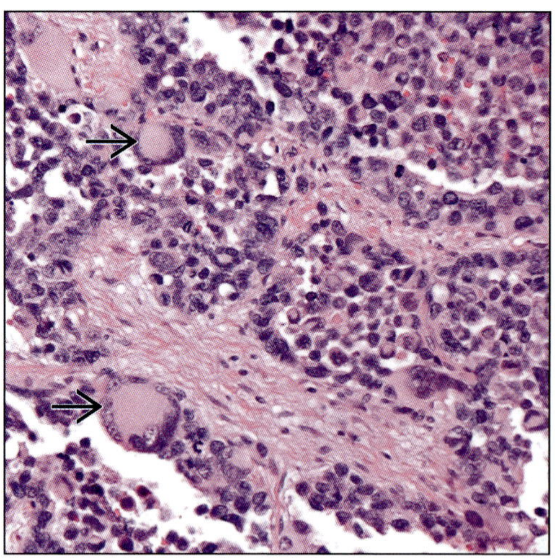

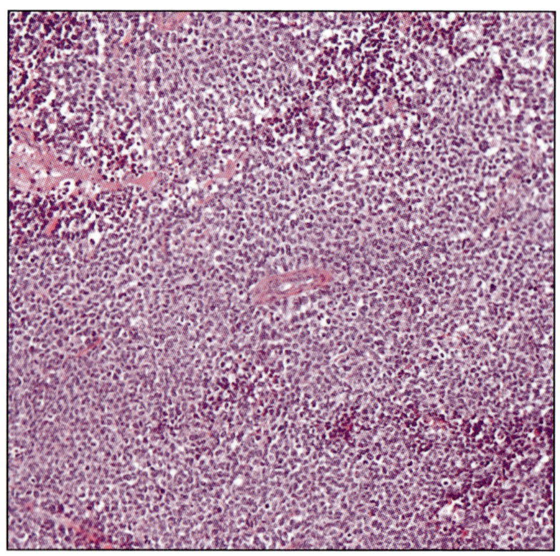

Microscopic Features

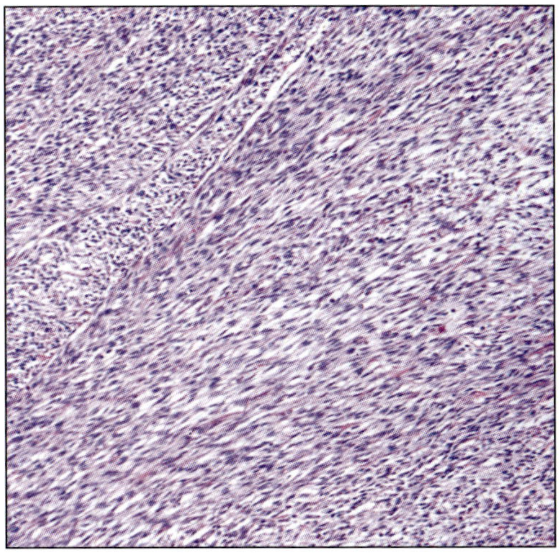
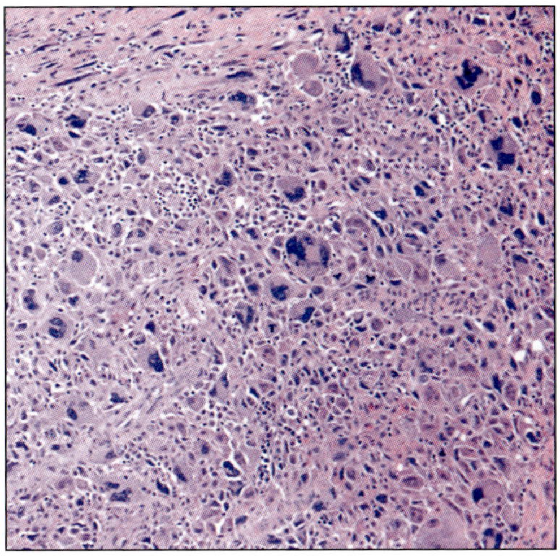

(Left) *Spindle cell RMS is composed of spindled neoplastic cells arranged in fascicles and loose storiform arrays. Rhabdomyoblasts are generally present but are often focal. These tumors have a predilection for the head and neck region.* ***(Right)*** *Pleomorphic RMS is usually characterized by diffuse cytologic anaplasia and is often impossible to distinguish from other pleomorphic sarcomas without IHC. Notably, pleomorphic RMS most commonly occurs in older adults.*

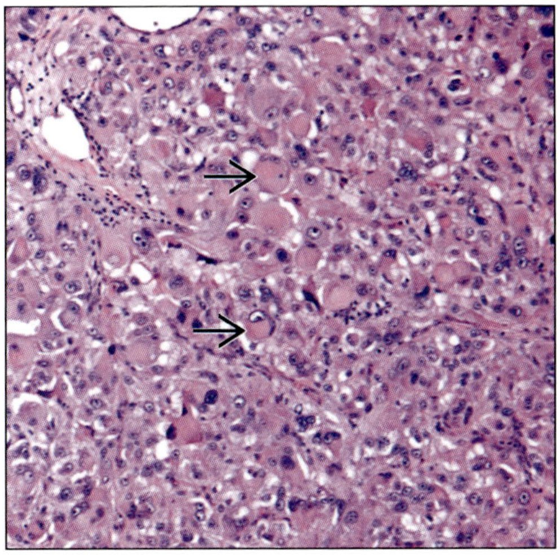
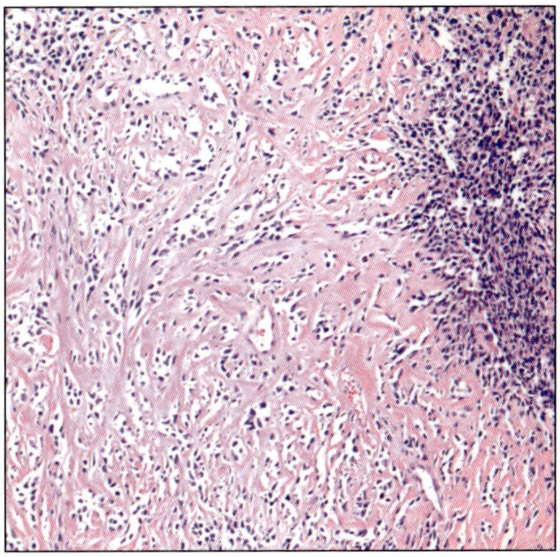

(Left) *Some pleomorphic RMS show sheets of large, eosinophilic rhabdoid cells with prominent cytoplasmic inclusions →. Immunohistochemistry is usually necessary to distinguish this tumor from other similar malignancies.* ***(Right)*** *The sclerosing subtype of RMS shows small hyperchromatic cells within a sclerotic to myxochondroid stromal matrix. The sclerosis may be so prominent that it mimics a vascular neoplasm (particularly angiosarcoma) or other sclerosing malignancy.*

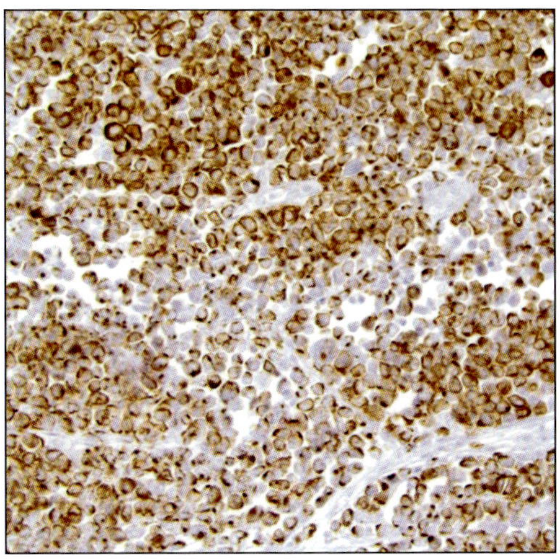
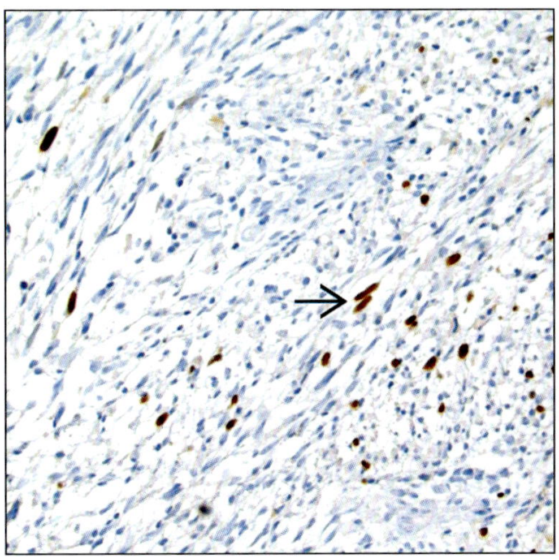

(Left) *Desmin is expressed to some degree in essentially all forms of RMS and is a good screening marker. One particular subtype (sclerosing RMS) is known to show a characteristic perinuclear dot-like pattern of expression.* ***(Right)*** *Myogenin (MYO D1) is a specific marker of skeletal muscle derivation and is helpful in confirming a diagnosis of RMS. Expression may be very focal to diffuse. Most importantly, only nuclear expression → is significant.*

SCHWANNOMA

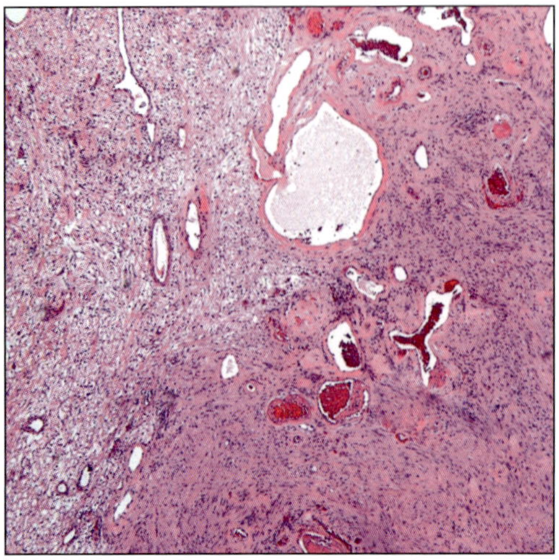

Schwannoma is a common soft tissue neoplasm that occurs most often in the superficial extremities and characteristically shows areas of varying cellularity with a prominent vascular background.

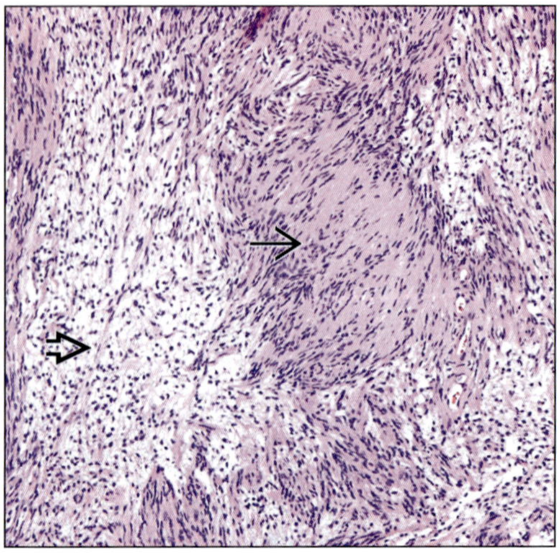

Schwannoma is classically described as having both cellular (Antoni A) ➔ and hypocellular (Antoni B) ➲ regions. Antoni B zones often contain degenerative changes.

TERMINOLOGY

Definitions

- Encapsulated, benign peripheral nerve sheath tumor composed predominantly of Schwann cells

ETIOLOGY/PATHOGENESIS

Molecular Aberrations

- Somatic *NF2* gene mutations present in most tumors
- Bilateral vestibular schwannomas occur in setting of germline *NF2* gene mutations

CLINICAL ISSUES

Epidemiology

- Incidence
  - 90% are sporadic
  - 10% are syndromic
    - ~ 3% with neurofibromatosis type 2 (NF2)
    - 2% with schwannomatosis
    - 5% with multiple meningiomas
    - Rarely in association with neurofibromatosis type 1 (NF1)
- Age
  - All ages
  - Common between 20 and 50 years
- Gender
  - Affects males and females equally

Site

- Head & neck
- Upper and lower extremities
- Deep-seated tumors occur in mediastinum and retroperitoneum

Presentation

- Slow growing
- Painless mass
  - Large tumors may be painful
- Cystic tumors may show fluctuation in size

Treatment

- Surgical excision is curative

Prognosis

- Excellent

Multiple Schwannoma Syndromes

- Neurofibromatosis type 2
  - Autosomal dominant condition
  - Incidence is ~ 1:30,000-40,000
  - Inactivating germline mutations of *NF2* gene on chromosome 22
  - Bilateral vestibular schwannomas are characteristic
  - Schwannomas involving other cranial nerves may be present
  - CNS tumors, such as meningioma, ependymoma, and gliomas, are also part of disease spectrum
  - Schwannomas in NF2 resemble their sporadic counterparts
- Schwannomatosis
  - Not associated with germline mutations in *NF1* or *NF2* genes
  - Autosomal dominant inheritance with incomplete penetrance
  - Both sexes affected equally
  - Patients do not develop bilateral vestibular schwannomas or CNS tumors as seen in NF2
  - Locus of disease has been mapped to chromosome 22 proximal to *NF2* gene
  - Morphology similar to sporadic schwannomas

MACROSCOPIC FEATURES

General Features

- Surrounded by true capsule consisting of epineurium

SCHWANNOMA

Key Facts

Terminology
- Encapsulated, benign peripheral nerve sheath tumor composed predominantly of Schwann cells

Clinical Issues
- Common between 20 and 50 years
- Affects males and females equally
- Surgical excision is curative

Macroscopic Features
- Typically presents as eccentric mass loosely attached to underlying nerve

Microscopic Pathology
- Hallmark: Variable amounts of hypercellular Antoni A and hypocellular Antoni B areas
- Spindle cells in short fascicles in Antoni A areas
- Loose matrix with cystic change and inflammatory cells in Antoni B areas
- Bland nuclear features in most instances; degenerative nuclear atypia in "ancient" schwannoma
- Cellular schwannoma may mimic MPNST
- Plexiform schwannoma usually seen in children
- Epithelioid schwannoma may be mistaken for smooth muscle tumor
- Melanotic psammomatous schwannoma often associated with Carney complex
- Schwannomas in NF2 and schwannomatosis are similar to sporadic tumors
- Microcystic/reticular schwannoma has predilection for visceral location

Ancillary Tests
- Diffuse, strong S100 positivity is characteristic

- Eccentric mass loosely attached to underlying nerve
- Small tumors may be fusiform in shape and mimic neurofibroma
- Dumbbell-shaped tumors occur in vertebral canal, usually in posterior mediastinum
- Cut surface is pink, white-yellow
- Large tumors may show cystic change, hemorrhage, or calcification

Size
- Variable

MICROSCOPIC PATHOLOGY

Histologic Features
- Uninodular mass with fibrous capsule
- Hallmark: Variable amounts of hypercellular Antoni A and hypocellular Antoni B areas
- Antoni A
  - Spindle cells in short fascicles
  - Plump nuclei, indistinct cytoplasmic borders
  - Intranuclear vacuoles in some tumors
  - Nuclear palisading or whorling
  - Verocay bodies
    - Compact rows of palisaded nuclei separated by fibrillary processes
- Antoni B
  - Spindle or oval cells
  - Loose matrix with cystic change and inflammatory cells
  - Large vessels with thick hyalinized walls and luminal thrombi
- Benign epithelial structures and glands may be present in rare instances

Cytologic Features
- Bland nuclear features in most instances

Variants
- **"Ancient" schwannoma**
  - Marked nuclear atypia of degenerative type
  - Usually seen in deep-seated large tumors of long duration
  - Cystic change, hemorrhage, calcification, and hyalinization present
  - Lacks mitotic activity
  - Behavior is similar to ordinary schwannoma
- **Cellular schwannoma**
  - Composed almost exclusively of hypercellular Antoni A areas, which lack Verocay bodies
  - More common in mediastinum and retroperitoneum
  - Encapsulated tumors; some may be multinodular or plexiform in architecture
  - Long sweeping fascicles of spindle-shaped cells
  - Mitotic activity is generally low (< 4/10 HPF)
  - Small foci of necrosis may be present
  - Diffuse strong S100 positivity distinguishes cellular schwannoma from malignant peripheral nerve sheath tumors (MPNSTs)
- **Plexiform schwannoma**
  - Usually involves skin
  - Infrequent in deeper locations
  - Encapsulated tumors with multinodular or plexiform architecture
  - Often more cellular than ordinary schwannoma
  - Association with neurofibromatosis is weak (unlike plexiform neurofibroma, which is almost pathognomonic of NF1)
- **Epithelioid schwannoma**
  - Small round Schwann cells with eosinophilic cytoplasm and sharp cell borders
  - Arranged in clusters, cords, or as single cells
  - Stroma is collagenous or myxoid
  - Foci of typical schwannoma may be present
  - Degenerative nuclear atypia may be seen
  - Lacks mitotic activity
  - Immunostains for S100 and type IV collagen are positive
- **Melanotic psammomatous schwannoma**

- Distinctive tumor of adults (average age ~ 33 years) that often arises in spinal or autonomic nerves near midline
- ~ 50% of patients have evidence of Carney complex (cardiac myxoma, spotty pigmentation, endocrine overactivity, acromegaly, or sexual precocity)
- Multiple tumors may be present in 20% of patients
- Pigmentation may be heavy and mask underlying tumor morphology
- Syncytial arrangement of spindle to ovoid cells with prominent nucleoli and intranuclear inclusions
- Psammoma bodies are present in most cases
- Tumors express not only S100 but also HMB-45
- Difficult to predict behavior since bland-appearing tumors have also been known to metastasize
- Overall, metastasis occurs in ~ 26% of cases

- **Neuroblastoma-like schwannoma**
  - Schwann cells are round and small in this variant and cluster around large collagen cores
  - Mimics rosettes seen in neuroblastoma
- **Pseudoglandular schwannoma**
  - Prominent cystic change
  - Cystic spaces are lined by small round tumor cells
  - Mimics epithelial neoplasm
- **Microcystic/reticular schwannoma**
  - Anastomosing strands of spindle cells in myxoid, fibrillary, or collagenous matrix
  - Predilection for visceral location
  - Mimics reticular perineurioma
- **Malignant transformation in schwannomas**
  - Extremely rare
  - Malignant change in schwannomas usually resembles epithelioid MPNST

ANCILLARY TESTS

Immunohistochemistry

- Diffuse, strong S100 positivity is characteristic
- LEU-7 and GFAP may be positive in some tumors

Electron Microscopy

- Transmission
  - Almost exclusively composed of Schwann cells
  - Basal lamina with electron-dense material lines surface of Schwann cells
  - Flat invaginated nucleus and attenuated cell processes
  - Increased lysosomes in Schwann cells in Antoni B areas

DIFFERENTIAL DIAGNOSIS

Leiomyoma

- Nuclear palisading is also seen in smooth muscle tumors and may mimic schwannoma
- Leiomyomas lack Antoni A and Antoni B areas
- Leiomyomas are positive for desmin and smooth muscle actin and are negative for S100

MPNST

- Cellular schwannomas may be mistaken for MPNST
- Plexiform schwannomas are also cellular and may be mistaken for MPNST arising in plexiform neurofibroma
- MPNSTs show greater nuclear atypia, necrosis, and only focal S100 positivity, unlike benign schwannoma variants, which are diffusely S100 positive

Malignant Melanoma

- Melanotic schwannomas may be mistaken for melanoma due to coexpression of S100 and HMB-45
- Melanotic schwannomas do not have degree of nuclear atypia or mitotic activity seen in malignant melanoma
- Psammoma bodies are present in melanotic schwannoma but not in metastatic melanomas

DIAGNOSTIC CHECKLIST

Pathologic Interpretation Pearls

- Encapsulated tumor with alternating hypercellular and hypocellular areas with diffuse strong S100 positivity

SELECTED REFERENCES

1. Liegl B et al: Microcystic/reticular schwannoma: a distinct variant with predilection for visceral locations. Am J Surg Pathol. 32(7):1080-7, 2008
2. MacCollin M et al: Diagnostic criteria for schwannomatosis. Neurology. 64(11):1838-45, 2005
3. Woodruff JM et al: Congenital and childhood plexiform (multinodular) cellular schwannoma: a troublesome mimic of malignant peripheral nerve sheath tumor. Am J Surg Pathol. 27(10):1321-9, 2003
4. McMenamin ME et al: Expanding the spectrum of malignant change in schwannomas: epithelioid malignant change, epithelioid malignant peripheral nerve sheath tumor, and epithelioid angiosarcoma: a study of 17 cases. Am J Surg Pathol. 25(1):13-25, 2001
5. Antinheimo J et al: Population-based analysis of sporadic and type 2 neurofibromatosis-associated meningiomas and schwannomas. Neurology. 54(1):71-6, 2000
6. Kindblom LG et al: Benign epithelioid schwannoma. Am J Surg Pathol. 22(6):762-70, 1998
7. Chan JK et al: Pseudoglandular schwannoma. Histopathology. 29(5):481-3, 1996
8. Goldblum JR et al: Neuroblastoma-like neurilemoma. Am J Surg Pathol. 18(3):266-73, 1994
9. Brooks JJ et al: Benign glandular schwannoma. Arch Pathol Lab Med. 116(2):192-5, 1992
10. Carney JA: Psammomatous melanotic schwannoma. A distinctive, heritable tumor with special associations, including cardiac myxoma and the Cushing syndrome. Am J Surg Pathol. 14(3):206-22, 1990
11. Fletcher CD et al: Cellular schwannoma: a distinct pseudosarcomatous entity. Histopathology. 11(1):21-35, 1987
12. Fletcher CD et al: Benign plexiform (multinodular) schwannoma: a rare tumour unassociated with neurofibromatosis. Histopathology. 10(9):971-80, 1986

Microscopic Features

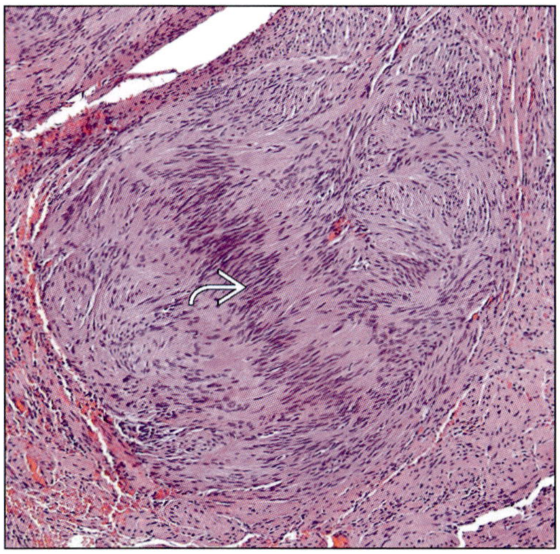

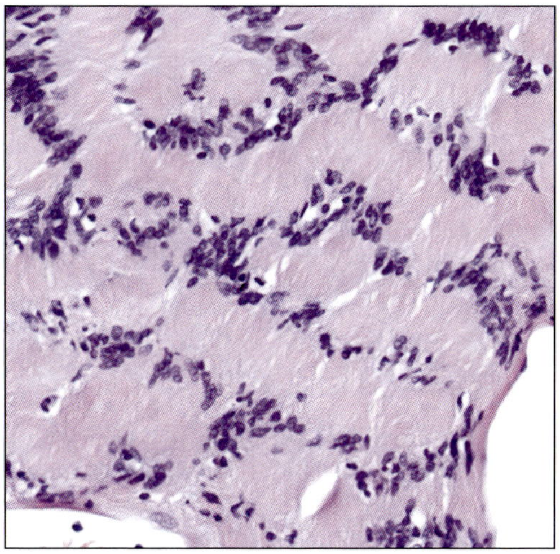

(Left) *A common finding in schwannomas is the formation of Verocay bodies within the cellular Antoni A zones, defined as palisading rows of nuclei around a pink fibrillary core. It is important to note, however, that nuclear palisading can be seen in a variety of other tumors and is therefore nonspecific.* ***(Right)*** *In some cases of schwannoma, Verocay bodies may be prominent and extensive. However, in other cases, they may be focal or even absent.*

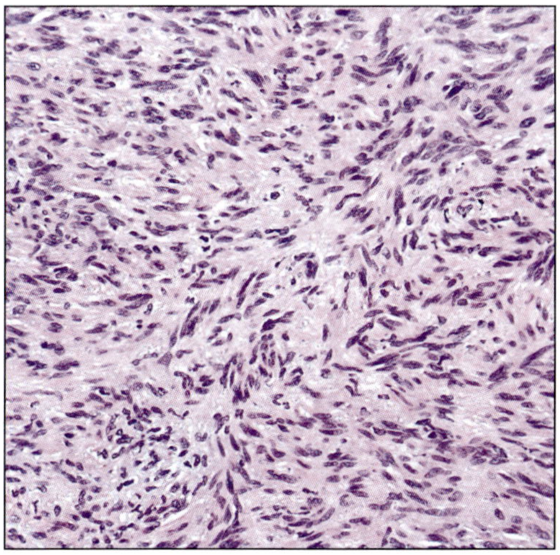

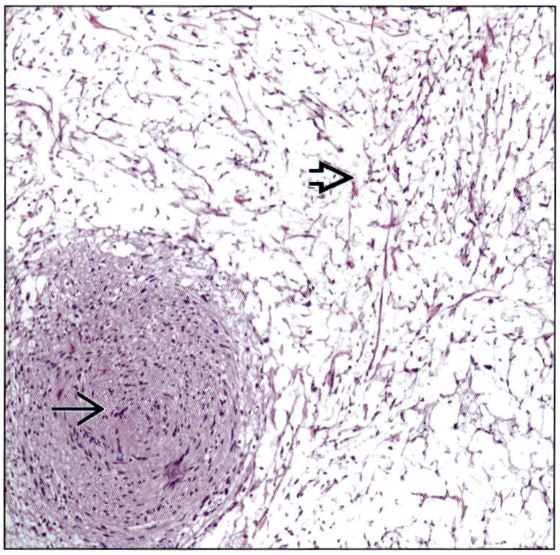

(Left) *Schwann cell nuclei are generally small, elongated, and wavy or "buckled," similar to what is seen in other neural tumors, although larger, rounder nuclei are not uncommon. Of note, prominent nuclear pleomorphism and mitotic activity are not features of this neoplasm.* ***(Right)*** *The interface between Antoni A and Antoni B areas is often quite abrupt in many cases of schwannoma and is a helpful clue to at least suggest the diagnosis.*

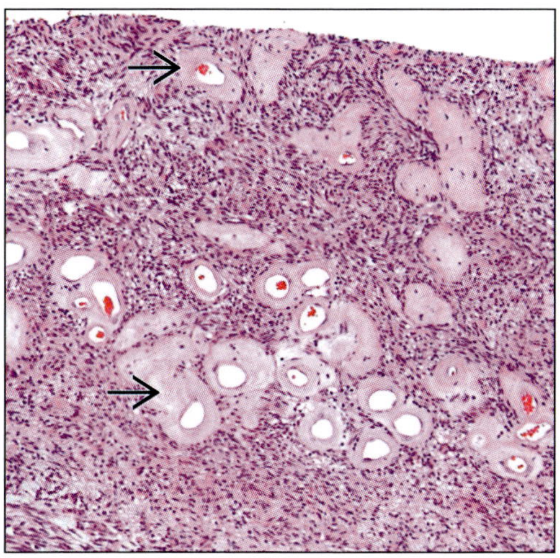

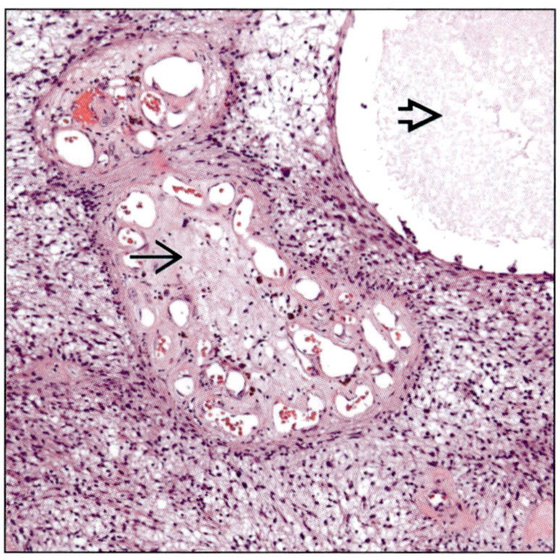

(Left) *Thick, hyalinized blood vessels are common in schwannoma, particularly in Antoni B zones. This finding is in no way pathognomonic, but it should prompt consideration of diagnosis.* ***(Right)*** *Antoni B zones in schwannoma typically contain a variety of degenerative changes including hyalinized vessels, xanthomatous (foamy) and chronic inflammation, and cystic stromal degeneration. Some tumors may appear to completely lack Antoni A zones.*

SCHWANNOMA

Variant Microscopic Features

*(**Left**) Schwannoma is 1 of the few encapsulated soft tissue neoplasms. Note the thick fibrous capsule → overlying the main tumor ⇨. (**Right**) A common finding in Antoni B areas is the presence of enlarged, hyperchromatic, "smudgy" nuclei →, which may be focal or extensive. Although alarming at first, this change is a degenerative phenomenon and should not suggest malignancy. Furthermore, mitoses are rare to nonexistent in these tumors, supporting their benign nature.*

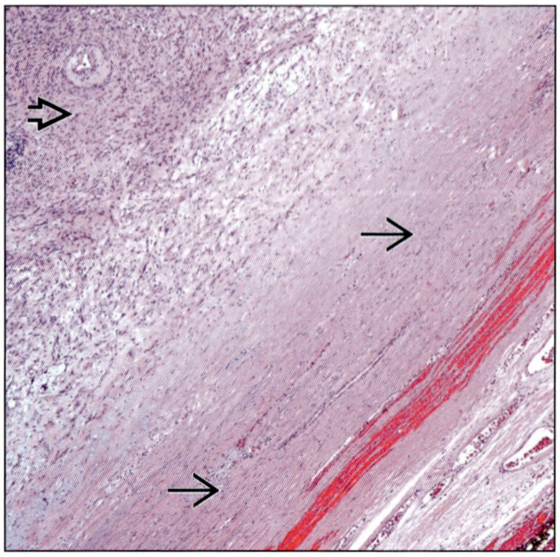

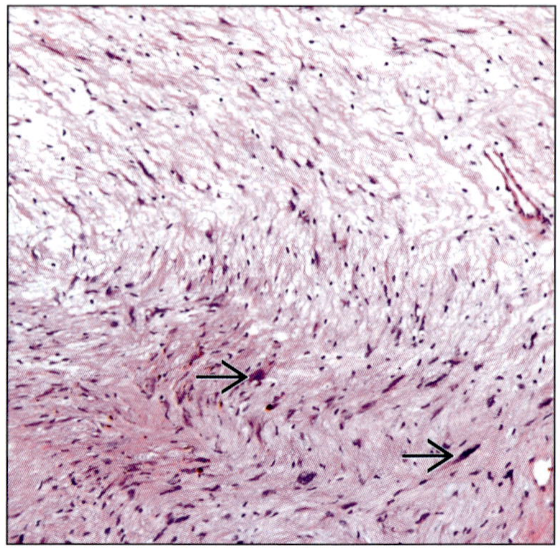

*(**Left**) The degenerative, "smudgy" quality of the nuclei → is better appreciated at higher magnification. This finding has also been described as "ancient change." (**Right**) A subset of schwannomas are composed almost entirely (> 90%) of Antoni A areas and are classified as cellular schwannomas. This variant can simulate a malignant peripheral nerve sheath tumor, but other typical features of schwannoma (e.g., small size, encapsulation, strong S100 protein expression) are often present.*

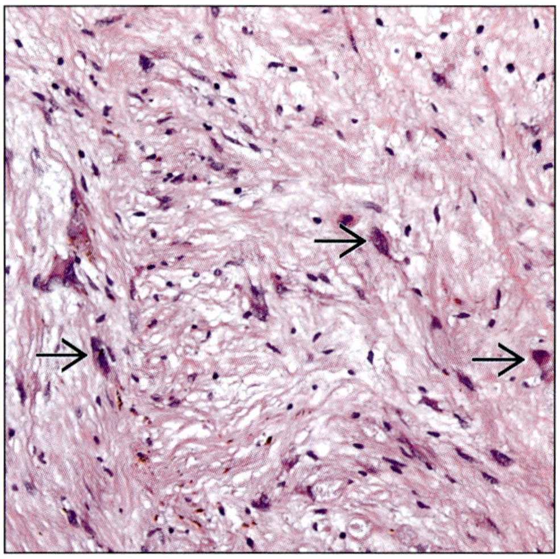

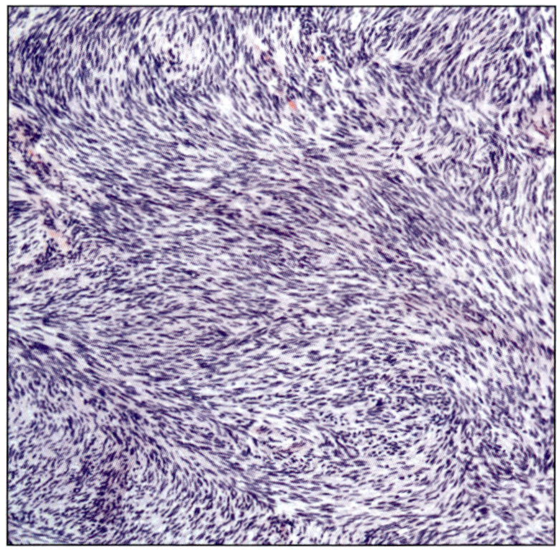

*(**Left**) Many cellular schwannomas (particularly visceral cases) demonstrate a lymphocytic cuff → at the periphery, which is often patchy. This finding can be very useful in suggesting a diagnosis of schwannoma in difficult cases with unusual morphologies. (**Right**) An epithelioid morphology can also be seen in some cases of schwannoma and may be focal or extensive (epithelioid schwannoma). The epithelioid Schwann cells often cluster together in small aggregates.*

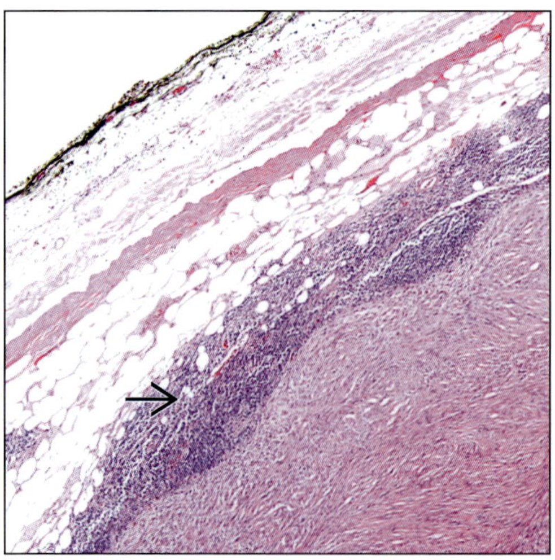

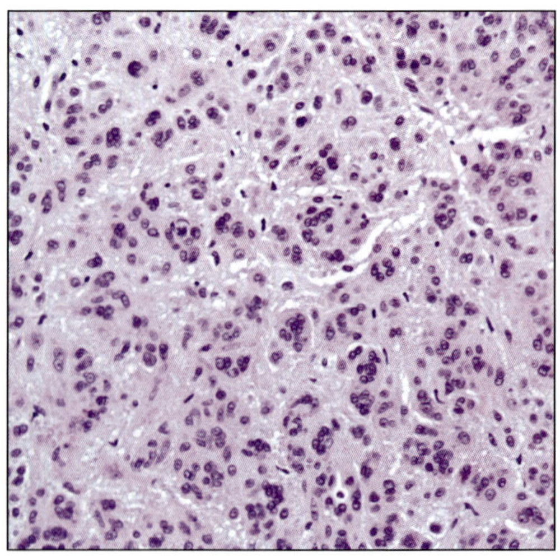

Microscopic Features

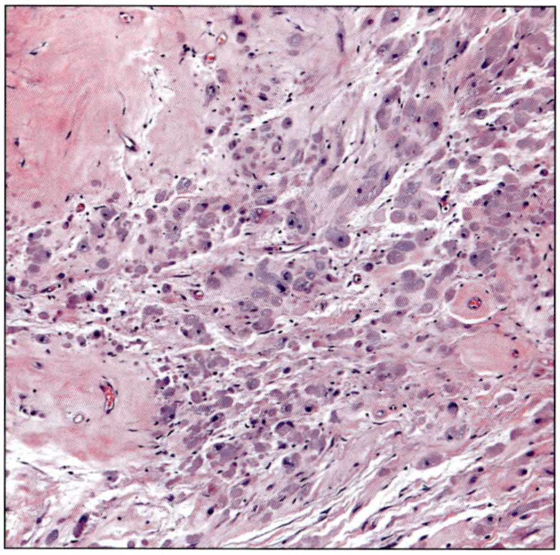

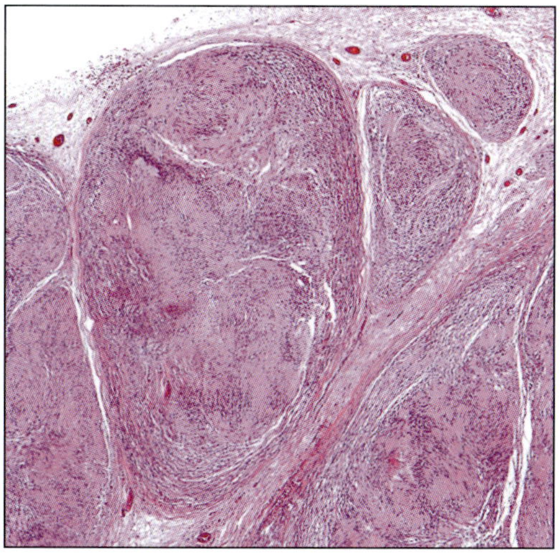

(Left) *In some cases of epithelioid schwannoma, the cells may be larger than usual with prominent nucleoli, similar to epithelioid malignant peripheral nerve sheath tumor. Importantly, the former contain few, if any, mitoses.* ***(Right)*** *Plexiform schwannomas contain many features of ordinary or cellular schwannoma but show a unique multinodular growth pattern. They are also more likely to occur in cutaneous locations and have no association with neurofibromatosis.*

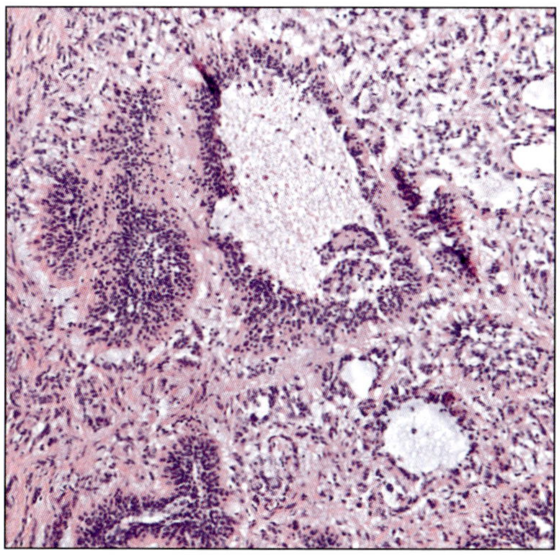

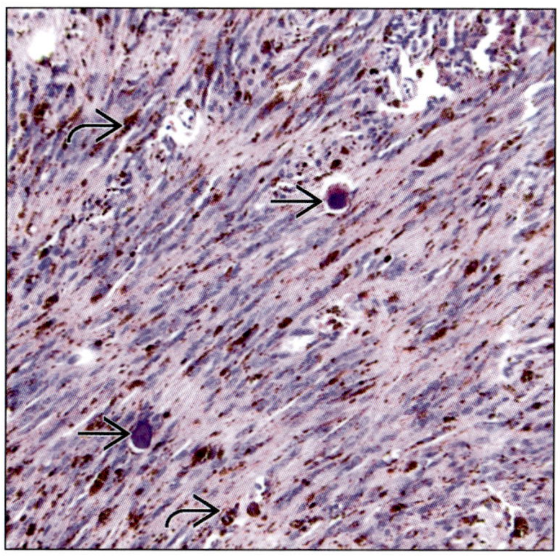

(Left) *Pseudoglandular schwannoma is a rare variant that may be mistaken for an epithelial neoplasm. Fortunately, they often contain more conventional areas of schwannoma, and they may show a peripheral lymphocytic cuff.* ***(Right)*** *Melanotic psammomatous schwannoma is an unusual variant associated with Carney complex. In contrast to conventional schwannoma, this tumor contains extensive melanin pigmentation* ↪ *and often shows psammomatous calcifications* →.

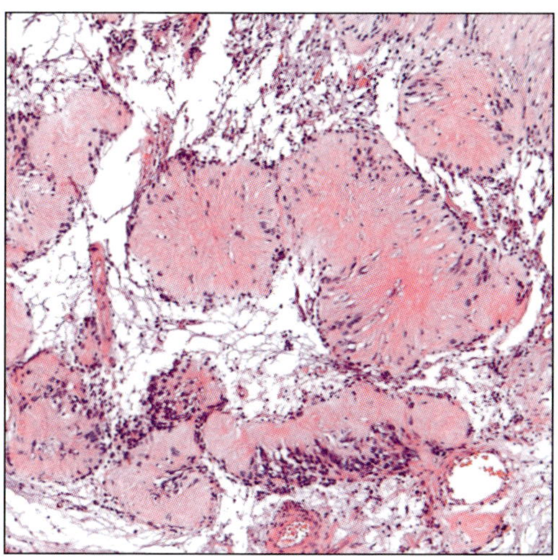

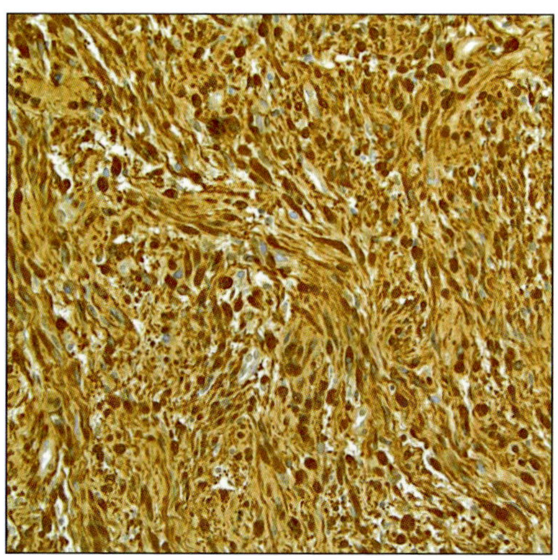

(Left) *An interesting but rare variant of schwannoma demonstrates the formation of hyalinized rosettes, similar to what is seen in neuroblastoma. As in other schwannoma variants, this tumor may show areas of conventional morphology.* ***(Right)*** *Strong and diffuse cytoplasmic and nuclear expression of S100 protein is a highly characteristic and reliable finding in schwannoma and all of its morphologic variants. This strong expression is uncommon in malignant neural tumors.*

Head and Neck

SQUAMOUS CELL CARCINOMA, HEAD AND NECK

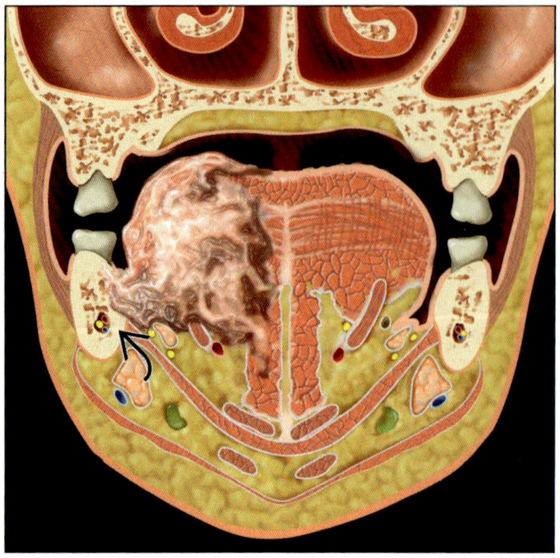

Coronal view through the mid oral cavity shows a lateral dorsal squamous cell carcinoma (SCC) that has grown into the deep muscles of the tongue and into the cortical bone of the mandible ➔.

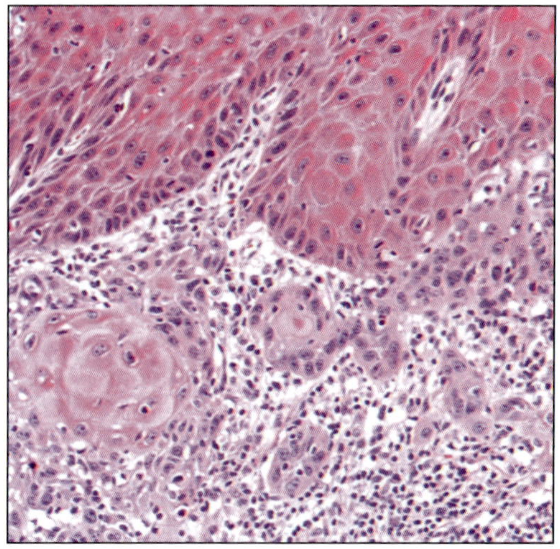

Well-differentiated SCC shows basement membrane violation with islands of malignant cells arising from the overlying epithelium invading into the lamina propria as a single or a group of cells with focal keratinization.

TERMINOLOGY

Abbreviations

- Squamous cell carcinoma (SCC)

Synonyms

- Epidermoid carcinoma (general for head and neck carcinomas)
- Sinonasal carcinoma
- Transitional carcinoma
- Respiratory epithelial carcinoma
- Cylindrical cell carcinoma

Definitions

- Malignant neoplasm characterized by squamous cell differentiation arising from squamous epithelium

ETIOLOGY/PATHOGENESIS

Genetic Predisposition for Head and Neck Squamous Cell Carcinoma

- **Dyskeratosis congenita**
  - *TERT*, *TERC*, *DKC1*, *TINF2*, and other genes involved in telomere maintenance
  - Squamous cell carcinoma of head and neck and squamous cell carcinoma of tongue
  - Other manifestations
    - Skin cancer, anorectal carcinoma, gastric carcinoma, lung carcinoma, colonic carcinoma, esophageal carcinoma, Hodgkin lymphoma, and retinoblastoma, among others
- **Fanconi anemia**
  - 13 separate genes (FANCx) comprise the Fanconi anemia pathway
  - Squamous cell carcinoma of head and neck
  - Other manifestations
    - Short stature
    - Eye abnormalities
    - Wilms tumor
    - Hematologic neoplasms: Cumulative incidence of hematologic malignancy is 25% by age 45; predominantly myeloid malignancies, acute myeloid leukemia, and other hematopoietic abnormalities; 600x increased risk of acute myeloid leukemia (AML), 5,000x increased risk of myeloplastic syndrome (MDS)
    - Solid tumors as squamous cell carcinoma (esophagus, anogenital, and cervix)
    - Hepatocellular carcinoma
    - Brain tumors
    - Breast cancer susceptibility
- **Xeroderma pigmentosum (XP)**
  - Genes involved in nucleotide excision repair of ultraviolet light-induced damage: *XPA-XPG*
  - Squamous cell carcinoma of tongue (100,000x increase in XP patients; disease manifests 20 years earlier than in general population)
  - Other manifestations
    - Carcinomas and sarcomas of skin
    - Melanomas
    - Ocular cancer
    - Brain tumors (medulloblastomas and glioblastomas)
    - Spinal cord astrocytomas
    - Carcinomas of lung, uterus, breast, stomach, kidney, and testicular
    - Leukemias
    - Multiple benign tumors
- **Bloom syndrome**
  - *BLM*: Tumor-suppressor gene that belongs to family of RecQ DNA helicase
  - Squamous cell carcinoma of head and neck
  - Other manifestations
    - Up to 50% of patients will develop a malignancy
    - Hematolymphoid malignancies predominant in the first 2 decades of life

SQUAMOUS CELL CARCINOMA, HEAD AND NECK

Key Facts

Terminology
- Malignant neoplasm characterized by squamous cell differentiation arising from squamous epithelium

Etiology/Pathogenesis
- Genetic
  - Dyskeratosis congenita
  - Fanconi anemia
  - Xeroderma pigmentosum
  - Bloom syndrome
- Iron deficiency (Plummer-Vinson syndrome) associated with elevated risk of squamous cell carcinoma (SCC)
- Tobacco use, alcohol consumption, gastroesophageal reflux, chronic inflammation, nickel exposure
- Oncogenic viruses: Human papillomavirus (HPV) and Epstein-Barr virus (EBV)

Microscopic Pathology
- SCC is generally divided into multiple categories
  - Histologic categories: In situ, superficially invasive, or deeply invasive
  - Histologic grade includes well-, moderately, and poorly differentiated SCC
  - Divided into keratinizing and nonkeratinizing

Top Differential Diagnoses
- Nasal cavity SCC
  - Schneiderian papillomas
  - *NUT* midline carcinoma
- Tongue and laryngeal SCC
  - Pseudoepitheliomatous hyperplasia
  - Necrotizing sialometaplasia
  - Radiation changes

    - Carcinomas predominant after first 2 decades of life and arise in varied sites, including skin, head and neck, lung, uterus, breast, and gastrointestinal tract, including esophagus (both squamous cell carcinoma and adenocarcinoma), stomach, and colon
    - Medulloblastoma
    - Wilms tumor
    - Osteosarcoma
- Other syndromes

Environmental Exposure
- Laryngeal SCC
  - Tobacco use (e.g., cigarette, cigar, pipe, smokeless)
  - Alcohol consumption: Independent of tobacco but multiplicative if both are used
    - Maté drinking is a suggested risk factor
  - Gastroesophageal reflux or laryngopharyngeal reflux (chronic inflammation as a mutagen)
  - Radiation exposure (therapeutic and environmental)
  - Occupational factors/exposures
  - Protective effect by high intake of fruits and vegetables
- Tongue SCC
  - Tobacco use
  - Alcohol consumption
  - Nutritional deficiencies
    - Iron deficiency (Plummer-Vinson syndrome) associated with elevated risk of SCC
  - Betel quid (a.k.a. paan): Combination of betel leaf and 1 or more other ingredients (e.g., areca palm nuts, slaked lime, tobacco)
  - Radiation exposure (ultraviolet and therapeutic)
- Nasal
  - Nickel exposure
  - Textile dust
  - Tobacco smoking
  - Prior Thorotrast use

Infectious Agents
- Tongue SCC
  - Oncogenic virus: HPV, high-risk type associated with development of tonsil and base of tongue cancer
    - Relationship to oral SCC is not as convincing
  - Can develop from area of leukoplakia or erythroplakia
  - Malignant transformation of severe dysplasia or carcinoma in situ
- Laryngeal SCC
  - HPV, human herpesvirus 8 (HHV-8), EBV may have a minor causative role
- Nasal and sinonasal SCC
  - HPV

Developmental
- Nasal SCC: May develop from sinonasal (schneiderian) papilloma
  - Majority transform to keratinizing SCC
  - Majority arise in association with inverted-type sinonasal papilloma

CLINICAL ISSUES

Presentation
- Depending on location of head and neck SCC
  - Glottic tumors: Hoarseness is earliest symptom
  - Supraglottic &/or hypopharyngeal tumors: Dysphagia, changes in phonation, foreign body sensation in throat, and odynophagia
  - Subglottic tumors: Dyspnea and stridor most common
  - Tracheal tumors: Dyspnea, stridor, cough, and hemoptysis
  - Neck mass (lymph nodes) more common in transglottic tumors
  - Tongue: Difficulty eating and swallowing, sore that does not heal, dentures that fit poorly, loose teeth
  - Nasal cavity: Unilateral obstruction, nonhealing sore, rhinorrhea, epistaxis, mass, or pain
  - Maxillary sinus: Early symptoms often confused with sinusitis resulting in delay in diagnosis; with progression of disease, grouped in 5 categories

SQUAMOUS CELL CARCINOMA, HEAD AND NECK

- Oral: Referred pain including upper premolar and molar teeth, ulceration, loosening of teeth, and fistula
- Nasal: Nasal obstruction, mass, persistent purulent rhinorrhea, nonhealing sore/ulcer, epistaxis
- Facial: Swelling, facial asymmetry
- Ocular: Eyelid swelling, proptosis/exophthalmos
- Neurologic: Numbness, paraesthesia, pain, cranial neuropathy

MACROSCOPIC FEATURES

General Features

- Gross findings vary depending on origin and location of tumor

MICROSCOPIC PATHOLOGY

Histologic Features

- SCC is generally divided into multiple categories
  - **Histologic categories**:
    - Squamous cell carcinoma in situ
    - Squamous cell carcinoma, superficially invasive
    - Squamous cell carcinoma, deeply invasive
  - **Histologic grade includes well-, moderately, and poorly differentiated SCC**
    - **Grade 1 (well differentiated)**: Resembles normal squamous epithelium but shows invasion
    - **Grade 2 (moderately differentiated)**: Easily identified nuclear pleomorphism, loss of polarity, disorganization, increased mitotic activity, usually less keratinization
    - **Grade 3 (poorly differentiated)**: Immature cells predominate, high nuclear to cytoplasmic ratio, limited keratinization, numerous typical and atypical mitoses
  - **Keratinization: Absent or present and divided into**
    - Squamous cell carcinoma, keratinizing
    - Squamous cell carcinoma, nonkeratinizing

Variants of SCC

- Verrucous carcinoma
- Basaloid SCC
- Spindle cell squamous carcinoma
- Adenosquamous carcinoma
- Papillary SCC
- Lymphoepithelial carcinoma
- Acantholytic squamous cell carcinoma (pseudoglandular or adenoid)
- Carcinoma cuniculatum

ANCILLARY TESTS

Cytogenetics

- **Molecular genetics of oral SCC**
  - Loss of heterozygosity commonly noted at 3p (*FHIT*), 9p (*CDKN2A*), 17p (*TP53*)
  - Mutations in *TP53*, a tumor suppressor gene, increases with tobacco smoking
  - Overexpression of cyclooxygenase-2 (COX-2) may play a future role for targeted molecular therapy
- **Molecular genetics of laryngeal SCC**
  - *TP53* mutations are early event in SCC but not a prognostic marker
  - *EGFR* may be amplified, but it is not overexpressed
  - Cytogenetics and comparative genomic hybridization show +3q21-29 and -3p
  - *CCND1* is amplified and overexpressed; expression is lower in metastatic tumors
  - MMP13 expression and MMP14 overexpression are associated with advanced tumors
  - Losses at 8p, 9q, and 13 are more frequent in metastatic than in primary tumors

DIFFERENTIAL DIAGNOSIS

Nasal Cavity SCC

- Schneiderian papillomas
- *NUT* midline carcinoma
- Sinonasal undifferentiated carcinoma (SNUC)

Tongue SCC

- Pseudoepitheliomatous hyperplasia
- Necrotizing sialometaplasia
- Radiation changes

Laryngeal SCC

- Pseudoepitheliomatous hyperplasia (PEH)
- Radiation changes
- Squamous papilloma
- Necrotizing sialometaplasia

SELECTED REFERENCES

1. Boscolo-Rizzo P et al: New insights into human papillomavirus-associated head and neck squamous cell carcinoma. Acta Otorhinolaryngol Ital. 33(2):77-87, 2013
2. Lin BM et al: Long-term prognosis and risk factors among patients with HPV-associated oropharyngeal squamous cell carcinoma. Cancer. 119(19):3462-71, 2013
3. McBride SM et al: Mutation frequency in 15 common cancer genes in high-risk head and neck squamous cell carcinoma (HNSCC). Head Neck. Epub ahead of print, 2013
4. Saba NF et al: Acetylated tubulin (AT) as a prognostic marker in squamous cell carcinoma of the head and neck. Head Neck Pathol. Epub ahead of print, 2013
5. Takahashi Y et al: Comprehensive assessment of prognostic markers for sinonasal squamous cell carcinoma. Head Neck. Epub ahead of print, 2013
6. Wilson GA et al: Integrated virus-host methylome analysis in head and neck squamous cell carcinoma. Epigenetics. 8(9), 2013

SQUAMOUS CELL CARCINOMA, HEAD AND NECK

Diagrammatic Features

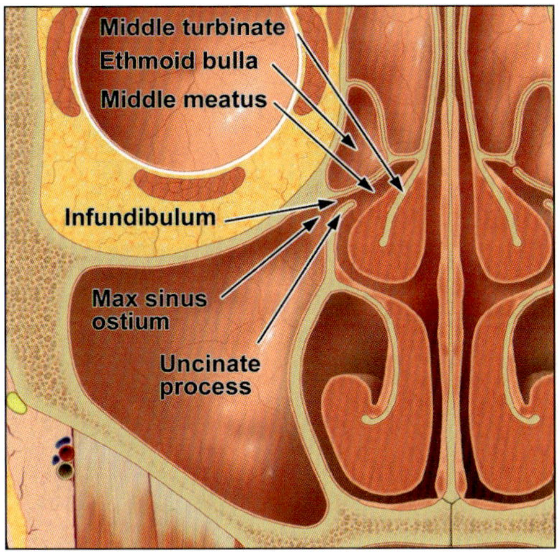

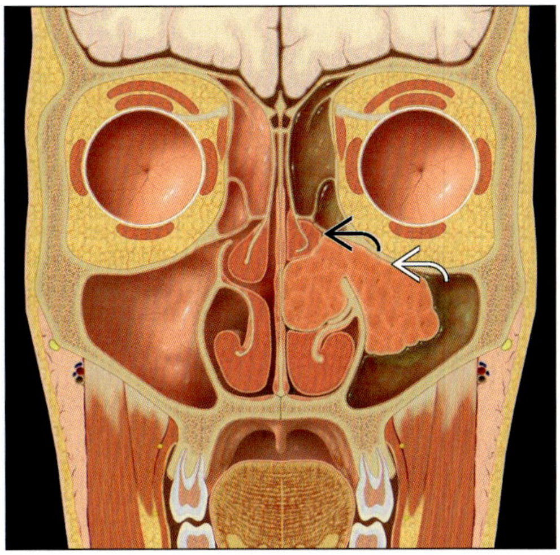

(Left) Squamous cell carcinoma can arise from nasal cavity and paranasal sinus. This coronal graphic illustrates the anatomic separations of the maxillary sinus from the nasal cavity, ethmoid sinus, and orbit. ***(Right)*** *This coronal graphic illustrates the presence of a lobular inverted papilloma centered at the middle meatus. The lesion enters the maxillary sinus via an enlarged infundibulum. This may be a precursor lesion of SCC.*

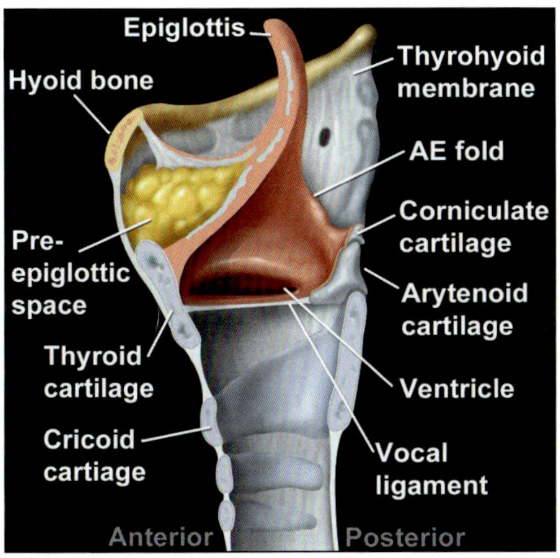

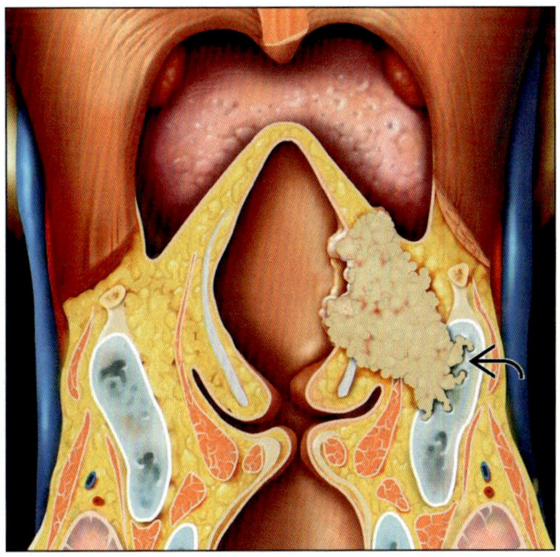

(Left) *Basic anatomic landmarks of the larynx are used in accurate classification and separation of specific tumors into location and stage. The vocal cords are used to separate tumors into supraglottic, glottic, and subglottic regions, one of the most useful staging parameters. Extension into cartilage or across membranes also changes tumor stage.* ***(Right)*** *A large supraglottic tumor fills the laryngeal side of the epiglottis with expansion into thyroid cartilage and bone.*

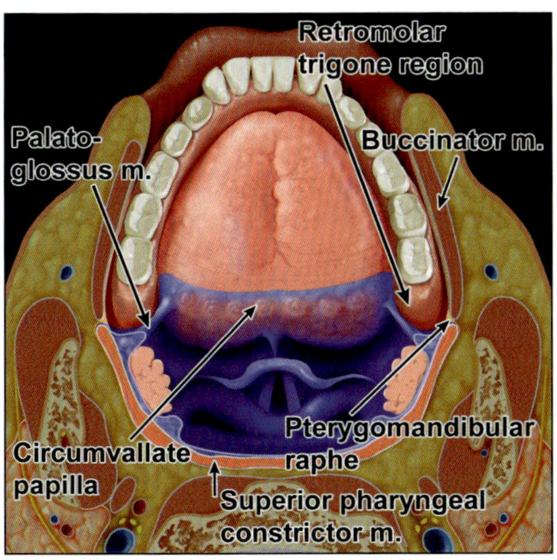

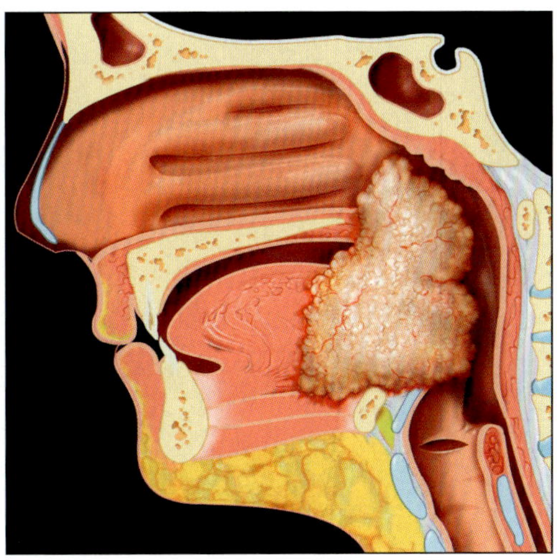

(Left) *The oropharynx, highlighted in purple, includes the base of tongue (posterior 1/3), vallecula, tonsil, tonsillar fossa and pillars, inferior surface of the soft palate and uvula, and posterior wall of the pharynx.* ***(Right)*** *This oropharyngeal SCC is large and extends from the base of tongue to vallecul, involves the oropharynx and nasopharynx, and extends into the posterior nasal cavity. SCC of the tongue may be associated with dyskeratosis congenita and xeroderma pigmentosum.*

SQUAMOUS CELL CARCINOMA, HEAD AND NECK

Nasal Cavity Squamous Cell Carcinoma

(Left) *Coronal graphic demonstrates a tumor involving the maxillary sinus with extension into bone. This squamous cell carcinoma may develop from a sinonasal papilloma and be associated with a few familial syndromes.* ***(Right)*** *Patients with hereditary retinoblastoma develop diverse neoplasms and may also develop an SCC of nasal cavity. This is a typical microscopic feature of nonkeratinizing SCC formed by sheets of basaloid cells with sharply defined borders. No stromal reaction is seen in the tumor.*

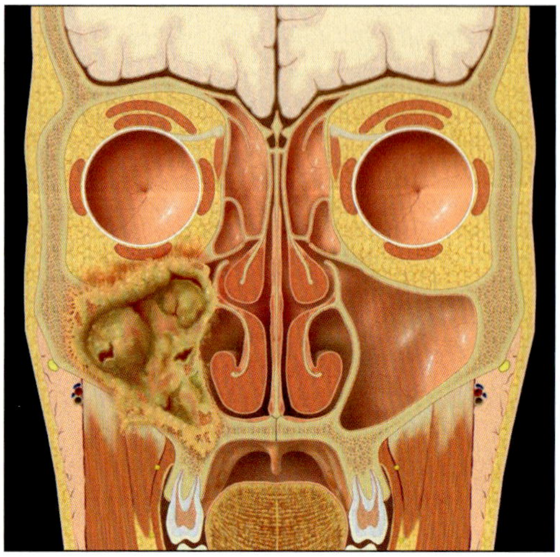

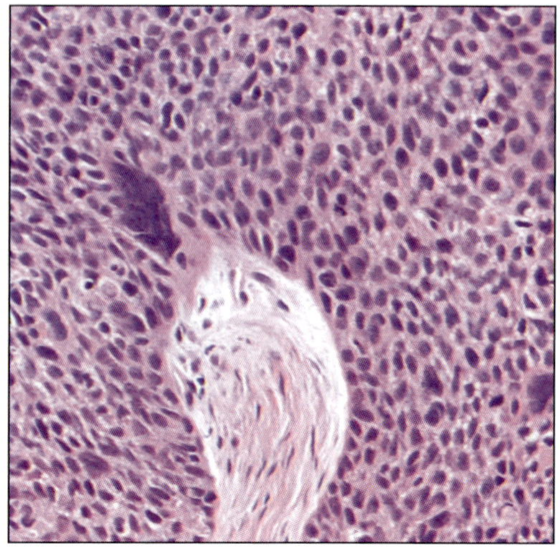

(Left) *Most of the SCC of nasal cavity and paranasal sinuses are of the well-differentiated keratinizing type and may be 1 of the neoplasms occurring in patients with hereditary retinoblastoma. This picture shows widened and downwardly growing rete, marked dysplastic cellular changes, and, focally, violation of the basement membrane by tumor cells.* ***(Right)*** *This picture illustrates p16 positivity in an SCC. HPV, high-risk type, may be associated with development of head and neck SCC.*

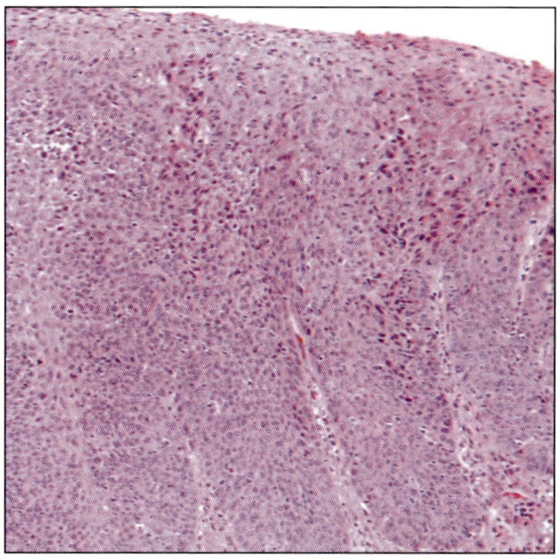

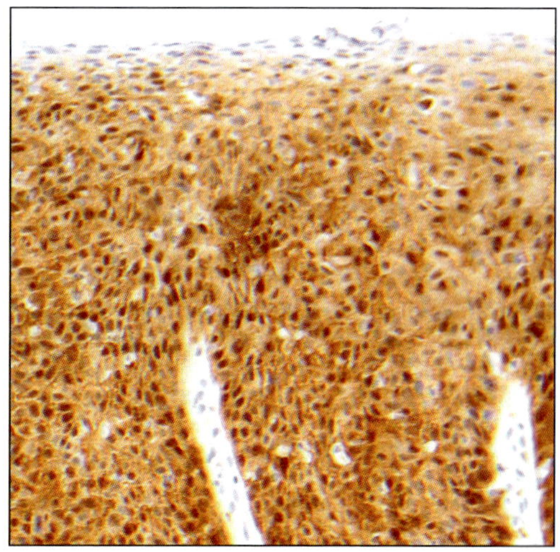

(Left) *Nonkeratinizing SCC originates from the surface epithelium, invades into the submucosa as broad bands of neoplastic epithelium growing down, and very frequently invades adjacent bone →.* ***(Right)*** *A sinonasal, invasive, keratinizing well-differentiated SCC shows a nest of carcinoma cells → within the bone and is associated with marked desmoplastic reaction.*

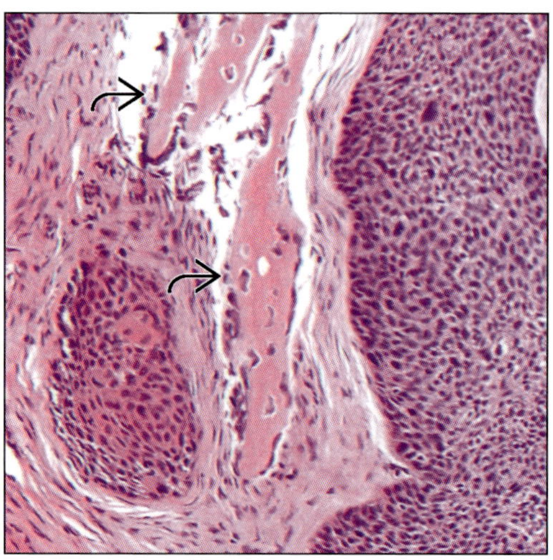

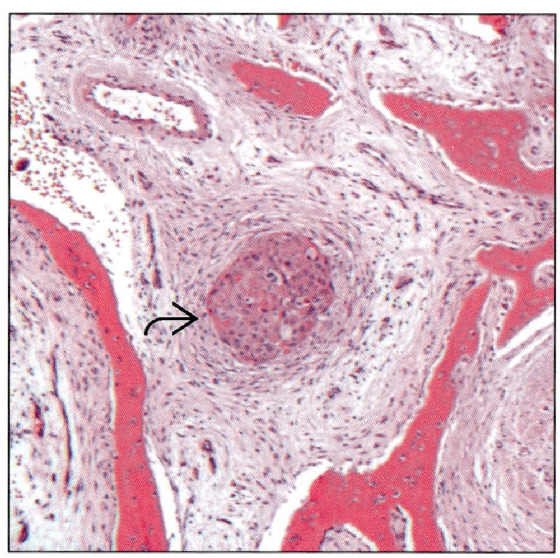

Oropharyngeal Squamous Cell Carcinoma

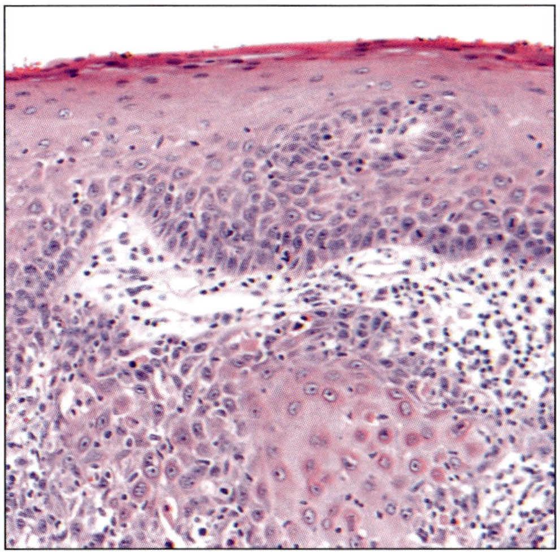
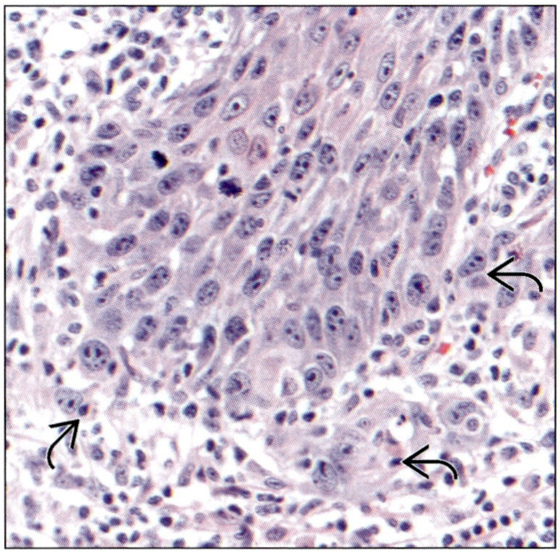

(Left) *SCC of head and neck may be associated with dyskeratosis congenita (DC) and Fanconi anemia. SCC of tongue is seen in patients with xeroderma pigmentosum (XP) and DC. This picture illustrates a keratinizing invasive SCC of tongue in a patient with DC.* ***(Right)*** *An invasive nonkeratinizing SCC may show only focal keratinization (< 10% of the tumor). Note that the basement membrane is violated and cells are present in lamina propria.*

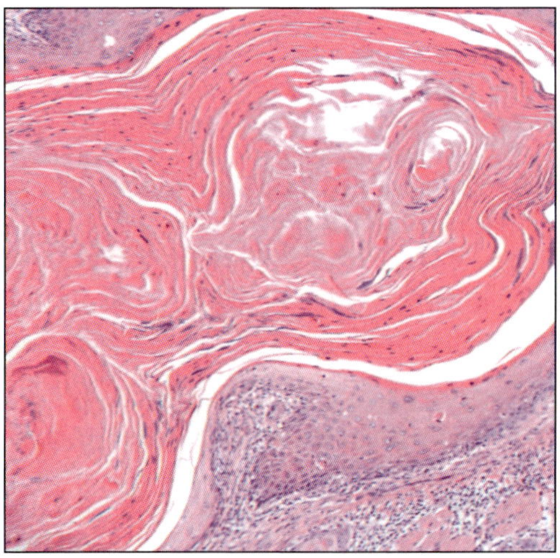
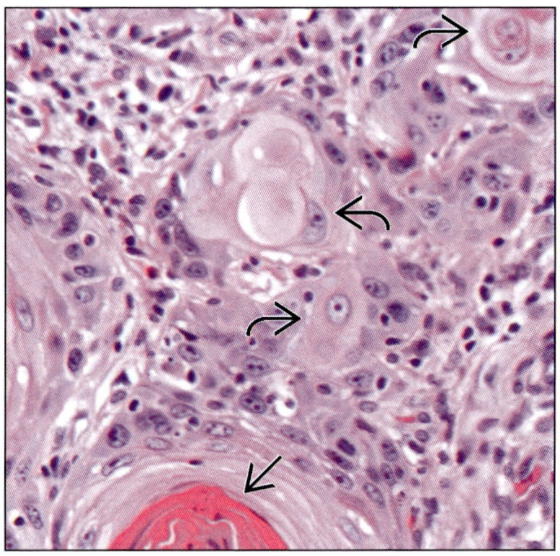

(Left) *This invasive, keratinizing, well-differentiated SCC shows islands of malignant epithelial cells invading into deeper tissues with extensive keratin pearl formation and formation of a large mass of keratin.* ***(Right)*** *Higher magnification of a well-differentiated SCC shows violation of the basement membrane by groups of malignant epithelial cells associated with inflammatory cell infiltrate. Dyskeratotic cells are seen throughout. A keratin pearl is present.*

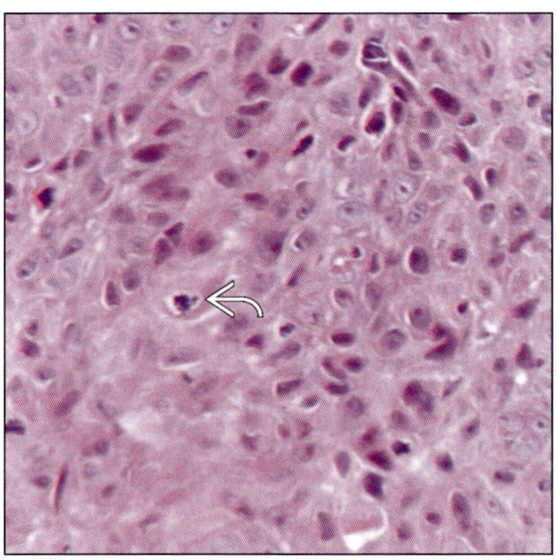
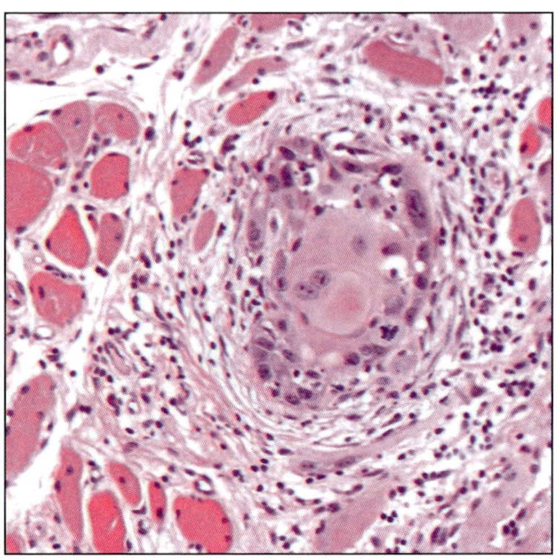

(Left) *Higher magnification of an SCC shows a large group of malignant epithelial cells with dyskeratotic cells. The tumor cells show nuclear atypia, prominent nucleoli, and mitosis.* ***(Right)*** *An invasive SCC of tongue in a patient with XP shows an island of keratinizing malignant cells infiltrating between the muscle fibers and surrounded by mixed inflammatory infiltrate and mild desmoplastic reaction.*

ENDOLYMPHATIC SAC TUMOR

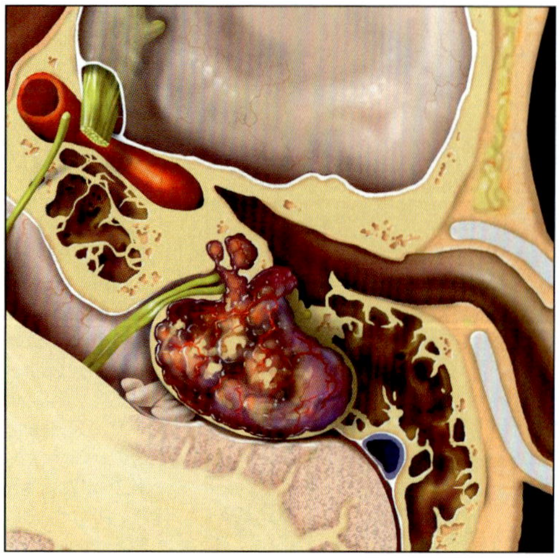

Axial graphic of temporal bone shows the typical appearance of endolymphatic sac tumor. The tumor is vascular, shows a tendency to fistulize the inner ear, and contains bone fragments within the tumor matrix.

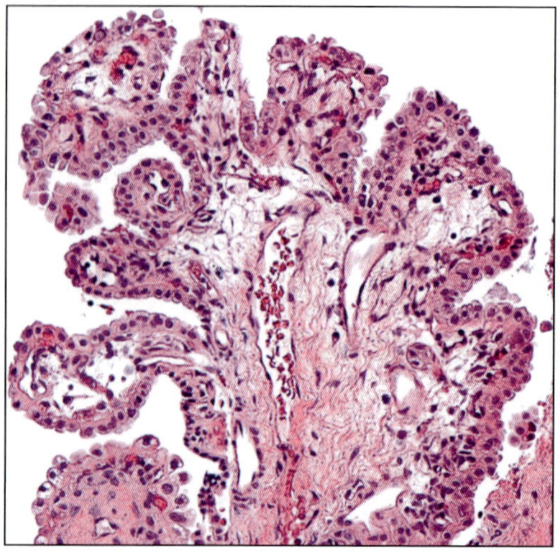

Endolymphatic sac tumors typically show a papillary architecture with fibrovascular cores and a single row of eosinophilic cuboidal epithelium. Nuclei are ovoid with fine chromatin.

TERMINOLOGY

Abbreviations

- Endolymphatic sac tumor (ELST)

Synonyms

- Endolymphatic sac papillary tumor
- Papillary adenoma of endolymphatic sac
- Adenoma/adenocarcinoma of temporal bone
- Low-grade adenocarcinoma of endolymphatic sac
- Aggressive papillary cystadenomas of endolymphatic sac
- Heffner tumor

Definitions

- Rare, slowly growing, locally invasive but nonmetastasizing papillary neoplasm arising from endolymphatic sac within temporal bone

ETIOLOGY/PATHOGENESIS

Genetic Predisposition

- von Hippel-Lindau (VHL) disease
  - Prevalence: 1 in 39,000 people
  - Autosomal dominant inheritance
  - Germline mutation in *VHL* tumor suppressor gene on chromosome 3p25
    - VHL protein (pVHL): E3 ubiquitin ligase that marks certain proteins (e.g., alpha subunits of hypoxia-inducible factors [HIF]) for degradation
  - Somatic inactivation or loss of remaining wild-type *VHL* allele leads to characteristic manifestations
    - Retinal & central nervous system hemangioblastomas
    - Pheochromocytoma
    - Renal cysts & renal cell carcinoma
    - Pancreatic cysts, cystadenomas, carcinomas, & islet cell tumors
    - Epididymal papillary cystadenoma (men)
    - Female adnexal tumor of probable wolffian origin (FATWO)
    - ELST
  - 2 types of VHL disease based on absence/presence of pheochromocytoma
    - Type 1 VHL: Pheochromocytoma absent
    - Type 2 VHL: Pheochromocytoma present
- ~ 10% of patients with ELSTs have VHL disease
  - Conversely, ~ 15% of patients with VHL disease have radiographically detectable ELSTs

Histogenesis

- Endolymphatic sac
  - Endolymph-filled, neuroectodermally derived, nonsensory component of membranous labyrinth
  - Paddle-shaped structure consisting of complex network of interconnecting tubules
  - Connected to utricular & saccular ducts by endolymphatic duct
- Specific precursor lesions for ELSTs: Not well characterized

CLINICAL ISSUES

Epidemiology

- Incidence
  - ELSTs are detected by MR or CT in ~ 15% of patients with VHL disease
    - 60% of VHL patients with vestibulocochlear symptoms may have microscopic ELSTs that are not visible by MR or CT imaging studies
  - Compared to sporadic cases, ELSTs in VHL patients are associated with the following (some features may be due to increased screening by imaging in VHL patients)
    - Younger patients
    - Less advanced
    - Bilateral tumors (30% of VHL patients with ELSTs have bilateral tumors)

ENDOLYMPHATIC SAC TUMOR

Key Facts

Terminology
- Rare, slowly growing, locally invasive but nonmetastasizing papillary neoplasm arising from endolymphatic sac within temporal bone

Clinical Issues
- Association with von Hippel-Lindau (VHL) disease
- Presentation: Meniere-like clinical syndrome of hearing loss, tinnitus, & vertigo; aural fullness; facial nerve dysfunction

Microscopic Pathology
- Papillary, tubular, &/or cystic structures lined by single layer of cuboidal/columnar cells with pale eosinophilic to clear cytoplasm

Ancillary Tests
- Positive: Cytokeratins (CK7, CK8, CK19, CAM5.2, 34bE12), vimentin, vascular endothelial growth factor (VEGF)
- Negative: CK10/13, CK20, chromogranin, synaptophysin

Top Differential Diagnoses
- Middle ear adenoma/carcinoid tumor
  - a.k.a. neuroendocrine adenoma of middle ear
- Ceruminous gland adenoma/adenocarcinoma
- Meningioma
- Paraganglioma
- Heterotopic or primary choroid plexus papillomas of cerebellopontine angle (CPA)
- Metastatic carcinoma

- Age
  - 2nd-8th decades of life
  - Rare pediatric cases have been reported
- Gender
  - 2x female predominance among VHL patients

Site
- Posteromedial region of petrous portion of temporal bone (site of normal endolymphatic sac)

Presentation
- VHL patients with evidence of ELST by imaging may show following symptoms
- Meniere-like clinical syndrome of hearing loss in 95%, tinnitus in 92%, & vertigo in 62%
  - Hearing loss: Usually irreversible; mean age of onset: 22 years
    - Typically sensorineural rather than conductive hearing loss
    - Acute & clinically significant in 43%
    - Subacute & progressive (over 3-6 months) in 43%
    - Gradual hearing loss in 14%
- Aural fullness in 29%
- Facial nerve dysfunction in 8%

Laboratory Tests
- VHL patients should undergo serial audiologic tests & high-resolution imaging studies for early detection of small ELSTs
- Conversely, all patients with ELSTs should be screened for other signs & symptoms of VHL disease

Treatment
- Early & complete surgical resection: Relieves hearing & vestibular symptoms, prevents permanent neurologic deficits

Prognosis
- Slowly growing tumor with potential for local destruction & extension into vital structures
- Invasion into posterior cranial fossa and brain can result in meningitis and death

IMAGE FINDINGS

CT and MR Findings
- Contrast-enhancing lytic lesion
- Typically 4-6 cm in greatest dimension
- Location: Posteromedial aspect of petrous portion of temporal bone
- Radiographic differential diagnosis includes inflammatory, cystic, & neoplastic lesions involving temporal bone

Angiography Findings
- Well-vascularized lesion with tumoral blush

MACROSCOPIC FEATURES

Size
- Variable; can measure up to several cm

MICROSCOPIC PATHOLOGY

Histologic Features
- Architecture: Papillary, tubular, &/or cystic structures lined by single layer of epithelial cells
  - Cystic structures may contain eosinophilic colloid-like fluid, resembling thyroid follicles
  - Variably cellular stroma ± small blood vessels ± fibrosis
  - Hemorrhage, hemosiderin, cholesterol clefts, & chronic inflammatory cells may be present

Cytologic Features
- Cuboidal to columnar cells with pale eosinophilic to clear cytoplasm
- Typically uniform, ovoid nuclei ± intranuclear pseudoinclusions
- Finely granular chromatin

ENDOLYMPHATIC SAC TUMOR

Differential Diagnosis of Endolymphatic Sac Tumor

Tumor	Site	Architecture	Cytology	IHC: Positive	IHC: Negative
ELST	Petrous portion of temporal bone	Papillary, tubular, cystic	Cuboidal to columnar cells; pale eosinophilic to clear cytoplasm; uniform, ovoid nuclei with occasional pseudoinclusions	Various cytokeratins including CK7 and CAM5.2, vimentin, VEGF, S100, CD34, NSE, GFAP, EMA	CK20, chromogranin, synaptophysin
Middle ear adenoma (neuroendocrine adenoma of middle ear [NAME])	Middle ear cavity of temporal bone	Glandular, trabecular, cords, single cells	Dual-cell population of flattened luminal and cuboidal/columnar basal cells; neuroendocrine "salt-and-pepper" chromatin pattern	Luminal cells (pankeratin, CAM5.2, CK7); basal cells (pankeratin, CAM5.2, synaptophysin, chromogranin)	S100, GFAP, EMA
Ceruminous adenoma	External auditory canal, outer portion	Glandular and cystic	Dual-cell population with secretory-type luminal cells and basal layer of myoepithelial cells; yellow-brown ceroid pigment in cytoplasm	Luminal cells (pankeratin, EMA, CK7); basal cells (pankeratin, EMA, CK5/6, p63, S100, CD117)	CK20, chromogranin
Meningioma	Jugular foramen and internal auditory canal region of temporal bone	Infiltrative lobules and nests with whorled, syncytial pattern	Epithelioid cells with ill-defined cell borders, ovoid nuclei, fine chromatin, and occasional intranuclear pseudoinclusions	Pankeratin, CAM5.2, EMA, S100 (weak)	Chromogranin, synaptophysin
Paraganglioma	Middle ear (glomus tympanicum paraganglioma) or jugular foramen (glomus jugulotympanicum paraganglioma) regions of temporal bone	Ball-like clusters of tumor cells ("zellballen" architecture)	Granular, basophilic cytoplasm, round nuclei, delicate to coarse chromatin	Chromogranin, synaptophysin, NSE, CD56; S100 and GFAP positive in sustentacular cells	Pankeratin
Choroid plexus papilloma	Extraventricular tumors can occur at the cerebellopontine angle	Papillary, tubular, glandular	Cuboidal to columnar cells, eosinophilic to clear cytoplasm, bland nuclear features	Pankeratin, vimentin; variable staining with transthyretin, S100, GFAP, synaptophysin	
Metastatic carcinoma	Variable	Variable	Variable	Distinguishing markers include TTF-1 (thyroid or lung), RCC antigen (kidney), and CD10 (kidney)	

ANCILLARY TESTS

Histochemistry

- Periodic acid-Schiff (PAS)-diastase
  - Reactivity: PAS(+)/diastase-sensitive glycogen globules
  - Staining pattern
    - Intracytoplasmic

Immunohistochemistry

- Positive: Cytokeratins (CK7, CK8, CK19, CAM5.2, 34bE12), vimentin, vascular endothelial growth factor (VEGF)
  - Weak &/or focal: S100 (nuclear and cytoplasmic), CD34, neuron-specific enolase (NSE), glial fibrillary acidic protein (GFAP), and epithelial membrane antigen (EMA)
- Negative: CK10/13, CK20, chromogranin, synaptophysin

Molecular Genetics

- In patients with germline mutations in *VHL*, fluorescence in situ hybridization (FISH) can show loss of remaining wild-type *VHL* allele (genetic "second hit" leading to tumor formation) in ELSTs

Electron Microscopy

- Scant microvilli, luminal glycocalyx, intercellular junctions, and basement membrane formation
- Abundant cytoplasmic glycogen, filaments, rough endoplasmic reticulum, & few secretory granules

SELECTED REFERENCES

1. Bisceglia M et al: Endolymphatic sac papillary tumor (Heffner tumor). Adv Anat Pathol. 13(3):131-8, 2006
2. Choo D et al: Endolymphatic sac tumors in von Hippel-Lindau disease. J Neurosurg. 100(3):480-7, 2004
3. Lonser RR et al: Tumors of the endolymphatic sac in von Hippel-Lindau disease. N Engl J Med. 350(24):2481-6, 2004
4. Horiguchi H et al: Endolymphatic sac tumor associated with a von Hippel-Lindau disease patient: an immunohistochemical study. Mod Pathol. 14(7):727-32, 2001
5. Heffner DK: Low-grade adenocarcinoma of probable endolymphatic sac origin A clinicopathologic study of 20 cases. Cancer. 64(11):2292-302, 1989

ENDOLYMPHATIC SAC TUMOR

Microscopic Features

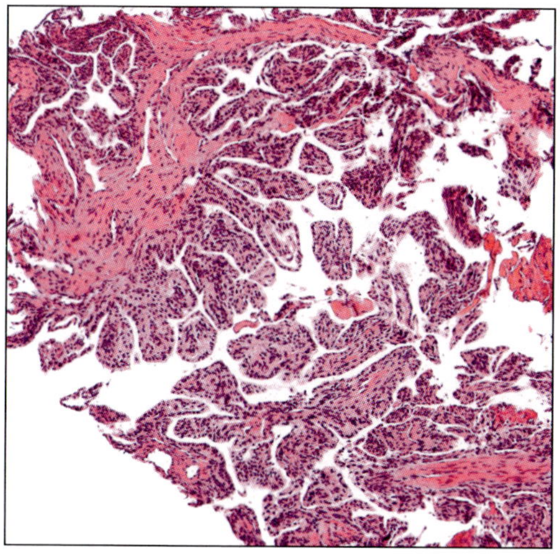
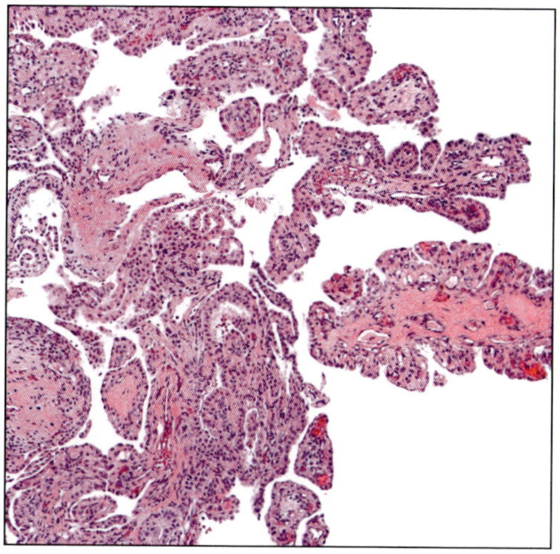

*(**Left**) This low-magnification view highlights the papillary architecture of endolymphatic sac tumors (ELSTs) with their branching fibrovascular cores and single layer of cuboidal epithelium. (**Right**) Another low-magnification view of an ELST demonstrates the characteristic papillary architecture.*

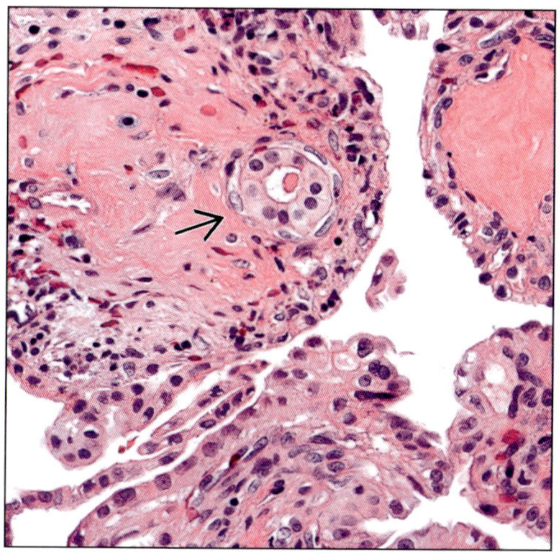
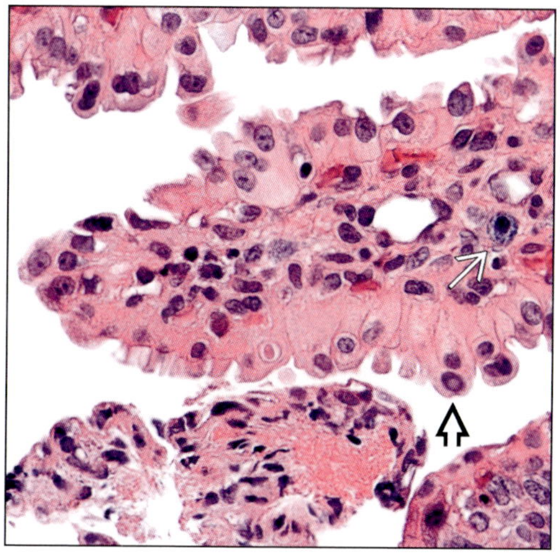

*(**Left**) A glandular structure with colloid-like material in the lumen is shown →. The epithelium is cuboidal with pale cytoplasm and uniform, ovoid nuclei. (**Right**) The papillae of this ELST is lined by columnar epithelium with pale eosinophilic cytoplasm. Mast cells ➔ can occasionally be seen in the fibrovascular cores. Nuclei are ovoid with fine chromatin, variably prominent nucleoli, and scattered intranuclear pseudoinclusions ⇨.*

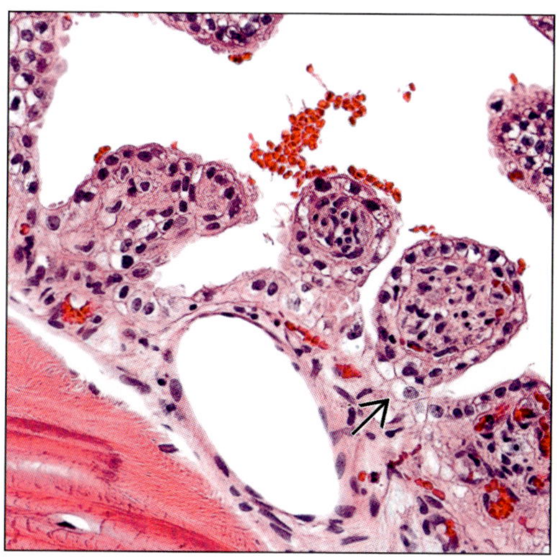
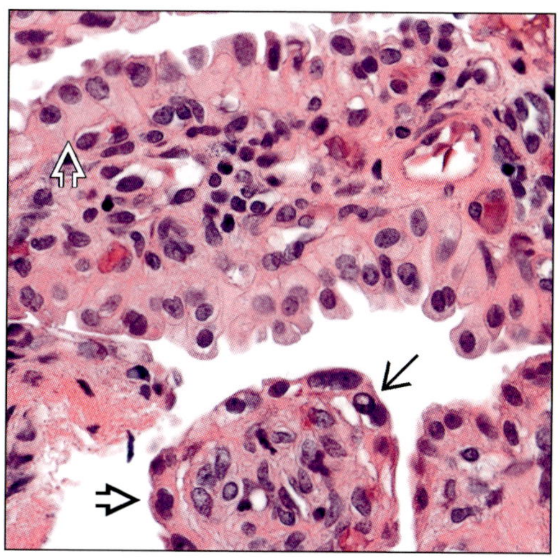

*(**Left**) A portion of the temporal bone is shown in the lower left corner. The cytoplasm of ELSTs ranges from clear → to pale eosinophilic. (**Right**) High-magnification image shows the cuboidal ⇨ to columnar ➔ epithelium characteristic of ELSTs. Occasional intranuclear pseudoinclusions are present →.*

Endocrine

ADRENAL CORTICAL ADENOMA

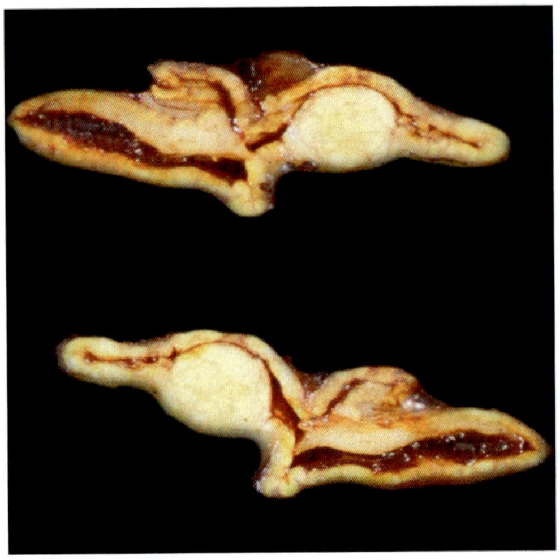

This cross section of an adrenal gland shows classical features of aldosterone-producing tumor. A round, small, well-circumscribed mass has the characteristic yellow cut surface.

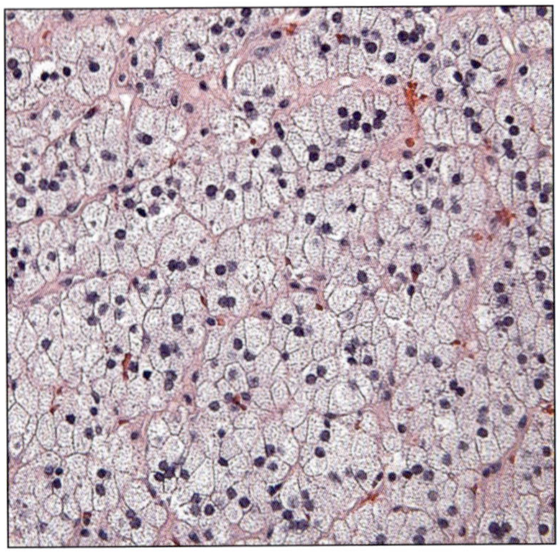

High-magnification view of an aldosterone-secreting adenoma shows a nesting pattern (one of the characteristic patterns), as well as large lipid-rich cells, which are usually the predominant cell type.

TERMINOLOGY

Abbreviations

- Adrenal cortical adenoma (ACA)

Synonyms

- Cortisol-producing adrenocortical adenoma
- Aldosterone-producing adrenal adenoma
- Cushing syndrome
- Functional and nonfunctional adrenal adenoma

Definitions

- Benign neoplasm arising from adrenal cortical cells ± hormone hypersecretion

ETIOLOGY/PATHOGENESIS

Syndromes Associated With Adrenal Cortical Adenoma

- Multiple endocrine neoplasia 1 (MEN1)
- McCune-Albright syndrome
- Carney complex
- Beckwith-Wiedemann syndrome
- Congenital adrenal hyperplasia
- Carney triad

Sporadic

- Most ACA cases are considered sporadic

CLINICAL ISSUES

Epidemiology

- Incidence
  - True incidence is unknown
  - According to some literature, incidence of adrenal cortical adenomas is low if incidentalomas are excluded
  - Typically unilateral, solitary, and benign
- Age
  - Can occur in any age group
- Gender
  - Slight female predilection

Presentation

- Nonfunctional, detected more often by imaging studies
- Most common presentation is associated with hormonal production
  - Glucocorticoid
    - Weight gain (central obesity)
    - Supraclavicular and dorsocervical fat pads
    - Facial rounding (moon face) and plethora
    - Easy bruising and poor wound healing
    - Purple striae and hirsutism
    - Proximal muscle weakness
    - Osteoporosis
  - Mineralocorticoid
    - Hypertension and hypokalemia
  - Androgens
    - Virilization in women
    - Excess testosterone in men
  - Estrogens
    - Gynecomastia in men
    - Menstrual irregularities in women

Treatment

- Surgical unilateral adrenalectomy

IMAGE FINDINGS

MR Findings

- Homogeneous
- Signal intensity less than fat but greater than muscle
- Similar intensity to liver on T1 and T2

CT Findings

- Well defined with smooth borders, homogeneous

ADRENAL CORTICAL ADENOMA

Key Facts

Terminology
- Benign neoplasm arising from adrenal cortical cells with cortisol hypersecretion

Etiology/Pathogenesis
- Associated with syndromes
  - Multiple endocrine neoplasia 1 (MEN1)
  - McCune-Albright syndrome
  - Carney complex
  - Beckwith-Wiedemann syndrome
  - Congenital adrenal hyperplasia
  - Carney triad
- Sporadic

Microscopic Pathology
- Smooth pushing borders without well-defined fibrous capsule
- Clear cytoplasm that is finely vacuolated due to intracytoplasmic lipid droplets
- Cells are larger than in normal adrenal and have pleomorphic nuclei
- Nuclei are single, round/oval, with chromatin margination and single dot-like nucleolus
- Mixed pattern with oxyphilic and clear cells
- Mixed composition of pale-staining lipid-rich cells and cells with lipid-poor compact cytoplasm

Ancillary Tests
- Positive for adrenal cortical markers, such as inhibin and Melan-A
- Adenomas and carcinomas are monoclonal

Top Differential Diagnoses
- Pheochromocytoma

- Attenuation values less than normal adrenal tissue
- May enhance after contrast administration

MACROSCOPIC FEATURES

General Features
- Generally solitary, unilateral, and unicentric
- Rarely bilateral (contralateral adenoma is sometimes nonhyperfunctional)
- Cross section: Yellow, golden yellow, or brown
- Geographic or mottled zones of dark pigmentation may be present
  - Due to lipid depletion of neoplastic cells as well as lipofuscin accumulation
- Necrosis, coarse lobulation, and cystic changes are rare (as compared to carcinomas)
- When diffusely dark brown or black: Black adenoma

Size
- Average diameter: 3.6 cm (range: 1.5-6 cm)
- Usually < 50 g
- If > 100 g, considered carcinoma until proven otherwise

MICROSCOPIC PATHOLOGY

Histologic Features
- Smooth pushing borders without well-defined fibrous capsule
- Broad fields of pale-staining, lipid-rich cells with uniform nuclei
- Architectural patterns are cells in nesting or alveolar arrangement with delicate intersecting vasculature and areas of short cords
- Distinct cell borders mimicking cells of normal adrenal
- Mixed pattern with oxyphilic and clear cells
  - Mixed composition of pale-staining lipid-rich cells and cells with lipid-poor compact cytoplasm
- May have areas of lipomatous or myelolipomatous metaplasia
- Mitotic figures are very rare
- Some may have degenerative features: Fibrosis, organizing fibrin-rich thrombi within sinusoids, dystrophic calcification, or even metaplastic bone
- Myxoid changes are rare; however, when present, they should prompt suspicion of borderline or malignant tumor

Cytologic Features
- Clear or eosinophilic cytoplasm which, at higher magnification, is finely vacuolated due to intracytoplasmic lipid droplets
- Cells are larger than in normal adrenal and have pleomorphic nuclei
- Nuclei are single, round/oval, with chromatin margination and single dot-like nucleoli
  - Intranuclear inclusions may be present

ANCILLARY TESTS

Serologic Testing
- According to the European Network for the Study of Adrenal Tumors (ENSAT), tests should be performed when a functional adenoma is suspected
  - Fasting blood glucose
  - Potassium
  - Cortisol
  - ACTH
  - 24-hour urinary free cortisol
  - Fasting serum cortisol at 8 am following 1 mg dose of dexamethasone at bedtime
  - Adrenal androgens (e.g., dehydroepiandrostrone sulfate [DHEAS], androstenedione, testosterone, 17-OH progesterone)
  - Serum estradiol in men and postmenopausal women

Immunohistochemistry
- Used to confirm diagnosis, to differentiate from pheochromocytoma, or when tumors occur in unusual locations in abdomen or spinal canal

ADRENAL CORTICAL ADENOMA

- Positive for adrenal cortical markers, such as inhibin and Melan-A
- Can also be positive for synaptophysin and neuron-specific enolase (NSE) (do not mistake for pheochromocytoma!)
- Negative for chromogranin
- Negative for cytokeratin

Electron Microscopy

- Abundant amount of intracytoplasmic lipid droplets
- Some may have little or no lipid
- Abundant smooth endoplasmic reticulum
- Mitochondria can be prominent with cristae that have tubular or vesicular profile (similar to normal cells of zona fasciculata)

Cytogenetics

- Genetic background is poorly understood
- Adenomas and carcinomas both appear to be monoclonal
- Mean number of comparative genomic hybridization (CGH) changes in carcinomas is 7.6 (range: 1-15) whereas adenomas have a mean of 1.1 changes (range: 0-4)
- Chromosomal loci implicated in adrenal cortical tumorigenesis include
  - Activation of oncogenes on chromosomes 5 and 12
  - Inactivation of tumor suppressor genes on chromosome arms 1p and 17p

DIFFERENTIAL DIAGNOSIS

Adrenal Cortical Carcinoma

- Differentiation is based on numerous morphological criteria, including
  - Capsular invasion, lymphovascular invasion, invasion into adjacent structures, presence of necrosis, mitosis, and metastases
  - Weight and size of tumor
- Clinical symptoms specific for each hormone will help in differential; carcinomas are usually nonfunctional

Pheochromocytoma

- Negative for inhibin, Melan-A, and positive for chromogranin

Metastatic Carcinoma

- Most metastatic carcinomas to adrenal are originally from lung or kidney
- Immunohistochemistry differentiates these tumors
  - Negative for inhibin and Melan-A and positive for cytokeratin

DIAGNOSTIC CHECKLIST

Pathologic Interpretation Pearls

- Unilateral
- Solitary
- Usually benign neoplasms
- Cross section: Yellow or golden yellow
- Geographic or mottled zones of dark pigmentation may be present
- Smooth pushing borders
- Broad fields of pale-staining, lipid-rich cells with uniform nuclei
- Clear cytoplasm that is finely vacuolated due to intracytoplasmic lipid droplets
- Mixed cell population with small compact eosinophilic cells and pale-staining lipid-rich cells
- Positive for inhibin and Melan-A
- Negative for cytokeratin and chromogranin

SELECTED REFERENCES

1. Carney JA et al: Adrenal cortical adenoma: the fourth component of the carney triad and an association with subclinical cushing syndrome. Am J Surg Pathol. 37(8):1140-9, 2013
2. Jamilloux Y et al: A MEN1 syndrome with a paraganglioma. Eur J Hum Genet. Epub ahead of print, 2013
3. Lloyd RV: Adrenal cortical tumors, pheochromocytomas and paragangliomas. Mod Pathol. 24 Suppl 2:S58-65, 2011
4. Zhang Y et al: Endocrine tumors as part of inherited tumor syndromes. Adv Anat Pathol. 18(3):206-18, 2011
5. Yaneva M et al: Genetics of Cushing's syndrome. Neuroendocrinology. 92 Suppl 1:6-10, 2010
6. McNicol AM: A diagnostic approach to adrenal cortical lesions. Endocr Pathol. 19(4):241-51, 2008
7. Stratakis CA: Cushing syndrome caused by adrenocortical tumors and hyperplasias (corticotropin- independent Cushing syndrome). Endocr Dev. 13:117-32, 2008
8. Giordano TJ: Molecular pathology of adrenal cortical tumors: separating adenomas from carcinomas. Endocr Pathol. 17(4):355-63, 2006
9. Cassarino DS et al: Spinal adrenal cortical adenoma with oncocytic features: report of the first intramedullary case and review of the literature. Int J Surg Pathol. 12(3):259-64, 2004
10. Tung SC et al: Bilateral adrenocortical adenomas causing ACTH-independent Cushing's syndrome at different periods: a case report and discussion of corticosteroid replacement therapy following bilateral adrenalectomy. J Endocrinol Invest. 27(4):375-9, 2004
11. Sugawara A et al: A case of aldosterone-producing adrenocortical adenoma associated with a probable post-operative adrenal crisis: histopathological analyses of the adrenal gland. Hypertens Res. 26(8):663-8, 2003
12. Zhang PJ et al: The role of calretinin, inhibin, melan-A, BCL-2, and C-kit in differentiating adrenal cortical and medullary tumors: an immunohistochemical study. Mod Pathol. 16(6):591-7, 2003
13. Loy TS et al: A103 immunostaining in the diagnosis of adrenal cortical tumors: an immunohistochemical study of 316 cases. Arch Pathol Lab Med. 126(2):170-2, 2002
14. Sidhu S et al: Comparative genomic hybridization analysis of adrenocortical tumors. J Clin Endocrinol Metab. 87(7):3467-74, 2002
15. Munro LM et al: The expression of inhibin/activin subunits in the human adrenal cortex and its tumours. J Endocrinol. 161(2):341-7, 1999
16. Pelkey TJ et al: The alpha subunit of inhibin in adrenal cortical neoplasia. Mod Pathol. 11(6):516-24, 1998
17. Neville AM et al: Histopathology of the human adrenal cortex. Clin Endocrinol Metab. 14(4):791-820, 1985
18. Bertagna C et al: Clinical and laboratory findings and results of therapy in 58 patients with adrenocortical tumors admitted to a single medical center (1951 to 1978). Am J Med. 71(5):855-75, 1981

ADRENAL CORTICAL ADENOMA

Immunohistochemistry

Antibody	Reactivity	Staining Pattern	Comment
Inhibin	Positive	Cell membrane & cytoplasm	
Mart-1	Positive	Cytoplasmic	
Melan-A103	Positive	Cytoplasmic	
Chromogranin-A	Negative		Helps to discriminate from pheochromocytoma
CK7	Negative		Helps to discriminate from other epithelial tumors
CK20	Negative		Helps to discriminate from other epithelial tumors
AE1/AE3	Negative		Helps to discriminate from other epithelial tumors
EMA	Negative		Helps to discriminate from other epithelial tumors
CD10	Negative		Helps to discriminate from renal cell carcinoma
Hep-Par1	Negative		Helps to discriminate from hepatocellular carcinoma
HMFG	Negative		
RCC	Negative		Helps to discriminate from renal cell carcinoma
HMB-45	Negative		

Differential Diagnosis of Adrenal Cortical Adenoma

Neoplasm	Inhibin	Melan-A	Chromo	Syn	Hep-Par1	CD10
Adrenal cortical adenoma	Positive	Positive	Negative	Positive (57%)	Negative	Negative
Pheochromocytoma	Negative	Negative	Positive	Positive	Negative	Negative
Hepatocellular carcinoma	Negative	Negative	Negative	Negative	Positive	Positive (61%)
Renal cell carcinoma	Negative	Negative	Negative	Negative	Negative	Positive

Chromo: Chromogranin; Syn: Synaptophysin.

Criteria for Differentiation Between Adenoma and Carcinoma

Criteria	Adenoma	Carcinoma
Hormonal production	Often functional	Usually nonfunctional
Gross	Weight < 50 g	Weight > 100 g
Tumor gross color	Variable	Variable; does not differentiate
Circumscription	Well circumscribed	Invasive
Hemorrhage	Absent	Frequent
Necrosis	Absent	Frequent
Capsular invasion	Absent	Usually present
Invasion into adjacent tissues	Absent	Usually present
Intratumoral fibrosis	May be present	May be present
Myxomatous degeneration	May be present	May be present
Cytology	May have cytologic atypia	Cytologic atypia present
Histology	Atypia may be present	Atypia present
Necrosis	Necrosis absent	Present; confluent necrosis
Mitosis	Rare	> 5/50 HPF
Venous invasion	Absent	Present

Adrenal Cortical Lesions Associated With Syndromes

Adrenal Pathology	Syndromes Associated With Adrenal Pathology
Adrenal cortical adenoma	MEN1, McCune-Albright syndrome, Beckwith-Wiedemann syndrome, congenital adrenal hyperplasia, Carney complex, Carney triad
Adrenal cortical carcinoma	MEN1, Beckwith-Wiedemann syndrome, Li-Fraumeni syndrome
Macronodular hyperplasia	MEN1, McCune-Albright syndrome, Beckwith-Wiedemann syndrome, congenital adrenal hyperplasia
Primary pigmented adrenocortical disease (PPNAD)	Carney complex

MEN1: Multiple endocrine neoplasia 1.

ADRENAL CORTICAL ADENOMA

Gross and Microscopic Features

(Left) Cross section from a cortisol-secreting adenoma shows the typical round, well-circumscribed ➡, golden yellow appearance. This tumor has foci of dark discoloration ➡ that can be attributed to an old hemorrhage, an area of lipid depletion of the tumor cells, or increased lipofuscin pigment. ***(Right)*** The tumor cells in cortisol-producing adrenal adenomas are arranged in a solid pattern with cytoplasmic lipofuscin pigment ➡, gradation in cell size, and a varying amount of lipid.

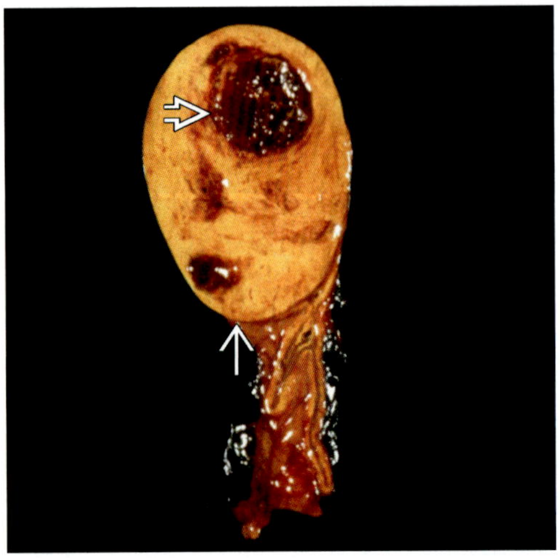

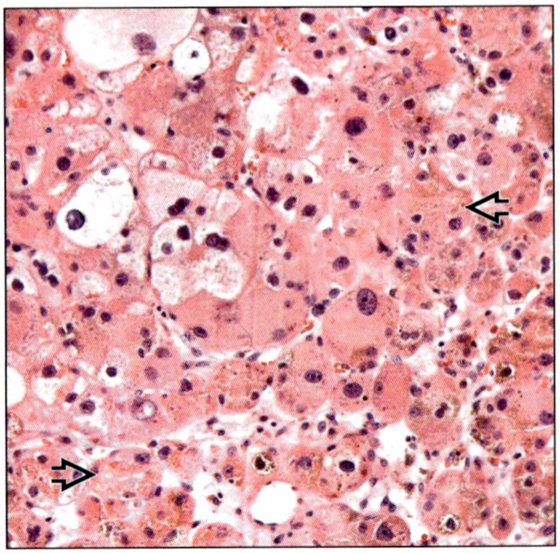

(Left) Adrenal cortical adenoma in Cushing syndrome has a yellow-orange surface and mottled zones of dark pigmentation ➡ due to accumulation of lipofuscin and lipid depletion of the neoplastic cells. ***(Right)*** This cortisol-producing adrenal cortical adenoma is composed of large cells with eosinophilic cytoplasm and enlarged hyperchromatic nuclei. Some cells show a prominent intranuclear inclusion ➡.

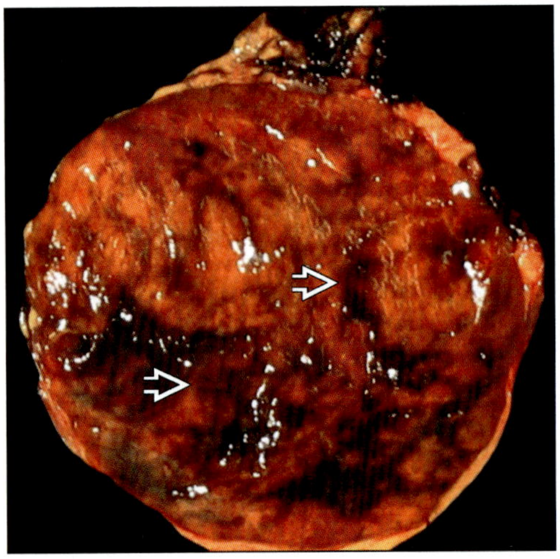

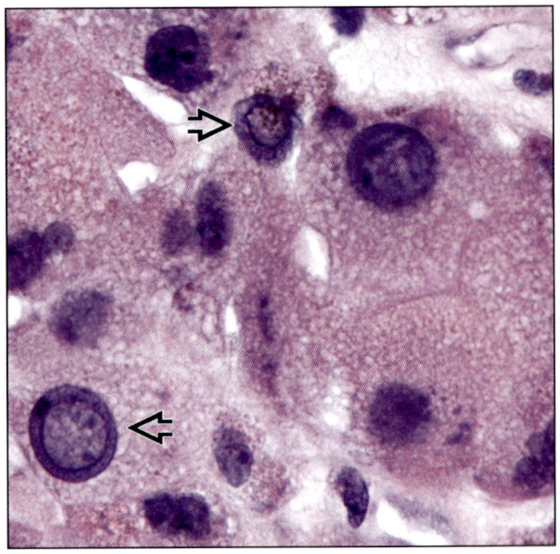

(Left) Close view of adenoma highlights the mottled zones of dark pigmentation ➡. These areas are composed of lipid-depleted cells and cells with accumulation of lipofuscin pigment. Note the marked atrophy of the residual adrenal cortex ➡. ***(Right)*** Cortisol-secreting adrenal cortical adenomas are usually composed of cells with eosinophilic cytoplasm with enlarged hyperchromatic nuclei, some with prominent nucleoli. The cytoplasm contains pigmented granular lipofuscin ➡.

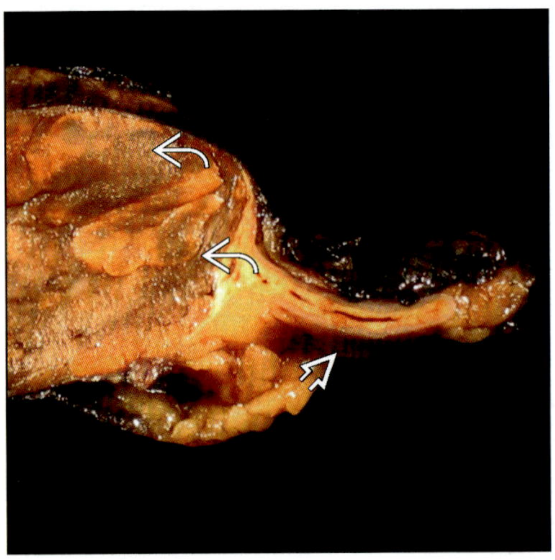

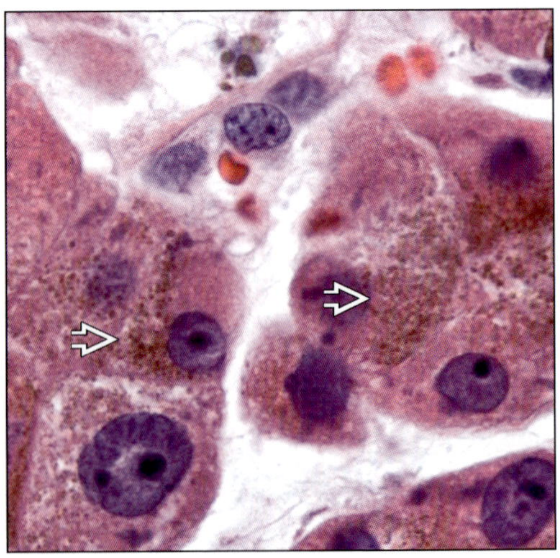

ADRENAL CORTICAL ADENOMA

Gross and Microscopic Features

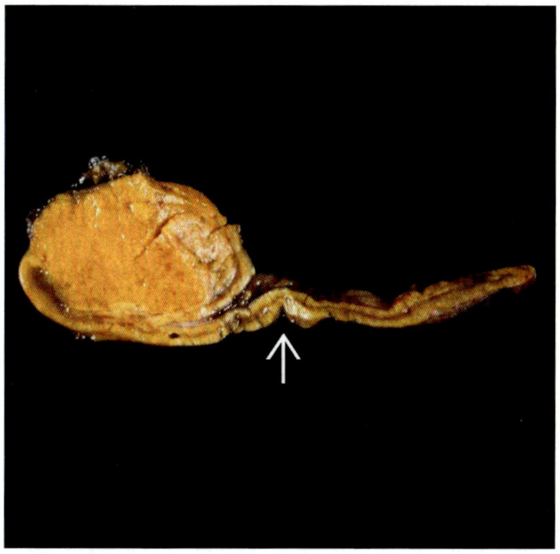
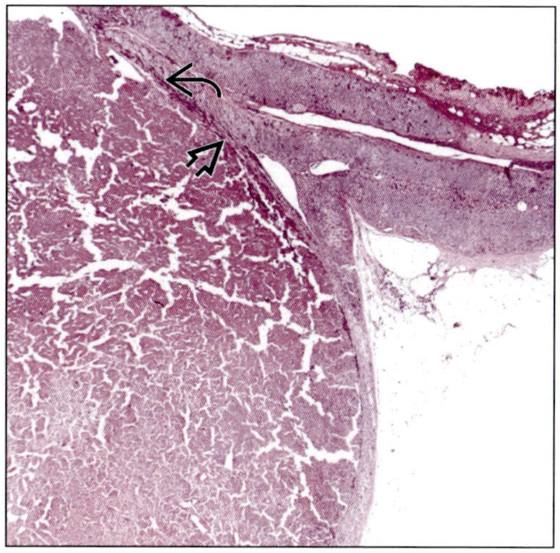

(Left) *This well-circumscribed adenoma has a homogeneous yellow cut surface, and there is marked atrophy of the attached adrenal cortex. Adrenal cortical adenomas can be present in patients with MEN1 syndrome, McCune-Albright syndrome, Carney complex, and Beckwith-Wiedemann syndrome.* ***(Right)*** *This view of an adrenal cortical adenoma shows a sharp demarcation between the normal adrenal parenchyma, contrasting with the pushing borders of the adenoma.*

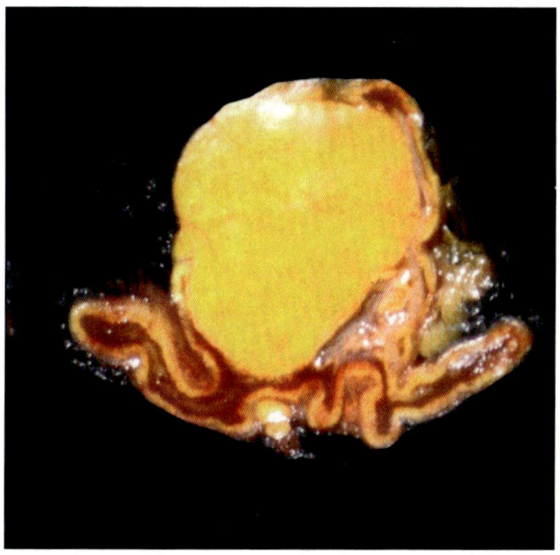
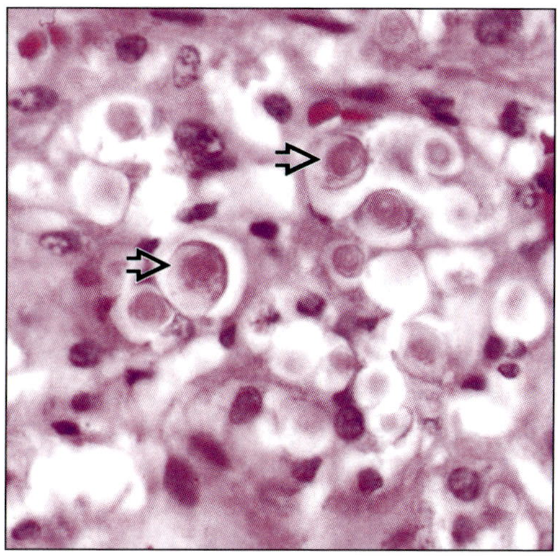

(Left) *Cross section through an adrenal mass shows the classic canary-yellow color of an aldosterone-secreting adenoma. Another characteristic of these tumors is the pushing borders.* ***(Right)*** *High-magnification view of an aldosterone-producing adenoma has the characteristic spironolactone bodies, which are small intracytoplasmic eosinophilic inclusions with a laminated appearance surrounded by a clear halo, which appear in patients treated with spironolactone.*

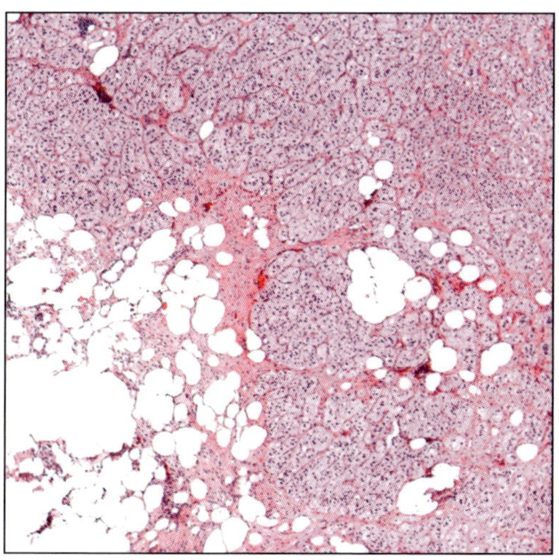
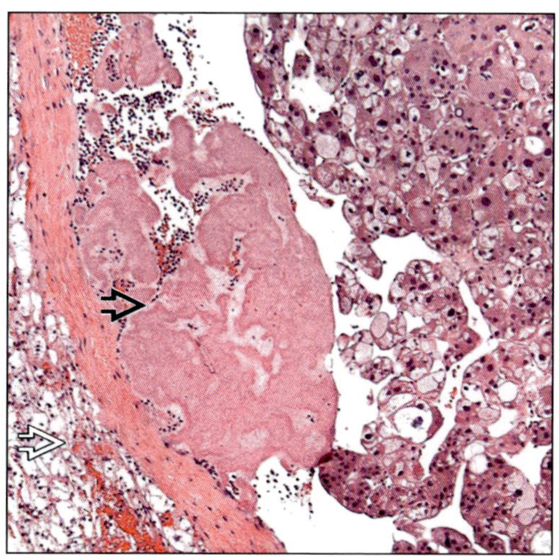

(Left) *This photomicrograph of an aldosterone-secreting adenoma shows lipomatous metaplasia intermixed with tumoral cells, which are arranged in a diffuse architecture. Central degenerative changes can be seen in large tumors.* ***(Right)*** *The tumor cells in this cortisol-producing adrenal cortical adenoma are present within the central vein. There is an associated fibrin thrombus within the lumen, compressing the adjacent normal adrenal cortex.*

ADRENAL CORTICAL ADENOMA

Microscopic Features

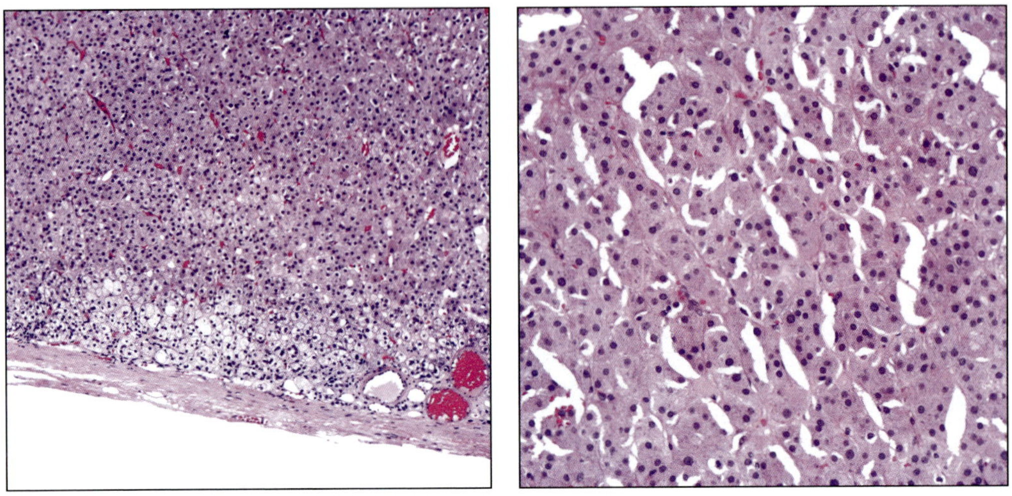

(Left) *Low-power magnification shows a well-circumscribed corticoadrenal neoplasm. A thick fibrous capsule can be seen.* ***(Right)*** *High magnification shows an adrenal cortical adenoma that secretes sex steroids. This picture shows eosinophilic cells with abundant cytoplasm that resemble the cells in the zona reticularis.*

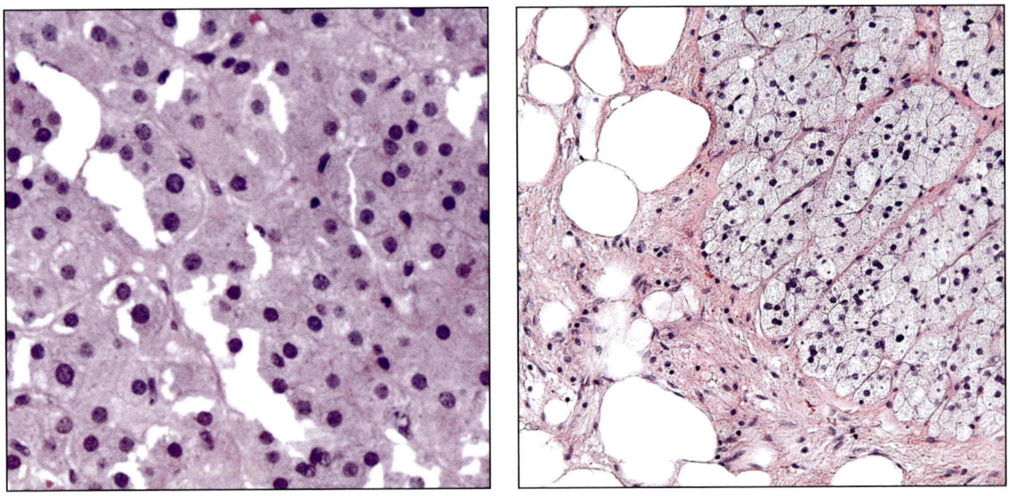

(Left) *High-power photomicrograph shows eosinophilic cells with abundant cytoplasm, characteristic of a sex-steroid-producing adenoma.* ***(Right)*** *This photomicrograph of an aldosterone-secreting adenoma has several characteristic features seen in these tumors. Lipomatous metaplasia is intermixed with tumoral cells in a diffuse architecture or different morphological patterns and may coexist as nesting pattern and cords.*

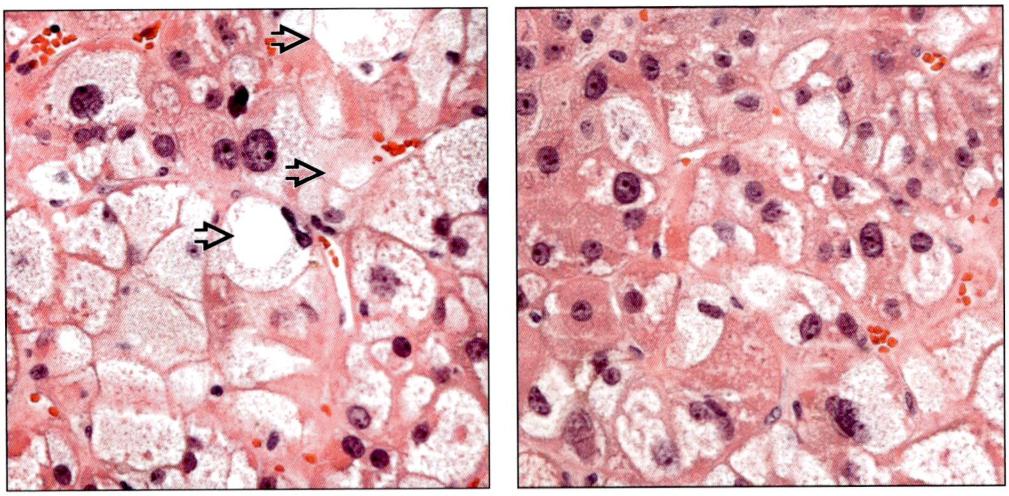

(Left) *The tumor cells are arranged in short cords or clusters. Individual tumor cells contain abundant lipid, which appears as numerous clear vacuoles ⮚. There is variation in nuclear size.* ***(Right)*** *The tumor cells are arranged in a solid pattern with a gradation in tumor cell size and a varying amount of lipid. There is a mixture of oncocytic cells and clear cells in this adrenal cortical adenoma.*

Immunohistochemical Features

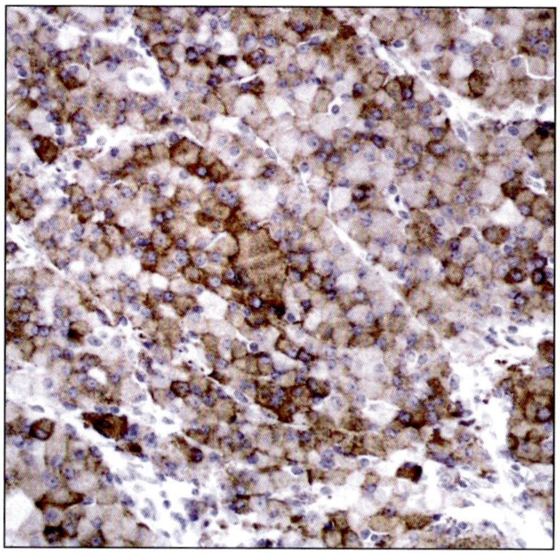

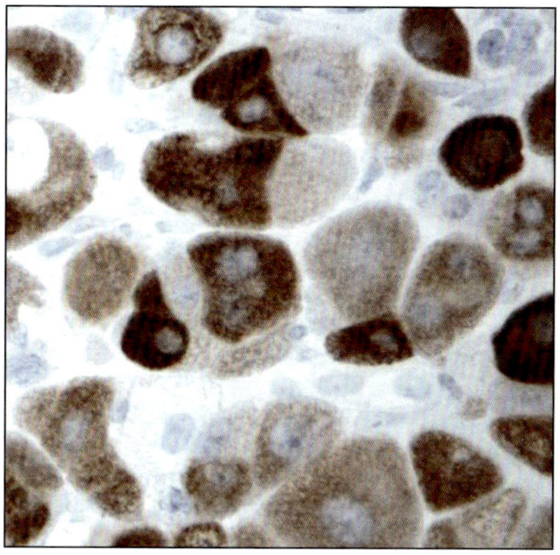

(Left) *This picture shows positivity for synaptophysin, which is 1 of the characteristics of adrenal cortical neoplasms. There is positive cytoplasmic staining in this case of sex-steroid-producing adrenal cortical adenoma.* ***(Right)*** *Immunoreactivity for α-inhibin as well as for Melan-A is sensitive but not specific for adrenal cortical tumors. This photomicrograph illustrates that the tumor cells have variably intense cytoplasmic granular immunopositivity for MART-1.*

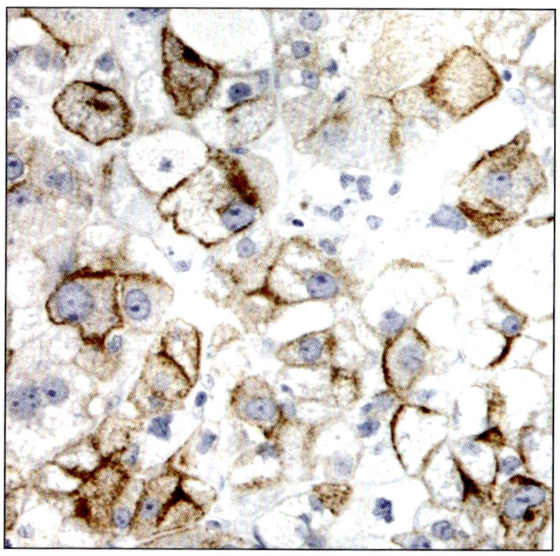

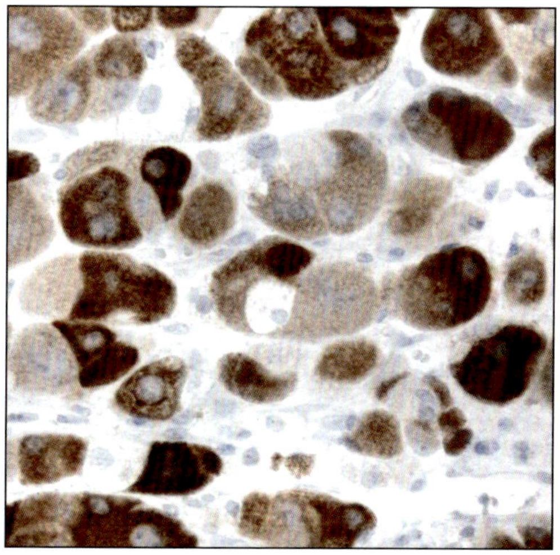

(Left) *Synaptophysin is present in adrenal cortical tumors in a moderately weak membranous and cytoplasmic pattern. This positivity is usually less intense than in pheochromocytoma.* ***(Right)*** *Immunoreactivity for α-inhibin as well as for Melan-A is sensitive but not specific for adrenal cortical tumors. The tumor cells have variably intense cytoplasmic granular immunopositivity for inhibin. In contrast with other epithelial tumors, the tumor cells are negative for cytokeratin and EMA.*

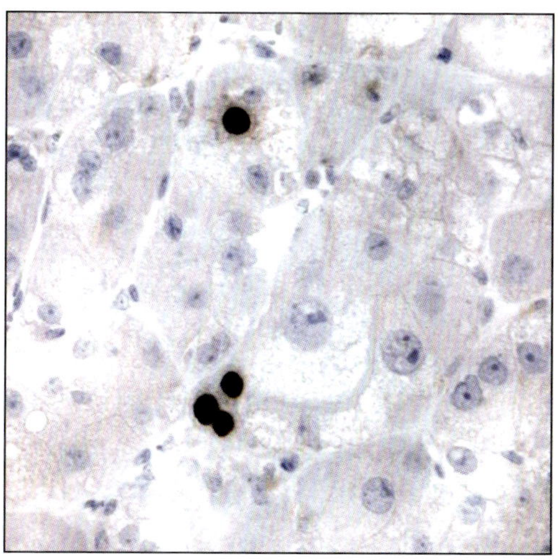

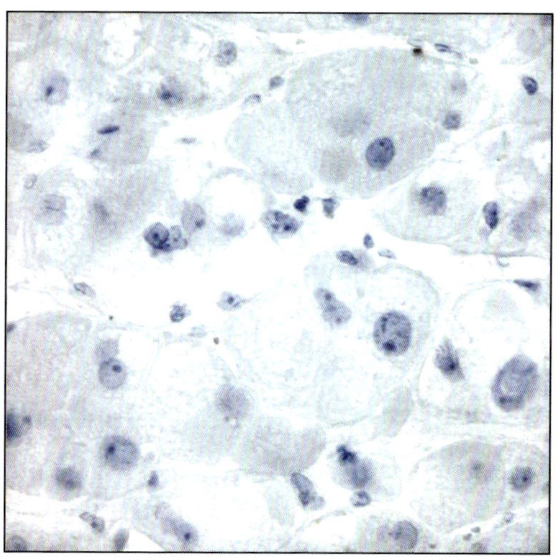

(Left) *Immunohistochemistry for Ki-67 reveals a low proliferative index in the benign cortisol-secreting adrenal cortical adenomas. These findings correlate with a very low mitotic index.* ***(Right)*** *Immunohistochemistry in adrenal cortical adenoma is characteristically negative for chromogranin. The tumor cells in these tumors are also negative for CK7, CK20, AE1/AE3, S100, and CD10, aiding in the differential diagnosis with other epithelial neoplasms.*

ADRENAL CORTICAL CARCINOMA

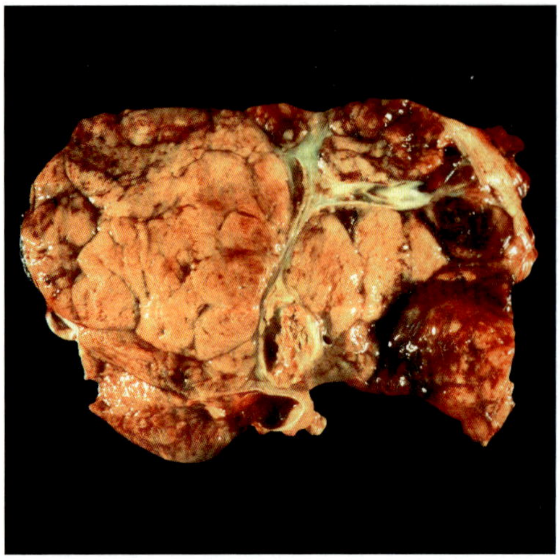

This adrenal cortical carcinoma presented as an irregularly shaped, bulky, unilateral mass. The cut surface shows extensive regressive changes, necrosis, hemorrhage, fibrosis and degeneration, and calcification.

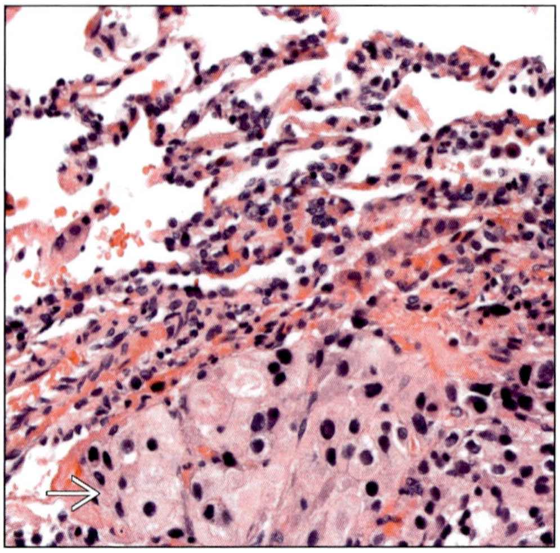

Adrenal cortical carcinoma metastatic to lung exhibits tumor cells ➡ with abundant, granular, oncocytic cytoplasm with round, uniform, hyperchromatic nuclei. Nuclear pleomorphism can be seen among tumor cells.

TERMINOLOGY

Abbreviations

- Adrenal cortical carcinoma (ACC)

Synonyms

- Adrenocortical carcinoma

Definitions

- Malignant epithelial neoplasm of adrenal cortical cells

ETIOLOGY/PATHOGENESIS

Possible Multistep Process

- Adrenal cortical hyperplasia and adenoma may represent precursor lesions

Syndrome Association

- Beckwith-Wiedemann (autosomal dominant)
  - Gene locus includes *IGF2* and *P57/KIP2* genes
  - Involves chromosome 11p15.5 in ~ 80% of cases
- Li-Fraumeni syndrome (autosomal dominant)
  - Germline mutations in tumor suppressor gene *TP53* (17p13.1)
- Multiple endocrine neoplasia 1 (MEN1)
  - *MEN1* gene in chromosome 11q13
- Carney complex
  - *PRKAR1A* in chromosome 17q22-24
  - 2p15-16
- Congenital adrenal hyperplasia
  - Autosomal recessive
- Lynch syndrome

CLINICAL ISSUES

Epidemiology

- Incidence
  - 1-2 cases per 1 million people
  - Comprises ~ 3% of endocrine neoplasms
  - No gender or ethnicity predilection
- Age
  - Bimodal age distribution
    - Primary peak: 60-70 years
    - Secondary peak: Early childhood

Presentation

- Nonfunctional tumors are detected more often as radiographic techniques improve
- Most common presentation is associated with hormone oversecretions
  - Glucocorticoid
    - Cushing syndrome
    - Central obesity
    - Moon facies
    - Protein wasting, striae, and skin thinning
    - Muscle atrophy, osteoporosis
    - Diabetes, hypertension, gonadal dysfunction
    - Psychiatric disorders
  - Mineralocorticoid
    - Hypertension and hypokalemia
  - Androgens
    - Virilization in women
    - Excess testosterone in men
  - Estrogens
    - Very rare, yielding gynecomastia in men
    - Menstrual irregularities in women
- Mass
  - Flank pain due to compressive symptoms

Laboratory Tests

- Serum or urinary hormone quantification
  - Hormones may not be bioactive
  - May require special methods for detection
  - Deoxycorticosterone, hydroxyprogesterone
  - Androstenedione, estrogens
  - Urine 17-ketogenic steroids or 17-ketosteroids may be elevated
  - Dehydroepiandrosterone sulfate (DHEAS)

ADRENAL CORTICAL CARCINOMA

Key Facts

Terminology
- Malignant epithelial neoplasm of adrenal cortical cells

Etiology/Pathogenesis
- Familial
  - Beckwith-Wiedemann syndrome
  - Li-Fraumeni syndrome
  - Multiple endocrine neoplasia 1
  - Carney complex
  - Congenital adrenal hyperplasia
- Sporadic

Clinical Issues
- Bimodal age distribution
- Overall 5-year survival: 70%

Macroscopic Features
- Bulky tumors with red-brown and fleshy, firm appearance
  - 3-40 cm
  - Usually > 200 g

Microscopic Pathology
- No single feature is diagnostic of carcinoma
- Multiple systems used for diagnosis (Weiss, Hough, van Slooten)

Ancillary Tests
- Positive for inhibin, Melan-A, calretinin, and SF1

Top Differential Diagnoses
- Adrenal cortical adenoma, metastatic tumors, renal cell carcinoma, and pheochromocytoma

- Dexamethasone suppression test

Treatment
- Options, risks, complications
  - Complications due to pituitary-hypothalamus-adrenal axis suppression
- Surgical approaches
  - Complete, radical surgical resection is treatment of choice
- Drugs
  - Mitotane
    - May help prolong recurrence-free survival after radical surgery
    - Can be used after incomplete resection or for metastatic disease
    - In patients not eligible for surgery
  - Chemotherapy regimens reported
    - Etoposide, doxorubicin, cisplatin, and mitotane
    - Streptozotocin and mitotane
    - Failure possibly due to high rate of multidrug resistance protein 1 (*MDR1*) gene expression
- Radiation
  - Radiotherapy can help control residual disease

Prognosis
- Overall 5-year survival: 50-70%
- Disease-free 5-year survival: 30%
- Dependent on age and stage
  - Children have better prognosis than adults
  - Stage 1 and stage 2 tumors have better prognosis than stage 3 or stage 4
- Majority of cases present with stage 4 disease
- Key prognostic factor is feasibility of complete tumor resection
- Local recurrence is frequent
- Nearly 40% have distant metastases at presentation
  - Most common metastases to liver, lung, lymph nodes, and bone

IMAGE FINDINGS

Radiographic Findings
- Inhomogeneous masses with irregular borders and necrosis
- Usually show low tumor fat content
  - Distinctly different from adenomas, which have high fat content

MR Findings
- Carcinoma tends to be large (> 5 cm)
- Irregular or invasive borders
- Decreased intracellular lipid and macroscopic fat
- Signal heterogeneity and necrosis
- Vena cava extension/invasion may be seen

CT Findings
- Heterogeneous, enhancing large mass
- Typically > 5 cm
- Frequently with displacement or invasion of adjacent organs
- Calcifications present in 30% of cases

PET Scan
- Helpful in determining distant metastases

MACROSCOPIC FEATURES

General Features
- Bulky tumors with red-brown and fleshy, firm appearance
- Typically unilateral
  - If bilateral, consider contralateral metastasis

Sections to Be Submitted
- Sample foci of hemorrhage &/or necrosis
- Usually 1 section per cm, up to 15 sections

Size
- Range: 3-40 cm (mean: 12 cm)

ADRENAL CORTICAL CARCINOMA

Weight
- Usually > 200 g
- Can be 10-5,000 g

MICROSCOPIC PATHOLOGY

Histologic Features
- May resemble normal adrenal
- Patternless sheets or nests of cells
- Broad trabeculae and fine sinusoids
- Myxoid change may be present
- Necrosis may be absent or abundant
- In children, these features may not indicate malignancy
- Benign cortical tumors with oncocytic change can have some of these features

Cytologic Features
- Cells have clear to eosinophilic cytoplasm
- Nuclei range from bland to highly atypical
- Variable mitotic rate

ANCILLARY TESTS

Cytology
- Unable to separate benign from malignant adrenal cortical lesions
- High nuclear pleomorphism, chromatin irregularities, and prominent nucleoli favor carcinoma
- FNA can be diagnostic for metastatic tumors

Histochemistry
- Reticulin
  - Reactivity: Quantitative changes in ACC with extensive loss and disruption of fibers
  - Staining pattern
    - Detect the presence of reticulin fiber disruptive changes

Immunohistochemistry
- Positive for inhibin, Melan-A, calretinin, synaptophysin, CD99, steroidogenic factor-1 (SF1)

Molecular Genetics
- Adrenocorticotrophic hormone-cAMP-protein kinase A and Wnt pathways are implicated
- Overexpression of *IGF2*
- Somatic mutations of *TP53* or *RB*
- Low expression of *P57*, *H19*, and *MYC*

Electron Microscopy
- Features of steroidogenesis
  - Abundant rough and smooth endoplasmic reticulum
  - Many mitochondria
  - Intracytoplasmic lipid droplets

DIFFERENTIAL DIAGNOSIS

Adrenal Cortical Adenoma
- Tends to be smaller and weigh < carcinoma
- Often lacks mitotic figures, necrosis, and invasion
- Diagnosis of pediatric adrenal cortical tumors is difficult

Metastatic Tumors
- More likely to be bilateral
- Glandular, squamous, or small cell histology

Hepatocellular Carcinoma
- Confirm biopsy site
- Trabecular pattern, bile pigment, glandular arrangement
- Positive keratin, CEA, and Hep-Par1

Renal Cell Carcinoma
- Pseudoalveolar pattern
- Extravasated erythrocytes
- Clear cytoplasm, prominent cell borders
- Positive for keratin, CD10, and EMA

Pheochromocytoma
- Different radiographic appearance, especially with scintigraphic studies
- Nested and zellballen pattern
- Basophilic cytoplasm, bizarre, isolated, atypical nuclei
- Positive for chromogranin, synaptophysin, and CD56 in paraganglia cells
- S100 protein positive sustentacular cells

DIAGNOSTIC CHECKLIST

Distinction Between Benign and Malignant Adrenal Cortical Neoplasms
- No single feature is diagnostic of carcinoma
- Multiple systems used for diagnosis (Weiss, Hough, van Slooten)
- Most significant histologic features
  - High nuclear grade (analogous Fuhrman grade 4)
  - > 5 mitotic figures/50 HPF
  - Atypical mitotic figures
  - < 25% of tumor cells with clear/vacuolated cytoplasm
  - Diffuse architecture (> 1/3 of tumor)
  - Confluent tumor necrosis
  - Venous invasion (of smooth muscle-walled vessels)
  - Sinusoidal invasion (no smooth muscle in vessel wall)
  - Capsular invasion
  - Acellular, fibrous connective tissue bands

STAGING

Recently Adopted AJCC and UICC Staging Systems
- Stage 1: Confined to gland, ≤ 5 cm
- Stage 2: Confined to gland, > 5 cm
- Stage 3: Extends beyond gland but not into adjacent organs
- Stage 4: Distant metastases or adjacent organ involvement

ADRENAL CORTICAL CARCINOMA

Immunohistochemistry

Antibody	Reactivity	Staining Pattern	Comment
Vimentin	Positive	Cytoplasmic	
Inhibin	Positive	Cytoplasmic	Nondiscriminating between adenoma and carcinoma
Melan-A103	Positive	Cytoplasmic	Nondiscriminating between adenoma and carcinoma
Calretinin	Positive	Nuclear & cytoplasmic	
SF1	Positive	Nuclear	
CK-PAN	Equivocal	Cytoplasmic	< 5% of tumor cells are reactive

Histologic Criteria for Distinguishing Benign From Malignant Adrenal Cortical Neoplasms

Weiss Criteria*	van Slooten System**
High nuclear grade; Fuhrman criteria used	Histologic criteria and weight
> 5 mitoses/50 HPF	Extensive regressive changes (necrosis, hemorrhage, fibrosis, calcification)/**5.7**
Atypical mitotic figures	Loss of normal structure/**1.6**
< 25% of tumor cells are clear cells	Nuclear atypia (moderate to marked)/**2.1**
Diffuse architecture (> 33% of tumor)	Nuclear hyperchromasia (moderate to marked)/**2.6**
Necrosis	Abnormal nucleoli/**4.1**
Venous invasion (smooth muscle in wall)	Mitotic activity (≥ 2/10 HPF)/**9.0**
Sinusoidal invasion (no smooth muscle in wall)	Vascular or capsular invasion/**3.3**
Capsular invasion	

**Presence of 3 or more criteria highly correlates with malignant behavior. **Histologic index > 8 correlates with malignant behavior.*

System of Hough for Distinguishing Benign From Malignant Adrenal Cortical Neoplasms

Histologic Criteria/Value*	Nonhistologic Criteria/Value*
Diffuse growth pattern/**0.92**	Tumor mass > 100 g/**0.60**
Vascular invasion/**0.92**	Urinary 17-ketosteroids (10 mg/g creatinine/24 h)/**0.50**
Tumor cell necrosis/**0.69**	Response to ACTH (17-hydroxysteroids increased 2x after 50 mg ACTH IV)/**0.42**
Broad fibrous bands/**1.00**	Cushing syndrome with virilism, virilism alone, or no clinical manifestations/**0.42**
Capsular invasion/**0.37**	Weight loss (10 lb/3 months)/**2.00**
Mitotic index (1/10 HPF)/**0.60**	
Pleomorphism (moderate and marked)/**0.39**	

**Mean histologic index of malignant tumors is 2.91, indeterminate tumors 1.00, and benign tumors 0.17.*

SELECTED REFERENCES

1. Duregon E et al: The reticulin algorithm for adrenocortical tumor diagnosis: A multicentric validation study on 245 unpublished cases. Am J Surg Pathol. Epub ahead of print, 2013
2. Raymond VM et al: Adrenocortical carcinoma is a Lynch syndrome-associated cancer. J Clin Oncol. Epub ahead of print, 2013
3. McNicol AM: Lesions of the adrenal cortex. Arch Pathol Lab Med. 132(8):1263-71, 2008
4. Volante M et al: Pathological and molecular features of adrenocortical carcinoma: an update. J Clin Pathol. 61(7):787-93, 2008
5. Sasano H et al: Recent advances in histopathology and immunohistochemistry of adrenocortical carcinoma. Endocr Pathol. 17(4):345-54, 2006
6. Wieneke JA et al: Adrenal cortical neoplasms in the pediatric population: a clinicopathologic and immunophenotypic analysis of 83 patients. Am J Surg Pathol. 27(7):867-81, 2003
7. Stratakis CA: Genetics of adrenocortical tumors: Carney complex. Ann Endocrinol (Paris). 62(2):180-4, 2001
8. Weiss LM et al: Pathologic features of prognostic significance in adrenocortical carcinoma. Am J Surg Pathol. 13(3):202-6, 1989
9. Weiss LM: Comparative histologic study of 43 metastasizing and nonmetastasizing adrenocortical tumors. Am J Surg Pathol. 8(3):163-9, 1984
10. Hough AJ et al: Prognostic factors in adrenal cortical tumors. A mathematical analysis of clinical and morphologic data. Am J Clin Pathol. 72(3):390-9, 1979

ADRENAL CORTICAL CARCINOMA

Imaging, Gross, and Microscopic Features

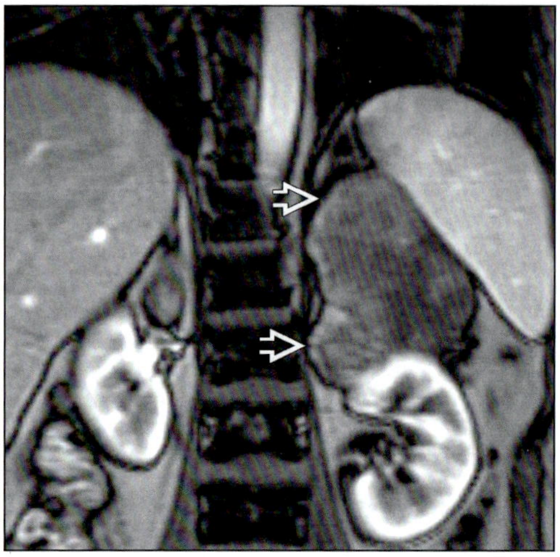
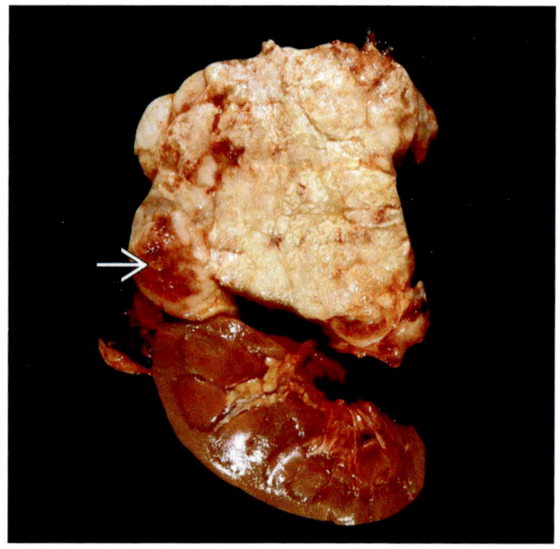

(Left) *Radiologic image shows a large left adrenal gland mass* ➔ *pushing the kidney down and compressing the adjacent spleen. The interior is mottled and shows mixed intensity.* ***(Right)*** *Adrenal cortical carcinomas tend to appear grossly as large solid masses in the suprarenal region, typically measuring > 5 cm. Focal areas of necrosis and hemorrhage* ➔ *are usually present.*

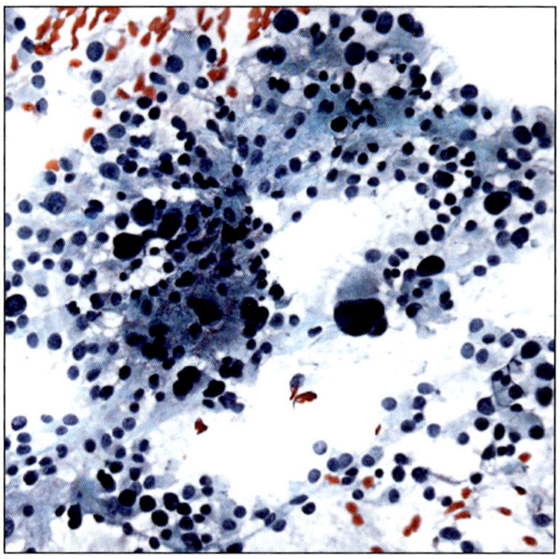
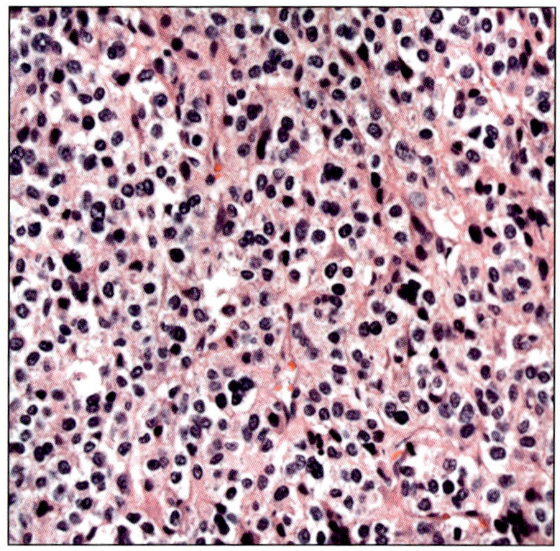

(Left) *Cytologic diagnosis of adrenal cortical carcinoma can be challenging. The degree of polymorphism and nuclear irregularity shown in this cytology favors carcinoma, confirmed on histological examination.* ***(Right)*** *This adrenal cortical carcinoma (ACC) shows an alveolar and solid pattern composed of relatively uniform small round cells with clear cytoplasm. The differential diagnosis of this morphological variant includes metastatic carcinomas, such as renal cell carcinoma or hepatocellular carcinoma.*

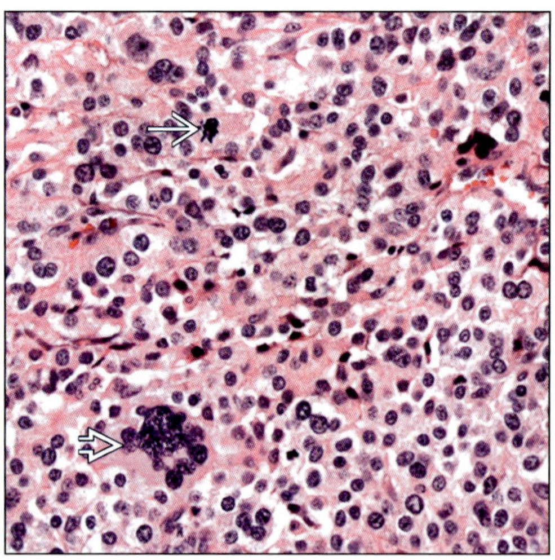
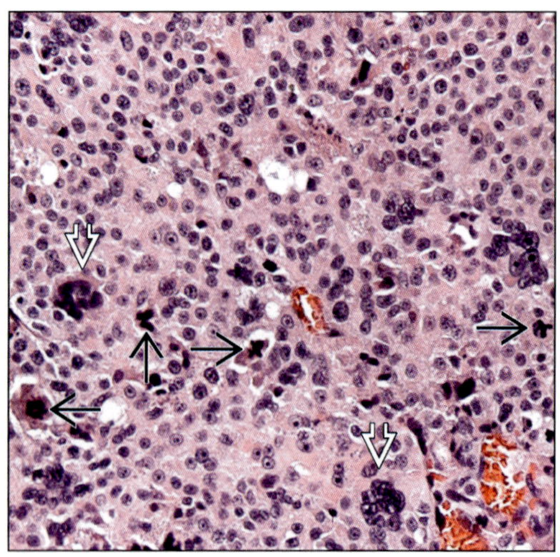

(Left) *High-magnification view of an ACC shows a tumor composed of slightly pleomorphic round cells with both clear and eosinophilic cytoplasm. An atypical mitotic figure* ➔ *and a multinucleated giant cell are indicated* ➔*.* ***(Right)*** *This picture shows an ACC composed of small, compact eosinophilic cells, some with prominent nucleoli intermixed with scattered, bizarre multinucleated cells* ➔*. Several mitotic figures, including atypical mitoses* →*, are present in this field.*

Microscopic Features

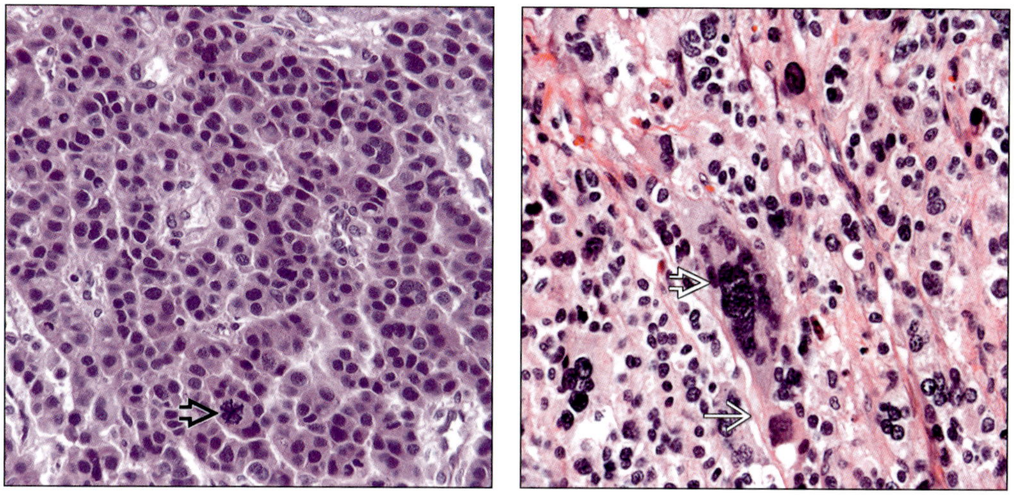

(Left) *Hematoxylin & eosin shows small trabeculae composed of neoplastic cells with a high nuclear to cytoplasmic ratio. Mitotic figures are noted, including an atypical form.* ***(Right)*** *High magnification shows cells in a trabecular arrangement separated by thin fibrovascular bands. Scattered large bizarre multinucleated cells intermixed with small cells may be present.*

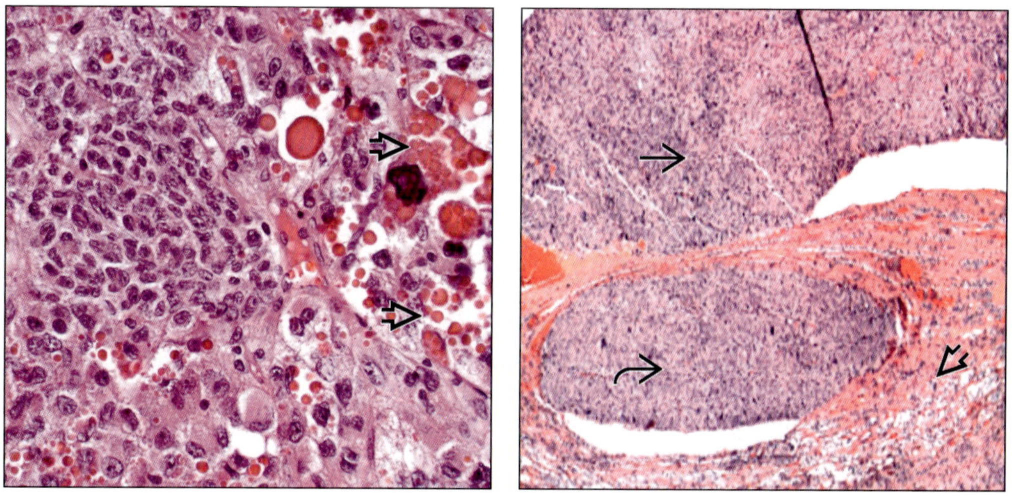

(Left) *Small cells with a high nuclear to cytoplasmic ratio are juxtaposed with larger cells. Intracellular and extracellular eosinophilic globules can be seen in adrenal cortical carcinoma cells.* ***(Right)*** *Low-magnification view shows an area of juxtaposition between an adrenal cortical carcinoma composed of small uniform cells and the residual normal adrenal tissue. Tumor invasion of a large intraparenchymal vessel is shown.*

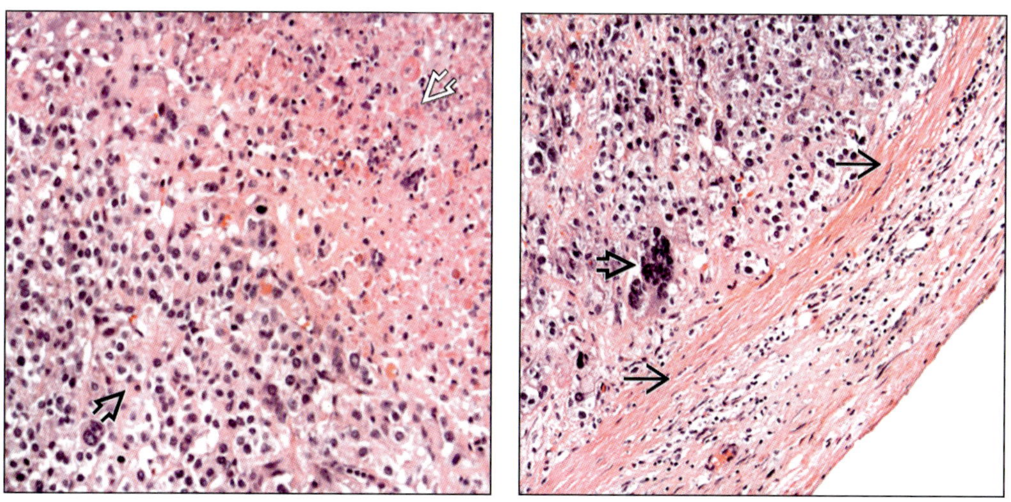

(Left) *Viable tumor and necrosis are depicted. Tumor necrosis is an important histologic criterion in all schemes for differentiation between benign and malignant adrenal cortical neoplasms.* ***(Right)*** *This tumor invades a vessel wall and is composed of small, uniform cells with clear cytoplasm. Atypical cells with large irregular nuclei and a large bizarre multinucleated cell are also shown.*

ADRENAL CORTICAL CARCINOMA

Beckwith-Wiedemann Syndrome

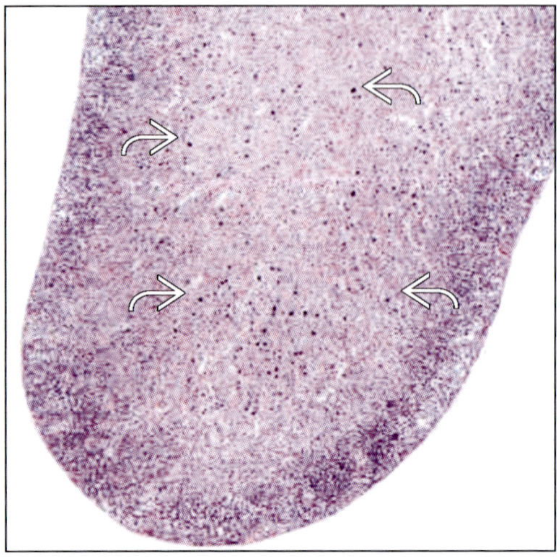

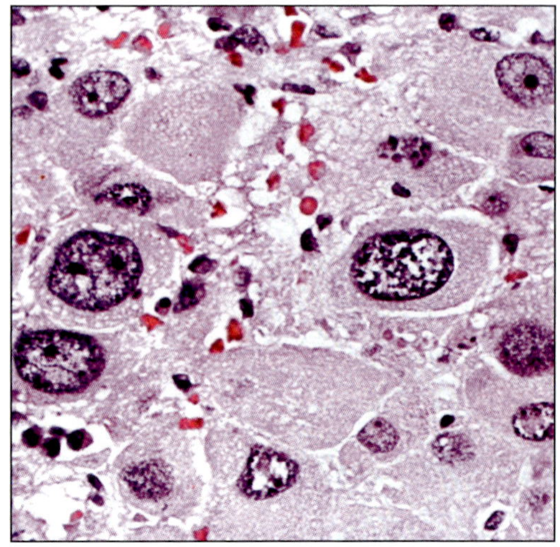

(Left) *The adrenal cortical cells in children with Beckwith-Wiedemann syndrome are composed by a mixture of small cells and large polyhedral cells with markedly enlarged nuclei, also observed at a low magnification.* ***(Right)*** *Adrenal cortical cytomegaly is usually present in children with Beckwith-Wiedemann syndrome. The adrenal cortical cells are composed of a mixture of large polyhedral cells with markedly enlarged nuclei and small cells with small round nuclei.*

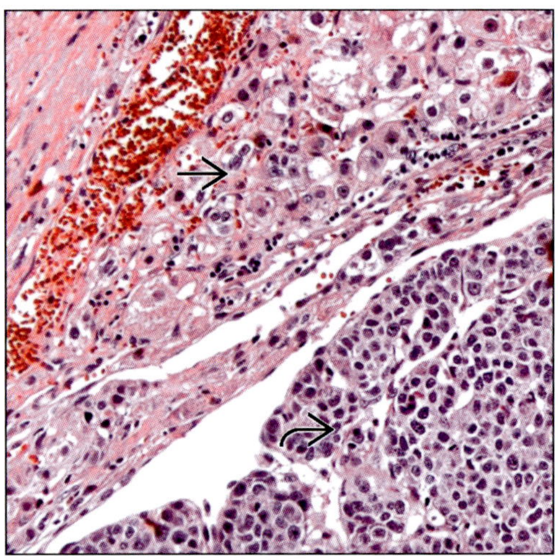

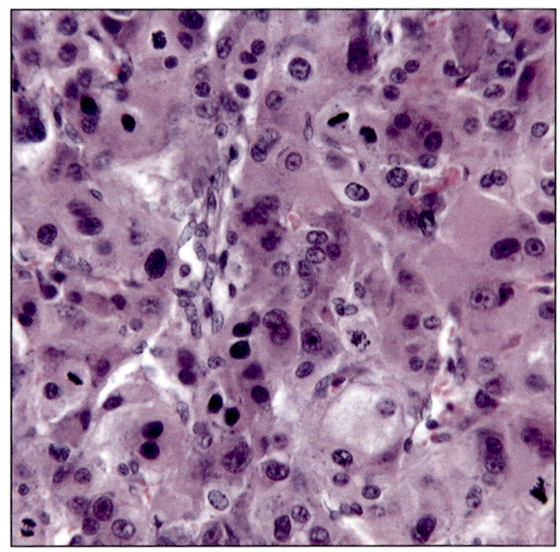

(Left) *H&E shows the interface between 2 distinct areas of an adrenal cortical carcinoma. One area of the tumor is made up of sheets of small, compact round cells with scant cytoplasm. There is a sharp contrast in the cell size of the 1st component compared to the 2nd component.* ***(Right)*** *Adrenal cortical carcinoma in a child with Beckwith-Wiedemann syndrome shows that the tumor is composed of large cells with nuclear pleomorphism, prominent nucleoli, and numerous mitotic figures.*

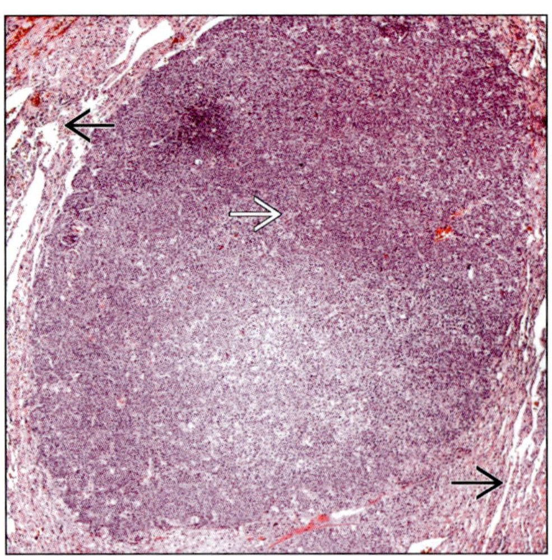

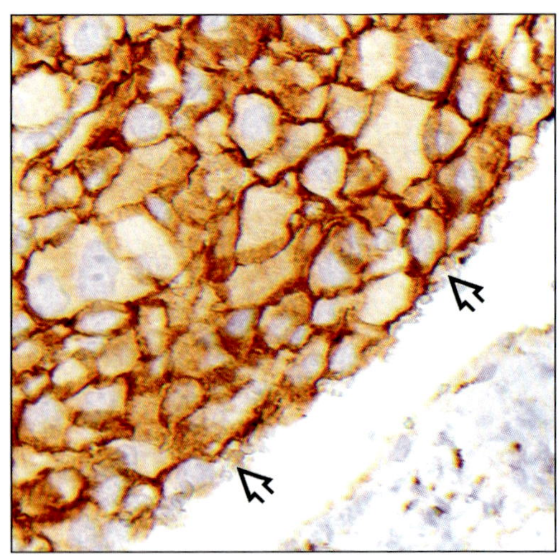

(Left) *H&E shows metastatic adrenal cortical carcinoma to lung parenchyma. The tumor mass is composed of small, compact eosinophilic cells and is surrounded by lung parenchyma.* ***(Right)*** *Extensive lymphovascular invasion may be present in adrenalectomy specimens of pediatric adrenal cortical carcinoma. Immunohistochemistry for CD99 in this photomicrograph highlights the intravascular tumor in a child with Beckwith-Wiedemann syndrome producing steroids.*

Tumor Staging Graphics

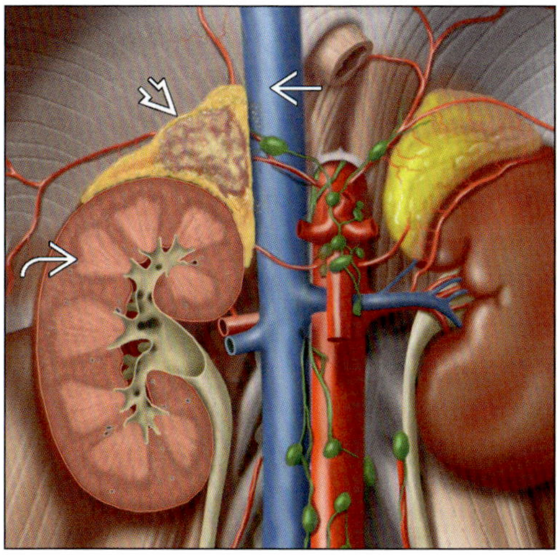
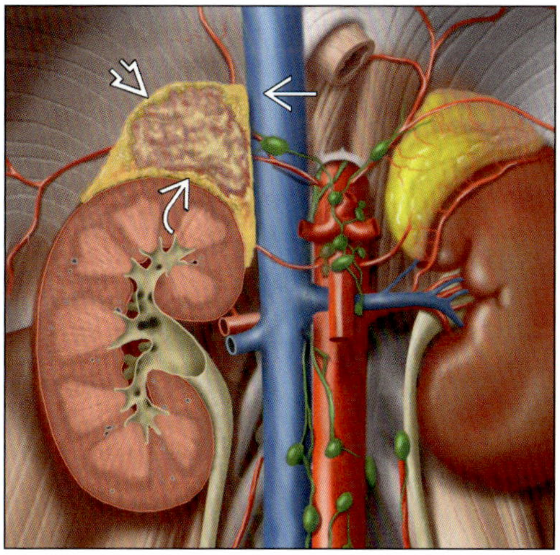

*(**Left**) Coronal graphic demonstrates T1 disease. The primary tumor is ≤ 5 cm in greatest dimension, without invasion of adjacent organs, including kidney or inferior vena cava. (**Right**) Coronal graphic demonstrates T2 disease. The primary tumor is > 5 cm in greatest dimension, without invasion of adjacent organs, including kidney or inferior vena cava.*

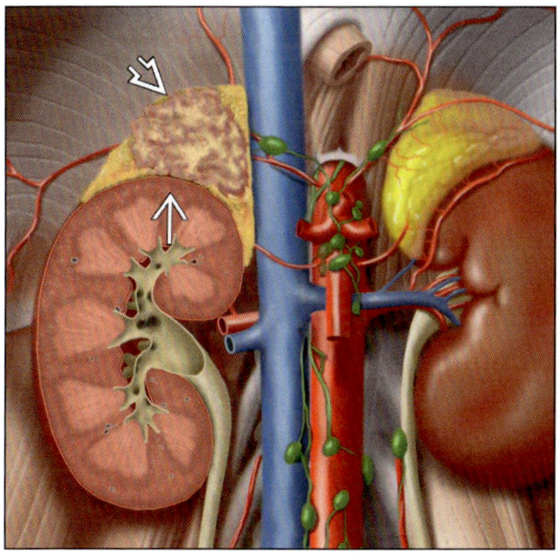
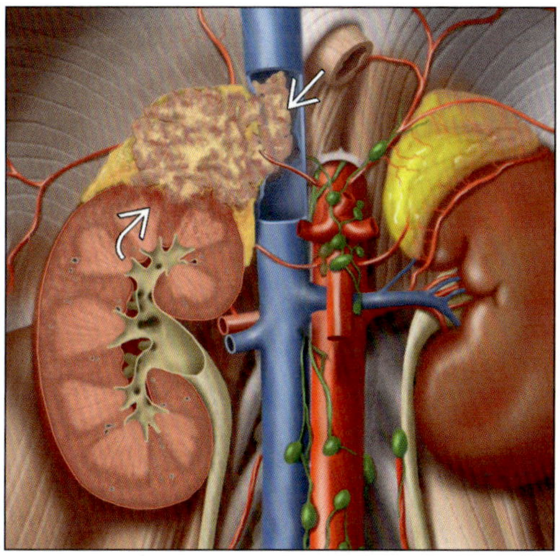

*(**Left**) Coronal graphic demonstrates T3 disease. The primary tumor may be any size, with local invasion beyond the adrenal capsule, shown in the superolateral margin, but no involvement of adjacent organs such as the kidney. (**Right**) Coronal graphic demonstrates T4 disease. The primary tumor can be any size, with local invasion beyond the confines of the adrenal capsule and into adjacent organs, including the kidney. Direct extension into the inferior vena cava is seen.*

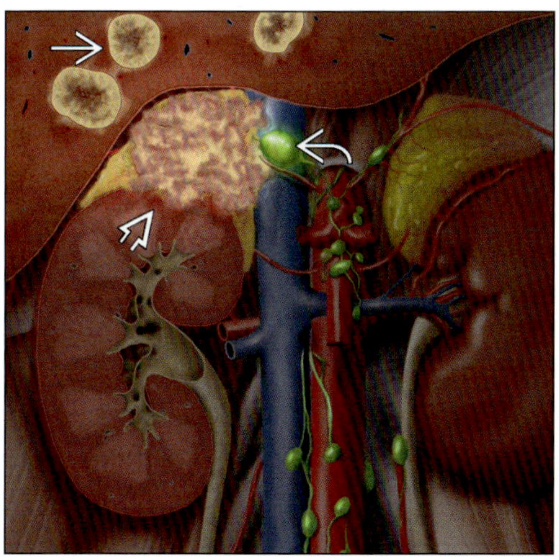
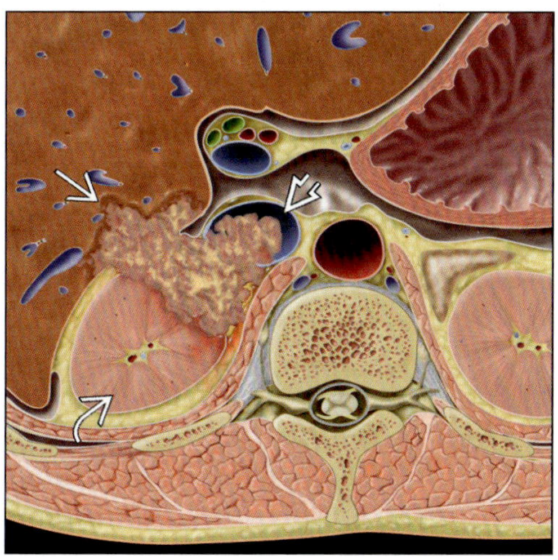

*(**Left**) Coronal graphic shows primary adrenal cortical carcinoma with invasion into the adjacent kidney. N1 and M1 disease is illustrated via an involved paraaortic lymph node and multifocal hepatic metastases. (**Right**) Axial graphic demonstrates T4 right-sided adrenal cortical carcinoma invading adjacent organs, including the right kidney, the liver, and the inferior vena cava.*

ADRENAL CORTICAL NEOPLASMS IN CHILDREN

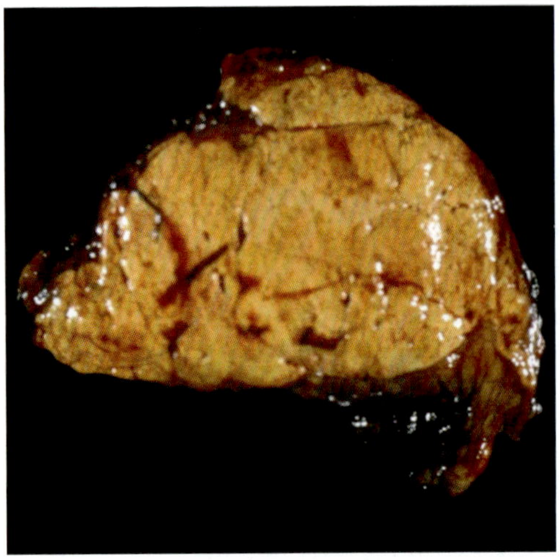

Gross photo shows a cross section of a large adrenal mass replacing the adrenal parenchyma in a young child. This adrenal cortical carcinoma is yellow-tan, has irregular borders and necrosis, and weighs over 100 g.

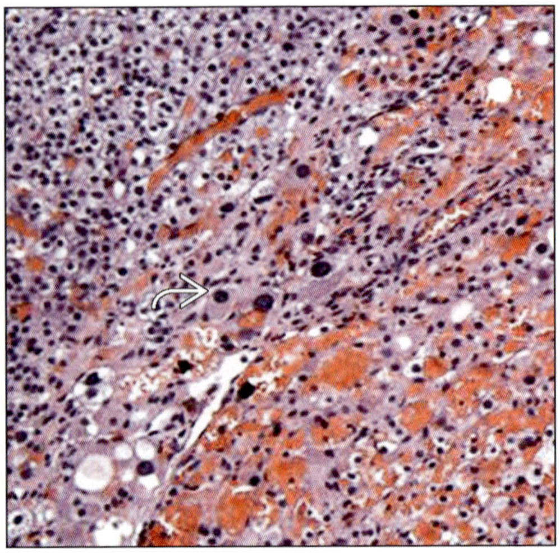

Adrenal cortex shows numerous enlarged and bizarre polyhedral cells with eosinophilic granular cytoplasm and large hyperchromatic nuclei ➔ in a patient with Beckwith-Wiedemann syndrome.

TERMINOLOGY

Abbreviations

- Adrenal cortical neoplasm (ACN)

Synonyms

- Adrenal cortical adenoma (ACA)
- Adrenal cortical carcinoma (ACC)
- Adrenal cortical tumor

Definitions

- Neoplasms arising from the adrenal cortical cells

ETIOLOGY/PATHOGENESIS

Beckwith-Wiedemann Syndrome (BWS)

- Involves chromosome 11p15.5 in ~ 80% of cases
  - *IGF2* and *KCNQ1OT1* are normally expressed from paternal allele
  - *H19*, *CDKN1C*, and *KCNQ1* are normally expressed from maternal allele
- Characterized by adrenal cytomegaly
- Associated with adrenal cortical neoplasms
- Characterized by embryonal tumor in childhood
  - Main tumors associated with BWS are nephroblastoma, ACC, and hepatoblastoma
- Characteristic facies in early childhood (often normal by adulthood)
- Somatic overgrowth
- Classic triad
  - Exomphalos
  - Gigantism
  - Macroglossia

Li-Fraumeni Syndrome

- A.k.a. SBLA syndrome: **S**arcoma; **b**reast and **b**rain tumors; **l**eukemia, **l**aryngeal carcinoma, and **l**ung cancer; **a**drenal cortical carcinoma
- Endometrial carcinoma
- Autosomal dominant mode of inheritance
- Alterations in *P53* tumor suppressor gene have been detected
- Most common associated neoplasms are soft tissue sarcomas, bone sarcomas, and breast carcinoma

Congenital Adrenal Hyperplasia

- ACA and ACC have been associated with congenital adrenal hyperplasia (CAH)(adrenogenital syndrome)
- Associated with testicular tumors of adrenal cortical type

Hemihypertrophy

- Adrenal cortical neoplasms have been associated with hemihypertrophy in children
- Adrenal neoplasms are not necessarily located ipsilateral to hemihypertrophy
- Other associated tumors are Wilms tumor, hepatoblastoma, and pheochromocytoma

Other Syndromes

- Multiple endocrine neoplasia type 1 (MEN1)
- Carney complex
- McCune-Albright syndrome
- Neurofibromatosis type 1 (NF1)
- Familial adenomatous polyposis; Lynch syndrome
- Hereditary nonpolyposis colorectal cancer (HNPCC)

Sporadic

- Rare cases in children are nonsyndromic

CLINICAL ISSUES

Epidemiology

- Incidence
  - ~ 20 new ACC cases per year
  - ~ 25 new cases of ACA per year in United States in patients < 20 years of age
  - Annual incidence is 3:1,000,000 patients < 20 years old

ADRENAL CORTICAL NEOPLASMS IN CHILDREN

Key Facts

Etiology/Pathogenesis
- Beckwith-Wiedemann syndrome
  - Characterized by adrenal cytomegaly
  - Associated with adrenal cortical neoplasms
- Li-Fraumeni syndrome
- Congenital adrenal hyperplasia
  - ACA and ACC have been associated with adrenogenital syndrome
- Hemihypertrophy
  - Adrenal cortical neoplasms have been associated with hemihypertrophy in children
- Multiple endocrine neoplasia type 1
- Carney complex
- Familial adenomatous polyposis; Lynch syndrome
- Neurofibromatosis type 1 (NF1)
- McCune-Albright syndrome

Clinical Issues
- Most cases occur in patients < 5 years old
- > 90% of children with adrenal cortical neoplasms present with symptoms of endocrine syndrome
- Most common presentation is virilization
- Adrenal cortical tumors in children more frequently show adverse histologic features in clinically benign tumors as compared to adult tumors

Microscopic Pathology
- Different architectural patterns are seen
  - Alveolar: Most common pattern in ACA
  - Trabecular: Commonly seen in ACC
  - Solid
- Confluent necrosis is a histologic feature; adverse prognostic finding if > 25%

  - Females have higher incidence until 5 years of age, after which sex difference disappears
  - Adrenal cortical neoplasms constitute 0.2% of all malignancies observed in children
- Age
  - Average at presentation: 8 years old
    - Most cases occur in patients < 5 years old

Presentation
- > 90% of children with adrenal cortical neoplasms present with symptoms of endocrine syndrome
- Functionally active tumors account for > 80%
- Most common presentation is virilization
  - Expressed in females
    - Increased muscle mass, clitoromegaly, facial hair, pubic hair, deepening of voice
  - Expressed in males
    - Penile enlargement, pubic hair
- May present with Cushing syndrome
  - If so, syndrome is usually associated with virilization

Prognosis
- Adrenal cortical tumors in children more frequently show adverse histologic features in clinically benign tumors vs. adult tumors
- Adverse prognostic factors in pediatric tumors
  - Older age at diagnosis: > 5 years of age
  - Average tumor size: 12 cm
  - Tumor weight: > 400 g
  - Mitotic count: > 30 per 50 HPF
  - Average tumor necrosis: 60%
  - Vascular &/or capsular invasion
  - Tumor ploidy has been shown **not** to correlate with outcome
- Most frequent sites of metastases are lung and liver; other places are peritoneum, pleura/diaphragm, abdominal lymph nodes, and kidneys

Associated Neoplasms
- BWS
  - Wilms tumor
  - Hepatoblastoma
  - Rhabdomyosarcoma
  - Neuroblastoma
- Li-Fraumeni syndrome (a.k.a. SBLA syndrome)
  - Endometrial carcinoma

MACROSCOPIC FEATURES

General Features
- Mostly unilateral; bilateral tumors are extremely rare

Size
- Wide range: 2.5-20 cm
- Tumors with better prognosis have average size of 6 cm, whereas those with worse prognosis have average size of 12 cm

MICROSCOPIC PATHOLOGY

Histologic Features
- Pediatric tumors differ from adult adrenal cortical neoplasms in that those features associated with malignancy in adults can sometimes be seen in clinically benign tumors in children
  - Capsular invasion
  - Confluent necrosis (adverse prognostic finding if > 25%)
  - Vascular invasion
- Different architectural patterns are seen
  - Alveolar pattern is most common pattern in ACA
  - Trabecular (commonly seen in malignant neoplasms)
  - Solid

Cytologic Features
- Nuclear pleomorphism
- Some can have oncocytic features
- Nuclear hyperchromasia
- Mitosis: Few figures can be seen in clinically benign tumors; sign of malignancy if numerous (> 30 per 50 HPF)
- Intracytoplasmic hyaline globules

ADRENAL CORTICAL NEOPLASMS IN CHILDREN

Adrenal Cortical Tumor as Part of Inherited Tumor Syndromes

Syndrome	Gene	Adrenal Pathology
Beckwith-Wiedemann syndrome	*CDKN1C, NSD1*	Adrenal cortical carcinoma, adenoma, and hyperplasia
Li-Fraumeni syndrome	*TP53*	Adrenal cortical carcinoma
McCune-Albright syndrome	*GNAS1*	Adrenal nodular hyperplasia, adenoma and carcinoma
Multiple endocrine neoplasia 1 (MEN1)	*MEN1*	Adrenal cortical adenoma and carcinoma
Congenital adrenal hyperplasia	*CYP21*	Adrenal nodular hyperplasia; adrenal cortical adenoma and carcinoma
Carney complex	*PRKAR1A*	Primary pigmented adrenal nodular disease (hyperplasia)
Neurofibromatosis 1	*NF1*	Adrenal cortical carcinoma
Familial adenomatous polyposis	*APC*	Adrenal cortical adenoma and carcinoma
HNPCC	*MLH1, MSH2, MSH6, PMS2*	Adrenal cortical carcinoma

ANCILLARY TESTS

Immunohistochemistry

- Positive for adrenal cortical markers such as inhibin, synaptophysin, chromogranin, and Melan-A
- Negative for cytokeratin (rarely may be positive)

DIFFERENTIAL DIAGNOSIS

Pheochromocytoma

- Positive for chromogranin; negative for inhibin and MART-1

Renal Cell Carcinoma

- Negative for chromogranin

Other Primary or Metastatic Neoplasms

- Neuroblastoma, Wilms tumor, hepatoblastoma

SELECTED REFERENCES

1. Choufani S et al: Molecular findings in Beckwith-Wiedemann syndrome. Am J Med Genet C Semin Med Genet. 163(2):131-40, 2013
2. Kantaputra PN et al: A novel mutation in CDKN1C in sibs with Beckwith-Wiedemann syndrome and cleft palate, sensorineural hearing loss, and supernumerary flexion creases. Am J Med Genet A. 161A(1):192-7, 2013
3. Sidhu A et al: Infantile adrenocortical tumor with an activating GNAS1 mutation. J Clin Endocrinol Metab. 98(1):E115-8, 2013
4. Carney JA et al: Massive neonatal adrenal enlargement due to cytomegaly, persistence of the transient cortex, and hyperplasia of the permanent cortex: findings in Cushing syndrome associated with hemihypertrophy. Am J Surg Pathol. 36(10):1452-63, 2012
5. Malkin D: Li-fraumeni syndrome. Genes Cancer. 2(4):475-84, 2011
6. Michalkiewicz E et al: Clinical and outcome characteristics of children with adrenocortical tumors: a report from the International Pediatric Adrenocortical Tumor Registry. J Clin Oncol. 22(5):838-45, 2004
7. Ribeiro RC et al: Childhood adrenocortical tumours. Eur J Cancer. 40(8):1117-26, 2004
8. Wieneke JA et al: Adrenal cortical neoplasms in the pediatric population: a clinicopathologic and immunophenotypic analysis of 83 patients. Am J Surg Pathol. 27(7):867-81, 2003
9. Ribeiro RC et al: An inherited p53 mutation that contributes in a tissue-specific manner to pediatric adrenal cortical carcinoma. Proc Natl Acad Sci U S A. 98(16):9330-5, 2001
10. Teinturier C et al: Clinical and prognostic aspects of adrenocortical neoplasms in childhood. Med Pediatr Oncol. 32(2):106-11, 1999
11. Lack EE et al: Adrenal cortical neoplasms in the pediatric and adolescent age group. Clinicopathologic study of 30 cases with emphasis on epidemiological and prognostic factors. Pathol Annu. 27 Pt 1:1-53, 1992
12. Medeiros LJ et al: New developments in the pathologic diagnosis of adrenal cortical neoplasms. A review. Am J Clin Pathol. 97(1):73-83, 1992
13. Weiss LM et al: Pathologic features of prognostic significance in adrenocortical carcinoma. Am J Surg Pathol. 13(3):202-6, 1989
14. Li FP et al: A cancer family syndrome in twenty-four kindreds. Cancer Res. 48(18):5358-62, 1988
15. Cagle PT et al: Comparison of adrenal cortical tumors in children and adults. Cancer. 57(11):2235-7, 1986
16. Weiss LM: Comparative histologic study of 43 metastasizing and nonmetastasizing adrenocortical tumors. Am J Surg Pathol. 8(3):163-9, 1984
17. Li FP et al: Soft-tissue sarcomas, breast cancer, and other neoplasms. A familial syndrome? Ann Intern Med. 71(4):747-52, 1969
18. Fraumeni JF Jr et al: Primary carcinoma of the liver in childhood: an epidemiologic study. J Natl Cancer Inst. 40(5):1087-99, 1968
19. Fraumeni JF Jr et al: Adrenocortical neoplasms with hemihypertrophy, brain tumors, and other disorders. J Pediatr. 70(1):129-38, 1967

Clinical, Gross, Graphic, and Microscopic Features

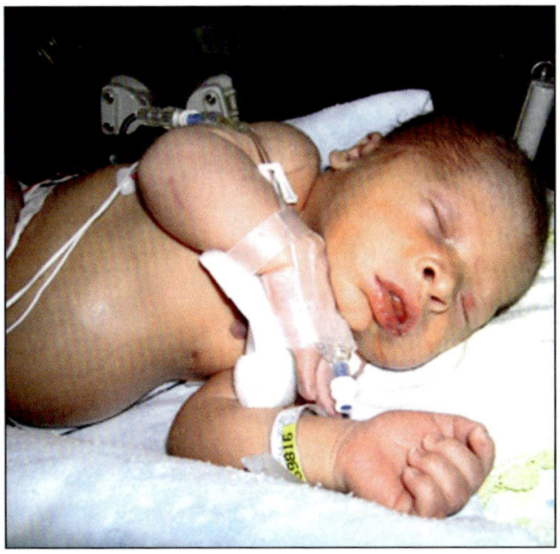

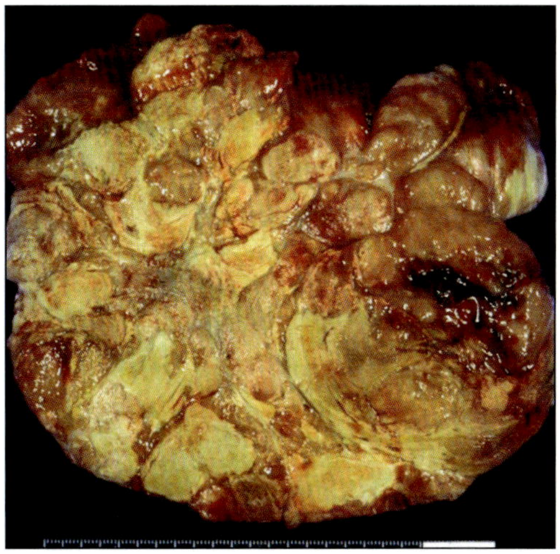

(Left) *This term infant with Beckwith-Wiedemann syndrome (BWS) has a protuberant abdomen, secondary to enlarged liver and kidneys, and a large mouth with macroglossia. (Courtesy J. L. B. Byrne, MD.)* ***(Right)*** *Adrenal cortical carcinomas tend to appear grossly as large solid masses in the suprarenal region, typically measuring > 5 cm. Focal areas of necrosis and hemorrhage are usually present.*

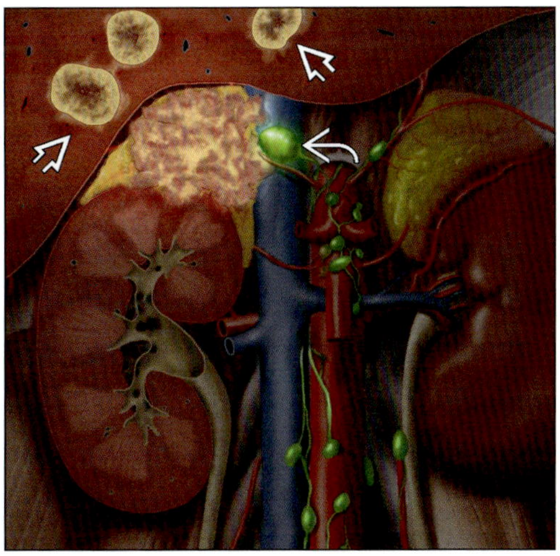

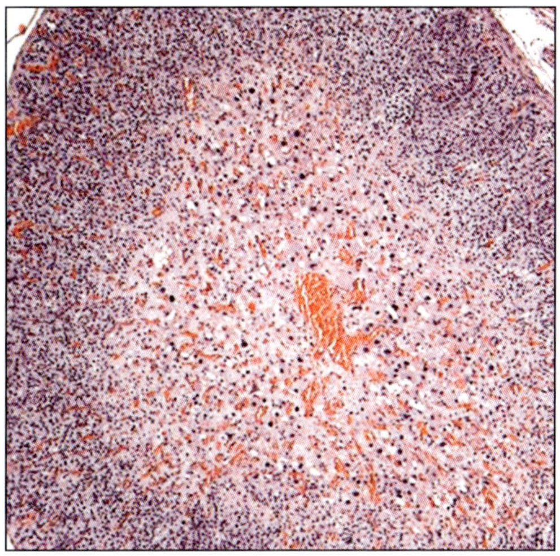

(Left) *Coronal graphic shows primary adrenal cortical carcinoma with invasion into adjacent kidney. N1 and M1 disease is illustrated via an involved paraaortic lymph node and multifocal hepatic metastases.* ***(Right)*** *Low-power view shows an adrenal gland with adrenal cortical cell cytomegaly in a patient with Beckwith-Wiedemann syndrome. This syndrome is frequently associated with cytomegaly.*

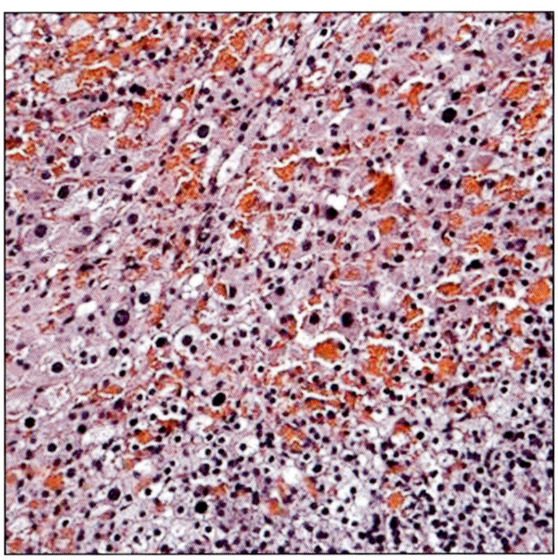

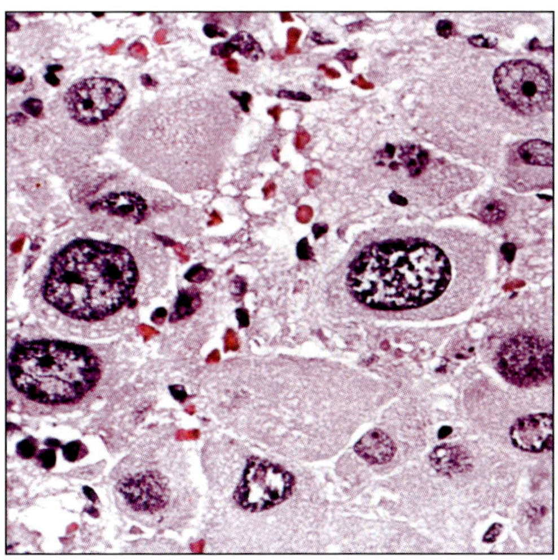

(Left) *Adrenal cytomegaly is characterized by the presence of large polyhedral cells with eosinophilic granular cytoplasm and enlarged nuclei in the adrenal cortex. This is frequently associated with BWS.* ***(Right)*** *Photomicrograph shows adrenal cortical cytomegaly, a characteristic finding in Beckwith-Wiedemann syndrome. There are large polyhedral cells with hyperchromatic nuclei.*

ADRENAL CORTICAL NEOPLASMS IN CHILDREN

Microscopic Features

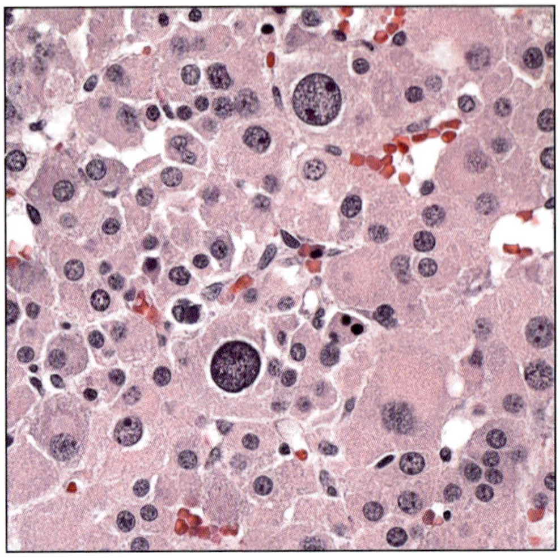
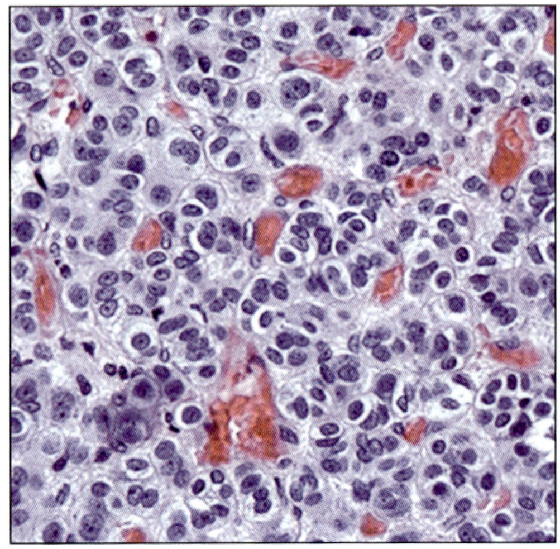

(Left) *Adrenal cortical carcinoma (ACC) in a child with Beckwith-Wiedemann syndrome shows residual numerous large bizarre cells with nuclei 3-5x the size of nuclei of adjacent cells.* ***(Right)*** *High-power magnification shows an adrenal cortical carcinoma in a patient with Beckwith-Wiedemann syndrome. In these patients, the adrenal neoplasms are usually associated with pleomorphism.*

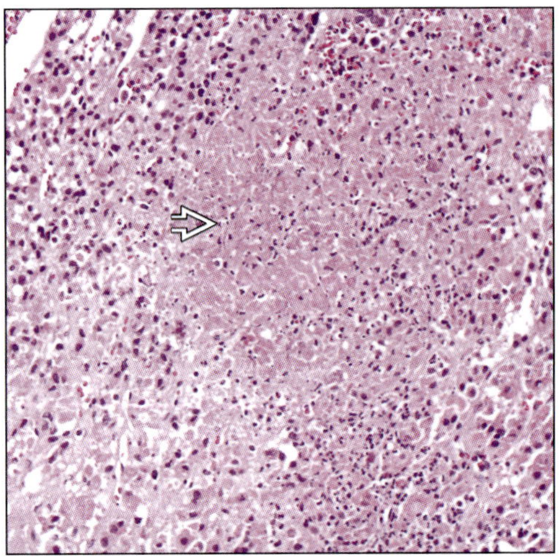
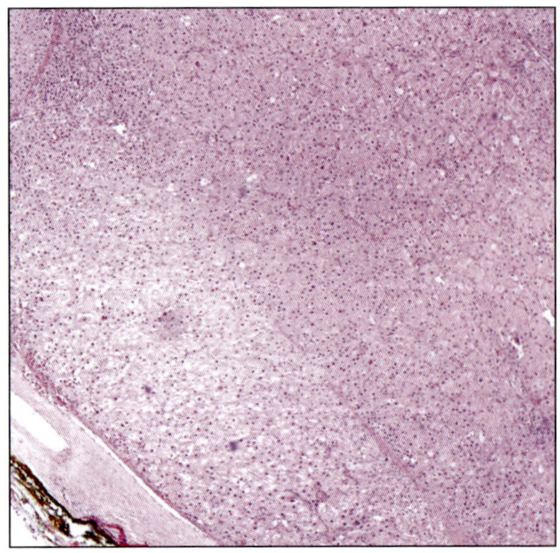

(Left) *High-magnification view shows an area of virilizing ACC with necrosis ➡ in the center of the field. Necrosis of > 50-60% is a feature seen in adrenal cortical carcinomas.* ***(Right)*** *This tumor from a 6-year-old female with virilizing adrenal cortical carcinoma shows a well-circumscribed mass; however, the tumor also had multiple atypical mitosis and necrosis (not shown). All these features are suggestive of carcinoma (ACC).*

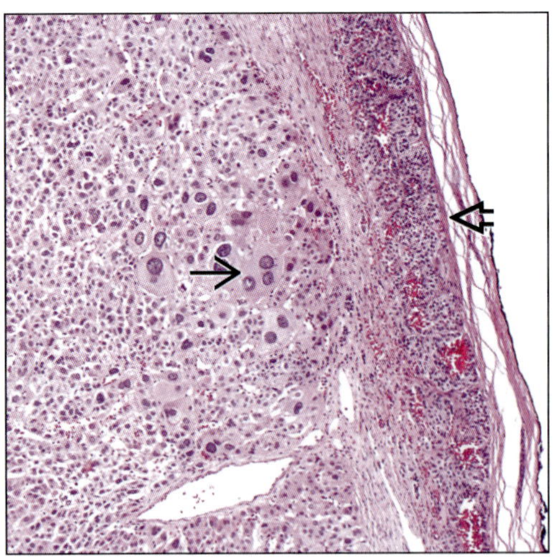
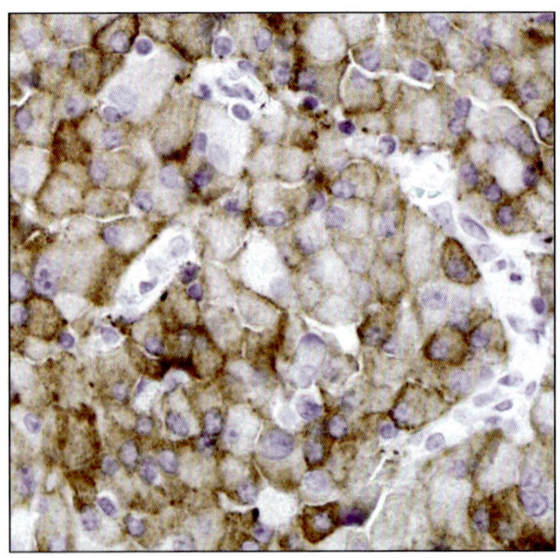

(Left) *Higher magnification view of virilizing adrenal cortical carcinoma shows the residual adrenal gland ⇨. There are numerous bizarre and multinucleated giant cells →, some with intranuclear inclusions. This lesion has several features of malignancy.* ***(Right)*** *Adrenal cortical carcinomas usually have immunopositivity for synaptophysin, calretinin, Melan-A, and inhibin. Synaptophysin is present in these tumors in the cytoplasm and in cellular membranes and can be very weak in some tumors.*

Variant Microscopic Features

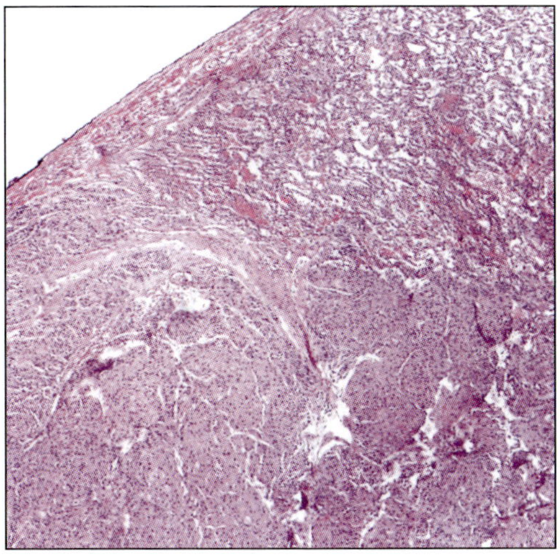
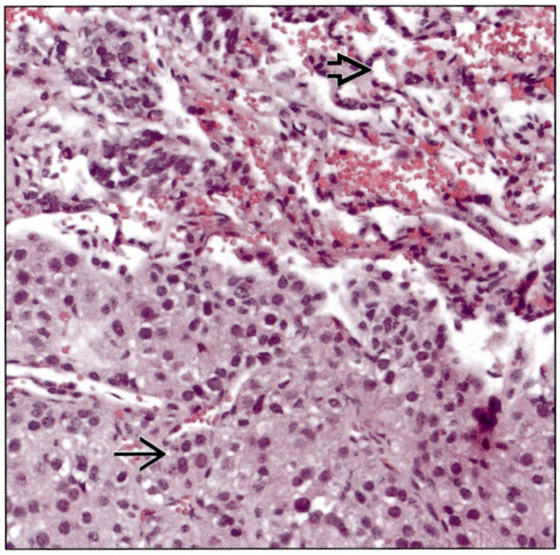

(Left) *H&E shows lung metastasis from an ACC from a 6-year-old female. The patient presented with multiple lesions in her lungs a few months after the diagnosis of ACC. Biopsy of those lesions showed metastatic carcinoma that was morphologically and immunophenotypically similar to the originally diagnosed ACC.* ***(Right)*** *Higher magnification shows a metastatic ACC* → *in the lung of a 6-year-old female. Note the lung parenchyma* ⇨*.*

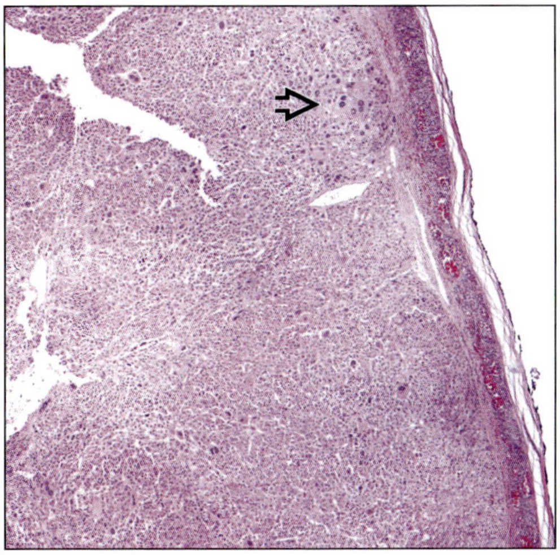
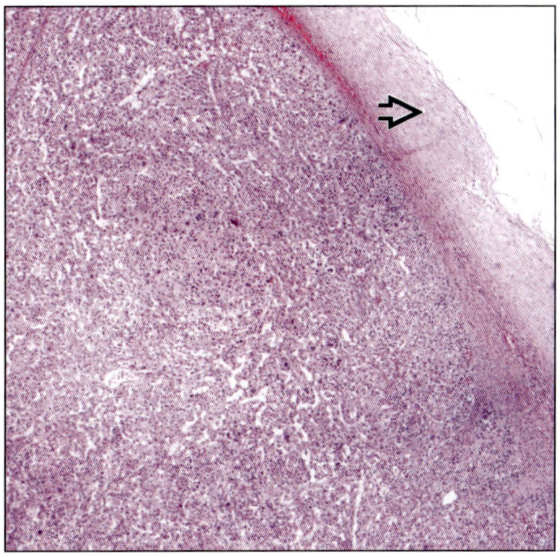

(Left) *Photomicrograph shows a moderately well-circumscribed lesion with areas of necrosis and multiple enlarged cells with atypical nuclei* ⇨ *in a 20-day-old male with an adrenal mass.* ***(Right)*** *This adrenal mass from a 20-day-old female is surrounded by a thick fibrous capsule* ⇨*. The tumor is composed of cells with predominantly eosinophilic cytoplasm with a solid and trabecular pattern. The cytoplasm is compact and eosinophilic.*

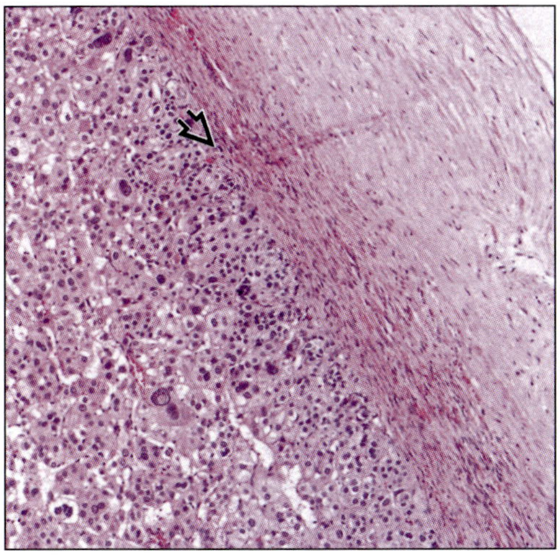
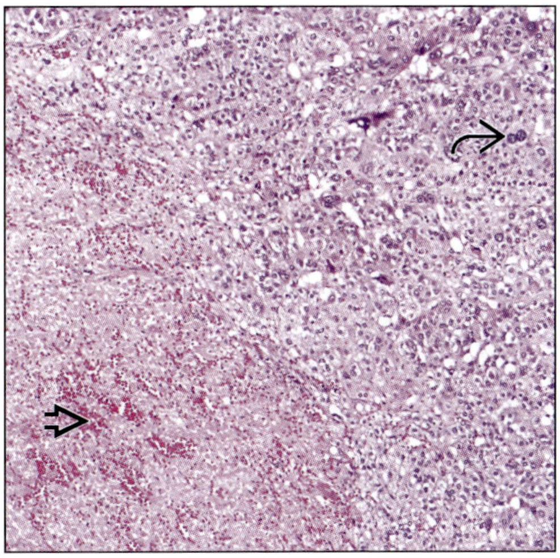

(Left) *Higher magnification of an ACC shows the interface* ⇨ *between the tumor and the fibrous capsule. The tumor has a predominantly trabecular and solid pattern and is composed of compact cells with nuclear atypia and focal nuclear pleomorphism.* ***(Right)*** *H&E shows an area of ACC with focal necrosis* ⇨*. The tumor cells have an eosinophilic cytoplasm with nuclear pleomorphism, atypia, and mitosis. Some of the cells are multinucleated* ↷*.*

PRIMARY PIGMENTED NODULAR ADRENOCORTICAL DISEASE

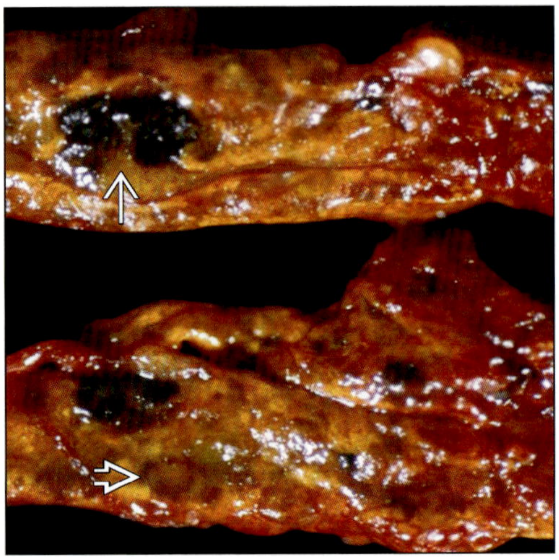

These bilateral adrenal glands show pigmented nodules that are jet black to gray-brown ⇨. These nodules are usually small, however, some are macronodules resulting from a confluence of smaller nodules ⇨.

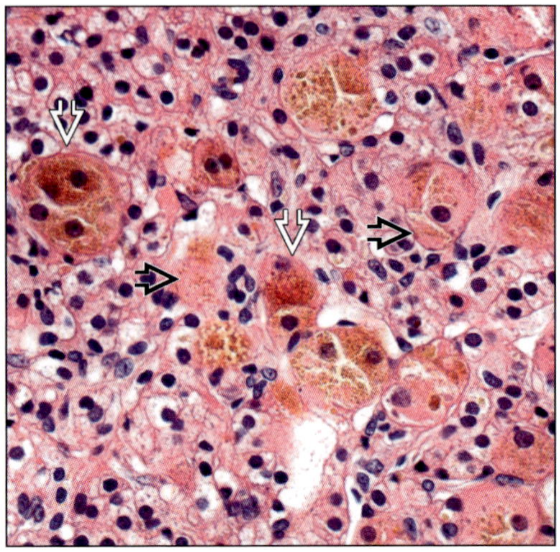

The intranodular cells in primary pigmented nodular adrenocortical disease (PPNAD) have lipid-depleted, compact, eosinophilic cytoplasm. Some have abundant, finely granular cytoplasmic lipofuscin pigment ⇨ with focal accumulation of pigment ⇨.

TERMINOLOGY

Abbreviations

- Primary pigmented nodular adrenocortical disease (PPNAD)

Synonyms

- Primary pigmented nodular adrenal disease
- Isolated or sporadic primary pigmented nodular adrenocortical disease (iPPNAD)
- PPNAD associated with Carney complex (C-PPNAD)
- Adrenocortical dysplasia
- Bilateral micronodular hyperplasia

Definitions

- Rare form of primary bilateral adrenal disease that is often associated with adrenocorticotropic hormone (ACTH)-independent Cushing syndrome (CS)
- Characterized by bilateral micronodular adrenocortical hyperplasia
- Can be inherited in autosomal dominant manner associated with Carney complex (CNC)
- Nonfamilial, or isolated or sporadic (iPPNAD) forms also exist

ETIOLOGY/PATHOGENESIS

Etiology

- Unknown
- **Familial**
  - Can occur in familial form, inherited as autosomal dominant trait when associated with CNC
    - Known genetic heterogeneity in CNC
    - PPNAD is the most frequent endocrine manifestation of CNC, occurring in about 1/4 of patients
- **Sporadic**
  - Can occur as nonfamilial isolated or sporadic form (iPPNAD)
- **Autoimmune origin**
  - May result from adrenal-stimulating antibodies, which stimulate corticotropin receptor sites in adrenal cortex

Genetic Abnormality

- Disorder has been mapped to genomic loci on chromosomes 2q15-16 and 17q22-24
- Inactivating mutations of *PRKAR1A* gene on 17q22-24 have been reported in most patients with CNC
- Inactivating mutations of phosphodiesterase 11A (*PDE11A*) located at 2q31-2q35 have been identified in sporadic PPNAD
- Despite the known genetic heterogeneity in CNC, in most cases, PPNAD in its sporadic or isolated forms (iPPNAD) is caused by inactivating heterozygous mutations of *PRKAR1A* gene
  - Polypyrimidine tract mutation of *PRKAR1A* gene leading to a probable mild alteration of PRKAR1A mRNA splicing
  - Compared with mutations described for *PRKAR1A* gene, exon 7 IVS del([-]7 → [-]2) has a low penetrance and is almost exclusively associated with iPPNAD
- Strong genotype-phenotype correlation in CNC &/or PPNAD for *PRKAR1A* mutation

Pathogenesis

- All genetic events lead to constitutive activation of cAMP/PKA pathway, which results in hyperglucocortisolism and adrenocortical hyperplasia

CLINICAL ISSUES

Epidemiology

- Age
  - Patients with PPNAD in both sporadic and familial forms usually present in late childhood/early adulthood

Key Facts

Terminology
- Rare cause of ACTH-independent Cushing syndrome that may occur sporadically or in autosomal dominant familial form associated with CNC
- Characterized by bilateral adrenocortical hyperplasia

Etiology/Pathogenesis
- All genetic events lead to constitutive activation of cAMP/PKA pathway, which results in hyperglucocortisolism and adrenocortical hyperplasia

Clinical Issues
- Corticotropin-independent Cushing syndrome
- Familial form as part of CNC; sporadic cases are rare

Macroscopic Features
- Small to normal-sized adrenal glands with multiple small pigmented nodules; similar in both forms

Microscopic Pathology
- Nodules are composed of cells with compact eosinophilic cytoplasm and abundant brown, granular pigment (lipofuscin)
- Findings are similar in familial and sporadic cases

Top Differential Diagnoses
- Cushing syndrome caused by primary cortisol-producing adrenocortical adenoma
- Corticotropin (ACTH)-independent bilateral macronodular adrenal hyperplasia (AIMAH)
- Cushing disease
- Malignant melanoma

- Gender
  - Slight female predominance

Presentation
- Most patients with PPNAD also have a multiple neoplasia syndrome within CNC
- PPNAD in its sporadic or isolated forms is rare
- **Familial form as part of CNC: Autosomal dominant**
  - In addition to PPNAD, which is the most common endocrine manifestation, CNC patients have
    - Myxomas
    - Spotty skin pigmentation
    - Cutaneous abnormalities
    - Schwannomas
    - Testicular tumors, including Leydig cell tumor and large cell calcifying Sertoli cell tumors
    - Mammary myxoid fibroadenoma
    - Pituitary macroadenoma
    - Psammomatous melanotic schwannoma
- **Sporadic or isolated corticotropin-independent Cushing syndrome (iPPNAD)**
  - Establishing diagnosis of PPNAD can be challenging, particularly when PPNAD is the only manifestation of disease; a few signs are
    - Weight gain
    - Fatigue
    - Muscle weakness
    - Moon face
    - Facial flushing
    - Buffalo hump

Laboratory Tests
- Plasma cortisol is usually moderately elevated without diurnal rhythm
- Plasma ACTH is low or undetectable
- Hypercortisolism is resistant to high-dose dexamethasone suppression test (HDDST), metyrapone stimulation, and corticotropin-releasing hormone stimulation

Treatment
- Surgical approaches
  - Bilateral adrenalectomy is treatment of choice for PPNAD in patients with Cushing syndrome

Prognosis
- Most tumors are slow growing without malignant potential
- Life span is decreased in patients with CNC due to increased incidence of sudden death caused by heart myxoma or its complications

IMAGE FINDINGS

CT Findings
- Bilateral irregular adrenal margins with nodules
- Size of adrenal can be normal

MACROSCOPIC FEATURES

General Features
- Small to normal-sized adrenal glands
  - Rarely, slight increase in adrenal gland size
- Multiple small cortical nodules, 0.1-0.3 cm in diameter involving both glands
- Nodules may be pigmented, either brown or black
  - Some nodules may be pale to bright yellow

MICROSCOPIC PATHOLOGY

Histologic Features
- Nodules composed of cells with compact eosinophilic cytoplasm and abundant brown, granular pigment (lipofuscin)
- Cell nuclei are vesicular and may contain prominent eosinophilic nucleoli
- Intervening cortical tissue is atrophic

ANCILLARY TESTS

Serologic Testing

- Elevated basal cortisol
- Low ACTH
- High 24-hour urinary free cortisol
- Nonsuppressed cortisol after HDDST suggests ACTH-independent Cushing syndrome

Immunohistochemistry

- Increased expression of glucocorticoid receptor

Molecular Genetics

- PPNAD in its sporadic or isolated forms (iPPNAD) is caused by inactivating heterozygous mutations of *PRKAR1A* gene, encoding regulatory subunit type I-α of the cAMP-dependent protein kinase A (PKA)
  - Compared with other mutations described for the *PRKAR1A* gene, exon 7 IVS del([-]7 → [-]2) has a low penetrance and is almost exclusively associated with iPPNAD
- Loss of heterozygosity of *PRKAR1A* gene or nonsense mutation
- Mutations of *PDE11A* and *PDE8B* genes

DIFFERENTIAL DIAGNOSIS

Corticotropin (ACTH)-Independent Bilateral Macronodular Adrenal Hyperplasia (AIMAH)

- Associated with tumefactive enlargement of both adrenal glands
- Also associated with bilateral adrenocortical nodules, but nodules are much larger
- Associated with markedly enlarged adrenal glands
- Marked distortion of cortical architecture composed of lipid-rich cells with some lipid-depleted cells showing atrophy between nodules

Cushing Syndrome Caused by Primary Cortisol-Producing Adrenocortical Adenoma

- Patient presents with Cushing syndrome
- Lab: High cortisol, low ACTH
- Well-demarcated tumor lesion inside adrenal gland
- Gross: Single tumor nodule with expansile appearance, adjacent to grossly normal adrenal gland

Cushing Disease

- ACTH-dependent hypercortisolism caused by pituitary adenoma
- Lab: High cortisol, high ACTH
- MR shows mass in anterior pituitary gland
- Diffuse enlargement of adrenal cortex
- Microscopically, diffuse adrenocortical hyperplasia without pigment deposition

Metastatic Malignant Melanoma

- Both diseases involve both adrenal glands
  - Immunohistochemistry for S100, HMB-45, Melan-A can readily separate both diseases

DIAGNOSTIC CHECKLIST

Pathologic Interpretation Pearls

- Adrenal glands usually normal in size
- Scattered small pigmented nodules ranging from light gray, gray-brown, dark brown, to jet black
- Histologically, pigmented nodules are round or oval; sporadic and familial forms have similar findings
- Unencapsulated nodules of mixed lipid-rich and lipid-depleted adrenocortical cells with expansile borders
- Intracytoplasmic pigment is lipofuscin

SELECTED REFERENCES

1. Almeida MQ et al: Activation of cyclic AMP signaling leads to different pathway alterations in lesions of the adrenal cortex caused by germline PRKAR1A defects versus those due to somatic GNAS mutations. J Clin Endocrinol Metab. 97(4):E687-93, 2012
2. Anselmo J et al: A large family with Carney complex caused by the S147G PRKAR1A mutation shows a unique spectrum of disease including adrenocortical cancer. J Clin Endocrinol Metab. 97(2):351-9, 2012
3. Rauschecker M et al: Molecular genetics of adrenocortical tumor formation and potential pharmacologic targets. Minerva Endocrinol. 37(2):133-9, 2012
4. da Silva RM et al: Children with Cushing's syndrome: primary pigmented nodular adrenocortical disease should always be suspected. Pituitary. 14(1):61-7, 2011
5. LibØR et al: Frequent phosphodiesterase 11A gene (PDE11A) defects in patients with Carney complex (CNC) caused by PRKAR1A mutations: PDE11A may contribute to adrenal and testicular tumors in CNC as a modifier of the phenotype. J Clin Endocrinol Metab. 96(1):E208-14, 2011
6. Zhang Y et al: Endocrine tumors as part of inherited tumor syndromes. Adv Anat Pathol. 18(3):206-18, 2011
7. Peck MC et al: A novel PRKAR1A mutation associated with primary pigmented nodular adrenocortical disease and the Carney complex. Endocr Pract. 16(2):198-204, 2010
8. Bertherat J et al: Mutations in regulatory subunit type 1A of cyclic adenosine 5'-monophosphate-dependent protein kinase (PRKAR1A): phenotype analysis in 353 patients and 80 different genotypes. J Clin Endocrinol Metab. 94(6):2085-91, 2009
9. Groussin L et al: Mutations of the PRKAR1A gene in Cushing's syndrome due to sporadic primary pigmented nodular adrenocortical disease. J Clin Endocrinol Metab. 87(9):4324-9, 2002
10. Carney JA: Carney complex: the complex of myxomas, spotty pigmentation, endocrine overactivity, and schwannomas. Semin Dermatol. 14(2):90-8, 1995
11. Carney JA et al: The complex of myxomas, spotty pigmentation, and endocrine overactivity. Medicine (Baltimore). 64(4):270-83, 1985
12. Shenoy BV et al: Bilateral primary pigmented nodular adrenocortical disease. Rare cause of the Cushing syndrome. Am J Surg Pathol. 8(5):335-44, 1984

PRIMARY PIGMENTED NODULAR ADRENOCORTICAL DISEASE

Clinical and Microscopic Features

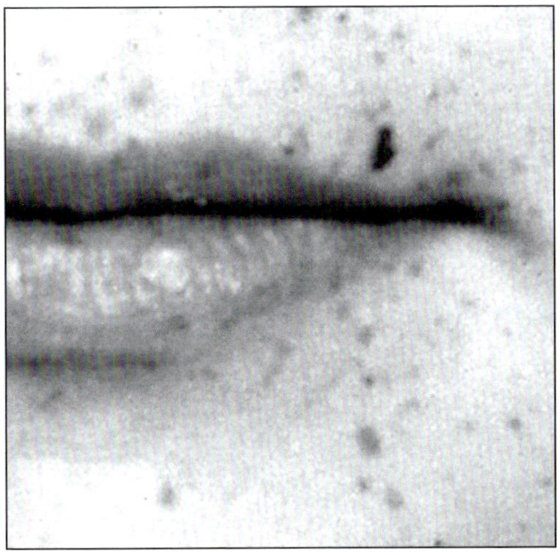

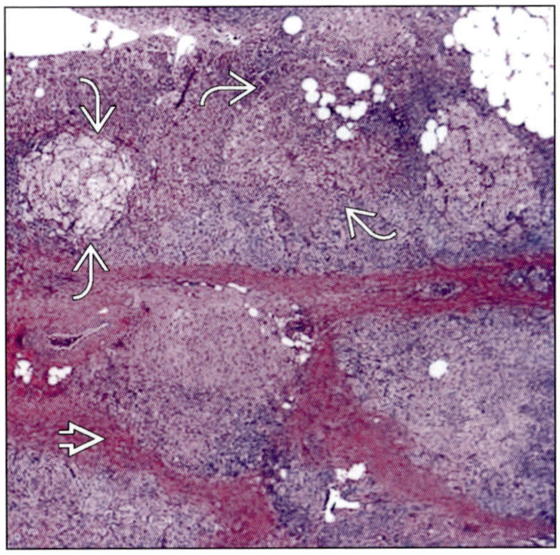

(Left) *In addition to PPNAD, which is the most common endocrine manifestation, CNC patients have the characteristic findings of spotty skin pigmentation in the mucocutaneous regions around eyes and lips. (Courtesy J.A. Carney, MD.)* ***(Right)*** *The normal adrenal gland architecture in PPNAD is replaced by multiple nodules, most of which are unencapsulated but some with a thin fibrous capsule. The adjacent adrenal is atrophic.*

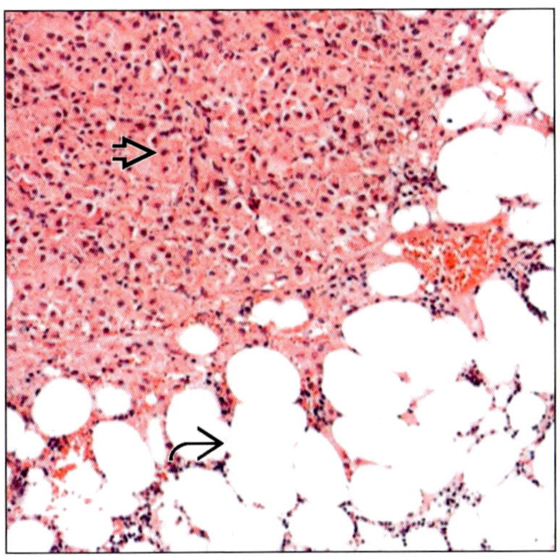

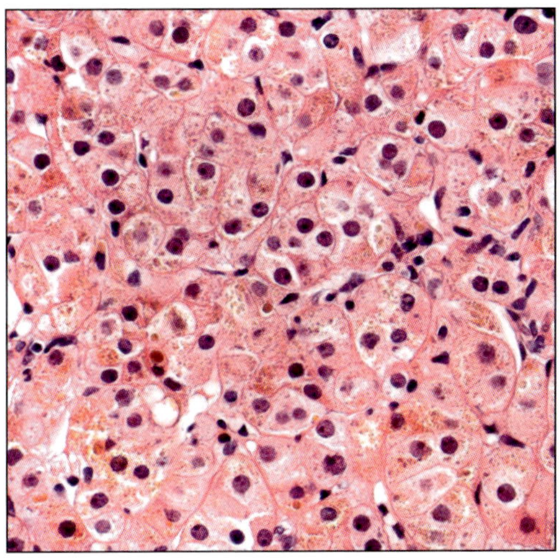

(Left) *Low power of an adrenal gland from a patient with PPNAD shows a nodule composed of cells with lipid-depleted cytoplasm containing a small amount of finely granular lipofuscin pigment. Lipomatous metaplasia is also present.* ***(Right)*** *Intranodular cells in PPNAD have lipid-depleted cytoplasm with finely granular to focally coarse cytoplasmic lipofuscin. The pigmented nodule cells may have pleomorphic nuclei and prominent nucleoli.*

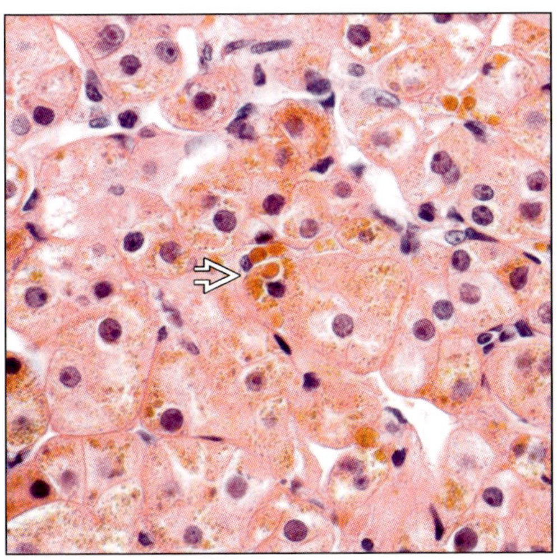

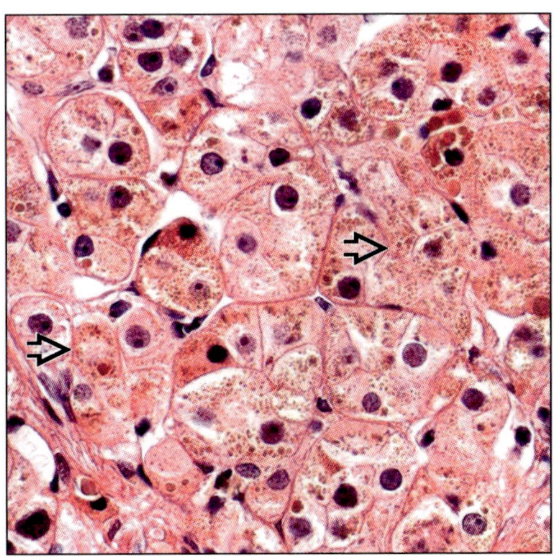

(Left) *The lipid-depleted, compact, and eosinophilic cells in PPNAD may have abundant, finely granular, cytoplasmic, orange-brown lipofuscin pigment with focal globular pigment formation.* ***(Right)*** *Cytologically, the cells are uniform, although occasional binucleated or cells with enlarged nuclei and prominent nucleoli can be seen. The lipid-poor eosinophilic cytoplasm may contain a finely granular, orange-brown lipofuscin pigment with focal globular pigment.*

ADRENAL MEDULLARY HYPERPLASIA

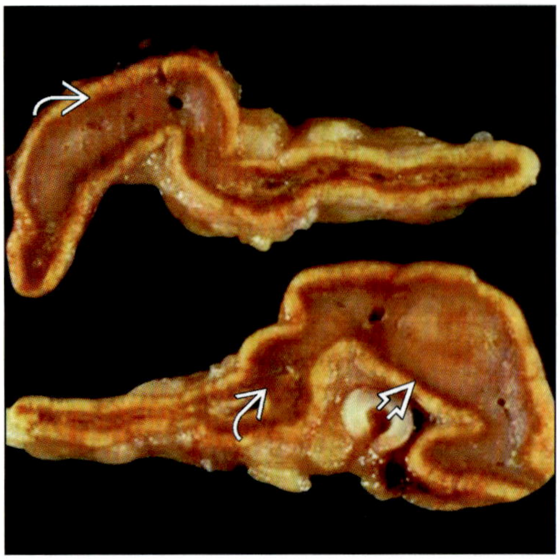

This adrenal gland from a patient with multiple endocrine neoplasia type 2A (MEN2A) shows diffuse medullary expansion, characteristic of adrenal medullary hyperplasia, and a well-defined nodule.

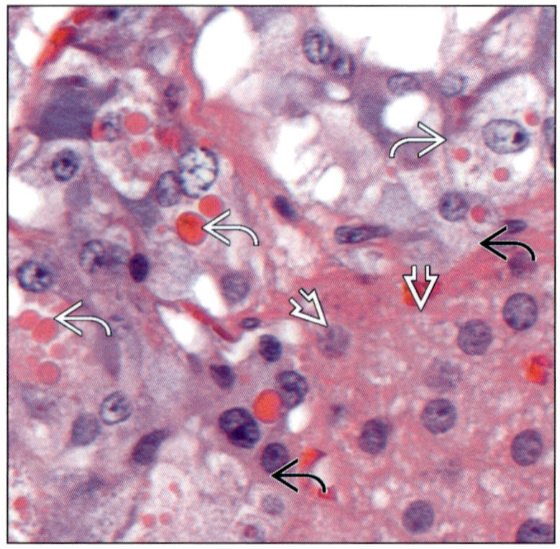

Adrenal medullary hyperplasia in a patient with MEN2 syndrome shows medullary cells within the adrenal cortex. The presence of hyaline granules is usually present in MEN2.

TERMINOLOGY

Abbreviations

- Adrenal medullary hyperplasia (AMH)

Definitions

- Increase in mass of adrenal medullary cells and expansion of these cells into areas of gland where they are not normally present
- Benign change in adrenal gland characterized by disproportionate enlargement of medulla compared with cortex
  - Considered an adrenal cortex to medulla ratio of < 10:1
- Arbitrarily, lesions of < 1 cm in diameter are called adrenal medullary hyperplasia
  - It should be expected that majority of these are early lesions and, if left in situ, would grow to a pheochromocytoma
- Increased cell number in sympathoadrenal or parasympathetic paraganglia

ETIOLOGY/PATHOGENESIS

Familial Medullary Hyperplasia

- Known to be a precursor lesion of MEN2 syndromes
- Other predisposing genetic syndromes are not typically associated with adrenal medullary hyperplasia
  - Identification of adrenal medullary hyperplasia has been considered to be diagnostic of MEN2 syndrome
  - Recently, there was a report of bilateral diffuse adrenal medullary hyperplasia in a patient with *SDHB* mutation

Hyperplasia Associated With Genetic Disorders

- Bilateral adrenal medullary hyperplasia was first described in 1966
  - Its significance was not understood until identification of *RET* proto-oncogene
    - Now, the association of AMH and MEN2 syndromes is well established
- Adrenal medullary hyperplasia is a precursor of pheochromocytomas in MEN2 syndrome
  - AMH is common in multiple endocrine neoplasia 2A and 2B (MEN2A and MEN2B)
- AMH is known to be absent or very rare in other pheochromocytoma/paraganglioma syndromes
  - Report of bilateral diffuse adrenal medullary hyperplasia in a patient with *SDHB* mutation
- AMH and hyperplasia of extraadrenal sympathetic paraganglia in Beckwith-Wiedemann syndrome (BWS) noted by Beckwith in 1969 description
  - Now seems less consistent than cortical abnormalities
- Mature chromaffin cell nodules (sometimes present in fetuses with BWS) suggest extraadrenal paraganglia developing within adrenals

As Precursor Lesion

- Because of the link between *RET* mutations and adrenal medullary hyperplasia, it is hypothesized that medullary hyperplasia is a precursor lesion that will eventually develop into pheochromocytoma given enough time
  - Similar pattern of progression from hyperplasia to malignancy is seen in other endocrine tumors, such as medullary thyroid cancer and adrenal cortical tumors

Sporadic Adrenal Medullary Hyperplasia

- Sporadic AMH reported in different settings
  - In patients with cystic fibrosis

ADRENAL MEDULLARY HYPERPLASIA

Key Facts

Terminology

- Increase in mass of adrenal medullary cells and expansion of these cells into areas of gland where they are not normally present

Etiology/Pathogenesis

- Adrenal medullary hyperplasia is a precursor of pheochromocytomas in MEN2 syndrome
- AMH is common in multiple endocrine neoplasia 2A and 2B
  - Absent or very rare in other pheochromocytoma/paraganglioma syndromes

Macroscopic Features

- Adrenal medulla normally confined to central region (body) of gland
  - Medullary hyperplasia often identifiable by gross extension of gray medullary tissue into alae and tail
- Patients with MEN2 syndromes usually have diffuse and nodular hyperplasia involving both glands
- Nodules are gray to tan and may compress adjacent cortex

Microscopic Pathology

- Nodules can occur with little or no diffuse hyperplasia
- Histology shows medullary hyperplasia composed of proliferation of cells containing normal cellular architecture
  - As opposed to nests of cytologically atypical polygonal cells that characterize pheochromocytoma

  - In infants dying of sudden infant death syndrome (SIDS)
  - Cushing syndrome
  - In sporadic forms of Beckwith-Wiedemann syndrome
  - Other rare causes

Compensatory Physiological Hyperplasia

- Extensively documented in parasympathetic paraganglia; mostly carotid body, sometimes vagal
  - Presumed association with hypoxia: Occurs in humans and animals living at high altitude; also reported in lung disease, cystic fibrosis, and cyanotic heart disease
  - Controversial association of hyperplastic paraganglia with SIDS

CLINICAL ISSUES

Presentation

- AMH may present with signs of catecholamine excess or be discovered incidentally after adrenalectomy for pheochromocytoma
- Hyperplasia of extraadrenal paraganglia usually studied in autopsy series of patients dying from other causes

MACROSCOPIC FEATURES

General Features

- Patients with MEN2 syndromes usually have diffuse and nodular hyperplasia involving both glands
  - Characteristically in these patients, medullary hyperplasia involves the tail
- Nodules are gray to tan and may compress adjacent cortex
- Adrenal medulla normally confined to central region (body) of gland
  - AMH often identifiable by gross extension of gray medullary tissue into alae and tail
  - Nodules often superimposed on diffuse hyperplasia
  - Mild diffuse hyperplasia may require morphometry for confirmation (usually not done in practice)
- On gross examination, as well as radiologic imaging, medullary hyperplasia has poorly defined nodules
  - Unlike pheochromocytoma, which usually presents as an enlarged adrenal nodule arising from medulla
- Hyperplasia of other paraganglia usually not identifiable macroscopically

Size

- Morphometrically calculated weight of 1 normal adrenal medulla: 0.3-0.5 g (~ 10% of total adrenal weight)
  - AMH often begins as diffuse ↑ in volume and weight
- Carotid body weight ↑ with age
  - Average normal combined weight in adults: < 15 mg (> 30 mg suggests hyperplasia)

MICROSCOPIC PATHOLOGY

Histologic Features

- Shows medullary hyperplasia composed by proliferation of cells containing normal cellular architecture
  - As opposed to nests of cytologically atypical polygonal cells that characterize pheochromocytoma
  - In MEN2-associated medullary hyperplasia, hyaline globules may be present
  - Hyperplastic medullary cells may show various growth patterns: Alveolar, diffuse or solid, and trabecular
  - Sometimes, hyperplastic cells are arranged in small nests separated by thin fibrous tissue
- Presence of adrenal medullary tissue in tail indicates presence of adrenal medullary hyperplasia
- Classic AMH shows diffuse medullary expansion with increasing atypia and superimposed nodules
- Adrenal medullary nodules can occur with little or no diffuse hyperplasia

ADRENAL MEDULLARY HYPERPLASIA

- Medulla does not represent > 1/3 of gland thickness, with cortex on each side comprising the other 2/3
  - However, significant cortical atrophy, usually due to exogenous steroid administration, alters ratio and can mimic medullary hyperplasia
    - Careful evaluation of cortical anatomy and cytology is required before diagnosis of AMH
- Normal carotid body is divided by thick fibrous septa into variable number of lobes
  - Lobes are further divided by thin septa into lobules
    - Lobules contain clusters (zellballen) of chief cells with peripheral sustentacular cells
  - Carotid body hyperplasia at high altitude
    - ↑ number of lobes and larger lobes with ↑ cellularity caused by chief cell hyperplasia
  - Studies variably report proportionate or disproportionate ↑ of sustentacular cells, especially in hyperplasia unrelated to high altitude

ANCILLARY TESTS

Immunohistochemistry

- Neuroendocrine markers highlight medullary cells
  - Chromogranin-A
  - Synaptophysin
  - Neuron-specific enolase (NSE)
  - CD56
  - S100 stain identifies sustentacular cells
- SDHA and SDHB immunostains help identify *SDHx*-associated inherited cases

DIFFERENTIAL DIAGNOSIS

Pheochromocytoma

- Distinction between AMH and pheochromocytoma can be challenging
  - Cutoff of 1 cm to differentiate pheochromocytoma from hyperplastic nodule is arbitrary
    - Some pheochromocytomas may be < 1.0 cm
    - Benign adrenal nodules in patients with MEN2B can be monoclonal
    - Both AMH and pheochromocytoma are often monoclonal
    - Best to consider nodular hyperplasia and small pheochromocytomas as part of continuum of same disease process
- Presence of unilateral vs. bilateral disease may be helpful in distinguishing AMH from pheochromocytoma (PCC)
  - Unilateral AMH has been reported in isolated and familial AMH
- Altered macroscopic appearance and histology probably more meaningful
- Pheochromocytomas have the characteristic alveolar pattern (zellballen) with variably sized nests of tumor cells surrounded by thin-walled vessels and thin bands of fibrous tissue
- Some pheochromocytomas lack the organoid pattern and instead may show a diffuse growth pattern
- Some pheochromocytomas show a mosaic-like pattern of often large cells with granular basophilic cytoplasm admixed with cells that have amphophilic to slightly eosinophilic cytoplasm
- Some pheochromocytomas are formed by small cells with ample eosinophilic cytoplasm with occasional bizarre cells

Metastatic Carcinoma

- Can be distinguished by characteristic morphological features
- Distinguished by immunohistochemical profile
  - Positivity for chromogranin, synaptophysin, NSE, and CD56 in AMH
  - Characteristic positivity for S100 in sustentacular cells, when present, helps identifying AMH

DIAGNOSTIC CHECKLIST

Pathologic Interpretation Pearls

- Adrenals removed for pheochromocytoma should be carefully examined for additional nodules as clue to presence of MEN2

SELECTED REFERENCES

1. Mete O et al: Precursor lesions of endocrine system neoplasms. Pathology. 45(3):316-30, 2013
2. Grogan RH et al: Bilateral adrenal medullary hyperplasia associated with an SDHB mutation. J Clin Oncol. 29(8):e200-2, 2011
3. van Nederveen FH et al: Precursor lesions of the adrenal gland. Pathobiology. 74(5):285-90, 2007
4. Powers JF et al: Ret protein expression in adrenal medullary hyperplasia and pheochromocytoma. Endocr Pathol. 14(4):351-61, 2003
5. Diaz-Cano SJ et al: Clonal patterns in phaeochromocytomas and MEN-2A adrenal medullary hyperplasias: histological and kinetic correlates. J Pathol. 192(2):221-8, 2000
6. Tischler AS et al: Adrenal medullary nodules in Beckwith-Wiedemann syndrome resemble extra-adrenal paraganglia. Endocr Pathol. 7(4):265-272, 1996
7. Lack EE et al: Carotid body hyperplasia in cystic fibrosis and cyanotic heart disease. A combined morphometric, ultrastructural, and biochemical study. Am J Pathol. 119(2):301-14, 1985
8. Carney JA et al: Adrenal medullary disease in multiple endocrine neoplasia, type 2: pheochromocytoma and its precursors. Am J Clin Pathol. 66(2):279-90, 1976
9. DeLellis RA et al: Adrenal medullary hyperplasia. A morphometric analysis in patients with familial medullary thyroid carcinoma. Am J Pathol. 83(1):177-96, 1976
10. Beckwith JB: Macroglossia, omphalocele, adrenal cytomegaly, gigantism and hyperplastic visceromegaly. Birth Defects: Original Article Series, 5: 188-96, 1969

ADRENAL MEDULLARY HYPERPLASIA

Gross and Microscopic Features

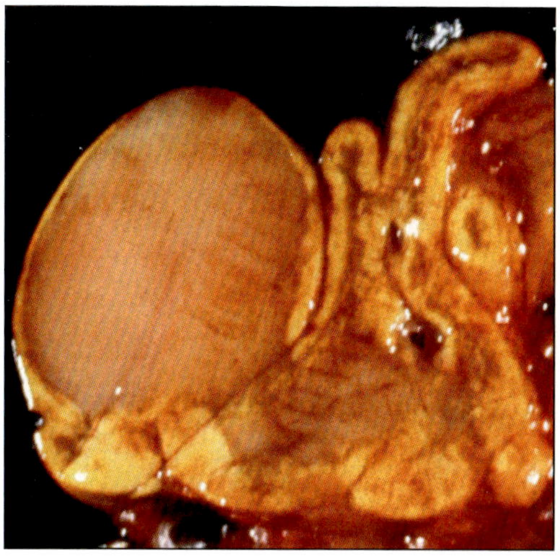

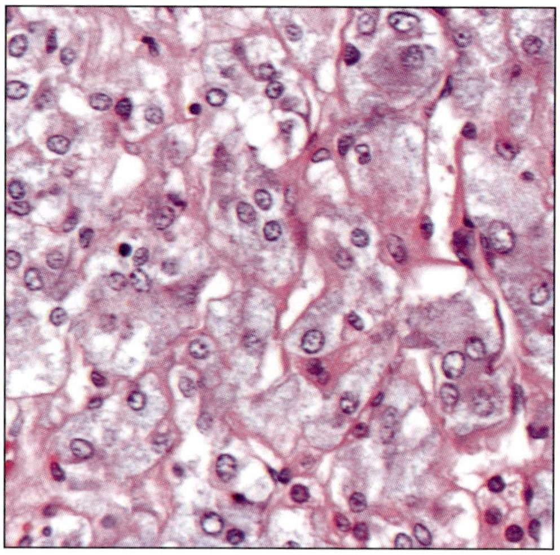

(Left) *Familial medullary hyperplasia is most commonly present in patients with MEN2A and MEN2B and associated with pheochromocytoma. The involvement is usually bilateral, diffuse, and nodular, and often extends to both alae and the tail of the adrenal gland.* ***(Right)*** *The hyperplastic medullary cells may show various growth patterns: Alveolar, solid, or trabecular. This example of adrenal medullary hyperplasia shows an alveolar growth pattern.*

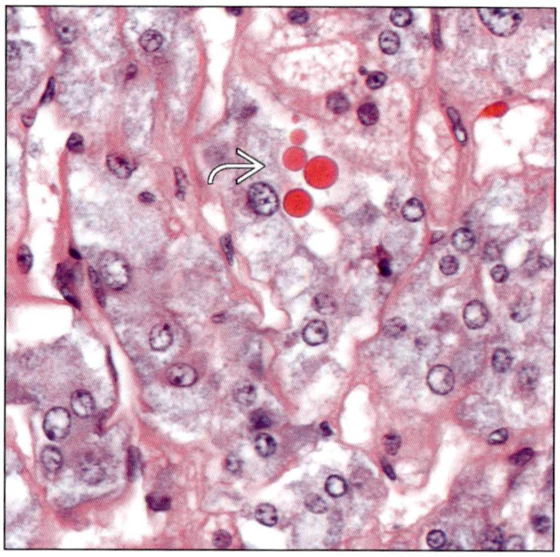

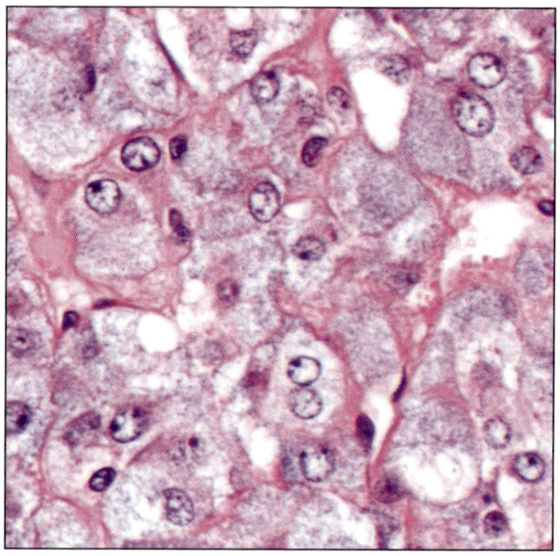

(Left) *This photomicrography shows an area of adrenal medullary hyperplasia in a patient with MEN2 with a mixed alveolar-trabecular growth pattern. Note the presence of hyaline granules* ↪*, usually present in MEN2.* ***(Right)*** *In areas of adrenal medullary hyperplasia, the hyperplastic cells may be arranged in small nests of cells, or as single cells, separated by thin fibrous tissue.*

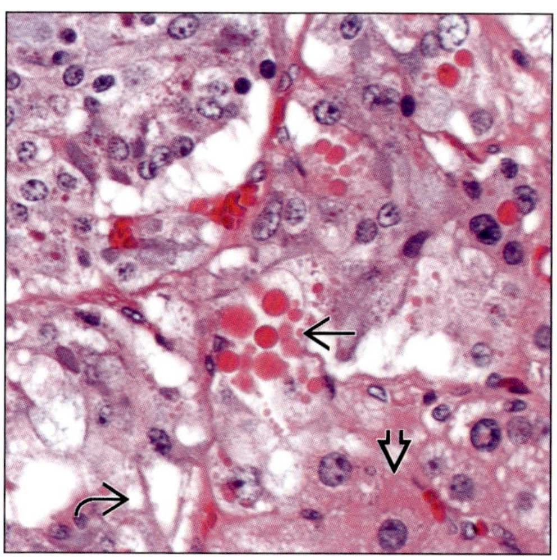

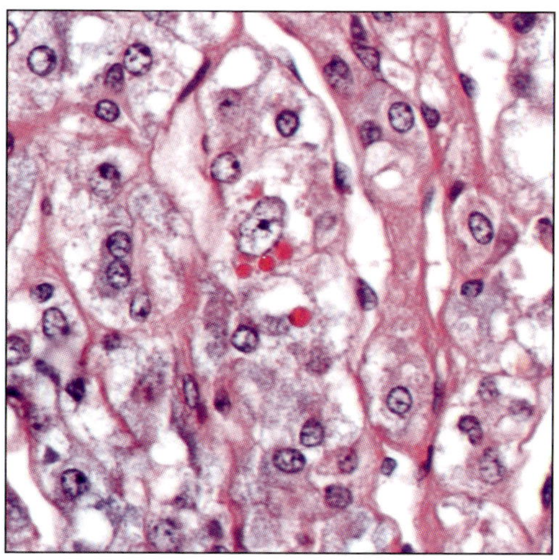

(Left) *Patients with MEN2 syndrome may have diffuse and nodular adrenal medullary hyperplasia. This picture shows medullary cells* ↪ *within the adrenal cortex* ⇩*. The presence of hyaline granules* → *is usually present in MEN2.* ***(Right)*** *H&E shows that diffuse adrenal medullary hyperplasia has cells arranged in cords and is composed of medullary cells with ample granular basophilic cytoplasm and small nuclei. There is mild nuclear pleomorphism.*

NEUROBLASTOMA

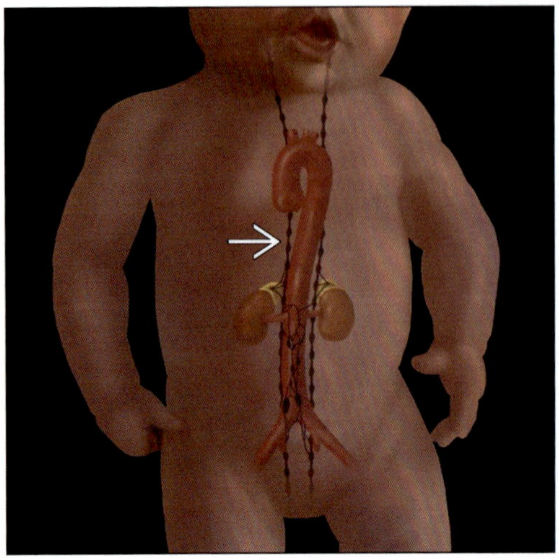

Neuroblastoma (NB) can arise anywhere along the sympathetic chain ➡ from the cervical region through the mediastinum and abdomen, including the adrenal gland, to the inferior pelvis.

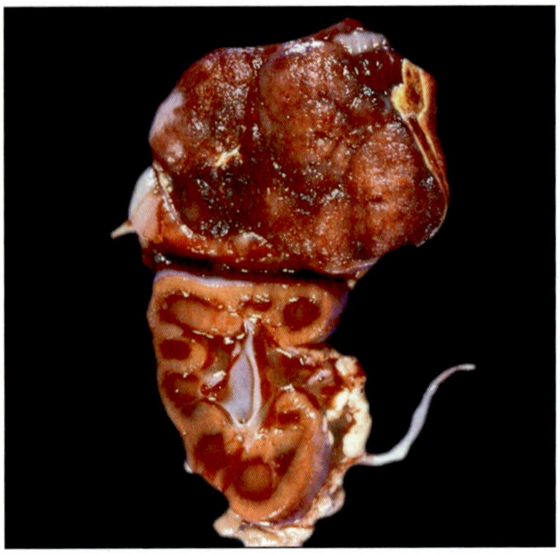

Gross image shows a large mass arising from the adrenal gland and compressing the upper pole of the kidney. NB is often grossly hemorrhagic with areas of necrosis.

TERMINOLOGY

Abbreviations

- Neuroblastoma (NB)
- Ganglioneuroblastoma (GNB)

Synonyms

- Peripheral neuroblastic tumor
- Schwannian stroma-poor neuroblastic tumor

Definitions

- Malignant tumor derived from primordial neural crest cells
  - NB is less differentiated
  - GNB is moderately differentiated, showing variable cytodifferentiation into ganglion cells

ETIOLOGY/PATHOGENESIS

Developmental Anomaly

- Derived from primordial neural crest cells
  - Migrate from spinal cord to adrenal medulla and sympathetic ganglia
- Hereditary
  - Inherited cases represent ~ 2-3.5% of new cases
  - Heterogeneous etiology
    - Autosomal dominant
    - *ALK* mutations
    - *MYCN* amplification
    - Heterozygous mutations in the *PHOX2B* on 4p12
    - Found in 2 people with nonsyndromic NB
  - Potential susceptibility loci at 16p12-p31, 4p16, 2p21-p25.1, 12p12.1-p13.33
    - Suggests a possible oligogenic model in which 2 loci have a synergistic effect on NB
  - Patients with familial NB have 20% risk of developing bilateral adrenal and multifocal primary tumors
    - Patients may have associated ganglioneuroma

CLINICAL ISSUES

Epidemiology

- Incidence
  - 4th most common malignant tumor in children
  - Usually sporadic
    - Some autosomal dominant familial cases have been seen
- Age
  - Most cases of familial NB are diagnosed before 1 year of age
  - 1/2 of patients diagnosed by 2 years of age
  - 85% of patients < 5 years of age
  - ~ 20-30% congenital (some detected on ultrasound during pregnancy)
- Ethnicity
  - Less common in African Americans (very low incidence in "Burkitt lymphoma belt" in Africa)

Site

- Follows distribution of sympathetic ganglia
  - Abdomen (54%)
    - Adrenal (36%)
    - Extraadrenal (18%)
  - Thorax (14%)
  - Neck (5%)
  - Pelvis (5%)
  - Unknown/others (22%)

Presentation

- Depends on age of patient, location of tumor, and associated clinical syndromes
- Most have nonspecific symptoms
  - e.g., fever, weight loss, diarrhea, anemia, hypertension
- Fetuses may have hydrops
- Palpable mass
- ~ 2/3 have metastasis on presentation
- "Blueberry muffin" baby

NEUROBLASTOMA

Key Facts

Terminology
- Malignant tumor derived from primordial neural crest cells

Etiology/Pathogenesis
- Hereditary
  - Inherited cases represent ~ 2-3.5% of new cases
  - Heterozygous mutations in the *PHOX2B* on 4p12
  - *ALK* mutations
  - *MYCN* amplification
- Potential susceptibility loci at 16p12-p31, 4p16,2p21-p25.1, 12p12.1-p13.33
- Patients with familial NB have 20% risk of developing bilateral adrenal and multifocal primary tumors

Clinical Issues
- 85% of patients < 5 years of age
- 4th most common malignant tumor in children
- Follows distribution of sympathetic ganglia
- About 2/3 have metastases on presentation

Microscopic Pathology
- International Neuroblastoma Pathology Committee (INPC) classification
  - Undifferentiated NB
  - Poorly differentiated NB
  - Differentiating NB
  - Nodular ganglioneuroblastoma (GNB)
  - Intermixed GNB

Diagnostic Checklist
- Worse prognosis
  - *MYCN* amplification
  - Loss of heterozygosity of 1p and 11q

  - Blue-red cutaneous lesions in infants
- Opsoclonus/myoclonus syndrome (dancing eyes, dancing feet)

Laboratory Tests
- Urine catecholamine metabolites and dopamine have been used for screening
- Lactate dehydrogenase
  - > 1,500 IU/L associated with worse clinical outcome
- Ferritin
  - > 142 ng/mL associated with worse clinical outcome
- Neuron-specific enolase (NSE)
  - > 100 ng/mL associated with worse clinical outcome

Natural History
- Some cases undergo spontaneous regression, including stage IV-S
  - Most in children < 1 year of age

Treatment
- Low risk
  - Surgery or observation alone
- Intermediate risk
  - Surgery and adjuvant chemotherapy
- High risk
  - Induction chemotherapy
  - Delayed tumor resection
  - Radiation of primary site
  - Myeloablative chemotherapy with stem cell recovery
- Metastases
  - Bone
  - Lymph nodes
  - Liver
  - Skin

Prognosis
- 5-year survival based on stage at time of diagnosis
  - Stage I: > 90%
  - Stage II: 70-80%
  - Stage III: 40-70%
  - Stage IV
    - < 1 year old: > 60%
    - 1-2 years old: 20%
    - > 2 years old: 10%
  - Stage IV-S: > 80%
- Adverse factors
  - Older age at diagnosis
  - Advanced stage of disease (except IV-S)
  - High histologic grade of tumor
  - Diploid DNA value
  - *MYCN* oncogene amplification
  - Cytogenetic abnormalities of chromosomes 1 and 17
  - Pattern of urinary catecholamine excretion
  - Increased levels of ferritin, NSE, LDH, creatine kinase BB or chromogranin-A
  - Abnormalities in ganglioside composition
  - Lack of high affinity nerve growth factor receptors

IMAGE FINDINGS

General Features
- Extensive radiographic evaluation is required to determine extent of disease and identify metastatic foci
- Calcifications often seen in central portion of tumor

Bone Scan
- Radiolabeled metaiodobenzylguanidine (MIBG) incorporates into catecholamine-secreting cells and can detect neuroblastoma

MACROSCOPIC FEATURES

General Features
- Color and consistency depend on amount of stroma present (stroma-poor vs. stroma-rich tumors) and presence of hemorrhage and necrosis
- Usually solitary masses
- Cystic degeneration and calcification can be seen

NEUROBLASTOMA

MICROSCOPIC PATHOLOGY

Histologic Features

- Neuroblasts
  - Small round blue cells with very scant cytoplasm
- Homer Wright rosettes or pseudorosettes (uncommon)
  - Nuclei grouping in ring-like structures around central cores of tangled neuritic cell processes
- Ganglionic differentiation
  - Cells are enlarged
  - Increased eosinophilic or amphophilic cytoplasm
  - Vesicular chromatin pattern
  - Must have synchronous differentiation of cytoplasm and nucleus
- Neuropil
  - Fibrillar eosinophilic matrix
- Mitotic-karyorrhectic index (MKI), applicable for stroma-poor tumors
  - Count of cells undergoing mitosis or karyorrhexis (per 5,000 cells)
    - Low: < 100 cells
    - Intermediate: 100-200 cells
    - High: > 200 cells

International Neuroblastoma Pathology Committee (INPC) Classification

- a.k.a. Shimada classification
- **Undifferentiated NB**
  - No ganglionic differentiation
  - No neuropil
  - No or minimal schwannian stroma
  - Often requires immunohistochemistry for accurate diagnosis
- **Poorly differentiated NB**
  - < 5% of tumor cells showing ganglionic differentiation
  - Most cells appear undifferentiated
  - Neuropil background
  - No or minimal schwannian stroma
- **Differentiating NB**
  - > 5% of tumor cells showing ganglionic differentiation
  - More abundant neuropil
  - Usually more prominent schwannian stroma
    - Must be < 50%
- **Nodular GNB**
  - Grossly identifiable nodules will be neuroblastoma
  - Abrupt demarcation between stroma-poor neuroblastoma and stroma-rich component
  - Fibrous pseudocapsule often seen surrounding NB component
  - > 50% schwannian stroma
- **Intermixed GNB**
  - Microscopic nests of neuroblastoma within schwannian stroma
  - > 50% schwannian stroma
- Do not classify post-treatment resections
  - "Neuroblastoma with treatment effect" is sufficient
- May classify metastatic disease if resection/biopsy is pretreatment

ANCILLARY TESTS

Immunohistochemistry

- NSE
- NB84(+) in almost all NBs
  - Not specific; occasionally positive in other small round cell tumors
- S100 protein
- Other useful positive immunostains include
  - Chromogranin
  - Synaptophysin
  - Protein gene product 9.5 (PGP9.5)
  - CD56

Cytogenetics

- *MYCN*
  - Amplification is associated with worse prognosis
  - Usually seen in advanced disease
- DNA ploidy
  - Near-diploidy or tetraploidy is associated with worse prognosis
  - Hyperdiploidy is associated with better prognosis
- Loss of heterozygosity of 1p and 11q
  - Both associated with worse prognosis
- TrkA (high-affinity nerve growth factor receptor)
  - Increased expression associates with better prognosis

Electron Microscopy

- Wide range of cytologic differentiation
- Dense core of neurosecretory granules
  - Found in elongated cell processes
  - 100 nm in diameter
  - Dense core surrounded by clear halos and delicate outer membranes

DIFFERENTIAL DIAGNOSIS

Ganglioneuroma

- Differs from intermixed GNB in having single cells instead of nests of cells within schwannian stroma

Ewing Sarcoma/Primitive Neuroectodermal Tumor (PNET)

- Usually older patients
- Cells have finely stippled chromatin and glycogen-filled cytoplasm
- CD99 positivity
- Specific gene fusions, most commonly *EWSR1-FLI1*

Alveolar Rhabdomyosarcoma

- Cells with more pleomorphism and abundant cytoplasm
- Immunoreactivity for muscle markers (desmin, myogenin)
- t(1;13) or t(2;13) with *PAX-FOXO1* fusion

Lymphoma

- Lymphoid immunomarkers (CD45, CD3, CD20)

NEUROBLASTOMA

Favorable vs. Unfavorable Histology in Neuroblastic Tumors

Classification	Subclass	MKI	Age at Diagnosis	Histologic Category
Neuroblastoma (NB)	Undifferentiated	Any MKI	Any age	Unfavorable histology
	Poorly differentiated	High MKI	Any age	Unfavorable histology
		Low or intermediate MKI	> 1.5 years	Unfavorable histology
			< 1.5 years	Favorable histology
	Differentiating	High MKI	Any age	Unfavorable histology
		Intermediate MKI	> 1.5 years	Unfavorable histology
			< 1.5 years	Favorable histology
		Low MKI	> 5 years	Unfavorable histology
			< 5 years	Favorable histology
Ganglioneuroblastoma (GNB)	Nodular	*	*	Unfavorable or favorable histology

*The determination of favorable vs. unfavorable histology in nodular GNB is based on the NB component. Mitosis-karyorrhexis index (MKI).

Neuroblastoma Staging System

Stage	Definition
I	Localized confined tumor; complete gross excision; ipsilateral and contralateral nodes negative
IIA	Unilateral tumor; incomplete gross excision; identifiable ipsilateral and contralateral nodes negative
IIB	Unilateral tumor ± complete gross excision; identifiable ipsilateral nodes positive, identifiable ipsilateral and contralateral nodes negative
III	Tumor infiltrating across midline without positive nodes or unilateral tumor with positive contralateral nodes
IV	Distant metastases to nodes, bone, bone marrow, liver, skin, &/or other organs not stage IV-S
IV-S	Localized primary tumor (stages 1 or 2) with metastases limited to liver, skin, &/or bone marrow

DIAGNOSTIC CHECKLIST

Clinically Relevant Pathologic Features

- Gross appearance
  - Cystic degeneration and calcification can be seen
- Microscopy
  - Small round blue cells with very scant cytoplasm
  - Homer Wright rosettes or pseudorosettes
  - Ganglionic differentiation
- Mitotic-karyorrhectic index (MKI), applicable for stroma-poor tumors
  - Count of cells undergoing mitosis or karyorrhexis (per 5,000 cells)

Pathologic Interpretation Pearls

- To assess classification based on degree of tumor differentiation
- High importance of cytogenetics
  - *MYCN* amplification is associated with worse prognosis
  - Loss of heterozygosity of 1p and 11q associated with worse prognosis

SELECTED REFERENCES

1. Suganuma R et al: Peripheral neuroblastic tumors with genotype-phenotype discordance: a report from the Children's Oncology Group and the International Neuroblastoma Pathology Committee. Pediatr Blood Cancer. 60(3):363-70, 2013
2. Capasso M et al: Genetics and genomics of neuroblastoma. Cancer Treat Res. 155:65-84, 2010
3. Maris JM: Recent advances in neuroblastoma. N Engl J Med. 362(23):2202-11, 2010
4. Ambros PF et al: International consensus for neuroblastoma molecular diagnostics: report from the International Neuroblastoma Risk Group (INRG) Biology Committee. Br J Cancer. 100(9):1471-82, 2009
5. Cohn SL et al: The International Neuroblastoma Risk Group (INRG) classification system: an INRG Task Force report. J Clin Oncol. 27(2):289-97, 2009
6. Shimada A et al: Expression of KIT and PDGFR is associated with a good prognosis in neuroblastoma. Pediatr Blood Cancer. 50(2):213-7, 2008
7. Sano H et al: International neuroblastoma pathology classification adds independent prognostic information beyond the prognostic contribution of age. Eur J Cancer. 42(8):1113-9, 2006
8. Attiyeh EF et al: Chromosome 1p and 11q deletions and outcome in neuroblastoma. N Engl J Med. 353(21):2243-53, 2005
9. Shimada H: The International Neuroblastoma Pathology Classification. Pathologica. 95(5):240-1, 2003
10. Shimada H et al: International neuroblastoma pathology classification for prognostic evaluation of patients with peripheral neuroblastic tumors: a report from the Children's Cancer Group. Cancer. 92(9):2451-61, 2001
11. Shimada H et al: Terminology and morphologic criteria of neuroblastic tumors: recommendations by the International Neuroblastoma Pathology Committee. Cancer. 86(2):349-63, 1999
12. Shimada H et al: The International Neuroblastoma Pathology Classification (the Shimada system). Cancer. 86(2):364-72, 1999

NEUROBLASTOMA

Clinical, Gross, and Microscopic Features

(Left) *Child has bilateral orbital masses, clinically presenting with proptosis and ecchymosis.* ***(Right)*** *This is a typical appearance of a nodular ganglioneuroblastoma (GNB). The hemorrhagic nodule is stroma-poor NB whereas the tan, fleshy rim is either ganglioneuroma or intermixed GNB. The diagnosis of nodular GNB requires gross visible nodules.*

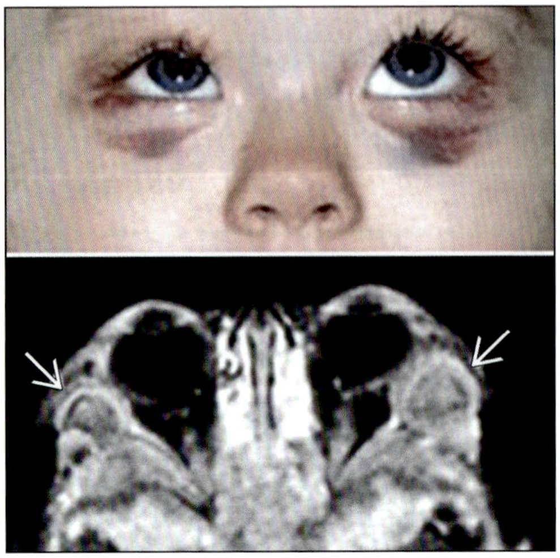

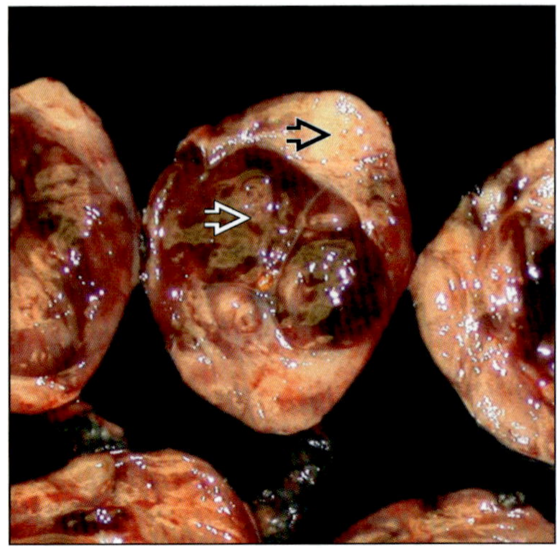

(Left) *This is a GNB from the mediastinum. This image depicts a tumor with a tan firm cut surface, but the gross appearance of GNB depends on how much of the tumor is neuroblastic.* ***(Right)*** *This specimen of liver shows diffuse involvement and extensive replacement by multiple deposits of metastatic NB. There are several foci of hemorrhage.*

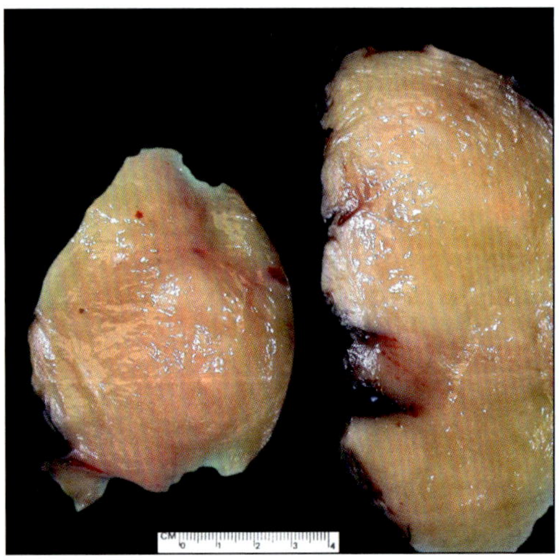

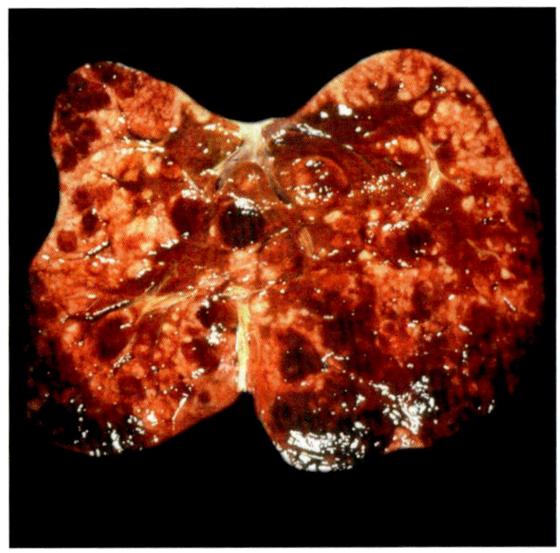

(Left) *Undifferentiated NB shows cells with scant cytoplasm with round and hyperchromatic nuclei. The differential diagnosis should include other small blue round cell tumors.* ***(Right)*** *The mitotic-karyorrhectic index (MKI) is determined by counting the number of mitoses and karyorrhectic cells per 5,000 tumor cells. MKI counts should be averaged over the entire tumor and not assessed in only the worst-looking areas.*

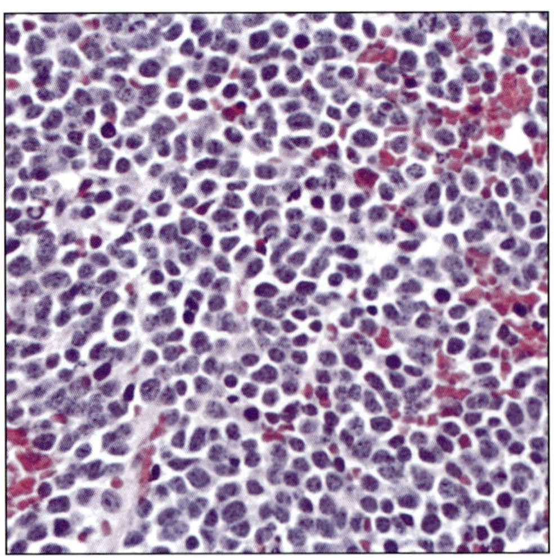

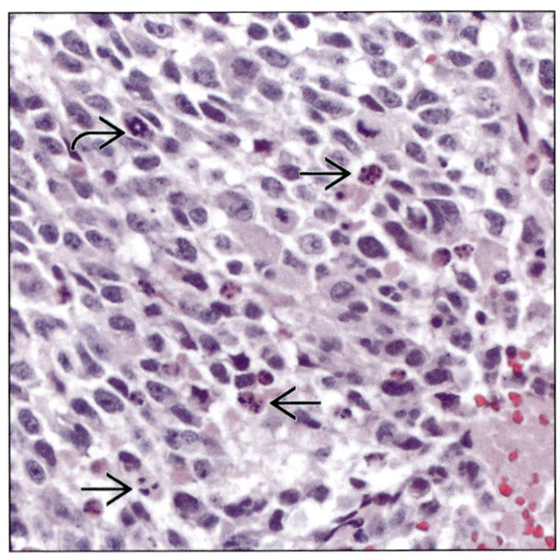

NEUROBLASTOMA

Microscopic Features

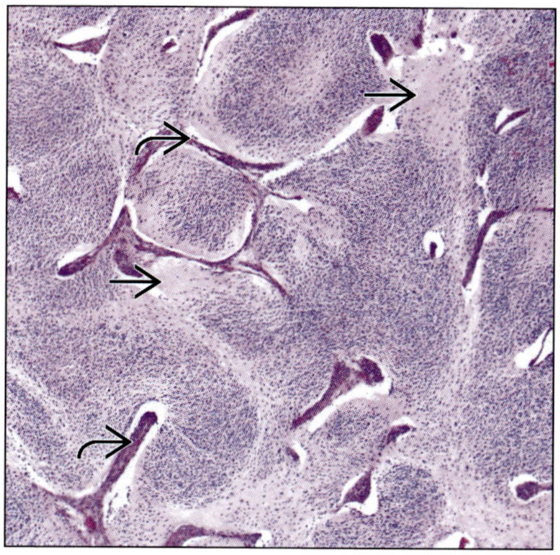

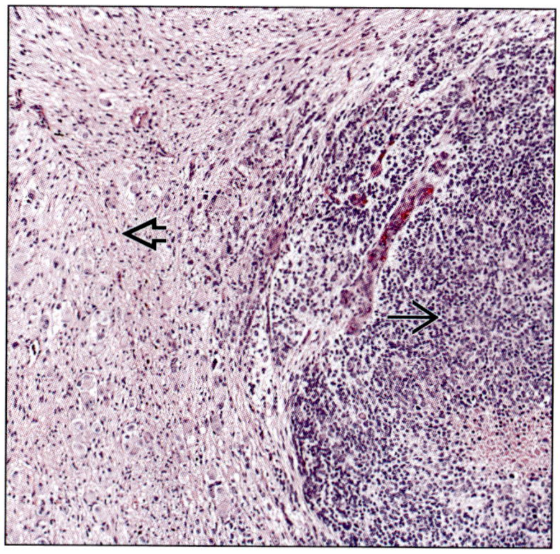

(Left) *Low-power view of a poorly differentiated NB shows thin septa composed of schwannian stroma ↷. Pale, eosinophilic neuropil → is seen in places between the nodules or nests of neuroblastoma cells.* ***(Right)*** *This nodular GNB shows the pushing border between the stroma-poor NB component → and the ganglioneuroma component ⇨. Even with this histologic picture, a grossly visible nodule is required to diagnose nodular GNB.*

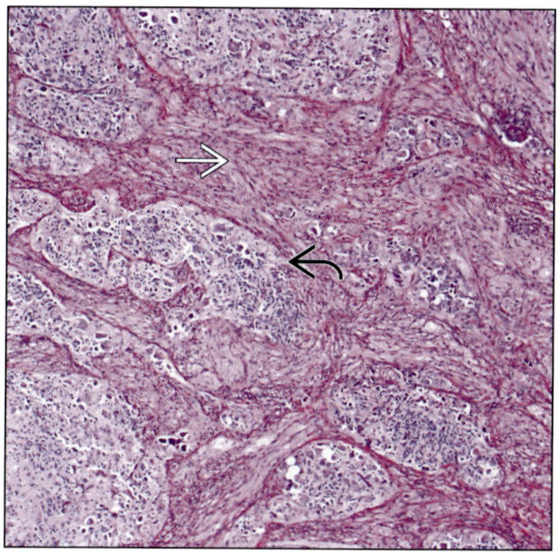

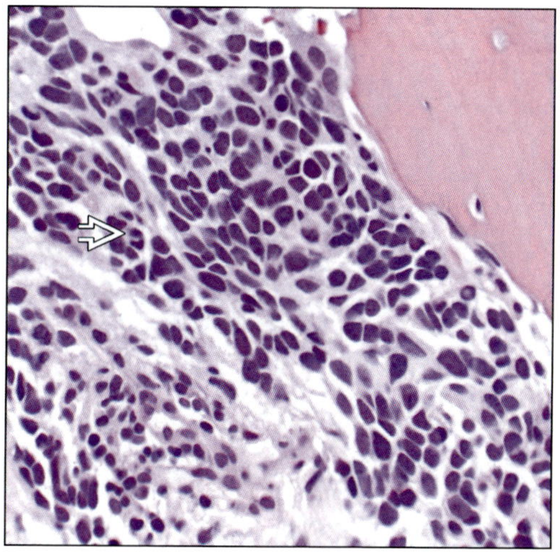

(Left) *This intermixed GNB shows well-defined nests ↷ of maturing neuroblasts, ganglion cells, and neuropil within a schwannian stroma ➡.* ***(Right)*** *This is a focus of metastatic NB in a core biopsy specimen of bone. The marrow has been extensively replaced by sheets of metastatic small round cell tumor ⇨ and shows no areas with normal trilineage hematopoiesis.*

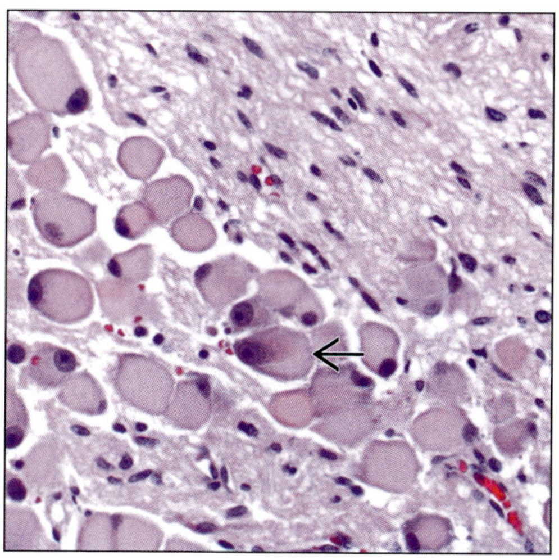

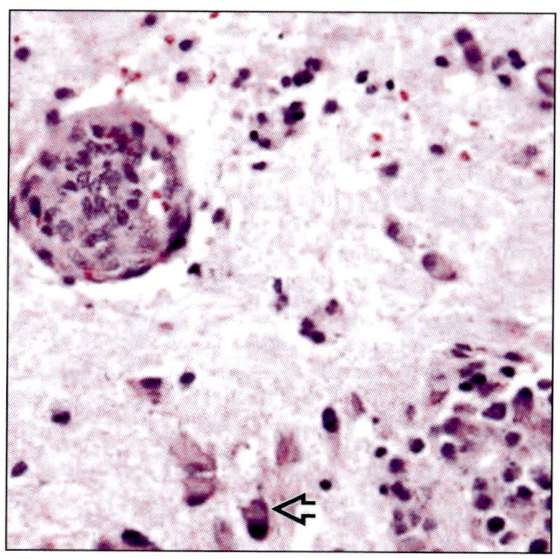

(Left) *Mature ganglion cells → are characterized by abundant eosinophilic to amphophilic cytoplasm, eccentric nuclei, and prominent nucleoli. Nissl substance may or may not be present. Focally, these cells are admixed with a schwannian stroma.* ***(Right)*** *High-power view of a GNB highlights the maturing ganglion cells ⇨ in a background of neuropil. The neuropil is composed of a dense tangle of fibrillary, eosinophilic cytoplasmic processes.*

NEUROBLASTOMA

Microscopic Features

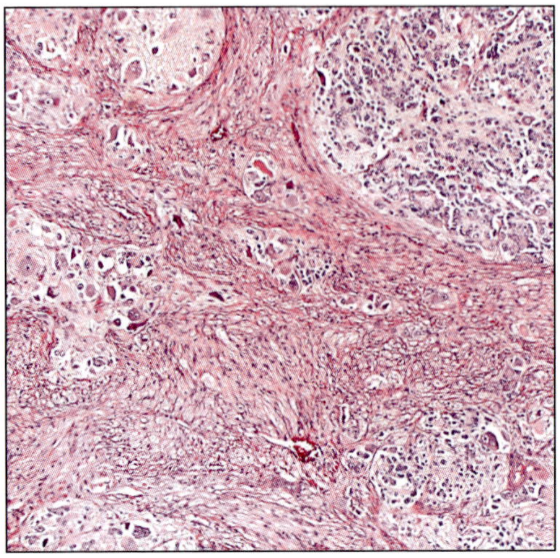
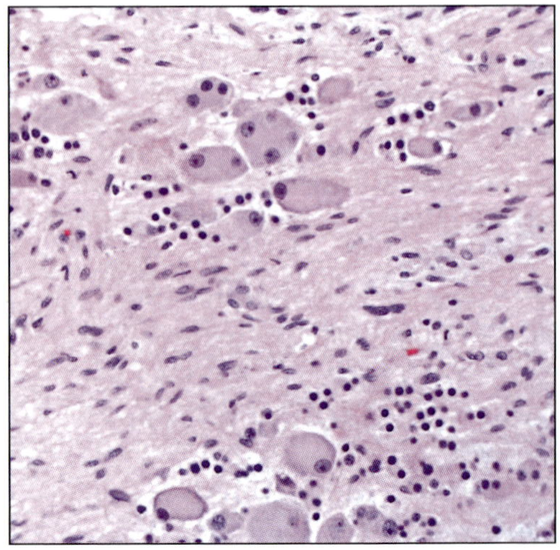

(Left) *In intermixed-type GNB, at least 50% of the tumor must be schwannian stroma. This is characterized by spindled, wavy cells in bundles of varying densities.* ***(Right)*** *This section from an intermixed GNB could be mistaken for a maturing ganglioneuroma (GN). In maturing GN, the tumor is mainly composed of schwannian stroma, and individual neuroblastic cells merge into the schwannian stroma instead of forming distinct nests.*

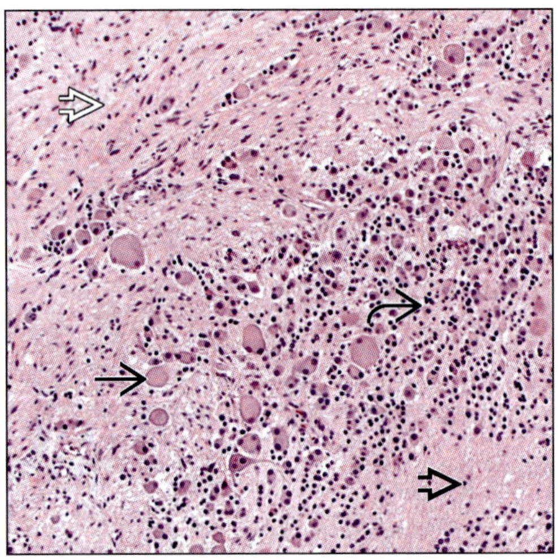
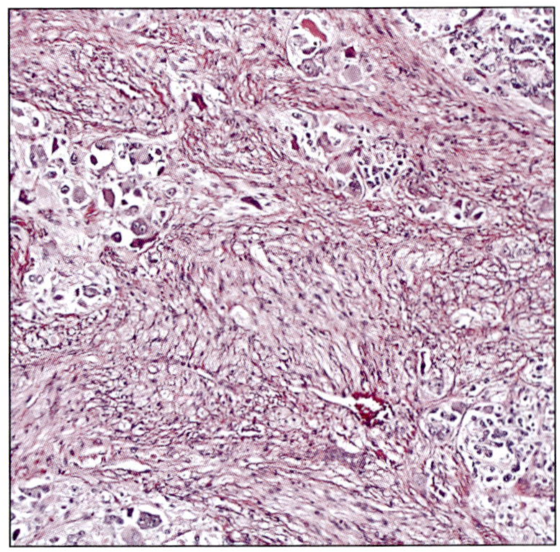

(Left) *Low-power view of an intermixed GNB shows maturing ganglion cells →, neuroblasts ↪, and neuropil ⇨ admixed with schwannian stroma ➡.* ***(Right)*** *At least 50% of the tumor must be composed of schwannian stroma to make the diagnosis of intermixed GNB. This is characterized by spindled, wavy cells in bundles of varying cellularity. The Schwann cells demonstrate nuclear immunoreactivity for S100 protein.*

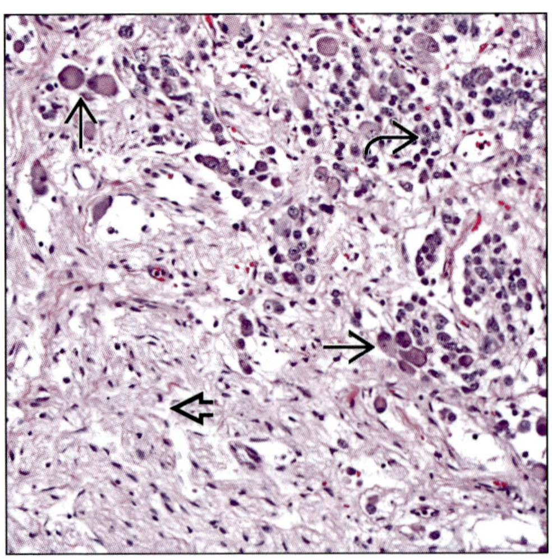
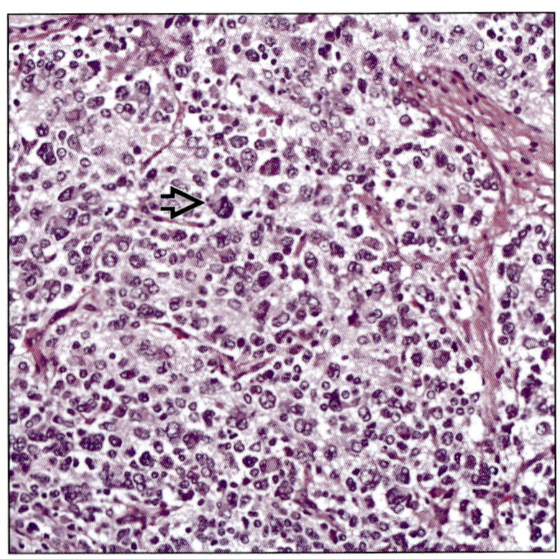

(Left) *A typical intermixed GNB is seen in this image. The tumor is composed of a mixture of maturing ganglion cells →, neuroblasts ↪, and abundant schwannian stroma ⇨.* ***(Right)*** *This is an example of differentiating NB, in which > 5% of the neuroblasts show differentiation with increased cytoplasm and vesicular nuclei ⇨.*

Ancillary Techniques

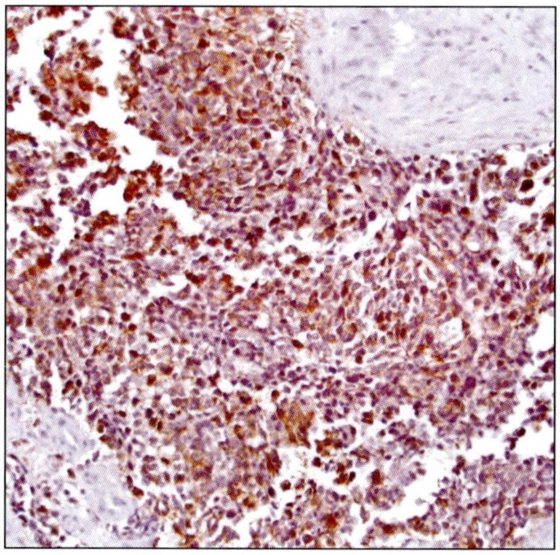

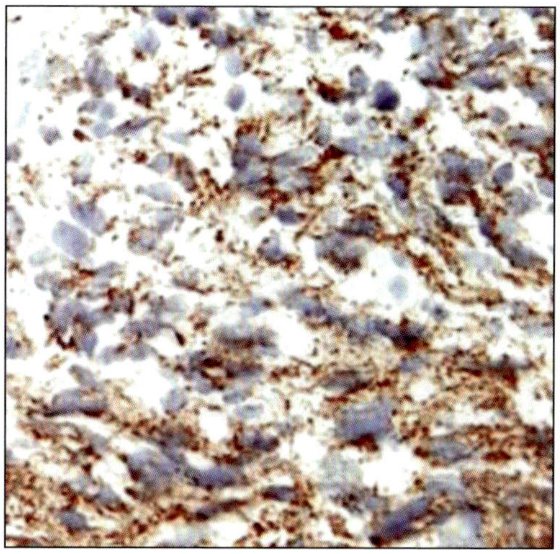

(Left) *NSE IHC staining in NBs shows strong diffuse cytoplasmic positivity. NSE is a sensitive marker for NB, although nonspecific.* ***(Right)*** *Immunohistochemistry for synaptophysin shows membranous staining. Although not specific, it can be used for differential diagnosis of other small round blue cell tumors of childhood, such as lymphoma, rhabdomyosarcoma, or Ewing sarcoma. These tumors are also positive for chromogranin and CD56.*

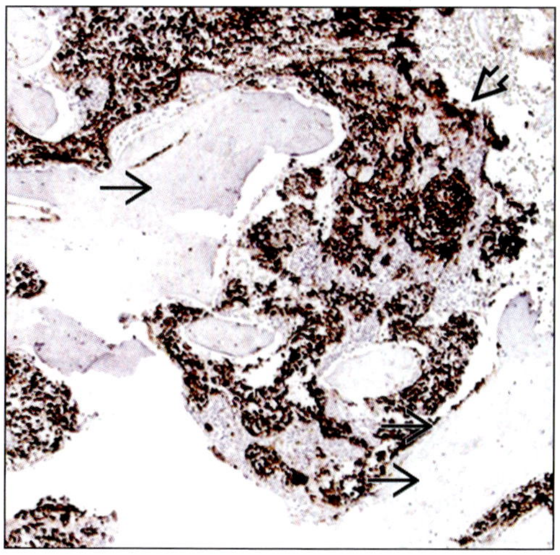

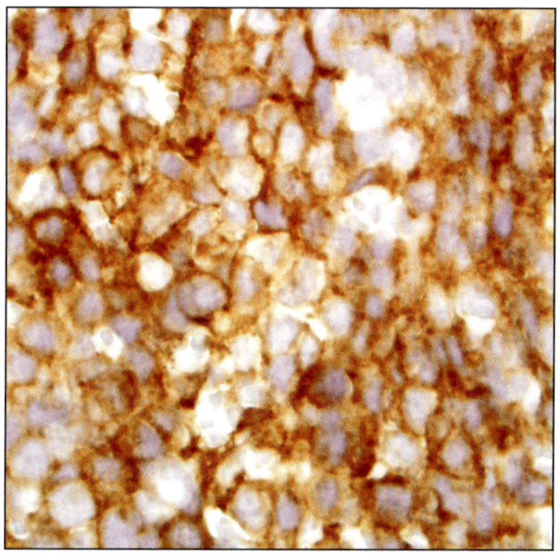

(Left) *In this bone marrow trephine specimen, there is diffuse immunoreactivity for NB antigen (NB84) in metastatic deposits of NB ⇨ that extend between bony trabeculae →.* ***(Right)*** *Immunohistochemical staining for ALK1 in NB shows strong membranous staining. Activating mutations in the ALK gene have been reported in NB and provide a potential therapeutic target.*

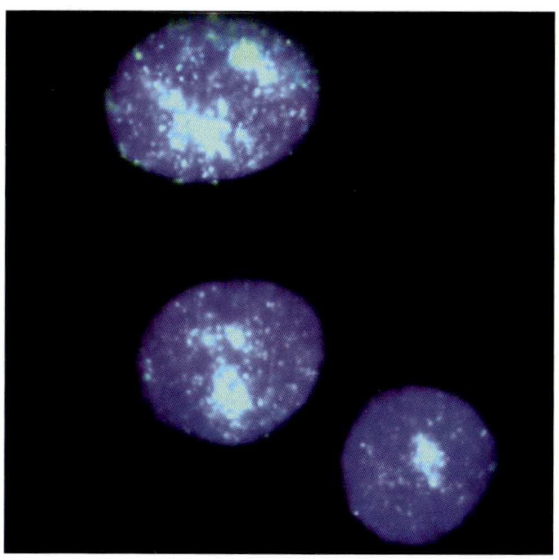

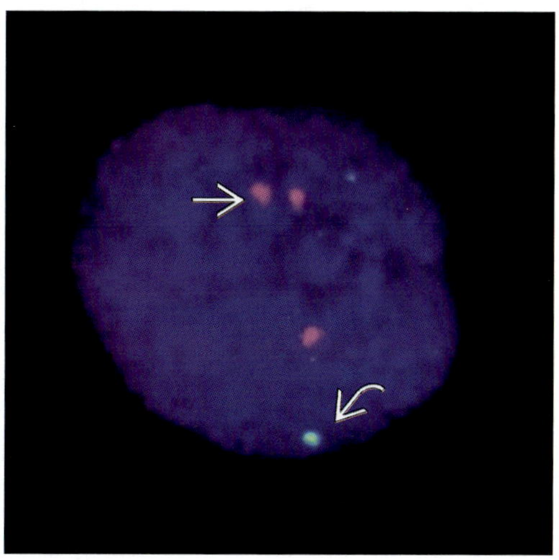

(Left) *Fluorescence in situ hybridization (FISH) of NB shows marked amplification of N-Myc (multiple confluent green dots). The degree of N-Myc amplification, higher or lower, is not correlated with a worse outcome.* ***(Right)*** *Deletion of 1p might be seen on 70-80% of NB. Here, red dots represent the chromosome 1 centromere →, and the green dot represents 1p36 ↗ (only 1 chromosomal copy is present).*

PHEOCHROMOCYTOMA/PARAGANGLIOMA

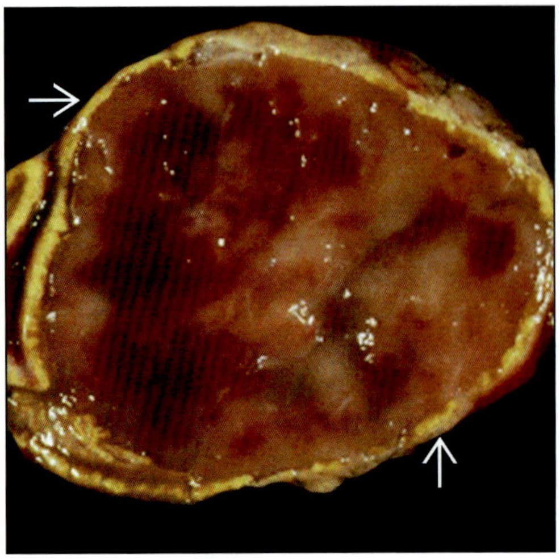

The typical pheochromocytoma has a gray-pink cut surface with areas of hemorrhage, which distinguishes it from the yellow-brown of adrenal cortex ➔.

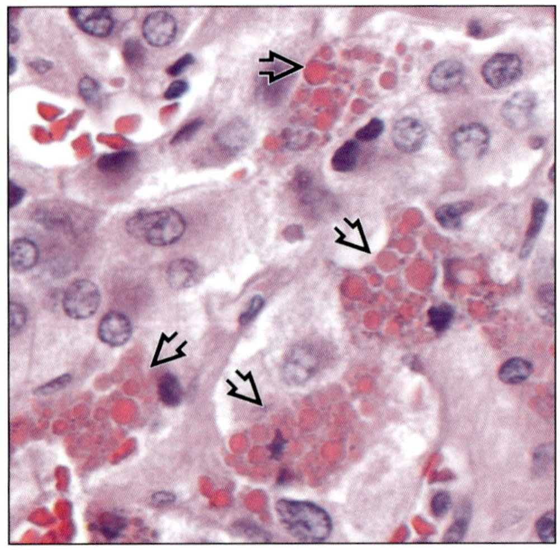

Pheochromocytomas in patients with multiple endocrine neoplasia type 2 (MEN2) syndromes may have numerous hyaline globules ⇨ that are particularly conspicuous in pheochromocytomas of these patients.

TERMINOLOGY

Abbreviations

- Pheochromocytoma (PCC)
- Paraganglioma (PGL)

Definitions

- Normal paraganglia consist of neural crest-derived neuroendocrine cells associated with sympathetic and parasympathetic nerves
  - Adrenal medulla and organ of Zuckerkandl are major sympathetic paraganglia; others are microscopic
  - Carotid bodies are major parasympathetic paraganglia; others are microscopic
- PCC and PGL are catecholamine-secreting tumors of neural crest origin that arise from the adrenal medulla or extraadrenal sympathetic paraganglia, respectively
- World Health Organization definitions of 2004 arbitrarily established terminology for tumors of paraganglia to eliminate previous inconsistent usage
  - PCC: Neuroendocrine tumor arising from chromaffin cells of adrenal medulla
  - Similar tumors in other locations are extraadrenal PGL (often abbreviated in practice to just PGL)
    - Sympathetic (sympathoadrenal) PGLs arise in vicinity of sympathetic chains and along sympathetic nerve branches in pelvic organs and retroperitoneum
    - Parasympathetic PGL (a.k.a. head and neck PGL [HNP]) arise mainly from branches of vagus and glossopharyngeal nerves in head and neck, sometimes mediastinum
    - PCC is an intraadrenal sympathetic PGL

ETIOLOGY/PATHOGENESIS

Hereditary PCC/PGL

- Over the last decade, extensive genetic heterogeneity of these tumors came to light with identification of multiple susceptibility genes
- Most striking feature is genetic diversity
- ≥ 1/3 of PCCs/PGLs are hereditary
  - These mutations account for ≥ 1/3 of PCC and PGL
    - Highest inheritable proportion of any known human tumor
  - Occult germline mutations of susceptibility genes common in patients with apparently sporadic tumors
  - ≥ 10 susceptibility genes now established
- Most attributable to mutations in *RET, VHL, NF1, SDHA, SDHB, SDHC, SDHD, SDHAF2, KIF1B, TMEM127,* and *MAX*
- Most recently identified hereditary forms of PCC and PGL are *SDHx*, transmembrane-encoding gene, *TMEM127,* and *MYC*-binding partner, *MAX*
  - Greater understanding of molecular signals transduced by these genes and their respective mutants has advanced our understanding of kinase signaling pathways, hypoxia regulation, and link between metabolic disruptions and cell growth
- Multiple endocrine neoplasia type 2 (MEN2)
  - Autosomal dominant syndrome caused by mutation of *RET* proto-oncogene
  - Activating *RET* mutations predispose to PCCs, which are often recurrent and bilateral but typically have a low risk of malignancy
  - PCC are bilateral in 50-80% of cases but are almost always benign
- Familial PGL/PCC syndromes
  - PGL syndromes encompass a group of inherited syndromes which involve mutations in the genes that encode components of the succinate

Key Facts

Terminology
- Use of term pheochromocytoma restricted to adrenal medulla
- Malignancy is defined by documentation of metastases to sites where normal paraganglia are not present

Etiology/Pathogenesis
- At least 30% of PCCs are hereditary; at least 10 susceptibility genes are now known
- Most attributable to mutations in *RET*, *VHL*, *NF1*, *SDHA*, *SDHB*, *SDHC*, *SDHD*, *SDHAF2*, *KIF1B*, *TMEM127*, and *MAX*
- *SDH*x mutations account for up to 80% of familial PCC/PGL aggregations, 30% of pediatric tumors, and ~ 50% of malignant tumors
- *SDHB* mutation associated with extraadrenal abdominal location, high probability of metastasis, and poor prognosis

Clinical Issues
- Identification of patients with hereditary PCC involves clinical assessment, biochemical testing, and pathology leading to directed genetic testing

Microscopic Pathology
- Classic pattern is small nests (zellballen) of neuroendocrine cells with interspersed small blood vessels

Ancillary Tests
- Immunohistochemistry for SDHB and SDHA can triage patients for appropriate genetic testing

dehydrogenase (SDH) mitochondrial enzyme complex 2
    - SDH is composed of 4 subunits: A, B, C, and D
  - Germline mutations in *SDHx* genes give rise to familial PCC/PGL syndrome, sometimes only referred to as familial PGL
  - Associated with germline mutations in genes encoding subunits of SDH enzyme complex in context of familial PGL syndromes
    - PGL1, PGL 2, PGL3, and PGL4 caused by mutations in the *SDHD, SDHAF2, SDHC,* and *SDHB* genes, respectively
    - Familial PGL syndrome, PGL2, is caused by mutations in *SDHAF2/SDH5,* which encodes for a molecule that is an accessory to the function of the SDH enzyme and its SDHA subunit
    - SDHA-related PGLs are rare and are caused by loss-of-function mutation in *SDHA*
- Carney triad
  - Mean age of presentation of PGL/PCC: 28 years
    - Only 16% present with PCC
- von Hippel-Lindau syndrome (VHL)
  - Autosomal dominant disorder caused by mutation of *VHL*
  - About 10-26% of VHL patients develop PCC or PGL, but risk varies between different families
  - Frequency of PCC in individuals with VHL is 10-20%
  - Mean age of onset of PCC in VHL: ~ 30 years
- Neurofibromatosis type 1 (NF1)
  - Autosomal dominant disorder caused by mutation of *NF1*
  - PCCs occur in 20-50% of individuals with NF1 and hypertension
  - NF1-associated PCCs and PGLs typically have characteristics similar to those of sporadic tumors, with a relatively late mean age of onset and about 10% risk of malignancy
  - Gangliocytic duodenal PGL may occur in patients with NF1
  - Approximately 84% of PCC are unilateral
- Carney-Stratakis dyad
  - Inherited predisposition to gastrointestinal stromal tumor (GIST) and PGL caused by inactivating germline mutations in *SDHB, SDHC,* or *SDHD*
  - Only rare cases reported to be associated with PCC
- Most recently identified hereditary forms of PCC and PGL are transmembrane-encoding gene, *TMEM127,* and *MYC*-binding partner, *MAX*
  - So far, no specific syndrome has been described for *TMEM127*
  - *MAX* mutations occur in families with PCC, but no specific syndrome has been described yet

Sporadic PCC/PGL
- Majority of PCCs appear to arise sporadically
- Only occasionally harbor somatic mutations except for NF1, which is mutated in > 25% of sporadic tumors
  - Germline mutations in known susceptibility genes may be seen in up to 16% of sporadic-appearing cases
- Changes in copy number of hereditary susceptibility genes may be present

Environmental Influences
- High-altitude PGL in people and cattle living in mountainous areas of some countries
  - Mostly carotid PGL

CLINICAL ISSUES

Site
- ~ 98% of sympathetic PGLs are located in abdomen or pelvis; 90% are adrenal PCCs
- Most parasympathetic PGLs are carotid, jugulotympanic, or vagal

Presentation
- Depends on tumor location
  - Sympathoadrenal PCCs/PGLs usually cause signs and symptoms of catecholamine excess

    - Tumors with *SDHB* gene mutation are more likely than other sympathoadrenal PCCs/PGLs to be clinically silent
  - Parasympathetic PGLs are usually clinically silent mass lesions
- Hereditary PCC/PGL often found after other stigmata point to hereditary tumor syndrome (usually MEN2, VHL, NF1)
- Gastrointestinal stromal tumors are important component of several new syndromes with mutated *SDHx*
- Variants of some hereditary syndromes can cause only PCC/PGL (VHL type 2C)
- Mutations of some genes (e.g., *TMEM127*) cause hereditary but nonsyndromic PCC/PGL (no associated abnormalities)
- Affected by genotype
  - Sporadic tumors solitary, usually in adults
  - Multiple tumors or tumors presenting in children suggest hereditary disease
  - Tumors with *RET* or *NF1* mutations almost always intraadrenal
  - Abdominal PGL or combination of sympathetic and parasympathetic PCC/PGL suggests *SDH*x mutation
- *SDHD*- and *SDHAF2*-related PGL show parent-of-origin dependent expression; tumor development only with paternal inheritance
- Identification of patients with hereditary PCC/PGL involves clinical assessment, biochemical testing, and pathology leading to directed genetic testing

Laboratory Tests

- Plasma metanephrine and normetanephrine more sensitive than corresponding catecholamines for tumor detection
  - Methoxytyramine: New marker sometimes produced by clinically nonfunctional tumors, especially with *SDH* mutations
- PCC can be adrenergic or noradrenergic; extraadrenal PGL almost always noradrenergic; HNP can lack ability for catecholamine biosynthesis
- Genotype affects biochemical function
  - Noradrenergic PCC raises suspicion of VHL

Treatment

- Complete surgical excision is only cure
- Unresectable primary tumors and metastases can have long doubling time; watchful waiting often a viable option

Prognosis

- Most patients with metastases eventually die from complications of excess catecholamines or destructive local growth

Malignancy

- World Health Organization 2004 defines malignancy by presence of metastasis
  - Must be to sites where normal paraganglia are not present to avoid confusion with new primary tumor
- Currently, no generally accepted histological criteria to predict whether primary PCC or PGL will metastasize
  - Extensive local invasion alone is poor predictor of metastasis
  - Predictive value of tumor size is controversial
- Risk of metastasis and prognosis vary with tumor location and genotype
  - ~ 10% metastasis for PCCs, > 20% for PGLs
  - Best predictor of metastasis is presence of *SDHB* mutation (> 30%)
  - After metastases occur, worst prognosis is for tumors caused by *SDHB* mutation
- Metastases can develop years or decades after resection of primary tumor
  - Currently recommended that no PCC/PGL be signed out as benign; all patients receive lifelong follow-up

IMAGE FINDINGS

General Features

- Anatomic imaging
  - MR: Very intense T2-weighted image (light bulb sign) is classic but not always present
  - Contrast-enhanced CT
- Functional imaging
  - More specific because based on specific aspects of tumor phenotype
  - More sensitive for small tumors or metastases in bone
  - Efficacy of different functional imaging techniques varies according to tumor genotype

MACROSCOPIC FEATURES

General Features

- Cut surface usually pink-gray to tan, distinguishes PCCs from yellow-gold of most adrenal cortical tumors
- Occasional tumors show patchy or diffuse brown pigmentation
- Cystic degeneration and necrosis sometimes present
- Medullary hyperplasia, when present, may indicate hereditary form of the disease

MICROSCOPIC PATHOLOGY

Histologic Features

- Classic pattern is small nests (zellballen) of neuroendocrine cells (chief cells) with interspersed small blood vessels
- Numerous variant and combined patterns exist, including diffuse growth, large zellballen, spindle cells, cell cords
- Sustentacular cells variably present, best seen with IHC
  - Possibly nonneoplastic cell type induced or attracted by tumor-derived factors
- Cavernous blood vessels sometimes prominent, especially in HNP

Cytologic Features

- Tumor cells smaller or larger than normal chromaffin cells, inconspicuous or large nucleoli

- Nuclear pseudoinclusions, embracing cells, extracellular hyaline globules variably present
- Basophilic, amphophilic, or clear cytoplasm
  - Clear cytoplasm particularly likely in parasympathetic PGL
- Extreme pleomorphism and hyperchromasia can be seen in benign tumors
- Mitoses usually rare

ANCILLARY TESTS

Immunohistochemistry

- Generic neuroendocrine markers chromogranin (CgA or CgB) and synaptophysin are usually positive in chief cells; keratins are usually negative
  - Parasympathetic PGL can be negative for CgA and positive for CgB
- Sustentacular cells stain for S100
- Tyrosine hydroxylase (TYH) identifies ability to synthesize catecholamines; can be negative, especially in parasympathetic PGL
  - Elevated metanephrine after resection of TYH(-) PGL suggests 2nd primary, not metastasis
- SDHB and SDHA important new surrogate markers to triage patients for genetic testing
  - SDHB protein lost in PCC/PGL with *SDHA*, *SDHB*, *SDHC*, or *SDHD* mutations; SDHA protein lost only when *SDHA* is mutated
  - Sustentacular and endothelial cells serve as intrinsic positive controls for SDHB

Molecular Genetics

- Major genes causing hereditary PCCs/PGLs are *RET* (causes MEN2A and MEN2B), *VHL*, *NF1*, *SDH*x
- *SDH*x mutations account for up to 80% of familial PCC/PGL aggregations, 30% of pediatric tumors, > 40% of malignant tumors

Gene Expression Profiling

- Tumors with *VHL* or *SDH*x mutations have hypoxia-associated gene expression profile
- Tumors with *RET* and *NF1* mutations characterized by expression of genes that mediate kinase signaling, translation initiation, protein synthesis, anabolic functions of activated *RAS*
  - Sporadic tumors or those with other mutations often segregate with 1 or other gene profile cluster

DIFFERENTIAL DIAGNOSIS

Adrenal Cortical Carcinoma

- Synaptophysin immunoreactivity present in both cortical and medullary tumors and should not be used in this differential diagnosis
- Chromogranin (-), TYH(-), inhibin (+)

Other Neuroendocrine Tumors (NETs)

- Neuroendocrine carcinomas and carcinoids, pancreatic endocrine tumors, medullary thyroid carcinoma
- Chromogranin and keratins are positive
- TYH usually negative but positive in some intestinal neuroendocrine tumors
- Tissue-specific hormones (e.g., calcitonin in medullary thyroid carcinoma, serotonin in intestinal NETs) are helpful but some can be produced ectopically in PCC/PGL

Hepatocellular Carcinomas

- Absence of neuroendocrine markers, presence of keratins &/or tissue-specific markers

Renal Cell Carcinoma (RCC)

- Absence of neuroendocrine markers, presence of keratins &/or CD10, RCC, and other tissue-specific markers

Alveolar Soft Part Sarcomas

- Absence of neuroendocrine markers, presence of soft tissue-specific marker: TFE3

Glomus Tumors and Glomangiomas

- Location: Outside adrenal
- Presence of neuroendocrine markers, S100, GFAP

Squamous Cell Carcinomas

- Absence of neuroendocrine markers, presence of keratins &/or p63

SELECTED REFERENCES

1. Dahia PL: Novel hereditary forms of pheochromocytomas and paragangliomas. Front Horm Res. 41:79-91, 2013
2. Dahia PL: The genetic landscape of pheochromocytomas and paragangliomas: somatic mutations take center stage. J Clin Endocrinol Metab. 98(7):2679-81, 2013
3. Rao JU et al: Genotype-specific abnormalities in mitochondrial function associate with distinct profiles of energy metabolism and catecholamine content in pheochromocytoma and paraganglioma. Clin Cancer Res. 19(14):3787-95, 2013
4. Rattenberry E et al: A comprehensive next generation sequencing-based genetic testing strategy to improve diagnosis of inherited pheochromocytoma and paraganglioma. J Clin Endocrinol Metab. 98(7):E1248-56, 2013
5. Toledo RA et al: In vivo and in vitro oncogenic effects of HIF2A mutations in pheochromocytomas and paragangliomas. Endocr Relat Cancer. 20(3):349-59, 2013
6. Burnichon N et al: MAX mutations cause hereditary and sporadic pheochromocytoma and paraganglioma. Clin Cancer Res. 18(10):2828-37, 2012
7. Gimenez-Roqueplo AP et al: An update on the genetics of paraganglioma, pheochromocytoma, and associated hereditary syndromes. Horm Metab Res. 44(5):328-33, 2012
8. Janeway KA et al: Defects in succinate dehydrogenase in gastrointestinal stromal tumors lacking KIT and PDGFRA mutations. Proc Natl Acad Sci U S A. 108(1):314-8, 2011
9. Jiang S et al: Minireview: the busy road to pheochromocytomas and paragangliomas has a new member, TMEM127. Endocrinology. 152(6):2133-40, 2011

PHEOCHROMOCYTOMA/PARAGANGLIOMA

Tumor Distributions in Major Familial Paraganglioma Syndromes

Syndrome	Gene (Chromosome)	Adrenal	Other Sympathetic	Head & Neck	Other Tumors
MEN2A and MEN2B	*RET* (10q11)	+++	+/-	+/-	**Medullary thyroid carcinoma**, parathyroid adenoma (MEN2A only)
VHL	*VHL* (3p25-26)	+++	++	+/-	RCC, **hemangioblastoma**, endolymphatic sac tumor, neuroendocrine tumor (carcinoid), pancreatic endocrine tumor
NF1	*NF1* (17q11.2)	+++	+/-	+/-	**Neurofibroma**, gastrointestinal stromal tumor (GIST), neuroendocrine tumor (carcinoid)
PGL1	*SDHD* (11q23)	++	++	++	
PGL2	*SDHAF2* (assembly factor for *SDH* complex)		+/-		
PGL3	*SDHC* (1q21-23)	+/-	+/-	+++	GIST
PGL4	*SDHB* (1p36)	++	+++	+	RCC, GIST
SDHA related	*SDHA*		+		GIST
Carney-Stratakis dyad	*SDHB*, *SDHC*, or *SDHD*	++	+	+	GIST
Familial pheochromocytoma 2q	*TMEM127* (membrane protein involved in protein trafficking)	+	+/-	+/-	
MAX related	*MAX*	+			
KIF1Bβ related	*KIF1Bβ*				Neuroblastoma, medulloblastoma

GIST: Gastrointestinal stromal tumor; RCC: Renal cell carcinoma.

10. King KS et al: Functional imaging of SDHx-related head and neck paragangliomas: comparison of 18F-fluorodihydroxyphenylalanine, 18F-fluorodopamine, 18F-fluoro-2-deoxy-D-glucose PET, 123I-metaiodobenzylguanidine scintigraphy, and 111In-pentetreotide scintigraphy. J Clin Endocrinol Metab. 96(9):2779-85, 2011
11. Korpershoek E et al: SDHA immunohistochemistry detects germline SDHA gene mutations in apparently sporadic paragangliomas and pheochromocytomas. J Clin Endocrinol Metab. 96(9):E1472-6, 2011
12. Neumann HP et al: Germline mutations of the TMEM127 gene in patients with paraganglioma of head and neck and extraadrenal abdominal sites. J Clin Endocrinol Metab. 96(8):E1279-82, 2011
13. Burnichon N et al: SDHA is a tumor suppressor gene causing paraganglioma. Hum Mol Genet. 19(15):3011-20, 2010
14. Cerecer-Gil NY et al: Mutation of SDHB is a cause of hypoxia-related high-altitude paraganglioma. Clin Cancer Res. 16(16):4148-54, 2010
15. Boedeker CC et al: Head and neck paragangliomas in von Hippel-Lindau disease and multiple endocrine neoplasia type 2. J Clin Endocrinol Metab. 94(6):1938-44, 2009
16. Pasini B et al: SDH mutations in tumorigenesis and inherited endocrine tumours: lesson from the phaeochromocytoma-paraganglioma syndromes. J Intern Med. 266(1):19-42, 2009
17. Stratakis CA et al: The triad of paragangliomas, gastric stromal tumours and pulmonary chondromas (Carney triad), and the dyad of paragangliomas and gastric stromal sarcomas (Carney-Stratakis syndrome): molecular genetics and clinical implications. J Intern Med. 266(1):43-52, 2009
18. van Nederveen FH et al: An immunohistochemical procedure to detect patients with paraganglioma and phaeochromocytoma with germline SDHB, SDHC, or SDHD gene mutations: a retrospective and prospective analysis. Lancet Oncol. 10(8):764-71, 2009
19. Wu D et al: Observer variation in the application of the Pheochromocytoma of the Adrenal Gland Scaled Score. Am J Surg Pathol. 33(4):599-608, 2009
20. Amar L et al: Succinate dehydrogenase B gene mutations predict survival in patients with malignant pheochromocytomas or paragangliomas. J Clin Endocrinol Metab. 92(10):3822-8, 2007
21. Pacak K et al: Pheochromocytoma: recommendations for clinical practice from the First International Symposium. October 2005. Nat Clin Pract Endocrinol Metab. 3(2):92-102, 2007
22. Dahia PL et al: A HIF1alpha regulatory loop links hypoxia and mitochondrial signals in pheochromocytomas. PLoS Genet. 1(1):72-80, 2005
23. DeLellis RA et al: Pathology & Genetics: Tumours of Endocrine Organs. World Health Organization Classification of Tumours. Lyon: IARC Press, 2004
24. Douwes Dekker PB et al: Multiparameter DNA flow-sorting demonstrates diploidy and SDHD wild-type gene retention in the sustentacular cell compartment of head and neck paragangliomas: chief cells are the only neoplastic component. J Pathol. 202(4):456-62, 2004

Associated Tumors and Lesions

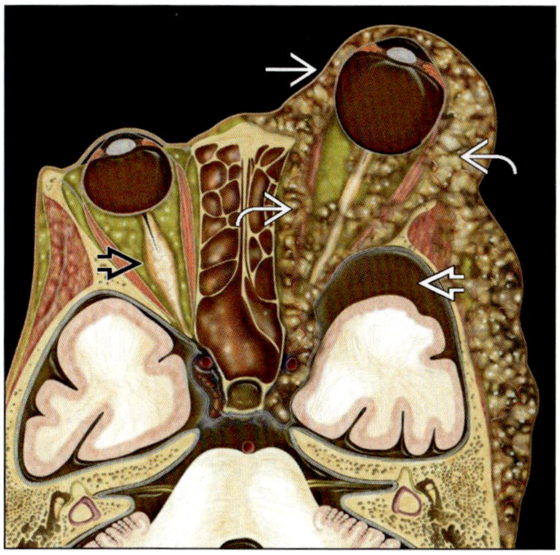

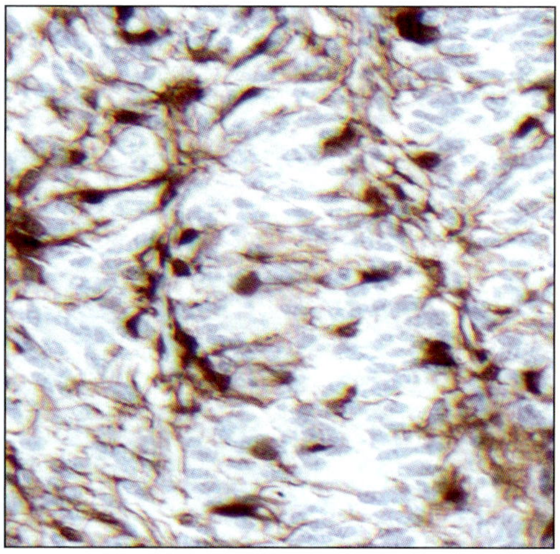

(Left) *Neurofibromatosis (NF) is characterized by involvement of the neural crest and bony dysplasia. This axial graphic depicts sphenoid dysplasia with arachnoid cyst, optic nerve glioma, buphthalmos, and multiple plexiform NFs. PCC occurs in 20-50% of NF1 patients.* ***(Right)*** *Patients with NF1 may develop duodenal gangliocytic paraganglioma (PGL). S100 stain shows staining of sustentacular cells, which sometimes have conspicuous cytoplasmic processes.*

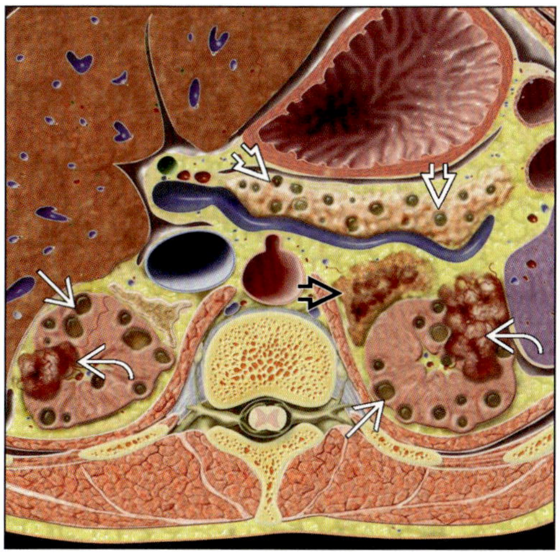

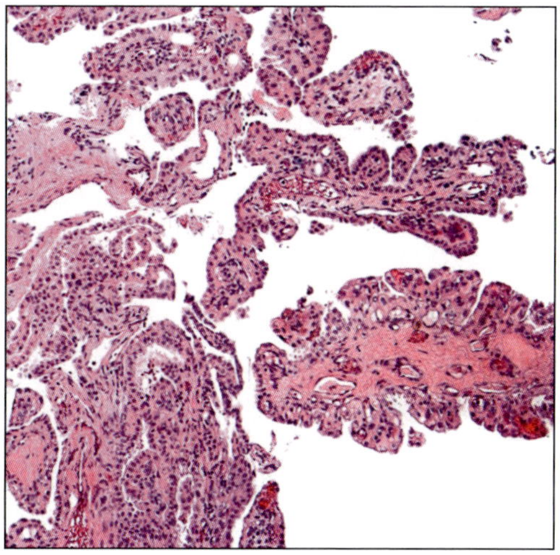

(Left) *Graphic representation of abdominal lesions in von Hippel-Lindau (VHL) syndrome shows multiple bilateral renal cysts, renal tumors, pancreatic cysts, and pheochromocytoma (PCC). PCC or PGL occurs in about 10-26% of VHL patients.* ***(Right)*** *Endolymphatic sac tumors typically show a papillary architecture with fibrovascular cores and a single row of columnar epithelium with pale eosinophilic cytoplasm. These tumors are usually present in VHL syndrome.*

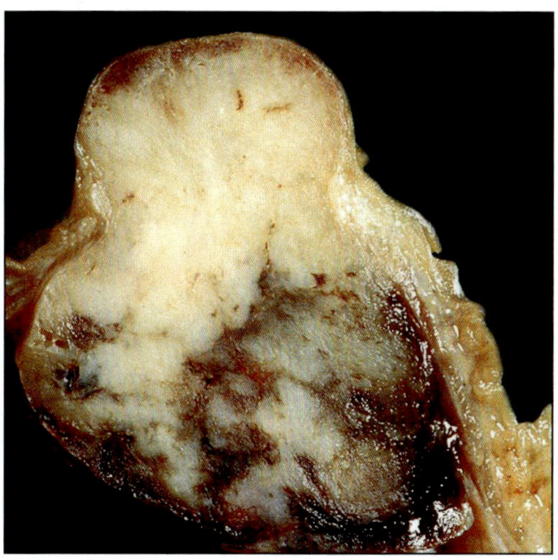

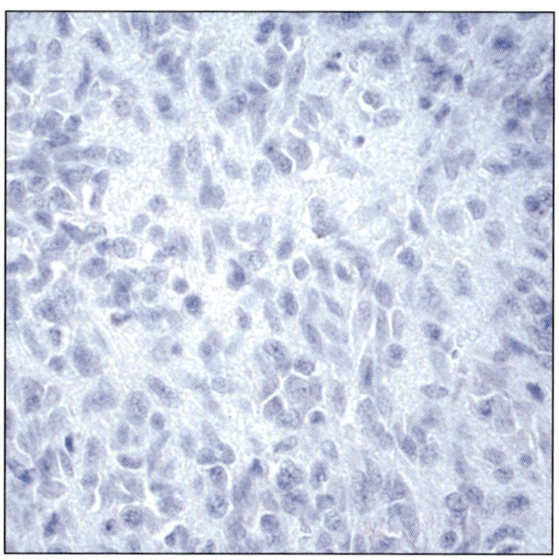

(Left) *Gross photograph shows a small intestinal gastrointestinal stromal tumor (GIST). These tumors may be associated with pheochromocytomas &/ or paragangliomas in some familial PGL/PCC syndromes.* ***(Right)*** *GISTs associated with paragangliomas in some syndromes are negative for SDHB, with preservation of SDHA. Pediatric GISTs may have the same phenotype.*

PHEOCHROMOCYTOMA/PARAGANGLIOMA

Gross and Imaging Features

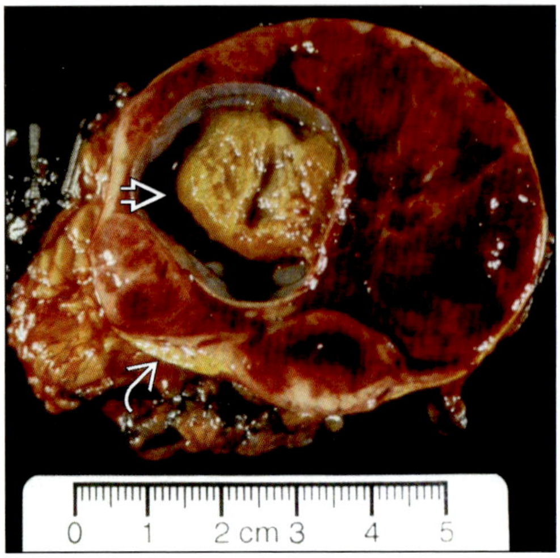

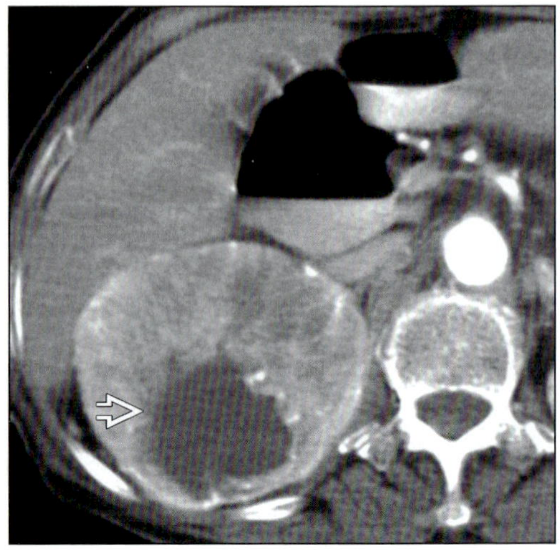

(Left) *Gross image shows the cut surface of a well-circumscribed adrenal pheochromocytoma with a central area of necrosis ➔ and with hemorrhage. Note small amount of residual adrenal cortex ➔.* ***(Right)*** *Axial CECT shows a large, well-circumscribed, moderately enhancing right adrenal pheochromocytoma with a hypodense area of necrosis ➔.*

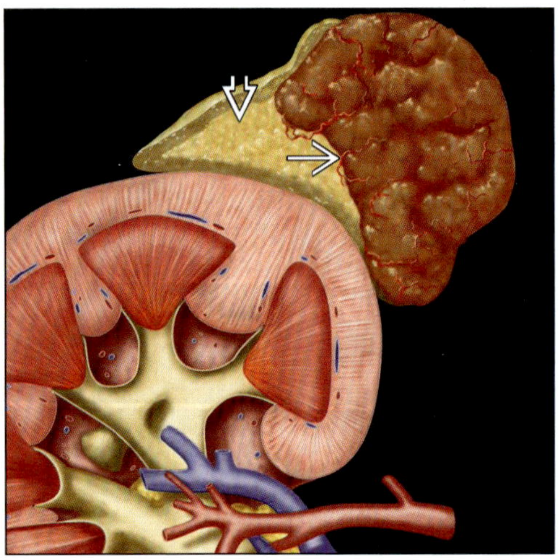

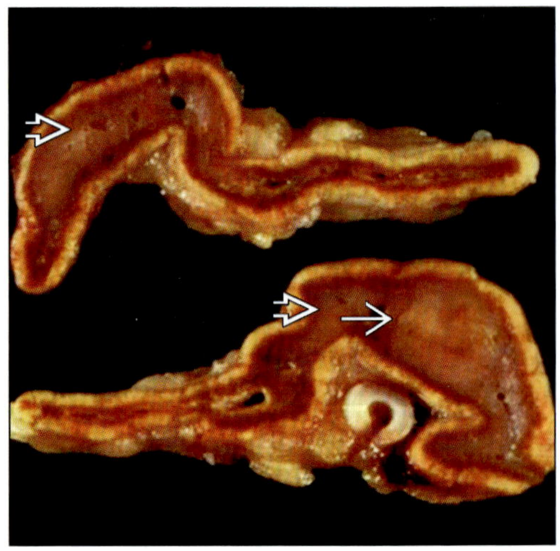

(Left) *This graph shows both adrenal medullary hyperplasia ➔ and MEN2 pheochromocytoma ➔. Adrenal medullary hyperplasia is characteristic of MEN2.* ***(Right)*** *This adrenal gland shows both MEN2-associated adrenal medullary hyperplasia ➔ and a pheochromocytoma ➔. Adrenal medullary hyperplasia is characteristic of MEN2.*

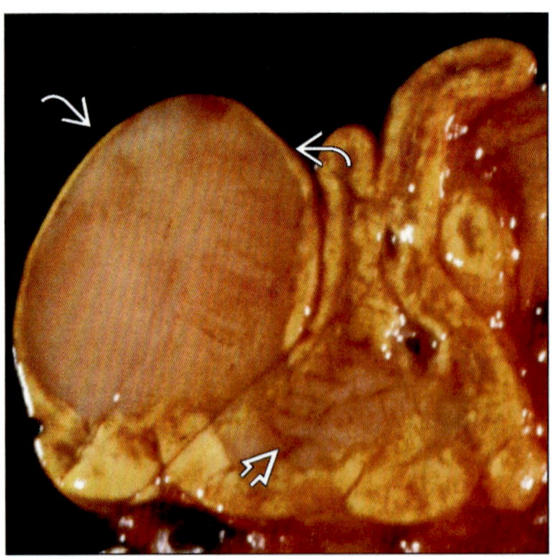

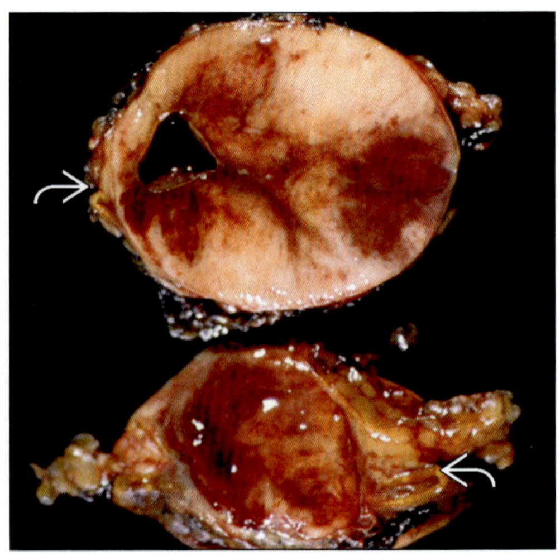

(Left) *This adrenal gland shows both MEN2-associated pheochromocytoma and adrenal medullary hyperplasia ➔, which is characteristic of MEN2. The cut surface is gray-pink, which distinguishes it from the yellow adrenal cortex ➔.* ***(Right)*** *Gross photograph shows the cut surface of a well-circumscribed adrenal pheochromocytoma with an area of hemorrhage. The gross appearance of pheochromocytomas is variable and may mimic other tumors. Small residual adrenal cortex is present ➔.*

Variant Microscopic Features

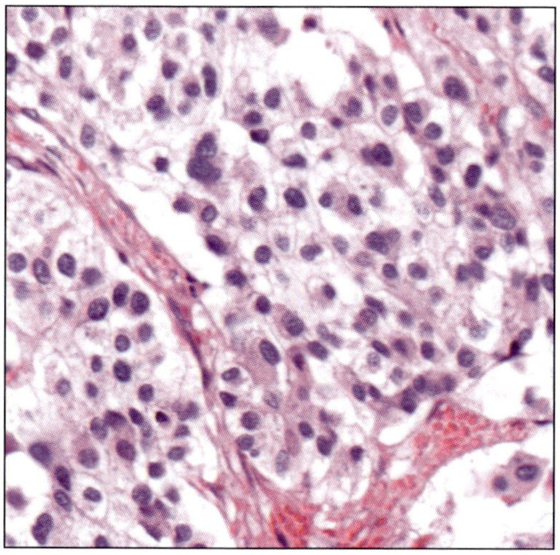
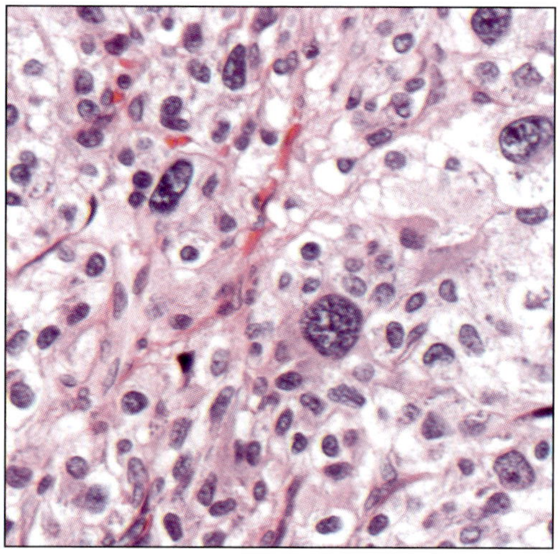

(Left) *The classic histologic pattern of pheochromocytoma is a small zellballen cellular arrangement. The group of cells is surrounded by a thin fibrovascular core. The cells have both eosinophilic and pale cytoplasm.* ***(Right)*** *The growth of this PCC is patternless with thin fibrous septae, but lacking the zellballen cellular arrangement. There is marked variability in cell size, with scattered pleomorphic cells surrounded by tumor cells with clear cytoplasm.*

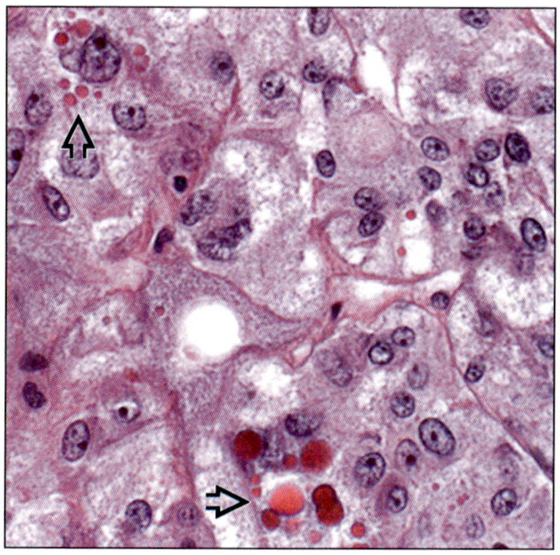
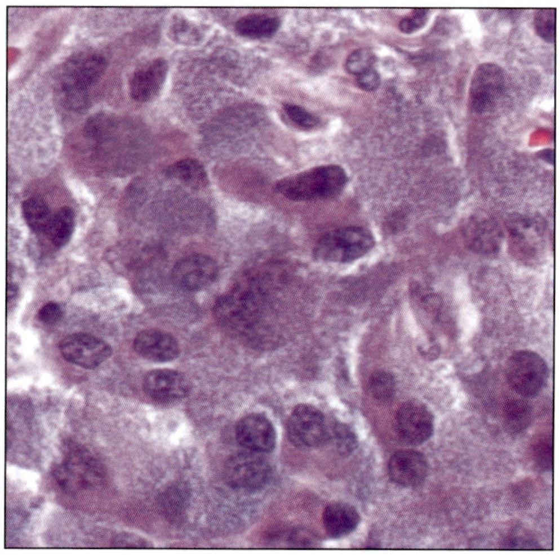

(Left) *The classic histologic pattern of pheochromocytoma is a small zellballen cellular arrangement. Hyaline globules ⇨ are particularly conspicuous in pheochromocytomas of patients with MEN2.* ***(Right)*** *Pheochromocytoma may contain cells with ample basophilic, amphophilic, or clear cytoplasm. This figure highlights the characteristic basophilic granular cytoplasm of some of these tumors.*

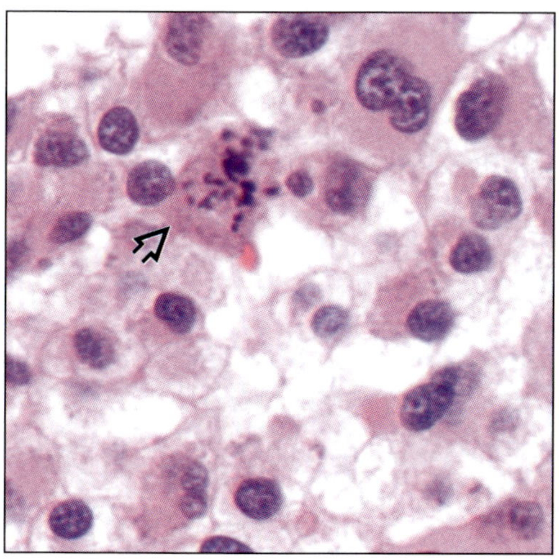
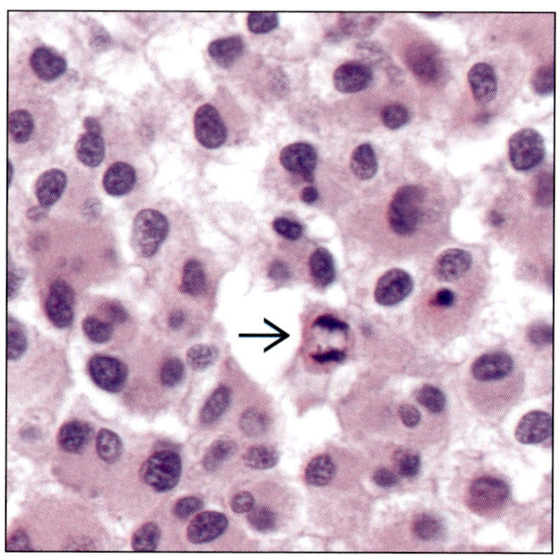

(Left) *A mitotic figure ⇨ is present in this malignant pheochromocytoma with a diffuse pattern, lacking the classic zellballen pattern. This tumor is composed of compact eosinophilic cells, which may be associated with more aggressive behavior.* ***(Right)*** *Although the classic histologic pattern of pheochromocytoma is a zellballen pattern, numerous variants and combined patterns exist, including diffuse growth, large zellballen, spindle cells, and cell cords. Note the mitotic figure →.*

SDHB and SDHA Immunohistochemical Features

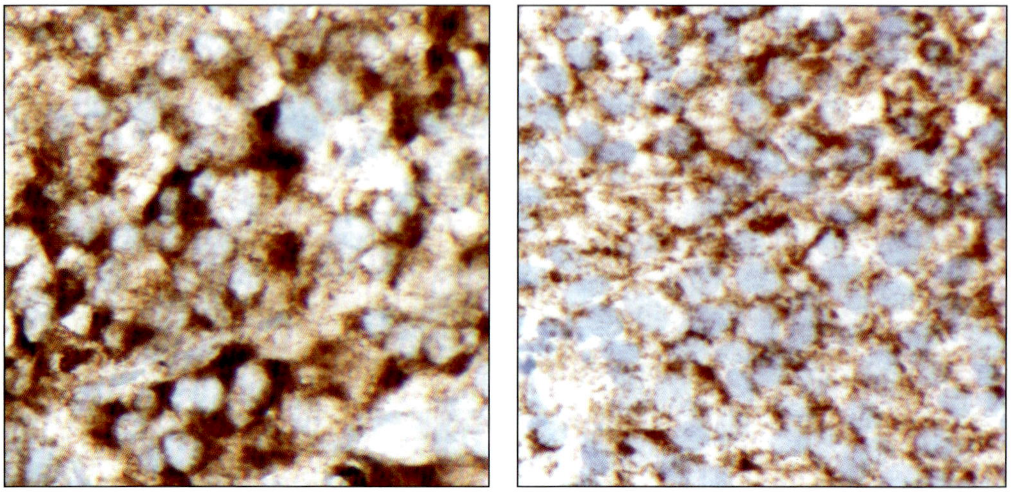

(Left) *Familial PCCs in syndromes other than those with mutations of SDHx genes show maintained coarse granular immunoreactivity of tumor cell cytoplasm for SDHB. Patients with VHL may have decreased or even absent immunoexpression of SDHB.* ***(Right)*** *Familial PCCs without mutations of SDHx genes but with other inherited familial pheochromocytoma show coarse granular immunoreactivity of tumor cell cytoplasm for SDHA and SDHB proteins.*

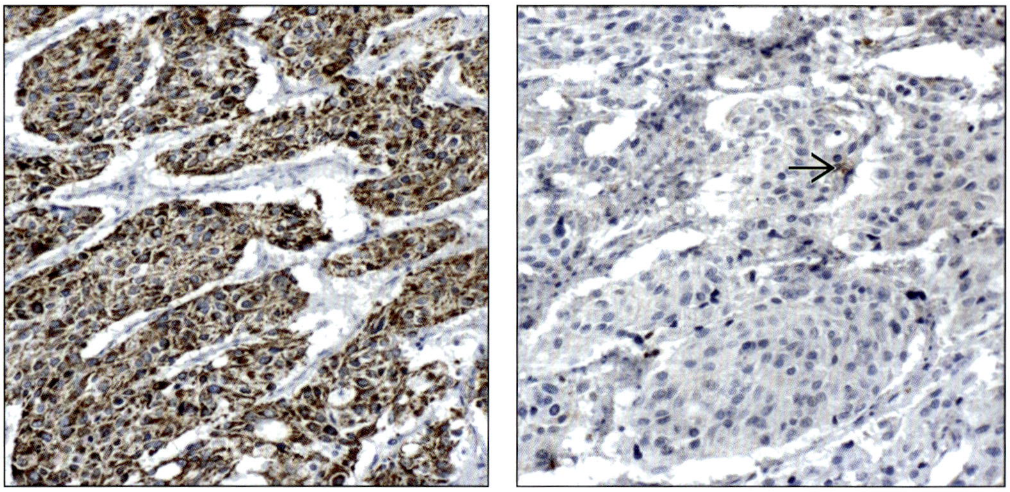

(Left) *Familial pheochromocytomas without mutations of SDHx genes and with other mutations show coarse granular immunoreactivity of tumor cell cytoplasm for SDHB protein.* ***(Right)*** *Tumor cells in PCC with mutations of the SDHA, SDHB, SDHC, or SDHD genes are negative for SDHB protein whereas sustentacular cells → and endothelial cells serve as intrinsic positive controls.*

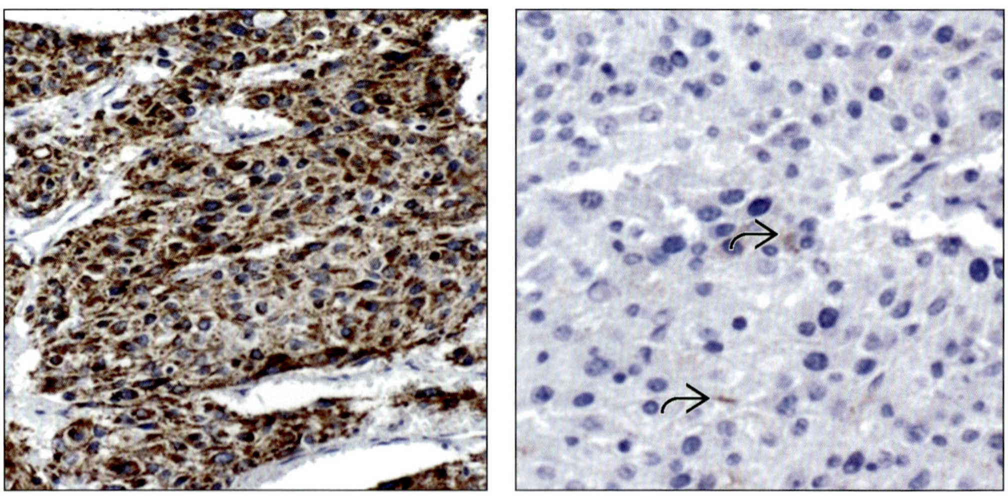

(Left) *Pheochromocytomas and other paragangliomas without mutations of SDHx genes show immunoreactivity of tumor cell cytoplasm for SDHB protein. The staining is coarsely granular because the protein is localized to mitochondria.* ***(Right)*** *Tumor cells in PCC with mutations of the SDHA gene are negative for SDHA protein. Rare cases have been reported. The sustentacular cells and endothelial cells ↪ serve as intrinsic positive controls.*

Ancillary Techniques

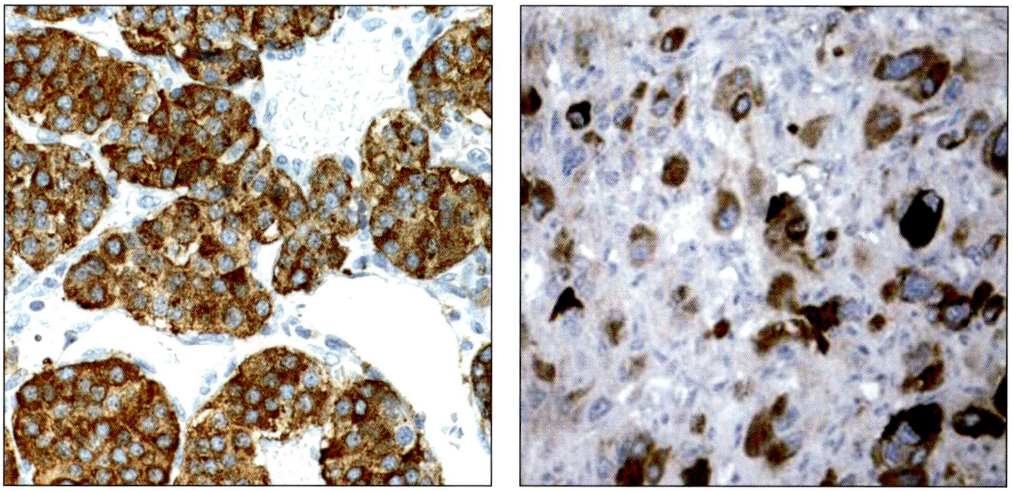

(Left) *Chromogranin-A immunostain shows granular immunoreactivity in the neuroendocrine cell nests between cavernous blood vessels in a carotid PGL. Note the negativity of the endothelial cells for this marker.* ***(Right)*** *Chromogranin-A immunostain may show great variability of staining in pheochromocytomas. There is variable granular immunoreactivity in the neuroendocrine cell nests.*

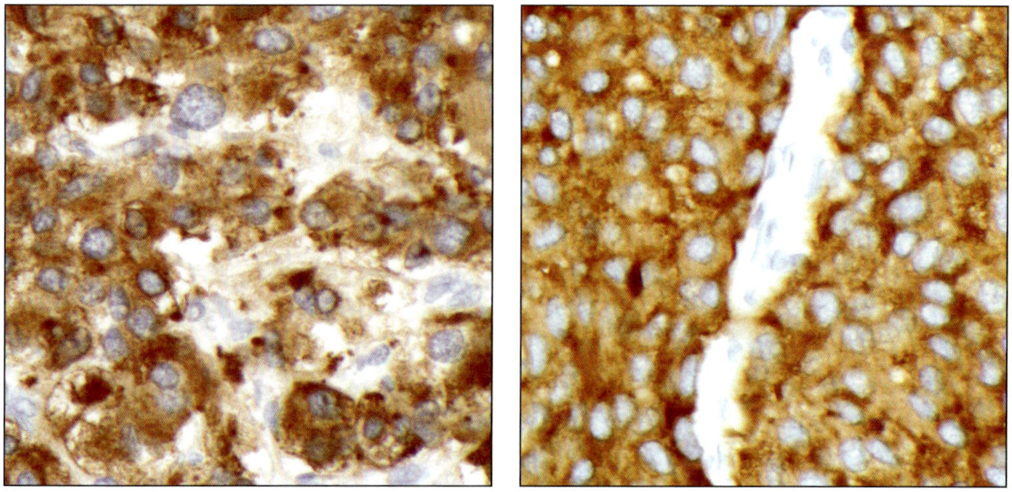

(Left) *Synaptophysin immunostain shows granular immunoreactivity in the nests of neuroendocrine cells of a pheochromocytoma in a patient with MEN2A.* ***(Right)*** *Synaptophysin immunostain shows homogeneous, finely granular immunoreactivity throughout the tumor, with less variability in staining in the neuroendocrine cells of a pheochromocytoma in a patient with MEN2A.*

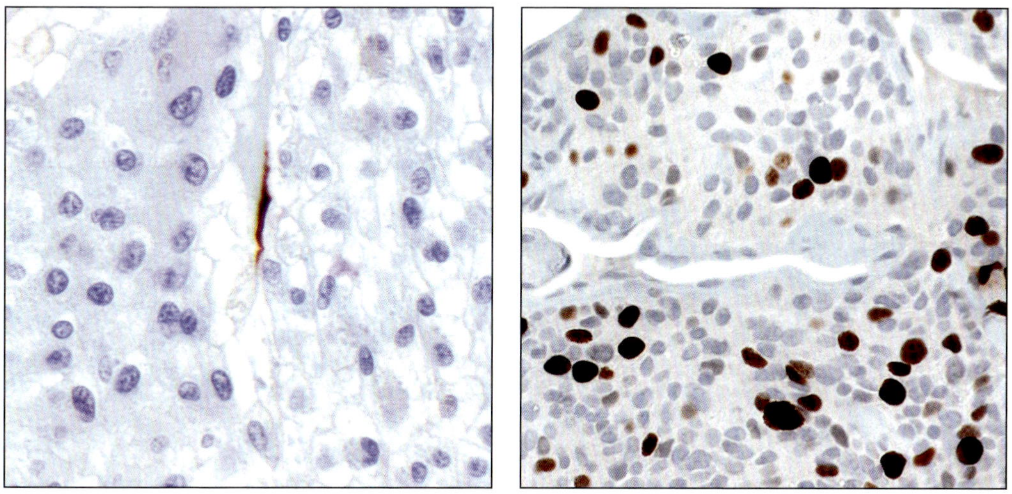

(Left) *S100 stain shows nuclear and cytoplasmic staining of sustentacular cells, which sometimes have conspicuous cytoplasmic processes. The chief cells are usually negative for this marker but sometimes may show weak staining.* ***(Right)*** *A high Ki-67 labeling index is unusual in PCC/PGL and, when present, may be associated with aggressive tumor behavior. This carotid PGL showed angioinvasion and soft tissue infiltration. (Courtesy A. Tischler, MD.)*

PARAGANGLIOMA

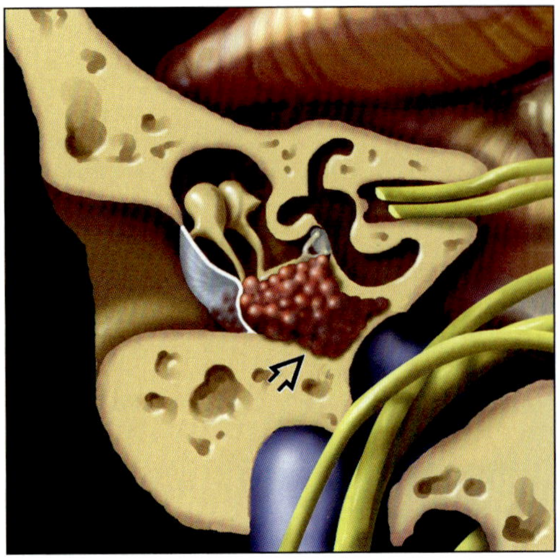

This coronal graphic shows a highly vascular glomus tympanicum paraganglioma extending out of the cochlear promontory, filling the middle ear cavity, and subtly expanding into the bony floor ⊳.

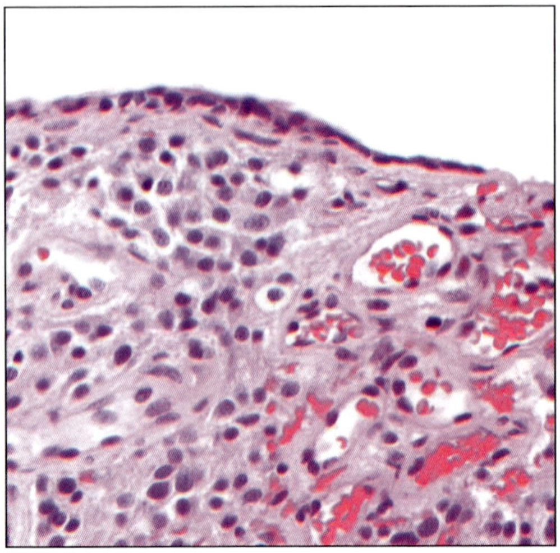

This highly vascular glomus tympanicum paraganglioma shows nests of tumor cells intermixed with vascular channels. These richly vascularized tumors may show large hemorrhagic areas.

TERMINOLOGY

Abbreviations

- Paraganglioma (PGL)

Synonyms

- Hereditary paraganglioma/pheochromocytoma (PGL/PCC) syndromes

Definitions

- Pheochromocytomas (PCCs) and PGLs are neuroendocrine tumors that arise in adrenal medulla or extraadrenal sympathetic and parasympathetic paraganglia
- PGLs arise from neuroendocrine tissues symmetrically distributed along paravertebral axis from their predominant location at base of skull and neck to pelvis
- **Paragangliomas** are classified by location and secretory status
  - **Sympathetic**: Hypersecrete catecholamines
    - Arise from chromaffin cells of paraganglia along the sympathetic chains and are usually located in the chest, abdomen, or pelvis
  - **Parasympathetic**: Do not hypersecrete catecholamines
    - Arise from the glomera that are distributed along parasympathetic nerves in the head, neck, and upper mediastinum and are therefore also referred to as head and neck PGLs
- **Pheochromocytomas** are catecholamine-secreting PGLs confined to adrenal medulla
  - a.k.a. adrenal chromaffin tumors
    - Another term for any sympathetic (catecholamine-secreting) neuroendocrine cell/tumor regardless of location
    - Chromaffin refers to brown-black color that results from oxidization and polymerization of catecholamines contained in cells/tumors by chromium salts, such as potassium dichromate
- Occurs sporadically or as part of different hereditary tumor syndromes
- > 30% of PCCs and PGLs are currently believed to be caused by germline mutations, and several novel susceptibility genes have recently been discovered
- Genes *RET*, *VHL*, *NF1*, *SDHA*, *SDHB*, *SDHC*, *SDHD*, *SDHAF2*, *KIF1B*, *TMEM127*, and *MAX* have been associated with hereditary PCC or PGL
- Hereditary PGL/PCC syndromes should be considered in all individuals with PGL or PCC with the following findings
  - Multiple tumors, including bilateral tumors
  - Recurrent PGLs and PCCs
  - Early onset (age < 40 years)
  - Multifocal with multiple synchronous or metachronous tumors
  - Family history of such tumors
- **Simplex cases:** Many individuals with a hereditary PGL/PCC syndrome may present with solitary tumor of head or neck, thorax, abdomen, adrenal, or pelvis and no family history of the disorder

ETIOLOGY/PATHOGENESIS

Inherited

- Most attributable to mutations in *RET*, *VHL*, *NF1*, *SDHA*, *SDHB*, *SDHC*, *SDHD*, *SDHAF2*, *KIF1B*, *TMEM127*, and *MAX*
- **Syndromes characterized by susceptibility to pheochromocytoma and paraganglioma**
  - Multiple endocrine neoplasia type 2 (MEN2), von Hippel-Lindau (VHL) disease, and neurofibromatosis type 1 (NF1)
  - Small fraction associated with other syndromes, including Carney triad, Carney-Stratakis syndrome, and MEN1

PARAGANGLIOMA

Key Facts

Etiology/Pathogenesis

- **Syndromes characterized by susceptibility to pheochromocytoma and paraganglioma**
  - Multiple endocrine neoplasia type 2 (MEN2)
  - von Hippel-Lindau (VHL) disease
  - Neurofibromatosis type 1 (NF1)
  - Mutations in genes encoding different subunits of *SDH* complex have been linked to familial pheochromocytoma/paraganglioma (PCC/PGL) syndrome (PGL1, 2, 3, and 4)
  - Small fraction associated with other syndromes, including Carney triad, Carney-Stratakis syndrome, and MEN1
  - Several other genes, such as *KIF1B*, *EGLN1/PHD2*, *TMEM127*, and *MAX* have recently been added to list

Clinical Issues

- Up to 50% of people with malignant extraadrenal PGLs have a germline *SDHB* mutation

Macroscopic Features

- Multifocal, bilateral, with multiple synchronous or metachronous tumors

Microscopic Pathology

- Histological features of familial paragangliomas are similar to those of tumors that occur sporadically

Ancillary Tests

- SDHB immunostain is decreased &/or absent in tumors of patients with *SDHB* or *SDHD* mutation

---

- Mutations in genes encoding different subunits of succinate dehydrogenase (SDH) complex have been linked to familial PCC/PGL syndrome (PGL1, 2, 3, and 4)

Multiple Endocrine Neoplasia Type 2 (MEN2)

- Autosomal dominant syndrome caused by mutation of *RET* proto-oncogene
- Mean age at PCC presentation: 36 years
- Clinically, it can be divided into 3 types: MEN2A (55% of all cases), MEN2B (5-10%), and familial medullary thyroid carcinoma (FMTC, 35-40%)
- ~ 50% of individuals with MEN2A and MEN2B develop PCC
- Activating *RET* mutations predispose patients to PCCs, which are often recurrent and bilateral, but typically have a low risk of malignancy
- PCCs are bilateral in 50-80% of cases but are almost always benign
- PGLs very rare in MEN2, and only a few cases of sympathetic and parasympathetic PGL have been described

PGL/PCC Syndromes

- Germline mutations in the *SDH*x genes give rise to familial PCC/PGL syndrome, sometimes only referred to as familial PGL
- Hereditary PGL/PCC syndromes caused by mutation in 1 gene encoding 3 of 4 subunits of SDH are within differential diagnosis for all individuals with PGL and PCC
- Prevalence of PCC/PGL syndrome is unknown, but a review of ~ 13% of all PCC/PGL cases gives an estimate of 1:50,000 to 1:20,000

VHL Syndrome

- Autosomal dominant disorder caused by mutation of *VHL*
- ~ 10-26% of VHL patients develop PCC or PGL, but risk varies between different families
  - Frequency of PCC in individuals with VHL is 10-20%
- Mean age of onset of PCC in VHL: ~ 30 years
- *VHL* mutations predispose to unilateral or bilateral PCCs and, much less frequently, to sympathetic or parasympathetic PGLs
- ~ 5% of VHL-related catecholamine-secreting tumors become malignant, most commonly extraadrenal sympathetic PGL
- Mean age at diagnosis of PCC/PGL: 29 years

Neurofibromatosis Type 1 (NF1)

- Autosomal dominant disorder caused by mutation of *NF1*
- PCCs and PGLs are not among most common manifestations of NF1 but occur in 0.1-5.7% of patients
- PCCs occur in 20-50% of individuals with NF1 and hypertension
- Gangliocytic PGL of duodenum occurs in patients with NF1
- NF1-associated PCCs and PGLs typically have characteristics similar to those of sporadic tumors, with a relatively late mean age of onset and ~ 10% risk of malignancy
- Up to 84% of PCCs are unilateral

Carney Triad

- Extremely rare disorder that primarily affects young women
- Mean age at presentation with PGL/PCC: 28 years
  - ~ 85-90% present with PGL, including both sympathetic and parasympathetic tumors, and 10-15% present with PCC
- Metastasis occurs in ~ 1% of patients

Carney-Stratakis Syndrome

- Inherited predisposition to gastrointestinal stromal tumor (GIST) and PGL that is caused by inactivating germline mutations in *SDHB*, *SDHC*, or *SDHD*
  - Association of PGL and GISTs (dyad)
- PGLs occur in head and neck, thorax, and abdomen
- 100% had PGL and 1 patient also presented with unilateral PCC

PARAGANGLIOMA

- Mean age of presentation: 33 years
- Multiple PGLs in ~ 75% of patients

Other Syndromes

- MEN1: No cases of PGL and only 7 cases of PCC in MEN1 syndrome have been reported in the literature
- Several other genes have recently been added to list of genes associated with unknown hereditary PGL/PCC
  - Kinesin family member 1B (*KIF1B*)
  - EGL 9 homolog 1 (*EGLN1*), also termed *PHD2*
  - Transmembrane protein 127 (*TMEM127*)
  - *MYC*-associated factor X (*MAX*)
- No specific syndrome has been attributed yet, but patients with germline *KIF1Bβ* mutations seem to be predisposed to at least PCCs and neuroblastomas
  - Ganglioneuroma, leiomyosarcoma, and lung adenocarcinoma have also been reported in a family with *KIF1Bβ* mutations
- Only 1 PGL patient, suffering from recurrent PGL and erythrocytosis, has been reported to have a germline mutation in *EGLN1*
  - Presentation with sympathetic PGL and a recurrent tumor was diagnosed 3 years later, but no metastases have been reported
- So far, no specific syndrome has been described for *TMEM127*
  - *TMEM127* mutations were identified in 2% of cases considered sporadic, all of which had PCC
  - 96% of patients have PCC, and 39% have bilateral PCC
- *MAX* mutations segregate with disease in families with PCC, but no specific syndrome has been described yet
  - Usually bilateral tumors, early age of onset, &/or familial antecedents with disease
  - Notably, 25% of patients showed metastasis at diagnosis, suggesting that *MAX* mutations are associated with high risk of malignancy
  - So far, no studies on PGLs have been reported

CLINICAL ISSUES

Epidemiology

- Incidence
  - Annual incidence has been reported to be 2-10 per million
  - Prevalence is unknown but has been estimated to be between 1:6,500 and 1:2,500 in the United States
  - Autopsy series have revealed a higher prevalence of ~ 1:2,000, suggesting that many tumors remain undiagnosed
- Age
  - Tumors may occur in all ages but have the highest incidence between 40 and 50 years, with an approximately equal sex distribution

Presentation

- Diagnosis of PGL and PCC is based on physical examination, imaging studies, biochemical testing, and pathology findings
- Clinical presentation, including localization, malignant potential, and age of onset varies depending on genetic background of tumors
- Symptoms of PGL/PCC result from either
  - Mass effect
  - Catecholamine hypersecretion: Sustained/paroxysmal elevations in blood pressure, headache, episodic sweating, palpitations, pallor, and anxiety
- PCCs and sympathetic PGLs are very similar histologically as well as functionally: Produce large amounts of catecholamines, mainly adrenaline and noradrenaline
  - Tumors usually cause hypertension, which may be either paroxysmal or sustained
- Up to 10% of patients have minor or no signs of clinical symptoms
- Increasing number of tumors are incidentally found during imaging studies
- Parasympathetic PGLs are histologically similar to PCCs and sympathetic PGLs, but parasympathetic PGLs are usually not functional and many patients are nonsymptomatic
- Majority of PCCs and PGLs are benign
- Malignancy is defined as presence of distant metastases and occurs in 5-13% of PCCs
  - Most common sites for metastasis are bone, liver, and lung
  - Prognosis of malignant PCC and PGL is poor, with a 5-year mortality rate > 50%

Laboratory Tests

- Catecholamines hypersecreted by PGL/PCC can be epinephrine (adrenaline), norepinephrine (noradrenaline), or dopamine
- When a catecholamine-secreting tumor is suspected, plasma &/or 24-hour urinary fractionated metanephrine or catecholamines are evaluated for catecholamine hypersecretion
- Measurement of fractionated metanephrine concentrations in plasma or urine is preferred
- False-positive results may be reduced by follow-up testing for plasma chromogranin-A &/or urine fractionated metanephrine levels
- Secretion of norepinephrine with little or no epinephrine suggests extraadrenal PGL or PCC associated with von Hippel-Lindau syndrome

Treatment

- Treatment of manifestations
  - For secretory tumors including PCC: Antagonism of catecholamine excess followed by surgery
  - For nonsecretory head and neck PGL: Surgical resection
  - PGL/PCCs identified in *SDHB*-mutation-positive individuals require prompt resection due to high risk of malignant transformation

IMAGE FINDINGS

General Features

- **MR/CT**
  - PGLs may be identified anywhere along paravertebral axis from head to pelvis, including paraortic sympathetic chain and urinary bladder

- Common sites of neoplasia are near renal vessels and in organ of Zuckerkandl
- Multiple tumors can be present

MACROSCOPIC FEATURES

General Features

- Fairly well circumscribed, tan, rubbery-firm mass with fibrous pseudocapsule

MICROSCOPIC PATHOLOGY

Histologic Features

- Inherited tumors are similar to sporadically occurring tumors
- Classic pattern is small nests of cells (zellballen) with interspersed small blood vessels
  - Numerous other patterns and combined patterns: Diffuse growth, large zellballen, spindle cells, cell cords
- Tumor cells smaller or larger than normal chromaffin cells, inconspicuous or large nucleoli

ANCILLARY TESTS

Immunohistochemistry

- Features similar to those of sporadic tumors
  - Chromogranin and synaptophysin (neuroendocrine markers) positive; keratins usually negative
- SDHA and SDHB are important surrogate markers to triage patients for genetic testing
  - SDHB immunostain is decreased &/or absent in tumors of patients with *SDHB, SDHC,* or *SDHD* mutation
  - SDHA immunostain is decreased/absent in tumors of patients with *SDHA* mutation

DIFFERENTIAL DIAGNOSIS

Sporadic PGL/PCC

- Sporadic tumors constitute majority of PCCs and PGLs
- Patients are generally somewhat older at onset
- Patients with sporadic PGLs/PCCs have a lower rate of multiple tumors than do those with familial disease
- Rate of inherited mutations in patients with negative family history has been reported to be 11-24%
- Of patients with apparently sporadic PCC or PGL, 73% have PCC, and 29% have PGL (9% sympathetic and 20% parasympathetic PGL)
- Bilateral PCC was seen in 6% of patients and multiple PGLs in only 1%
- Average age at presentation: 48 years
- 9% of patients had malignant disease
- Negative for mutations in *RET*, *VHL*, *SDHB*, *SDHC*, and *SDHD* and showed no clinical signs of NF1 syndrome

SELECTED REFERENCES

1. Crona J et al: MAX mutations status in Swedish patients with pheochromocytoma and paraganglioma tumours. Fam Cancer. Epub ahead of print, 2013
2. Dahia PL: Novel hereditary forms of pheochromocytomas and paragangliomas. Front Horm Res. 41:79-91, 2013
3. Elston MS et al: Novel mutation in the TMEM127 gene associated with phaeochromocytoma. Intern Med J. 43(4):449-51, 2013
4. Fishbein L et al: Inherited mutations in pheochromocytoma and paraganglioma: why all patients should be offered genetic testing. Ann Surg Oncol. 20(5):1444-50, 2013
5. Welander J et al: Germline SDHA mutation detected by next-generation sequencing in a young index patient with large paraganglioma. J Clin Endocrinol Metab. Epub ahead of print, 2013
6. Janeway KA et al: Defects in succinate dehydrogenase in gastrointestinal stromal tumors lacking KIT and PDGFRA mutations. Proc Natl Acad Sci U S A. 108(1):314-8, 2011
7. Korpershoek E et al: SDHA immunohistochemistry detects germline SDHA gene mutations in apparently sporadic paragangliomas and pheochromocytomas. J Clin Endocrinol Metab. 96(9):E1472-6, 2011
8. Burnichon N et al: SDHA is a tumor suppressor gene causing paraganglioma. Hum Mol Genet. 19(15):3011-20, 2010
9. Opocher G et al: Genetics of pheochromocytomas and paragangliomas. Best Pract Res Clin Endocrinol Metab. 24(6):943-56, 2010
10. van Nederveen FH et al: An immunohistochemical procedure to detect patients with paraganglioma and phaeochromocytoma with germline SDHB, SDHC, or SDHD gene mutations: a retrospective and prospective analysis. Lancet Oncol. 10(8):764-71, 2009
11. Dahia PL et al: A HIF1alpha regulatory loop links hypoxia and mitochondrial signals in pheochromocytomas. PLoS Genet. 1(1):72-80, 2005

PARAGANGLIOMA

Diagrammatic, Imaging, and Microscopic Features

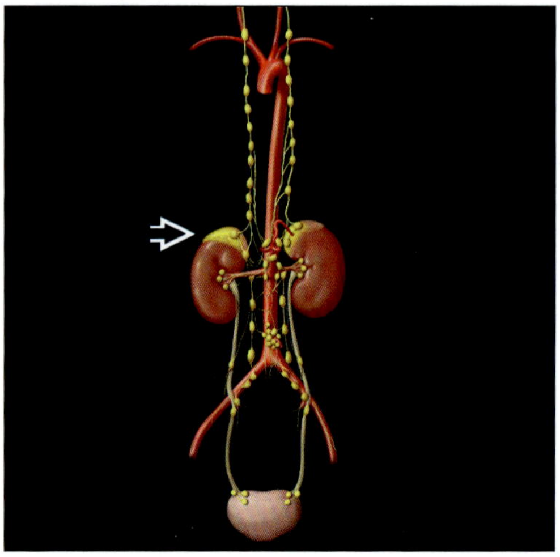

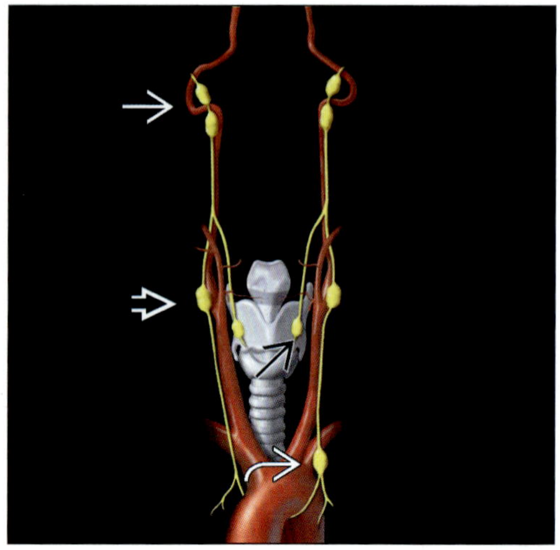

(Left) *Graphic shows paraganglia and neuroendocrine tissues symmetrically distributed along the paravertebral axis from the base of the skull to the pelvis, including the adrenal medulla →.* ***(Right)*** *Graphic shows paraganglia in head, neck, and upper thorax that are associated with arteries or cranial nerves. They include aortic → and carotid bodies → and jugulotympanic →, vagal, and laryngeal → paraganglia.*

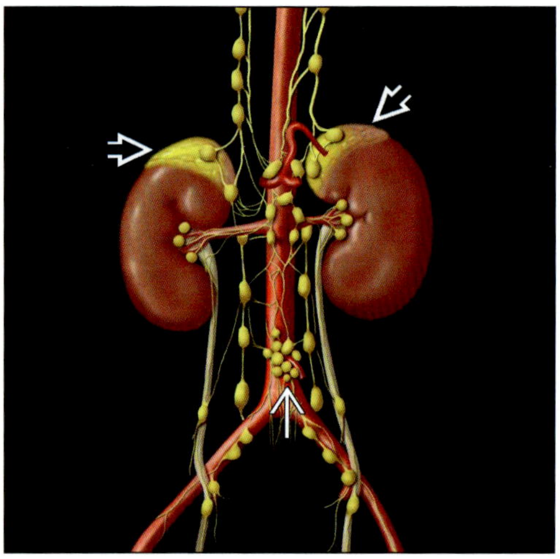

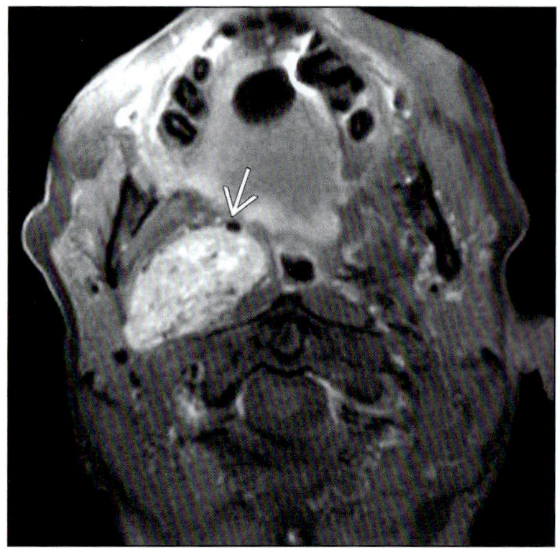

(Left) *Graphic shows paraganglia and neuroendocrine tissues symmetrically distributed along the paravertebral axis in the abdomen, including the organ of Zuckerkandl → and the adrenal medulla →.* ***(Right)*** *Axial T2WI MR with fat suppression shows a large glomus vagale paraganglioma as a hyperintense right carotid space mass with subtle internal flow voids. Internal carotid artery → on the anterior surface is shown.*

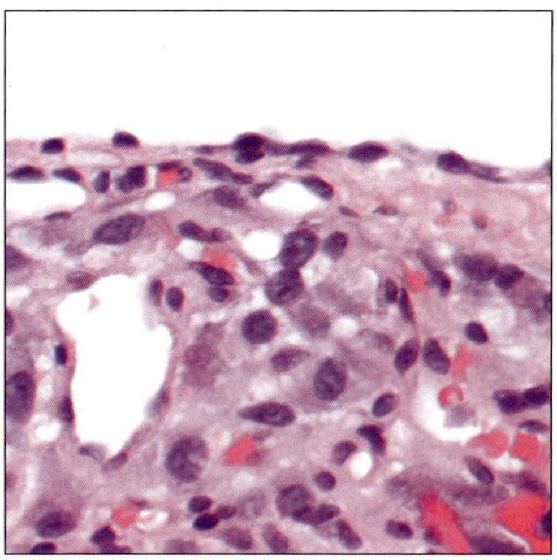

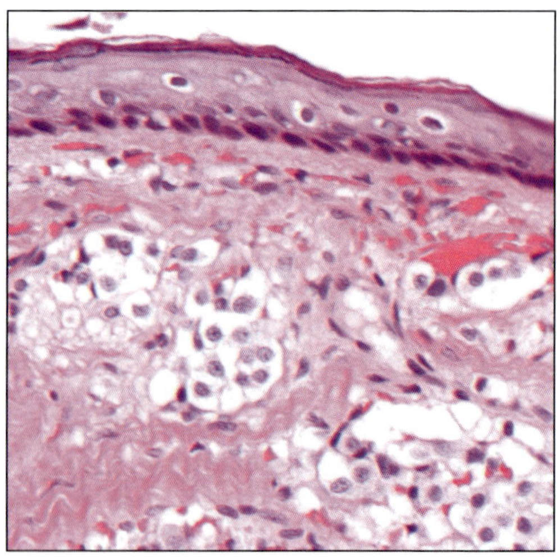

(Left) *This richly vascularized paraganglioma shows vascular channels interspersed with nests of paraganglioma cells. In this picture, the classic zellballen paraganglioma features are missing.* ***(Right)*** *This photomicrograph shows an intact squamous epithelium subtended by a nested neoplastic proliferation associated with a rich vascularized network and fibrous proliferation.*

PARAGANGLIOMA

Paraganglia and Paraganglioma

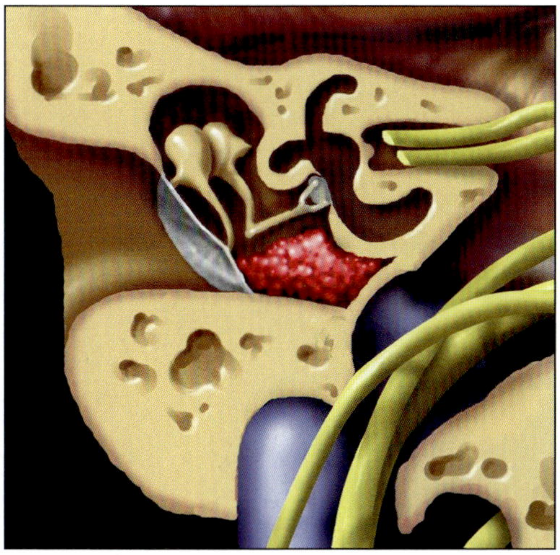

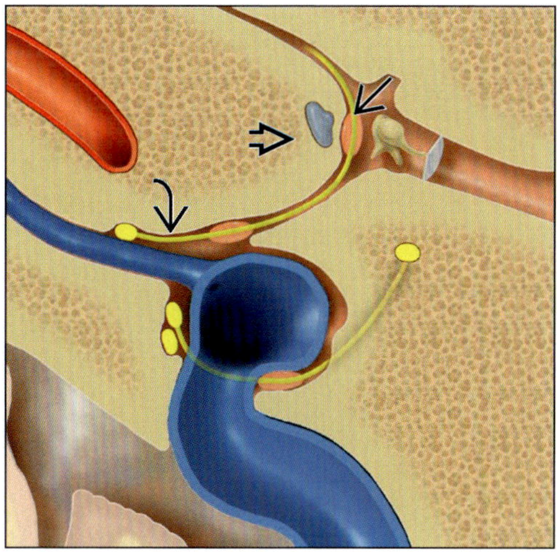

(Left) *This coronal graphic shows a highly vascular glomus tympanicum paraganglioma filling a portion of the middle ear cavity without involving adjacent structures and bone.* ***(Right)*** *This axial graphic shows glomus bodies → along the course of the inferior tympanic nerve (branch of Jacobsen →) on the cochlear promontory. Glomus tympanicum tumors arise from this normal cellular collection. Also note the cochlea →.*

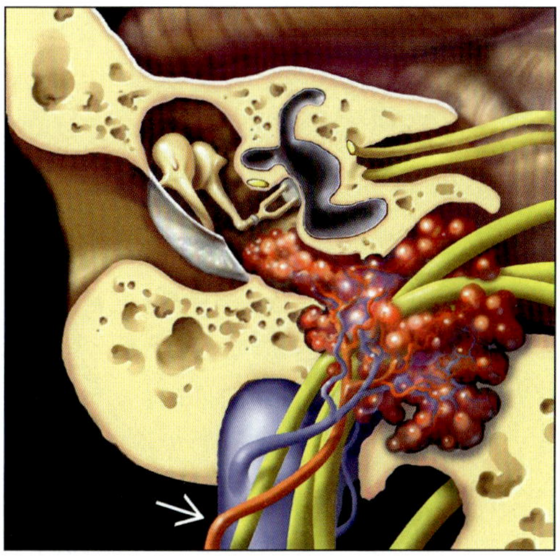

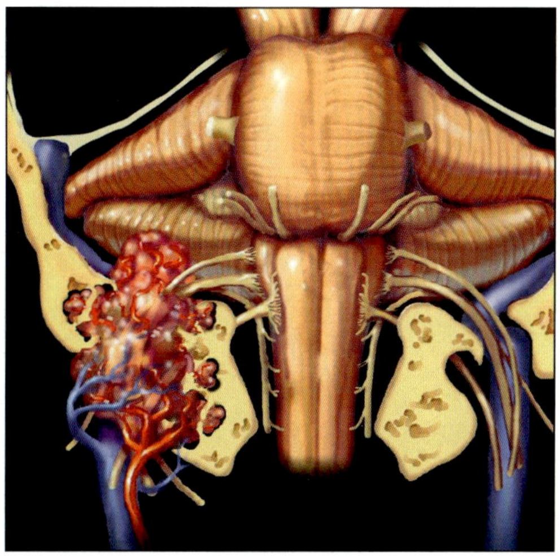

(Left) *This coronal graphic shows a glomus jugulare paraganglioma centered in the jugular foramen with superolateral extension into the middle ear. The ascending parapharyngeal artery → is feeding this vascular tumor.* ***(Right)*** *This coronal graphic shows a large glomus jugulare paraganglioma arising from the jugular foramen, engulfing the jugular vein and CN9-12, and infiltrating the adjacent skull base.*

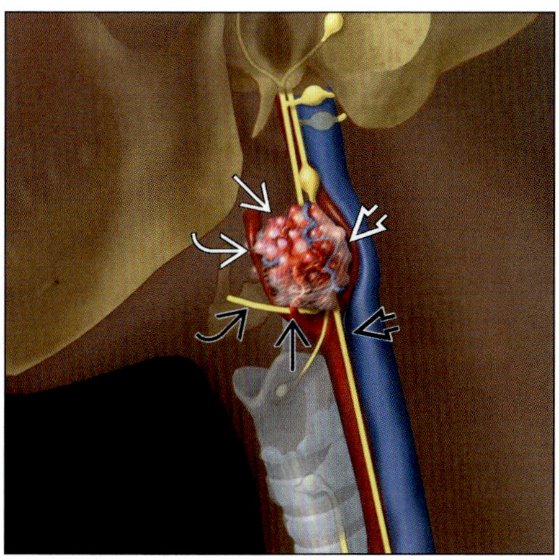

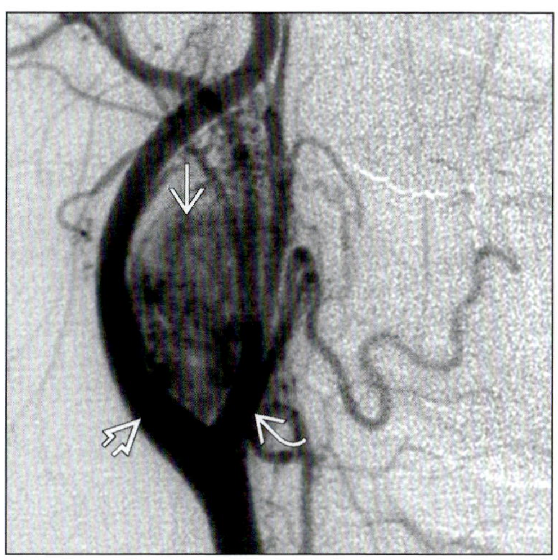

(Left) *This lateral graphic depicts a carotid body paraganglioma at the carotid bifurcation →, splaying the ICA → and ECA →. The main arterial feeder is the ascending pharyngeal artery →. The vagus → and hypoglossal → nerves are in close proximity.* ***(Right)*** *Lateral common carotid angiogram in late arterial phase demonstrates intense tumor blush → between the external → and internal → carotid arteries.*

PARAGANGLIOMA

Microscopic Features

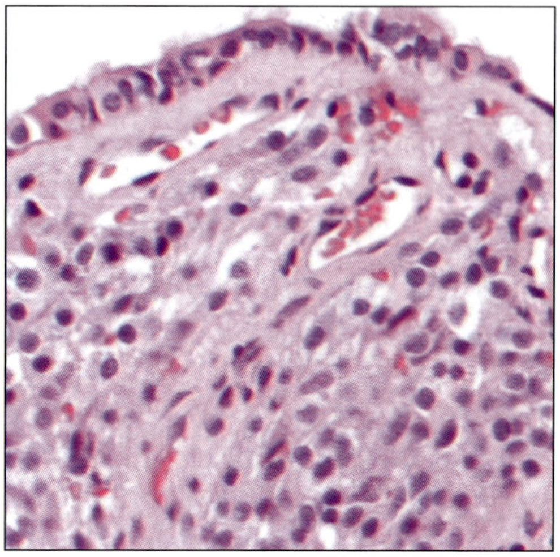

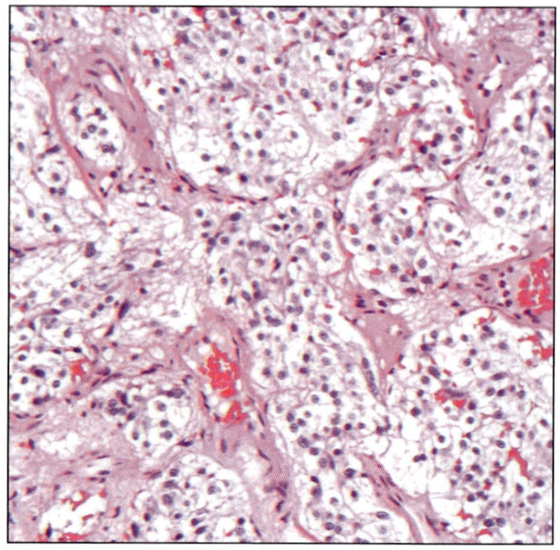

(Left) *This highly vascular paraganglioma underneath an intact mucosa shows scattered and nested neoplastic cells interspersed around vascular channels.* ***(Right)*** *This paraganglioma shows the classic zellballen nested cellular arrangement with variably sized nests of tumor cells. The small nests are surrounded by a thick fibrous vascular tissue.*

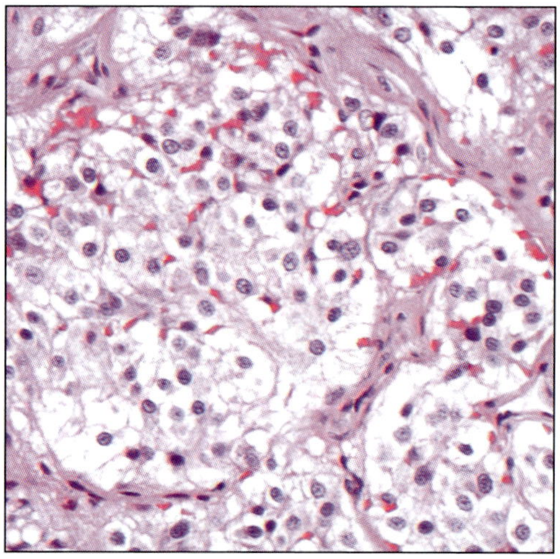

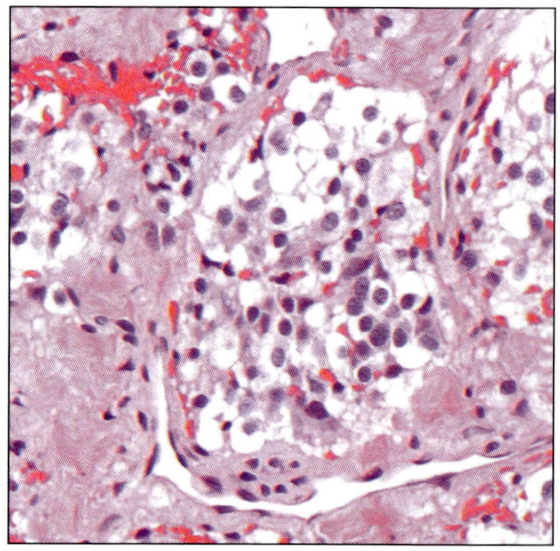

(Left) *The characteristic alveolar pattern (zellballen) with variably sized nests of tumor cells surrounded by thin-walled vessels is seen in this metastasizing paraganglioma from an SDHB mutation-positive patient.* ***(Right)*** *This photomicrograph shows the characteristic alveolar pattern (zellballen) with a nest of tumor cells surrounded by vessels and thick fibrous bands.*

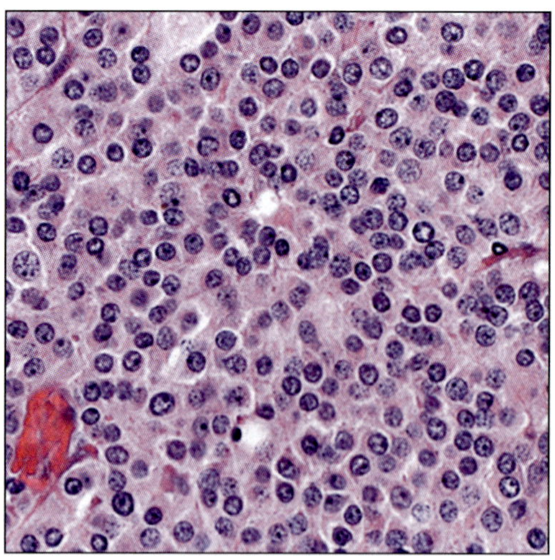

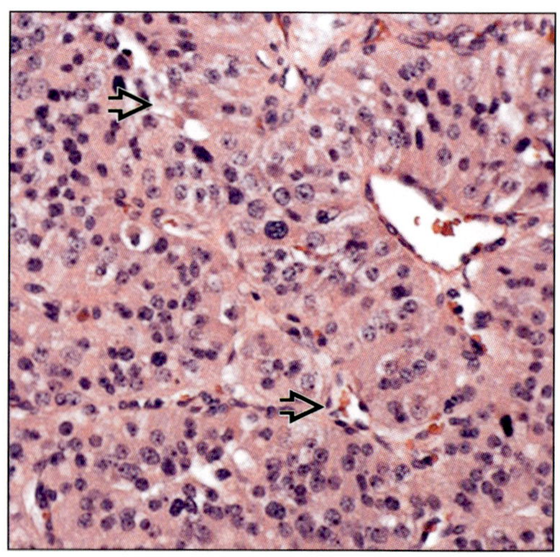

(Left) *Some PGLs lack the typical pattern of small nests (zellballen) of neuroendocrine cells with interspersed small blood vessels and instead may show a diffuse growth pattern, as in this case.* ***(Right)*** *This high-power view of a paraganglioma shows an alveolar pattern with variably sized nests of tumor cells surrounded by thin-walled vessels ⇨. Focally, this tumor has a solid, patternless component with large sheets of tumor cells.*

Gross, Microscopic, and Immunohistochemical Features

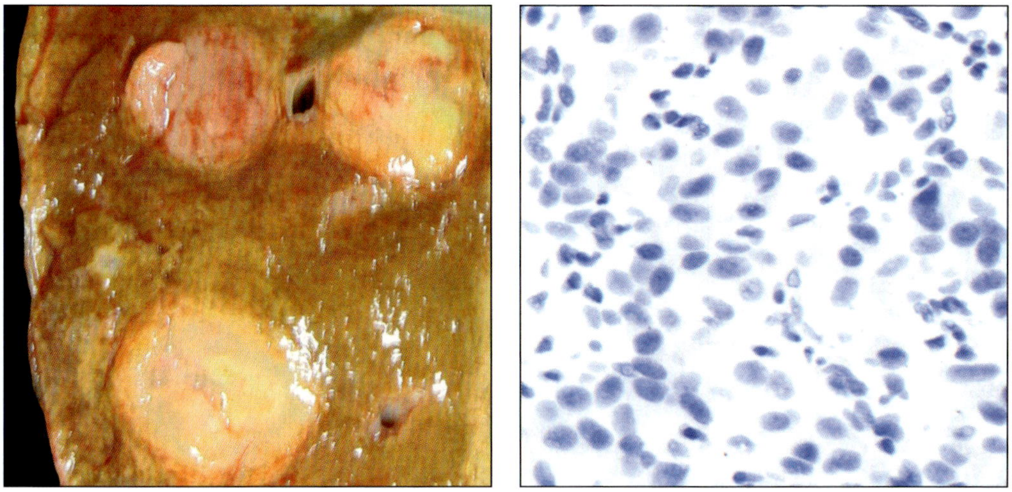

(Left) *This gross cut surface of a liver from a patient with a hereditary SDHB-associated malignant middle ear paraganglioma shows multiple well-circumscribed, firm, pale pink metastatic nodules. This patient also had metastases to the pancreas.* ***(Right)*** *SDHB immunostaining reveals loss of immunoreactivity in a patient with SDHB-associated hereditary middle ear paraganglioma. The patient presented with metastatic disease.*

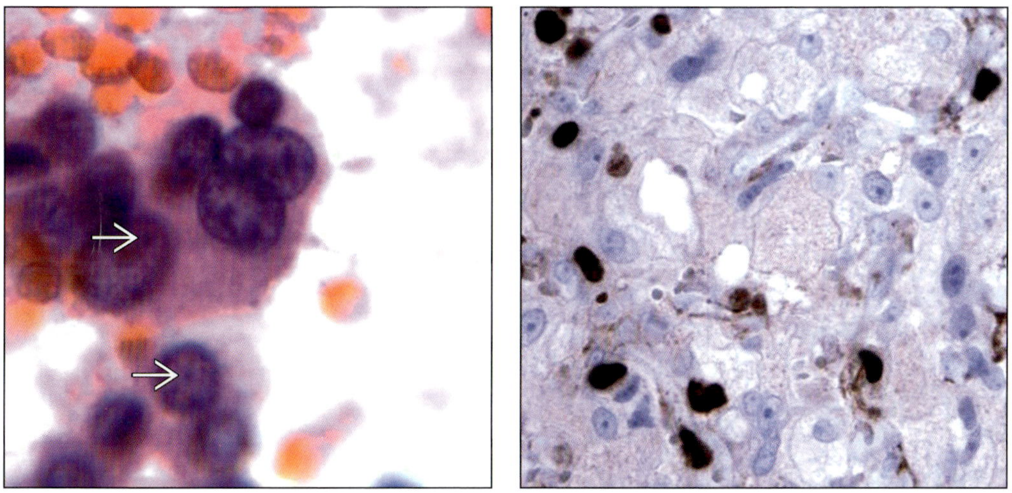

(Left) *A smear from a cardiac paraganglioma shows a homogeneous population of cells with pale eosinophilic cytoplasm and round to oval nuclei with regular nuclear membranes and stippled chromatin. Minute nucleoli* ➔ *can be identified in this picture.* ***(Right)*** *A metastatic focus of a malignant paraganglioma shows a high proliferative index by Ki-67 stain, as depicted in this photograph. The original paraganglioma had a lower proliferative index when compared with the metastases.*

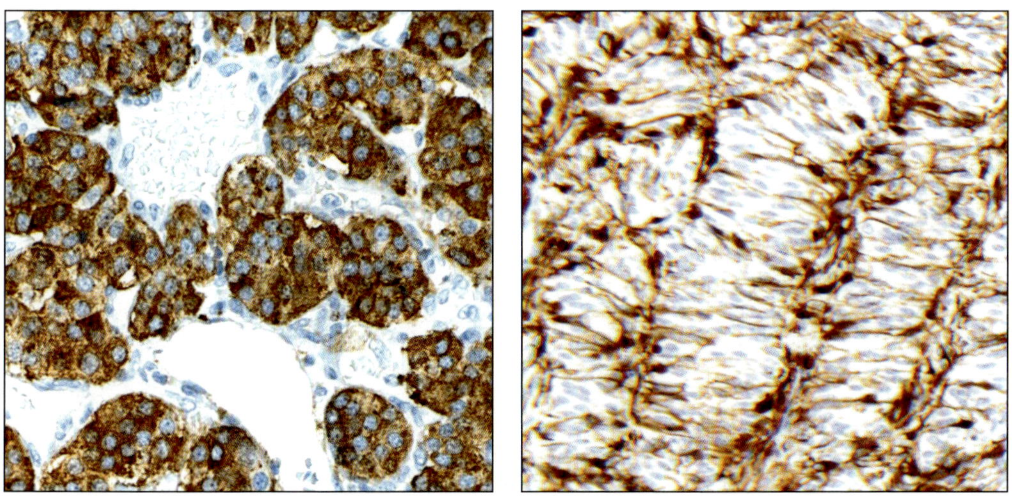

(Left) *Chromogranin-A immunostain shows granular immunoreactivity in the neuroendocrine cell nests between cavernous blood vessels in a carotid PGL. Note the negativity of the endothelial cells for this marker.* ***(Right)*** *S100 stain in a duodenal gangliocytic paraganglioma of a patient with NF1 shows nuclear and cytoplasmic staining of sustentacular cells, which sometimes have conspicuous cytoplasmic processes.*

PARAGANGLIOMA

Microscopic Features

(Left) *Underneath an intact mucosa, the characteristic alveolar pattern (zellballen) with variably sized nests of tumor cells surrounded by thin-walled vessels is seen in this paraganglioma.* **(Right)** *SDHB immunostaining reveals maintenance of immunoreactivity in a paraganglioma in a patient with a MEN2-associated hereditary paraganglioma, without SDHB or SDHD mutation.*

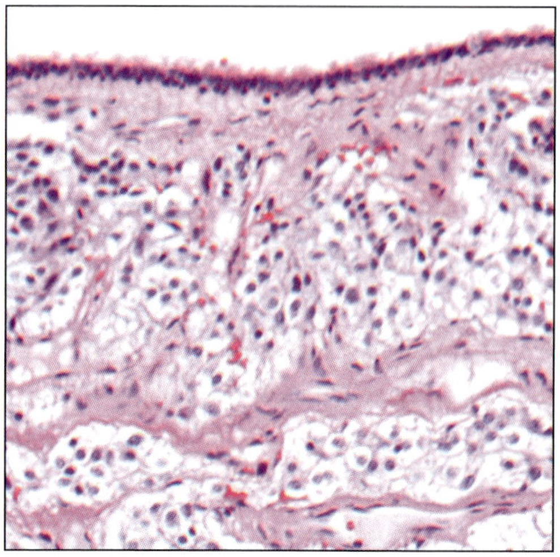

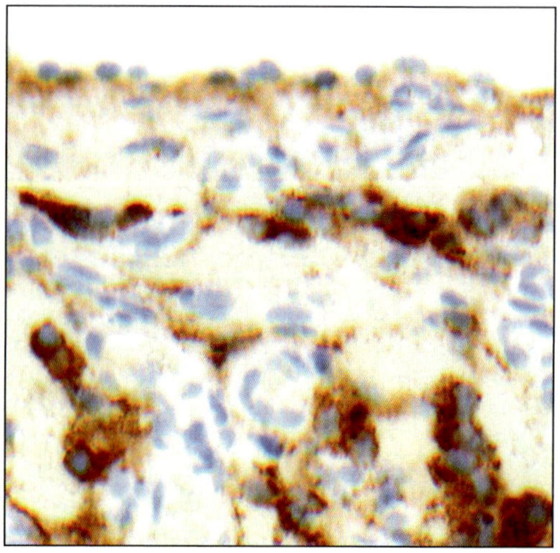

(Left) *Cytokeratin stains the overlying epithelium but is negative in the paraganglioma cells. The tumor is composed of variably sized tumor cells in a solid arrangement.* **(Right)** *Neuroendocrine markers highlight the paraganglioma cells. The usual neuroendocrine markers include synaptophysin (shown), chromogranin, CD56, and NSE, among others.*

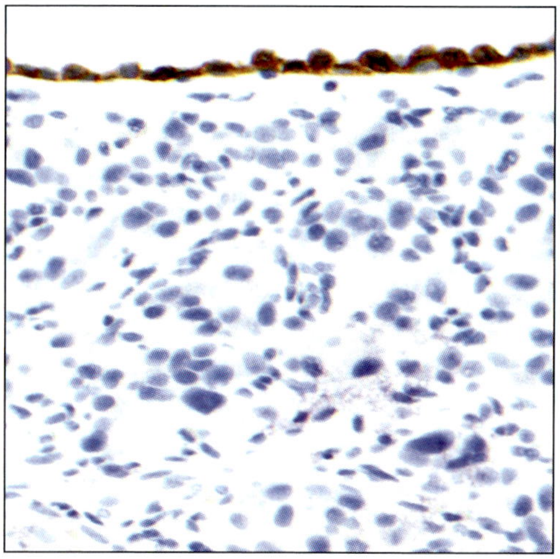

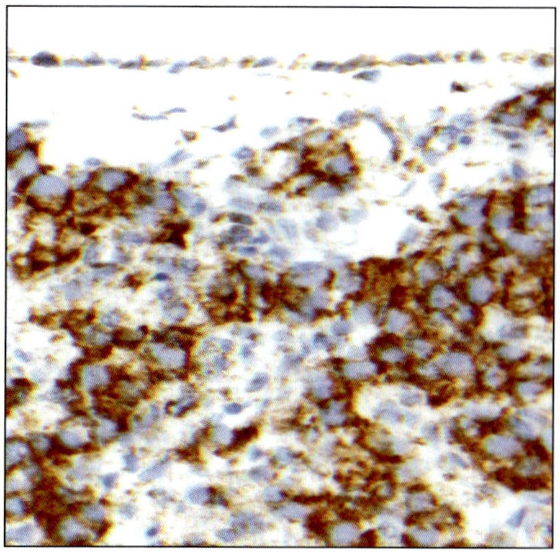

(Left) *High-power view shows an intact mucosa and a paraganglioma in the submucosa with the characteristic alveolar pattern (zellballen) with variably sized nests of tumor cells surrounded by thin-walled vessels.* **(Right)** *Chromogranin-A immunostain shows granular immunoreactivity in the neuroendocrine cell nests between cavernous blood vessels in a middle ear paraganglioma. The endothelial cells are negative for this marker.*

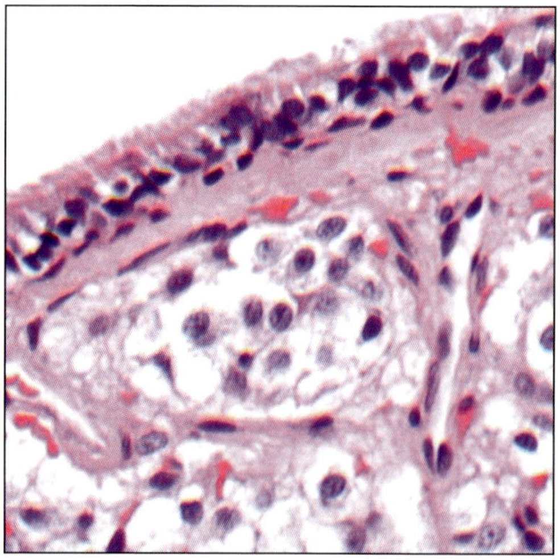

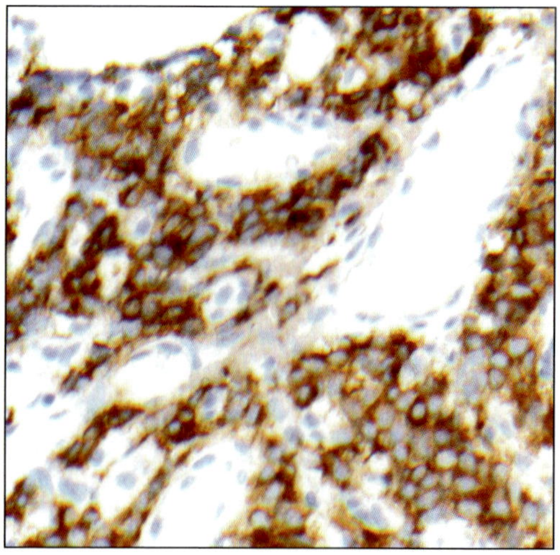

SDH Paraganglioma

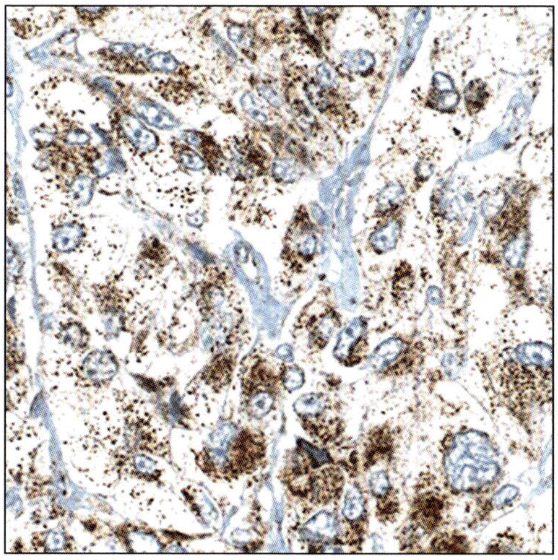

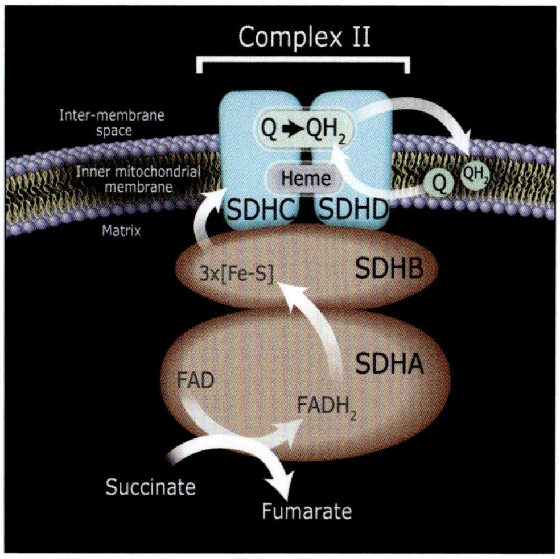

(Left) *Pheochromocytomas and other paragangliomas without mutations of SDHx genes show immunoreactivity of tumor cell cytoplasm for SDHB protein. The staining is coarsely granular as the protein is localized to mitochondria.* ***(Right)*** *This graphic of part of the mitochondrial respiratory chain complex II shows the relationship between the succinate ubiquinone oxidoreductase subunits (SDHA → SDHD). Inactivating mutations result in hereditary paraganglioma.*

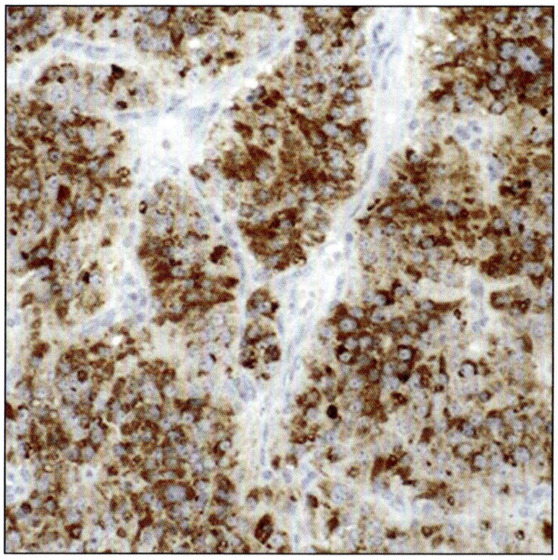

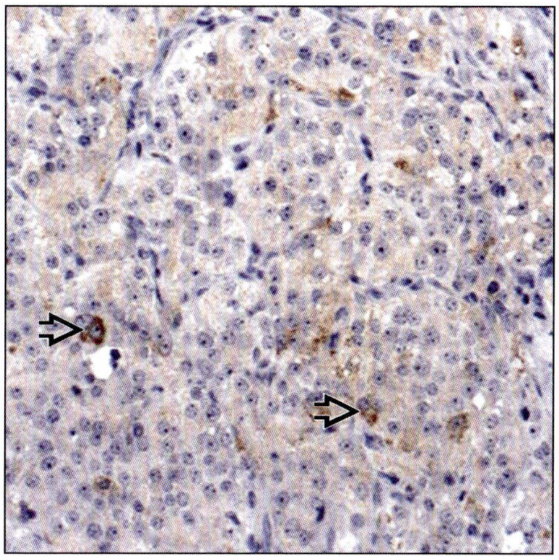

(Left) *Immunostaining for SDHA is preserved in the cytoplasm of paragangliomas of patients with an SDHB or SDHD mutation. This stain is used as a control for the SDHB stain. Note the granular brown deposits present in the cytoplasm of the tumor cells.* ***(Right)*** *SDHB immunostaining reveals the near-complete loss of immunoreactivity in a paraganglioma in a patient with SDHB mutation. Only endothelial cells display immunoreactivity ➪.*

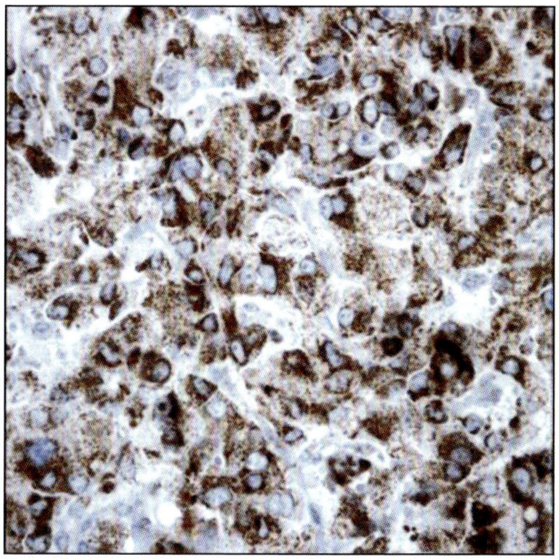

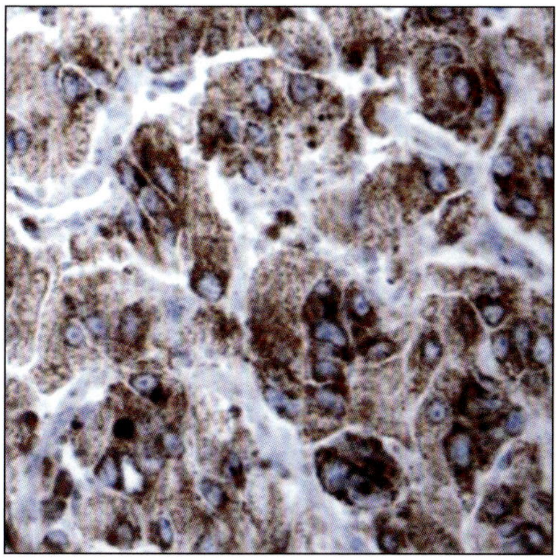

(Left) *Immunostaining for SDHA is preserved in the cytoplasm of paragangliomas in patients with an SDHB or SDHD mutation. SDHA can be used as a control for the SDHB stain. Note the granular brown deposits present in the cytoplasm of the tumor cells.* ***(Right)*** *SDHB immunostaining reveals maintenance of granular cytoplasmic immunoreactivity in a patient with MEN2-associated paraganglioma, without SDHB or SDHD mutation.*

PANCREATIC ENDOCRINE TUMOR

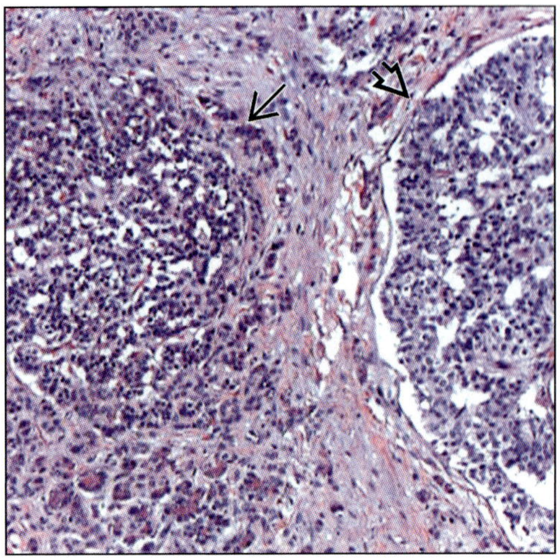

Two distinct pancreatic endocrine cell proliferations are shown in a case of MEN1. The lesion on the left side of this figure ⇒ has irregular borders, and the lesion on the right side ⇨ is well demarcated and larger.

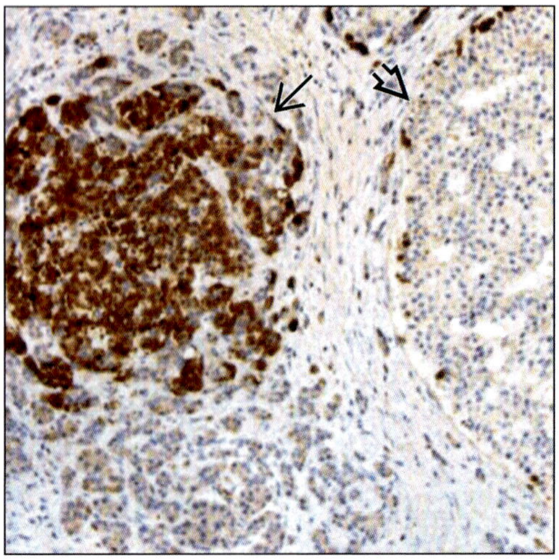

The smaller pancreatic endocrine lesion ⇒ is uniformly positive for glucagon (microadenoma), whereas the larger lesion ⇨ shows a pattern of distribution of glucagon similar to a normal islet, indicating hyperplasia.

TERMINOLOGY

Abbreviations

- Pancreatic endocrine tumor (PET)

Synonyms

- Pancreatic neuroendocrine tumor (PNET)
- Pancreatic endocrine neoplasm (PEN)
- Gastroenteropancreatic neuroendocrine tumors (GEP-NETs)

Definitions

- Functional or nonfunctional neoplasm arising from endocrine cells of pancreas
- PETs can be classified as sporadic or inherited
- WHO classifies PETs into 3 broad categories
  - **Well-differentiated endocrine tumors**
    - Benign: Confined to pancreas; no angioinvasion, no perineural invasion, < 2 cm, < 2 mitoses/10 HPF, < 2% Ki-67 proliferative index
    - Uncertain: Confined to pancreas; 1 or more of the following features: > 2 cm, 2-10 mitoses/10 HPF, > 2% Ki-67 proliferative index, angioinvasion, perineural invasion
  - **Well-differentiated endocrine carcinomas**: Gross local invasion, metastases
  - **Poorly differentiated endocrine carcinoma** (small cell carcinoma): High-grade malignancy, > 10 mitoses/10 HPF
  - Endocrine microadenoma (< 0.5 cm)
    - Nonfunctional, discovered incidentally (surgery, radiographic, autopsy)
    - Pancreatic head affected most commonly
    - Often coexpress > 1 peptide
    - Multiple microadenomas are present in MEN1 syndrome

ETIOLOGY/PATHOGENESIS

Syndromic

- Associated with multiple endocrine neoplasia type 1 (MEN1), von Hippel-Lindau (VHL), tuberous sclerosis (TS), and neurofibromatosis type 1 (NF1) syndromes
- PETs associated with syndromes are associated with characteristic genetic abnormalities
- **MEN1**
  - *MEN1* gene
  - 80% of cases have PETs
    - PETs are diagnosed clinically in ~ 80% of patients with MEN1
    - This number approaches 100% in autopsy studies
  - Patients with MEN1 have a unique profile of hormonal function: 50% are gastrin-producing and 20% are insulin-producing tumors
    - In MEN1, duodenal gastrin-producing NETs are more common than those arising in pancreas
  - MEN1 involvement of pancreas initially involves development of multiple small PETs, often microadenomas, associated with foci of nesidioblastosis or ductuloinsular complexes
  - Presence of peliosis in islets and adenomas is a curious feature
  - Islet dysplasia, defined as normal-sized or slightly enlarged islets containing cells with mild cytologic atypia
    - Readily confirmed by immunohistochemistry that shows loss of normal spatial and quantitative arrangement of the 4 main cell types
  - Once islet dysplasia attains a size of 0.5 mm, it is classified as microadenoma; islet dysplasia is most frequently associated with MEN1
  - MEN1 is diagnosed in ~ 25% of patients who have a gastrinoma and in ~ 5% of those who have an insulin-producing PET
  - In contrast to sporadic PETs, those associated with MEN1 tend to present at an earlier age (30-50 years),

PANCREATIC ENDOCRINE TUMOR

Key Facts

Etiology/Pathogenesis

- **Precursor lesions**: Neuroendocrine cell proliferations in both ducts and islets in familial pancreatic NETs in patients with MEN1 and VHL
- Familial PETs are associated with MEN1, VHL, TS, and NF1 syndromes
- **MEN1**: 80% have PETs
  - 50% are gastrin-producing and 20% are insulin-producing tumors
  - Development of multiple, small PETs, often microadenomas, associated with foci of nesidioblastosis or ductuloinsular complexes
- **VHL**: Benign cysts and microcystic or serous adenomas, which occur in 35-70% of VHL patients
  - There is association of nesidioblastosis and microadenomas with VHL
  - Up to 60% of the tumors contain clear cells or multivacuolated lipid-rich cells
- **Tuberous sclerosis**: Rare PETs
- **NF1**: Pancreatic somatostatinomas are more rare than those of duodenal origin
- Majority of PETs are nonsyndromic (sporadic)

Clinical Issues

- 2-4% of clinically detected pancreatic neoplasms
- Body and tail most common
- Clinical syndromes related to excessive or inappropriate hormone or biogenic amine production
- Behavior depends on tumor size, functional status, hormone produced, and extent of local invasion
  - > 2 cm, > 2 mitoses/10 HPF, > 2% Ki-67
- Multifocal tumors more common in MEN1 and less frequently in VHL

have a higher rate of postoperative recurrence, and are a common cause of death in these patients
  - MEN1-associated PETs display a wide variety of molecular abnormalities including chromosomal loss, chromosomal loss with duplication, mitotic recombination, or point mutation of the wild-type MEN1 allele
  - Similar to their sporadic counterparts, they exhibit inter- and intratumoral genetic heterogeneity indicating chromosomal instability
- **VHL**
  - *VHL* gene
  - Pancreatic pathology in VHL usually takes the form of benign cysts and microcystic or serous adenomas
    - Occur in 35-70% of VHL patients
    - Occur in young patients, are multiple, and located anywhere in the pancreas
    - Tumors are said to be functionally inactive, although immunohistochemistry does show focal positivity for pancreatic polypeptide, somatostatin, glucagon, &/or insulin in 30-40% of cases
    - Initially reported to not be associated with either microadenomas (endocrine cell foci, 0.5 cm in diameter) or nesidioblastosis; however, there is association of these findings with VHL
  - VHL-associated PETs tend to be arranged in trabeculae, glandular configurations, and solid foci
  - Characteristically, up to 60% of the tumors contain clear cells or multivacuolated lipid-rich cells in varying proportions
  - There are no data on VHL genotypic predisposition to PETs
  - Pancreatic tumors in patients with this disorder have been documented to exhibit loss of heterozygosity of normal VHL allele
- **Tuberous sclerosis** (TS)
  - *TSC1* and *TSC2* genes
  - Rare PETs have been reported in patients with TS
    - It is not clear if this is a causal or a casual association
  - Malignant PETs have been described in children
  - Functional PETs have been reported to produce both insulin and gastrin
  - TSC1 (hamartin) is highly expressed in normal islet cells; loss of this tumor suppressor is speculated to have an etiologic role in these lesions
- **NF1**
  - *NF1* gene
  - Somatostatinomas of pancreas are rarer than those of duodenal origin
    - 16x less common than duodenal somatostatinomas
  - Duodenal somatostatinomas occur in NF1 patients
    - NF1 accounted for 48% of duodenal somatostatinomas reported in the literature
  - Occasional NF1 patients may have pancreatic gastrinoma, insulinoma, and nonfunctioning PET

Precursor Lesions

- Although no precursor lesions have so far been described in sporadic PNETs, there is evidence of neuroendocrine cell proliferations in both ducts and islets as precursor lesions of familial PNETs in patients with MEN1 and VHL
- **Pancreatic neuroendocrine cell ductular proliferations**, a distinct phenomenon called nesidioblastosis or ductuloinsular complexes, is seen in both MEN1 and VHL
  - However, these changes may also be found in several other conditions, including chronic pancreatitis and ductal obstruction
- Alterations in islets of Langerhans, including islet hyperplasia and islet dysplasia, is seen only in setting of inherited pancreatic NETs
- **Islet dysplasia** refers to slightly enlarged islets (< 0.5 mm) that contain neuroendocrine cells arranged in trabeculae that display mild atypia and show loss of normal spatial and quantitative arrangement of normal 4 main cell types
  - Islet dysplasia is most frequently associated with MEN1

PANCREATIC ENDOCRINE TUMOR

- **Pancreatic neuroendocrine microadenoma** is when an islet cell dysplasia attains a size > 0.5 mm
- Microadenoma > 5 mm is classified as PNET
- Pancreatic microadenomatosis, the presence of multiple pancreatic neuroendocrine microadenomas, is linked to MEN1 syndrome and also seen in association with VHL disease
  - At molecular level, microadenomas in MEN1 syndrome show loss of MEN1 wild-type allele, proving their neoplastic nature
  - Pancreatic microadenomatosis has also been described in a patient with oculofaciocardiodental syndrome
- Characteristically, VHL-related NETs contain clear cells or multivacuolated lipid-rich cells in varying proportions
- Ductuloinsular complexes and islet hyperplasia/ dysplasia are precursor premalignant lesions since they may give rise to the development of pancreatic neuroendocrine microadenomas and NETs in the setting of familial disease
- In addition to ductuloinsular complexes, islet dysplasia, and microadenomas, peliotic change of islets can also be seen in MEN1- or VHL-related lesions

Sporadic

- Majority of cases are nonsyndromic (sporadic)
- There are no defined precursor lesions in sporadic pancreatic NETs
- Somatic mutations of *MEN1* gene are identified in ~ 20% of sporadic PETs and up to 68% harbor losses of 11q13 &/or more distal parts of long arm of chromosome 11

CLINICAL ISSUES

Epidemiology

- Incidence
  - 1-2% of clinically detected pancreatic neoplasms
    - 1 per 100,000 people per year (USA)
    - 2-4 per million people per year for insulinoma
    - Asymptomatic type found in up to 1.5% of autopsies
  - ~ 20% of PET are MEN1 associated
  - Relative increase due to more sensitive diagnostic approaches
- Age
  - Peak: 30-60 years (mean: 50 years)
  - Syndrome-associated tumors (MEN1) tend to occur earlier (10-30 years)
- Gender
  - Equal distribution
    - Exception for somatostatinoma: F > M (2:1)
    - Exception for gastrinoma: M > F (1.2:1)

Site

- Entire pancreas may be affected; most common sites are body and tail
  - Somatostatinomas: More common in head
  - Gastrinoma: Head, duodenum, gastric antrum, and peripancreatic soft tissues
  - Glucagonoma: Tail most common
  - Vasoactive intestinal peptide (VIP)-oma: Most common in tail

Presentation

- **Functional**: Clinical syndromes related to excessive or inappropriate hormone or biogenic amine production
  - ~ 60%
  - Ectopic hormone: Gastrin, vasoactive intestinal peptide, pancreatic polypeptide (PP), and neurotensin
  - Pancreatic hormone: Insulin, glucagon, somatostatin
  - **Insulinoma syndrome** (~ 25%)
    - Whipple triad includes the following 3 characteristics
    - Symptoms of hypoglycemia
    - Plasma glucose levels < 3.0 mmol/L
    - Relief of symptoms with administration of glucose
  - **Glucagonoma syndrome**
    - Skin rash (necrolytic migratory erythema): 70% of patients
    - Rash usually starts in groin/perineum and migrates to distal extremities
    - Associated with angular stomatitis, cheilitis, atrophic glossitis, alopecia, onycholysis, vulvovaginitis, and urethritis
    - Marked weight loss (65%), mild diabetes mellitus (glucose intolerance) (50%), anemia (33%), diarrhea, depression (20%), deep vein thrombosis (12%)
  - **Somatostatinoma syndrome**
    - Nonspecific findings, although diabetes mellitus, hypochlorhydria, gallbladder disease (cholelithiasis), diarrhea, steatorrhea, anemia, and weight loss may be present
    - Markedly elevated somatostatin serum/tumor levels define the syndrome
  - **Gastrinoma syndrome** (~ 15%)
    - Zollinger-Ellison syndrome
    - Increased gastrin results in gastric or duodenal ulcers, resulting in abdominal pain, diarrhea, vomiting, and weight loss
    - 25% of patients are found to have MEN1 syndrome
  - **VIPoma syndrome**
    - a.k.a. Verner-Morrison syndrome
    - VIP excess produces voluminous watery diarrhea, hypokalemia, achlorhydria, and metabolic acidosis
    - Accounts for 80% of diarrheagenic tumors
- **Nonfunctional**: Inactive, nonsyndromic, incidentally discovered
  - ~ 40%
  - May have elevated hormone levels, but not a distinct syndrome
  - Large abdominal mass, abdominal or back pain, obstructive symptoms, pancreatitis
  - Jaundice may develop in large tumors located in head of pancreas
  - Large tumors are usually nonfunctional

PANCREATIC ENDOCRINE TUMOR

Laboratory Tests

- **Insulinoma**
  - Elevated plasma insulin and proinsulin concentrations by radioimmunoassay
    - Combined measures of insulin, proinsulin, C-peptide, and blood glucose help exclude factitious hyperinsulinemia
- **Glucagonoma**
  - Elevated fasting plasma glucagon concentration (usually 10-20x)
  - Tolbutamide or arginine stimulation tests may be used
  - ~ 20% will also have increased plasma gastrin levels
- **Somatostatinoma**
  - Elevated plasma somatostatin levels
- **Gastrinoma**
  - Secretin stimulation test (measures evoked gastrin levels)
  - 3 separate elevated fasting gastrin levels
  - Gastric acid secretion and pH

Treatment

- Options, risks, complications
  - Multidisciplinary approach is mandatory
  - Before surgery, important to separate MEN1-associated tumors from solitary, nonsyndrome-associated, and malignant tumors
  - Management of hormone production is critical
- Adjuvant therapy
  - Usually employed for high-stage, malignant, &/or metastatic tumors
  - Includes chemoembolization for liver metastases

Prognosis

- Routine morphologic examination does not always predict behavior
  - Locally infiltrative disease, perineural and vascular invasion seen more often in malignant tumors
- Up to 30% of patients already have metastatic disease at diagnosis
  - ~ 65% will develop metastatic disease at some point during disease course
- Survival depends on tumor size, functional status, and extent of local invasion
  - Nonfunctional: 65% 5-year survival; 45% 10-year survival
  - Functional: 45% 5-year survival (except insulinoma)
- Tumor behavior is associated with functional status and specific hormone produced
  - Nonfunctional tumors are nearly all malignant (90%)
  - **Insulinoma**: Has best prognosis
    - Vast majority are benign (~ 8% malignant)
    - Early detection, as a result of symptoms while still small
  - **Glucagonoma**
    - ~ 60-70% have metastases at time of diagnosis
  - **Somatostatinoma**
    - Generally large at time of diagnosis
    - ~ 70% have metastases at time of diagnosis
- Adverse prognostic factors
  - Metastasis to regional lymph nodes &/or liver
  - Gross invasion into adjacent organs
  - Angiolymphatic invasion and perineural invasion
  - Rule of 2: > 2 cm, > 2 mitoses/10 HPF, > 2% proliferation index (Ki-67)
  - Necrosis
  - Functioning tumor (except insulinoma)

IMAGE FINDINGS

Ultrasonographic Findings

- Endoscopic ultrasonography: 20-65% sensitivity

MR Findings

- MR imaging: 25-60% sensitivity

Somatostatin Receptor Scintigraphy (SRS) &/or Positron Emission Tomography (PET)

- Somatostatin analogues attach with high-affinity binding to receptors overexpressed by tumors
- Allows for detection of very small tumors
- Gastrinoma, somatostatinoma, glucagonoma, and VIPoma are usually detected
- Insulinoma usually not detected

MACROSCOPIC FEATURES

General Features

- Vast majority are well demarcated, discrete/circumscribed, and solitary
  - Multifocal tumors more common in MEN1

Size

- Overall range: < 0.5 up to 35 cm
- Microinsulinomas in MEN1 usually functionally silent, especially when there are multiple lesions
- Size as it relates to functional status and hormone produced
  - Functional: Usually < 2 cm
    - **Insulinomas**: < 2 cm
    - **Somatostatinomas**: Mean = 5-6 cm
    - **Glucagonomas**: Mean = 7 cm
  - Nonfunctional: > 2 cm
  - Microadenoma: < 0.5 cm but are nearly always nonfunctioning

MICROSCOPIC PATHOLOGY

Histologic Features

- Wide architectural and cytomorphologic appearance
  - Ribbon-like, trabecular, festooned, or gyriform
  - Solid, trabecular, glandular, tubuloacinar, or pseudorosette
- Cells are relatively uniform
- Lipid-rich, clear cell (in von Hippel-Lindau), oncocytic, and rhabdoid subtypes rare
- Nuclei show salt-and-pepper chromatin distribution
- Stroma and fibrosis are variably present
  - Amyloid seen in insulinoma
  - Psammoma bodies seen in somatostatinoma
- Invasion can be seen

PANCREATIC ENDOCRINE TUMOR

Criteria for Clinicopathological Classification of Tumors of Endocrine Pancreas

WHO Tumor Type	Criteria for Clinicopathological Classification
Well-differentiated endocrine tumor: Benign behavior	Confined to pancreas; < 2 cm in diameter; < 2 mitoses/10 HPF, < 2% Ki-67 proliferative index; no lymphovascular invasion; no perineural invasion
Well-differentiated endocrine tumor: Uncertain behavior	Confined to pancreas, and 1 or more of the following features: > 2 cm in diameter; 2-10 mitoses/10 HPF, > 2% Ki-67 proliferative index; lymphovascular invasion, perineural invasion
Well-differentiated endocrine carcinoma	Gross local invasion &/or metastases; low-grade malignant
Poorly differentiated endocrine carcinoma (small cell carcinoma)	High-grade malignant; > 10 mitoses/10 HPF
Mixed endocrine-exocrine carcinoma	Malignant mixed neoplasm in which endocrine and exocrine cells are intimally admixed (each component comprises at least 1/3 of tumor)

WHO Histological Classification of Tumors of the Endocrine Pancreas.

- Mitotic figures are usually sparse (< 2/10 HPF)
  - Ki-67 required to document proliferation index

Well-Differentiated PET

- Functioning
  - **Insulinoma** (most common type): β-cell derived
    - Nonfunctioning and microtumors not encapsulated
    - Amyloid is unique to this tumor type (islet amyloid polypeptide [IAPP] or amylin)
  - **Gastrinoma** (2nd most common)
    - Many times, no primary tumor is identified in spite of having lymph node metastases
    - High risk of malignant behavior, irrespective of size
  - **Glucagonoma** (3rd most common): α-cell derived
    - Glucagonomas commonly occur in tail of pancreas or attached to surface of pancreas
  - **VIPoma** (4th most common)
    - Often react with other markers (growth hormone release hormone, α-human chorionic gonadotropin, pancreatic polypeptide)
  - **Somatostatinoma** (least common): δ-cell derived
    - Tend to have glands and psammoma bodies

Well-Differentiated Endocrine Carcinoma

- Functional or nonfunctional
- Gross local invasion (fat or organs)
- Regional lymph nodes (peripancreatic, coeliac, periaortic) involved first
- Metastases to liver

Poorly Differentiated Neuroendocrine Carcinoma

- **Small cell variant**: Diffuse sheet-like arrangements of cells, geographic necrosis, mitotic figures > 10/10 HPF
  - Resembles small cell carcinoma of lung
- **Large cell neuroendocrine variant**
  - Resembles large cell neuroendocrine carcinoma of lung

ANCILLARY TESTS

Immunohistochemistry

- Variety of neuroendocrine markers are positive
  - Synaptophysin, chromogranin, neuron-specific enolase
- Specific hormone products/prohormones can be found
  - Insulin, glucagon, somatostatin, gastrin, VIP, PP
- In addition to usual pancreatic peptides, others can also be seen
  - Adrenocorticotrophic hormone (ACTH), parathyroid-like hormone, calcitonin, growth hormone releasing hormone, serotonin

SELECTED REFERENCES

1. Chou A et al: von Hippel-Lindau syndrome. Front Horm Res. 41:30-49, 2013
2. Hatipoglu E et al: Von Hippel Lindau disease with metastatic pancreatic neuroendocrine tumor causing ectopic Cushing's syndrome. Neuro Endocrinol Lett. 34(1):9-13, 2013
3. Liu TC et al: Comparison of WHO Classifications (2004, 2010), the Hochwald grading system, and AJCC and ENETS staging systems in predicting prognosis in locoregional well-differentiated pancreatic neuroendocrine tumors. Am J Surg Pathol. 37(6):853-9, 2013
4. Thakker RV: Multiple endocrine neoplasia type 1 (MEN1) and type 4 (MEN4). Mol Cell Endocrinol. Epub ahead of print, 2013
5. Klöppel G: Classification and pathology of gastroenteropancreatic neuroendocrine neoplasms. Endocr Relat Cancer. 18 Suppl 1:S1-S16, 2011
6. Zhang Y et al: Endocrine tumors as part of inherited tumor syndromes. Adv Anat Pathol. 18(3):206-18, 2011
7. Klöppel G et al: The ENETS and AJCC/UICC TNM classifications of the neuroendocrine tumors of the gastrointestinal tract and the pancreas: a statement. Virchows Arch. 456(6):595-7, 2010
8. Hofer MD et al: Immunohistochemical and clinicopathological correlation of the metastasis-associated gene 1 (MTA1) expression in benign and malignant pancreatic endocrine tumors. Mod Pathol. 22(7):933-9, 2009

PANCREATIC ENDOCRINE TUMOR

Microscopic Features

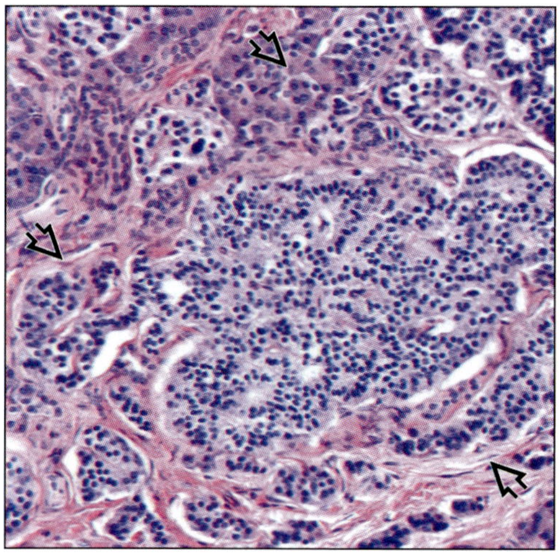

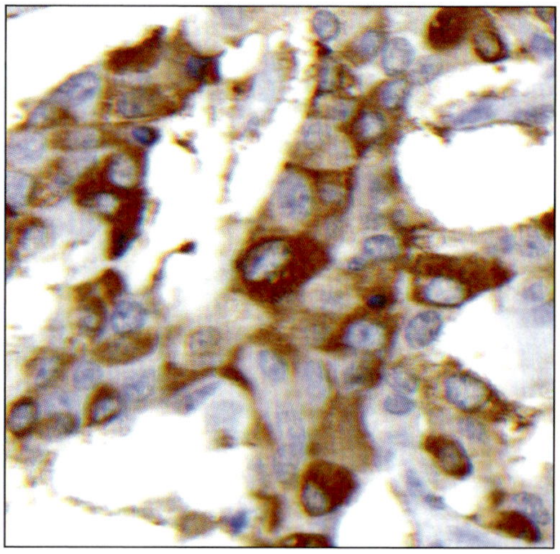

(Left) *In the pancreata of patients with MEN1, there are typically multiple small (< 5 mm) neuroendocrine tumors, a finding that has been referred to as microadenomatosis. Note the irregular borders of the endocrine components ⇨.* ***(Right)*** *Multiple pancreatic microadenomas (< 5 mm) seen in patients with MEN1 and NF are often accompanied by 1 or more macroadenomas (diameter > 5 mm), some of which may become insulinomas, as seen in this picture.*

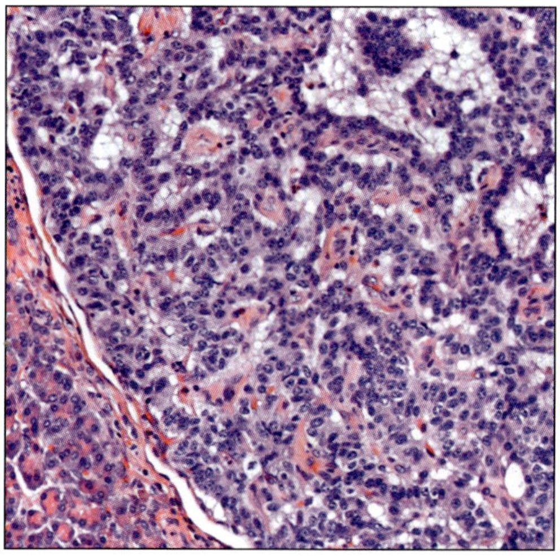

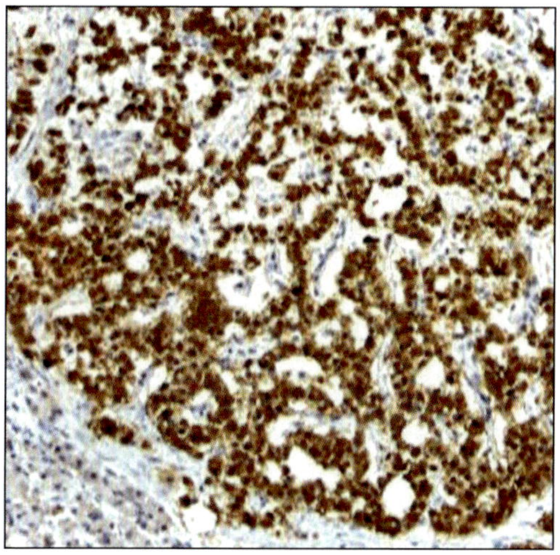

(Left) *Islet dysplasia refers to slightly enlarged islets that contain neuroendocrine cells arranged in trabeculae that display mild atypia and show loss of the normal spatial distribution and numbers of the normal main cell types. This is usually present in patients with MEN1 and VHL.* ***(Right)*** *Immunohistochemistry for chromogranin-A in a pancreas of a patient with MEN1 shows a markedly enlarged islet. The pancreas also had multiple microadenomas, adenomas, and hyperplasia/dysplasia.*

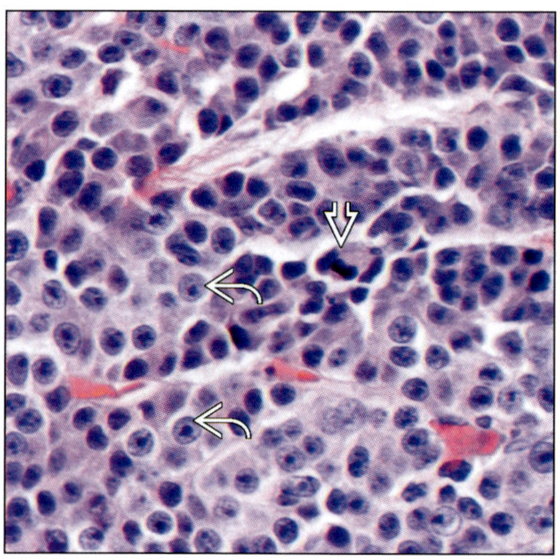

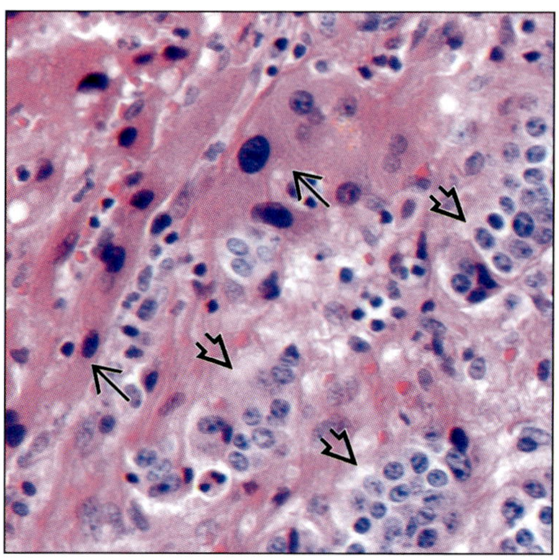

(Left) *This pancreatic endocrine tumor in a 17-year-old boy with MEN1 was large and associated with islet cell hyperplasia. Note prominent nucleoli ➡ and mitoses ➡.* ***(Right)*** *This photomicrograph from a liver in a 17-year-old boy with MEN1 shows metastases from the pancreatic endocrine tumor ⇨ compressing the adjacent liver parenchyma →. Metastases was present at diagnosis.*

PARATHYROID ADENOMA

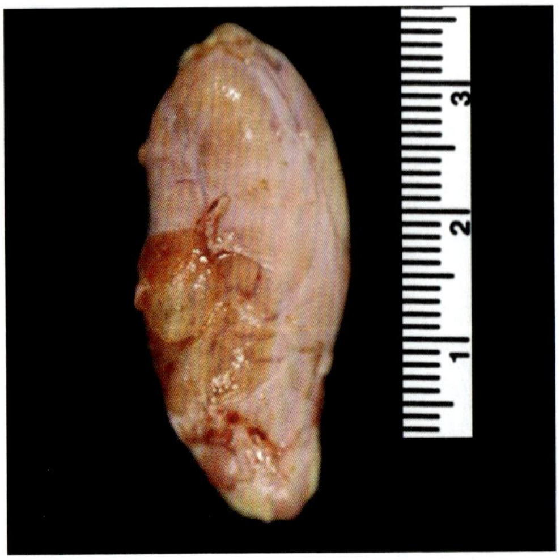

Parathyroid adenoma is a single enlarged parathyroid gland with a tan-yellow appearance. The surface is usually homogeneous and covered by a thin fibrous capsule.

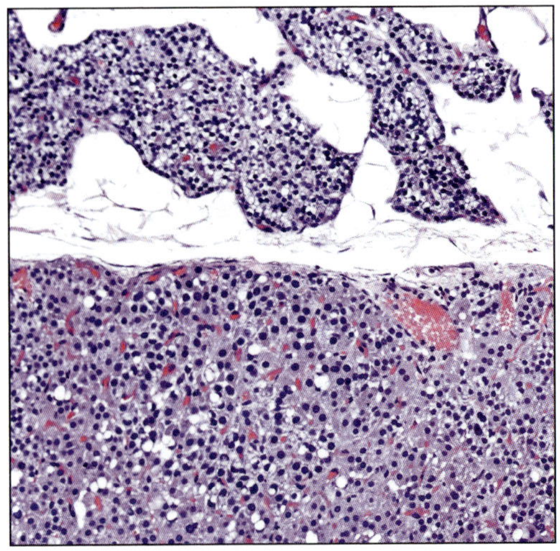

Chief cell parathyroid adenoma shows a rim of normal parathyroid tissue. Rims of normal parathyroid tissue are identified in 50-60% of parathyroid adenomas.

TERMINOLOGY

Abbreviations

- Parathyroid adenoma (PTA)

Definitions

- Benign neoplasm composed of chief cells, oncocytic cells, transitional cells, water-clear cells, or a mixture of cell types generally affecting a single parathyroid gland

ETIOLOGY/PATHOGENESIS

Sporadic Parathyroid Adenomas

- Predisposing factors poorly understood; possible association with prior ionizing radiation

Hereditary Parathyroid Adenomas

- Hereditary hyperparathyroidism is less common than sporadic hyperparathyroidism
- ~ 5-10% of cases of primary hyperparathyroidism are associated with familial syndromes
  - Study of this group has provided great insight into the genetic and molecular changes that underlie the neoplastic transformation of parathyroid tissue
- Most common genetic syndromes associated with primary hyperparathyroidism are multiple endocrine neoplasia types 1 and 2A (MEN1, MEN2A), hyperparathyroidism-jaw tumor syndrome (HPT-JT), familial isolated hyperparathyroidism (FIHP), and familial hypocalciuric hypercalcemia (FHH)
- **HPT-JT**
  - Autosomal dominant, inactivating mutations in *HRPT2* (1q21-q31) tumor suppressor gene that encodes parafibromin
  - Hyperparathyroidism, fibroosseous jaw tumors, kidney cysts, hamartomas, and Wilms tumors
  - Parathyroid hyperplasia or adenoma and increased risk of parathyroid carcinoma
  - Germline *HRPT2* mutations identified in subset of patients with mutation-positive carcinomas thought to be sporadic
- **Familial isolated hyperparathyroidism (FIHP)**
  - Autosomal dominant, 1% of primary hyperparathyroidism (parathyroid is only endocrine organ involved), adenoma or hyperplasia, and increased risk of parathyroid carcinoma
  - Cause unknown in most families, but *HRPT2* gene, *MEN1* gene, and area on chromosome 2 implicated
- **MEN1**
  - Autosomal dominant, high-penetrance germline mutation in *MEN1* tumor suppressor gene (11q13) encoding menin protein
  - Parathyroid adenomas and carcinomas occur in MEN1 but are less common than hyperplasia (multiglandular parathyroid disease)
  - Other MEN1 features
    - Endocrine: Pituitary adenomas; neuroendocrine tumors of pancreas, duodenum, thymus and lung; gastrinomas; adrenal cortical adenomas and hyperplasia
    - Nonendocrine: Angiofibromas, collagenomas, café au lait macules, lipomas, gingival papules, meningiomas, ependymomas, leiomyomas
- **MEN2A**
  - Autosomal dominant, high-penetrance germline *RET*-activating proto-oncogene (10q11.2) mutation
  - 20-30% of MEN2A is associated with parathyroid hyperplasia or adenomas; may also have medullary thyroid carcinoma &/or pheochromocytomas
- **Neonatal severe primary hyperparathyroidism**

CLINICAL ISSUES

Epidemiology

- Incidence
  - Most common cause of primary hyperparathyroidism (80-85%), followed by

PARATHYROID ADENOMA

Key Facts

Terminology
- Benign neoplasm of chief, oncocytic, transitional, water-clear, or mixture of cells

Etiology/Pathogenesis
- Most are sporadic
- ~ 5-10% of cases of primary hyperparathyroidism are associated with familial syndromes
- Most common genetic syndromes
  - Hyperparathyroidism-jaw tumor syndrome (HPT-JT)
  - Familial isolated hyperparathyroidism (FIHP)
  - Multiple endocrine neoplasia types 1 and 2A (MEN1, MEN2A)
  - Familial hypocalciuric hypercalcemia (FHH)

Clinical Issues
- Often asymptomatic or vague symptoms, identified with serum calcium screening

Microscopic Pathology
- Parathyroid adenoma is composed of chief, oxyphilic, transitional, clear cells, or mixtures of cell types

Ancillary Tests
- Positive for chromogranin, synaptophysin, CAM5.2, and PTH; negative for TTF-1 and thyroglobulin
- Chromosome 11: Frequent loss in adenomas and frequent gain in carcinomas

Top Differential Diagnoses
- Parathyroid hyperplasia, parathyroid carcinoma, thyroid tumor

parathyroid hyperplasia (15%) and carcinoma (1-2%)
  - Incidence has been increasing for 3 decades, attributable to introduction of automatic serum calcium screening
- Age
  - Any age, but most commonly in patients 50-60 years
  - Familial cases occur at younger ages (20-25 years)
- Gender
  - F:M = 3:1
  - Females and males equally affected in familial cases

Site
- Single parathyroid gland involved; lower parathyroids involved slightly more often than upper parathyroids
  - 10% in other locations: Intrathyroidal, mediastinum, thymus, soft tissue behind esophagus & pharynx
  - Exceptionally rare "double adenoma," but asymmetric hyperplasia more common

Presentation
- Usually asymptomatic or vague symptoms of fatigue, weakness, gastrointestinal symptoms, depression
- Historical symptoms of nephrolithiasis and severe bone disease (osteitis fibrosa cystica) less common today

Treatment
- Surgical approaches
  - Bilateral neck exploration with excision of adenoma is the classic approach, although minimally invasive surgery guided by noninvasive imaging and intraoperative parathyroid hormone (PTH) monitoring is gaining favor in nonfamilial cases
  - Subtotal parathyroidectomy is indicated in familial syndromes, such as MEN1 and FIHP
  - Using a surgical approach in HPT-JT is controversial because of the increased risk of parathyroid cancer, but subtotal parathyroidectomy with close postoperative biochemical monitoring for recurrence is currently recommended over prophylactic total parathyroidectomy
  - Resection of single gland (parathyroid adenoma), often with assistance of intraoperative PTH monitoring
    - ≥ 50% drop in intraoperative PTH from baseline at 10 minutes after gland excision is helpful to ensure that abnormal gland(s) has been removed
- Medical therapy with calcimimetics is useful for patients with primary hyperparathyroidism who are poor surgical candidates or have non-localizable tumors or an inoperable disease

IMAGE FINDINGS

General
- Tc-99m sestamibi and ultrasound are commonly used to localize site of adenoma
- May use computed tomography (CT), magnetic resonance (MR) imaging, etc.

MACROSCOPIC FEATURES

Parathyroid Adenoma Macroscopic Features
- Single enlarged gland: Usually 0.2 to > 1 g, tan to red-tan, encapsulated, ± rim of normal tissue
- Cystic change may occur in adenomas, particularly larger adenomas and in those with HPT-JT syndrome
- Parathyroid adenoma is ectopic in up to 10% (intrathyroidal, mediastinum, thymus, soft tissue behind esophagus and pharynx)
- Rare double adenomas (exercise caution as asymmetric hyperplasia is much more common)

MICROSCOPIC PATHOLOGY

Histologic Features
- **Parathyroid adenoma histology**

PARATHYROID ADENOMA

- Proliferation of parathyroid parenchymal chief cells, oxyphil cells, transitional cells, clear cells, or mixtures of cell types
- May have thin connective tissue capsule
- 50-60% have rim of normal parathyroid tissue
  - Rim more often identified in small adenomas
  - Rim often separated from adenoma by connective tissue capsule, but not always
  - Parathyroid parenchymal cells within rim are typically smaller than those within adenoma
  - Suppressed parathyroid parenchymal cells within rim have larger and more fat droplets than in adenoma cells, which have less lipid and more dispersed lipid than cells in the rim
  - Parathyroid hyperplasia can occasionally also have rims of normal tissue
- Fat cells sparse (scattered or nested) or absent
- Often a mixture of growth patterns: Follicular, acinar, cords, solid, rosette-like, but rarely papillae
- Scattered mitoses in up to 70% of adenomas (more in parathyroid carcinoma)
- No atypical mitoses
- Cysts and cystic change and degeneration common, especially in large adenomas and HPT-JT cases
- Parathyroid adenomas in MEN1 are histologically similar to sporadic parathyroid adenomas

ANCILLARY TESTS

Frozen Sections

- **Assessing cellularity in small biopsies can be difficult**
  - Cellularity is difficult to assess in small biopsies because it is variable within parathyroid glands and among glands within a single individual
  - Polar regions of parathyroid are more cellular than are central regions
  - Cellularity decreases with age and varies with gender, ethnicity, and body habitus
- **Features helpful in differentiating parathyroid from thyroid**
  - Parathyroid cells have well-defined cytoplasmic membranes (very helpful feature in differentiating parathyroid from thyroid)
  - Cytoplasmic lipid (fat droplets) common in parathyroid cell cytoplasm (not in thyroid)
  - Parathyroid cells are smaller and more vacuolated than thyroid cells
  - Parathyroid nuclei have rounder and denser chromatin than thyroid nuclei
  - Parathyroid lacks birefringent calcium oxalate crystals seen in thyroid
  - Parathyroid lacks colloid

Immunohistochemistry

- Positive for neuroendocrine markers chromogranin and synaptophysin
- Positive for keratin (CAM5.2 is most helpful keratin for neuroendocrine tumors)
- Negative for TTF-1, thyroglobulin, calcitonin (usually, but calcitonin can be variable in staining, thus panel of immunostains is often helpful)
- Positive for parathyroid hormone but less intense staining in adenomas compared to normal parathyroid or rim of normal parathyroid
- Increased p27 (cyclin-dependent kinase inhibitor protein) in parathyroid adenomas compared to carcinomas
- Adenomas are positive for p27, Bcl-2, and MDM2, and have low Ki-67 labeling index (< 4%)
- Carcinomas often low/absent p27, MDM2, and higher Ki-67 labeling index (> 4%)
- Parafibromin (encoded by *HRPT2*)
  - Loss of nuclear parafibromin in *HRPT2*-associated parathyroid carcinomas and adenomas
  - Sporadic adenomas are usually positive for parafibromin, and many carcinomas show loss of parafibromin
  - Parathyroid carcinomas in hemodialysis patients can show staining in parathyroid carcinomas and metastasis
  - Parafibromin immunostaining shows some promise, but reproducibility and variability in interpretation of this immunostain needs to be confirmed

Cytogenetics

- Chromosome 11: Frequent loss in adenomas and frequent gain in carcinomas

Molecular Genetics

- Study of uncommon familial syndromes has helped to define the pathophysiology of both familial and sporadic parathyroid neoplasms
  - Tumor suppressor genes *MEN1* and *HRPT2* were discovered through genetic analysis of kindreds with MEN1 and HPT-JT
  - Somatic mutations in *MEN1* and *HRPT2* are frequent events in the clonal development of sporadic parathyroid adenomas and carcinomas, respectively
- *HRPT2* mutation (tumor suppressor gene, 1q21-q31, encodes parafibromin)
  - Germline *HRPT2*-inactivating mutation in HPT-JT syndrome-associated parathyroid adenoma or hyperplasia and increased risk of parathyroid carcinoma
  - Germline *HRPT2* mutations have been identified in subset of patients with mutation-positive carcinomas (consider genetic testing in patients with parathyroid carcinoma)
  - Somatic *HRPT2* mutations are common in sporadic parathyroid carcinomas and rare in sporadic adenomas
  - Strong association with *HRPT2* mutation and familial and sporadic parathyroid cancer
- Cyclin-D1/*CCND1* oncogene (11q13)
  - 5-8% of parathyroid adenomas have genetic alterations in cyclin-D1/*CCND1* (parathyroid adenoma) gene
  - Cyclin-D1/*CCND1* encodes cyclin-D1, a cell cycle regulator from G1 to S phase transition

Parathyroid Adenoma vs. Carcinoma

Feature	Parathyroid Adenoma	Parathyroid Carcinoma
Symptoms	Usually asymptomatic or vague	Often symptomatic
Serum calcium	Elevated	Markedly elevated (> 13 mg/dL)
Palpable mass	Unusual	Yes
Tumor size	Enlarged	Larger but may overlap
Invasion into adjacent structures	No (but can have irregular growth and cells in capsule due to degenerative features)	Yes
Fibrous bands	Can be present due to degenerative features	Yes
Perineural invasion	No	Yes
Vascular invasion	No	Yes
Growth pattern	Patterns of growth (follicular, acinar, etc.)	Monotonous, sheet-like growth
Cellular features	Often mixed cell types, can show endocrine atypia	Often monotonous cytomorphology, prominent nucleoli
Mitoses	Few, scattered	Yes, more numerous mitoses than adenomas
Proliferation markers (Ki-67/MIB-1)	Low	Moderate to high

Parathyroid and Thyroid Immunohistochemistry

Tissue	Keratin	TTF-1	PTH	Chro	Syn	Calcitonin
Parathyroid cells and tumors	Positive (particularly low molecular weight keratins, e.g., CAM5.2)	Negative	Positive (but often not an overly robust stain)	Positive	Positive	Negative
Thyroid follicular cells and neoplasms	Positive	Positive (strong nuclear staining)	Negative	Negative	Negative	Negative
Medullary thyroid carcinoma	Positive (particularly low molecular weight keratins, e.g., CAM5.2)	Positive (nuclear staining, may not be as strong as in follicular cells and neoplasms)	Negative	Positive	Positive	Positive

Chro: Chromogranin; Syn: Synaptophysin.

  - Cyclin-D1 protein overexpression observed in up to 40% of adenomas
- *MEN1* mutation (tumor suppressor gene, 11q13, results in truncated menin protein)
  - Parathyroid adenomas and carcinomas occur in MEN1, but parathyroid hyperplasia occurs more commonly
  - Up to 40% of sporadic parathyroid adenomas have loss of 1 *MEN1* allele, and 1/2 of these have inactivating mutation in 2nd allele
- *RET* mutation (proto-oncogene, 10q11.2)
  - Germline *RET*-activating mutation in MEN2A (95% mutation in exon 10 or 11, codon 634)
  - 30% of patients with MEN2A have parathyroid hyperplasia, but adenomas can also occur
  - *RET* mutation is generally not identified in sporadic parathyroid disease

DIAGNOSTIC CHECKLIST

Clinically Relevant Pathologic Features

- Often asymptomatic, identified by screening calcium
- Serum calcium elevated, but markedly elevated serum calcium (> 13 mg/dL) worrisome for carcinoma

Pathologic Interpretation Pearls

- Composed of chief, oxyphilic, transitional, clear, or mixtures of cell types
- Parathyroid (unlike thyroid) has well-demarcated cytoplasmic membranes, cytoplasmic lipid, round nuclei, and dense chromatin and lacks colloid and calcium oxylate crystals
- Normal parathyroid tissue shows significant variation in cellularity within and among glands
- Rims of normal tissue in 50-60% of adenomas, but can be seen in hyperplasia

SELECTED REFERENCES

1. DeLellis RA: Parathyroid tumors and related disorders. Mod Pathol. 24 Suppl 2:S78-93, 2011
2. Zhang Y et al: Endocrine tumors as part of inherited tumor syndromes. Adv Anat Pathol. 18(3):206-18, 2011
3. Chow LS et al: Parathyroid lipoadenomas: a rare cause of primary hyperparathyroidism. Endocr Pract. 12(2):131-6, 2006
4. Prasad KK et al: Water-clear cell adenoma of the parathyroid gland: a rare entity. Indian J Pathol Microbiol. 47(1):39-40, 2004
5. DeLellis RA et al: Paraneoplastic endocrine syndromes: a review. Endocr Pathol. 14(4):303-17, 2003

PARATHYROID ADENOMA

Gross and Microscopic Features

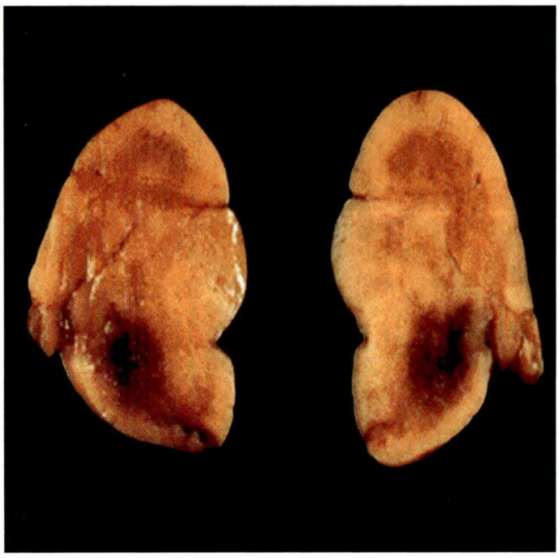

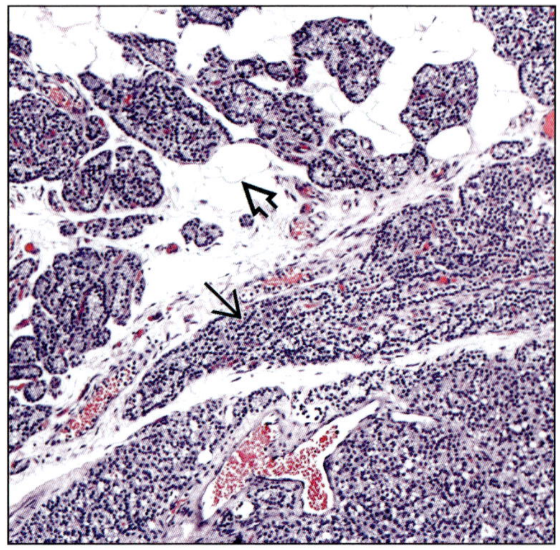

(Left) *Parathyroid adenoma is a single enlarged parathyroid gland, usually 0.2 to > 1 g. The cut surface of a parathyroid adenoma is usually homogeneous tan-yellow to tan-red with focal areas of hemorrhage.* ***(Right)*** *Chief cell parathyroid adenoma* → *shows adjacent rim of normal* ⇨ *parathyroid tissue, a feature often identified in smaller rather than larger adenomas. The rim is often separated from the adenoma by connective tissue.*

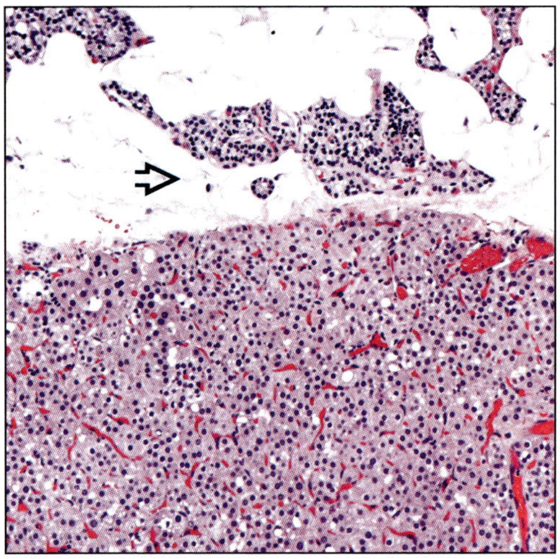

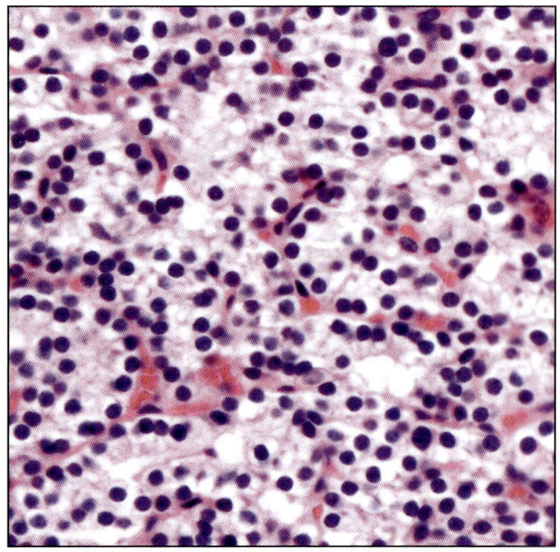

(Left) *Oxyphil parathyroid adenoma shows a rim of normal parathyroid* ⇨*. Oxyphil adenomas are usually functional tumors and are associated with levels of serum calcium that are similar to those seen in chief cell adenomas.* ***(Right)*** *This chief cell parathyroid adenoma has a nested growth pattern and prominent vascularity. The nuclei are round. The cytoplasm of the chief cells is eosinophilic to amphophilic. The cells do not show significant nuclear pleomorphism or mitotic activity.*

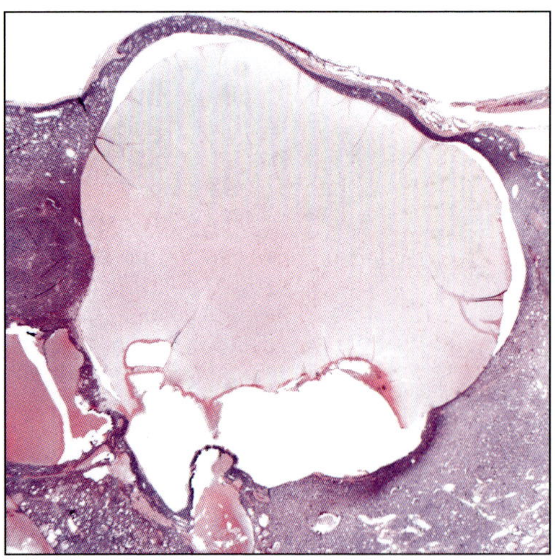

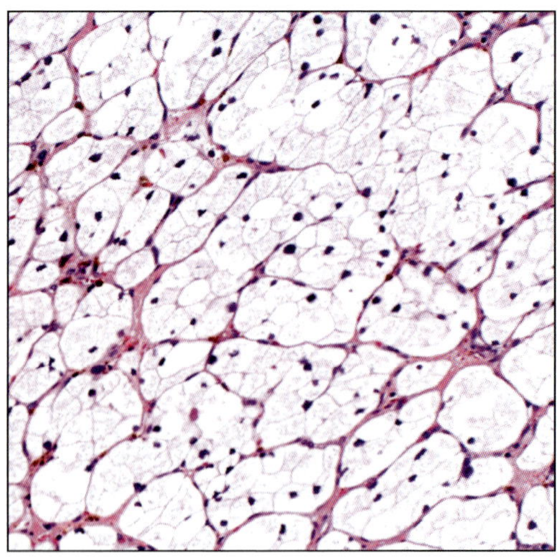

(Left) *Varying degrees of cystic change can be seen in parathyroid adenomas. Cystic change is particularly common in larger parathyroid adenomas and those associated with hyperparathyroidism-jaw tumor syndrome (HPT-JT). HPT-JT is an autosomal dominant disorder caused by inactivating mutations in HRPT2 gene that encodes parafibromin.* ***(Right)*** *This clear (water-clear/wasserhelle) cell parathyroid adenoma is composed of large polyhedral cells with distinct plasma membranes and extensively vacuolated cytoplasm.*

Microscopic Features

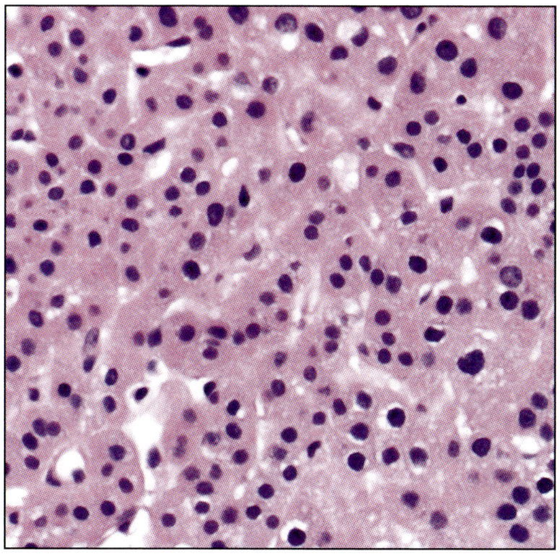
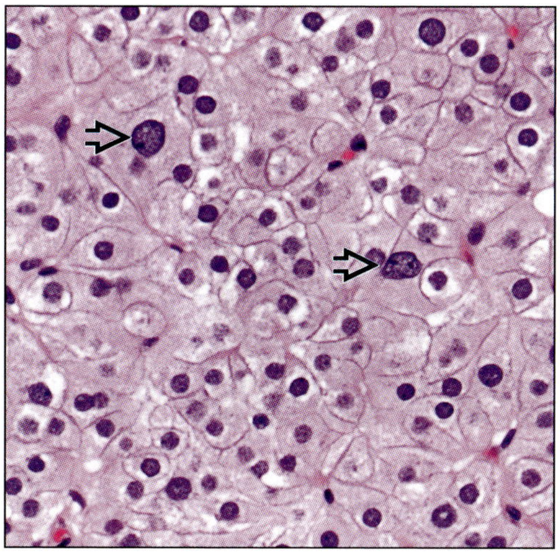

(Left) *Oxyphil cells (10-20 μm) are larger than chief cells (10 μm) and have abundant eosinophilic granular cytoplasm. Oxyphil cell adenomas are uncommon, comprising approximately 3-6% of parathyroid adenomas.* ***(Right)*** *Foci of nuclear pleomorphism (endocrine atypia) ⇨ can be seen in oxyphil cell adenomas. Well-defined cytoplasmic membranes of parathyroid cells help to differentiate parathyroid from thyroid.*

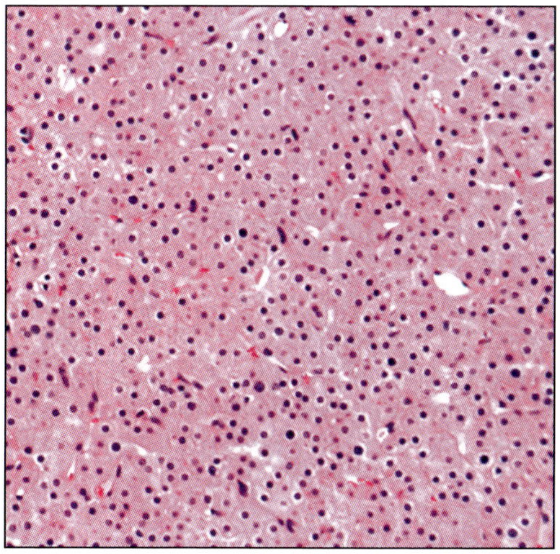
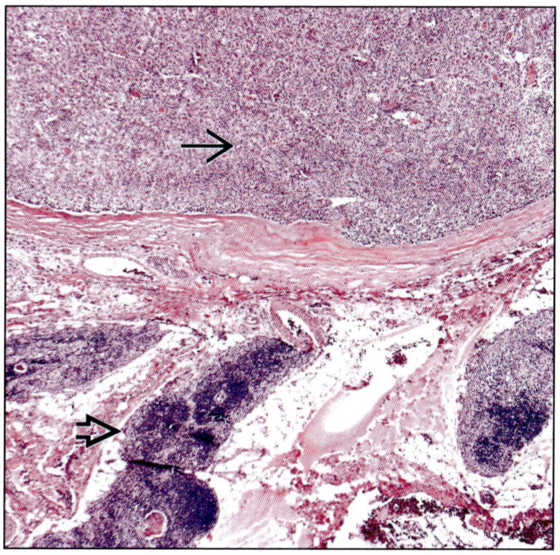

(Left) *Oxyphil adenomas are composed exclusively or predominantly (> 90%) of mitochondrion-rich oxyphil cells. Although originally thought to be nonfunctional, oxyphil adenomas are now recognized as usually functional tumors.* ***(Right)*** *This parathyroid chief cell adenoma → is present within the thymus ⇨. Approximately 10% of parathyroid adenomas occur in unusual locations, such as intrathyroidal or within mediastinum, thymus, or soft tissues behind the esophagus and pharynx.*

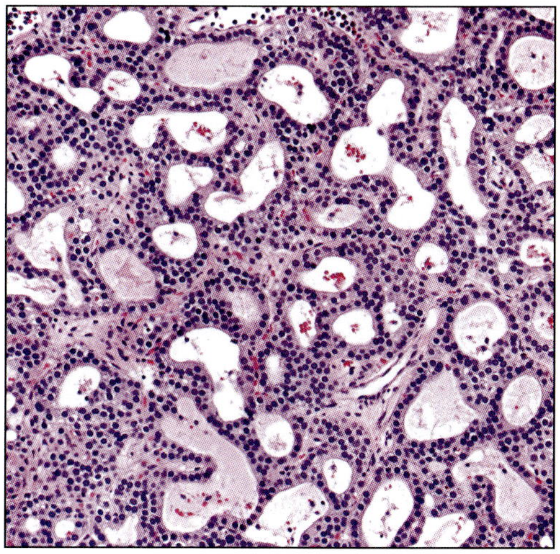
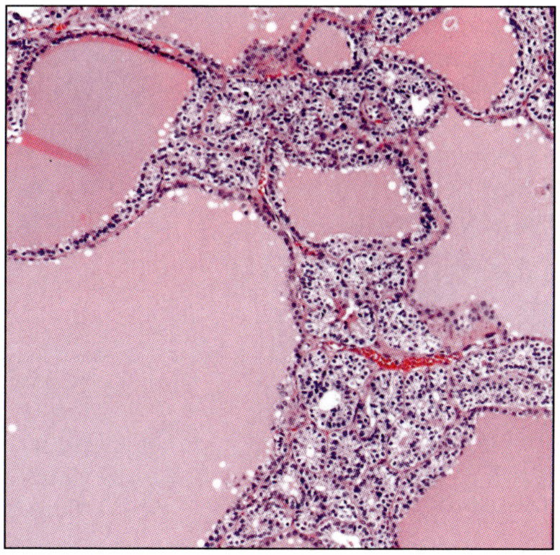

(Left) *This chief cell adenoma has a follicular growth pattern. Patterns such as this are commonly seen in parathyroid adenomas, unlike the monotonous or trabecular growth of parathyroid carcinomas.* ***(Right)*** *Follicular patterns are relatively common in parathyroid adenoma. Occasionally, parathyroid adenomas may show large follicular-like spaces with proteinaceous fluid and can be mistaken for thyroid follicles. (Courtesy L. Erickson, MD.)*

PARATHYROID CARCINOMA

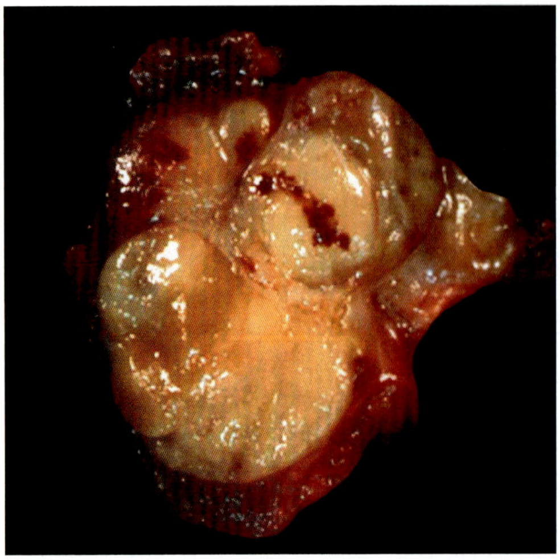

Cut section of a parathyroid carcinoma shows a firm yellow-gray, nodular cut surface invading into adjacent structures. (Courtesy L. Erickson, MD.)

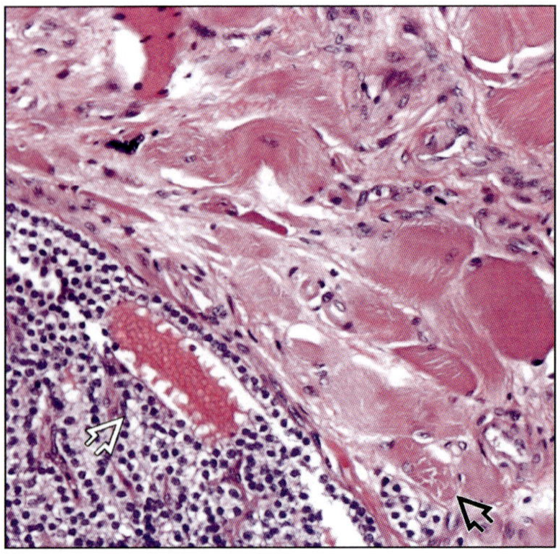

Parathyroid carcinoma ➡ is invading into the sternocleidomastoid muscle ⇨. Invasive growth is diagnostic of malignancy in parathyroid.

TERMINOLOGY

Abbreviations

- Parathyroid carcinoma (PC)

Definitions

- Malignant neoplasm of parathyroid parenchymal cells (chief cells, oxyphilic cells, transitional cells, water/ clear cells, or mixtures of cell types)

ETIOLOGY/PATHOGENESIS

Inherited

- Most parathyroid carcinomas are sporadic but increased incidence in patients with hyperparathyroidism-jaw tumor syndrome (HPT-JT)

HPT-JT

- Autosomal dominant disorder of hyperparathyroidism, fibroosseous jaw tumors, kidney cysts, hamartomas, and Wilms tumors
- Inactivating mutation tumor suppressor gene *HRPT2* (1q21-q31) that encodes parafibromin
- Parathyroid hyperplasia, adenoma, or carcinoma
  - 15% with HPT-JT develop parathyroid carcinoma
- Germline *HRPT2* mutations identified in a subset of patients with *HRPT2* mutation-positive carcinomas

Familial Isolated Hyperparathyroidism (FIH)

- Autosomal dominant, accounts for 1% of primary hyperparathyroidism (parathyroid is only endocrine organ involved), adenoma, or hyperplasia
- Increased risk of parathyroid carcinoma has been reported but may be due to inclusion of HPT-JT cases
- Cause unknown in most families, but *HRPT2* gene, *MEN1* gene, and area on chromosome 2 implicated

Multiple Endocrine Neoplasia Type 1 (MEN1)

- Autosomal dominant, high penetrance, germline mutation in *MEN1* tumor suppressor gene (11q13); results in truncated menin protein
- 20% of patients with primary parathyroid hyperplasia have MEN1, but only rare case of parathyroid carcinoma reported in MEN1
- Loss of heterozygosity and somatic *MEN1* mutations identified in some parathyroid carcinomas
- Somatic *MEN1* mutations occur in 15-20% of sporadic adenomas and occasionally in sporadic carcinomas

Multiple Endocrine Neoplasia 2A (MEN2A)

- 20-30% with MEN2A have parathyroid hyperplasia or adenoma (only rare reports of carcinoma)

Sporadic

- Predisposing factors poorly understood, possible association with prior ionizing radiation
- Reports of parathyroid carcinoma occurring in setting of secondary parathyroid hyperplasia

CLINICAL ISSUES

Epidemiology

- Incidence
  - 1-2% of primary hyperparathyroidism (parathyroid adenoma: 80-85%; parathyroid hyperplasia: 15%)
  - Reports: Up to 5% of hyperparathyroidism due to carcinoma in Italy and Japan
- Age
  - Middle-aged and older adults (mid 40s to mid 50s; 1 decade earlier than parathyroid adenomas)
- Gender
  - Males and females are equally affected (unlike adenomas, which are more frequent in females)

Site

- Arises in site of parathyroid gland

PARATHYROID CARCINOMA

Key Facts

Terminology
- Malignant parathyroid parenchymal neoplasm

Etiology/Pathogenesis
- Most parathyroid carcinomas are sporadic, but increased incidence in patients with HPT-JT
- **HPT-JT**: Autosomal dominant disorder of hyperparathyroidism, fibroosseous jaw tumors, kidney cysts, hamartomas, and Wilms tumors
- **FIH**: Autosomal dominant, accounts for 1% of primary hyperparathyroidism: Adenoma or hyperplasia
- **MEN1**: Autosomal dominant; only rare case of parathyroid carcinoma reported in MEN1
- **MEN2A**: 20-30% with MEN2A have parathyroid hyperplasia or adenoma with only rare reports of carcinoma

Clinical Issues
- Markedly elevated serum calcium (> 13 mg/dL), PTH, alkaline phosphatase
- *HRPT2* mutations in familial and some sporadic, can be new germline mutation

Microscopic Pathology
- Require invasive growth with capsular, vascular, perineural, or invasion into adjacent structures
- Histologic features in sporadic and HPT-JT parathyroid lesions similar, but HPT-JT lesions may be cystic

Ancillary Tests
- Positive for chromogranin, synaptophysin, CAM5.2, PTH; negative for TTF-1, thyroglobulin, calcitonin
- Loss of parafibromin nuclear staining in many

  - Similar to parathyroid adenomas, carcinomas can also occur in ectopic sites
  - Slightly more common in lower parathyroid glands

Presentation
- Most parathyroid carcinomas are functional and patients are symptomatic, but nonfunctional tumors occur
- Palpable neck mass (unusual for adenoma)
- Local recurrence of a parathyroid adenoma is worrisome for carcinoma but can be parathyromatosis

Laboratory Tests
- Extremely high serum calcium levels (> 13 mg/dL) more common in carcinoma
- Markedly elevated PTH levels (> 1,000 ng/L)
- High serum alkaline phosphatase activity (> 200 IU/L)

Natural History
- Usually recur 1st in neck then metastasize to cervical and mediastinal lymph nodes, lung, bone, and liver

Treatment
- Surgical approaches
  - First-line treatment is en block resection of parathyroid tumor and surrounding structures, usually ipsilateral thyroid lobe at 1st surgery (better local control and disease-free survival)
  - Risk progression associated with margin status
- Drugs
  - Inoperable parathyroid carcinoma management may include calcimimetics to control hypercalcemia and bisphosphonates to control bone resorption
  - Chemotherapy effectiveness unclear
  - Few reports of immunomodulating therapeutic approaches with vaccines
- Radiation
  - Patients treated with surgery and postoperative radiation may have lower risk of locoregional progression and improved cause-specific survival

Prognosis
- 5-year survival up to 85%, 10-year survival is 49%

IMAGE FINDINGS

General Features
- Tc-99m sestamibi scintigraphy or sonography identifies location but does not separate adenoma from carcinoma
- Mass noted on CT and MR, often no specific features

MACROSCOPIC FEATURES

General Features
- Firm tumors, may be adherent to or invasive into adjacent structures
  - Caution as large parathyroid adenomas, especially with cystic change, can become fibrotic and adhere to adjacent structures
  - May be grossly encapsulated and resemble adenomas

Size
- Large tumors (mean = 6.7 g, range from 1.5-27 g); larger than adenomas but overlap in size

MICROSCOPIC PATHOLOGY

Histologic Features
- Hypercellular parathyroid with invasive growth (invasion into adjacent structures, capsular, vascular, or perineural invasion)
- Capsular invasion of tumor beyond thickened capsule identified in 60%
- Fibrous bands common (up to 90%) but not specific
- Invasion of vessels in thickened capsule or surrounding soft tissue (most specific feature for carcinoma but seen in 15% of cases)
- Perineural invasion
- Solid growth pattern with sheets of cells or closely packed nests or trabecular growth but can show follicular or other growth patterns

PARATHYROID CARCINOMA

- Cellular monotony is common, but occasional cases are pleomorphic
- Mitotic figures identified in at least 80% of carcinomas but also in up to 70% of adenomas
- Atypical mitoses limited to parathyroid carcinoma
- Suggested that triad of macronucleoli, > 5 mitoses per 50 high-power fields, and necrosis is associated with aggressive behavior in parathyroid carcinoma
- Histologic features in sporadic and HPT-JT parathyroid lesions similar, but HPT-JT lesions may be cystic
- Parathyroid carcinomas can be composed entirely of oxyphil (oxyphil parathyroid carcinoma) or clear cells (clear cell parathyroid carcinoma)
  - Same criteria used to diagnose these variants

ANCILLARY TESTS

Immunohistochemistry

- Positive for chromogranin and synaptophysin
- Positive for keratin (CAM5.2 most helpful keratin for neuroendocrine tumors)
- Positive for parathyroid hormone
- Negative for TTF-1, thyroglobulin, calcitonin (usually)
- Ki-67 (MIB-1) elevated > 4 (higher than in adenomas)
- p27 (cyclin-dependent kinase inhibitor protein) decreased expression in parathyroid carcinomas compared to adenomas
- Carcinomas often low/absent p27, MDM2, and higher Ki-67 labeling index
  - Adenomas often positive for p27, Bcl-2, and MDM2 and low Ki-67 labeling index
- Keratin 14 reported negative in oxyphil carcinomas and positive in oxyphil adenomas
- Parafibromin
  - *HRPT2* encodes parafibromin
  - Loss of nuclear parafibromin in *HRPT2*-associated parathyroid carcinomas and adenomas
  - Sporadic parathyroid adenomas are usually positive for parafibromin whereas many carcinomas show loss of parafibromin
  - Parathyroid carcinomas in hemodialysis patients can show staining in primary and metastasis
  - Parafibromin shows some promise, but reproducibility and variability in interpretation need to be confirmed

Cytogenetics

- Loss of 1p and 13q relatively common in parathyroid carcinomas whereas loss of 11q (*MEN1* gene location) most common abnormality in parathyroid adenoma
- Loss of chromosome 11 common in parathyroid adenoma; gain of chromosome 11 in carcinoma, particularly in those who died of disease
- Loss of heterozygosity on 13q (*RB* and *BRCA2* gene location) in carcinomas, but specific abnormalities of *RB* or *BRCA2* not identified by sequencing

Molecular Genetics

- *HRPT2* mutation (tumor suppressor gene, 1q21-q31, encodes parafibromin)
  - Strong association *HRPT2* mutation in familial and sporadic parathyroid cancer
    - *HRPT2* mutation uncommon in sporadic adenomas but identified in 20% of sporadic cystic adenomas
  - 15% with HPT-JT (caused by germline *HRPT2* inactivating mutation) develop parathyroid carcinoma
  - Germline *HRPT2* mutations identified in a subset of patients with mutation-positive carcinomas
    - Consider genetic testing in patients with parathyroid carcinoma
- *MEN1* mutation (tumor suppressor gene, 11q13, results in truncated menin protein)
  - Somatic *MEN1* mutations in 15-20% of sporadic adenomas and some sporadic carcinomas
  - Loss of heterozygosity and somatic *MEN1* mutations in some parathyroid carcinomas
  - Only a rare case of parathyroid carcinoma identified in MEN1
- *RET* mutation (proto-oncogene, 10q11.2)
  - Only rare case reports of parathyroid carcinomas in setting of MEN2A
- Cyclin-D1/*CCND1* (11q13)
  - Genetic alterations in cyclin-D1/*CCND1* (parathyroid adenoma) gene, 11q13, in 5-8% of parathyroid neoplasms
  - Loss of chromosome 11 frequent in parathyroid adenomas, and frequent chromosomal gain in parathyroid carcinomas in FISH studies
  - Cyclin-D1/*CCND1* encodes cyclin-D1 (regulator of cell cycle progression from G1 to S phase), and cyclin-D1 overexpression observed in neoplastic parathyroid
    - Lack of definitive genotype-phenotype correlation limits utility

SELECTED REFERENCES

1. DeLellis RA: Parathyroid tumors and related disorders. Mod Pathol. 24 Suppl 2:S78-93, 2011
2. Fang SH et al: Parathyroid cancer. Endocr Pract. 17 Suppl 1:36-43, 2011
3. Witteveen JE et al: Downregulation of CASR expression and global loss of parafibromin staining are strong negative determinants of prognosis in parathyroid carcinoma. Mod Pathol. 24(5):688-97, 2011
4. Zhang Y et al: Endocrine tumors as part of inherited tumor syndromes. Adv Anat Pathol. 18(3):206-18, 2011
5. Okamoto T et al: Parathyroid carcinoma: etiology, diagnosis, and treatment. World J Surg. 33(11):2343-54, 2009
6. Delellis RA: Challenging lesions in the differential diagnosis of endocrine tumors: parathyroid carcinoma. Endocr Pathol. 19(4):221-5, 2008
7. Erickson LA et al: Oxyphil parathyroid carcinomas: a clinicopathologic and immunohistochemical study of 10 cases. Am J Surg Pathol. 26(3):344-9, 2002
8. Sandelin K et al: Prognostic factors in parathyroid cancer: a review of 95 cases. World J Surg. 16(4):724-31, 1992

Microscopic Features

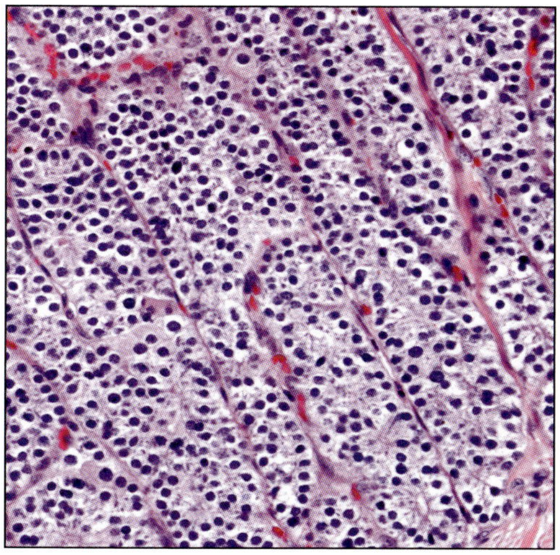
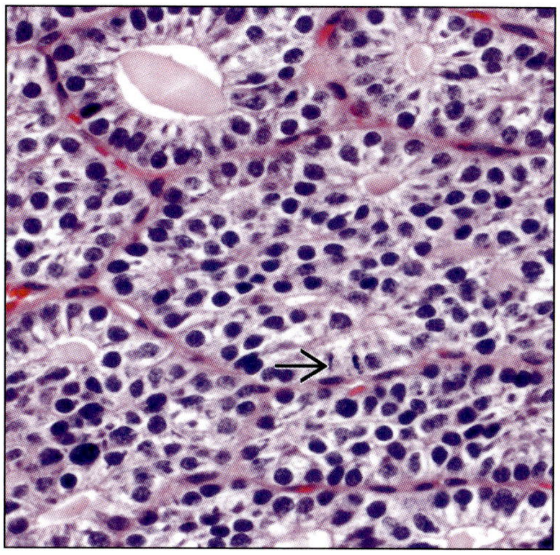

(Left) *Parathyroid carcinoma shows a trabecular growth pattern. Parathyroid carcinomas usually have monotonous or trabecular growth. Other patterns of growth (follicular, acinar) are less common. The cytomorphology of the constituent cells is generally monotonous.* ***(Right)*** *Nested and acinar growth is shown in parathyroid carcinoma with a mitotic figure →. Mitoses are commonly identified in parathyroid carcinoma but can also be found in adenomas.*

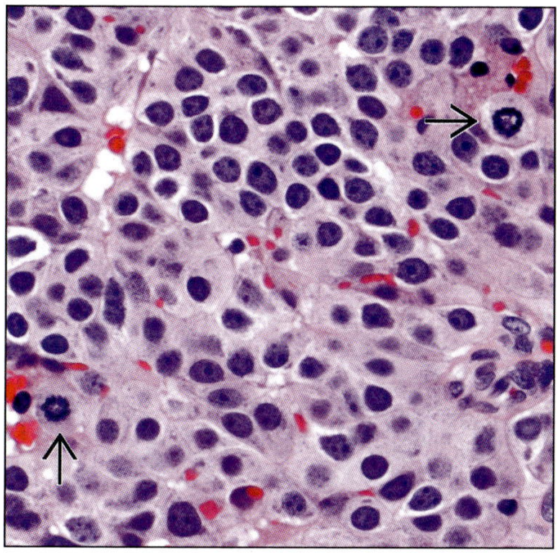
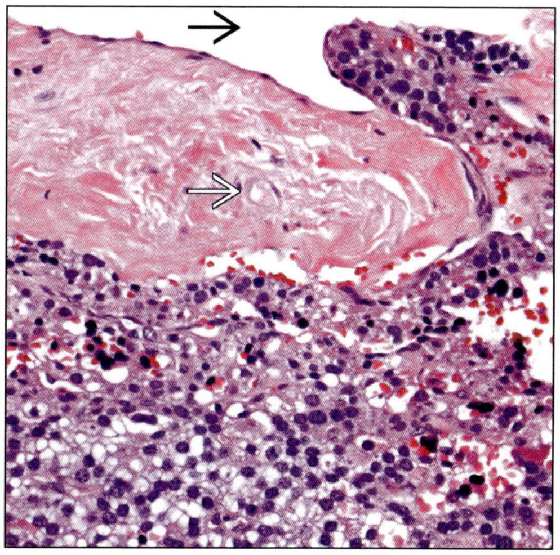

(Left) *Parathyroid carcinoma shows mitotic figures →. Oxyphil carcinomas are usually functional and much larger than oxyphil adenomas. Similar to conventional parathyroid carcinomas, invasion is required to diagnose malignancy.* ***(Right)*** *Parathyroid carcinoma invades through the capsule ➔ into a vascular space →. (Courtesy L. Erickson, MD.)*

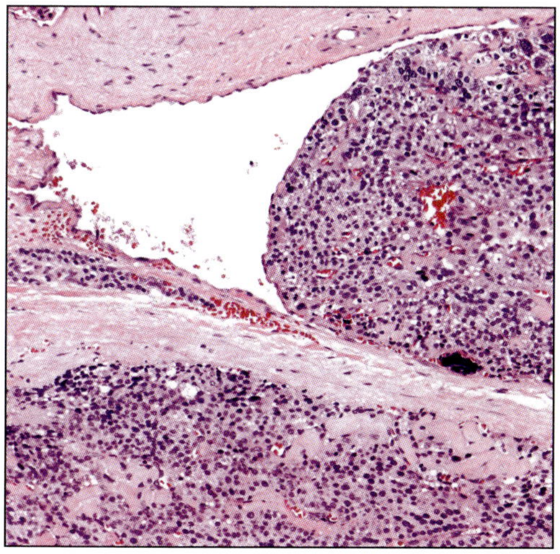
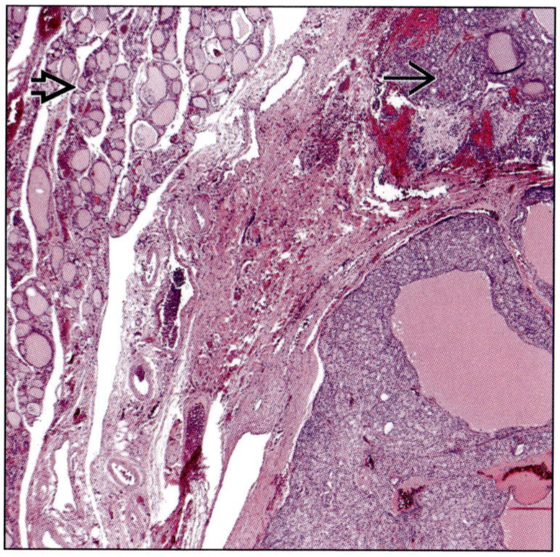

(Left) *Tumor thrombus is seen in a vessel within the thickened capsule of a parathyroid carcinoma. Vascular invasion is essentially diagnostic of malignancy in parathyroid.* ***(Right)*** *Parathyroid carcinoma → is invading into the perithyroidal tissue (thyroid parenchyma ⇨). Invasive growth, including invasion into adjacent structures, is diagnostic of malignancy in parathyroid carcinoma. (Courtesy L. Erickson, MD.)*

PARATHYROID HYPERPLASIA

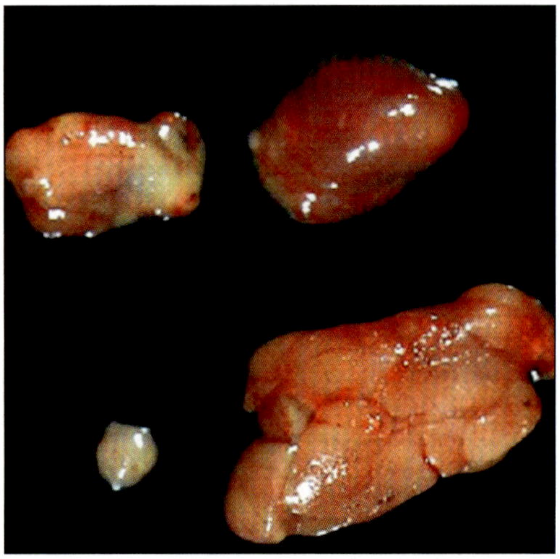

This picture shows 4 enlarged parathyroid glands with a great variability in glandular size (asymmetric hyperplasia), which can distinguish parathyroid hyperplasia from adenoma.

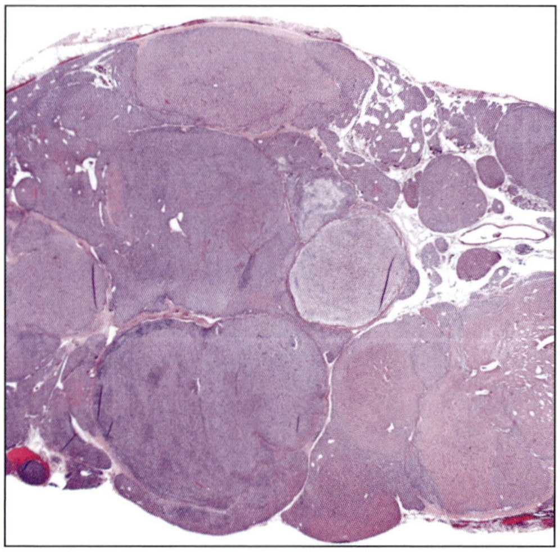

Asymmetric hyperplasia, a.k.a. pseudoadenomatous variant of hyperplasia with marked variation in extent of glandular involvement, is easily confused with adenoma or multiple adenomas.

TERMINOLOGY

Synonyms

- Nodular hyperplasia
- Primary parathyroid hyperplasia
- Secondary parathyroid hyperplasia
- Multiple adenomatosis

Definitions

- Absolute increase in parathyroid parenchymal mass resulting from proliferation of chief, oxyphil, and transitional cells in multiple parathyroid glands in absence of recognized stimulus for parathyroid hormone (PTH) secretion

ETIOLOGY/PATHOGENESIS

Sporadic Primary Hyperparathyroidism

- Etiology of sporadic primary hyperplasia is unclear

Familial Hyperparathyroidism

- Hereditary hyperparathyroidism is less common than primary sporadic hyperparathyroidism
- Most common hereditary hyperparathyroidism includes
  - Multiple endocrine neoplasia type 1 (MEN1), multiple endocrine neoplasia type 2A (MEN2A), familial hypocalciuric hypercalcemia, neonatal severe primary hyperparathyroidism, hyperparathyroidism-jaw tumor syndrome (HPT-JT), and familial isolated hyperparathyroidism
- **MEN1**
  - Autosomal dominant due to germline mutation *MEN1* tumor suppressor gene (11q13)
    - Encodes menin (truncated with *MEN1* mutation)
    - Sporadic MEN1 cases due to new mutations
  - MEN1 equally affects females and males; no ethnic or geographic differences
  - Primary parathyroid hyperplasia (multiglandular parathyroid tumors) is the most common manifestation of MEN1
  - 90% of patients with MEN1 have primary parathyroid hyperplasia, and 20% of patients with primary parathyroid hyperplasia have MEN1
  - MEN1-associated hyperparathyroidism has onset of 20-25 years of age and affects males and females equally
  - Parathyroid adenomas and rare report of carcinoma in MEN1, but much less common than hyperplasia
- **MEN2A**
  - Autosomal dominant, high penetrance, germline *RET*-activating proto-oncogene mutation (10q11.2)
  - 20-30% of MEN2A cases are associated with parathyroid hyperplasia (or adenomas; rare report of carcinoma)
  - MEN2A is diagnosed clinically by occurrence of at least 2 specific endocrine tumors
    - Medullary thyroid carcinoma, pheochromocytoma, or parathyroid hyperplasia/adenoma in individual or close relatives
- **HPT-JT**
  - Autosomal dominant, inactivating mutations in putative tumor suppressor gene *HRPT2* (1q21-q31) that encodes parafibromin
  - Disorder of hyperparathyroidism, fibroosseus jaw tumors, kidney cysts, hamartomas, and Wilms tumors
  - Parathyroid hyperplasia or adenoma and increased risk of parathyroid carcinoma
- **Familial isolated hyperparathyroidism**
  - Autosomal dominant
  - 1% of primary hyperparathyroidism (parathyroid is only endocrine organ involved)
    - Adenoma or hyperplasia and suggested increased risk of parathyroid carcinoma (but may be due to inclusion of HPT-JT cases)

PARATHYROID HYPERPLASIA

Key Facts

Terminology

- Absolute increase in parathyroid parenchymal mass resulting from proliferation of chief, oxyphil, and transitional cells in multiple parathyroid glands in absence of recognized stimulus for parathyroid hormone (PTH) secretion

Etiology/Pathogenesis

- Hereditary hyperparathyroidism is less common than primary sporadic hyperparathyroidism
- **Hyperparathyroidism jaw-tumor syndrome**
  - Autosomal dominant, inactivating mutations in putative tumor suppressor gene *HRPT2* that encodes parafibromin
- **Multiple endocrine neoplasia type 1 (MEN1)**
  - Autosomal dominant; germline mutation *MEN1* tumor suppressor gene that encodes menin
- **Familial isolated hyperparathyroidism**
  - Autosomal dominant; parathyroid only endocrine organ involved; adenoma or hyperplasia, and suggested increased risk of parathyroid carcinoma
- **Multiple endocrine neoplasia type 2A (MEN2A)**
  - Autosomal dominant; germline *RET*-activating proto-oncogene mutation
- **Calcium-sensing receptor** (*CASR*) **mutation**
  - Inactivating *CASR* (3q13.3-21) mutation causes decreased calcium sensitivity of parathyroid and kidney and results in PTH-dependent hypercalcemia
  - **Familial hypocalciuric hypercalcemia**
  - **Familial autosomal dominant hypoparathyroidism and familial hypocalcemia**
  - **Neonatal severe hyperparathyroidism**

  - Cause is unknown in most families, but *HRPT2* gene, *MEN1* gene, and area on chromosome 2 have been implicated
- Calcium-sensing receptor (*CASR*) mutation
  - Inactivating *CASR* (3q13.3-21) mutation causes decreased calcium sensitivity of parathyroid and kidney and results in PTH-dependent hypercalcemia
  - CASRs detect extracellular calcium levels that regulate PTH release
    - Present in parathyroid, kidney, thyroid C cells, intestine, and bone
  - **Neonatal severe primary hyperparathyroidism**
    - Homozygous inactivating *CASR* mutations
    - Life-threatening disorder with markedly hypercellular, hyperplastic parathyroid glands
    - Autosomal recessive
  - **Familial hypocalciuric hypercalcemia**
    - Heterozygous inactivating *CASR* mutations in familial hypocalciuric hypercalcemia
  - **Familial autosomal dominant hypoparathyroidism and familial hypocalcemia**
    - Activating *CASR* mutations in familial autosomal dominant hypoparathyroidism and familial hypocalcemia
  - **Hypocalciuric hypercalcemia**
    - Caused by autoantibodies directed at *CASR* and can simulate familial hypocalciuric hypercalcemia

Secondary Hyperparathyroidism

- Secondary to numerous stimuli
  - Most commonly seen secondary to renal failure

CLINICAL ISSUES

Epidemiology

- Incidence
  - Primary parathyroid hyperplasia accounts for 15% of primary hyperparathyroidism (parathyroid adenomas, 80-85%; carcinomas, 1%)
  - Incidence increased in past 3 decades with increased calcium screening with multichannel autoanalyzer
  - Parathyroid hyperplasia occurs in 90% of patients with MEN1 and in 30% with MEN2A
  - 20% of patients with primary parathyroid hyperplasia have MEN 1 or MEN2A
  - Prevalence of 7% in autopsy study (patients had elevated serum calcium but no bone disease)
- Age
  - Sporadic form typically presents in 5th decade but can manifest during a wide age range
  - Familial cases occur earlier (often 20-25 years of age)

Presentation

- Primary hyperparathyroidism (HPT) results from excessive secretion of parathyroid hormone from parathyroid tumors
- Most HPT cases are sporadic, but a minority of cases are associated with a familial syndrome
- HPT in its hereditary variants assumes special forms, has special associations, and requires special managements
- Familial hypocalciuric hypercalcemia (FHH) and neonatal severe primary hyperparathyroidism (NSHPT) reflect heterozygous and homozygous mutations, respectively, in the calcium-sensing receptor
  - FHH represents mildest variant of HPT whereas NSHPT represents severest form of HPT
  - Both FHH and NSHPT cause hypercalcemia from birth and atypical HPT that always and uniquely persists after subtotal parathyroidectomy
  - HPT resulting from FHH and NSHPT is likely polyclonal and nonneoplastic
- In contrast, monoclonal or oligoclonal parathyroid neoplasia underlies most other HPT variants: MEN1, MEN2A, and HPT-JT

Treatment

- Surgical approaches
  - Subtotal parathyroidectomy with 3 glands removed, leaving vascularized remnant of 4th gland, **or**
  - Total parathyroidectomy with autotransplantation of portion of parathyroid gland into neck or forearm

PARATHYROID HYPERPLASIA

  - Rapid intraoperative PTH measurements decrease risk of missing multiglandular disease and help confirm removal of diseased parathyroid gland(s)
  - Difficult or impossible to differentiate primary hyperplasia from adenoma based only on intraoperative examination of 1 gland
 - Residual tissue may become hyperplastic, requiring additional surgery
 - Concurrent transcervical thymectomy is also suggested at time of parathyroidectomy

MACROSCOPIC FEATURES

General Features

- Some reports indicate that 50% of cases show symmetric enlargement of all 4 glands; however, other studies report that in ~ 66% of cases, only 2 glands appear enlarged
- Asymmetric hyperplasia or pseudoadenomatous variant of hyperplasia with marked variation in parathyroid glands size
- Surgeons and pathologists must be cautious in evaluating parathyroid glands in relation to size and cellularity as these parameters can vary greatly within a single patient with parathyroid hyperplasia
  - Asymmetrically enlarged gland can be misinterpreted as parathyroid adenoma

MICROSCOPIC PATHOLOGY

Histologic Features

- **Primary parathyroid hyperplasia histology**
- Increase in parenchymal cell mass of multiple parathyroid glands
- Chief cell is predominant, but oxyphil, transitional, and clear cells may be present
- Asymmetric hyperplasia or pseudoadenomatous variant of hyperplasia with marked variation in extent of glandular involvement is easily confused with adenoma or multiple adenomas
  - Parathyroid hyperplasia in MEN1 usually involves increased numbers of chief cells that may have nodular or diffuse pattern
  - MEN1-associated hyperplasia is often asymmetric
  - Histologic features in HPT-JT-associated cases are similar to sporadic lesions, but HPT-JT cases are often cystic
- Hyperplastic chief cells are arranged in cords, nests, sheets, or follicular structures
- Scattered mitotic figures may be seen, but more mitoses and atypical mitoses are present in carcinoma
- Cells show slight variation in size and shape
  - Foci of endocrine atypia with pleomorphism and hyperchromasia (more common in adenomas)
- Stromal fat is decreased, but regional variations in stromal fat are present even among glands in a single individual (pitfall in evaluating small biopsies)
- Nodular or diffuse growth
  - Nodular is most common pattern in primary hyperplasia
- Rim of normal parathyroid tissue can rarely be seen but this feature is more common in adenoma
- Fibrosis and hemosiderin, especially in markedly enlarged glands or glands with cystic degeneration
- Cystic change is uncommon but can be seen in markedly enlarged glands
- No capsular, vascular, or perineural invasion or invasion into adjacent structures
- **Primary parathyroid hyperplasia variants**
- **Clear (water-clear) cell hyperplasia**
  - Multiple enlarged parathyroid glands associated with hyperplasia with parenchymal cells having abundant, vacuolated, clear cytoplasm
- **Lipohyperplasia**
  - Enlarged parathyroid glands with hyperparathyroidism, but abundant stromal fat of lipohyperplasia (or lipoadenoma) can be confused with normal parathyroid tissue

ANCILLARY TESTS

Immunohistochemistry

- Positive for PTH, chromogranin, and synaptophysin
- Positive for keratin (CAM5.2 most helpful keratin for neuroendocrine tumors)
- Negative for TTF-1, thyroglobulin, variable calcitonin
- Ki-67 lower in hyperplasia and adenomas than carcinomas

Molecular Genetics

- Parathyroid hyperplasia is often polyclonal, but monoclonality has been identified, particularly in nodular areas and in MEN1 (multiglandular parathyroid tumors)
- Somatic mutations in *MEN1* and *HRPT2* tumor suppressor genes are now recognized as frequent events in sporadic parathyroid adenomas and carcinomas, respectively
- Specific genetic abnormalities in idiopathic primary parathyroid hyperplasia are not as well defined as in hereditary forms of hyperparathyroidism
- *CCND1/PRAD1* oncogene was discovered by analysis of sporadic parathyroid tumors
- *RET* mutation test became essential in management of MEN2A
- *MEN1* test is less urgent because it rarely leads to a major patient benefit
  - *MEN1* germline mutation testing should be offered to index patients with MEN1 and their 1st-degree relatives
    - This includes relatives who are either asymptomatic or who have clinical manifestations of MEN1
  - *MEN1* germline mutation testing should be recommended in individuals with an atypical MEN1 phenotype, e.g., multigland hyperparathyroidism
- *CASR* test, perhaps the least urgent, has largely been unavailable
- Studies of familial isolated hyperparathyroidism and analysis of chromosomal loss and gain in

parathyroid tumors suggest that other genes relevant to parathyroid neoplasia await identification
- Study of these syndromes has helped define the pathophysiology of both familial and sporadic parathyroid neoplasms
- *HRPT2* mutation (tumor suppressor gene, 1q21-q31, encodes parafibromin)
  - Germline *HRPT2*-inactivating mutation in HPT-JT-associated hyperplasia, adenoma, and carcinoma
  - Strong association between *HRPT2* mutations and familial and sporadic parathyroid cancer
  - Germline *HRPT2* mutations identified in subset of patients with mutation-positive carcinomas
- *MEN1* mutation (tumor suppressor gene, 11q13, results in truncated menin protein)
  - Primary parathyroid hyperplasia (multiglandular parathyroid tumors) is most common manifestation of MEN1 (90% of MEN1 cases have hyperplasia)
    - Autosomal dominant; germline mutation in *MEN1* tumor suppressor gene (11q13)
    - Encodes menin
    - Sporadic MEN1 cases due to new mutations
    - Although classically referred to as parathyroid hyperplasia, recent studies demonstrated clonality (multiglandular parathyroid tumors)
  - Somatic *MEN1* mutations occur in 15-20% of sporadic parathyroid adenomas and some sporadic parathyroid carcinomas
- *RET* mutation (proto-oncogene, 10q21)
  - *RET* germline activating proto-oncogene mutation in MEN2A
    - Autosomal dominant, with high penetrance, 95% patients have mutation in exon 10 or 11, codon 634
    - 20-30% of MEN2A associated with parathyroid hyperplasia or adenoma
  - *RET* mutation is generally not identified in sporadic parathyroid disease
- Cyclin-D1/*CCND1*
  - Encodes cyclin-D1, a cell cycle regulator from G1 to S phase
  - Cyclin-D1 overexpression has been observed in hyperplastic parathyroid glands, but lack of definitive correlation limits utility
- Familial isolated hyperparathyroidism
  - Cause is unknown in most cases, but *HRPT2, MEN1* gene, and area on chromosome 2 have been implicated
- *CASR* mutation
  - Inactivating *CASR* (3q13.3-21) mutation causes decreased calcium sensitivity of parathyroid and kidney, resulting in PTH-dependent hypercalcemia
  - Familial hypocalciuric hypercalcemia
    - Heterozygous inactivating *CASR* mutations
  - Familial autosomal dominant hypoparathyroidism and familial hypocalcemia
    - Activating *CASR* mutations
  - Neonatal severe hyperparathyroidism
    - Homozygous inactivating *CASR* mutations
  - *CASR* mutations are generally not seen in sporadic parathyroid disease

DIAGNOSTIC CHECKLIST

Clinically Relevant Pathologic Features

- 20% of primary hyperplasia cases are associated with MEN1
- Mild, nonspecific symptoms or asymptomatic and identified by screening serum calcium

Pathologic Interpretation Pearls

- Normal parathyroid has significant variation in cellularity in and among glands (use caution when evaluating small biopsies)
- Distinguishing parathyroid tissue from thyroid: Well-demarcated cytoplasmic membranes; lack colloid, lack cytoplasmic lipid; rounder nuclei; denser chromatin
- Symmetric enlargement of all 4 glands only in subset of cases; many show enlargement of < 4 glands
  - Be very cautious in attempting to diagnose multiple adenomas (most likely asymmetric hyperplasia)
- Rims of normal tissue occasionally are seen in parathyroid hyperplasia
- Be aware of parathyroid hyperplasia variants (lipohyperplasia and clear cell hyperplasia)

SELECTED REFERENCES

1. Alevizaki M: Management of hyperparathyroidism (PHP) in MEN2 syndromes in Europe. Thyroid Res. 6 Suppl 1:S10, 2013
2. Rejnmark L et al: Further insights into the pathogenesis of primary hyperparathyroidism: a nested case-control study. J Clin Endocrinol Metab. 98(1):87-96, 2013
3. Tamiya H et al: A large functioning parathyroid cyst in a patient with multiple endocrine neoplasia type 1. Endocr J. 60(6):709-14, 2013
4. Vulpio C et al: Histology and immunohistochemistry of the parathyroid glands in renal secondary hyperparathyroidism refractory to vitamin D or cinacalcet therapy. Eur J Endocrinol. 168(6):811-9, 2013
5. DeLellis RA: Parathyroid tumors and related disorders. Mod Pathol. 24 Suppl 2:S78-93, 2011
6. Zhang Y et al: Endocrine tumors as part of inherited tumor syndromes. Adv Anat Pathol. 18(3):206-18, 2011
7. DeLellis RA et al: Primary hyperparathyroidism: a current perspective. Arch Pathol Lab Med. 132(8):1251-62, 2008
8. Delellis RA: Challenging lesions in the differential diagnosis of endocrine tumors: parathyroid carcinoma. Endocr Pathol. 19(4):221-5, 2008
9. Chow LS et al: Parathyroid lipoadenomas: a rare cause of primary hyperparathyroidism. Endocr Pract. 12(2):131-6, 2006
10. DeLellis RA: Parathyroid carcinoma: an overview. Adv Anat Pathol. 12(2):53-61, 2005

PARATHYROID HYPERPLASIA

Normal Parathyroid, Adenoma, and Carcinoma

(Left) *The graphic depicts normal parathyroid glands ➔ and their relationship to adjacent organs and structures.* **(Right)** *The normal parathyroid gland is composed predominantly of chief cells and can show a significant variation in cellularity, even in a single patient. The normal parathyroid cellularity is variable, distributed unevenly, is high in children and infants, and decreases proportionally with age.*

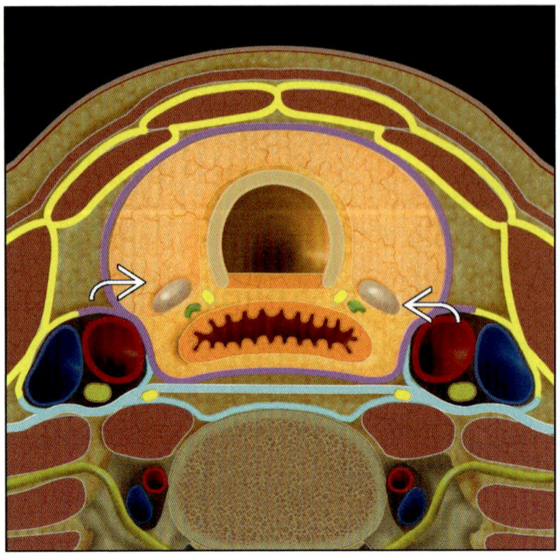

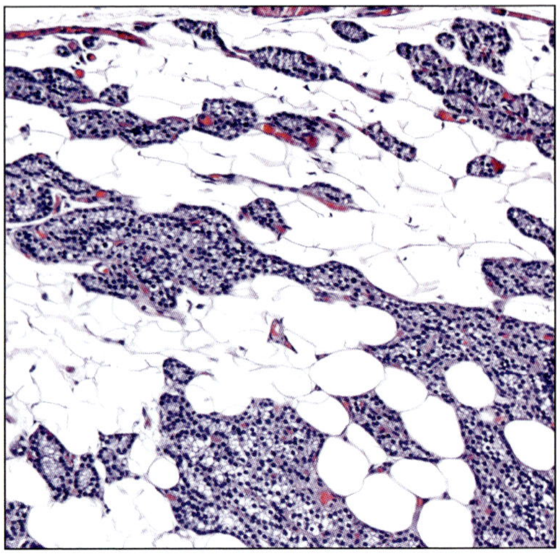

(Left) *Parathyroid adenoma usually involves only 1 gland. The other parathyroid glands are normal in size. Asymmetric hyperplasia or pseudoadenomatous variant of hyperplasia with marked variation in extent of glandular involvement is easily confused with multiple adenomas.* **(Right)** *Parathyroid adenomas consist of a monomorphic proliferation of chief cells in a diffuse pattern. The diagnosis of adenoma is made by the involvement of 1 gland and by the presence of a rim of normocellular parathyroid ➲.*

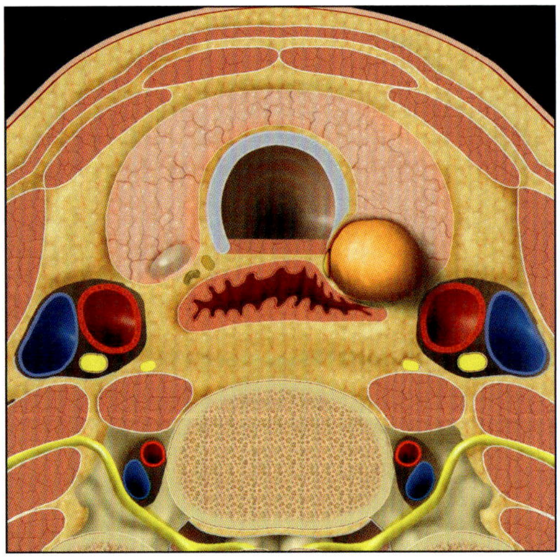

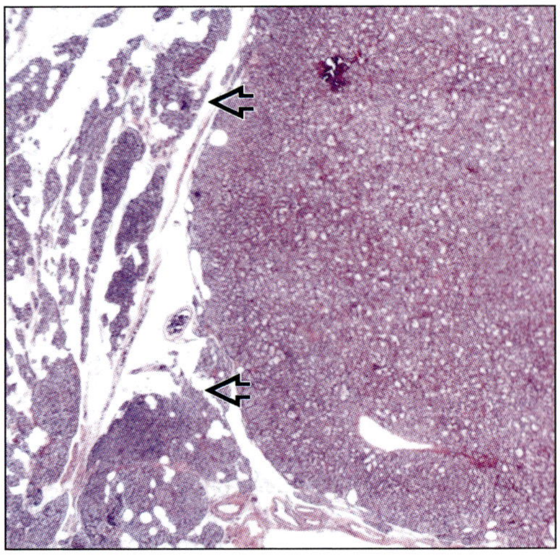

(Left) *A gross photograph of a parathyroid gland with multigland parathyroid hyperplasia shows a pale pink multilobulated outer surface. In contrast to a parathyroid adenoma, hyperplasia is characterized by heterogeneous enlargement of the 4 parathyroid glands.* **(Right)** *Parathyroid hyperplasia in MEN1 usually involves increased numbers of chief cells that may have a nodular or diffuse pattern. The nodular pattern is usually characteristic of parathyroid hyperplasia.*

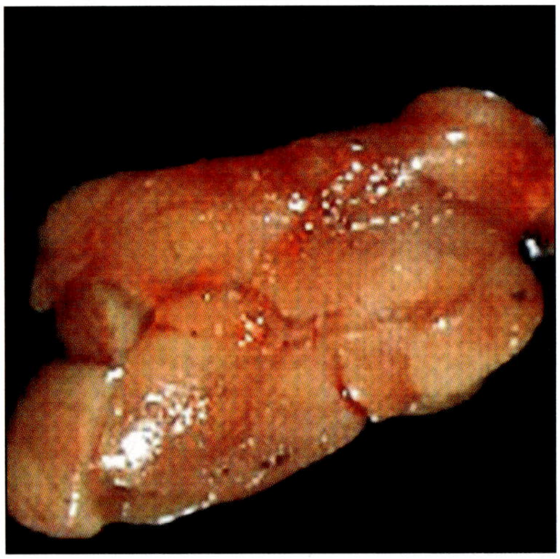

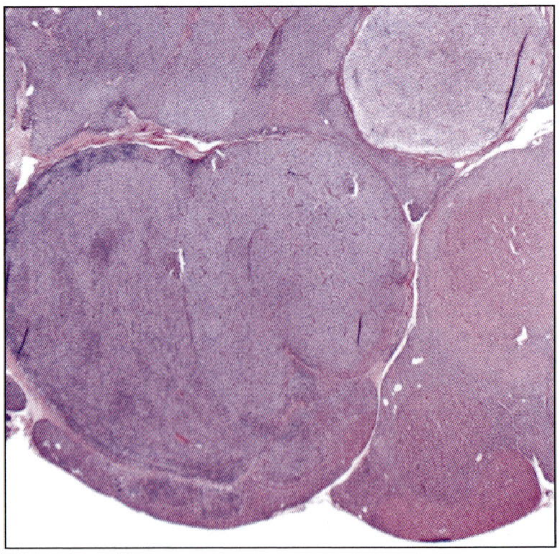

Microscopic Features of Parathyroid Hyperplasia

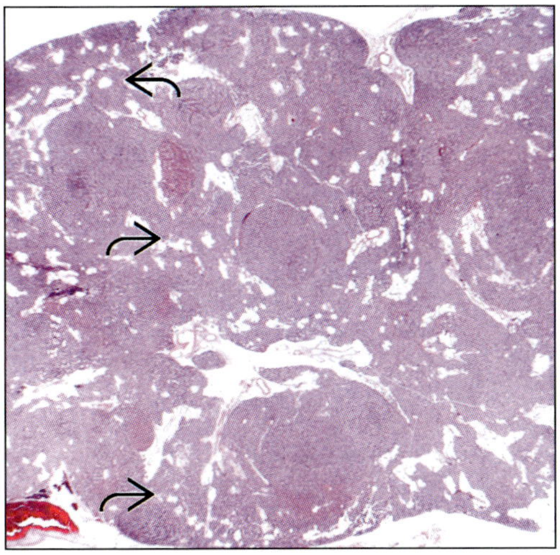

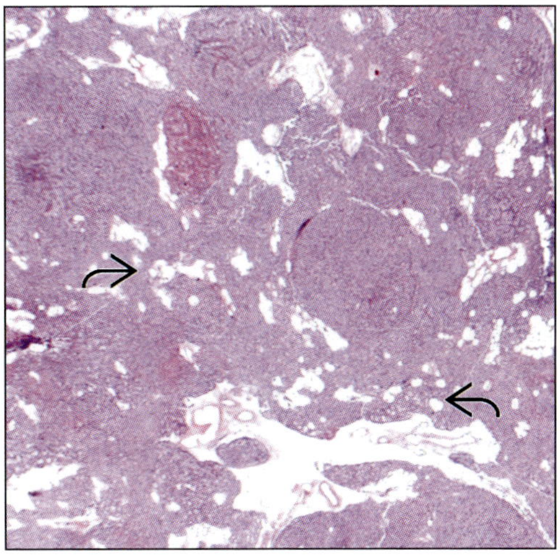

(Left) *Low-power view of a parathyroid gland with parathyroid nodular hyperplasia shows the presence of multiple irregular nodules of chief cells with intermixed residual fat cells* ⮫*.* ***(Right)*** *Parathyroid hyperplasia in MEN1 has an increase in the parenchymal cell mass of multiple parathyroid glands. Chief cells are predominant, but oxyphil, transitional, and clear cells may also be present. Stromal fat* ⮫ *is decreased, with marked variability within the gland.*

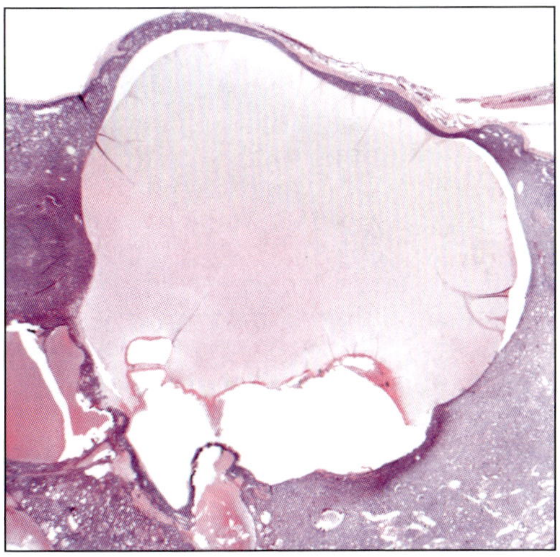

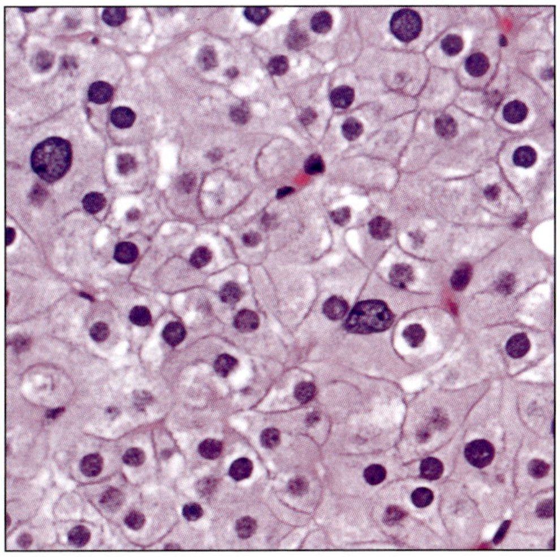

(Left) *Histologic features usually found in HPT-JT-associated parathyroid lesions include a cystic adenoma and parathyroid carcinoma. Parathyroid hyperplasia is not seen in patients with HPT-JT.* ***(Right)*** *Although foci of endocrine atypia with pleomorphism and hyperchromasia are more common in adenomas, they can be present in parathyroid hyperplasia.*

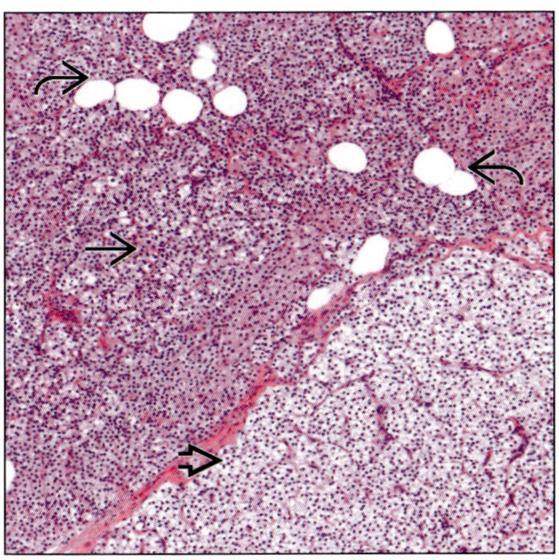

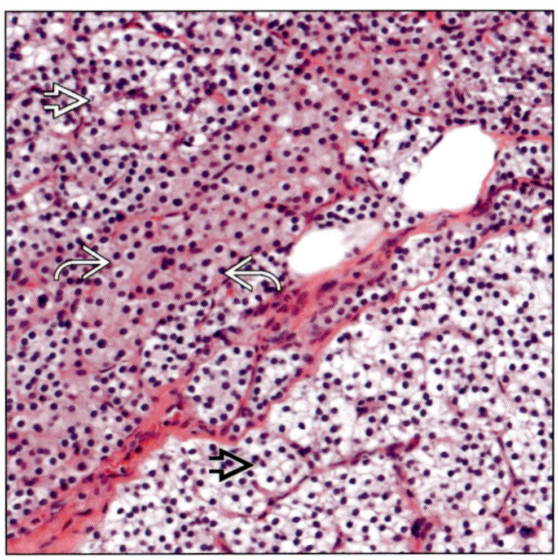

(Left) *Parathyroid hyperplasia in MEN1 has an increase in parenchymal cell mass. Chief cells* ➔ *are predominant, but oxyphil, transitional, and clear cells* ➯ *may also be present. Residual fat cells are present* ⮫*.* ***(Right)*** *High-power view of a parathyroid hyperplasia shows an increase in parenchymal cell mass with clear cells* ➯*, chief cells* ➯*, and a few oncocytic cells* ⮫*.*

PITUITARY ADENOMA

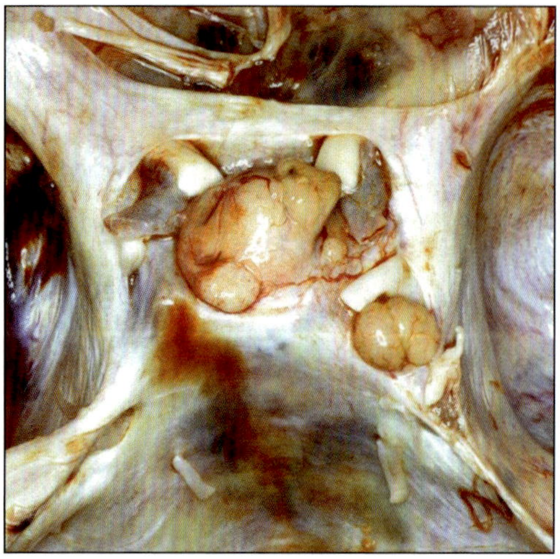

Gross image shows a pituitary macroadenoma that extends upward into the suprasellar cistern and laterally into the cavernous sinus. Pituitary adenomas are common findings in MEN1 syndrome patients.

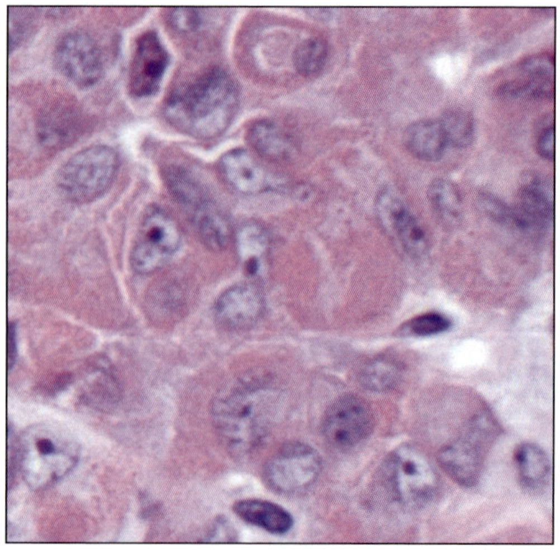

This image shows an acidophilic pituitary adenoma composed of cells that exhibit bright cytoplasmic eosinophilia, associated with a familial growth hormone-producing adenoma.

TERMINOLOGY

Abbreviations

- Pituitary adenoma (PA)

Definitions

- Benign clonal epithelial neoplasms derived from adenohypophyseal cells
- Usually arise in sella turcica and, occasionally seen as ectopic lesion

ETIOLOGY/PATHOGENESIS

Etiology

- Genetic, epigenetic factors, hormonal stimulation, growth factors, and their receptors implicated in pituitary tumorigenesis

Pathogenesis

- Most adenomas are sporadic
- **Hormone regulatory pathways**
  - Hormonal stimulus or impaired feedback inhibition on hypothalamic-pituitary-target organ axes may underlie pathogenesis of PAs
    - Excess GHRH, CRH, TRH, or GnRH production
    - Target organ failure resulting in increased stimulation of hypothalamic-pituitary axes
- **Somatic genetics**
  - Pituitary gland is rarely affected by activating mutations of common oncogenes
  - Cell type-specific genetic changes are common
  - Epigenetically silenced tumor suppressors are found in sporadic PAs
  - Dysregulation of FGFRs may play important role in pathogenesis of PAs

Associated Syndromes

- **Multiple endocrine neoplasia type 1 (MEN1)**
  - Autosomal dominant disorder associated with germline mutation of *MEN1* tumor suppressor gene that encodes menin
  - Affected individuals usually develop growth hormone (GH) &/or prolactin (PRL)-producing PAs
- **McCune-Albright syndrome (MAS)**
  - Mosaic mutations of *GNAS* gene (Gαs protein; Gsp)
  - Affected patients develop somatotroph hyperplasia or somatotroph PAs
- **Familial isolated pituitary adenoma (FIPA)**
  - Autosomal dominant disease with variable penetrance
    - 20% of patients affected by germline mutations in tumor suppressor aryl hydrocarbon receptor interacting protein (*AIP*)
    - No gene abnormality has been identified to date in majority of the FIPA families
  - Cyclin-dependent kinases inhibitor (CDKI) gene mutations have been described in a small number of other familial PAs
  - *AIP* mutation-positive patients have a characteristic clinical phenotype with usually young- or childhood-onset GH &/or PRL-secreting adenomas
    - It can be seen in cases with no apparent family history as well
  - Understanding tumorigenic process in *AIP*(+) and *AIP*(-) FIPA patients could result in better diagnostic and treatment options for both familial and sporadic cases
- **Isolated familial somatotropinoma syndrome (IFS)**
  - ~ 50% of IFS kindreds exhibit mutations in *AIP* gene
- **Carney complex (CC)**
  - Autosomal dominant disorder associated with germline mutations in *PRKAR1A* gene that encodes protein kinase-A regulatory subunit 1α
- MEN4
  - *CDKN1B*
  - Rare reported cases of GH-producing pituitary adenoma associated with hyperparathyroidism

PITUITARY ADENOMA

Key Facts

Terminology
- Benign epithelial neoplasms derived from adenohypophyseal cells exhibiting loss of reticulin network

Etiology/Pathogenesis
- Pituitary adenomas (PAs) may be sporadic or as part of an inherited tumor syndrome
  - Familial pituitary tumors are increasingly recognized
- Pituitary adenomas may be associated with the following familial syndromes
  - Multiple endocrine neoplasia type 1 (MEN1)
  - McCune-Albright syndrome (MAS)
  - Familial isolated pituitary adenoma (FIPA)
  - Isolated familial somatotropinoma syndrome (IFS)
  - Carney complex (CC)
  - Genetic, epigenetic factors, hormonal stimulation, growth factors, and their receptors implicated in pituitary tumorigenesis

Clinical Issues
- Occur in almost 20% of general population

Microscopic Pathology
- Chromophobic, acidophilic, or basophilic cells
- Architecture can predict cell type

Ancillary Tests
- Immunohistochemistry is most valuable tool in classification of PAs
- Immunopanel includes pituitary transcription factors, hormones, LMWK, and MIB-1
- Total breakdown of normal acinar architecture on reticulin stain is diagnostic of PA

CLINICAL ISSUES

Epidemiology
- Incidence
  - Common, occurring in almost 20% of general population
  - Uncommon in pediatric population
    - When present, suggests familial syndrome
  - Constitute 10-25% of all intracranial neoplasms
- Age
  - Incidence increases with age in autopsy studies; > 30% of individuals 50-60 years of age have clinically undetected PAs
  - FIPA families comprise approximately 2% of pituitary adenomas and represent a clinical entity with homogeneous or heterogeneous pituitary adenoma types occurring within same kindred

Presentation
- Hypersecretion of pituitary hormones
  - Adrenocorticotrophic (ACTH) excess presents with Cushing disease or Nelson syndrome
  - GH excess causes acromegaly, gigantism, or both
  - PRL excess presents with galactorrhea, amenorrhea, hypogonadism, and infertility
  - Thyrotropin (TSH) excess presents with hyperthyroidism and is sometimes associated with galactorrhea and hyperprolactinemia
  - Gonadotropin (FSH, LH) excess presents with gonadal dysfunction
- PAs present in 30-40% of MEN1 patients: PRL (20%), GH (10%)
- *AIP* mutations are usually associated with somatotropinomas, but prolactinomas, nonfunctioning pituitary adenomas, Cushing disease, and other adenoma types may occur
- PA in Carney complex is usually GH-producing adenoma
- Hypopituitarism due to compression of nontumorous anterior pituitary parenchyma
- Mass effects can be 1st sign, especially in clinically nonfunctioning adenomas

Prognosis
- Best prognosticator is classification of PAs based on hormone content and cell structure
- Some PA subtypes are usually associated with invasive or aggressive behavior

IMAGE FINDINGS

Radiographic Findings
- PAs are classified radiologically based on tumor size and degree of local invasion
  - Grade 1 (microadenomas) are intrapituitary lesions measuring up to 1 cm
  - Grade 2 (macroadenomas) are larger than 1 cm
  - Grade 3 PAs are locally invasive tumors associated with suprasellar extension and bone erosion
  - Grade 4 PAs involve extrasellar structures (bone, hypothalamus, cavernous sinus)

MACROSCOPIC FEATURES

General Features
- PAs are usually resected as multiple small pieces; majority of PAs exhibit soft white gross appearance

MICROSCOPIC PATHOLOGY

Histologic Features
- Solid, diffuse, trabecular, sinusoidal, papillary growth patterns are common
- Adenoma reveals breakdown of normal acinar architecture on Gordon-Sweet silver stain
  - This distinguishes neoplasia from hyperplasia that retains an acinar reticulin pattern
- Involvement of bone, posterior lobe, dura mater, or respiratory mucosa in invasive PAs

PITUITARY ADENOMA

Immunohistochemical Classification of Pituitary Adenomas

Adenoma Type	Transcription Factor	Hormones	LMWK
GH-Producing Adenomas			
Densely granulated somatotroph adenoma	PIT-1	GH, α-SU	Perinuclear
Sparsely granulated somatotroph adenoma	PIT-1	GH	Fibrous bodies
Mammosomatotroph adenoma	PIT-1, ER	GH, PRL, α-SU	
Mixed somatotroph and lactotroph adenoma	PIT-1, ER	GH, PRL, α-SU	
Plurihormonal GH-producing adenoma	PIT-1, ER	GH, PRL, α-SU, TSH-β	
PRL-Producing Adenomas			
Sparsely granulated lactotroph adenoma	PIT-1, ER	PRL (Golgi pattern)	
Densely granulated lactotroph adenoma	PIT-1, ER	PRL (diffuse)	
Acidophil stem cell adenoma	PIT-1, ER	PRL (diffuse), GH	Fibrous bodies (few)
TSH-Producing Adenoma			
Thyrotroph adenoma	PIT-1, GATA2	TSH-β, α-SU	
ACTH-Producing Adenomas			
Densely granulated corticotroph adenoma	Tpit	ACTH	
Sparsely granulated corticotroph adenoma	Tpit	ACTH	
Crooke cell adenoma	Tpit	ACTH	Ring-like
Gonadotropin-Producing Adenoma			
Gonadotroph adenoma	SF1, ER, GATA2	LH-β, FSH-β, α-SU	
Plurihormonal Adenomas			
Silent subtype 3 adenoma	PIT-1, ER	Multiple	
Unusual plurihormonal adenoma, NOS	Multiple	Multiple	
Hormone-Negative Adenoma			
Null cell adenoma	Absent	Absent	

- Invasive PAs exhibiting increased mitotic activity, MIB-1/Ki-67 proliferative index > 3%, or extensive p53 expression are considered "atypical adenomas"
- Periodic acid-Schiff (PAS) highlights secretory granules of corticotrophs, thyrotrophs, and gonadotrophs

ANCILLARY TESTS

Immunohistochemistry

- General neuroendocrine markers (chromogranin-A, synaptophysin, and neuron-specific enolase [NSE])
- Other markers: LMWK (CAM5.2), MIB-1, p53
- Most valuable tool in determination of cellular differentiation and classification of PAs
  - Hormones: GH, PRL, TSH-β, FSH-β, LH-β, ACTH, α-subunit

DIFFERENTIAL DIAGNOSIS

Pituitary Hyperplasia

- Adenoma reveals total breakdown of normal acinar architecture on silver stain

Paraganglioma

- Sometimes PAs can be negative for keratins

Spindle Cell Oncocytoma/Pituicytoma

- Positive for TTF-1, galactin-3, vimentin, S100, and EMA

Metastatic Neuroendocrine Carcinoma

- Negativity for pituitary transcription factors (PIT-1, Tpit, SF1) and positivity for other transcription factors (CDX-2, TTF-1, etc.) favors metastatic neuroendocrine carcinoma

SELECTED REFERENCES

1. Beckers A et al: Familial isolated pituitary adenomas (FIPA) and the pituitary adenoma predisposition due to mutations in the aryl hydrocarbon receptor interacting protein (AIP) gene. Endocr Rev. 34(2):239-77, 2013
2. Martucci F et al: Familial isolated pituitary adenomas: an emerging clinical entity. J Endocrinol Invest. 35(11):1003-14, 2012
3. Nosé V et al: Protocol for the examination of specimens from patients with primary pituitary tumors. Arch Pathol Lab Med. 135(5):640-6, 2011
4. Lee EB et al: Thyroid transcription factor 1 expression in sellar tumors: a histogenetic marker? J Neuropathol Exp Neurol. 68(5):482-8, 2009
5. Al Brahim NY et al: Complex endocrinopathies in MEN-1: diagnostic dilemmas in endocrine oncology. Endocr Pathol. 18(1):37-41, 2007

Diagrammatic, Imaging, and Microscopic Features

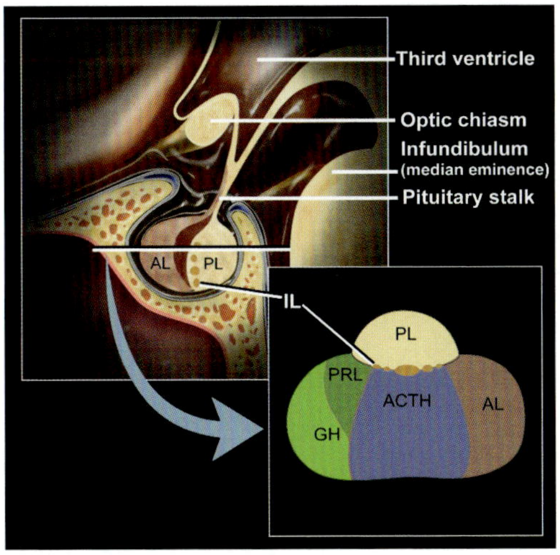

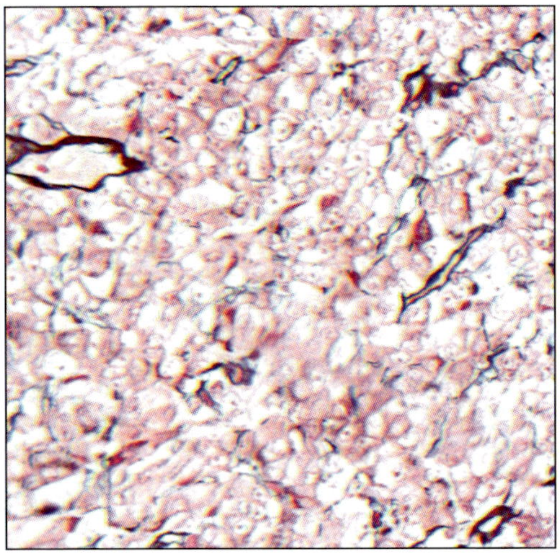

__(Left)__ The pituitary is composed of neuronal tissue forming the posterior pituitary (PL) and pituitary stalk, epithelial neuroendocrine tissue forming the anterior lobe (AL), and the cystic remnants of the intermediate lobe (IL). The anterior pituitary is composed of cells with production of diverse hormones. Normal distribution of cells is shown (inset). __(Right)__ Pituitary adenomas demonstrate a breakdown of normal acinar architecture, highlighted by the loss of silver stain.

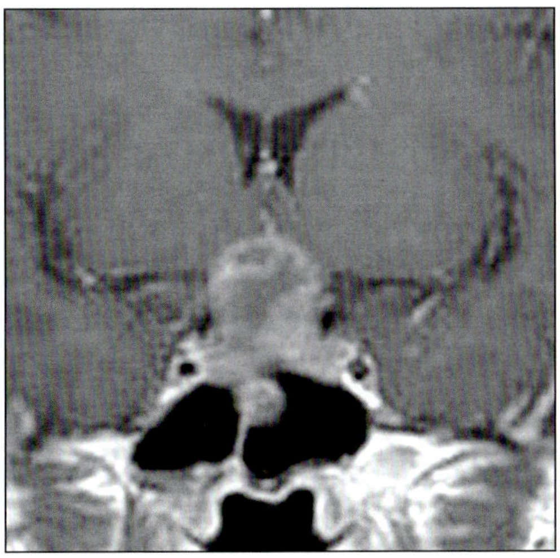

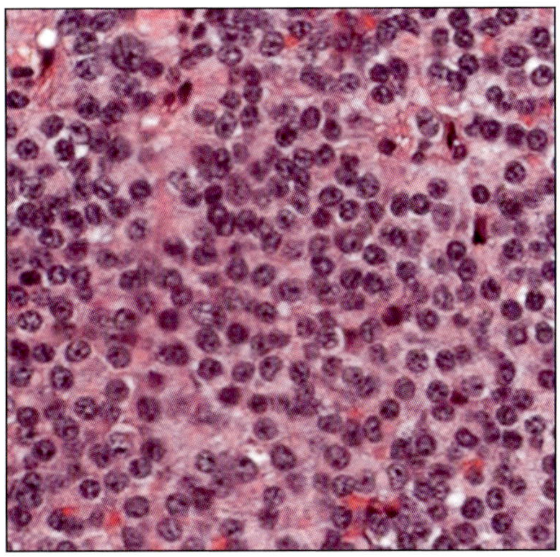

__(Left)__ MR shows invasive pituitary adenoma with sphenoid sinus and cavernous sinus invasion. __(Right)__ Cytoplasmic granularity gives 3 morphologically distinct cell types: Chromophobic, eosinophilic, and basophilic. This chromophobic pituitary adenoma is composed of cells that exhibit pale to light eosinophilic cytoplasm and small round nuclei.

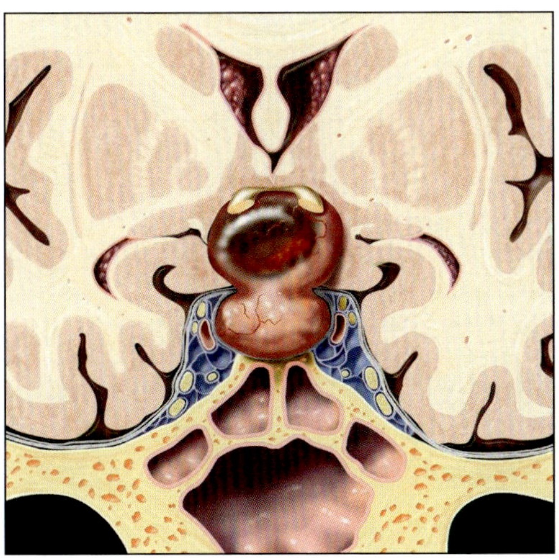

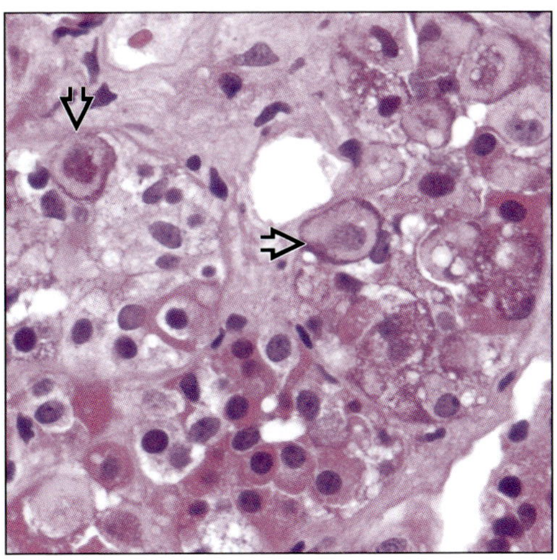

__(Left)__ Coronal graphic illustrates a large pituitary macroadenoma extending superiorly to compress the body of the chiasm, thus compressing the bulk of the crossing nasal retinal fibers. __(Right)__ Normal corticotrophs exposed to elevated glucocorticoids undergo Crooke hyaline change, which is characterized by the accumulation of glassy pink material (keratin) in the cell cytoplasm ➩.

PITUITARY CARCINOMA

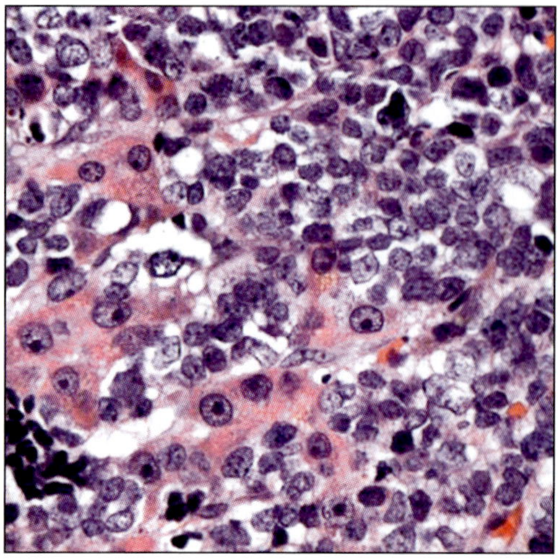

Partial hepatectomy specimen on a patient with history of pituitary tumor shows infiltration of liver parenchyma by a neuroendocrine neoplasm, with immunoreactivity similar to the pituitary tumor.

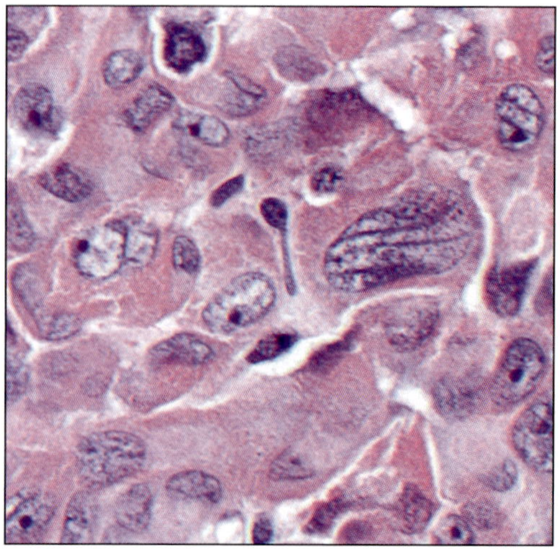

Pituitary carcinoma shows a solid arrangement of pleomorphic cells with an eosinophilic cytoplasm, nuclear pleomorphism, irregular nuclear membranes, and prominent nucleoli.

TERMINOLOGY

Abbreviations

- Pituitary carcinoma (PC)

Synonyms

- Pituitary adenocarcinoma
- Adenocarcinoma of pituitary

Definitions

- Tumor of adenohypophysis exhibiting cerebrospinal &/or systemic metastases
  - Conventional criteria of malignancy, such as nuclear atypia, pleomorphism, mitotic activity, necrosis, hemorrhage, &/or dural invasion are insufficient criteria for diagnosis
  - Local extension into adjacent structures is not criteria for malignancy
- Brain invasion is also indicative of malignancy

ETIOLOGY/PATHOGENESIS

Genetics

- **Inherited**
  - Minority may be associated with familial syndromes
    - Multiple endocrine neoplasia 1 (MEN1)
    - Carney complex
    - Familial isolated pituitary adenoma (FIPA)
    - Isolated familial somatotropinoma (IFS) syndrome
    - McCune-Albright syndrome
    - In comparison to sporadic tumors, incidence of PC is not increased in patients with syndromes
- Chromosomal gains were found in 4 cases
- Most common chromosomal gains (5, 7p, 14q)
- Chromosomal losses reported in 2 cases of PC comparative genomic hybridization (CGH)
- Clonality studies (X-linked gene analysis) show primary, recurrent, and metastatic carcinoma to have same allelic pattern
- Point mutations in *HRAS* in carcinomas but not their adenoma precursors
- *TP53* mutations are occasional

Pathophysiology

- Arise in transition from pituitary adenoma or de novo from previously normal adenohypophysial cells
- No evidence of pluripotent precursor cells involved in adenoma or carcinogenesis
- Invasion (e.g., dura) is common in adenomas, but malignant transformation is rare
- Latency from adenoma to carcinoma varies (longer latency for ACTH-secreting tumors > PRL)
- Spread to central nervous system by way of cerebrospinal fluid
- Direct infiltration of brain is rare
- Systemic metastases are hematogenous, associated with cavernous sinus/jugular vein involvement
- Lymph node metastases secondary to skull base and soft tissue involvement
- Unclear whether sellar surgery facilitates metastases

CLINICAL ISSUES

Epidemiology

- Incidence
  - Very rare; ~ 150 cases reported to date
  - 0.2% of operated adenohypophysial tumors
- Age
  - Adults; rarely adolescents
- Gender
  - Slight female predilection

Site

- Primary sellar; rarely ectopic
- Metastatic sites
  - Craniospinal leptomeninges
  - Systemic sites mainly liver, bone, lymph node, lung

PITUITARY CARCINOMA

Key Facts

Terminology
- Tumor of adenohypophysis exhibiting cerebrospinal &/or systemic metastases
- Conventional morphologic malignancy criteria (nuclear atypia, pleomorphism, mitotic activity, necrosis, hemorrhage, &/or dural invasion) are insufficient for diagnosis

Etiology/Pathogenesis
- Arise in transition from pituitary adenoma or de novo from previously normal adenohypophysial cells
- Inherited
  - Minority may be associated with familial syndromes
  - Multiple endocrine neoplasia 1 (MEN1)
  - Carney complex
  - Familial isolated pituitary adenoma (FIPA)
  - Isolated familial somatotropinoma (IFS) syndrome
  - McCune-Albright syndrome
  - In comparison to sporadic tumors, incidence of pituitary carcinoma is not increased in patients with syndromes
- Chromosomal gains were found in 4 cases
- Most common chromosomal gains (5, 7p, 14q)
- Point mutations in *HRAS* in carcinomas but not their adenoma precursors
- *P53* mutations occasional

Clinical Issues
- 0.2% of operated adenohypophysial tumors
- De novo malignancy adenoma

Top Differential Diagnoses
- Metastatic carcinoma from other organs

Presentation
- Diagnosis based on metastasis, often from multiple recurring, invasive adenoma
- De novo malignancy in adenoma
- Interval to metastasis: 4 months to 30 years (mean: 10 years)
- Malignant transformation rare in ectopic adenoma
- Majority (75%) endocrinologically functional
  - Prolactin and ACTH most frequent, followed by GH and TSH
  - Presentations: Hyperprolactinemia, Nelson syndrome, Cushing disease, acromegaly, hyperthyroidism
  - Nonfunctioning PCs are rare
- Pituitary hormone levels do not permit distinction of adenoma from carcinoma except for PRL (marked increase: 10-30,000 ng/mL)
- Early features of aggressive behavior: Infiltration of dura, bone, cavernous sinus, and cranial nerves
- Clinical signs specific to site of metastasis

Treatment
- Multimodality therapies (surgery, external beam radiotherapy, radiosurgery, adjuvant pharmacologic, and chemotherapy)
- Temozolomide therapy efficacious
- Dopamine agonist response temporary in PRL cell carcinomas

Prognosis
- Poor; mortality 6% at 1 year and 80% within 8 years
- Overall mean survival: 2 years; range: 0.25-8 years
- Survival shorter in systemic vs. craniospinal metastases (1 vs. 2.6 years)
- Long-term survival with benign histology, but poor survival with anaplasia
- Loss of MGMT immunoreactivity and promoter methylation of gene associated with high response to temozolomide therapy

IMAGE FINDINGS

CT and MR Findings
- No features unique to PC
- Bone metastases are usually osteolytic but may be osteoblastic
  - Mimic meningioma when presenting as dura-based masses
- Invasive sellar primary often extending into parasellar structures
  - Cranial nerves in cavernous sinus often affected
- Brain infrequently involved by primary tumor
- Multifocal craniospinal deposits affect leptomeninges and nerve roots, often in cauda equina

MACROSCOPIC FEATURES

General Features
- Primary tumor of macroadenoma size (> 1 cm); all invasive
- Metastatic deposits may be single or multiple, nodular or diffuse
- Metastasis of PC indistinguishable from metastases of carcinomas of other organs

Size
- Metastatic deposits vary from minute focus to macroscopic
- Metastasis to spinal axis are usually relatively small (< 2 cm)
- Metastatic deposits, particularly to liver, can be large

MICROSCOPIC PATHOLOGY

Histologic Features
- No combination of histologic features diagnostic of carcinoma
  - Presence of invasion, cellular pleomorphism, mitosis, or necrosis are not sufficient for diagnosis of malignancy

PITUITARY CARCINOMA

- Diagnosis of PC is dependent upon demonstration of metastases
- Nuclear atypia, cellular pleomorphism, mitotic activity, or necrosis may be present
  - Also present to varying degrees in nonmetastasizing adenohypophyseal tumors
- Most are not overtly malignant histologically or cytologically
- Mitotic activity is increased in carcinomas (up to 67%), but there is considerable overlap with adenomas
- Lack of acinar architecture on reticulin staining, such as adenomas

ANCILLARY TESTS

Immunohistochemistry

- Synaptophysin (+) in all tumors
- Chromogranin less often (+), usually (+) in glycoprotein-producing tumors
- All are hormone-producing tumors, even when clinically nonfunctional
- Ki-67 labeling index varies widely, up to 67%; often higher in metastases
- Topoisomerase-II, an indicator of proliferation rate, often exceeds 4%
- p27, cell cycle inhibitor widely expressed in normal pituitary, decreased in carcinomas
- p53 expressed in most PCs, staining in metastases higher than primary tumor
- VEGFR, related to angiogenesis, widely expressed
- Overexpression of HER2 rare

Electron Microscopy

- Does not distinguish adenoma from carcinoma

DIFFERENTIAL DIAGNOSIS

Metastatic Carcinoma From Other Organs

- Anaplasia more prominent in carcinoma
- Negative for pituitary hormones
  - Except for rare tumors secreting ACTH or GH
- Synaptophysin (+) only in neuroendocrine carcinomas
- Organ-specific markers positivity

Invasive Pituitary Adenoma

- Locally invasive tumor
- No metastases present
- Histological features, immunohistochemical profile, electron microscopy, and proliferation markers cannot distinguish benign from malignant tumors

DIAGNOSTIC CHECKLIST

Clinically Relevant Pathologic Features

- History of pituitary adenoma or invasive pituitary adenoma is helpful

Pathologic Interpretation Pearls

- Disseminating lesions present in carcinoma often arise in infiltrating adenoma
- Local infiltration is not, in itself, an indicator of carcinoma
- Useful to compare histological appearance and immunohistochemical profile of metastatic focus with primary pituitary tumor
- No histological, immunohistochemical, or ultrastructural finding conclusively separates pituitary adenomas from carcinomas

GRADING

Grading System

- No suitable grading system exists

SELECTED REFERENCES

1. Matsuno A et al: Molecular status of pituitary carcinoma and atypical adenoma that contributes the effectiveness of temozolomide. Med Mol Morphol. Epub ahead of print, 2013
2. Thakker RV: Multiple endocrine neoplasia type 1 (MEN1) and type 4 (MEN4). Mol Cell Endocrinol. Epub ahead of print, 2013
3. Zhou Y et al: Genetic and epigenetic mutations of tumor suppressive genes in sporadic pituitary adenoma. Mol Cell Endocrinol. Epub ahead of print, 2013
4. Moshkin O et al: Aggressive silent corticotroph adenoma progressing to pituitary carcinoma. The role of temozolomide therapy. Hormones (Athens). 10(2):162-7, 2011
5. Nosé V et al: Protocol for the examination of specimens from patients with primary pituitary tumors. Arch Pathol Lab Med. 135(5):640-6, 2011
6. Zada G et al: Atypical pituitary adenomas: incidence, clinical characteristics, and implications. J Neurosurg. 114(2):336-44, 2011
7. Zhang Y et al: Endocrine tumors as part of inherited tumor syndromes. Adv Anat Pathol. 18(3):206-18, 2011
8. Lau Q et al: MGMT immunoexpression in aggressive pituitary adenoma and carcinoma. Pituitary. 13(4):367-79, 2010
9. Salehi F et al: Biomarkers of pituitary neoplasms: a review (Part II). Neurosurgery. 67(6):1790-8; discussion 1798, 2010
10. Jeong KH et al: Expression of a gonadotropin-releasing hormone receptor-simian virus 40 T-antigen transgene has sex-specific effects on the reproductive axis. Endocrinology. 150(7):3383-91, 2009
11. Scheithauer BW et al: Multiple endocrine neoplasia type 1-associated thyrotropin-producing pituitary carcinoma: report of a probable de novo example. Hum Pathol. 40(2):270-8, 2009
12. Tanizaki Y et al: P53 gene mutations in pituitary carcinomas. Endocr Pathol. 18(4):217-22, 2007
13. Roncaroli F et al: Gonadotropic pituitary carcinoma: HER-2/neu expression and gene amplification. Report of two cases. J Neurosurg. 99(2):402-8, 2003
14. Nose-Alberti V et al: Adrenocorticotropin-producing pituitary carcinoma with expression of c-erbB-2 and high PCNA index: a comparative study with pituitary adenomas and normal pituitary tissues. Endocr Pathol. 9(1):53-62, 1998

Microscopic Features

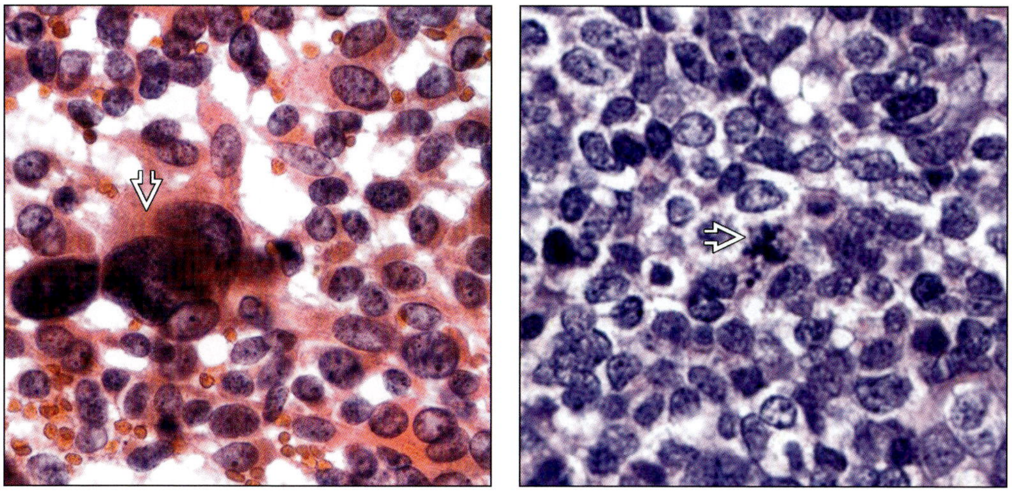

***(Left)** Smear from a liver nodule shows a highly cellular neoplasm composed of rare giant cells ➔ that are present in the background of a monotonous population of cells. The cells have scant cytoplasm and nuclei with a homogeneous appearance. **(Right)** Pituitary carcinoma metastatic to liver shows a solid arrangement of cells with mild atypia, cellular pleomorphism, apoptosis, and the presence of an atypical mitosis ➔.*

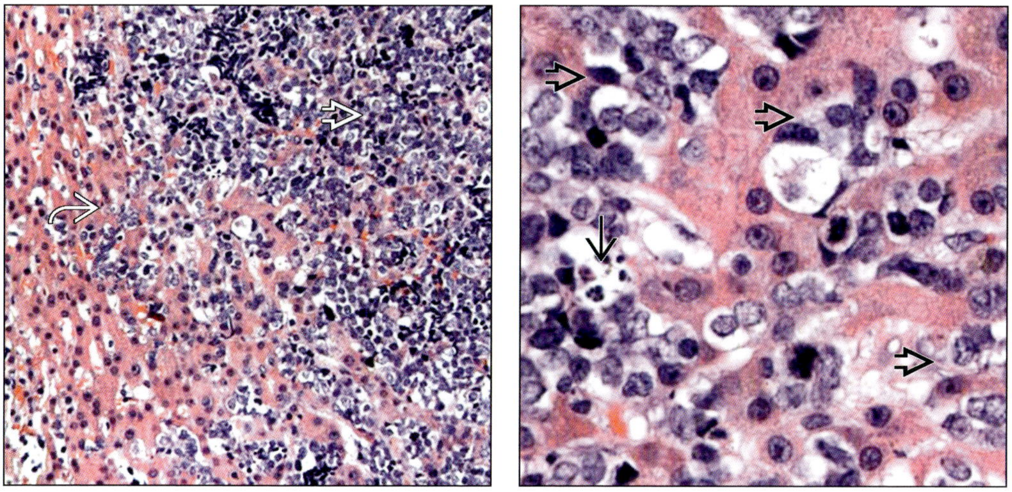

***(Left)** This low-power photomicrograph shows metastatic pituitary carcinoma in a liver. The tumor infiltrates the hepatic sinusoids ➔ and forms solid sheets of tumor cells ➔ with regular nuclei lacking pleomorphism. **(Right)** H&E from a liver with metastatic pituitary carcinoma shows diffuse infiltration of the hepatic sinusoids ➔ by tumor cells. There are apoptotic bodies ➔ present within the tumor.*

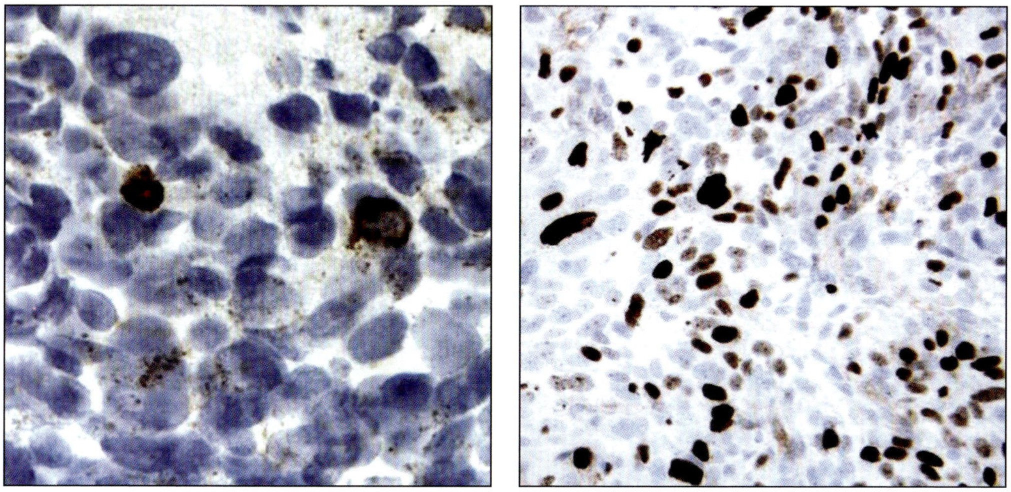

***(Left)** ACTH immunostain of a smear from a liver tumor nodule shows positivity in the cytoplasm of scattered tumor cells. This immunopositivity was also present in the pituitary tumor of this patient. **(Right)** Immunohistochemistry for Ki-67 (MIB-1) in a pituitary carcinoma metastatic to liver shows a high proliferative index. p53 immunoexpression is often high and usually higher in metastatic sites than in the primary tumor.*

FAMILIAL THYROID CARCINOMA

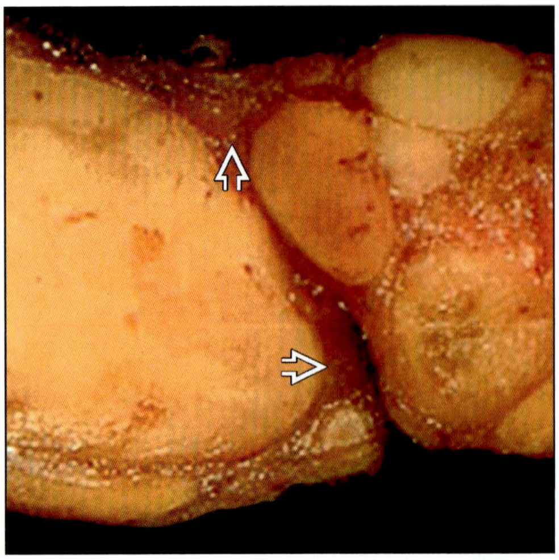

Gross cut surface of a thyroid from an 18-year-old woman with Cowden disease/PTEN hamartoma tumor syndrome shows multiple well-circumscribed nodules almost entirely replacing the thyroid parenchyma ⇨.

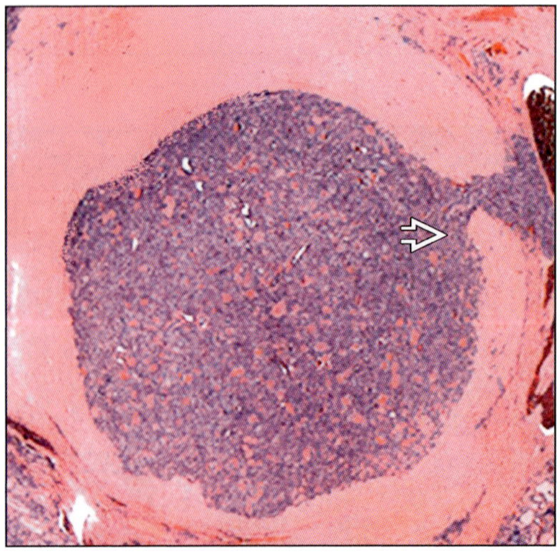

An encapsulated follicular carcinoma from a 12-year-old girl with Cowden syndrome shows complete capsular invasion ⇨. Follicular carcinoma is a major criterion for diagnosis of this syndrome.

TERMINOLOGY

Abbreviations

- Familial nonmedullary thyroid carcinoma (FNMTC)
- Familial medullary thyroid carcinoma (FMTC)

Definitions

- Thyroid carcinoma occurring in familial setting
  - Can be syndrome-associated or nonsyndromic
- Familial thyroid carcinomas are divided into 2 subgroups: FNMTC and FMTC
- **FNMTC or familial follicular cell tumors**, derived from thyroid follicular cells
  - Further subdivided into 2 subgroups
    - Familial tumor syndromes characterized by predominance of nonthyroidal tumors
    - Familial tumor syndromes characterized by predominance of nonmedullary thyroid carcinoma
- **FMTC**, derived from thyroid calcitonin-producing C cells
  - Occurs in 3 distinct settings
    - Familial medullary thyroid carcinoma (medullary thyroid carcinoma-only syndrome)
    - Multiple endocrine neoplasia 2A (MEN2A)
    - Multiple endocrine neoplasia 2B (MEN2B)

ETIOLOGY/PATHOGENESIS

Familial Follicular Cell Tumors or Familial Nonmedullary Thyroid Carcinoma (FNMTC)

- Rare tumors encompassing a heterogeneous group of diseases including both syndrome-associated and nonsyndromic tumors
- **Familial tumor syndromes characterized by predominance of nonmedullary thyroid carcinoma**
  - **PTEN-hamartoma tumor syndrome (PHTS)**: Cowden syndrome (CS) and Bannayan-Riley-Ruvalcaba syndrome (BRRS) are major entities composing PHTS
    - Caused by germline mutations of *PTEN* gene and inherited in autosomal dominant fashion
    - *PTEN* (phosphatase and tensin homolog deleted on chromosome 10) is tumor suppressor gene located on 10q23.3
  - **Familial adenomatous polyposis (FAP)**: Characterized by hundreds of adenomatous colonic polyps that develop during early adulthood
    - Inherited autosomal dominant syndrome caused by germline mutations in adenomatous polyposis coli (*APC*) gene on chromosome 5q21
  - **Carney complex**: Consists of myxomas, spotty pigmentation, and endocrine overactivity
    - Autosomal dominant condition
    - Most cases are classified as type 1 and are associated with mutation of protein kinase A regulatory subunit type 1α (*PRKAR1A*) gene, a probable tumor suppressor gene on chromosome 17q22-24
    - Type 2 patients have mutation on chromosome 2p16, which may be regulator of genomic stability
  - **Werner syndrome**: Rare premature-aging syndrome that begins in 3rd decade
    - Autosomal recessive disease
    - Caused by mutations in *WRN* gene on chromosome 8p11-p12
  - **Pendred syndrome**: Most common hereditary syndrome associated with bilateral sensorineural deafness
    - Also called deaf-mutism and goiter
    - Autosomal recessive trait
    - Result of mutations in *SLC26A4* (*PDS*) gene, which encodes pendrin protein and is located on chromosome 7q21-34
    - 100 mutations identified in *PDS* gene, and most are family specific

FAMILIAL THYROID CARCINOMA

Key Facts

Terminology

- Thyroid carcinoma derived from C cells or follicular cells, occurring in familial setting
- Familial follicular cell tumors are classified in 2 subgroups
  - Familial tumor syndromes characterized by predominance of nonthyroid tumors
  - Familial tumor syndromes characterized by predominance of nonmedullary thyroid carcinoma
- Familial medullary thyroid carcinoma occurs in 3 distinct settings
  - Multiple endocrine neoplasia 2A (MEN2A)
  - Multiple endocrine neoplasia 2B (MEN2B)
  - Medullary thyroid carcinoma only

Clinical Issues

- Presence of multiple benign nodules, high incidence of multifocality and bilateral disease, more aggressive behavior, and worse prognosis than sporadic thyroid cancer
- Incidence of familial medullary carcinoma is 25%
- Incidence of familial follicular cell tumors is ~ 5%

Microscopic Pathology

- Presence of lymphocytic thyroiditis, nodular hyperplasia, multiple follicular adenomas, multiple adenomatous nodules, follicular carcinoma, and PTC
- Presence of bilateral and multifocal PTC with local invasion and intrathyroid dissemination
- Familial PTC has no distinct histological characteristics

- **Familial tumor syndromes characterized by predominance of nonmedullary thyroid carcinoma**
  - Characterized by 3 or more 1st-degree relatives with follicular-derived nonmedullary thyroid carcinoma and occurs regardless of presence of another familial syndrome
  - Also includes
    - **Pure familial papillary thyroid carcinoma (PTC) ± oxyphilia**: Mapped to chromosomal region 19p13
    - **Familial PTC (FPTC) with papillary renal cell carcinoma**: Mapped to chromosomal region 1q21
    - **FNMTC type 1**: Mapped to chromosome 2q21
    - **FPTC with multinodular goiter**: Mapped to chromosomal region 14q

Familial Medullary Thyroid Carcinoma (FMTC)

- Refers to those neoplasms arising from calcitonin-producing C cells derived from neural crest
- MTCs occur in sporadic or hereditary (25% of cases) forms, as part of MEN2 syndrome, or as MTC-only syndrome
  - MEN2 syndrome consists of 3 variants: MEN2A, MEN2B, and FMTC
  - MEN2A is associated with pheochromocytoma and parathyroid hyperplasia
  - MEN2B is associated with marfanoid habitus, mucosal neuromas, ganglioneuromatosis, and pheochromocytoma
- ~ 85% of all *RET* mutations responsible for FMTC are known
- In majority of MEN2A and FMTC patients, *RET* mutations are clustered in 6 cysteine residues in *RET* cysteine-rich extracellular domain
- Mutations have been detected in ~ 95% of MEN2A and ~ 85% of FMTC families
- Somatic *RET* point mutations have been identified in ~ 50% of patients with sporadic MTC

CLINICAL ISSUES

Epidemiology

- Incidence
  - Thyroid cancer accounts for only 1% of all malignant tumors
    - Advances in molecular genetics have confirmed presence of several familial cancer syndromes that have familial nonmedullary thyroid cancers (FNMTCs)
  - 5% incidence of FNMTC in 95% of patients with well-differentiated thyroid cancer
  - Familial forms of follicular cell-derived tumors are rare and encompass a heterogeneous group of diseases, including both syndrome-associated and nonsyndromic tumors
    - Thyroid neoplasia has been reported with increased frequency in familial syndromes, such as familial adenomatous polyposis (FAP), Cowden disease/PTEN-hamartoma tumor syndrome, Carney complex type 1, Werner syndrome, Pendred syndrome
    - Among nonsyndromic tumors, predominant neoplasm is nonmedullary thyroid carcinoma, although other neoplasms may occur with increased frequency
  - Incidence of MTC in patients with familial disease is 25%
    - This group represents ~ 5% of all thyroid tumors and ~ 15% of all thyroid cancer-related deaths
- Age
  - **Familial follicular cell tumors or familial nonmedullary thyroid carcinoma**
    - Age of diagnosis varies, but tumors generally occur in younger patients as compared to their sporadic counterparts
  - **Medullary thyroid carcinoma**
    - MEN2A syndrome or Sipple syndrome: In late adolescence or early adulthood; peak incidence of medullary carcinoma in these patients is in 4th decade

FAMILIAL THYROID CARCINOMA

- MEN2B patients usually develop medullary carcinoma early in life, diagnosed in infancy or early childhood; males and females are equally affected
- Inherited medullary carcinoma without associated endocrinopathies: Similar to other types of thyroid cancers, peak incidence ranges from 40-50 years

Presentation: FNMTC

- **Syndrome-associated group**
- Has increased prevalence of follicular cell-derived tumors within familial cancer syndrome, with preponderance of nonthyroidal tumors
  - **PTEN-hamartoma tumor syndrome**
    - > 90% of individuals affected with CS manifest a phenotype by age 20 years
    - By end of or during 3rd decade, almost all patients (99%) develop at least pathognomonic mucocutaneous lesions
    - Affected individuals with CS develop both benign and malignant tumors in a variety of tissues, such as breast, uterus, and thyroid
    - Thyroid pathologic findings in this syndrome typically affect follicular cells
  - **Familial adenomatous polyposis (FAP)**
    - Extracolonic manifestations include osteomas, epidermal cysts, desmoid tumors, gastrointestinal tract polyps-hamartomas, congenital hypertrophy of retinal pigmented epithelium (CHRPE), hepatoblastomas
    - Papillary thyroid carcinoma in 2-12% of FAP patients
    - Young women with FAP are at particular risk of developing thyroid cancer; their chance of being affected is ~ 160x greater than that of normal individuals
    - PTC occurs with frequency of ~ 10x greater than that expected for sporadic PTC
  - **Carney complex**
    - Characterized by skin and mucosal pigmentation, diverse pigmented skin lesions, nonendocrine and variety of endocrine neoplasias: Pituitary adenoma, pigmented nodular adrenal disease, Sertoli and Leydig cell tumors, and thyroid tumors
    - Myxomas occur in heart, skin or soft tissue, external auditory canal, and breast
  - **Werner syndrome**
    - Elderly appearance with short stature, thin skin, wrinkles, alopecia, and muscle atrophy
    - Age-related disorders (e.g., osteoporosis, cataracts, diabetes, peripheral vascular disease, or malignancy) are present in these patients
    - Cardiac disease and cancer are most common causes of death in these patients
    - Mutations of the *WRN* gene are specifically associated with malignancies such as melanoma, soft tissue sarcoma, osteosarcomas, and well-differentiated thyroid carcinoma
  - **Pendred syndrome**: Thyroid disease in these patients may range from minimal enlargement to large multinodular goiter
    - Most patients are euthyroid
- **Familial tumor syndromes characterized by predominance of nonmedullary thyroid carcinoma (follicular cell-derived tumors)**
  - FNMTC is associated with multiple benign nodules, multifocality, bilateral disease, more aggressive clinical behavior, and worse prognosis than sporadic nonmedullary thyroid cancer
    - Diagnosed when ≥ 3 family members have nonmedullary thyroid cancer in absence of other known associated syndromes
    - Patients have shorter disease-free survival than do sporadic disease patients because of frequent locoregional recurrence
    - Individuals with FNMTC have increased risk of multifocal disease and are more likely to have intraglandular dissemination, local invasion, local or regional recurrence, and lymph node metastases
  - **Familial multinodular goiter (FMNG) syndrome** (mapped to 14q)
    - Some patients may develop associated PTC
  - **Familial nonmedullary thyroid carcinoma type 1 (FNMTC1) syndrome** (chromosomal region 2q21)
    - Characterized by PTC without any distinguishing pathologic features
  - **Familial PTC associated with papillary renal neoplasia syndrome (FPTC/PRN)** (mapped to chromosomal region 1q21)
    - Includes not only PTC and expected benign thyroid nodules but also papillary renal neoplasia
  - **Familial papillary thyroid carcinoma (FPTC)** (chromosomal region 19p13)
    - Characterized by multicentric tumors and multiple adenomatous nodules ± oxyphilia

Presentation: FMTC

- **MEN2A syndrome** or Sipple syndrome has bilateral medullary carcinoma or C-cell hyperplasia (CCH), pheochromocytoma, and hyperparathyroidism
  - Inherited in autosomal dominant manner, and males and females are equally affected
- **MEN2B** is associated with pheochromocytoma and alterations in nonendocrine tissue
  - Syndrome also has medullary carcinoma and pheochromocytoma, but only rarely hyperparathyroidism
  - Patients have unusual appearance, which is characterized by mucosal ganglioneuromas and marfanoid habitus
  - Inheritance is autosomal dominant as in MEN2A
- **FMTC or inherited medullary carcinoma without associated endocrinopathies**
  - Least aggressive form of medullary carcinoma
  - MTC usually develops in patients with no other clinical manifestations

FAMILIAL THYROID CARCINOMA

MACROSCOPIC FEATURES

General Features

- Familial tumors have high incidence of multifocality, more likely to be bilateral

MICROSCOPIC PATHOLOGY

Histologic Features

- **Familial tumor syndromes characterized by predominance of nonmedullary thyroid carcinoma**
  - Most tumors are PTC and have no distinct morphological findings to differentiate them from sporadic counterparts
  - Mutations in patients with FNMTC syndromes have not been as well defined as in MTC
  - Familial thyroid cancers are more aggressive than sporadic thyroid cancer, with predisposition for lymph node metastasis, extrathyroidal invasion, and younger age of onset
- **PTEN-hamartoma tumor syndrome**
  - 2/3 of CS patients develop thyroid tumors; pathologic findings in this syndrome have been described as involving follicular cells
  - Majority of thyroid lesions occurring in PHTS are characteristically multicentric and bilateral; benign and malignant thyroid lesions are observed in PHTS
  - Multiple adenomatous nodules are characteristic, with multiple distinct well-circumscribed nodules, firm yellow-tan cut surface, diffusely involving thyroid gland
  - Follicular adenomas are very common, occur at earlier age, and usually are multicentric
  - Follicular carcinoma is a major criterion and an important feature in PTEN-hamartoma tumor syndrome; these tumors are more frequently multicentric
  - PTC and C-cell hyperplasia have rarely been associated with this entity
- **Familial adenomatous polyposis (FAP)**
  - Thyroid tumors in FAP patients occur almost exclusively in young females; the tumors are bilateral, multifocal, and well differentiated
  - Among patients with FAP who have synchronous PTC, > 90% exhibit histologic features of cribriform-morular variant (CMV), which focally shows typical nuclear features of PTC
  - Characteristic cribriform pattern with solid areas and spindle cell component, associated with marked fibrosis and morular areas
  - Characteristic PTC morphology is associated with follicular, papillary, trabecular, solid, spindle cell, and squamoid areas
- **Carney complex**
  - Thyroid is multinodular and has multifocal and bilateral thyroid disease
  - Lymphocytic thyroiditis, nodular hyperplasia, multiple follicular adenomas, characteristic multiple adenomatous nodules, follicular carcinoma, and PTC, usually present in ~ 15% of patients
- **Werner syndrome**
  - Patients present at younger age and have ~ 3x ↑ risk for developing follicular carcinoma and 6x ↑ risk for anaplastic thyroid carcinoma
- **Pendred syndrome**
  - Association of thyroid cancer and Pendred syndrome may be related to untreated congenital hypothyroidism and chronic stimulation by thyroid-stimulating hormone
  - Progression from thyroid goiter to cancer is uncommon, and risk is likely related to longstanding untreated hypothyroidism

ANCILLARY TESTS

Immunohistochemistry

- Immunostains of CMV-PTC show positivity for ER and PR, Bcl-2, E-cadherin, and galectin-3
- CMV-PTC is characterized by aberrant nuclear and cytoplasmic expression of β-catenin
- Immunostain for PTEN may be lost in cases of PHTS
- All other familial tumors have similar immunophenotype to sporadic thyroid tumor counterparts

Molecular Genetics

- Germline point mutation in *RET* gene on chromosome 10q11.2 is responsible for hereditary MTC
- Most patients with FAP-associated PTC have *APC* germline mutations
- Most patients with PHTS have germline mutations on gene *PTEN*
- Genetic inheritance of FNMTC remains unknown, believed to be autosomal dominant
  - Chromosomal regions involved: 14q, 2q21, 1q21, 19p13

DIFFERENTIAL DIAGNOSIS

Follicular Cell Carcinoma

- **Sporadic follicular cell neoplasm**
  - Comprises almost 95% of cases
  - Usually single and unilateral
  - Morphologically indistinguishable from tumor occurring in the familial setting

Medullary Thyroid Carcinoma

- **Sporadic MTC**
  - Accounts for up to 75% of all cases of medullary thyroid cancer
  - Females outnumber males by 3:2
  - Peak of onset is 40-60 years of age, mean: 50 years
  - 1/3 present with intractable diarrhea
  - Typically unilateral
  - No associated endocrinopathies (not associated with disease in other endocrine glands)

FAMILIAL THYROID CARCINOMA

Familial Follicular Cell Carcinoma Classification

Disease	Histologic Subtype
Syndromic or Familial Tumor Syndrome With Preponderance of Nonthyroidal Tumors	
PTEN-hamartoma tumor syndrome (Cowden disease)	FTC associated with follicular adenomas, multiple adenomatous nodules, and C-cell hyperplasia
Familial adenomatous polyposis (FAP)-hamartoma tumor syndrome	PTC with cribriform and morular pattern with sclerosis
Carney complex	FTC associated with follicular adenomas, multiple adenomatous nodules, and PTC
Werner syndrome	FTC, PTC, and ATC
Pendred syndrome	FTC
Nonsyndromic or Familial Tumor Syndrome With Preponderance of Nonmedullary Thyroid Carcinoma	
Familial papillary thyroid carcinoma	PTC, usual variant
Familial papillary thyroid carcinoma with papillary renal cell neoplasia	PTC, usual variant
Familial nonmedullary thyroid carcinoma type 1	PTC, usual variant
Familial papillary thyroid carcinoma and multinodular goiter	PTC and nodular hyperplasia

PTC: Papillary thyroid carcinoma; FTC: Follicular thyroid carcinoma; ATC: Anaplastic thyroid carcinoma.

Familial Follicular Cell Cancer in Familial Cancer Syndromes

Syndrome	Inheritance	Gene	Gene Location	Thyroid Involvement (%)
PTEN-hamartoma tumor syndrome	Autosomal dominant	*PTEN*	10q23.2	50
Familial adenomatous polyposis	Autosomal dominant	*APC*	5q21	2-12
Carney complex	Autosomal dominant	*PRKAR1*-α	2p12-17q22-24	60; 4
Pendred syndrome	Autosomal recessive	*SLC26A4* (pendrin)	7q21-24	1
Werner syndrome	Autosomal recessive	*WRN*	8p11-p12	18

DIAGNOSTIC CHECKLIST

Clinically Relevant Pathologic Features

- Familial thyroid carcinoma has been shown to occur at younger age, be associated with presence of multiple benign nodules, have high incidence of multifocality and bilateral disease, have more aggressive clinical behavior, and have worse prognosis than its sporadic counterparts

SELECTED REFERENCES

1. Laury AR et al: Thyroid pathology in PTEN-hamartoma tumor syndrome: characteristic findings of a distinct entity. Thyroid. 21(2):135-44, 2011
2. Mukherjee S et al: RET codon 804 mutations in multiple endocrine neoplasia 2: genotype-phenotype correlations and implications in clinical management. Clin Genet. 79(1):1-16, 2011
3. Nosé V: Familial thyroid cancer: a review. Mod Pathol. 24 Suppl 2:S19-33, 2011
4. Smith JR et al: Thyroid nodules and cancer in children with PTEN hamartoma tumor syndrome. J Clin Endocrinol Metab. 96(1):34-7, 2011
5. Zhang Y et al: Endocrine tumors as part of inherited tumor syndromes. Adv Anat Pathol. 18(3):206-18, 2011
6. Almeida MQ et al: Solid tumors associated with multiple endocrine neoplasias. Cancer Genet Cytogenet. 203(1):30-6, 2010
7. Cameselle-Teijeiro J: The pathologist's role in familial nonmedullary thyroid tumors. Int J Surg Pathol. 18(3 Suppl):194S-200S, 2010
8. Farooq A et al: Cowden syndrome. Cancer Treat Rev. 36(8):577-83, 2010
9. Khan A et al: Familial nonmedullary thyroid cancer: a review of the genetics. Thyroid. 20(7):795-801, 2010
10. Nosé V: Familial follicular cell tumors: classification and morphological characteristics. Endocr Pathol. 21(4):219-26, 2010
11. Richards ML: Familial syndromes associated with thyroid cancer in the era of personalized medicine. Thyroid. 20(7):707-13, 2010
12. Rubinstein WS: Endocrine cancer predisposition syndromes: hereditary paraganglioma, multiple endocrine neoplasia type 1, multiple endocrine neoplasia type 2, and hereditary thyroid cancer. Hematol Oncol Clin North Am. 24(5):907-37, 2010
13. Dotto J et al: Familial thyroid carcinoma: a diagnostic algorithm. Adv Anat Pathol. 15(6):332-49, 2008
14. Etit D et al: Histopathologic and clinical features of medullary microcarcinoma and C-cell hyperplasia in prophylactic thyroidectomies for medullary carcinoma: a study of 42 cases. Arch Pathol Lab Med. 132(11):1767-73, 2008
15. Nosé V: Familial non-medullary thyroid carcinoma: an update. Endocr Pathol. 19(4):226-40, 2008
16. Yassa L et al: Long-term assessment of a multidisciplinary approach to thyroid nodule diagnostic evaluation. Cancer. 111(6):508-16, 2007
17. Zambrano E et al: Abnormal distribution and hyperplasia of thyroid C-cells in PTEN-associated tumor syndromes. Endocr Pathol. 15(1):55-64, 2004

C-Cell Hyperplasia and Neoplasia

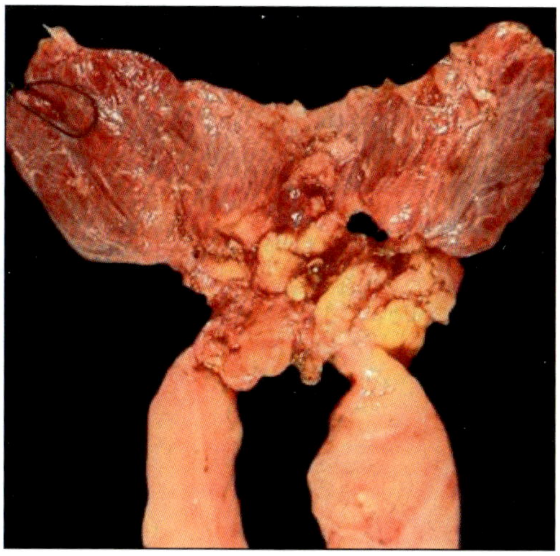
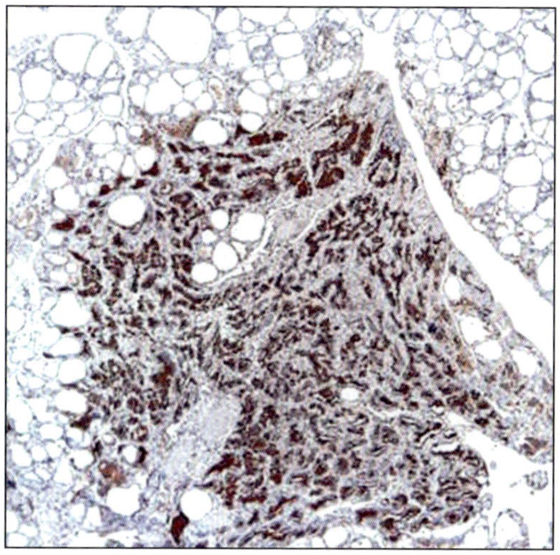

(Left) *Total prophylactic thyroidectomy plus thymectomy from a patient with a family history of MEN2 with RET mutation shows a grossly normal thyroid. The entirely submitted specimen showed CCH and 2 foci of medullary thyroid carcinoma.* ***(Right)*** *Patient with family history of MEN2B with RET mutation had prophylactic thyroidectomy, which showed CCH and 2 foci of medullary thyroid carcinoma. Calcitonin stain highlights the focus of carcinoma.*

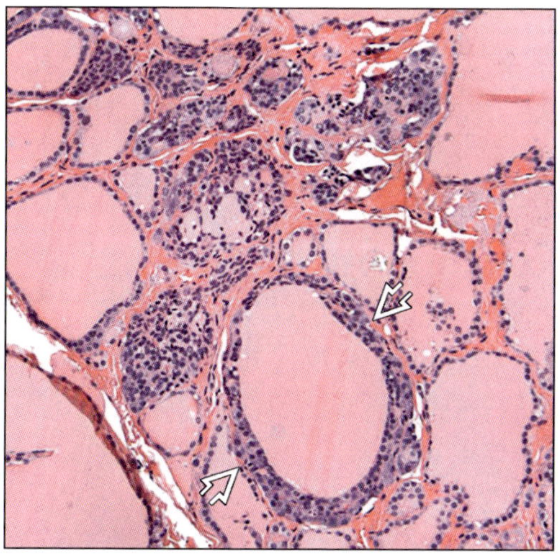
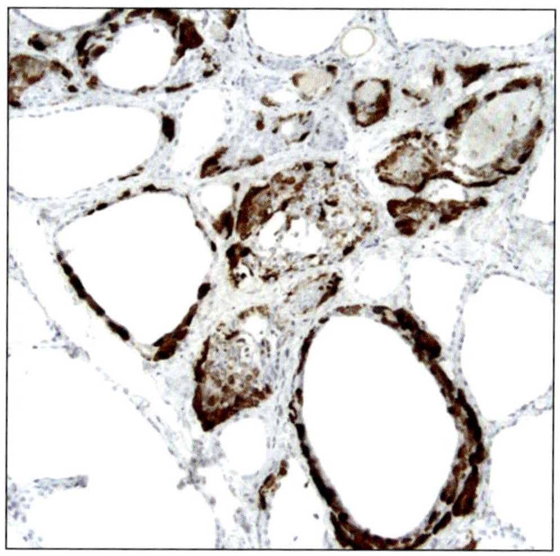

(Left) *C-cell hyperplasia is present in a patient with MEN2 syndrome, with C cells surrounding the entire thyroid follicle and replacing the follicular cells.* ***(Right)*** *Specimen from a patient with MEN2 syndrome who underwent prophylactic thyroidectomy shows C-cell hyperplasia, with calcitonin-positive C cells surrounding the thyroid follicle. Heritable medullary thyroid carcinoma is preceded by C-cell hyperplasia (called neoplastic C-cell hyperplasia).*

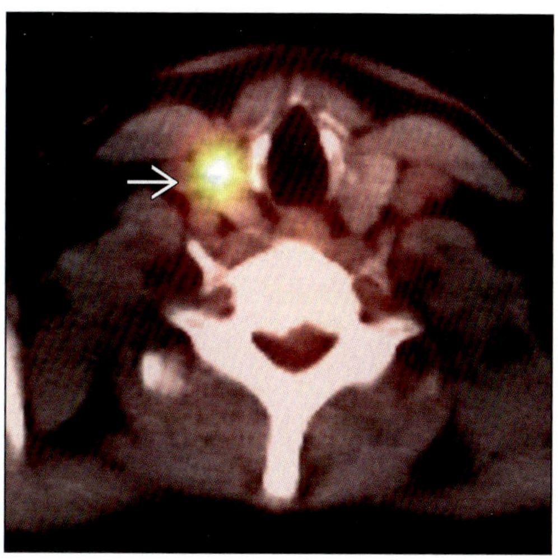
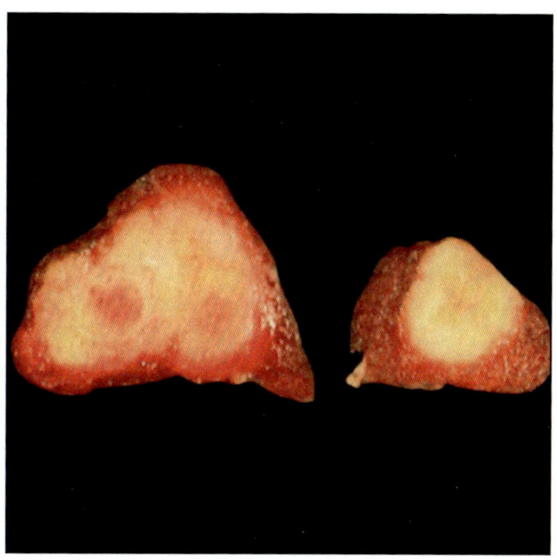

(Left) *Fused transaxial FDG PET/CT shows a focal hypermetabolic mass in the right thyroid lobe in a patient with medullary thyroid cancer.* ***(Right)*** *Gross cut surface of both thyroid lobes from a patient with MEN2A shows 2 well-circumscribed white-yellow thyroid tumor nodules. Medullary thyroid carcinomas are usually firm and gritty, and familial medullary thyroid carcinomas are usually bilateral and with associated C-cell hyperplasia.*

FAMILIAL THYROID CARCINOMA

Familial Medullary Thyroid Carcinoma

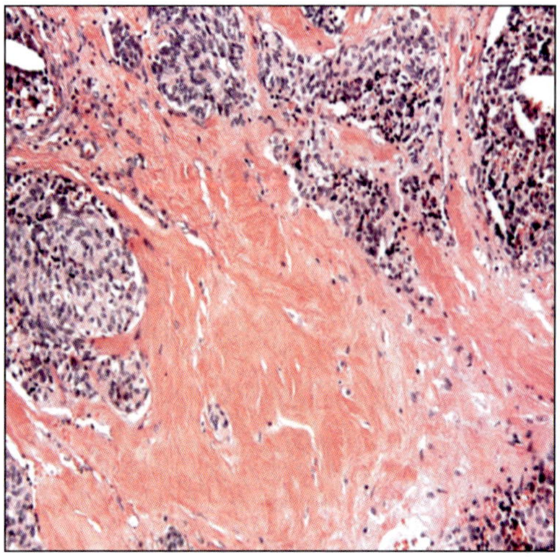

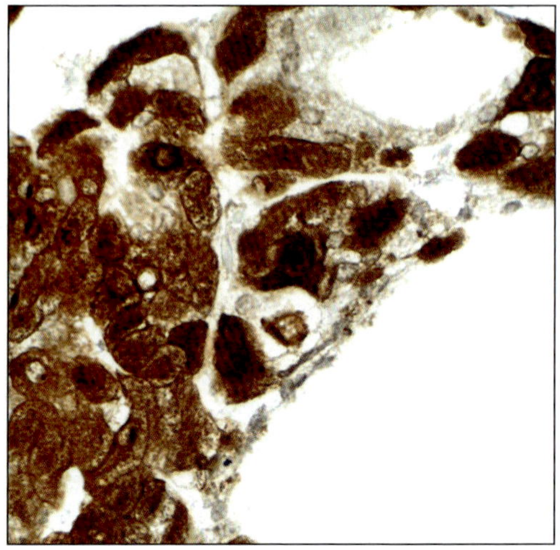

(Left) *H&E shows the characteristic histologic appearance of medullary thyroid carcinoma, a highly cellular tumor with a variable amount of fibrosis and amyloid deposition.* ***(Right)*** *Calcitonin immunostaining is usually strongly positive in the tumor cells whereas the areas of fibrosis or amyloid deposition are characteristically negative.*

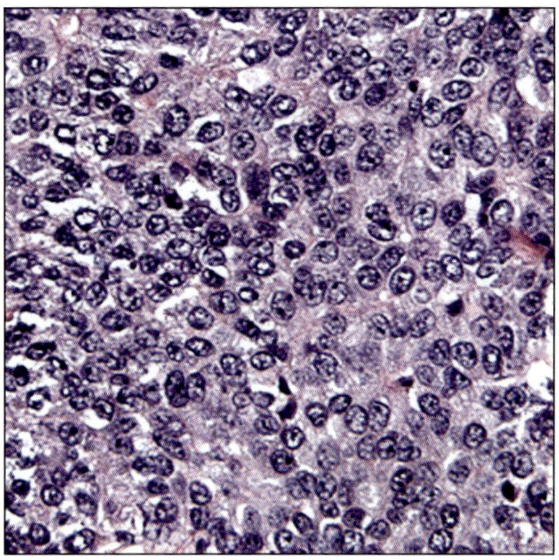

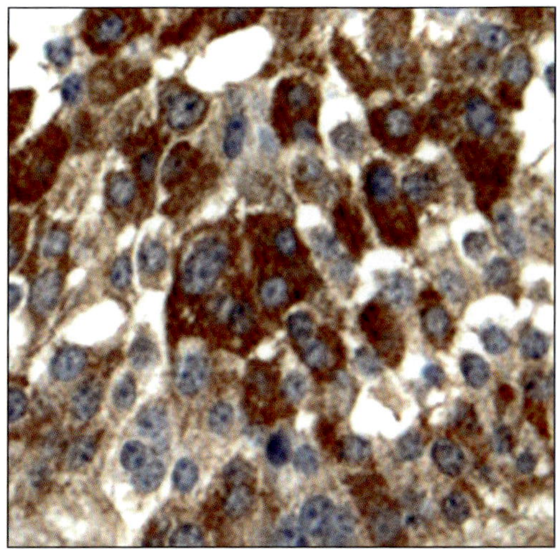

(Left) *The characteristic histopathological features of medullary thyroid carcinoma are solid sheets and groups of round to polygonal tumor cells separated by thin fibrovascular cores. There is a variable amount of cytoplasm, and the medium-sized nuclei have minimal nuclear pleomorphism. Mitoses are usually rare.* ***(Right)*** *Medullary thyroid carcinoma from a patient with familial medullary thyroid carcinoma syndrome shows variable cytoplasmic immunostaining for calcitonin.*

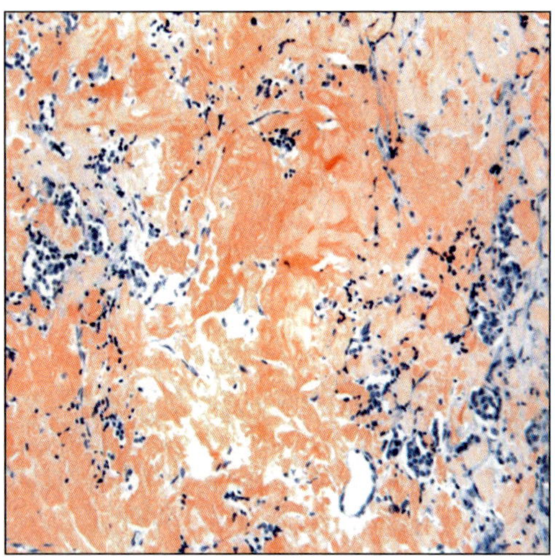

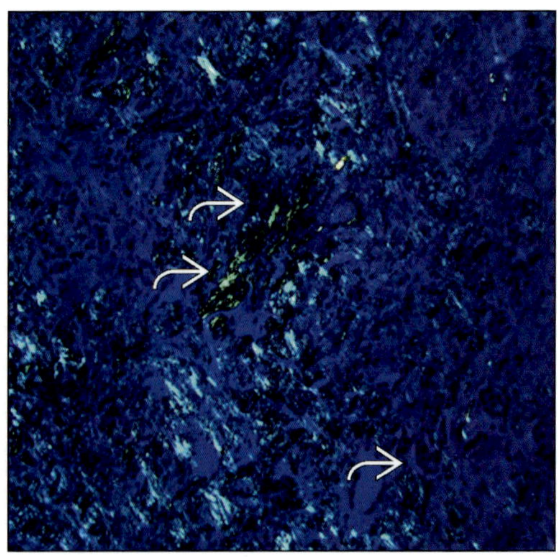

(Left) *This photomicrograph of a Congo red-stained tumor shows extensive deposition of amyloid. Although amyloid is not essential for the diagnosis of medullary thyroid carcinoma, most of these tumors have at least some amyloid deposition.* ***(Right)*** *Congo red-stained medullary thyroid carcinoma under polarized light reveals the characteristic apple-green birefringence ↪, confirming amyloid deposition.*

PTEN-Associated Thyroid Lesions

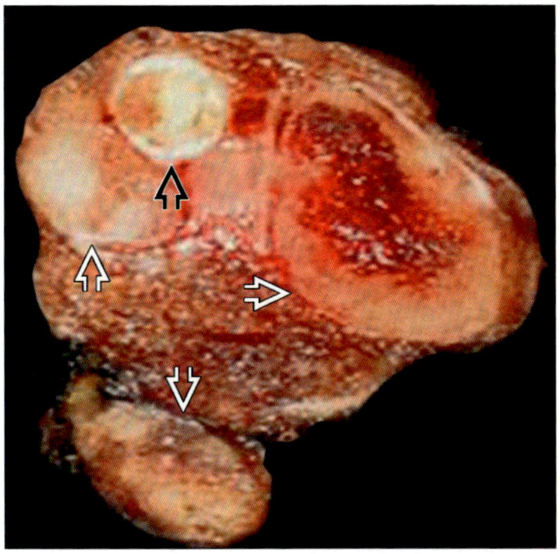

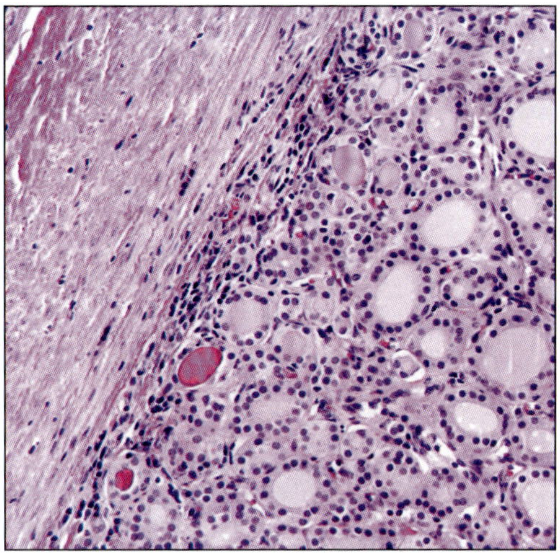

(Left) *Gross cut surface of a thyroid from a 12-year-old patient with Cowden syndrome/PTEN-hamartoma tumor syndrome (PHTS) shows multiple well-circumscribed nodules and 1 encapsulated nodule.* ***(Right)*** *This photomicrograph of thyroid tissue from a patient with Cowden disease shows a well-encapsulated follicular adenoma. These lesions are usually present in association with multiple adenomatous nodules.*

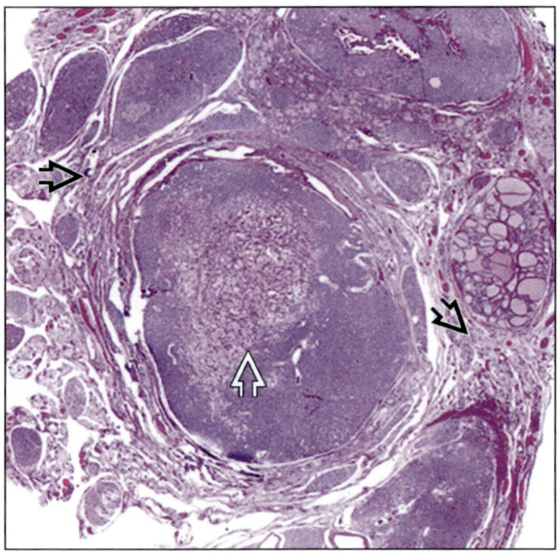

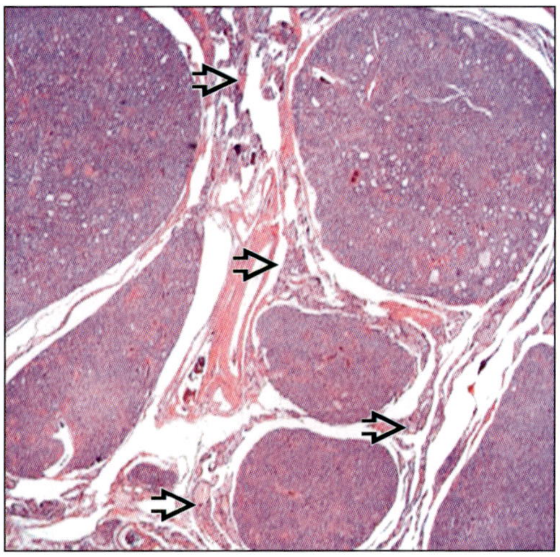

(Left) *H&E of the thyroid from a patient with Cowden disease shows diffuse involvement by diversely sized adenomatous nodules. The larger nodule shows focal central degenerative changes. Note compressed intervening thyroid parenchyma.* ***(Right)*** *H&E of the thyroid from an 18-year-old woman with Cowden disease shows multiple well-circumscribed adenomatous nodules with a small amount of compressed residual thyroid parenchyma.*

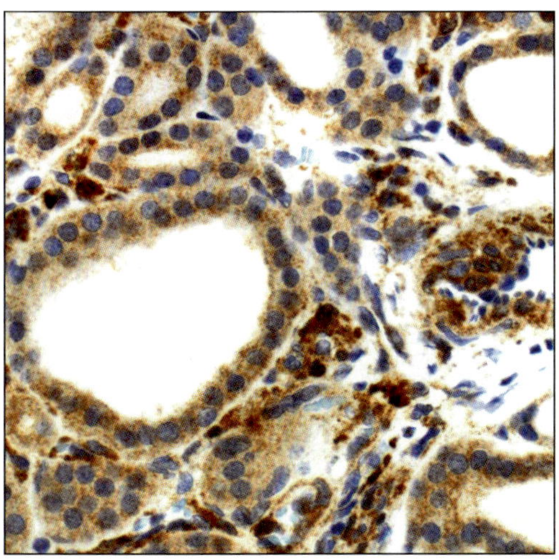

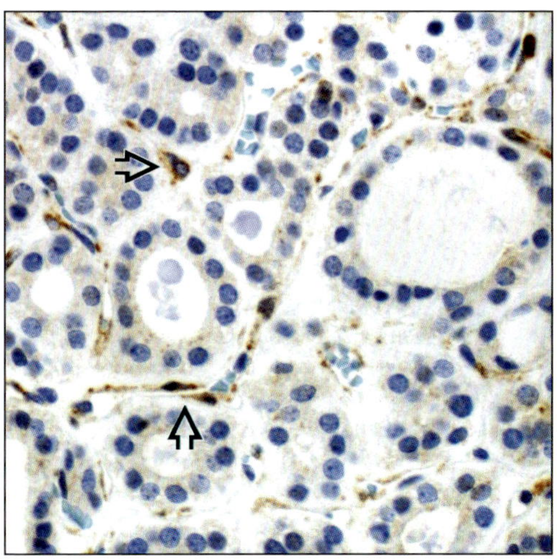

(Left) *Immunohistochemistry for PTEN shows preservation of the staining in the follicular cells in a patient with no known genetic abnormalities of the PTEN gene.* ***(Right)*** *Immunohistochemistry for PTEN in a thyroidectomy specimen from an 18-year-old woman with PHTS/Cowden disease shows loss of staining of the follicular cells with preservation of staining of the endothelial cells.*

FAMILIAL THYROID CARCINOMA

Familial Adenomatous Polyposis (FAP) Features

__(Left)__ This colectomy specimen from a 17-year-old girl with known thyroid tumor and familial adenomatous polyposis shows numerous polyps on the mucosal surface. This patient had multiple foci of cribriform-morular papillary thyroid carcinoma. __(Right)__ This image shows congenital hypertrophy of the pigmented retinal epithelium. This condition is benign, and it is found in up to 2/3 of patients who have FAP.

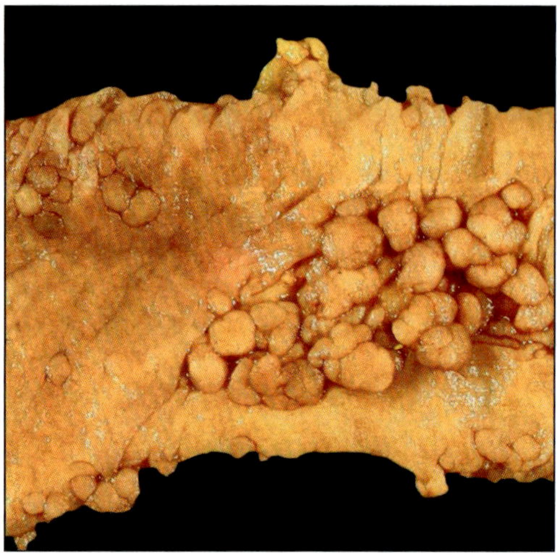

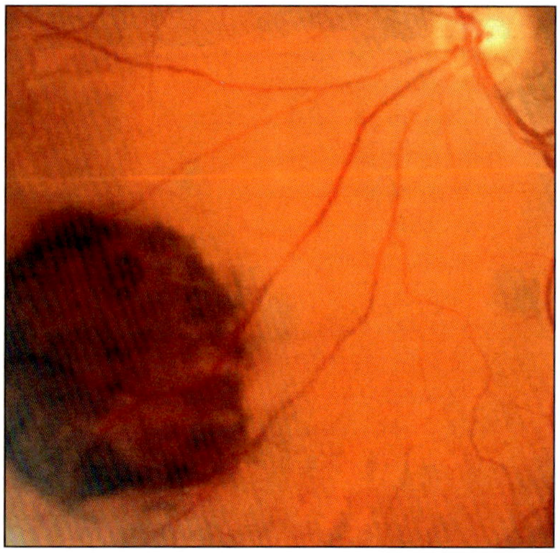

__(Left)__ Gross cut surface of a large PTC, cribriform-morular variant (CMV), shows irregular areas of fibrosis and a pale, soft, and friable tumor mass occupying most of the section. This variant usually has extensive fibrosis and a thick fibrous capsule. They are usually multiple and bilateral. __(Right)__ This image shows the cytologic features of tumor cells typically seen in the cribriform-morular variant. The cells are cuboidal with basophilic cytoplasm and hyperchromatic nuclei. Note the absence of classic PTC nuclei.

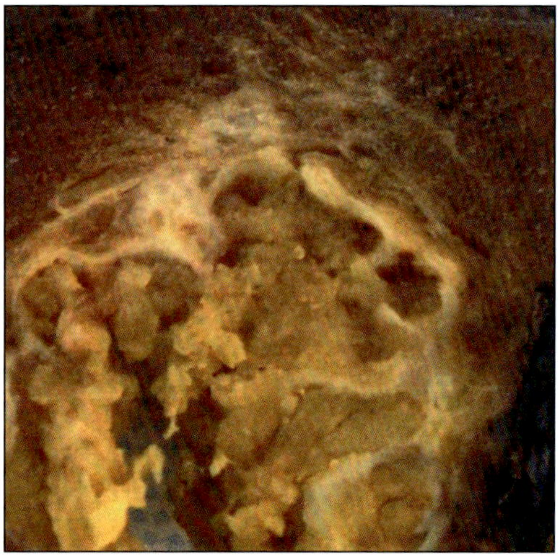

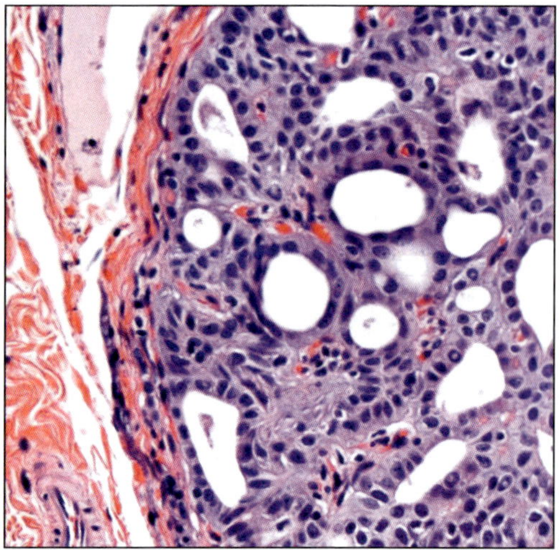

__(Left)__ Encapsulation is common in this variant of PTC. This particular example shows a thick fibrous band encapsulating the tumor. Note the papillary and cribriform architecture. Also shown are eosinophilic foci of sclerosis/hyalinization ⇨ within the stroma. This focus of tumor was < 1 cm. __(Right)__ This image shows a metastatic tumor focus in a lymph node, an unusual finding. The tumor deposit is largely cystic, though a small papillary structure with cribriform-appearing areas is present.

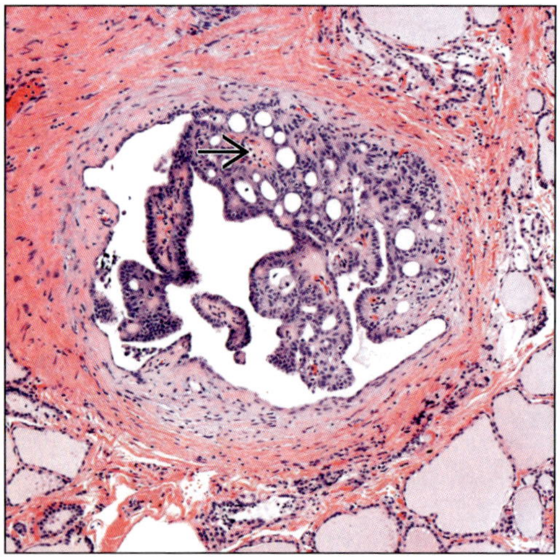

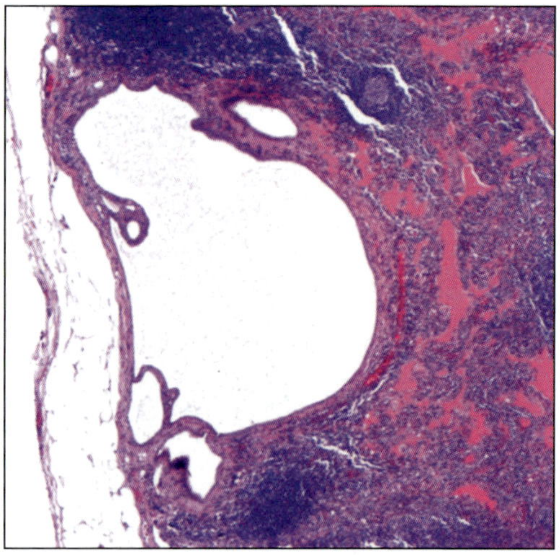

FAP-Associated Thyroid Tumors

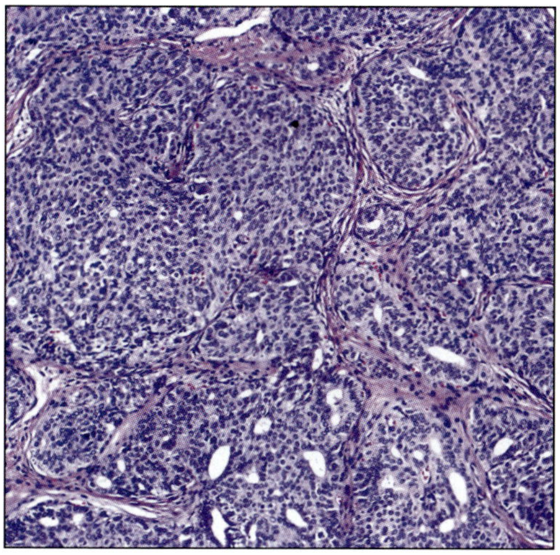

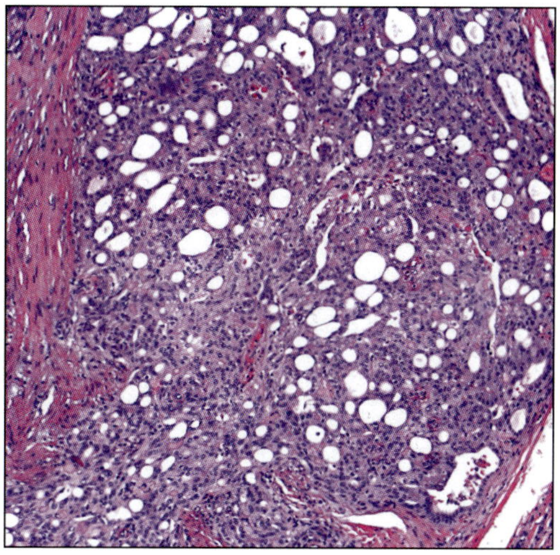

(Left) *This image demonstrates the solid pattern seen in cribriform-morular variant-papillary thyroid carcinoma (CMV-PTC). An area with the more common cribriform pattern is seen in the lower right-hand corner of the image.* ***(Right)*** *This photograph illustrates CMV-PTC and highlights the cribriform appearance of these types of tumors. This tumor shows areas of both cribriform pattern and solid pattern; however, this tumor has a predominantly cribriform architecture.*

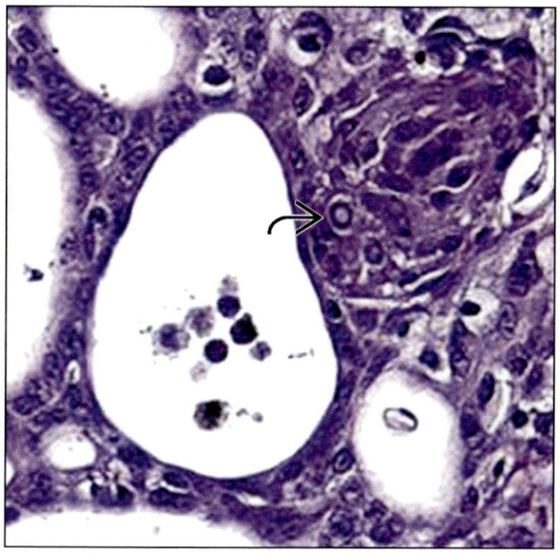

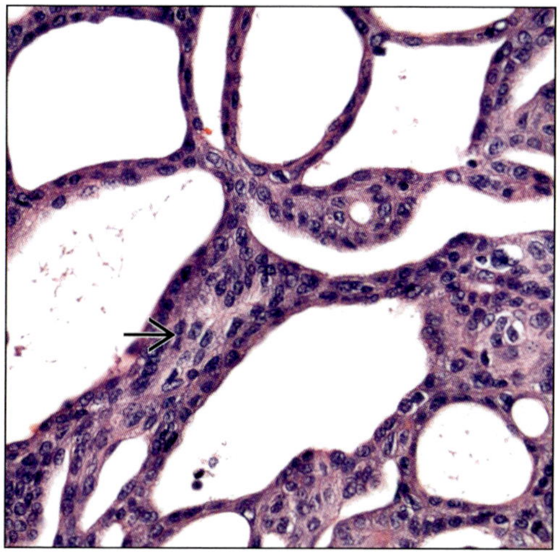

(Left) *High-power H&E stain demonstrates the characteristic peculiar nuclear clearing (PNC) → seen within some of the nuclei in CMV-PTC. These PNCs are characteristically found within squamous morules.* ***(Right)*** *A cribriform pattern tumor with focal solid areas and a spindle cell component → is seen in this high magnification. The cells are spindled with basophilic cytoplasm and hyperchromatic nuclei with absence of typical PTC nuclei.*

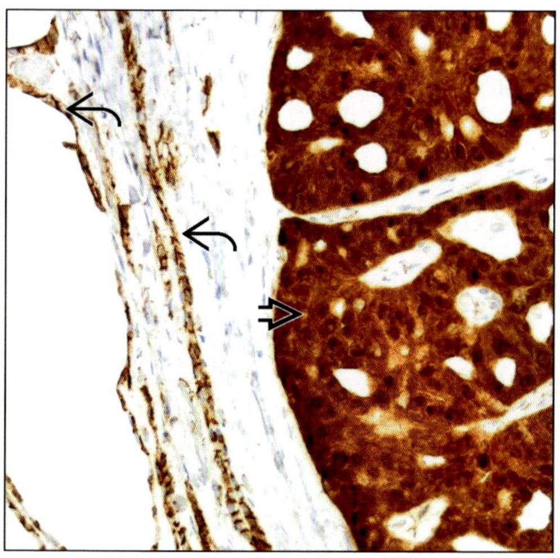

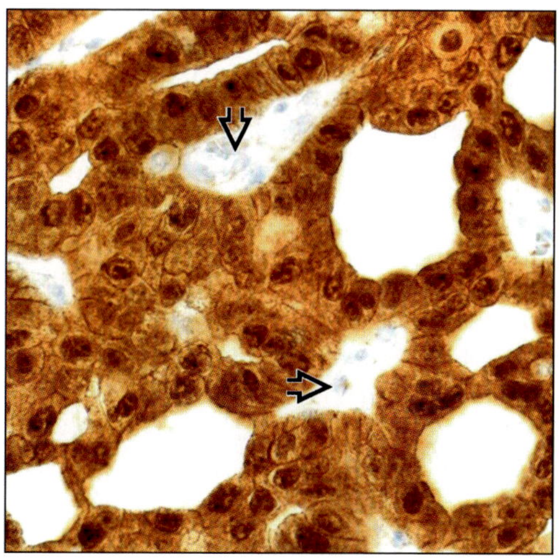

(Left) *β-catenin immunostain shows the characteristic cytoplasmic and nuclear staining → in CMV-PTC, as well as the cytoplasmic membrane staining in the adjacent compressed follicular cells →.* ***(Right)*** *High-power image of β-catenin immunostain in CMV-PTC demonstrates characteristic nuclear and cytoplasmic staining resulting from aberrant accumulation within the nucleus. Note the negativity of the endothelial cells →.*

FOLLICULAR CARCINOMA

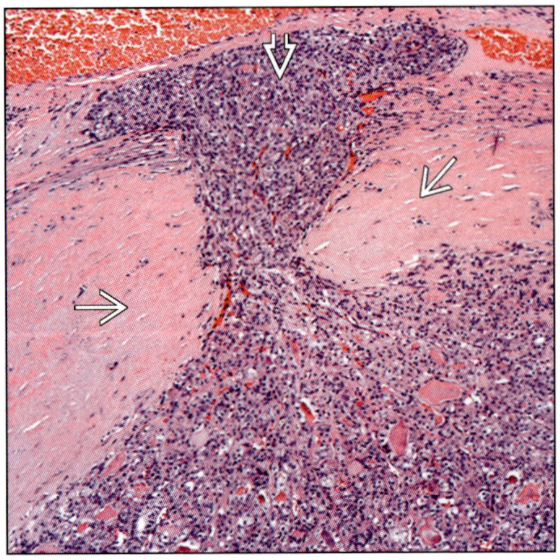

Photomicrograph depicts the classic "mushroom" sign, diagnostic of follicular thyroid carcinoma. The tumor cells are seen ➡ invading across the entire thickness of the fibrous capsule ➡.

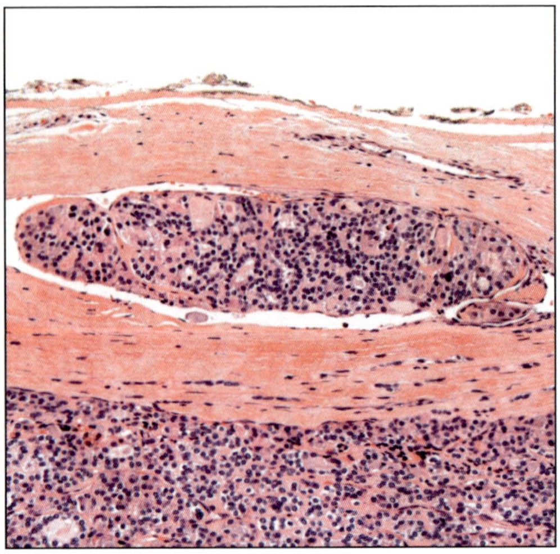

This image illustrates a hallmark in the diagnosis of follicular thyroid carcinoma. Vascular invasion is shown here with tumor cells present within a large capsular blood vessel.

TERMINOLOGY

Abbreviations

- Follicular carcinoma (FC)

Synonyms

- Follicular thyroid carcinoma
- Familial nonmedullary thyroid carcinoma
- Familial follicular thyroid carcinoma

Definitions

- Malignant epithelial follicular cell tumor of thyroid
  - Shows evidence of follicular cell differentiation
  - Lacks diagnostic features of papillary thyroid carcinoma
  - Occurs in a familial setting

ETIOLOGY/PATHOGENESIS

Inherited Tumor Syndromes

- Accounts for at least 5% of follicular thyroid carcinoma (FTC) in USA
- **PTEN-hamartoma tumor syndrome** (PHTS)
  - Cowden syndrome, Bannayan-Riley-Ruvalcaba syndrome (BRRS), Proteus syndrome, and Proteus-like syndrome
  - Germline mutation of *PTEN* gene transmitted in autosomal dominant fashion
  - Individuals may also develop multiple hamartomas of breast, colon, endometrium, brain, and ganglioneuromatous proliferations
    - Trichilemmomas
  - Affected individuals may develop benign and malignant tumors of breast, uterus, and thyroid
    - Breast cancer: Early onset; most women diagnosed between 38 and 46 years of age
  - May be associated with multiple follicular adenomas and carcinomas of the thyroid
    - Thyroid tumors are associated with multiple thyroid nodules in a young patient
    - Follicular thyroid carcinoma is a major diagnostic criteria for diagnosis of PHTS
- **Carney complex**
  - Autosomal dominant disorder caused by mutations in *PRKAR1A* gene
  - Carney complex includes cardiac myxomas, multiple endocrine neoplasms, and spotty cutaneous pigmentation
  - 75% of patients develop multiple thyroid nodules
    - ~ 5% of patients may present with follicular or papillary carcinoma
- **Werner syndrome**
  - Autosomal recessive
  - Caused by mutations in *WRN* gene
  - Age-related disorders are present early in patient's life including malignancies
    - Melanoma, soft tissue sarcoma, osteosarcoma
    - Up to 3% of patients will have thyroid disease, usually FTC
- **McCune-Albright syndrome**
  - Patients harbor postzygotic mutations in *GNAS1* gene with mosaic distribution
  - Triad of café au lait skin pigmentation, polyostotic fibrous dysplasia, and hyperfunctioning endocrinopathies
  - Associated with precocious puberty, hyperthyroidism, GH excess, and Cushing syndrome
    - Associated with FTC and papillary thyroid carcinomas
- **Li-Fraumeni syndrome**
  - Caused by germline mutation of *TP53*
  - Development of diverse sarcomas and carcinomas at a young age
  - Unusual thyroid follicular cell tumors with marked nuclear pleomorphism

FOLLICULAR CARCINOMA

Key Facts

Terminology
- Malignant epithelial tumor of thyroid showing evidence of follicular cell differentiation but lacking diagnostic features of papillary thyroid carcinoma

Etiology/Pathogenesis
- Familial follicular thyroid carcinoma (FTC) accounts for at least 5% of FTC in USA
- **PTEN-hamartoma tumor syndrome** (PHTS)
  - May be associated with multiple follicular adenomas and carcinomas
- **Carney complex**
  - 75% of patients develop multiple thyroid nodules
- **Werner syndrome**
  - Up to 3% of patients will have thyroid disease, usually FTC
- **McCune-Albright syndrome**
  - Associated with FTC and papillary thyroid carcinomas
- **Li-Fraumeni syndrome**
  - Unusual thyroid follicular cell tumors with marked nuclear pleomorphism

Macroscopic Features
- Usually multiple and bilateral in familial setting

Diagnostic Checklist
- Thyroid carcinoma in familial setting is usually multifocal and bilateral
- Familial cases are reportedly more aggressive than their sporadic counterparts and are usually associated with adenomatous nodules, multinodular hyperplasia, follicular adenomas, and lymphocytic thyroiditis

Preexisting Thyroid Disease
- Present in up to 15% of patients with FTC
- Dyshormonogenic goiter with chronic TSH stimulation may predispose to follicular neoplasms
- Associated with other thyroid tumors, mostly follicular adenoma
  - These tumors are identical histologically
  - Follicular adenoma may be the precursor of follicular carcinoma
    - Both harbor *RAS, PTEN,* and *PIK3CA* mutations
- Lymphocytic thyroiditis and FTC may coexist
- Association between lymphocytic thyroiditis and FTC remains unclear

CLINICAL ISSUES

Epidemiology
- Incidence
  - 10-20% of thyroid malignancies
- Age
  - Inherited syndrome-related FTC affects patients at earlier age than does sporadic FTC
    - Sporadic cases: 5th decade
- Gender
  - More common in women

Presentation
- Painless mass
- Slow growing
- Difficulty swallowing

Prognosis
- 70-80% cure rate if disease is confined to thyroid
- 20-30% recurrence when regional lymph node metastases are present
- 50-90% of patients who present with distant metastases will die

IMAGE FINDINGS

Ultrasonographic Findings
- In minimally invasive disease, usually a well-circumscribed nodule (> 1 cm)
- Cannot distinguish follicular adenoma from FTC
  - Carcinoma is usually associated with microcalcifications, hypoechogenicity, irregular margins or absent halo sign, solid aspect, intranodular vascularization, and shape (taller than wide)
- May be helpful in assessing lymph node involvement by thyroid carcinoma

Scintigraphy
- Scan shows "cold" nodule

MACROSCOPIC FEATURES

General Features
- Round to ovoid encapsulated tumors, tan to light brown
- Usually multiple and bilateral in familial setting
- Minimally invasive tumors: Thick irregular fibrous capsule and grossly similar or indistinguishable from follicular adenoma
- Widely invasive carcinomas: Lack of capsule or extensive permeation of capsule

Size
- Round to ovoid encapsulated tumors 1-10 cm in diameter

Categories of Tumor
- Minimally invasive follicular carcinoma
- Widely invasive follicular carcinoma
- Oncocytic follicular carcinoma
  - This subtype was formerly called oxyphil or Hürthle cell carcinoma

FOLLICULAR CARCINOMA

MICROSCOPIC PATHOLOGY

Histologic Features

- Tumors arise in a background of multiple adenomatous nodules, nodular hyperplasia, &/or lymphocytic thyroiditis
- Follicular carcinoma in familial diseases may be an incidental finding within a thyroid with multiple nodules
- Follicular carcinoma in inherited syndromes tends to be
  - Smaller than sporadic tumors
  - Multiple
  - Bilateral
- Criteria for capsular invasion
  - Tumor bud has invaded beyond outer contour of capsule
  - Tumor bud still clothed by thin capsule; however, it has extended through outer capsular surface
  - Presence of satellite nodule with cytoarchitectural and cellular features identical to those of tumor cells
  - Classic mushroom-like bud that has totally transgressed fibrous capsule
- Criteria for vascular invasion
  - Blood vessels should be of larger caliber with an identifiable wall the size of a vein, and involved blood vessels must be located within or outside fibrous capsule (i.e., not within tumor)
  - Intravascular polypoid tumor growth must protrude into lumen, be covered by endothelium, and be attached to wall of vessel and associated with a thrombus
  - Clusters of epithelial cells floating in vascular lumen and unattached to wall are not considered vascular invasion
- Nodal status
  - Metastasis present or absent, ipsilateral vs. contralateral, number with metastases, size of largest metastatic deposit
    - Metastases are reportedly more frequent in familial cases

ANCILLARY TESTS

Molecular Genetics

- Mutations in *PTEN, PRKAR1A, WRN, GNAS1,* and *TP53* genes
- Accumulation of additional mutations, such as *TP53,* may be associated with progression to poorly differentiated carcinomas
- **Testing families with a history of cancer**
  - Most useful to begin by testing the individual with cancer
    - If multiple affected individuals are present within a kindred, testing can establish linkage between the cancer(s) and the mutation
- **Predictive models**
  - *PTEN*: Available at http://www.lerner.ccf.org/gmi/ccscore/index.php

DIFFERENTIAL DIAGNOSIS

Sporadic Follicular Carcinoma

- Usually single
- Usually unilateral
- Background thyroid with no other pathological findings
- Less aggressive than familial counterpart

DIAGNOSTIC CHECKLIST

Pathologic Interpretation Pearls

- Pathologist's most important tasks are to
  - Demonstrate capsular or vascular invasion, as the diagnosis of FTC rests on identifying these
  - Differentiate between FTC and numerous variants of follicular adenoma and other benign or malignant neoplasms
  - Identify pathological characteristics of inherited tumor syndrome
- Thyroid carcinoma in familial setting is usually multifocal and bilateral
- Familial cases are reportedly more aggressive than their sporadic counterparts
- Familial cases are usually associated with other thyroid pathology: Adenomatous nodules, multinodular hyperplasia, follicular adenomas, and lymphocytic thyroiditis

SELECTED REFERENCES

1. Laury AR et al: Thyroid pathology in *PTEN*-hamartoma tumor syndrome: characteristic findings of a distinct entity. Thyroid. 21(2):135-44, 2011
2. Nosé V: Familial thyroid cancer: a review. Mod Pathol. 24 Suppl 2:S19-33, 2011
3. Paschke R et al: Thyroid nodule guidelines: agreement, disagreement and need for future research. Nat Rev Endocrinol. 7(6):354-61, 2011
4. Nosé V: Thyroid cancer of follicular cell origin in inherited tumor syndromes. Adv Anat Pathol. 17(6):428-36, 2010
5. Ohori NP et al: Contribution of molecular testing to thyroid fine-needle aspiration cytology of "follicular lesion of undetermined significance/atypia of undetermined significance". Cancer Cytopathol. 118(1):17-23, 2010
6. Dotto J et al: Familial thyroid carcinoma: a diagnostic algorithm. Adv Anat Pathol. 15(6):332-49, 2008
7. Rago T et al: Role of thyroid ultrasound in the diagnostic evaluation of thyroid nodules. Best Pract Res Clin Endocrinol Metab. 22(6):913-28, 2008
8. Serra S et al: Controversies in thyroid pathology: the diagnosis of follicular neoplasms. Endocr Pathol. 19(3):156-65, 2008
9. Rosai J et al: Pitfalls in thyroid tumour pathology. Histopathology. 49(2):107-20, 2006
10. Collins MT et al: Thyroid carcinoma in the McCune-Albright syndrome: contributory role of activating Gs alpha mutations. J Clin Endocrinol Metab. 88(9):4413-7, 2003
11. French CA et al: Genetic and biological subgroups of low-stage follicular thyroid cancer. Am J Pathol. 162(4):1053-60, 2003

FOLLICULAR CARCINOMA

Differential Diagnosis of Follicular Thyroid Carcinoma

Lesion	Characteristic Findings	Comments
Dominant nodule in nodular hyperplasia	Follicles have different sizes and shapes; colloid ranges from pale to dark red, and these nodules have irregular fibrosis and pseudocapsule	Capsule in follicular carcinoma is thick and surrounds entire nodule; colloid is homogeneous and dark red in follicular carcinoma
Adenomatous nodule	Usually multiple and nonencapsulated	Follicular carcinoma may occur in association with adenomatous nodules
Follicular adenoma	Usually single and surrounded by thin capsule	Fibrous capsule in follicular adenoma is usually thinner than in follicular carcinoma
Follicular variant of papillary thyroid carcinoma	Follicular-patterned neoplasm with focal nuclear features of papillary thyroid carcinoma	Usually main differential diagnosis with follicular carcinoma
Poorly differentiated thyroid carcinoma	Pattern of follicular cells is usually in solid, trabecular, and insular pattern, and presents with rare follicles	May show apoptosis, necrosis, and high mitotic rate; has higher Ki-67 proliferative index, and some are positive for p53
Hyalinizing trabecular tumor	This benign thyroid tumor is well circumscribed but lacks a fibrous capsule; has trabecular growth pattern and rarely forms follicles	Positive for TTF-1 and thyroglobulin; however, HTT has characteristic membranous staining for Ki-67/MIB-1
Medullary thyroid carcinoma, follicular patterned	Tumor cells in medullary thyroid carcinoma have ample eosinophilic granular cytoplasm and salt-and-pepper nuclei	Both tumors are positive for TTF-1; medullary thyroid carcinoma is positive for chromogranin, synaptophysin, calcitonin, and CEA

Follicular Thyroid Carcinoma in Familial Setting

Syndrome	Common Clinical Findings	Thyroid Pathology Findings
PTEN-hamartoma tumor syndrome	Mucocutaneous lesions, breast carcinoma, endometrial carcinoma, thyroid carcinoma, macrocephaly, gastrointestinal hamartomas, lipomas, and other tumors	Follicular carcinoma associated with multiple adenomatous nodules and multiple follicular adenomas
Carney complex	Myxomas, spotty mucocutaneous pigmentation, psammomatous melanotic schwannoma, breast ductal adenoma, multiple endocrine neoplasms including PPNAD, GH-producing adenoma, thyroid carcinoma	Small percentage (about 5%) of patients with this syndrome may develop follicular carcinoma, usually associated with other thyroid nodules
Werner syndrome	Bilateral cataracts, characteristic dermatological findings, short stature, osteoporosis, multiple neoplasms at a younger age	Small percentage (about 3%) of patients with this syndrome develop follicular carcinoma
McCune-Albright syndrome	GH excess, Cushing syndrome, precocious puberty	Patients may develop follicular carcinoma and papillary thyroid carcinoma
Li-Fraumeni syndrome	Sarcomas, brain tumor, adrenal cortical carcinoma, breast cancer, other tumors at a young age; rarely involves thyroid	Patients develop many thyroid nodules with nuclear pleomorphism and may develop follicular carcinoma

PPNAD = primary pigmented nodular adrenocortical disease.

FOLLICULAR CARCINOMA

Gross, Diagrammatic, and Microscopic Features

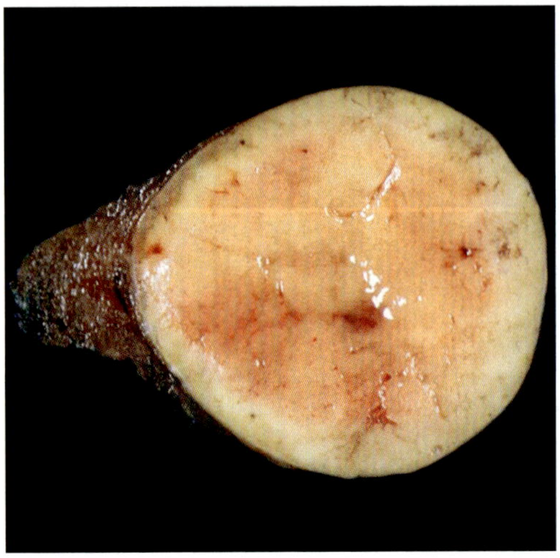
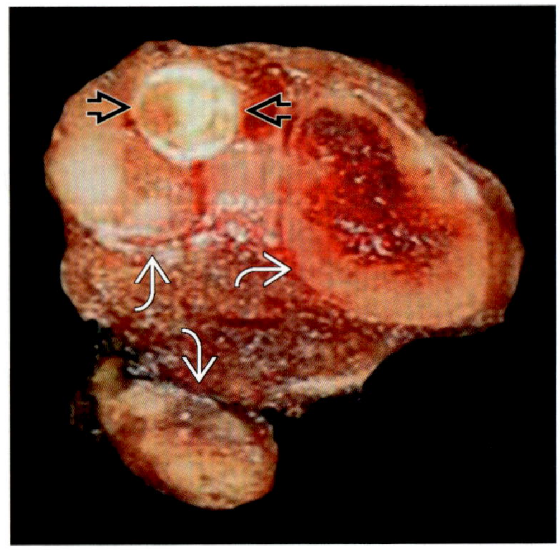

***(Left)** Gross photograph shows a minimally invasive follicular carcinoma presenting as a single nodule in a sporadic setting. The tumor is grossly indistinguishable from a follicular adenoma. Thorough examination of the capsule is crucial to identify foci of capsular invasion. **(Right)** Gross cut surface of a thyroid from a 12-year-old patient with PTEN-hamartoma tumor syndrome shows multiple adenomatous nodules ➔ and a follicular carcinoma ⇨, confirmed by histopathology.*

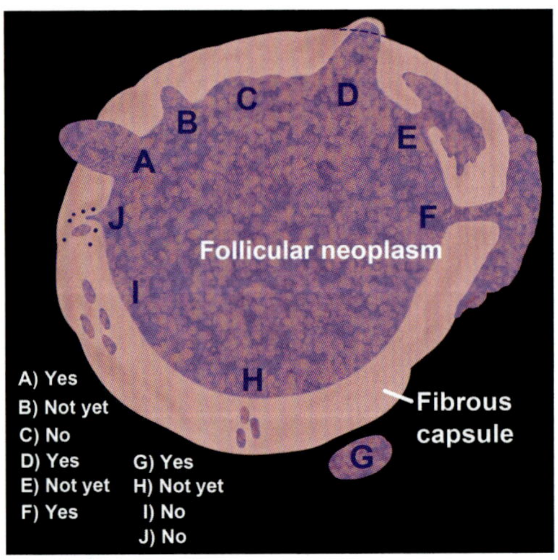

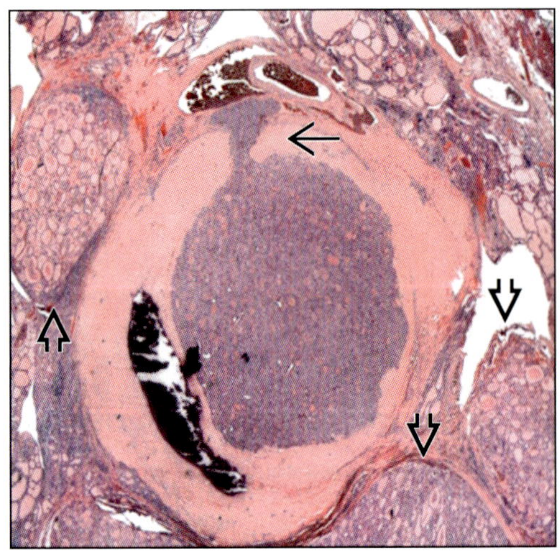

***(Left)** A schematic drawing illustrates the criteria necessary to interpret and diagnose a follicular neoplasm as follicular carcinoma based on capsular invasion. The follicular neoplasm is surrounded by a thick fibrous capsule with invasion on A, D, F, and G. **(Right)** Low-power photomicrograph shows multiple well-circumscribed adenomatous nodules ⇨ and a follicular carcinoma. Full-thickness capsular invasion is easily recognizable →. In this case, the patient has PTEN-associated thyroid disease.*

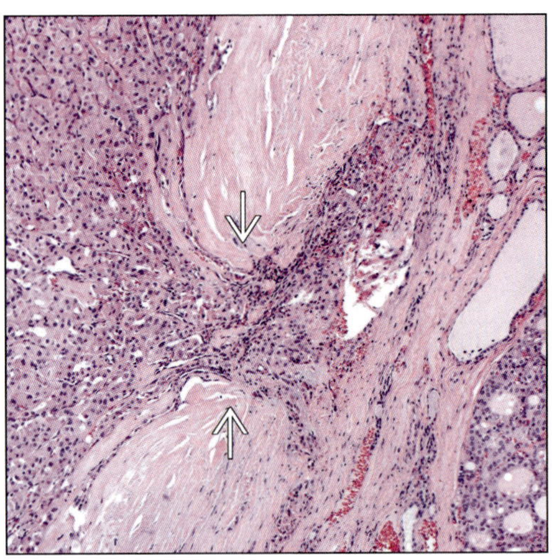
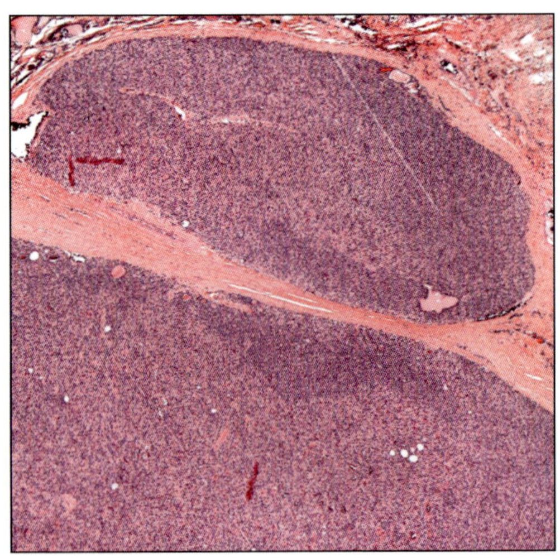

***(Left)** Minimally invasive follicular carcinoma shows the point of invasion. There is tumor capsule invasion ➔ through the entire capsule thickness, invading a large blood vessel along the way. **(Right)** Follicular carcinoma with cytologically identical satellite nodules indicates true capsular invasion, even without demonstration of the point of capsular penetration.*

Microscopic Features

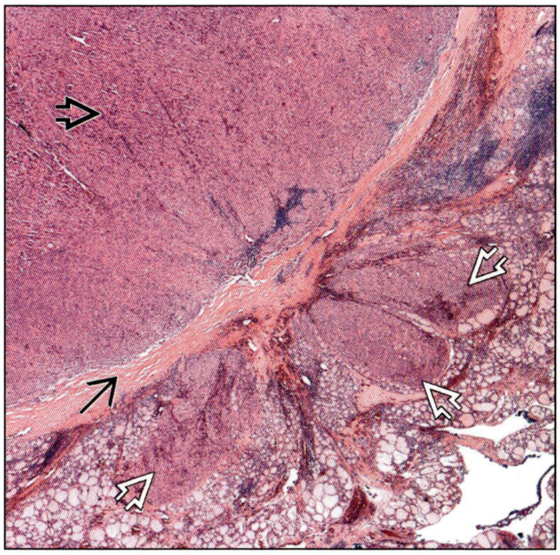

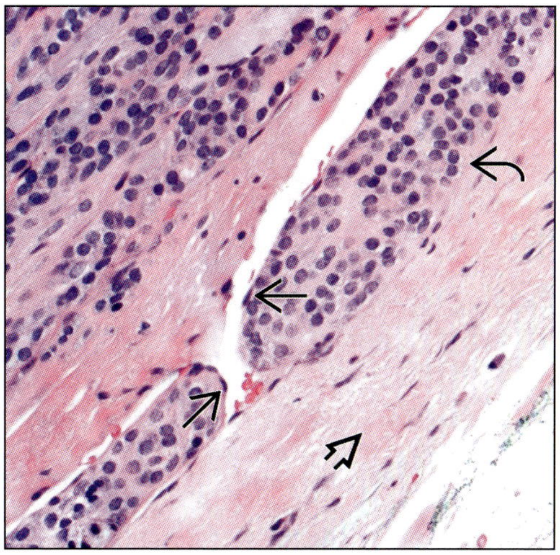

(Left) *Photomicrograph of a follicular carcinoma shows finger-like projections of the tumor protruding beyond the capsule into the surrounding thyroid parenchyma.* ***(Right)*** *High-power micrograph shows 2 groups of tumor cells in a vessel within the tumor capsule. The tumor cells are attached to the vessel wall. Endothelial cells can be seen lining both tumor thrombi.*

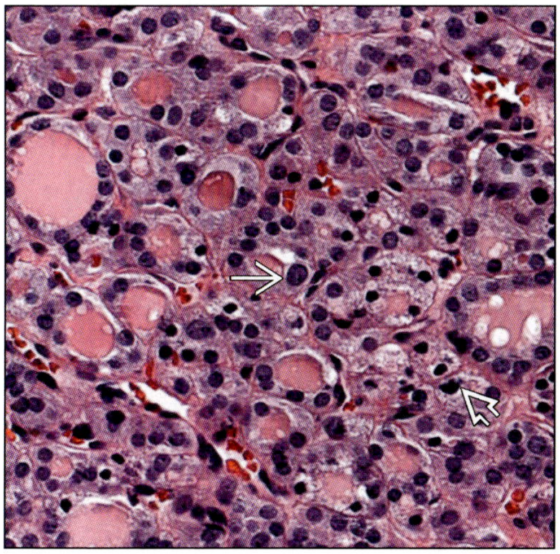

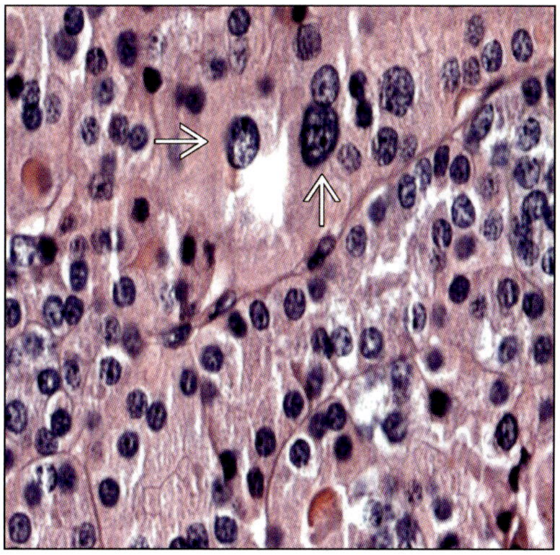

(Left) *Nuclear pleomorphism can be present to various degrees in follicular carcinoma. This case presents microfollicular architecture with a few large irregular nuclei that may show nucleoli. Colloid is present throughout the tumor. A mitotic figure is seen.* ***(Right)*** *High-power view of an FTC depicts pleomorphism and cellular atypia. The overall follicular architecture is preserved, but cells with pink granular cytoplasm and irregular large nuclei are present.*

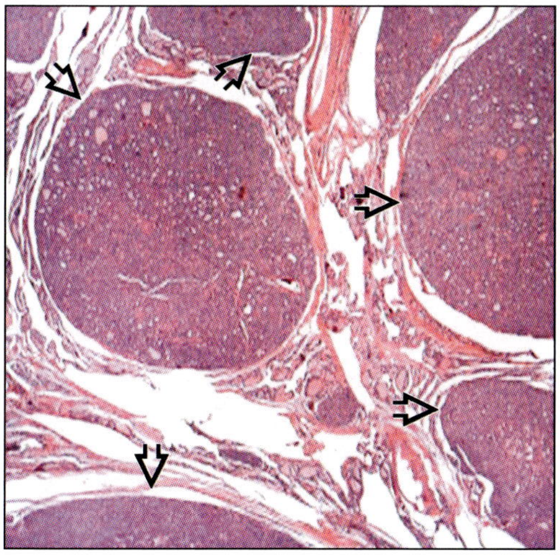

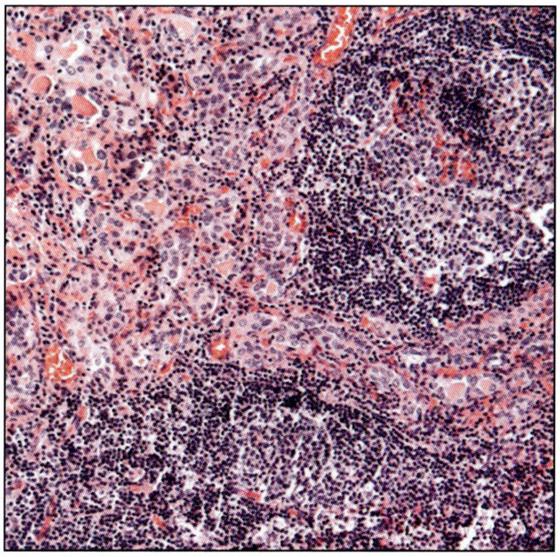

(Left) *Follicular thyroid carcinoma in a familial setting is usually associated with other thyroid diseases. In this patient with PTEN hamartoma tumor syndrome, the follicular carcinoma was found in a thyroid with multiple adenomatous nodules and lymphocytic thyroiditis.* ***(Right)*** *Patients with familial syndromes involving the thyroid usually have associated lymphocytic thyroiditis. This field shows prominent lymphoid aggregates with germinal center and focal oncocytic follicular cell changes.*

C-CELL HYPERPLASIA

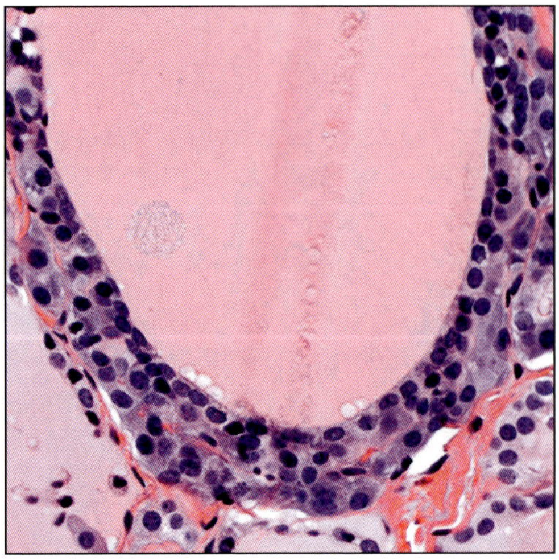

The hyperplastic C cells in this photomicrograph surround almost the entire thyroid follicle. The C-cell proliferation has a diffuse pattern and the C cells have an ample blue granular cytoplasm.

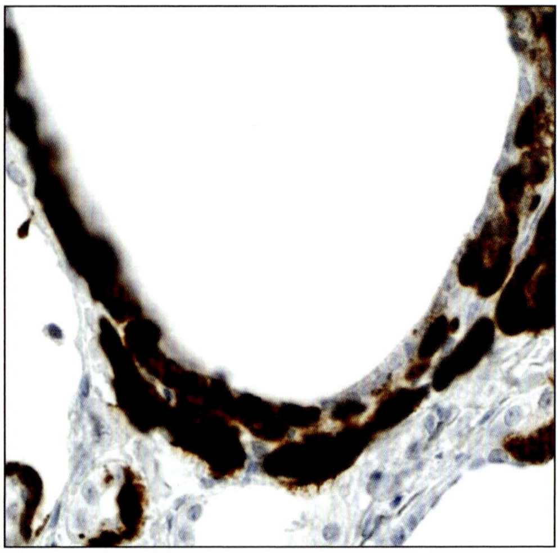

The thyroid follicular cells are almost completely replaced by an increased number of C cells, highlighted by calcitonin immunostaining. The C cells surround the thyroid follicle in a diffuse pattern.

TERMINOLOGY

Abbreviations

- C-cell hyperplasia (CCH)

Synonyms

- C-cell proliferation

Definitions

- C cells produce calcitonin and are normally found at junction of upper and middle 1/3 of thyroid lobes bilaterally
- CCH is an increase in C-cell population in thyroid due to reactive/physiologic or neoplastic process
- Proposed diagnostic criteria include
  - > 50 C cells per low-power field (WHO 2004)
  - > 50 C cells in 3 low-power fields (100x)
  - > 40 C cells/cm^2
  - For practical purposes, if C cells can be seen on H&E and confirmed by IHC, lesion should be reported as CCH
- **Neoplastic CCH**
  - Considered precursor lesion of familial medullary thyroid carcinomas (MTC)
    - Premalignant lesion; therefore, the term hyperplasia is a misnomer
  - Caused by mutations in *RET* protooncogene
  - Histopathology
    - Predominantly nodular or mixed nodular/diffuse
    - Usually easy to identify on conventional H&E
    - Cytomorphologically similar to medullary microcarcinomas
    - C-cell quantification not necessary for diagnosis
- **Reactive/physiologic CCH**
  - No clear malignant potential documented
  - Caused by stimuli external to C cell
  - Histopathology
    - Predominantly diffuse
    - Usually difficult to visualize on H&E stains
    - Calcitonin stain improves detection

CLINICAL ISSUES

Presentation

- **Neoplastic CCH**
  - Most cases are sporadic
  - 25-30% occur in context of multiple endocrine neoplasias (MEN2A and MEN2B) or familial MTC
  - Incidence rising due to increase in prophylactic thyroidectomies
    - Patients with family history of MTC and elevated serum calcitonin
    - Carriers of mutations in *RET* gene
- **Reactive CCH**
  - May be associated with hyperparathyroidism, Hashimoto thyroiditis, multinodular goiter, hyperthyroidism, and subtotal thyroidectomy
  - Can be seen in vicinity of large tumors of follicular cell origin or lymphomas

Treatment

- Surgical approaches
  - Prophylactic thyroidectomy appears to offer best chance of cure to patients with MEN2 and familial MTC
  - Thyroidectomy recommended to prevent progression to medullary microcarcinoma (MMC)
    - Recommended age of prophylactic thyroidectomy depends on *RET* mutation

Prognosis

- **Neoplastic CCH** is premalignant lesion often associated with MMC
  - Generally good prognosis with early detection and thyroidectomy
  - 10-year survival rates of 74-100% reported for MMC
- **Reactive CCH** is unlikely to represent premalignant lesion

C-CELL HYPERPLASIA

Key Facts

Terminology
- An increase in C-cell population in thyroid due to reactive/physiologic or neoplastic process
- For practical purposes, if C cells can be seen on H&E and confirmed by IHC, lesion should be reported as CCH
- **Reactive/physiologic CCH**
  - No clear malignant potential documented
  - Usually difficult to visualize on H&E stains
- **Neoplastic CCH**
  - Considered the precursor lesion to familial medullary thyroid carcinomas (MTC)

Clinical Issues
- 25-30% occur in context of multiple endocrine neoplasias (MEN2A and MEN2B) or familial MTC
- Prophylactic thyroidectomy appears to offer best chance of cure to patients with MEN2 and familial MTC
- Generally good prognosis with early detection and thyroidectomy
- 10-year survival rates of 74-100% reported for MMC

Microscopic Pathology
- Round and polygonal cells
- Slightly larger than adjacent follicular cells
- Granular to amphophilic cytoplasm
- Round nuclei, coarse granular or salt-and-pepper chromatin

Ancillary Tests
- C cells stain positively for calcitonin, chromogranin, synaptophysin, CRP, and CEA

  - Reports exist of MTC in patients thought to have reactive CCH, but with serum calcitonin > 50 pg/mL

IMAGE FINDINGS

General Features
- Due to diffuse nature or small size, CCH lesions may be easily overlooked on imaging studies

MACROSCOPIC FEATURES

General Features
- CCH is not usually grossly identified
- Associated MMC or MTC may be present as whitish, firm nodules typically in upper or middle 1/3 of lobe
- In at-risk patients who undergo thyroidectomy, entire gland should be submitted to identify areas of CCH

MICROSCOPIC PATHOLOGY

Histologic Features
- 4 histological patterns
  - **Nodular**: C-cell clusters between or filling a thyroid follicle
  - **Diffuse**: Cells are scattered between follicles
  - **Solitary**: Single focus of CCH
  - **Multifocal**: Foci of CCH throughout gland
- **Hereditary and neoplastic CCH**
  - More likely to be nodular, multifocal, and bilateral
  - Usually detectable on H&E sections
  - Presence of cytological atypia
  - Seen adjacent to medullary thyroid carcinoma
  - Usually bilateral
  - Can be nodular or diffuse
- **Reactive and sporadic CCH**
  - Tends to be solitary, diffuse, and unilateral
  - No cytologic atypia, not usually detectable on H&E-stained sections
  - Usually unilateral and diffuse
  - Seen in association with nodular thyroid disease

Cytologic Features
- Round and polygonal cells
- Slightly larger than adjacent follicular cells
- Granular to amphophilic cytoplasm
- Round nuclei, coarse granular or salt-and-pepper chromatin

ANCILLARY TESTS

Immunohistochemistry
- C cells stain positively for calcitonin, chromogranin, synaptophysin, CRP, and CEA

Molecular Genetics
- *RET* mutation analysis in familial cases

DIFFERENTIAL DIAGNOSIS

Benign Entities
- Squamous metaplasia, remnants of thymus, solid cell nests, palpation thyroiditis, intrathyroid parathyroid tissue, tangentially cut follicles

Neoplastic Processes
- Intrathyroid spread of MTC, MMC, follicular-derived neoplasms

Micromedullary Thyroid Carcinoma
- < 1 cm
- Can be sporadic or familial
- Incidental finding in patients undergoing thyroidectomies for nodular disease
- Detected by routine calcitonin screening in patients with nodular disease

Medullary Thyroid Carcinoma With Intrathyroidal Spread
- May be seen multifocally in areas where C cells are absent

C-CELL HYPERPLASIA

Immunohistochemistry

Antibody	Reactivity	Staining Pattern	Comment
CK-PAN	Positive	Cytoplasmic	
TTF-1	Positive	Nuclear	
Chromogranin-A	Positive	Cytoplasmic	
Synaptophysin	Positive	Cytoplasmic	
Calcitonin	Positive	Cytoplasmic	
CEA-M	Positive	Cytoplasmic	
Thyroglobulin	Negative		
S100	Negative		Positive in sustentacular cells of intrathyroidal paraganglioma
PTH	Negative		Used to differentiate from intrathyroidal parathyroid tissue
p63	Negative		Used in the differential diagnosis of solid cell nests
34bE12	Negative		Used in the differential diagnosis of solid cell nests
CD5	Negative		Used in the differential diagnosis of solid cell nests

Reactive/Physiologic vs. Neoplastic C-Cell Hyperplasia

Features	Reactive C-Cell Hyperplasia	Neoplastic C-Cell Hyperplasia
Detectable on H&E stains	No	Yes
Cytologic atypia	No	Yes
Seen adjacent to medullary thyroid carcinoma	No	Yes
Bilaterality	No	Yes
Staining with NCAM	No	Yes
Calcitonin reactivity	Yes	Yes
CEA reactivity	No	Yes/no
Chromogranin reactivity	Yes	Yes
Synaptophysin reactivity	Yes	Yes

- Present in lymphovascular spaces, most prominent at periphery

Solid Cell Nests
- Can be associated with C cells; finding in normal thyroid
- Positive for p63, CD5, 34bE12, and CEA

Tangentially Cut Follicles
- Smaller cells with small pale cytoplasm
- Absence of immunoexpression of chromogranin, synaptophysin, and calcitonin

Intrathyroid Parathyroid Tissue
- Small round nuclei
- Positive for PTH and negative for calcitonin and TTF-1

Palpation Thyroiditis
- Single or few follicles destroyed
- Presence of histiocytes and giant cells
- Random distribution throughout gland

DIAGNOSTIC CHECKLIST

Pathologic Interpretation Pearls
- Differentiation of nodular CCH from MMC represents a challenge
- Demonstration of breach of basement membrane and desmoplasia favor MMC

SELECTED REFERENCES

1. Diazzi C et al: The Diagnostic Value of Calcitonin Measurement in Wash-Out Fluid from Fine-Needle Aspiration of Thyroid Nodules in the Diagnosis of Medullary Thyroid Cancer. Endocr Pract. Epub ahead of print, 2013
2. Cameselle-Teijeiro J et al: C-cell hyperplasia and papillary thyroid carcinoma. Int J Surg Pathol. 20(6):643-4, 2012
3. Pirola S et al: C-cell hyperplasia in thyroid tissue adjacent to papillary carcinoma. Int J Surg Pathol. 20(1):66-8, 2012
4. Etit D et al: Histopathologic and clinical features of medullary microcarcinoma and C-cell hyperplasia in prophylactic thyroidectomies for medullary carcinoma: a study of 42 cases. Arch Pathol Lab Med. 132(11):1767-73, 2008
5. Ashworth M: The pathology of preclinical medullary thyroid carcinoma. Endocr Pathol. 15(3):227-31, 2004
6. Guyétant S et al: C-cell hyperplasia and medullary thyroid carcinoma: clinicopathological and genetic correlations in 66 consecutive patients. Mod Pathol. 16(8):756-63, 2003
7. Kaserer K et al: Recommendations for reporting C cell pathology of the thyroid. Wien Klin Wochenschr. 114(7):274-8, 2002
8. Baloch ZW et al: Neuroendocrine tumors of the thyroid gland. Am J Clin Pathol. 115 Suppl:S56-67, 2001
9. Krueger JE et al: Inherited medullary microcarcinoma of the thyroid: a study of 11 cases. Am J Surg Pathol. 24(6):853-8, 2000

Microscopic and Immunohistochemical Features

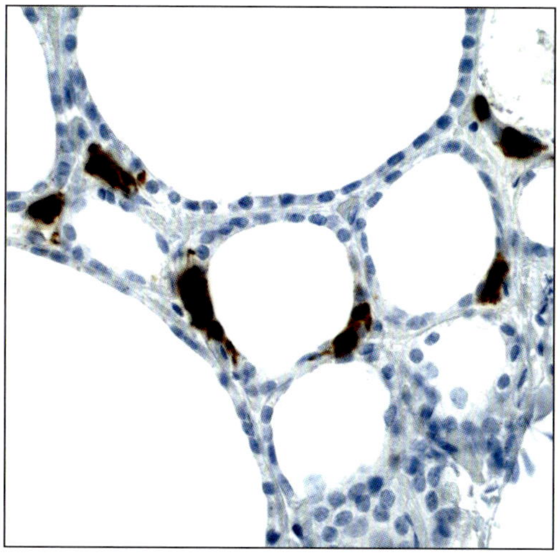
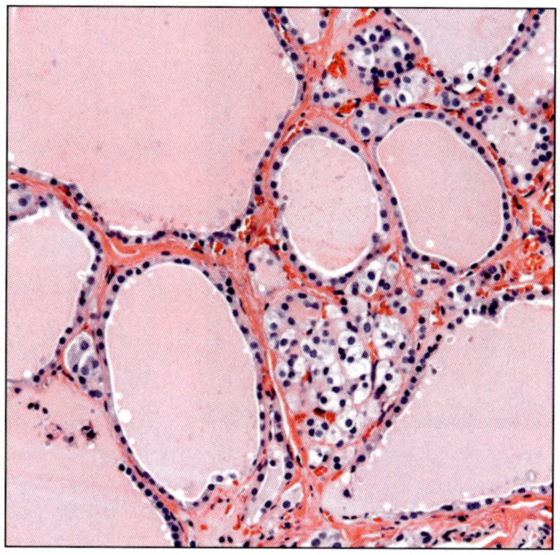

(Left) *Calcitonin stain highlights the normal C-cell distribution within the junction of the upper and middle 1/3 of the thyroid lobes. Normal C-cell population is characterized by < 50 calcitonin-positive cells per low-power field.* ***(Right)*** *An increased number of C cells can be seen adjacent to large thyroid nodules. The reactive C-cell proliferation is usually difficult to identify on H&E.*

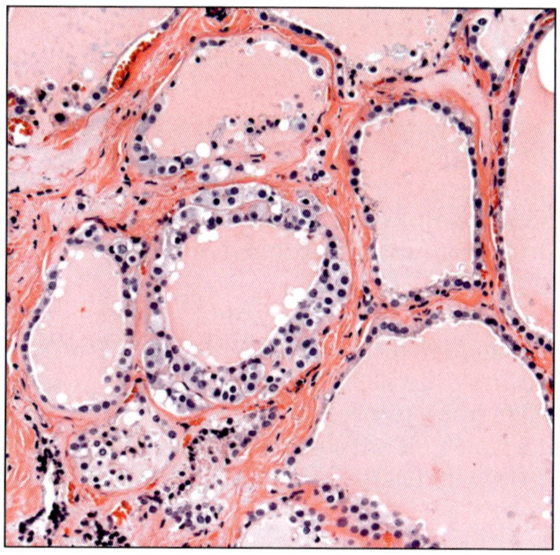
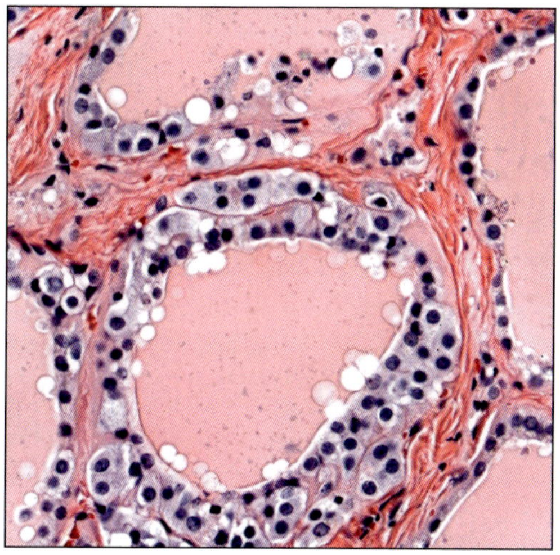

(Left) *Low-power photomicrograph shows a thyroid from a patient with multiple endocrine neoplasia syndrome type 2. The C-cell proliferation is easily identified by H&E. In inherited syndromes, the C-cell hyperplasia usually precedes neoplasia.* ***(Right)*** *The C-cell proliferation in this field is easily identified at this magnification. This finding is usually seen in cases of neoplastic C-cell hyperplasia.*

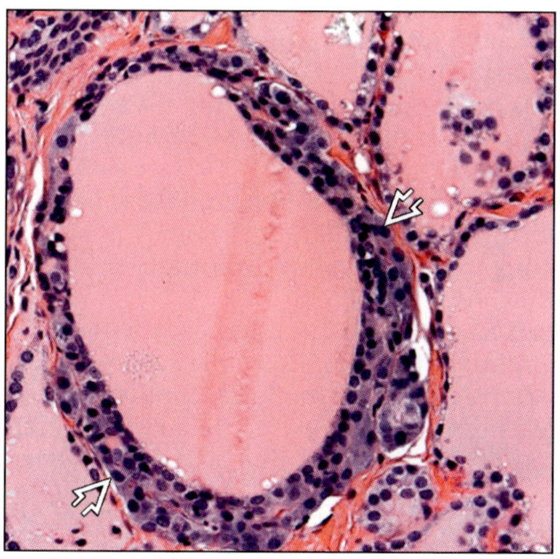
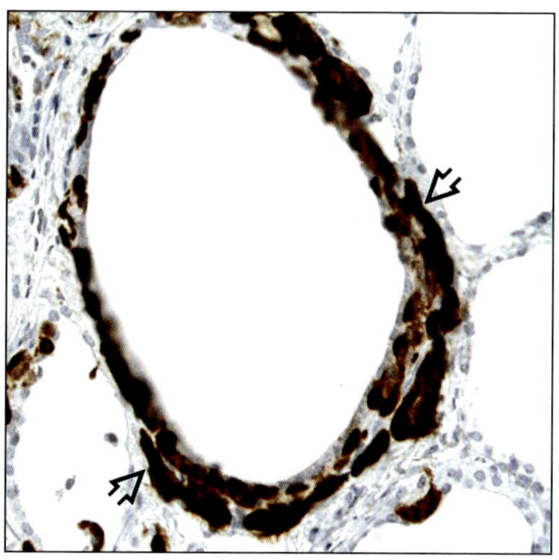

(Left) *The thyroid follicular cells are almost completely replaced by an increased number of C cells ➡, easily identified by H&E staining. The C cells have ample blue granular cytoplasm.* ***(Right)*** *C-cell hyperplasia highlighted by calcitonin staining shows the thyroid follicular cells replaced by an increased number of C cells ➡ that surround the entire follicle.*

MEDULLARY THYROID CARCINOMA

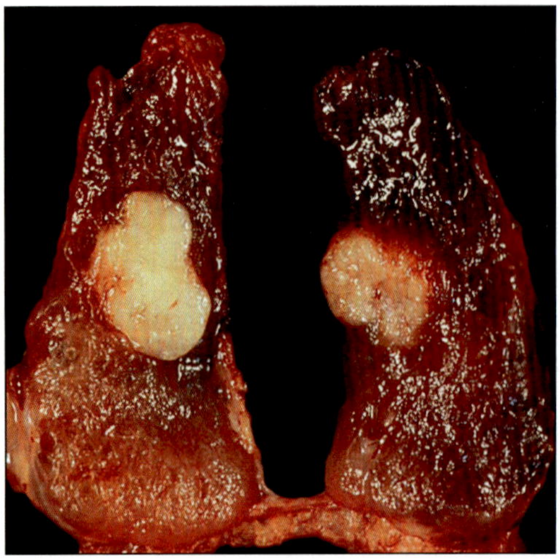

Bilateral medullary thyroid carcinoma from a patient with multiple endocrine neoplasia type 2A (MEN2A) shows the characteristic well-circumscribed cut surface. MEN-associated tumors are usually bilateral and multifocal.

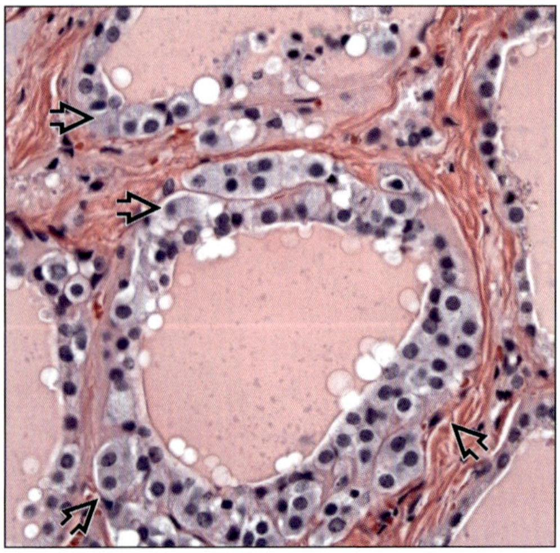

This photomicrograph shows a thyroid from a patient with multiple neoplasia type 2. The C-cell hyperplasia is easily identified by H&E ➯. In inherited syndromes, C-cell hyperplasia usually precedes neoplasia.

TERMINOLOGY

Abbreviations

- Medullary thyroid carcinoma (MTC)

Synonyms

- C-cell carcinoma
- Medullary carcinoma (MC) of thyroid
- Solid carcinoma with amyloid stroma
- Neuroendocrine carcinoma of thyroid

Definitions

- Neuroendocrine tumor derived from C cells of thyroid
- MTCs measuring < 1 cm in diameter are called medullary microcarcinomas (MMC)

ETIOLOGY/PATHOGENESIS

Genetic Predisposition

- Hereditary forms of MTC are transmitted as autosomal dominant traits, usually with high penetrance
- Multiple endocrine neoplasia type 2 (MEN2) syndrome and familial MTC (FMTC)-only syndrome are caused by mutations in *RET* gene
  - Commonly activating point mutations
  - Exon 10 codons 609, 611, 618, 620, and exon 11 codon 634 responsible for majority of MEN2A and of FMTC
    - MEN2A: Majority involve exon 11 codon 634
  - MEN2B: Majority is associated with exon 16 codon 918 mutation
  - Fusion genes with tyrosine kinase domain of *RET* also occur
    - *RET* chromosomal rearrangements also associated with papillary carcinoma (*RET/PTC*)
  - Somatic *RET* mutations also present in up to ~ 50% of sporadic MTCs
- MTC is seen in setting of MEN2 syndromes and familial MTC-only syndrome
  - **MEN2A**
    - MTC, parathyroid hyperplasia, pheochromocytoma, and pancreatic endocrine tumors
    - ~ 100% of individuals with MEN2A develop medullary thyroid carcinoma
  - **MEN2B**
    - MTC, pheochromocytoma, mucosal and soft tissue tumors (notably neuromas), marfanoid body habitus
    - Characterized by early development of aggressive form of medullary thyroid carcinoma in ~ 100% of affected individuals
  - **Familial MTC-only syndrome**
    - MTC not associated with other tumors
    - Comprises about 10-20% of MEN2 cases

Precursor Lesions

- **Neoplastic C-cell hyperplasia** (NCCH)
  - Precursor lesion in hereditary MTC
  - Clusters should have > 50 C cells
  - a.k.a. C-cell carcinoma in situ or medullary carcinoma in situ
  - These lesions harbor germline *RET* mutations
  - Postulated that CCH progresses to MMC and eventually to MTC
  - C-cell clusters surrounding or invading follicles
  - Found in vicinity of medullary carcinomas
  - Distinguishing CCH from MMC or intrathyroid spread of MTC may be difficult
- **Reactive C-cell hyperplasia**
  - Increase in number of C cells secondary to associated thyroid disorder (nodules, papillary or follicular carcinoma, inflammatory or autoimmune)
  - Lack pleomorphism, amyloid, fibrosis, or invasion of follicles
  - Difficult to visualize on H&E alone; requires calcitonin staining
- Role of CCH in sporadic MTC remains unknown

MEDULLARY THYROID CARCINOMA

Key Facts

Terminology
- Neuroendocrine tumor derived from C cells of thyroid
- MTCs measuring < 1 cm in diameter are called medullary microcarcinomas (MMC)

Etiology/Pathogenesis
- MTC is seen in setting of MEN2 and familial non-MEN MTC syndromes
- MEN2 is caused by mutations in *RET* gene
- Neoplastic C-cell hyperplasia (CCH) is precursor lesion in hereditary MTC

Clinical Issues
- 20-25% are hereditary
- Increased serum calcitonin and CEA levels
- *RET* gene mutation analysis
- In patients with hereditary MTC, recommended age for prophylactic thyroidectomy is according to *RET* mutations
- 5- and 10-year survivals of 60-80% and 40-70%, respectively

Microscopic Pathology
- In MEN2, age of transformation from CCH to MTC varies with different germline *RET* mutation

Ancillary Tests
- Positive for calcitonin and CEA

Diagnostic Checklist
- Desmoplasia and breaching of basement membrane helps differentiate CCH from MMC
- Finding CCH may serve as a morphological marker for MEN2-associated MTC

CLINICAL ISSUES

Epidemiology
- Incidence
  - 5-10% of all thyroid malignancies
    - 75-80% are sporadic
    - 20-25% are hereditary
  - Rising incidence due to calcitonin screening protocols and *RET* genetic testing
    - Increase in prophylactic thyroidectomies
    - Mostly MMC identified in familial cases
- Age
  - In sporadic cases: 50-60 years
  - Familial cases can present from early childhood
    - MTC in MEN2B: ~ 5 years
    - MTC in MEN2A: 25-30 years
    - MTC in FMTC: ~ 50 years
- Gender
  - 1:1 in familial cases

Presentation
- Often presents as painless "cold" nodule
- Up to 50% have nodal metastases
- Up to 20% may present with distant metastases
- Symptoms of carcinoid and Cushing syndromes may be present
- Large tumors may lead to dysphagia and upper airway obstruction
- Nonthyroid findings: Mucosal neuromas; parathyroid, adrenal, pituitary, and pancreatic tumors
- MTC tends to metastasize early: Liver, lungs, bone, soft tissue outside neck, brain, and bone marrow

Laboratory Tests
- Screening and monitoring tests are performed in patients at risk
  - History or presence of multiple endocrine neoplasias
  - Family history of MEN2 or familial MTC
  - Genetic counseling is recommended to assess patient-specific risk
  - Annual serum calcitonin screening should begin in children with MEN2B at 6 months, MEN2A at 3-5 years of age
- Increased serum calcitonin and CEA levels
- Abnormal pentagastrin-stimulated calcitonin response
- *RET* is the only gene associated with MEN2
- *RET* molecular genetic testing indicated in all individuals with
  - Diagnosis of MTC
  - Clinical diagnosis of MEN2
  - Primary C-cell hyperplasia
- *RET* gene mutation analysis
  - Most commonly exons 10, 11, 13, 14, and 16 in hereditary forms
  - Mutations in codons 768, 790, 791, and 804 may predispose to a milder form of MTC with low penetrance, late onset, and without family history
  - Most common somatic mutation in sporadic MTC is M918T
- MEN2A: ~ 100% of families have *RET* mutation in exon 10 or 11
- FMTC: Families have almost 100% *RET* mutation
- MEN2B: Individuals with features of this syndrome should have mutation analysis or sequencing of exons 15 or 16 to detect p.M918T and p.A883F mutations
- Rarely, germline *RET* mutation may not be detected in family with clinical diagnosis of MEN2A, MEN2B, or FMTC

Treatment
- Surgical approaches
  - Total thyroidectomy offers best chance of cure
  - Associated neck dissections considered for tumors > 1 cm
  - American Thyroid Association Guidelines Task Force has classified mutations based on risk for aggressive MTC
    - May be used in predicting phenotype and recommendations for age at which to perform prophylactic thyroidectomy and to begin biochemical screening for associated diseases
  - Prophylactic thyroidectomy

- Primary preventive measure for individuals with identified germline *RET* mutation
  - Prophylactic thyroidectomy recommendations for specific *RET* germline mutations
    - Codons 883, 918, or 922: Thyroidectomy by 1 year of age
    - Codons 609, 611, 618, 620, 630, or 634: Thyroidectomy before 5 years of age
    - Codons 786, 790, 791, 804, or 891: Consider surgery before age of 5; may delay surgery up to 10 years
    - Other mutations: Thyroidectomy once stimulated calcitonin screening turns abnormal
  - Thyroidectomy for C-cell hyperplasia, before progression to micromedullary carcinoma, may allow surgery to be limited to thyroidectomy alone, sparing of lymph nodes
- Adjuvant therapy
  - Targeted tyrosine kinase, hormone therapy, chemotherapy, and anti-CEA treatments can be considered
- Radiation
  - For residual disease and palliation

Prognosis

- Considerable variation
- Overall 5- and 10-year survivals of 60-80% and 40-70%, respectively
- 10-year survival by tumor stage
  - Stage I: Near 100%, stage II: 98%, stage III: 81%, stage IV: 28%
- Better prognostic factors are tumor stage, young age, women, and familial forms
- Poor prognostic factors are necrosis, squamous metaplasia, < 50% calcitonin immunoreaction, and CEA reactivity in absence of calcitonin

IMAGE FINDINGS

Scintigraphic Scan

- "Cold" nodule on iodine scan

MACROSCOPIC FEATURES

General Features

- Typically at junction of upper and middle 1/3 of lobe
- Sporadic tumors tend to present as solitary mass ± lymph node involvement
- Hereditary tumors seen in MEN are usually multicentric and bilateral
- Usually not encapsulated but well circumscribed
- Firm, yellow-white, gritty cut surface

Size

- Ranges from grossly undetectable to large, replacing entire lobe
- Small tumors often seen in prophylactic thyroidectomy specimens from MEN2 patients

Sections to Be Submitted

- In high-risk patients (MEN2 and familial MTC) who undergo prophylactic thyroidectomy, entire gland should be submitted to identify MMC and C-cell hyperplasia
- Specimen should be serially sectioned and submitted as a whole from superior to inferior
- C cells are normally situated in upper and middle portions of lobes; submit apparently normal thyroid for histological examination
  - Search for C-cell hyperplasia

MICROSCOPIC PATHOLOGY

Histologic Features

- MTC is diagnosed histologically when nests of C cells appear to extend beyond basement membrane and infiltrate and destroy thyroid follicles
- Finding C-cell hyperplasia may serve as a morphological marker for MEN2-associated MTC
- C-cell hyperplasia is diagnosed histologically by presence of increased number of diffusely scattered or clustered C cells
  - Immunohistochemistry for calcitonin expression may be performed as pathologic diagnosis adjunct
- In MEN2, age of transformation from CCH to MTC varies with different germline *RET* mutation
- Histologic appearance is quite variable
  - Most common morphology includes sheets, nests, trabeculae, or insular patterns
  - Cells are round, polygonal, or spindle-shaped, separated by thin fibrovascular cores
  - Cytoplasm can be clear, amphophilic, or eosinophilic
  - Nuclei are round to oval
  - Chromatin is fine, granular, and dispersed, typical of neuroendocrine tumors
  - Vacuoles with mucin have been frequently described
  - Psammoma-like concretions are occasionally seen
- May mimic other thyroid carcinomas (follicular, papillary, insular, anaplastic)
- 80% show calcitonin-positive amyloid in stroma

Histologic Variants

- Variants: Follicular, papillary, clear cell, oncocytic, small cell, giant cell, melanotic, paraganglioma-like and squamous cell
- Variant patterns of medullary thyroid carcinoma may resemble wide range of thyroid and extrathyroid tumors
- Staining for calcitonin is helpful in making distinction between MTC and other diverse tumors it may mimic

ANCILLARY TESTS

Cytology

- Aspirates are hypercellular with loosely cohesive to noncohesive cells
- Spindle, polygonal, or bipolar cells, often with eccentric nuclei

- Hyperchromatic nuclei with granular chromatin and moderate pleomorphism
- Amyloid may be seen in 50-70%
- Multinucleated giant tumor cells are common

Histochemistry

- Congo red
  - Reactivity: Positive
  - Staining pattern
    - Amyloid shows light green birefringence with polarization

Immunohistochemistry

- Hallmark of MTC is positivity for calcitonin
- Tumor cells are also positive for neuroendocrine markers (chromogranin, synaptophysin) and CEA
- TTF-1 and low molecular weight keratins may be positive
- Progesterone receptor and S100 (in peripheral sustentacular cells) can be positive in MTC

Cytogenetics

- Identify rearrangements involving *RET* gene

Molecular Genetics

- *RET* gene sequencing is important to determine prognosis and timing of prophylactic thyroidectomy
  - Exons 10, 11, 13, 14, 15, and 16 cover 95% of cases

Electron Microscopy

- Transmission
  - Presence of neurosecretory granules confirms neuroendocrine origin of tumor
    - Electron dense, membrane bound
  - Amyloid material is detected as fine fibrillary material within parenchymal space

DIFFERENTIAL DIAGNOSIS

Sporadic Medullary Thyroid Carcinoma

- There is only 1 genetic differential diagnosis for MTC: MEN2
- Important for medical management of individual and his/her family to distinguish MTC + MEN2 from truly sporadic MTC
- Germline mutations in *RET* gene in individuals with apparent sporadic MTC: 6-9.5%
- Usually solitary mass
- Usually unilateral
- Not associated with C-cell hyperplasia
- Histological findings: Same as familial

Intrathyroid Tumor

- **Metastatic neuroendocrine tumors**
  - Can be positive for calcitonin and CEA in rare cases
  - Clinical and radiologic correlation may help in differential
- **Paraganglioma**
  - Negative for calcitonin; zellballen with S100-positive sustentacular cells
- **Follicular carcinoma (FC)**
  - Thyroglobulin is positive
  - Nuclear features: Neuroendocrine chromatin in MTC compared to dark dense nuclei in FC
- **Undifferentiated carcinoma**
  - Hemorrhage, necrosis, and high mitotic activity seen in undifferentiated carcinoma
  - Negative for calcitonin
- **Papillary thyroid carcinoma**
  - Intranuclear inclusions can be seen in both MTC and PTC
  - Nuclear features usually unique to PTC
  - PTC is calcitonin negative and thyroglobulin positive
- **Hyalinizing trabecular tumor**
  - Thyroglobulin positive, calcitonin negative
  - Hyaline material is not amyloid when stained by Congo red under polarized light
- **Intrathyroid parathyroid tumors**
  - PTH positive; calcitonin and thyroglobulin negative
  - Clear cytoplasm, defined cell border

Tumor in Lymph Nodes

- MTC metastatic to lymph nodes may be misdiagnosed as melanoma or metastatic neuroendocrine tumors
- Calcitonin and CEA immunostains should be performed in any suspicious case

Benign Conditions

- **Amyloid goiter**
  - May infiltrate fat, and Congo red is positive
  - Involves thyroid gland diffusely
  - Calcitonin stain is negative

DIAGNOSTIC CHECKLIST

Pathologic Interpretation Pearls

- Finding C-cell hyperplasia may serve as a morphological marker for MEN2-associated MTC
- There is only 1 genetic differential diagnosis for MTC: MEN2
- Desmoplasia and breakage of follicular basement membrane helps differentiate C-cell hyperplasia from MMC

SELECTED REFERENCES

1. Maliszewska A et al: Differential gene expression of medullary thyroid carcinoma reveals specific markers associated with genetic conditions. Am J Pathol. 182(2):350-62, 2013
2. Agarwal S et al: MEN 2A family--prophylactic thyroidectomy for asymptomatic siblings with positive 634 codon mutation. J Assoc Physicians India. 60:127-9, 2012
3. Martucciello G et al: Multiple endocrine neoplasias type 2B and RET proto-oncogene. Ital J Pediatr. 38:9, 2012
4. Shankar RK et al: Medullary thyroid cancer in a 9-week-old infant with familial MEN 2B: Implications for timing of prophylactic thyroidectomy. Int J Pediatr Endocrinol. 2012(1):25, 2012
5. Marsh DJ et al: Multiple endocrine neoplasia: types 1 and 2. Adv Otorhinolaryngol. 70:84-90, 2011
6. Nosé V: Familial thyroid cancer: a review. Mod Pathol. 24 Suppl 2:S19-33, 2011

MEDULLARY THYROID CARCINOMA

Differential Diagnosis of Medullary Thyroid Carcinoma by Immunohistochemistry

	MTC	PTC	PDC	ATC	PA/C	Para	Met C
Cytokeratin	+	+	+	+/-	+	-	+
Thyroglobulin	-	+	+	-	-	-	-
TTF-1	+	+	+	-	-	-	-/+
Chromogranin	+	-	-	-	+	+	+/-
Synaptophysin	+	-	-	-	+/-	+	+/-
Calcitonin	+	-	-	-	-	-	-
PTH	-	-	-	-	+	-	-
S100	-	-	-	-	-	+	-

MTC: Medullary thyroid carcinoma; PTC: Papillary thyroid carcinoma; PDC: Poorly differentiated carcinoma; ATC: Anaplastic thyroid carcinoma; PA/C: Parathyroid adenoma/carcinoma; Para: Paraganglioma; Met C: Metastatic carcinoma.

Pathological Features Distinguishing Familial From Sporadic Medullary Thyroid Carcinoma

Characteristics	Familial Medullary Thyroid Carcinoma	Sporadic Medullary Thyroid Carcinoma
Gross features	Multicentric and bilateral	Solitary mass; unilateral
Tumor characteristics	Small tumors in prophylactic thyroidectomy specimens	Usually large tumors
Microscopic features	Associated with neoplastic C-cell hyperplasia	Association with C-cell hyperplasia unknown
Lymph node metastases	May be present at time of diagnosis	Usually present at time of diagnosis
RET mutation	Present in majority of hereditary forms	May be present up to 50% of sporadic cases

Differential Diagnosis of Micromedullary Thyroid Carcinoma

Characteristics	Familial	Sporadic
Multifocality	Frequent (~ 90%)	Rare (~ 10%)
Bilaterality	Common (~ 70%)	Rare (~ 10%)
Physiologic C-cell hyperplasia	Rare (~ 10%)	Common (~ 55%)
Neoplastic C-cell hyperplasia	Frequent (~ 90%)	Rare (~ 15%)

7. Waguespack SG et al: Management of medullary thyroid carcinoma and MEN2 syndromes in childhood. Nat Rev Endocrinol. 7(10):596-607, 2011
8. Eng C: Mendelian genetics of rare--and not so rare--cancers. Ann N Y Acad Sci. 1214:70-82, 2010
9. Pacini F et al: Medullary thyroid carcinoma. Clin Oncol (R Coll Radiol). 22(6):475-85, 2010
10. Phay JE et al: Targeting RET receptor tyrosine kinase activation in cancer. Clin Cancer Res. 16(24):5936-41, 2010
11. Richards ML: Familial syndromes associated with thyroid cancer in the era of personalized medicine. Thyroid. 20(7):707-13, 2010
12. Sadow PM et al: Mixed Medullary-follicular-derived carcinomas of the thyroid gland. Adv Anat Pathol. 17(4):282-5, 2010
13. Torino F et al: Medullary thyroid cancer: a promising model for targeted therapy. Curr Mol Med. 10(7):608-25, 2010
14. American Thyroid Association Guidelines Task Force et al: Medullary thyroid cancer: management guidelines of the American Thyroid Association. Thyroid. 19(6):565-612, 2009
15. Cakir M et al: Medullary thyroid cancer: molecular biology and novel molecular therapies. Neuroendocrinology. 90(4):323-48, 2009
16. Cerrato A et al: Molecular genetics of medullary thyroid carcinoma: the quest for novel therapeutic targets. J Mol Endocrinol. 43(4):143-55, 2009
17. Wells SA Jr et al: Targeting the RET pathway in thyroid cancer. Clin Cancer Res. 15(23):7119-23, 2009
18. Etit D et al: Histopathologic and clinical features of medullary microcarcinoma and C-cell hyperplasia in prophylactic thyroidectomies for medullary carcinoma: a study of 42 cases. Arch Pathol Lab Med. 132(11):1767-73, 2008
19. Tischler AS et al: Prophylactic thyroidectomy in multiple endocrine neoplasia type 2A. N Engl J Med. 353(26):2817-8; author reply 2817-8, 2005
20. Baloch ZW et al: Neuroendocrine tumors of the thyroid gland. Am J Clin Pathol. 115 Suppl:S56-67, 2001
21. Moline J, Eng C. Multiple endocrine neoplasia type 2. 1993-, 1999
22. DeLellis RA: Multiple endocrine neoplasia syndromes revisited. Clinical, morphologic, and molecular features. Lab Invest. 72(5):494-505, 1995

Imaging and Microscopic Features

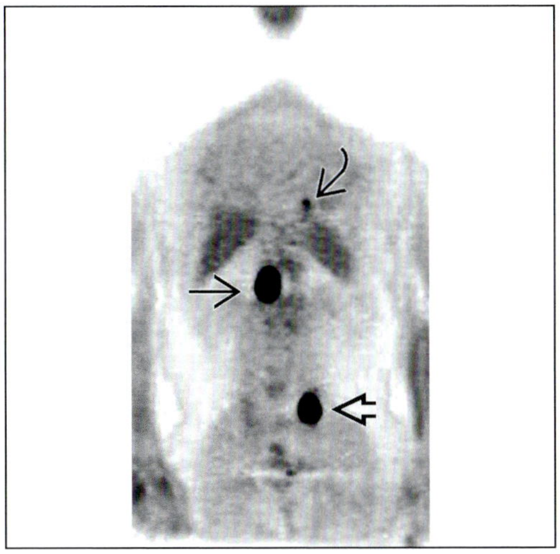
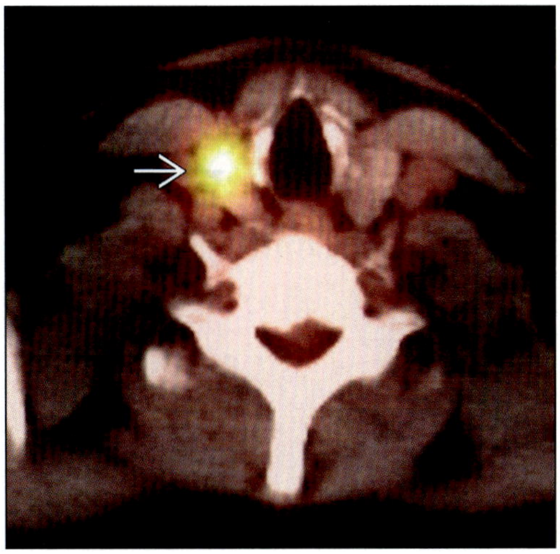

(Left) *Coronal FDG PET shows hypermetabolic foci in an upper lumbar vertebra →, left sacroiliac region →, and left lung → in a patient with metastatic medullary thyroid cancer. Up to 20% of patients may have distant metastases at the time of presentation.* ***(Right)*** *Fused transaxial fludeoxyglucose positron emission tomography/ computed tomography (FDG PET/CT) shows a focal hypermetabolic mass → in the right thyroid lobe in a patient with medullary thyroid cancer.*

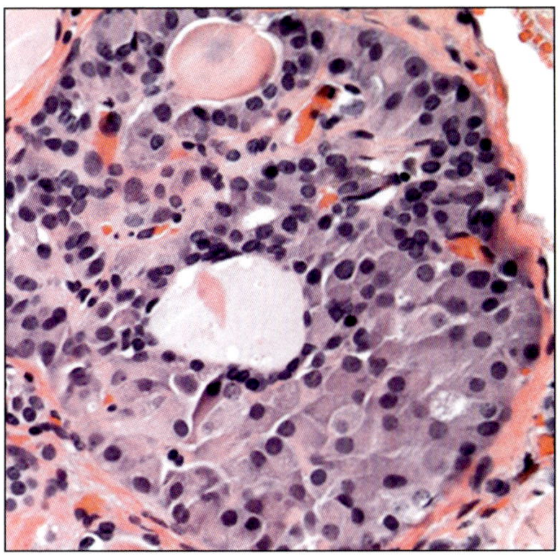
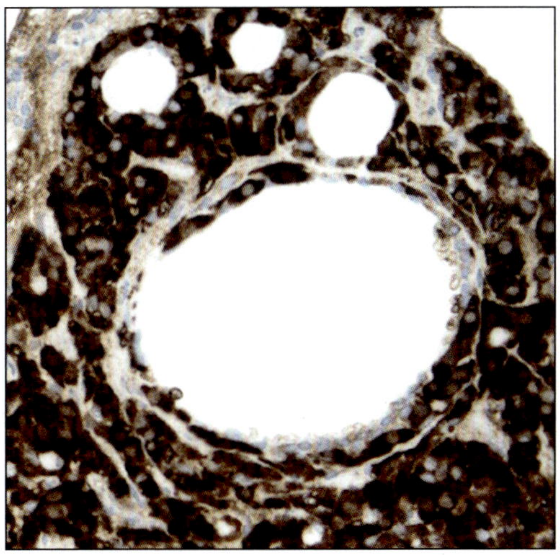

(Left) *Unlike sporadic medullary thyroid carcinoma, MEN2 is frequently accompanied by C-cell hyperplasia. C cells are usually identified by calcitonin staining; however, in many cases of MEN2, C cells are easily identified by H&E.* ***(Right)*** *In MEN2 patients, foci of C-cell hyperplasia are typically present in the vicinity of the tumor as well as in the contralateral lobe. This photomicrograph shows calcitonin stain highlighting CCH adjacent to a medullary thyroid carcinoma.*

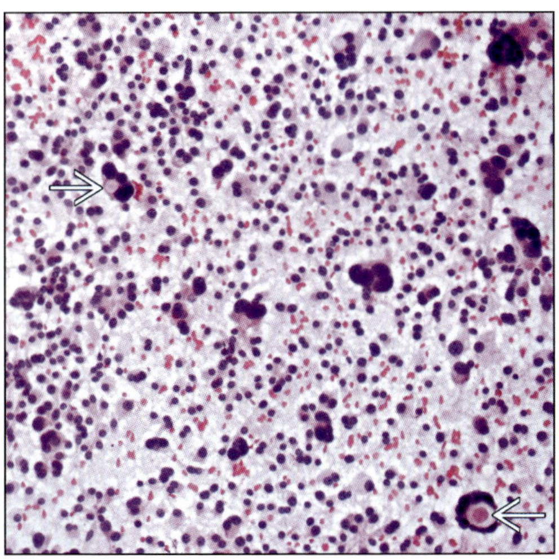
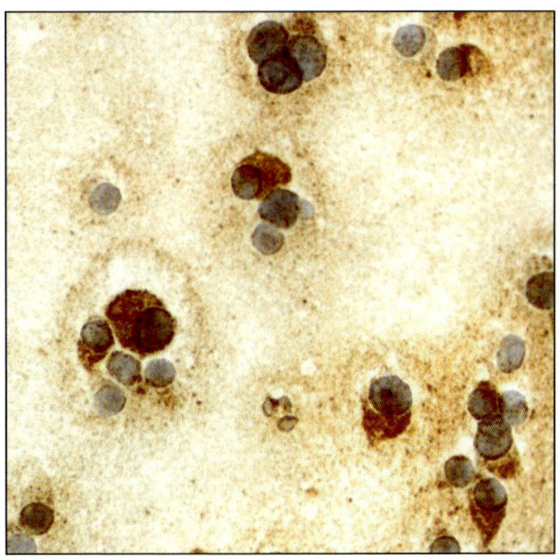

(Left) *FNA of an MTC shows a characteristic cellular specimen with clusters of loosely cohesive round to oval cells of variable sizes. Amyloid spheres → can be seen in the background or associated with clusters of malignant cells. Colloid is absent.* ***(Right)*** *Thyroid FNA specimen immunocytological staining for calcitonin shows coarse granular cytoplasmic staining. The MTC cells in this case demonstrate the characteristic coarse neuroendocrine-type nuclear chromatin.*

MEDULLARY THYROID CARCINOMA

Gross and Microscopic Features and Ancillary Techniques

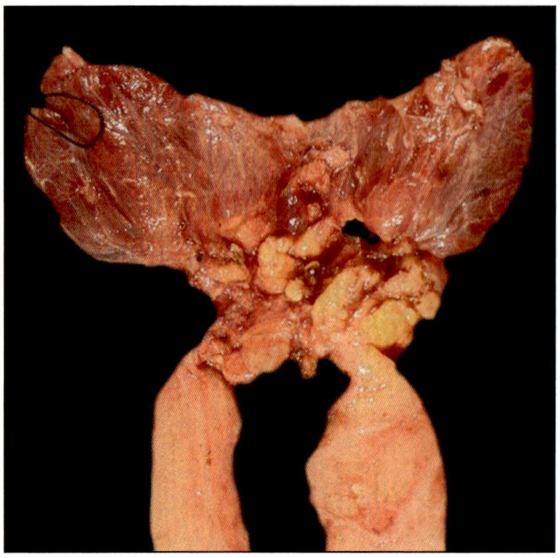

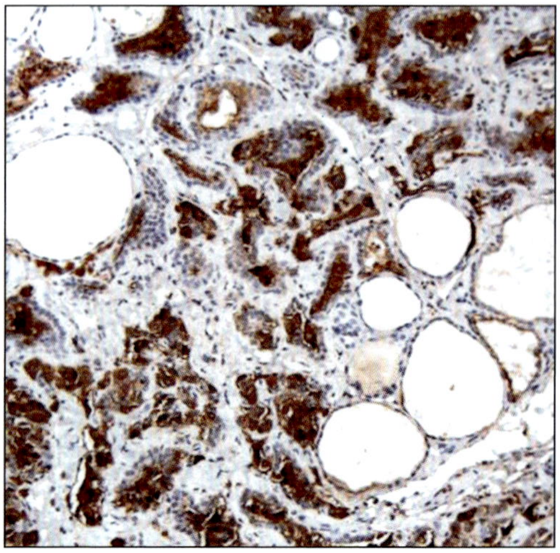

(Left) *Total prophylactic thyroidectomy with portion of thymus from a patient with MEN2B and with mutation of the RET gene shows a grossly normal thyroid. However, on histological examination, C-cell hyperplasia and a small medullary thyroid carcinoma were present.* ***(Right)*** *Calcitonin-stained thyroid section from a prophylactic thyroidectomy from a patient with RET mutation and family history of MEN2B shows C-cell hyperplasia and medullary thyroid microcarcinoma.*

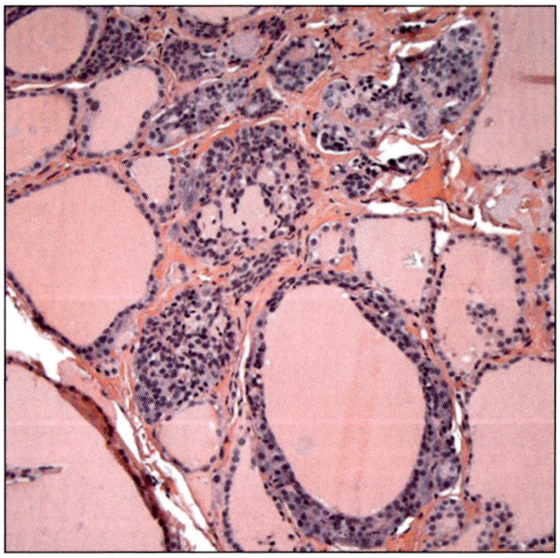

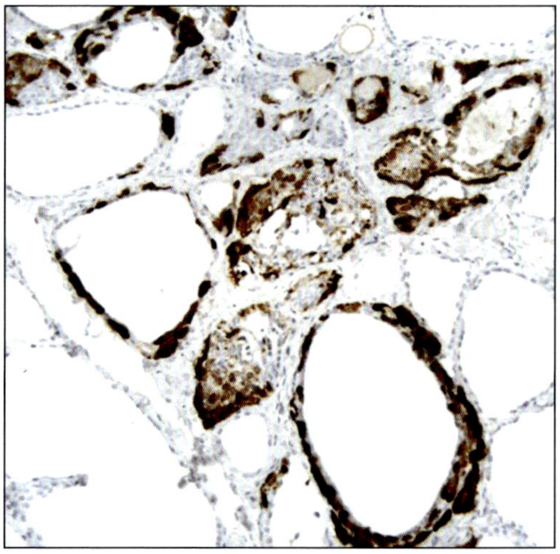

(Left) *Histological routine section reveals C-cell hyperplasia in a thyroid lobe of a patient with medullary thyroid carcinoma in the other lobe. Both were associated with MEN2 and RET mutation. C-cell hyperplasia can be easily identified on H&E section on heritable cases.* ***(Right)*** *C-cell hyperplasia highlighted by calcitonin staining shows the thyroid follicular cells replaced by an increased number of C cells.*

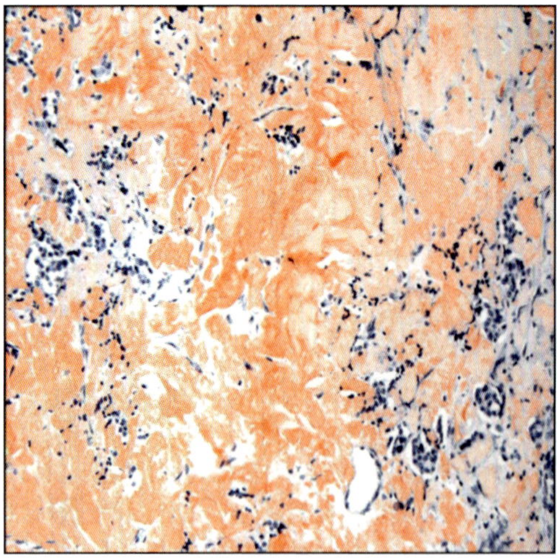

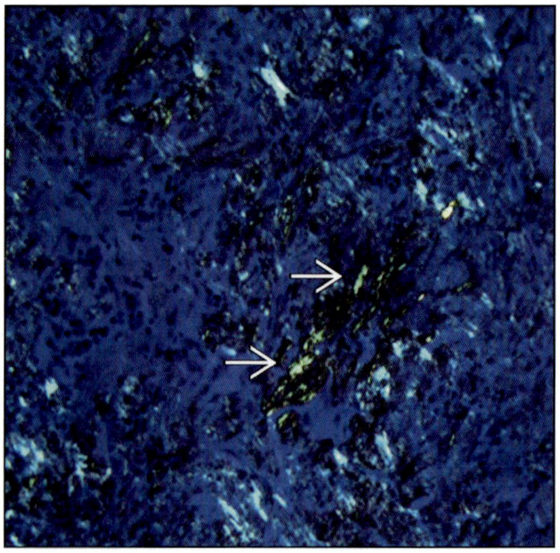

(Left) *This photomicrograph of a Congo red-stained tumor shows extensive deposition of dense amorphous material suggestive of amyloid. Although not essential for the diagnosis of medullary thyroid carcinoma, variable amounts of amyloid are commonly seen in these tumors.* ***(Right)*** *Congo red-stained medullary thyroid carcinoma under polarized light reveals the characteristic apple-green birefringence ➔ confirming amyloid deposition.*

Microscopic Features and Ancillary Techniques

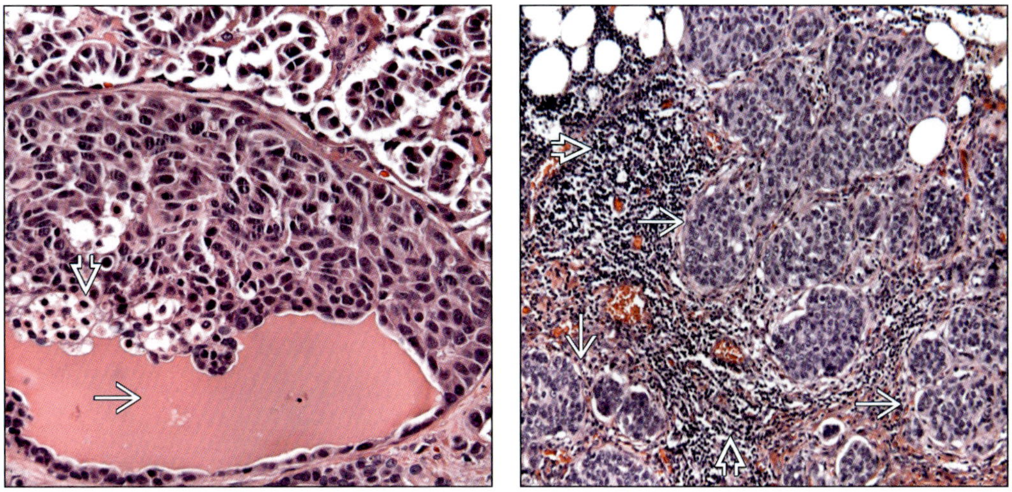

(Left) *Medullary thyroid carcinoma presents as a proliferation of epithelial cells with high nuclear to cytoplasmic ratio and moderate atypia. C-cell clusters* → *are shown surrounding and invading the follicular space* →*.* ***(Right)*** *MTC extending into extrathyroidal fibroadipose tissue shows multiple nests* → *of small cells with scant cytoplasm and regular round nuclei, associated with marked inflammatory infiltrate* →*.*

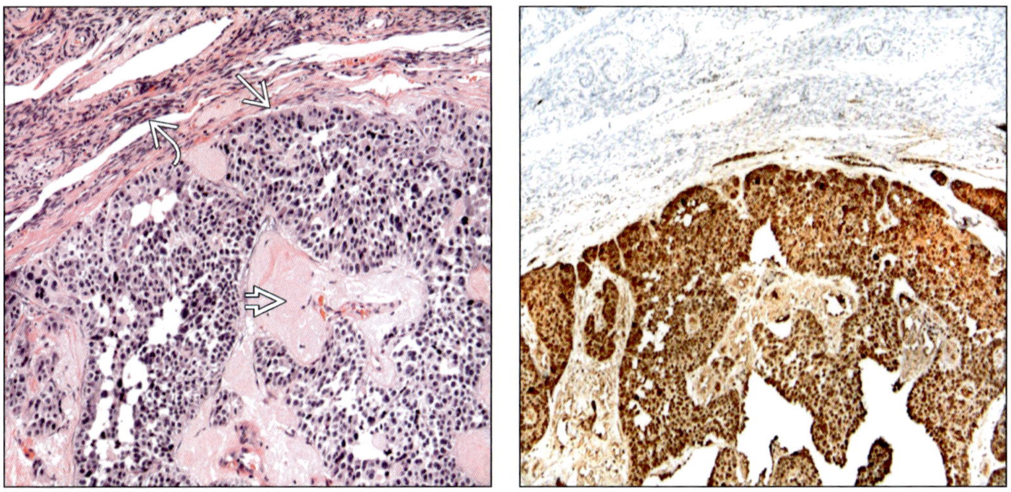

(Left) *This micrograph depicts an unusually aggressive case of medullary thyroid carcinoma metastatic to ovary. A well-defined nodule of tumor cells* → *with interspersed areas of amyloid deposition* → *can be seen. Compressed normal ovarian parenchyma* → *is present surrounding the tumor.* ***(Right)*** *Section of ovary stained for calcitonin highlights the neoplasm (positive staining) and confirms medullary thyroid carcinoma as the origin of this metastatic lesion.*

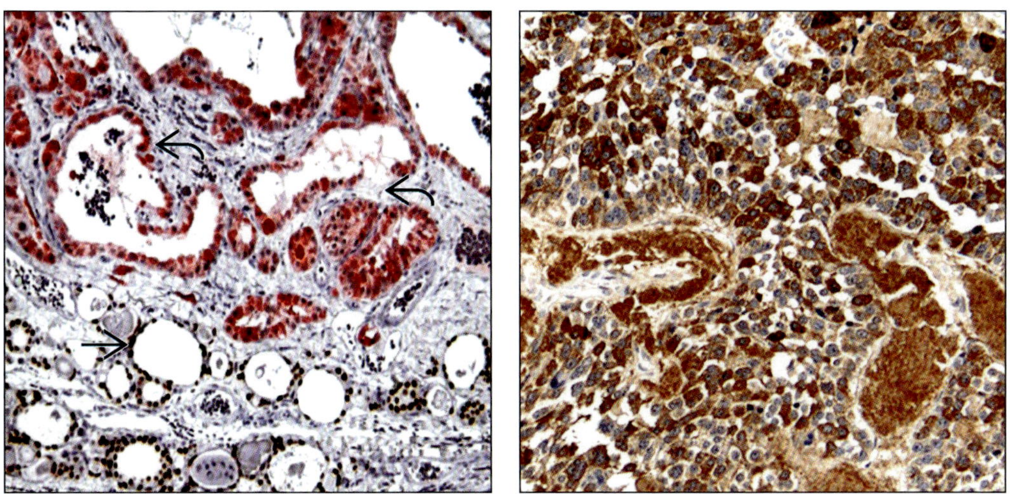

(Left) *Dual immunohistochemistry with chromogranin (red) and TTF-1 (brown) distinguishes the neuroendocrine-derived cells of a medullary thyroid carcinoma* → *from the normal adjacent TTF-1-positive follicular cells* →*. MTC cells have both TTF-1 and chromogranin positivity. The immunophenotypical distinction is especially important in cases with a follicular-patterned MTC morphology.* ***(Right)*** *Variable cytoplasmic calcitonin immunostaining is characteristic of MTC cells.*

Gastrointestinal

Gastrointestinal Tract

Hepatobiliary and Pancreas

COLON ADENOMA

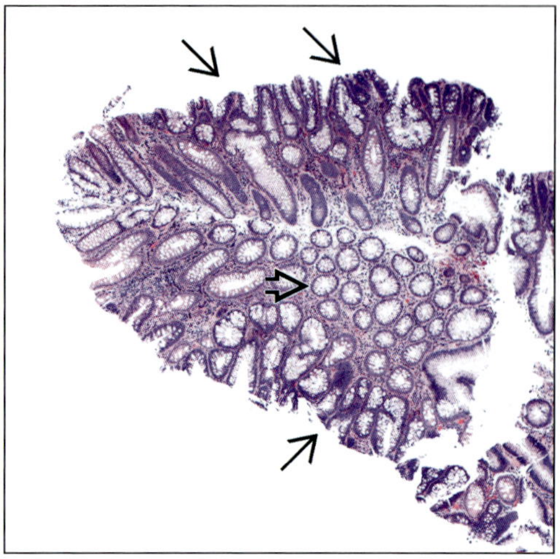

H&E shows a low-power view of an adenoma with crowded tubules of basophilic dysplastic epithelium ➙ overlying nonneoplastic tubules ➩.

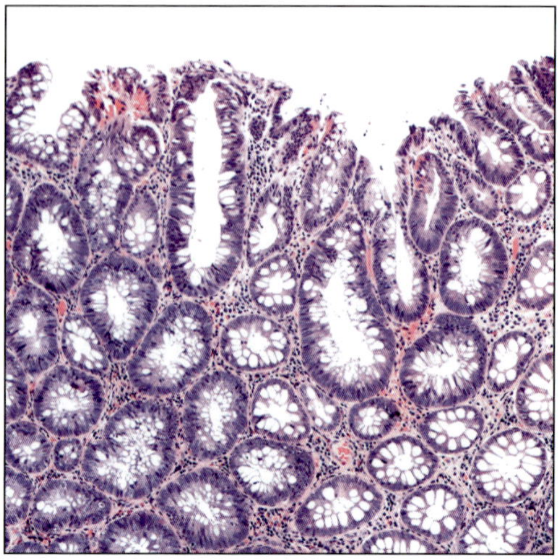

H&E shows a higher magnification view of a tubular adenoma (TA) with low-grade dysplasia. Note the "picket fence" arrangement of elongated hyperchromatic nuclei.

TERMINOLOGY

Synonyms

- Adenomatous polyp, intraepithelial neoplasia

Definitions

- Benign, premalignant (dysplastic), clonal (neoplastic) proliferation of colorectal epithelium
- Precursor lesions to colorectal carcinoma (CRC)
- Colorectal adenoma is by definition dysplastic
- Advanced adenomas
  - Any of following features
    - ≥ 1 cm, multiple (≥ 3), high-grade dysplasia, or any villous architecture
  - 3-5x ↑ CRC risk

ETIOLOGY/PATHOGENESIS

Adenoma to Carcinoma Sequence

- Monoclonal derivatives of mutated epithelial stem cell
  - Inherited or acquired genetic changes
  - May eventually produce malignant phenotype
  - Initiation: Inactivation of *APC*/β-catenin pathway
  - Step-wise accumulation of genetic mutations
    - Not always linear; occur over several years
- Aberrant crypt foci: Earliest recognizable alteration
  - Unicryptal adenomas can be found in familial adenomatous polyposis (FAP) patients
  - Adenomas grow in size by accelerated crypt fission
  - Early adenomas usually occupy mucosal surface
- Theories of histogenesis
  - Dysregulated proliferation zone (dysplastic cells)
    - Expansion upward to upper crypt/luminal surface
    - Highlighted with Ki-67 immunostain (MIB-1)
  - Rate of proliferation exceeds cell loss
  - Failed differentiation, cellular senescence/apoptosis
    - Altered expression of apoptotic genes *TGF*β, *BCL2*
- Lack of phenotypic/morphologic maturation

Family History

- Adenoma prevalence in CRC patients' relatives: 30-40%

Genetic Syndromes

- Familial adenomatous polyposis
  - Many (100-1,000) adenomas, present/diagnosed at younger age, germline *APC* mutation
  - Presence of unicryptal adenomas diagnostic
- Lynch syndrome
  - Fewer (< 10) adenomas, more/faster CRC progression
  - Adenomas often have increased numbers of adenoma-infiltrating lymphocytes

Nutritional Factors

- Implicated in colorectal neoplasia (adenoma and CRC)
  - Diet high in animal fat, low in fruits/vegetables/fiber
  - High caloric intake, obesity, sedentary lifestyle
  - Excessive smoking, alcohol

CLINICAL ISSUES

Epidemiology

- Incidence
  - 60-70% of endoscopically removed colorectal polyps
  - Lifetime prevalence of adenoma: 30-50% (Western countries)
    - Lifetime prevalence of CRC: 6% (USA)
- Age
  - Prevalence ↑ with age: 20-30% by 50, 40-50% by 60
  - Nonsyndromic patients: Sharp increase at 40 years
    - CRC generally develops 1-2 decades later
- Gender
  - M:F = 2:1
- Ethnicity
  - Adenoma, CRC: ↑ prevalence in African Americans

Site

- 60-75% of adenomas, CRC: Distal to splenic flexure

COLON ADENOMA

Key Facts

Etiology/Pathogenesis

- High-fat/low-fiber diet, obesity, smoking, sedentary
- Adenoma prevalence in CRC patients' relatives: 30-40%
- Familial adenomatous polyposis
  - Many (100-1,000) adenomas, present/diagnosed at younger age, germline *APC* mutation
- Lynch syndrome
  - Fewer (< 10) adenomas, more/faster CRC progression
  - Adenomas often have increased numbers of adenoma-infiltrating lymphocytes

Clinical Issues

- 60-70% of endoscopically removed colorectal polyps
- Advanced adenoma
  - ≥ 1 cm, multiple (≥ 3), high-grade dysplasia, or any villous component
- 3-5% of adenomas contain invasive CRC at diagnosis
- High-grade dysplasia and villous component

Microscopic Pathology

- Proliferating, crowded, hypercellular, colonic tubules
- "Picket fence": Elongated, hyperchromatic nuclei
- Low-grade dysplasia: No architectural complexity
  - Nuclei retain basal orientation (basal cytoplasm)
- High-grade dysplasia: Significant polymorphism
  - Marked nuclear stratification and loss of polarity
  - Architectural complexity: Back-to-back, cribriform
- TA (70-90% adenomas): < 20-25% villous component
- TVA (10-25%): Between 20-25% and 75-80% villous
- VA (~ 5% of adenomas): > 75-80% villous component
  - > 30% have high-grade dysplasia, 2% have CRC

  - With age, lesions become more proximal
- Hereditary nonpolyposis colorectal cancer (HNPCC): Mostly right-sided
- FAP: Mostly left-sided

Presentation

- Almost always asymptomatic, especially if < 1 cm
- Incidental at colonoscopy (screening or other reason)
- Overt or occult rectal bleeding (distal &/or > 1 cm)
- Bleeding risk increases with size and coexistent CRC
- Large polyps: Iron deficiency anemia, incontinence, prolapse, intussusception, partial bowel obstruction
- Cecal lesions mimic appendicitis (obstruct orifice)
- Large distal rectal VA: Watery diarrhea, hypokalemia
  - K^+ not reabsorbed (no more epithelium distally)
  - Abnormalities correct after adenoma removal

Endoscopic Findings

- Most accurate method of detecting polyps of all sizes
  - Safe electrocautery for biopsy &/or polypectomy
  - Allows for immediate diagnosis and removal
  - Better than barium radiography (misses up to 50%)
- Flexible sigmoidoscopy: Useful for distal neoplasms
  - Advanced adenoma in distal colon or rectum
    - Risk of proximal advanced adenoma: 11-12%
    - Follow-up with full colonoscopy
  - Small (< 1 cm) rectosigmoid adenoma
    - Risk of advanced proximal lesions: 0-7%
    - Decision for full colonoscopy individualized
- Endoscopic surveillance guidelines
  - Baseline colonoscopy: Starting at age 50 unless in high-risk group, such as those with a family history of adenomas or colon cancers, FAP, Lynch syndrome, irritable bowel disease (IBD)
- Gross findings at endoscopy
  - Redder than surrounding mucosa (lighter in melanosis coli)
  - Rarely multilobulated, filiform
  - Usually very friable, without architectural rigidity
  - Ulceration, depression, firmness: Possible CRC
  - Elevated sessile (no stalk) or pedunculated (long stalk of nonneoplastic tissue)
  - Larger, broad-based sessile lesions (usually VA)
    - Less well defined, harder to resect, tend to recur
  - Superficial, flat (nonprotruding), or depressed
    - Difficult to recognize; dyes may help
    - Mucosal erythema, subtle texture changes
    - Usually smaller, highlighted by formalin fixation
    - Often in HNPCC (right side, high-grade dysplasia, risk of synchronous or metachronous CRC)
- Complications of endoscopy
  - Perforation (0.2%), significant bleeding (1%)
  - In 5-10% of patients, colonoscope is not easily/safely passed to cecum
    - Diverticulosis, pelvic surgery adhesions
  - ~ 25% adenomas < 5 mm are missed (single colonoscopy)
  - Right-sided and ileocecal valve lesions easily missed

Natural History

- Well-established premalignant (CRC) precursors
  - ~ 1/2 of adenomas ↑ in size with time
  - Only some (5-10%) adenomas progress to CRC
    - Most small TA: Static, may even regress with time
    - 0.25% progress to CRC per year, usually slowly
    - 1% of advanced adenomas may progress per year
    - Estimated average of 10 years to transform to CRC
  - Endoscopic removal: Interruption of this sequence
    - Secondary prevention: ↓ CRC incidence by 70-90%
- Evidence for adenoma → carcinoma sequence
  - Similar anatomic distribution, frequently coexist
  - Epidemiologic prevalence/risk factors correlate
  - Direct transition areas can be seen
  - Similar and sequential molecular defects
  - But adenomas not always found in CRC vicinity
    - CRC has overgrown precursor vs. de novo (rare)

Treatment

- Complete removal (polypectomy) indicated for all
  - Regardless of size, dysplasia degree, villous component
  - Adequate margins evaluated at time of colonoscopy
  - Confirmed by pathology (when not piecemeal)

COLON ADENOMA

- Incomplete removal (advanced adenoma) or invasion (in sessile polyp or with unfavorable histology)
  - Resection indicated (surgical or endoscopic mucosal)
  - Weigh relative risks: Procedure vs. metastasis risk
- Surveillance (follow-up) intervals after polypectomy
  - Small, left-sided, hyperplastic polyps: 10 years
  - 1-2 low-risk adenomas: 5-10 years
  - Advanced adenomas, family history of CRC: 3 years
  - > 10 adenomas (possible genetic syndrome): < 3 years
  - Invasion in pedunculated adenoma: 0.5-1 year
    - If no unfavorable histologic features
  - Inadequately removed adenoma: 2-6 months
  - Large sessile adenoma: 2-6 months
  - Negative follow-up: May revert to 5-year frequency
- Chemoprevention: Indirect, inconclusive evidence
  - Vitamins A, C, D, E, folate, calcium
  - Aspirin, NSAIDs, selective COX-2 inhibitors
  - May reduce incidence of adenomas (mixed results)

Prognosis

- 5-7% of adenomas: High-grade dysplasia at presentation
  - More if ≥ 1 cm, ≥ 75% villous, age > 60, multiplicity
  - Adenomas < 5 mm: 1% risk of high-grade dysplasia
- 3-5% of adenomas contain invasive CRC at diagnosis
  - Size of adenoma: Best predictor of carcinoma risk
    - > 2 cm: 10-20%; 1-2 cm: 5%; < 1 cm: < 1%
  - High-grade dysplasia and villous component
    - Both are more likely with ↑ adenoma size
    - Unclear if independent prognostic factors
    - 30% of villous adenomas (VAs) > 5 mm have invasive CRC
- Multiplicity of adenomas at colonoscopy
  - 1 adenoma: 30-50% sync-/metachronous adenoma
    - ↑ risk: Larger lesions (advanced adenoma), CRC
  - 10-30% of patients have multiple (≥ 3) adenomas
    - Prevalence of multiple adenomas ↑ with age
    - 2x risk of villous component, high-grade dysplasia

MICROSCOPIC PATHOLOGY

Histologic Features

- Proliferating, crowded, hypercellular, colonic tubules
  - On surface (may have normal epithelium below)
  - Often abrupt transition to normal epithelium
  - Entire tubules replaced by dysplastic epithelium
  - No normal epithelial maturation toward surface
  - Mitotic activity extends upward (Ki-67 confirms)
- "Picket fence": Elongated, hyperchromatic nuclei
  - Also described as pencillate, cigar-shaped
  - Varying architectural complexity, stratified nuclei (polarity loss), cell maturation, and mucin content
  - Goblet cells may be seen: "Dystrophic" goblet cells
- Cystic dilatation, acute/chronic inflammation, hemorrhage, erosion (especially at surface)
  - Rupture: Extravasated mucin (if pedunculated)

Degree of Dysplasia

- Low-grade dysplasia (mild, moderate)
  - Crowded crypts, arranged in parallel, no complexity
    - No back-to-back, cribriform, or budding tubules
  - Nuclei retain basal orientation (bottom 1/2)
  - Absent or minimal: Atypical mitoses, significant loss of polarity, pleomorphism
- High-grade dysplasia (severe, carcinoma in situ)
  - Significant polymorphism (cytologically malignant)
    - Rounded (heaped up) cells, ↑ nuclear:cytoplasm ratio
    - Nuclei: "Open" chromatin, prominent nucleoli
  - Marked nuclear stratification and loss of polarity
    - Lost basal orientation, extend to luminal 1/2
  - Increased and atypical mitoses
  - Architectural complexity: Irregular, back-to-back tubules, cribriforming, solid nests
    - No definite breach of basement membrane
- Reactive changes (especially on surface)
  - May occur in preexisting adenoma
  - Focal loss of polarity, papillary tufting
  - Do not overinterpret as high-grade dysplasia
    - Associated inflammation helps distinguish
- Interobserver variability among pathologists
  - Inconsistent interpretation of dysplasia grade

Villous Component

- Elongated leaf-like projections of dysplastic epithelium
  - Length > 2x thickness of normal colonic mucosa
  - Arbitrary definition, subjective, not reproducible
  - Problematic distinction from long, separate tubules
  - 35-75% of adenomas > 1 cm have villous component
- % of adenoma surface area with villi defines type
  - TA (70-90% adenomas): < 20-25% villous component
    - Maintains original tubular architecture of mucosa
    - Most pedunculated, 2-3% lifetime malignancy risk
    - Dysplastic tubules over normal epithelium below
  - TVA (10-25%): Between 20-25% and 75-80% villous
    - Intermediate risk of malignant degeneration
  - VA (~ 5% of adenomas): > 75-80% villous component
    - Typically sessile, with hair-like surface
    - > 30% have high-grade dysplasia
    - ~ 2% invasive CRC at diagnosis (15-25% lifetime)

Intramucosal Carcinoma

- Neoplastic cells extend through basement membrane into surrounding lamina propria of mucosa but not through muscularis mucosae
- Single cell infiltrates, small irregular tubules, marked expansion of back-to-back cribriform glands in mucosa
- Nuclei become more rounded (rather than oval)
- Not shown to have metastatic risk
  - General paucity of lymphatics in colorectal mucosa
  - Some argue against use of the term "carcinoma" in this setting and suggest "adenoma with high-grade dysplasia" if no invasion
    - Avoids clinical overinterpretation of malignancy

Pseudoinvasion (Epithelial Misplacement)

- Misplaced (herniated) epithelium in submucosa
  - Pedunculated polyps, especially right-sided
- Can be mistaken for invasive carcinoma
  - Lacks desmoplastic stromal reaction

COLON ADENOMA

Flat or Depressed Adenoma

- Dysplastic lesions without polypoid component
- Slightly raised edges, typically centrally depressed
- Higher prevalence in patients with FAP
- Difficult to identify endoscopically
  - Usually smaller than raised (elevated) adenomas
  - Inaccurate assessment of prevalence, natural history
- Different molecular defect than classic adenomas
  - ↑ rate of high-grade dysplasia, carcinoma
  - Resulting flat/depressed CRC, no residual adenoma
  - ↑ incidence and significance in Japan, east Asia

Traditional Serrated Adenoma

- 1-5% of colorectal adenomas
- Commonly left-sided; large (> 1 cm) in right colon
- Serrated/sawtooth luminal/surface contour
  - Pattern reminiscent of hyperplastic polyp
  - Papillary infolding, budding, surface nuclear tufting
- Obvious cytologic dysplasia
  - Crowded, pseudostratified, elongated nuclei
  - Hypereosinophilic cytoplasm, prominent nucleoli
  - Lack of surface maturation
- Prominent mitoses anywhere along crypt axes
- May have distinct molecular abnormalities
  - *KRAS* > *BRAF* mutations; common MSI, CIMP

Other Types of Adenoma

- Villomicroglandular adenoma
  - VA with closely packed small tubules at sides of villi
- Hypersecretory adenoma
  - Usually rectal VA associated with hypokalemia
  - Pale mucus-filled cells line dysplastic villi
- Clear cell adenoma
  - Focal clear cell change in otherwise classic adenoma
  - Minimal cytologic atypia
    - Basal nuclei, abundant pale foamy cytoplasm

DIFFERENTIAL DIAGNOSIS

Reactive/Regenerative Epithelium

- Epithelium matures toward surface
  - Acquires more cytoplasm, mucin
  - Nuclei become smaller, more basal
- Usually associated with active inflammation
- Mitoses limited to crypt bases

Invasive Carcinoma

- Adenoma has reached beyond muscularis mucosae
  - Into underlying submucosa
- Dysplastic tubules mixed with submucosal structures
  - Medium-sized vessels, large lymphatics, fat, ganglia
- Accompanied by desmoplastic stromal reaction
  - Necessary for diagnosis of submucosal invasion

DIAGNOSTIC CHECKLIST

Clinically Relevant Pathologic Features

- Dysplasia (adenomatous change) can also occur in
  - Other preexisting lesions (hamartomatous polyps)
  - Other epithelial polyps (hyperplastic polyps)
    - Resulting in mixed adenoma-serrated polyps
  - Inflammatory bowel disease (ulceratice colitis, Crohn colitis)
- Multiple adenomas may be part of genetic syndrome

Pathologic Interpretation Pearls

- Dysplastic colorectal epithelium considered invasive
  - When through muscularis mucosae into submucosa
  - Otherwise, no clinically significant risk of metastases
- Desmoplasia strongly suggests invasive carcinoma
  - Should be interpreted as such in pathology report
  - Even absent cytologically malignant epithelium
    - Raises concern that invasive carcinoma present
    - Perhaps not properly sampled
  - Unless history of prior biopsy in same area
    - Difficult to distinguish desmoplasia from changes of prior biopsy site

REPORTING CONSIDERATIONS

Key Elements to Report

- Key facts to be included in pathology report
  - Extent of villous component, degree of dysplasia
  - If multiple pieces of adenoma (piecemeal removal)
    - Indicate as such (1 or multiple polyps)
    - Margin cannot be adequately evaluated
    - Attempt to account for each polyp removed
  - Large pedunculated polyp, removed in single piece
    - Bisect (or serially section) and properly orient
    - Comment on dysplasia at cauterized margin
    - Positive: Further removal &/or close follow-up
    - Cautery may actually destroy residual adenoma
  - If invasive carcinoma is present (desmoplasia)
    - Degree of differentiation
    - Lymphovascular invasion, if present
  - Invasive carcinoma in pedunculated polyp
    - Comment on any adverse histologic features
    - Poor differentiation, < 1-2 mm to margin, lymphovascular invasion, tumor budding
    - Any of these should prompt surgical resection
    - Significant risk of recurrence &/or metastases
    - Otherwise, complete polypectomy is curative if endoscopically and histologically confirmed
    - Invasion of stalk not unfavorable (if clean margin)

SELECTED REFERENCES

1. Del Vecchio Blanco G et al: Adenoma, advanced adenoma and colorectal cancer prevalence in asymptomatic 40- to 49-year-old subjects with a first-degree family history of colorectal cancer. Colorectal Dis. 15(9):1093-9, 2013
2. Jasperson KW et al: Serrated Polyposis: Colonic Phenotype, Extracolonic Features, and Familial Risk in a Large Cohort. Dis Colon Rectum. 56(11):1211-1216, 2013
3. Naini BV et al: Advanced precancerous lesions (APL) in the colonic mucosa. Best Pract Res Clin Gastroenterol. 27(2):235-56, 2013
4. Levine JS et al: Clinical practice. Adenomatous polyps of the colon. N Engl J Med. 355(24):2551-7, 2006

COLON ADENOMA

Microscopic Features

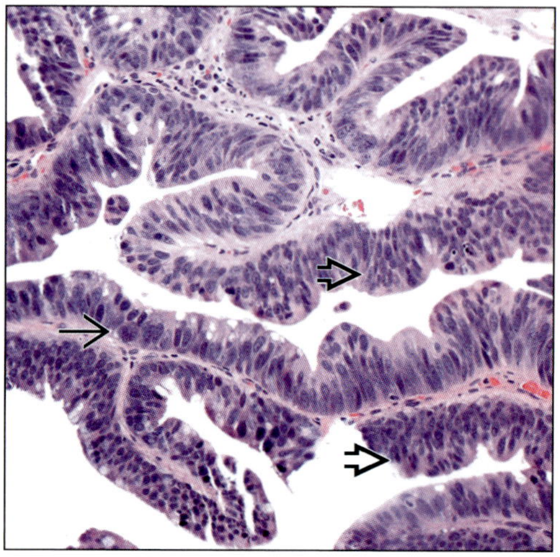
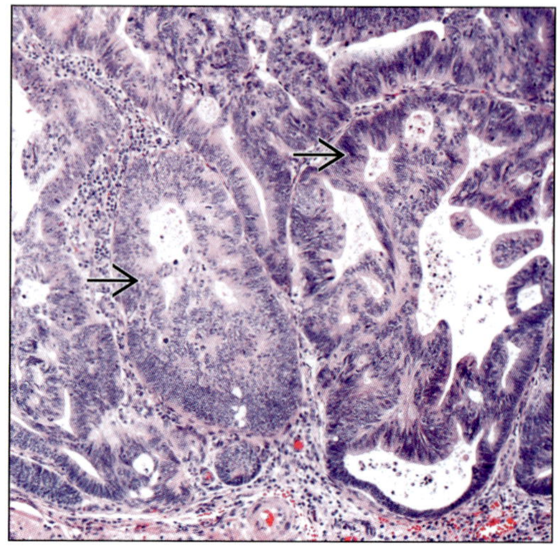

(Left) *H&E shows high-grade dysplasia. Note significant polymorphism and increased nuclear:cytoplasmic ratio and rounded-up cells ⇒. Marked nuclear stratification and extensive loss of polarity are also present ⇨.* ***(Right)*** *Hematoxylin & eosin shows extensive high-grade dysplasia, which some would classify as intramucosal carcinoma. There is increased architectural complexity with irregular back-to-back glands, often in cribriform shapes ⇒.*

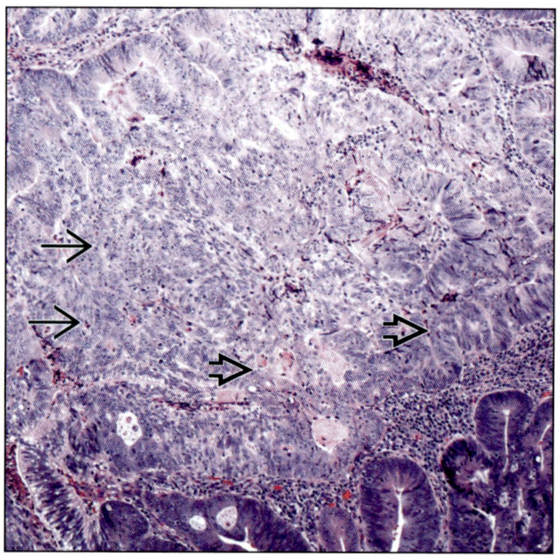
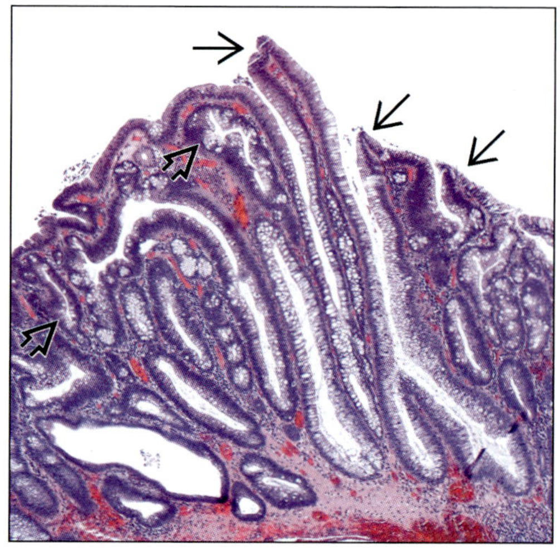

(Left) *H&E shows extensive high-grade dysplasia in an adenoma with solid nests of dysplastic cells ⇒ and back-to-back tubules ⇨. This would be classified as intramucosal carcinoma by some pathologists.* ***(Right)*** *H&E shows a tubulovillous adenoma (TVA) with some leaf-like villous projections of dysplastic epithelium ⇒. The dysplastic tissue occupies 25-75% of the adenoma, the rest consisting of tubular structures ⇨.*

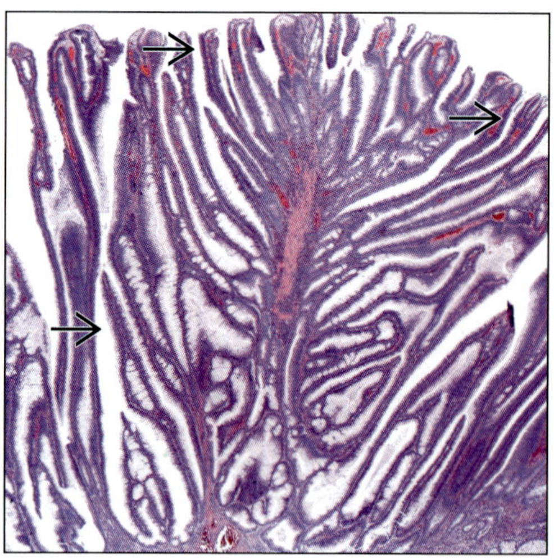
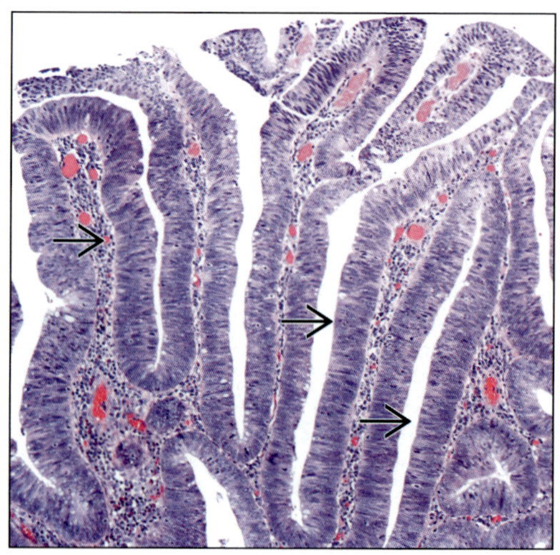

(Left) *H&E shows a villous adenoma (VA), almost entirely composed of villi, elongated, leaf-like projections of dysplastic epithelium ⇒ occupying > 75-80% of the adenoma.* ***(Right)*** *H&E shows a VA with high-grade dysplasia. VAs are more likely to have high-grade dysplasia, evidenced here by extensive nuclear stratification and loss of polarity ⇒.*

COLON ADENOMA

Microscopic Features

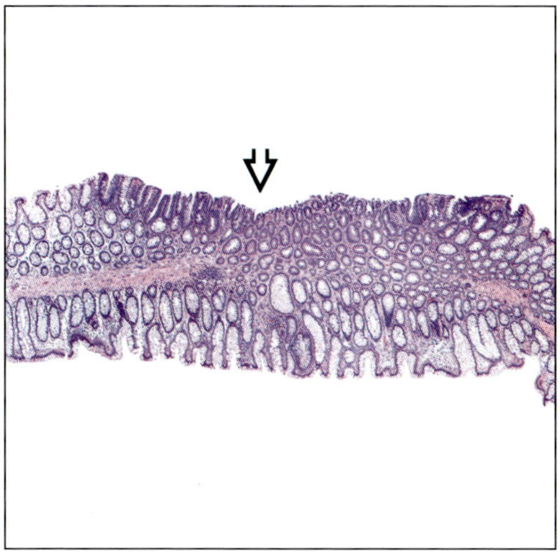

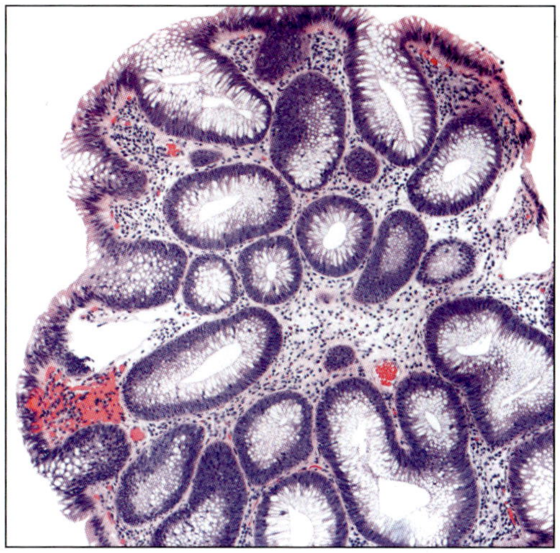

(Left) *H&E shows a flat adenoma that is depressed in the center ⇨. Mucosa width that is narrower than surrounding normal mucosa is typical of flat adenomas, making them difficult to identify endoscopically.* ***(Right)*** *H&E shows adenoma with very low-grade dysplasia. Tubules are not extensively proliferating or crowded and are thus hard to recognize as dysplastic. Overall basophilia helps identify the enlarged, hyperchromatic, and stratified nuclei.*

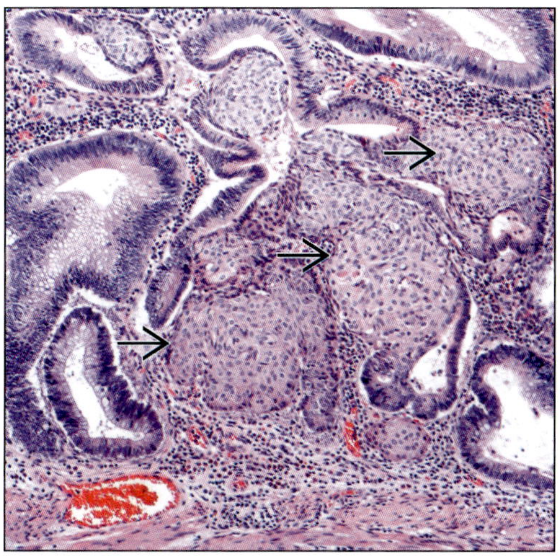

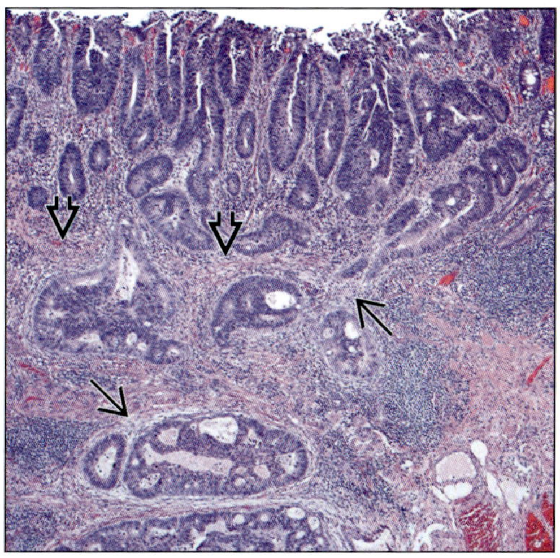

(Left) *H&E shows an adenoma with squamous metaplasia. The dysplastic glandular epithelium of the adenoma differentiates into morules of squamous epithelium →.* ***(Right)*** *H&E shows a tubular adenoma giving rise to an invasive adenocarcinoma. Typically arising from the base of the adenoma, invasive tubules elicit a desmoplastic stromal reaction → once they have invaded past the muscularis mucosae ⇨ into the submucosa.*

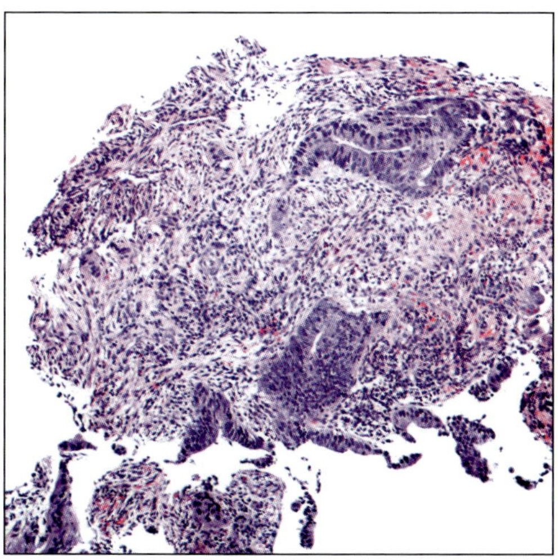

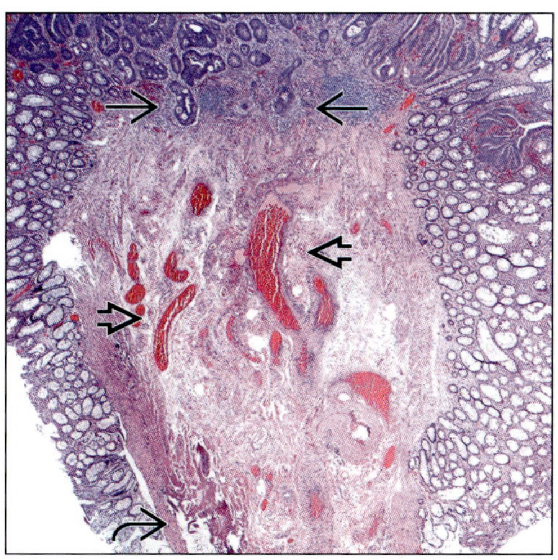

(Left) *H&E shows invasive carcinoma in a polyp biopsy. The presence of desmoplasia should raise concern for invasion, even if dysplastic tubules are not clearly seen invading the submucosa, as in this piecemeal specimen.* ***(Right)*** *H&E shows invasive adenocarcinoma arising from an adenoma at the head of a pedunculated polyp →. Large vessels ⇨ are present in the submucosa of the stalk. Invasive carcinoma is far from the cauterized polypectomy margin ↪.*

ESOPHAGEAL ADENOCARCINOMA

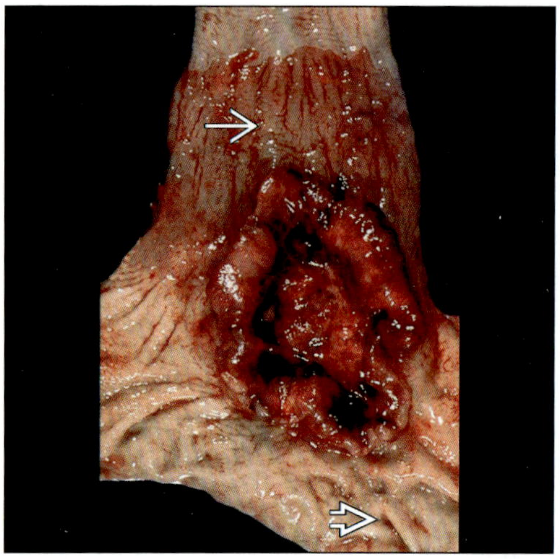

Gross pathology photograph shows an esophageal adenocarcinoma. The gastric folds are seen at the bottom of the field ⇨, and velvety background Barrett mucosa is readily identified →.

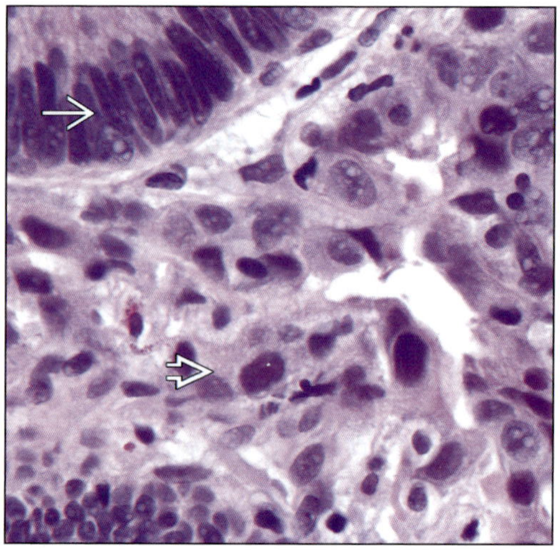

Hematoxylin & eosin shows a focus of intramucosal adenocarcinoma ⇨ adjacent to columnar epithelial dysplasia →.

TERMINOLOGY

Abbreviations

- Esophageal adenocarcinoma (EAC)

Definitions

- Malignant epithelial tumor of esophagus with glandular differentiation
- Arises predominantly in lower 1/3 of esophagus in association with Barrett esophagus

ETIOLOGY/PATHOGENESIS

Risk Factors

- Male gender
- Gastroesophageal reflux disease
- Obesity, smoking, alcohol

Familial

- Perhaps 5-10% of Barrett esophagus cases are familial
  - May be several rare autosomal dominant susceptibility genes with incomplete penetrance

CLINICAL ISSUES

Epidemiology

- Incidence
  - > 15,000 new cases annually in USA
  - Most rapidly increasing cancer in USA, especially among white males
- Age
  - Average age at presentation: 65 years
- Gender
  - About 80% of cases are in men

Presentation

- Dysphagia &/or retrosternal pain or epigastric pain

Treatment

- Endoscopic treatment for early lesions (T1, intramucosal, or superficial submucosal invasion)
  - Photodynamic therapy
  - Laser treatments
  - Endoscopic mucosal resection
- Chemoradiation and surgery for high-stage lesions

Prognosis

- Dependent on stage (most tumors detected at high stage)
  - Overall 5-year survival (20%)
  - For pT1 cancers, 5-year survival (65-80%)
  - 5-year survival for intramucosal carcinomas (invading only lamina propria) (> 90%)

MACROSCOPIC FEATURES

General Features

- Lower 1/3 of esophagus
- Background Barrett esophagus often present

MICROSCOPIC PATHOLOGY

Histologic Features

- Gland forming as per any adenocarcinoma

DIFFERENTIAL DIAGNOSIS

Gastric Cardiac Adenocarcinoma

- Epidemiology and immunoprofiles (CK7[+], CDX2[±], CK20 variable) show extensive overlap; some lesions cannot be separated
- If Barrett esophagus is detected, cancers at esophagogastric junction are labeled as esophageal cancers

ESOPHAGEAL ADENOCARCINOMA

Key Facts

Terminology
- Malignant epithelial tumor of esophagus with glandular differentiation
- Arises predominantly in lower 1/3 of esophagus in association with Barrett esophagus

Etiology/Pathogenesis
- Perhaps 5-10% of Barrett esophagus cases are familial
- Gastroesophageal reflux disease
- Obesity, smoking, alcohol

Clinical Issues
- Endoscopic treatment for early lesions (T1, intramucosal, or superficial submucosal invasion)
- Most rapidly increasing cancer in USA, especially among white males

Diagnostic Checklist
- Damaged muscularis mucosae duplicate and submucosal glands should be sought to determine invasion into submucosa

Histologic Grading of Esophageal Adenocarcinoma

Classification	Definition
Grade X	Grade cannot be assessed
Grade 1	Well differentiated (> 95% of tumor composed of glands)
Grade 2	Moderately differentiated (50-95% of tumor composed of glands)
Grade 3	Poorly differentiated (≤ 49% of tumor composed of glands)

Adapted from 6th Edition AJCC Staging Manual (2002).

- If bulk of neoplasm is in stomach, lesion is regarded as gastric and staged as such
  - Gastric cancers are staged as N0, N1, and N2 whereas esophageal cancers are staged as N0 or N1

Other Adenocarcinomas
- Metastases from other sites, direct spread from lung cancers
- Clinical history and application of immunohistochemistry
  - Thyroid transcription factor-1 (TTF-1) for lung and thyroid

Barrett High-Grade Dysplasia
- Typically lacks nucleoli, necrosis in glands, and syncytial growth pattern
- Necrosis in glands, back-to-back glands, and nucleoli are features of early intramucosal adenocarcinoma

DIAGNOSTIC CHECKLIST

Pathologic Interpretation Pearls
- Remember that damaged muscularis mucosae duplicate, and submucosal glands should determine invasion into submucosa

SELECTED REFERENCES

1. Kavanagh ME et al: The esophagitis to adenocarcinoma sequence; the role of inflammation. Cancer Lett. Epub ahead of print, 2013
2. Lagergren J et al: Recent developments in esophageal adenocarcinoma. CA Cancer J Clin. 63(4):232-48, 2013
3. Levine DM et al: A genome-wide association study identifies new susceptibility loci for esophageal adenocarcinoma and Barrett's esophagus. Nat Genet. Epub ahead of print, 2013

IMAGE GALLERY

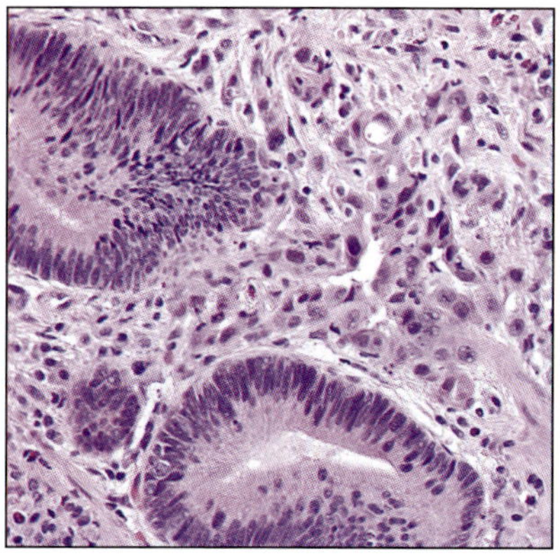

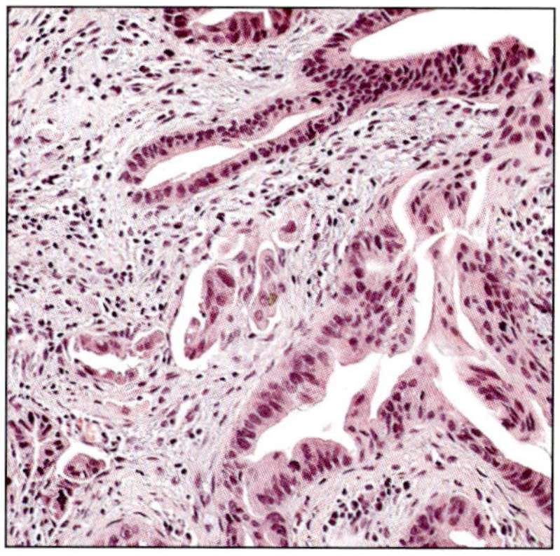

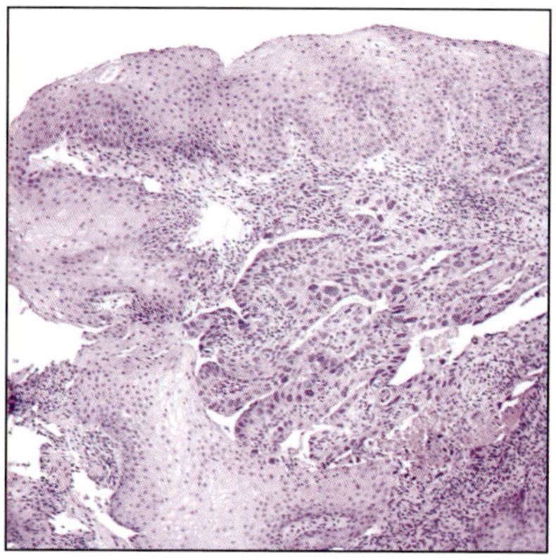

(Left) *Lower magnification H&E shows a contrasted background columnar epithelial dysplasia with the intramucosal carcinoma; the dysplasia lacks nucleoli in contrast to the invasive component.* ***(Center)*** *Hematoxylin & eosin shows the superficial portions of a deeply invasive adenocarcinoma. Note the well-developed desmoplasia.* ***(Right)*** *Hematoxylin & eosin shows an adenocarcinoma undermining squamous mucosa in the esophagus.*

ESOPHAGEAL SQUAMOUS CELL CARCINOMA

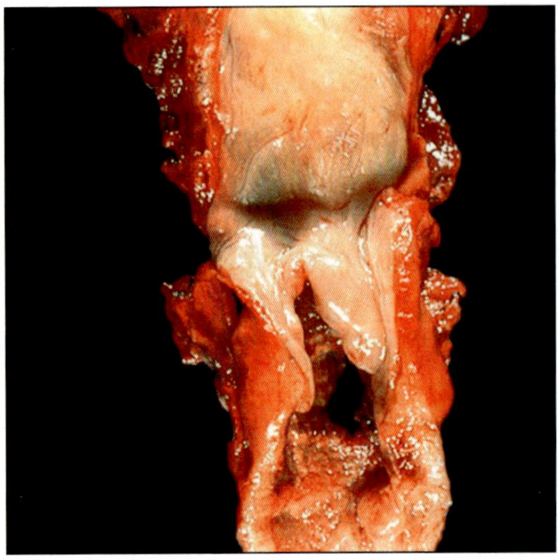

Gross pathology photograph shows an esophageal squamous cell carcinoma (SCCa) in the upper 1/3 of the esophagus. Most esophageal squamous carcinomas are identified in the middle 1/3.

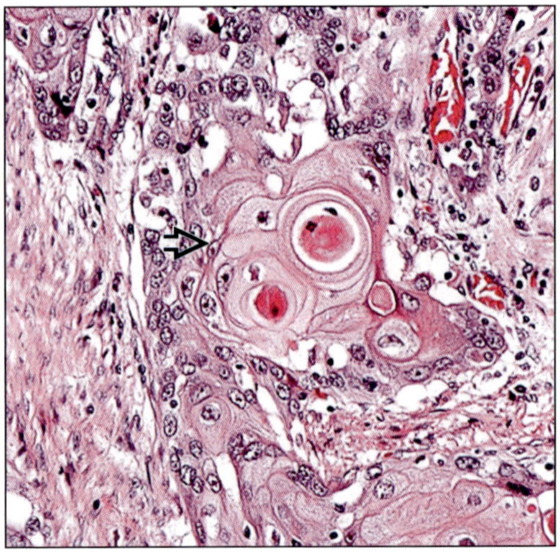

Hematoxylin & eosin shows SCCa of the esophagus. It has the same features as SCCa elsewhere. Note the abnormal keratinization in the keratin "pearl" ⇨.

TERMINOLOGY

Abbreviations

- Squamous cell carcinoma (SCCa)

Definitions

- Malignant epithelial neoplasm with squamous cell differentiation
  - Manifested as keratinocyte-like cells that may contain intercellular bridges &/or keratinization

ETIOLOGY/PATHOGENESIS

Risk Factors

- Tobacco
  - Accounts for majority of risk in Western countries
  - Potentiates risk associated with alcohol
- Alcohol
  - Northwest France and northern Italy; well studied and potentiated by tobacco use
- Nutrition
  - Nitrosamines in pickled or moldy foods
  - Vitamin deficiencies
- Ingestion of hot beverages: Thermal injury
  - Classic example: Mate tea in South America, consumed through a metal straw
- Human papillomavirus
  - Associated in endemic areas in China but rare in USA population
- Achalasia
- Prior corrosive ingestion
- Plummer-Vinson syndrome
  - Also called Paterson-Kelly syndrome or sideropenic dysphagia
  - Severe, long-term iron deficiency anemia with dysphagia due to esophageal webs

Genetic

- Tylosis
  - Also called focal nonepidermolytic palmoplantar keratoderma
  - Autosomal dominant skin disorder associated with familial early onset of esophageal SCCa
  - Abnormality localized to long arm of chromosome 17
    - Missense mutations in *RHBDF2* gene thought to be the cause
- Celiac disease
  - Risk of SCCa due to iron deficiency anemia, similar to Plummer-Vinson syndrome
- In Japanese alcoholics, associated with polymorphism in aldehyde dehydrogenase 2 (*ALDH2*) gene

CLINICAL ISSUES

Epidemiology

- Incidence
  - Varies by geography
    - Uncommon in USA: 5 per 100,000 men, 1 per 100,000 women
    - Normandy (northwest France) and Calvados (northern Italy): 30 per 100,000 men, 2 per 100,000 women
    - High-risk regions (China, Iran, Brazil, South Africa): > 100 per 100,000 men, 50 per 100,000 women
- Age
  - Rare before 30 years
  - Median age: 65 years
- Gender
  - Male predominance
- Ethnicity
  - In USA, 2-3x more common in African Americans than others

Presentation

- Difficulty swallowing

ESOPHAGEAL SQUAMOUS CELL CARCINOMA

Key Facts

Terminology
- Malignant epithelial neoplasm with squamous cell differentiation; manifested as keratinocyte-like cells that may contain intercellular bridges &/or keratinization

Etiology/Pathogenesis
- Plummer-Vinson syndrome
- Tylosis
- Celiac disease
- Tobacco, alcohol, others

Clinical Issues
- Varies by geography
- Uncommon in USA
  - 5 per 100,000 men, 1 per 100,000 women

Microscopic Pathology
- Appears as squamous cell carcinoma in other anatomic sites

Treatment
- Combined radiation and chemotherapy followed by surgery

Prognosis
- Stage specific: Typically poor since patients present at high stage

MACROSCOPIC FEATURES

General Features
- Typically mass in midesophagus

MICROSCOPIC PATHOLOGY

Histologic Features
- Appears as squamous cell carcinoma in other anatomic sites
  - Abnormal keratinization, "paradoxical maturation," squamous "pearls"
- Variants in esophagus
  - Basaloid: Appears as basaloid squamous carcinomas in other sites
  - Sarcomatoid variant often requires identification of in situ component to diagnose
  - Helpful to label with keratins and p63 to confirm

DIFFERENTIAL DIAGNOSIS

Pseudoepitheliomatous Hyperplasia
- Lacks "paradoxical maturation"
- Intact basal layer

Sarcomas and Spindle Cell Melanoma
- Sarcomas vanishingly rare in esophagus
- Immunohistochemistry for S100 protein for melanoma
- CD117 for gastrointestinal stromal tumor (very rare in esophagus)

Squamous Cell Carcinoma
- From lung with direct extension into esophagus
- Cannot be separated based on morphology or ancillary tests

SELECTED REFERENCES

1. Blaydon DC et al: RHBDF2 mutations are associated with tylosis, a familial esophageal cancer syndrome. Am J Hum Genet. 90(2):340-6, 2012
2. Hiyama T et al: Genetic polymorphisms and esophageal cancer risk. Int J Cancer. 121(8):1643-58, 2007
3. Enzinger PC et al: Esophageal cancer. N Engl J Med. 349(23):2241-52, 2003
4. Lauwers GY et al: Spindle cell squamous carcinoma of the esophagus: analysis of ploidy and tumor proliferative activity in a series of 13 cases. Hum Pathol. 29(8):863-8, 1998

IMAGE GALLERY

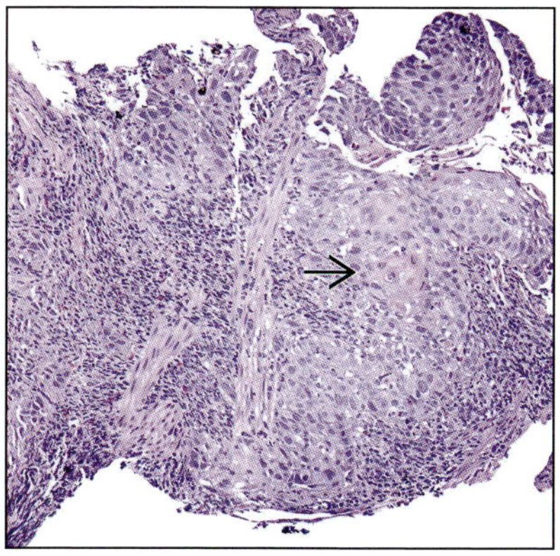

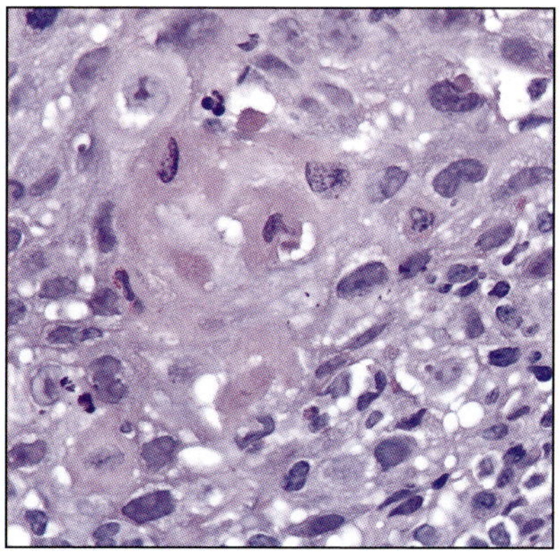

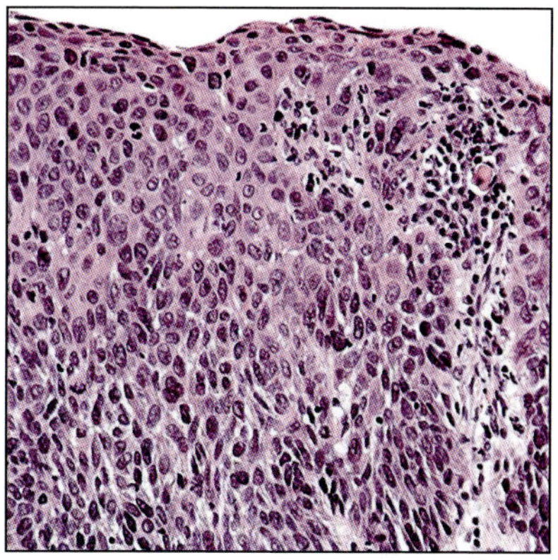

(Left) *Hematoxylin & eosin shows an esophageal SCCa (mucosal biopsy) with keratinization ⇒. The left side of the field appears more basaloid. These subtypes have little impact on outcome, which depends on stage.* ***(Center)*** *Hematoxylin & eosin shows higher magnification of the focus of overt squamous differentiation in the same neoplasm.* ***(Right)*** *Hematoxylin & eosin shows an area of high-grade squamous dysplasia in the resection sample from the same patient. Note the nucleoli and lack of keratinization.*

GASTRIC ADENOCARCINOMA

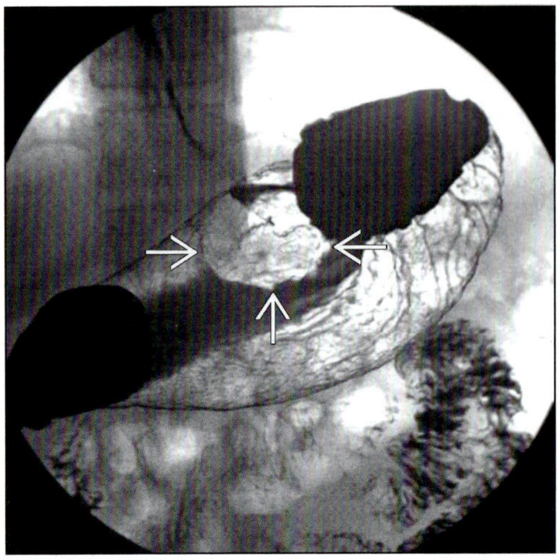

Upper GI study shows a large fungating mass ➔ located along the lesser curve of the stomach. Endoscopic biopsy demonstrated a gastric adenocarcinoma.

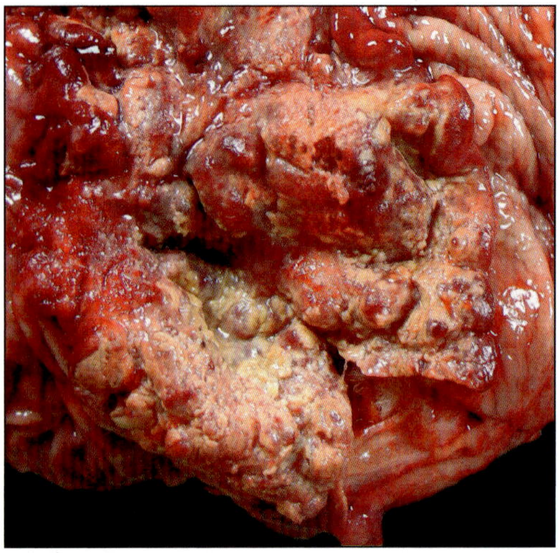

Gross photograph shows a large fungating gastric adenocarcinoma (Borrmann type 2).

TERMINOLOGY

Definitions

- Primary invasive epithelial gastric neoplasm
  - Early adenocarcinomas: Limited to mucosa and submucosa, irrelevant of lymph node status
  - Advanced adenocarcinomas: Invading muscularis propria and beyond

ETIOLOGY/PATHOGENESIS

Environmental Exposure

- Diet
  - Dried and salted foods
  - Low consumption of fresh fruits and vegetables
- Smoking

Infectious Agents

- *Helicobacter pylori*
  - Category 1 carcinogen
  - Infection leads to chronic inflammation and metaplastic changes, precursors of adenocarcinoma
  - Infection early in life
  - Variable risks associated with different strains

Hereditary Diffuse Gastric Cancer

- E-cadherin/*CDH1* gene

Previous Gastric Surgery

- Bile reflux and bacterial overgrowth are implicated

CLINICAL ISSUES

Epidemiology

- Incidence
  - Variable: 1.3 (Bangladesh) to 115 (Japan) per 100,000
    - Downward trend noticed in most industrialized nations
    - Early gastric adenocarcinomas encountered more frequently; represent 25-50% of all newly diagnosed gastric cancers
  - Increasing for adenocarcinomas of cardia
    - Geographically restricted; common in West but rare in Asia
    - Association with Barrett esophagus, gastroesophageal reflux disease, and intestinal metaplasia is debated
- Age
  - Primarily disease of late adulthood (5th decade and older)
  - Earlier presentation in syndromic patients with hereditary diffuse gastric cancer or hereditary intestinal gastric cancer
    - Look for multiple foci of early diffuse-type adenocarcinoma or signet ring cell carcinoma in situ in patients with hereditary diffuse gastric cancer
- Gender
  - M:F = 2:1

Presentation

- Abdominal pain
  - May mimic symptomatology related to peptic ulcer
- Anemia, vomiting, weight loss
- Young patients may present with intraabdominal dissemination and ascites
  - Females may present with metastatic ovarian lesions (Krukenberg tumors)

Endoscopic Findings

- Large polypoid mass
- Large ulcer
- Infiltrating with thickened gastric wall (linitis plastica)
- Early lesions may present as polyp, plaque, or mucosal erosion

GASTRIC ADENOCARCINOMA

Key Facts

Terminology
- Early adenocarcinomas are invasive neoplasms limited to mucosa and submucosa, irrelevant of lymph node status
- Advanced adenocarcinomas are neoplasms invading muscularis propria and beyond

Etiology/Pathogenesis
- *Helicobacter pylori*
- Diet
- Bile reflux and bacterial overgrowth are implicated
- E-cadherin/*CDH1* gene

Clinical Issues
- Decreasing incidence of distal adenocarcinomas
- Increasing incidence of cardial adenocarcinomas
- Currently, early adenocarcinomas are more commonly diagnosed
  - 90-100% survival at 5 years
- Endoscopic resection (mucosal or submucosal, depending on type and size)

Microscopic Pathology
- 2 main categories: Intestinal and diffuse
  - Intestinal type: Glandular or papillary structures of various degrees of differentiation
  - Diffuse type: Dyscohesive cells of plasmacytoid, histiocytic, or signet ring cell type

Top Differential Diagnoses
- Gastric dysplasia
- Gastric lymphoma
- Gastric xanthoma

Natural History
- Most early tumors progress to advanced carcinomas over months to years
- Lymphatic spread is common path of dissemination
- Transserosal coelomic extension common for diffuse-type adenocarcinomas with secondary ascites
  - Spread to ovaries produces Krukenberg tumor
- Hematogenous spread leads to liver and lung metastasis

Treatment
- Options, risks, complications
  - Endoscopic resection (mucosal or submucosal, depending on type and size)
- Surgical approaches
  - Gastrectomy
  - Associated with neoadjuvant and adjuvant therapies

Prognosis
- Early adenocarcinomas (T1) have good prognosis
  - > 90% survival at 5 years for mucosal tumors
    - Rate of lymph node metastasis is 0-7%
  - 80% survival at 5 years for submucosal tumors
    - Rate of lymph node metastasis is 8-25%
- Prognosis of advanced adenocarcinomas
  - T2: 65-81% survival at 5 years
  - T3: 35-44% survival at 5 years
  - T4: 16% survival at 5 years

MACROSCOPIC FEATURES

General Features
- Most cases diagnosed in antrum and antropyloric region
  - Preferentially on lesser curvature
- Multiple adenocarcinomas seen in 5% of patients

Size
- Microscopic to large bulky tumor several cm
  - Most early lesions measure 2-5 cm
  - 30% of advanced adenocarcinomas are 6-10 cm

Gross Appearance of Early Gastric Cancer
- Protruded (type 1)
- Superficial (type 2) (80% of cases)
  - 2a (elevated type)
    - Lesion is 2x as thick as normal mucosa
  - 2b (flat type)
  - 2c (mimics benign ulcer)
    - Most common subtype
    - May require multiple biopsies
- Excavated (type 3)

Gross Appearance of Advanced Cancer
- Borrmann classification for gastric carcinomas
  - Polypoid carcinoma (type 1)
    - ~ 25% of cases
    - More common in corpus, often on greater curvature
  - Fungating carcinoma (type 2)
    - ~ 35% of cases
    - Frequently found in antrum, along lesser curvature
  - Ulcerated carcinoma (type 3)
    - ~ 25% of cases
    - More common in corpus, often on greater curvature
  - Diffusely infiltrative carcinoma (type 4)
    - ~ 15% of cases
    - Known as linitis plastica when it involves entire stomach

DIFFERENTIAL DIAGNOSIS

Gastric Dysplasia
- May be hard to distinguish from early intramucosal adenocarcinoma
- Absence of desmoplasia
- Limited cytoarchitectural anomalies

Gastric Lymphoma
- May mimic poorly differentiated intestinal and diffuse adenocarcinoma

GASTRIC ADENOCARCINOMA

TNM Classification

Clinical	Stage Category Definitions
Primary tumor (T)	
TX	Primary tumor cannot be assessed
T0	No evidence of primary tumor
Tis	Carcinoma in situ: Intraepithelial tumor without invasion of lamina propria
T1	Tumor invades lamina propria, muscularis mucosae, or submucosa
T1a	Tumor invades lamina propria or muscularis mucosae
T1b	Tumor invades submucosa
T2	Tumor invades muscularis propria
T3	Tumor penetrates subserosal connective tissue without invasion of visceral peritoneum or adjacent structures*,**,***
T4	Tumor invades serosa (visceral peritoneum) or adjacent structures**,***
T4a	Tumor invades serosa (visceral peritoneum)
T4b	Tumor invades adjacent structures
Regional Lymph Nodes (N)	
NX	Regional lymph node(s) cannot be assessed
N0	No regional lymph node metastasis****
N1	Metastasis in 1-2 regional lymph nodes
N2	Metastasis in 3-6 regional lymph nodes
N3	Metastasis in ≥ 7 regional lymph nodes
N3a	Metastasis in 7-15 regional lymph nodes
N3b	Metastasis in 16 or more regional lymph nodes
Distant Metastasis (M)	
M0	No distant metastasis (no pathologic M0; use clinical M to complete stage group)
M1	Distant metastasis

**A tumor may penetrate the muscularis propria with extension into the gastrocolic or gastrohepatic ligaments, or into the greater or lesser omentum, without perforation of the visceral peritoneum covering these structures. In this case, the tumor is classified T3. If there is perforation of the visceral peritoneum covering the gastric ligaments or the omentum, the tumor should be classified T4. **The adjacent structures of the stomach include the spleen, transverse colon, liver, diaphragm, pancreas, abdominal wall, adrenal gland, kidney, small intestine, and retroperitoneum. ***Intramural extension to the duodenum or esophagus is classified by the depth of the greatest invasion in any of these sites, including the stomach. ****A designation of pN0 should be used if all examined lymph nodes are negative, regardless of the total number removed and examined. Adapted from 7th edition AJCC Staging Forms.*

Histologic Grading of Stomach Adenocarcinoma

Classification	Definition
Grade X	Cannot be assessed
Grade 1	Well differentiated (> 95% of tumor composed of glands)
Grade 2	Moderately differentiated (50-95% of tumor composed of glands)
Grade 3	Poorly differentiated (≤ 49% of tumor composed of glands)

- CD20 and CD45 (+); cytokeratin and CEA (-)

Gastric Xanthoma

- Foamy cytoplasm may mimic diffuse-type gastric cancer
- CD68(+), cytokeratin (-)

Whipple Disease

- May mimic diffuse-type gastric cancer
- Cytokeratin stain will be negative in Whipple disease
- CD68(+) stain in Whipple disease
- Bacteria (*Tropheryma whipplei*) observed on electron microscopy

SELECTED REFERENCES

1. Hidaka Y et al: Alteration in the Wnt/β-catenin signaling pathway in gastric neoplasias of fundic gland (chief cell predominant) type. Hum Pathol. Epub ahead of print, 2013
2. Marques M et al: Novel mutation identified in Cowden syndrome presenting as a gastric adenocarcinoma. Clin Res Hepatol Gastroenterol. Epub ahead of print, 2013
3. Wang LL et al: Clonality analysis of neuroendocrine cells in gastric adenocarcinoma. World J Gastroenterol. 19(32):5340-6, 2013
4. Chun N et al: Genetic testing by cancer site: stomach. Cancer J. 18(4):355-63, 2012

GASTRIC ADENOCARCINOMA

Diagrammatic and Microscopic Features

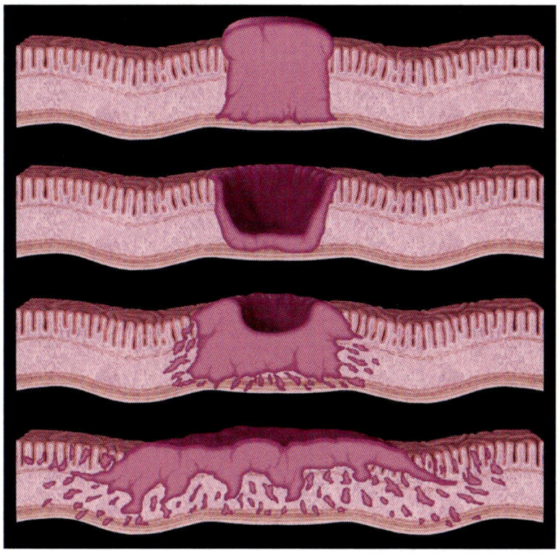

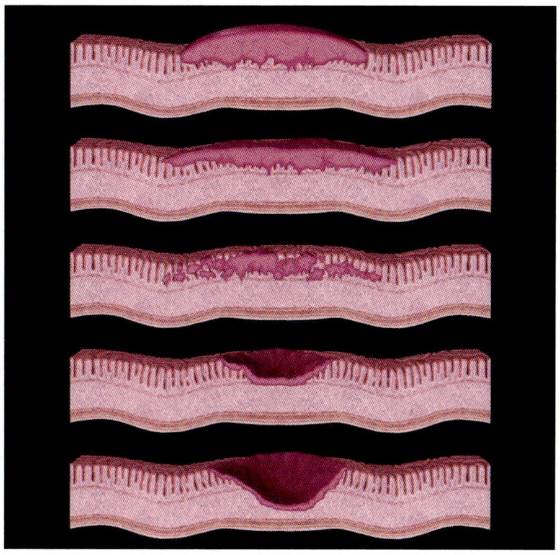

(Left) *From top to bottom, graphic shows the 4 types of advanced gastric adenocarcinoma in the Borrmann classification: Type 1 (polypoid), type 2 (fungating), type 3 (ulcerated), and type 4 (diffusely infiltrative).* ***(Right)*** *Graphic of the simplified endoscopic gross classification of early gastric adenocarcinoma shows 5 variants and subvariants, from top to bottom: Type 1 (polypoid), type 2a (elevated), type 2b (flat), type 2c (depressed), and type 3 (excavated).*

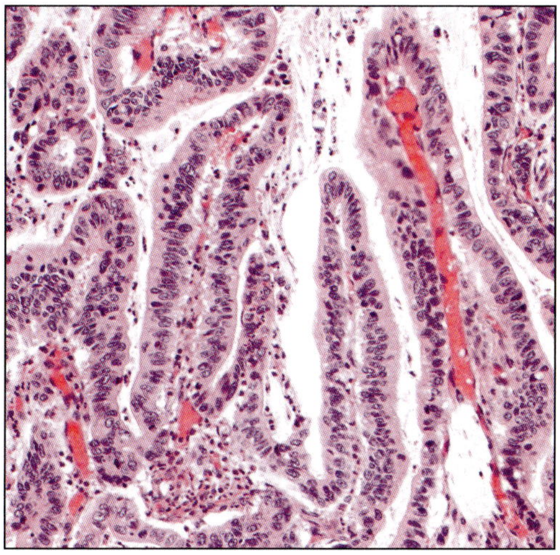

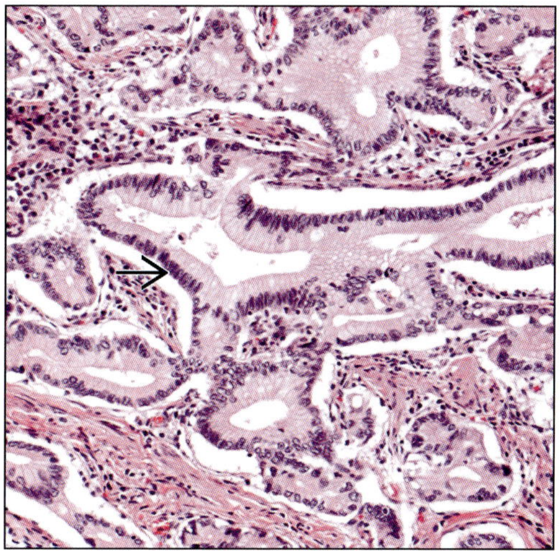

(Left) *Hematoxylin and eosin shows a well-differentiated papillary gastric adenocarcinoma.* ***(Right)*** *Hematoxylin and eosin shows a well-differentiated glandular adenocarcinoma. Cytologically, the tall clear neoplastic cells ⮕ are consistent with gastric foveolar phenotype.*

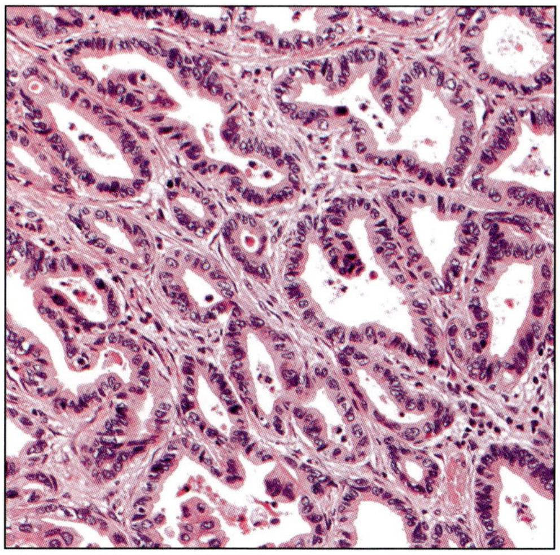

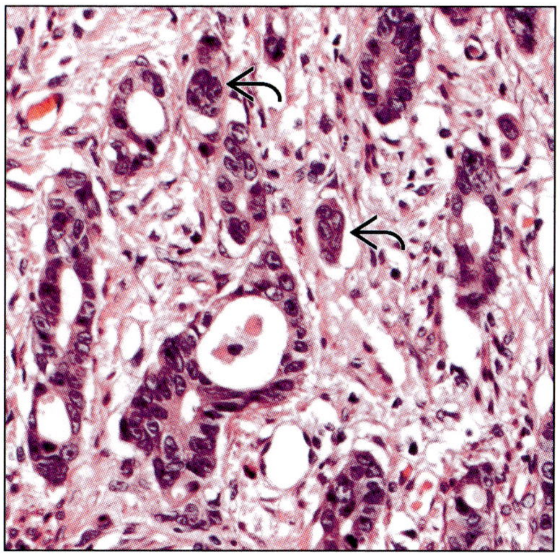

(Left) *Hematoxylin and eosin shows a moderately differentiated adenocarcinoma, glandular type. The glandular structures are irregular but remain easily identifiable.* ***(Right)*** *Hematoxylin and eosin shows an example of moderately differentiated adenocarcinoma. In this example, smaller dyscohesive groups of tumor cells ⮫ are seen invading the desmoplastic stroma.*

GASTRIC ADENOCARCINOMA

Microscopic and Imaging Features

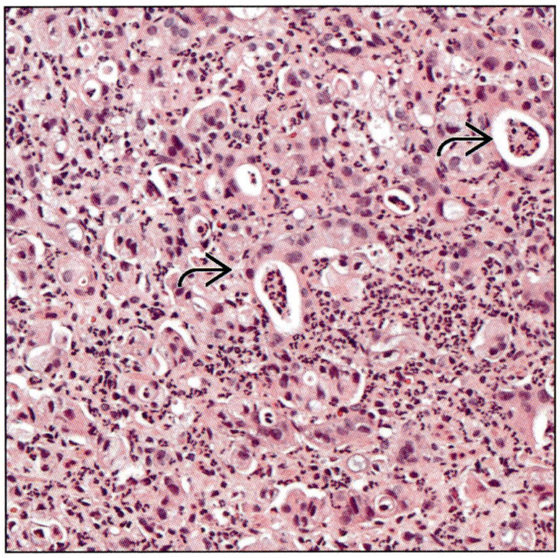

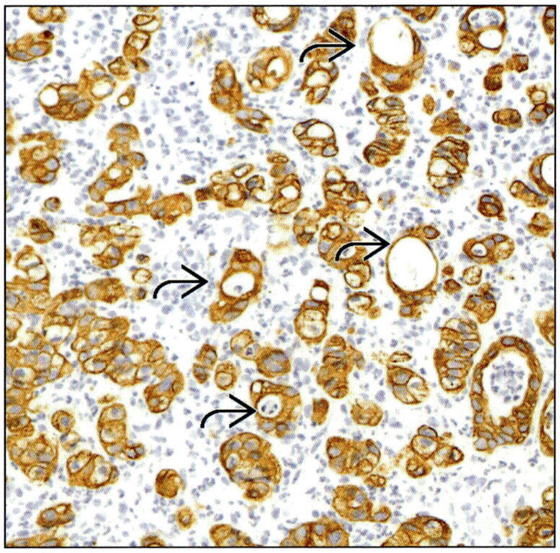

(Left) *Hematoxylin and eosin shows an example of a poorly differentiated intestinal-type adenocarcinoma. This case displays a sheet-like pattern of growth with only rare glandular structures* →. ***(Right)*** *Cytokeratin AE1/AE3 in the same case highlights the poorly formed glandular structures* →.

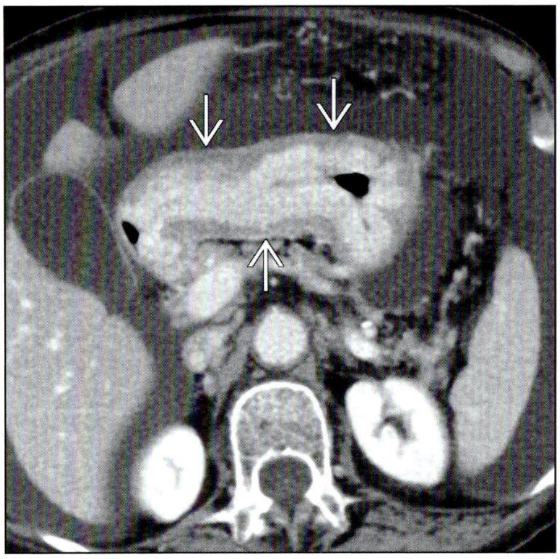

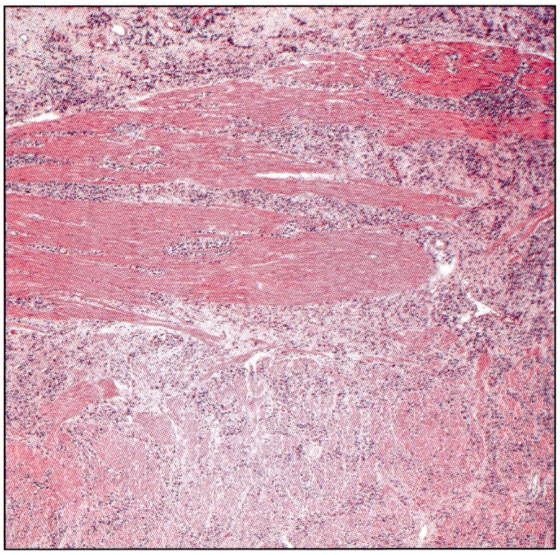

(Left) *Contrast-enhanced CT through the level of the gastric antrum shows diffuse thickening of the stomach wall* → *with lack of distensibility and narrowing of the lumen (linitis plastica). This appearance is typical for a diffusely infiltrating carcinoma.* ***(Right)*** *Hematoxylin and eosin shows a diffusely infiltrative adenocarcinoma. Sheets of dyscohesive tumors invade between the thick muscular fascicles of the muscularis propria.*

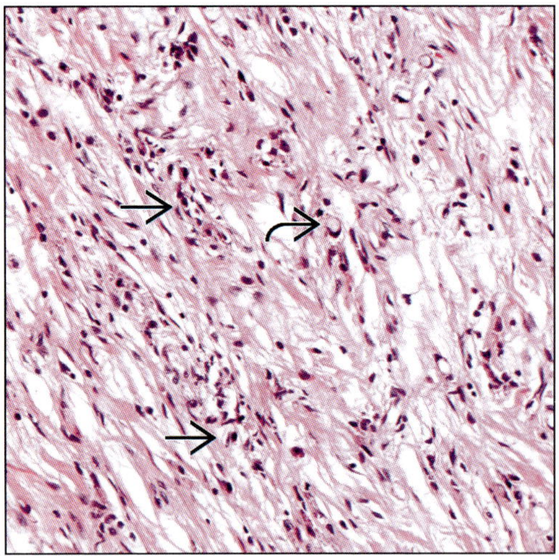

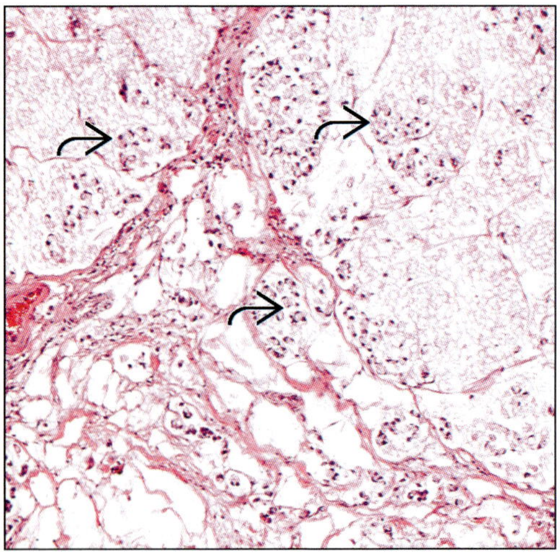

(Left) *Hematoxylin and eosin shows infiltrative diffuse-type tumor cells embedded in a thick desmoplastic stroma. Note that many assume a somewhat spindle-like appearance* →*, and only rare signet ring cells are seen* →. ***(Right)*** *Hematoxylin and eosin shows an infiltrative, diffuse-type adenocarcinoma with prominent mucin production. Note the clusters of tumor cells floating in the thick mucinous material* →.

Microscopic Features

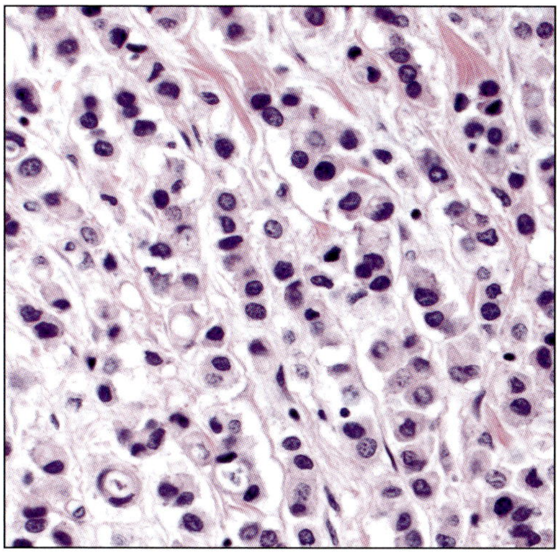
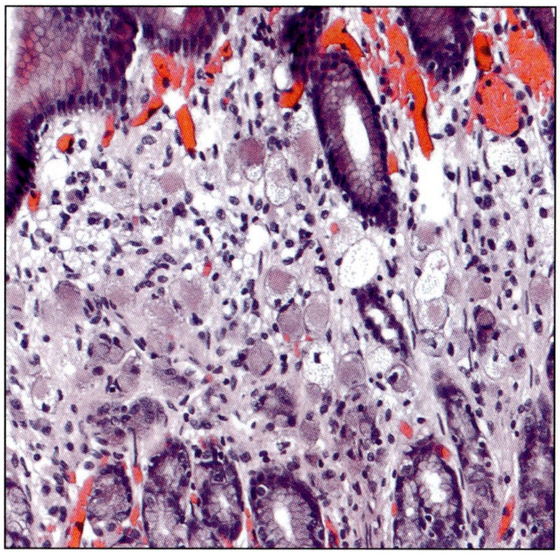

(Left) *Hematoxylin & eosin shows an "Indian file" infiltrative pattern in a case of diffuse-type adenocarcinoma. Caution should be exercised to not overlook a breast carcinoma metastatic to the stomach.* ***(Right)*** *Hematoxylin and eosin shows an early adenocarcinoma, diffuse type. The large mucin-rich cells should not be mistaken for a gastric xanthoma. Immunohistochemical stains, such as cytokeratin, can confirm the diagnosis.*

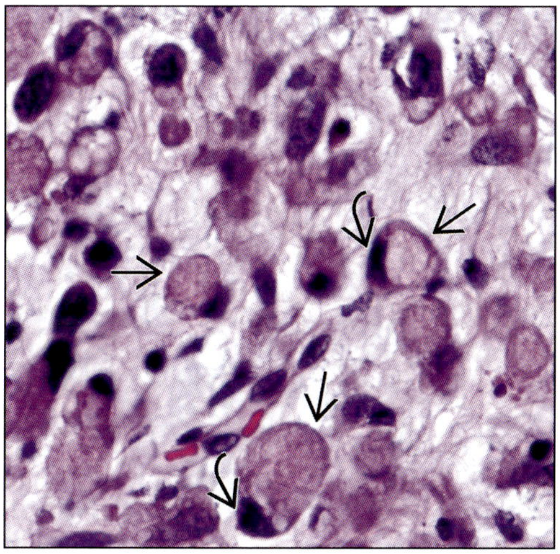
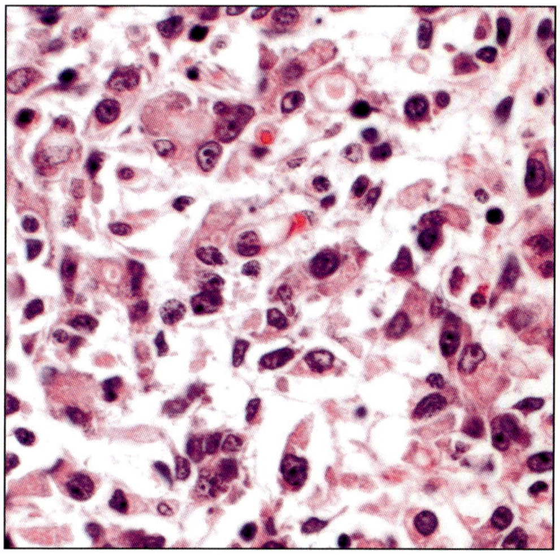

(Left) *High-power view of signet ring cells shows that the neoplastic cells are characterized by prominent mucin* ➔ *production; consequently, the nuclei are pushed to the side* ➚*.* ***(Right)*** *Hematoxylin and eosin shows another histologic variant of a diffuse-type gastric adenocarcinoma. The cells in this example have a vaguely histiocytic appearance.*

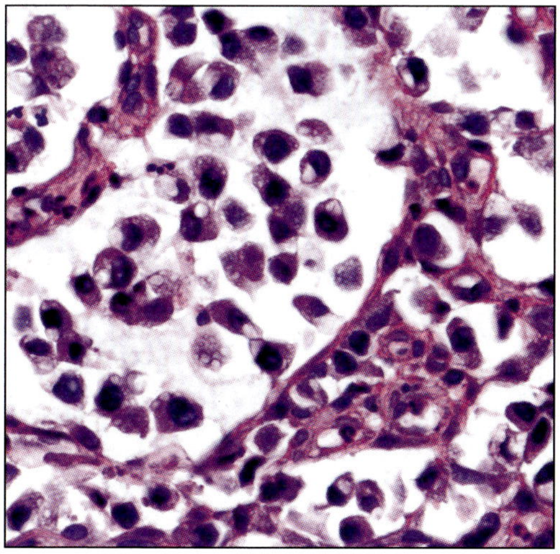
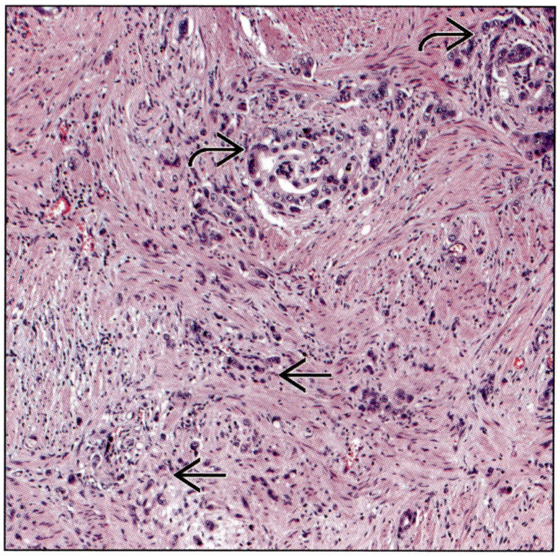

(Left) *Hematoxylin and eosin shows another histologic pattern of a diffuse type of gastric adenocarcinoma with a plasmacytoid appearance.* ***(Right)*** *Hematoxylin and eosin shows an example of gastric adenocarcinoma with mixed glandular* ➚ *and diffuse* ➔ *carcinoma. About 10% of gastric adenocarcinomas belong in this mixed category.*

GASTROINTESTINAL STROMAL TUMOR

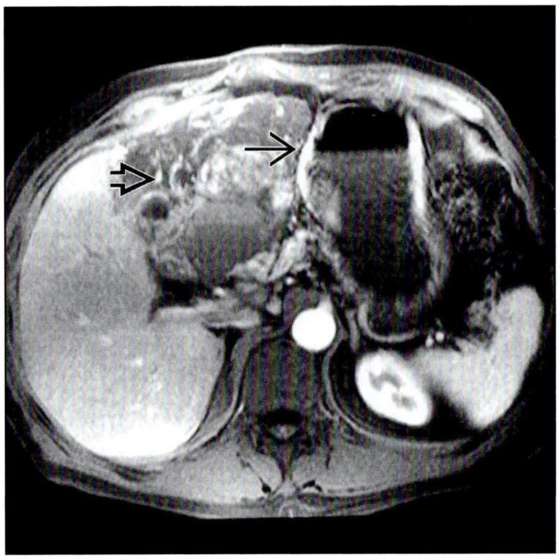

Radiologic image shows a large gastrointestinal stromal tumor (GIST) ⇨. The lesion compresses the liver but arises in association with the gastric wall →.

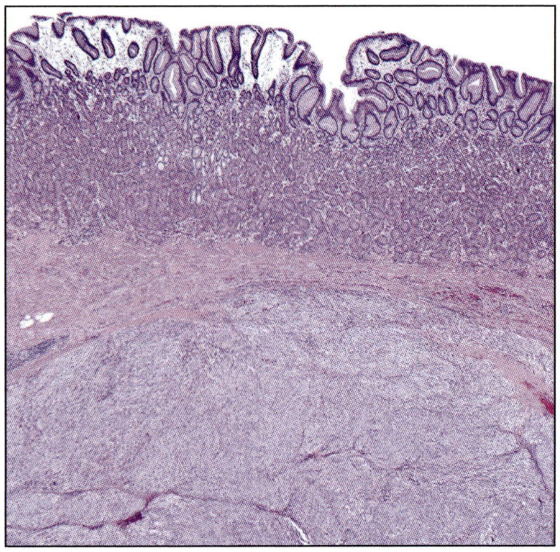

Hematoxylin & eosin shows low magnification of a gastric GIST that involved the muscularis propria of the gastric body. The lesion is lobulated and well marginated.

TERMINOLOGY

Abbreviations

- Gastrointestinal stromal tumor (GIST)

Synonyms

- Gastrointestinal smooth muscle tumors (used interchangeably in older literature)
- Gastrointestinal autonomic nerve tumor is now subsumed under GIST

Definitions

- Generally CD117(+) or *KIT* or *PDGFRA* mutation-driven mesenchymal tumors, usually of GI tract, with characteristic histologic features
  - Spindle cells
  - Epithelioid cells
  - Pleomorphic morphology (rare)
- Familial cases
  - Germline mutations of *KIT* gene, autosomal dominant
    - Relevant animal models are available for study
- Neurofibromatosis type 1 (NF1)
  - Interaction between *KIT* gene product and *NF1* gene product
  - Tumors have CD117 immunolabeling but no *KIT* gene mutations
- Carney triad
  - Epithelioid gastric GISTs, paraganglioma, pulmonary chondroma
- Carney-Stratakis syndrome
  - Epithelioid gastric GISTs and paraganglioma
  - Germline mutations in succinate dehydrogenase (SDH) complex B, C, and D subunits

CLINICAL ISSUES

Epidemiology

- Incidence
  - 14.5 per million people in Sweden, 11 per million people in Iceland, ~ 4,500 new cases per year in USA
  - Clinically silent lesions (studied in gastroesophageal resections for carcinomas) are common (10%)
    - Suggests that most lesions remain clinically insignificant and do not progress
- Age
  - Median is 60 years; rare in children and young adults
    - Familial examples present in middle age
    - Carney-Stratakis and Carney triad cases may present in childhood
    - Mean age for NF1-associated lesions is 49 years
- Gender
  - No predilection in most series
- Ethnicity
  - Overrepresentation of malignant examples reported in African Americans

Site

- Stomach is most common site (60%)
- Jejunum and ileum (30%)
  - NF1-associated lesions tend to occur in small bowel
- Duodenum (5%)
- Colorectum (< 5%)
- Esophagus and appendix (rare)
- Primary extraintestinal (mesentery, omentum, retroperitoneum) is rare
  - Most lesions in these sites are metastases/direct spread from GI tract

Presentation

- Gastrointestinal bleeding
  - Most common presentation
- GI obstruction
- Abdominal pain
- Incidental
  - During surgery, imaging studies, or endoscopy

GASTROINTESTINAL STROMAL TUMOR

Key Facts

Terminology
- Generally CD117(+) or *KIT* or *PDGFRA* mutation-driven mesenchymal tumors, usually of GI tract, with characteristic histologic features

Clinical Issues
- Molecular prognostication for GISTs
  - Not indicated for all cases
  - Best reserved for patients with advanced disease or disease refractory to treatment
- Both simple clinicopathologic features and molecular testing are prognostic
- Simple algorithms a function of size and mitotic counts
- Site is important risk factor
- 20-25% of gastric GISTs are malignant
- 40-50% of small intestinal GISTs are malignant
- Molecular analysis to determine likelihood of response to treatment
- *KIT* exon 11 (most common mutation type)
  - Complete remission (6%), partial response (61%), stable disease (25%), progressive disease (3%)
- *KIT* and *PDGFRA* wild type
  - Partial response (23%), stable disease (50%), progressive disease (19%)

Microscopic Pathology
- Uniform spindle cells or epithelioid cells arranged in lobules
- Nuclear pleomorphism is rare
- Eosinophilic cytoplasm
- Cytoplasmic vacuoles are common

Treatment
- Surgical approaches
  - Complete resection regardless of site
- Drugs
  - Imatinib mesylate (Gleevec): Inhibits tyrosine kinases (such as c-kit)
  - Newer drugs
    - Used for acquired resistance to imatinib (attributed to secondary *KIT* or *PDGFRA* mutations) or initial lack of response
    - Sunitinib malate (SU11248): Used for patients with *KIT* exon 9 mutations, others
    - Newer drugs in development

Prognosis
- Both simple clinicopathologic features and molecular testing are prognostic
  - Simple algorithms are function of size and mitotic counts
  - Site is important risk factor
    - 20-25% of gastric GISTs are malignant
    - 40-50% of small intestinal GISTs are malignant
- Small bowel criteria often applied for other sites of GISTs
- Molecular prognostication for GISTs
  - Not indicated for all cases
    - Best reserved for patients with advanced disease or disease refractory to treatment

MACROSCOPIC FEATURES

General Features
- Usually well-marginated lesions with their epicenter in muscularis propria

MICROSCOPIC PATHOLOGY

Histologic Features
- Uniform spindle cells or epithelioid cells arranged in lobules
  - Nuclear pleomorphism is rare
  - Occasional cases show dedifferentiated pattern with bland areas and high-grade areas in same neoplasm
  - Some cases have multinucleated cells
- Eosinophilic cytoplasm
- Cytoplasmic vacuoles common
- Minimal inflammation
- Inconspicuous vessels
- Can have myxoid or myxochondroid background
- Some cases have cystic spaces
- "Skeinoid" fibers (coarse, wire-like, haphazardly arranged collagen bundles) in small bowel tumors
- Occasional extension into mucosa (poor prognostic factor)
- Tumor necrosis uncommon (poor prognostic factor)

ANCILLARY TESTS

Immunohistochemistry
- Usually CD117(+)
  - Newer relatively specific markers
    - Protein kinase C8
    - *DOG1* (deleted on GIST-1)
  - Data accumulating on PDGFR-α antibodies

DIFFERENTIAL DIAGNOSIS

Solitary Fibrous Tumor
- Vanishingly rare in GI tract
- Spindle cell lesion, hemangiopericytoma-like vascular pattern
- CD34(+), Bcl-2(+), CD117(-)
- No *KIT* mutations

Schwannoma
- Usually in muscularis propria of stomach
- Prominent lymphoid cuff
- Intralesional lymphoplasmacytic inflammation
- S100(+), CD117(-)
- No *KIT* mutations

GASTROINTESTINAL STROMAL TUMOR

Fibromatosis

- Epicenter in mesentery with extension into muscularis propria
- Infiltrative growth pattern
- Pale cells, abundant collagen, prominent small vessels
- Usually CD34(-); some cases have cytoplasmic CD117, nuclear β-catenin (GISTs lack nuclear β-catenin)
- β-catenin and *APC* gene mutations
- No *KIT* mutations

Leiomyoma

- Usually in esophagus or in association with colonic muscularis mucosae
- Brightly eosinophilic cells with blunt-ended nuclei
- Desmin (+), actin (+), CD117(-)
- No *KIT* mutations

Leiomyosarcoma

- Brightly eosinophilic cells with blunt-ended nuclei
- Perpendicularly oriented fascicles
- Nuclear pleomorphism
- Desmin (+), actin (+), CD117(-)
- No *KIT* mutations

Melanoma

- Metastases tend to spread to small bowel; occasional anal and esophageal primaries
- Typically more pleomorphic than GIST
- CD117 often positive, but also S100, other melanocytic markers
- About 20% of mucosal melanomas have *KIT* mutations and respond to treatment with imatinib

Clear Cell Sarcoma of GI Tract

- Usually in small bowel
- Lobules of uniform cells with prominent nucleoli
- S100(+), most CD117(-)
- t(12;22), *EWS-ATF1* fusion, or *EWS-CREB1* fusion

Inflammatory Fibroid Polyp

- Submucosal based
- Bland proliferating cells, numerous eosinophils
- CD34(+), CD117(-)
- *PDGFRA* mutations, no *KIT* mutations

DIAGNOSTIC CHECKLIST

Pathologic Interpretation Pearls

- If considering GIST diagnosis when confronted with pleomorphic mesenchymal neoplasm in GI tract, first consider alternative diagnoses

SELECTED REFERENCES

1. Barnett CM et al: Gastrointestinal Stromal Tumors: Molecular Markers and Genetic Subtypes. Hematol Oncol Clin North Am. 27(5):871-888, 2013
2. Dwight T et al: Loss of SDHA expression identifies SDHA mutations in succinate dehydrogenase-deficient gastrointestinal stromal tumors. Am J Surg Pathol. 37(2):226-33, 2013
3. Miettinen M et al: Immunohistochemical loss of succinate dehydrogenase subunit A (SDHA) in gastrointestinal stromal tumors (GISTs) signals SDHA germline mutation. Am J Surg Pathol. 37(2):234-40, 2013
4. Nakamura M et al: Cowden syndrome complicated by a gastrointestinal stromal tumor. Dig Endosc. Epub ahead of print, 2013
5. Tenorio Jiménez C et al: Carney Stratakis syndrome in a patient with SDHD mutation. Endocr Pathol. 23(3):181-6, 2012
6. Gaal J et al: SDHB immunohistochemistry: a useful tool in the diagnosis of Carney-Stratakis and Carney triad gastrointestinal stromal tumors. Mod Pathol. 24(1):147-51, 2011
7. Janeway KA et al: Defects in succinate dehydrogenase in gastrointestinal stromal tumors lacking KIT and PDGFRA mutations. Proc Natl Acad Sci U S A. 108(1):314-8, 2011
8. Vaughan P et al: Cardiac paraganglioma and gastrointestinal stromal tumor: a pediatric case of Carney-Stratakis syndrome. Ann Thorac Surg. 92(5):1877-8, 2011
9. Almeida MQ et al: Solid tumors associated with multiple endocrine neoplasias. Cancer Genet Cytogenet. 203(1):30-6, 2010
10. Stratakis CA et al: The triad of paragangliomas, gastric stromal tumours and pulmonary chondromas (Carney triad), and the dyad of paragangliomas and gastric stromal sarcomas (Carney-Stratakis syndrome): molecular genetics and clinical implications. J Intern Med. 266(1):43-52, 2009
11. Antonescu CR: Targeted therapies in gastrointestinal stromal tumors. Semin Diagn Pathol. 25(4):295-303, 2008
12. Espinosa I et al: A novel monoclonal antibody against DOG1 is a sensitive and specific marker for gastrointestinal stromal tumors. Am J Surg Pathol. 32(2):210-8, 2008
13. Guler ML et al: Expression of melanoma antigens in epithelioid gastrointestinal stromal tumors: a potential diagnostic pitfall. Arch Pathol Lab Med. 132(8):1302-6, 2008
14. Heinrich MC et al: Primary and secondary kinase genotypes correlate with the biological and clinical activity of sunitinib in imatinib-resistant gastrointestinal stromal tumor. J Clin Oncol. 26(33):5352-9, 2008
15. Lasota J et al: Clinical significance of oncogenic KIT and PDGFRA mutations in gastrointestinal stromal tumours. Histopathology. 53(3):245-66, 2008
16. Miettinen M et al: Gastrointestinal stromal tumors in patients with neurofibromatosis 1: a clinicopathologic and molecular genetic study of 45 cases. Am J Surg Pathol. 30(1):90-6, 2006
17. Miettinen M et al: Gastrointestinal stromal tumors: review on morphology, molecular pathology, prognosis, and differential diagnosis. Arch Pathol Lab Med. 130(10):1466-78, 2006
18. Andersson J et al: NF1-associated gastrointestinal stromal tumors have unique clinical, phenotypic, and genotypic characteristics. Am J Surg Pathol. 29(9):1170-6, 2005
19. Miettinen M et al: Gastrointestinal stromal tumors of the stomach in children and young adults: a clinicopathologic, immunohistochemical, and molecular genetic study of 44 cases with long-term follow-up and review of the literature. Am J Surg Pathol. 29(10):1373-81, 2005
20. Miettinen M et al: Gastrointestinal stromal tumors of the stomach: a clinicopathologic, immunohistochemical, and molecular genetic study of 1765 cases with long-term follow-up. Am J Surg Pathol. 29(1):52-68, 2005
21. Tran T et al: The epidemiology of malignant gastrointestinal stromal tumors: an analysis of 1,458 cases from 1992 to 2000. Am J Gastroenterol. 100(1):162-8, 2005

Clinical Prognostication for GISTs From Largest Series (Untreated With Imatinib)

Size	Mitoses/50 HPF	Metastases	Risk
Gastric GISTs			
≤ 2 cm	≤ 5	None	None to negligible
> 2 and ≤ 5 cm	≤ 5	2%	Low
> 5 and ≤ 10 cm	≤ 5	4%	Low
> 10 cm	≤ 5	12%	Intermediate
≤ 2 cm	> 5	None	Low
> 2 and ≤ 5 cm	> 5	16%	Intermediate
> 5 and ≤ 10 cm	> 5	55%	High
> 10 cm	> 5	88%	High
Small Bowel GISTs			
≤ 2 cm	≤ 5	None	None to negligible
> 2 and ≤ 5 cm	≤ 5	4%	Low
> 5 and ≤ 10 cm	≤ 5	24%	Intermediate
> 10 cm	≤ 5	52%	High
≤ 2 cm	> 5	50%	High
> 2 and ≤ 5 cm	> 5	73%	High
> 5 and ≤10 cm	> 5	85%	High
> 10 cm	> 5	90%	High

Molecular Prognostication for GISTs

Mutation	Site	Prognosis	Likelihood of Response to Treatment
KIT exon 9	Typical of small bowel GISTs	Not a prognostic marker	Poor response to imatinib, improved by high-dose treatment; sunitinib malate (SU11248) can be used
KIT exon 11 deletions and substitutions	Found in all sites	May indicate poor prognosis	Complete remission (6%), partial response (61%), stable disease (25%), progressive disease (3%)
KIT exon 11 duplications	Gastric	May indicate improved prognosis	Complete remission (6%), partial response (61%), stable disease (25%), progressive disease (3%)
KIT exon 13 mutations	All sites	May indicate poor prognosis in gastric GISTs	Partial response, all cases (rare)
KIT exon 17 mutations	Small bowel	No prognostic significance	Variable, depending on specific mutation
PDGFRA exon 12 deletions and substitutions	Gastric	May indicate good prognosis	Most respond to imatinib
PDGFRA exon 14 substitutions	Gastric	May indicate good prognosis	No data available
PDGFRA exon 18 deletions and substitutions	Gastric	May indicate good prognosis	Variable and mutation specific
KIT and *PDGFRA* wild type	Typical of NF1 and Carney triad tumors	No prognostic significance	Partial response (23%), stable disease (50%), progressive disease (19%)

Microscopic Features

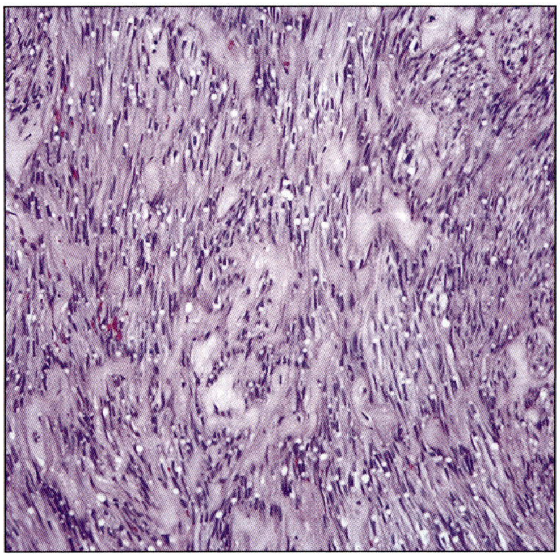
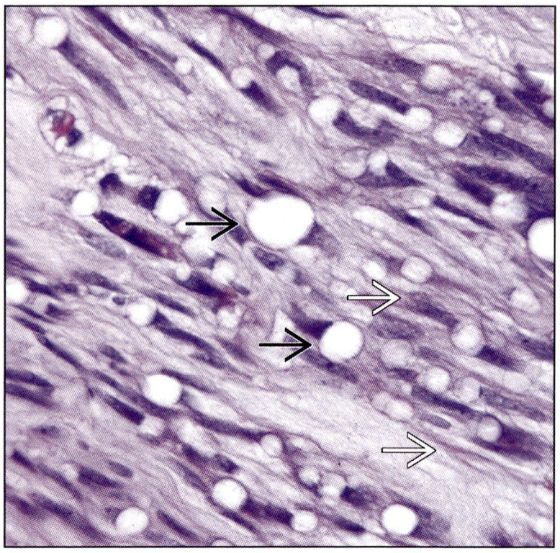

*(**Left**) Hematoxylin & eosin shows a spindle cell gastric GIST. Even at this low magnification, paranuclear vacuoles, usually associated with benign behavior, are numerous. (**Right**) Hematoxylin & eosin shows a high-power view of the previous image. In addition to prominent paranuclear vacuoles ⇨, note the brightly eosinophilic fibrillary cytoplasm ➡; both are reminiscent of smooth muscle differentiation. Such features led early pathologists to regard GISTs as smooth muscle neoplasms.*

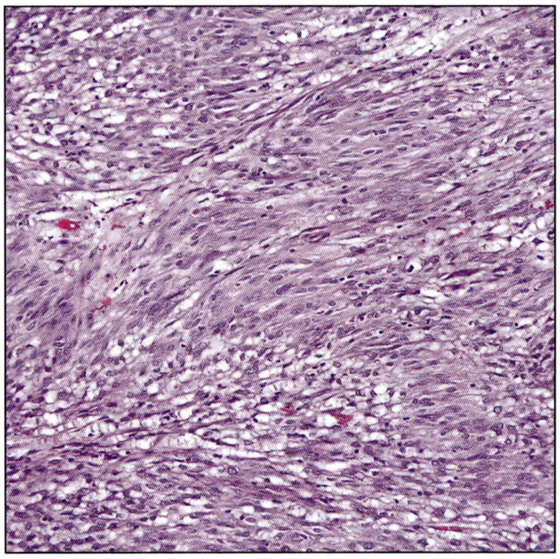
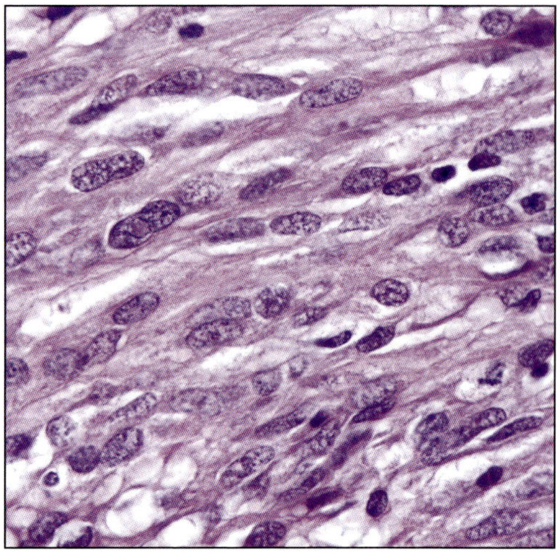

*(**Left**) Hematoxylin & eosin shows a spindle cell gastric GIST with enhanced cellularity in comparison to the previous lesion. Such appearances are often associated with an unfavorable outcome. (**Right**) Hematoxylin & eosin shows higher magnification of the same neoplasm. The lesional cells are very uniform, a feature of tumors associated with characteristic mutations.*

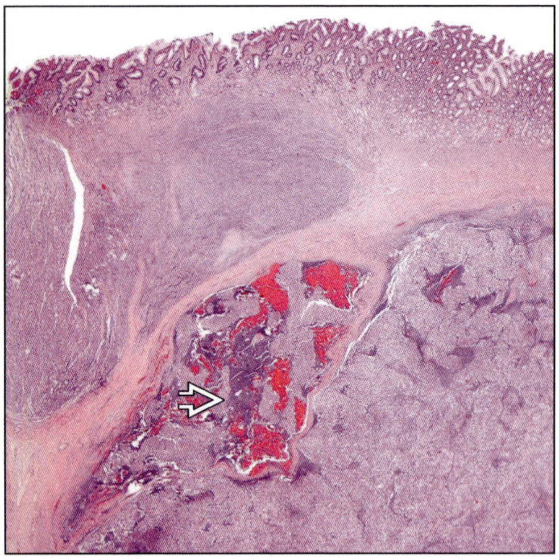
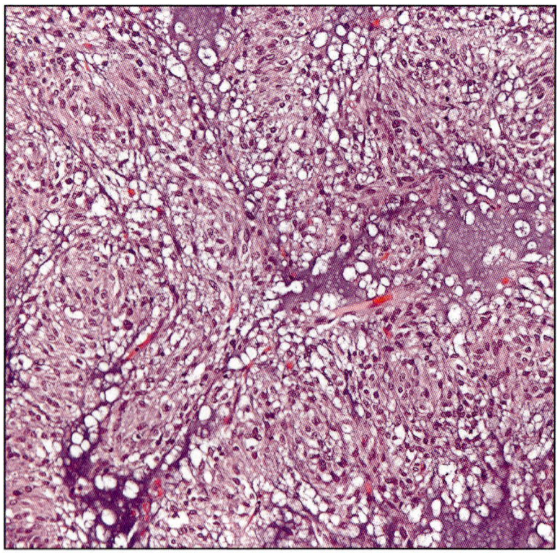

*(**Left**) Hematoxylin & eosin shows an epithelioid gastric GIST. It has a lobulated appearance with chondroid areas ➡. (**Right**) Hematoxylin & eosin shows an epithelioid GIST at intermediate magnification. There is a chondroid background, and the tumor cells have numerous cytoplasmic vacuoles. Epithelioid gastric GISTs such as this may be CD117 negative and have PDGFRA mutations.*

Microscopic and Gross Features

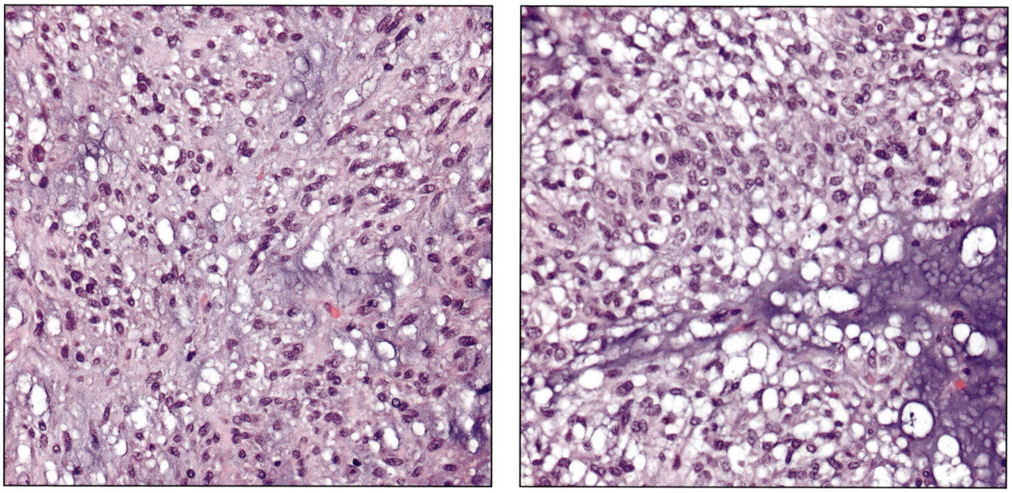

(Left) *Hematoxylin & eosin shows an epithelioid gastric GIST. This tumor has uniform epithelioid tumor cells with prominent vacuoles. There is minimal nuclear overlap. Patients whose tumors have such features typically have a favorable outcome.* ***(Right)*** *Hematoxylin & eosin shows the cytologic features of an epithelioid gastric GIST. The nuclei are uniform, and there is a chondromyxoid background.*

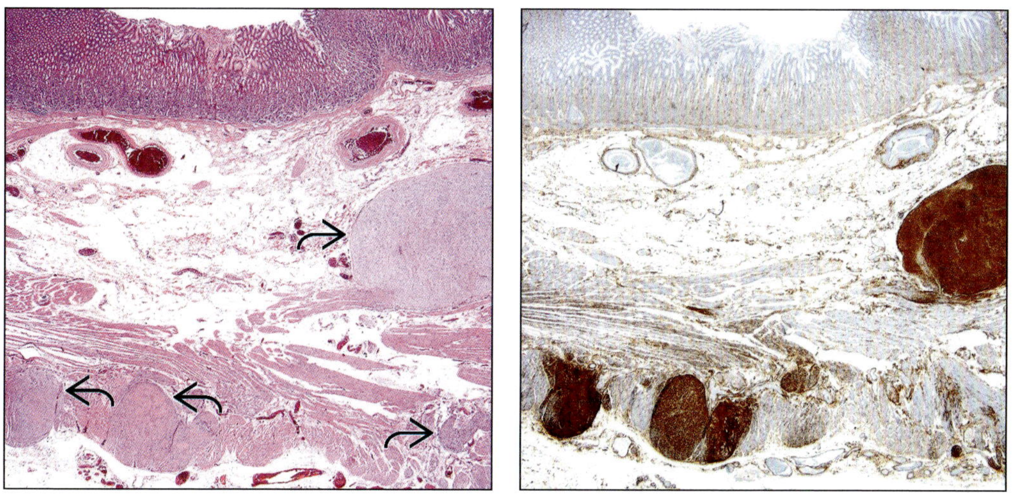

(Left) *Hematoxylin & eosin shows several tiny ("seedling") GISTs ➢ near the gastroesophageal junction. These were found incidentally in a resection performed for a separate gastric carcinoma.* ***(Right)*** *CD34 shows prominent staining in the small GISTs in the same patient. Such incidental tumors are common (~ 10% of esophagectomy samples contain them); since clinically evident GISTs are rare, few of these "seedling" lesions seem to progress.*

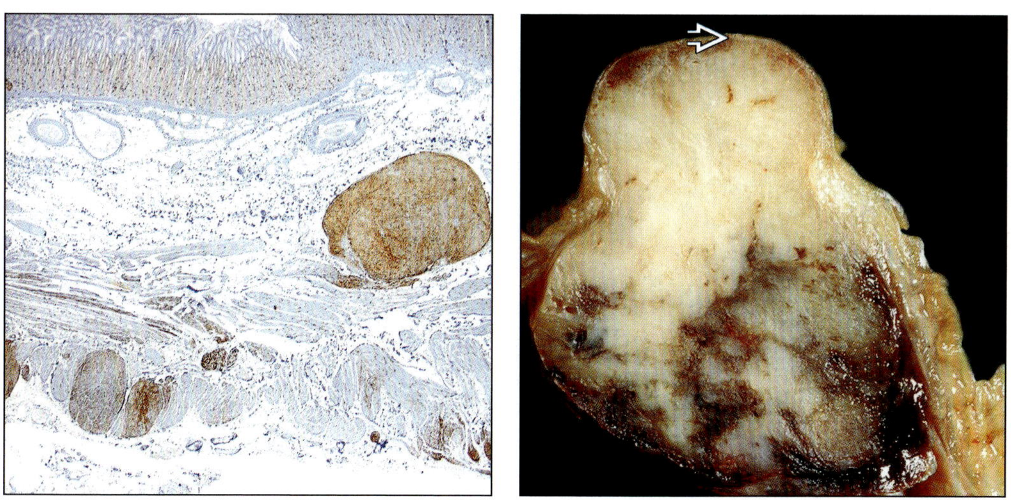

(Left) *CD117 shows labeling in "seedling" GISTs.* ***(Right)*** *Gross photograph shows a small intestinal GIST. The bulk of the tumor is in the muscularis propria, but the lesion has extended into the submucosa and was diagnosed by mucosal biopsy. Note the overlying mucosa ➡, which is eroded in places.*

GASTROINTESTINAL STROMAL TUMOR

Microscopic Features

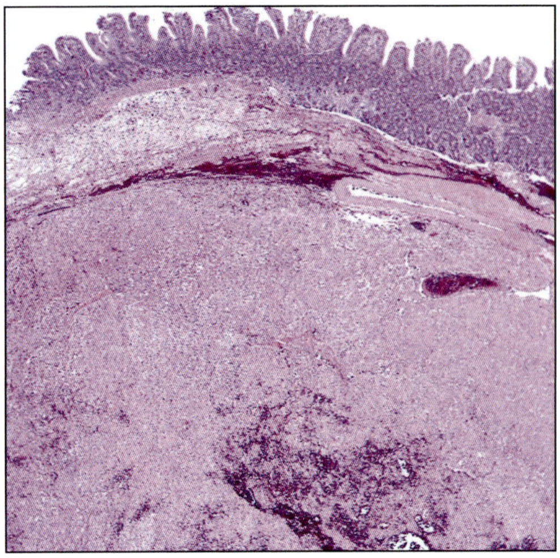
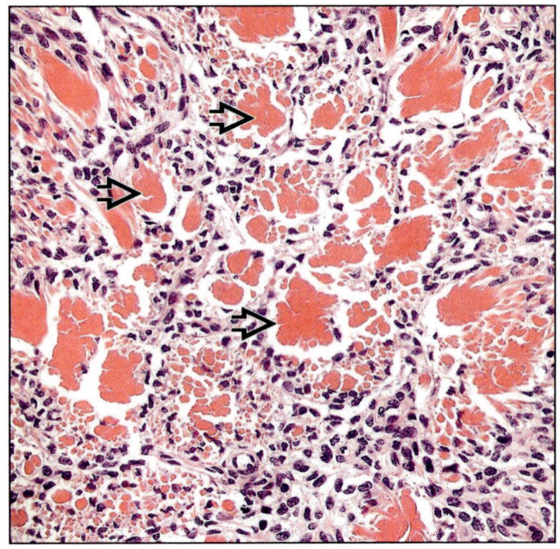

(Left) *Hematoxylin & eosin shows a small intestinal GIST at low magnification. The lesion has extended into the submucosa, and the overlying mucosa appears inflamed.* ***(Right)*** *Hematoxylin & eosin shows prominent "skeinoid" fibers ⇨ in a small intestinal GIST. These are principally found in small bowel GISTs, where they are associated with a favorable outcome.*

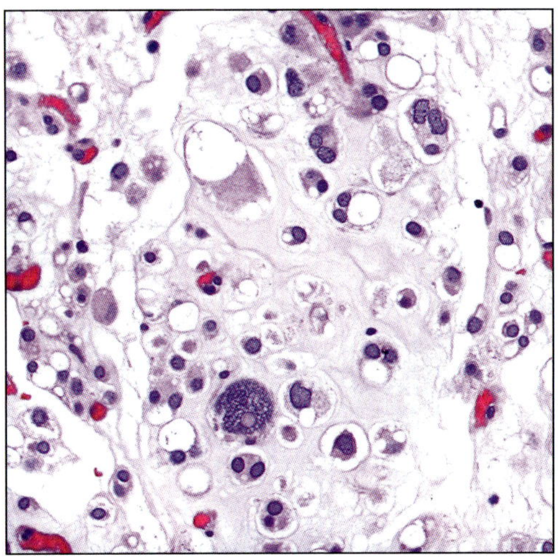
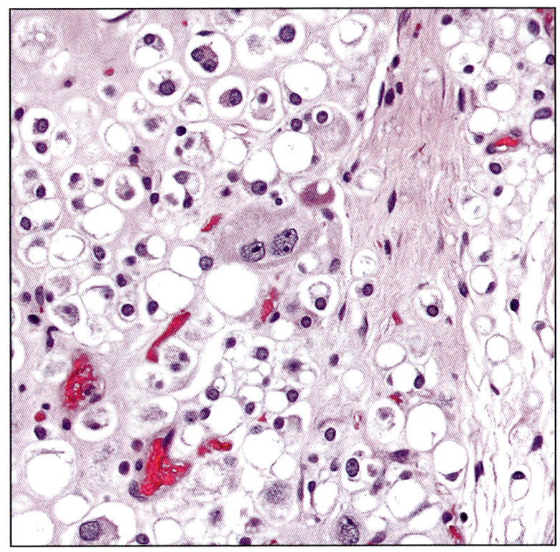

(Left) *Hematoxylin & eosin shows nuclear pleomorphism in an extraintestinal epithelioid GIST. Nuclear pleomorphism is unusual in GISTs, and its presence should prompt other diagnostic considerations.* ***(Right)*** *Hematoxylin & eosin shows striking cytoplasmic vacuoles in an extraintestinal epithelioid GIST. Cases such as this should be addressed as diagnoses of exclusion with an appropriate immunolabeling panel.*

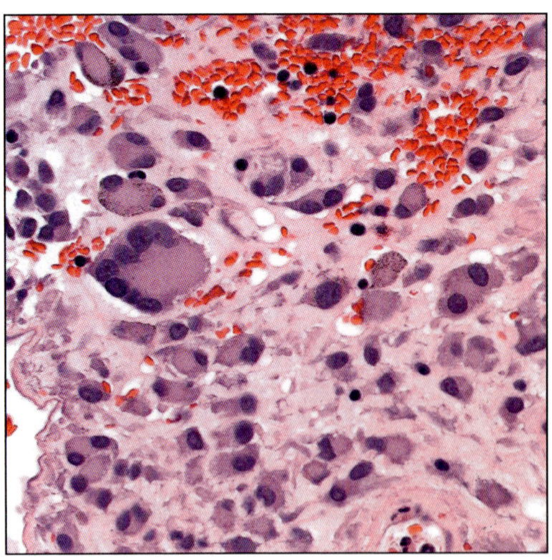
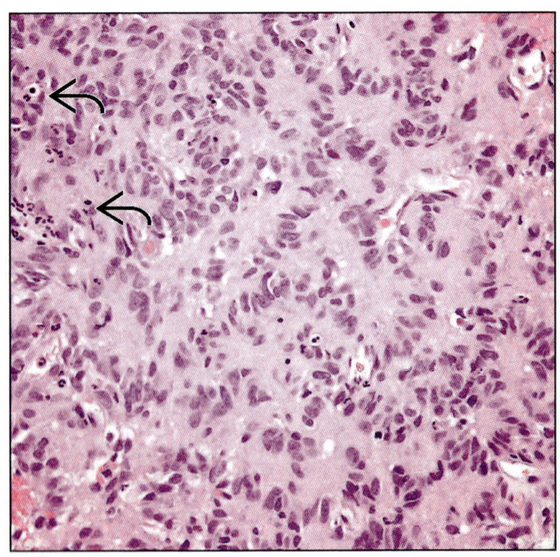

(Left) *Hematoxylin & eosin shows peculiar tumor giant cells and plasmacytoid features in a GIST, a variant pattern. Note that the background cells have rhabdoid appearances.* ***(Right)*** *Hematoxylin & eosin shows a palisaded pattern in a small intestinal GIST. This lesion displayed foci of individual tumor cell necrosis ↗. The patient presented with liver metastases. This lesion proved lethal, as is the case in ~ 40% of small bowel GISTs.*

Microscopic Features

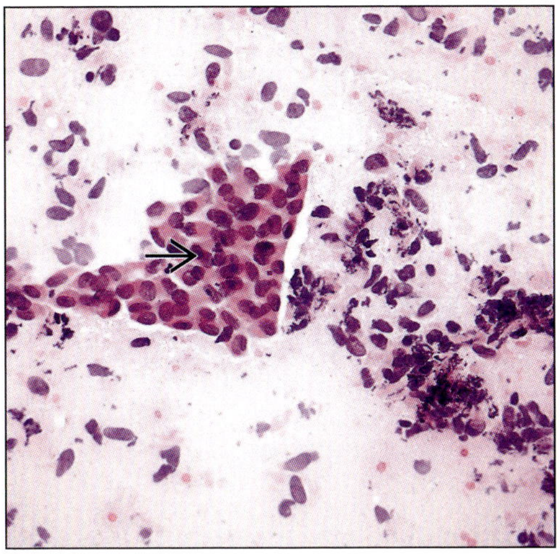

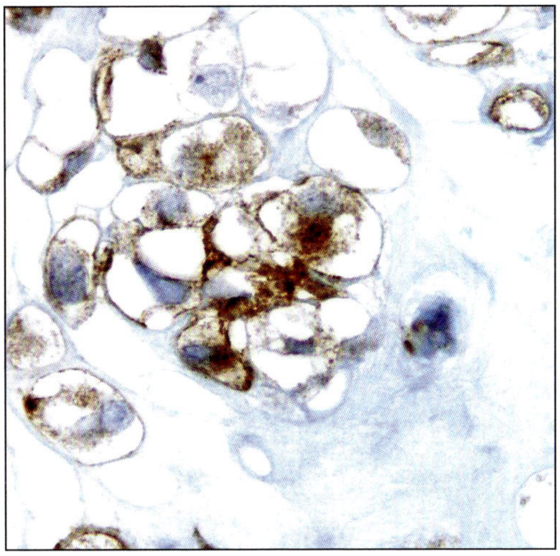

(Left) *Hematoxylin & eosin shows a smear prepared from an aspiration biopsy specimen of a malignant gastric GIST. There is a fragment of gastric mucosa* ⇒*. The lesional cells do not have diagnostic features; the diagnosis was made by performing immunohistochemistry on cell block material in this case.* ***(Right)*** *CD117 shows both Golgi zone and membranous labeling in this extraintestinal epithelioid GIST.*

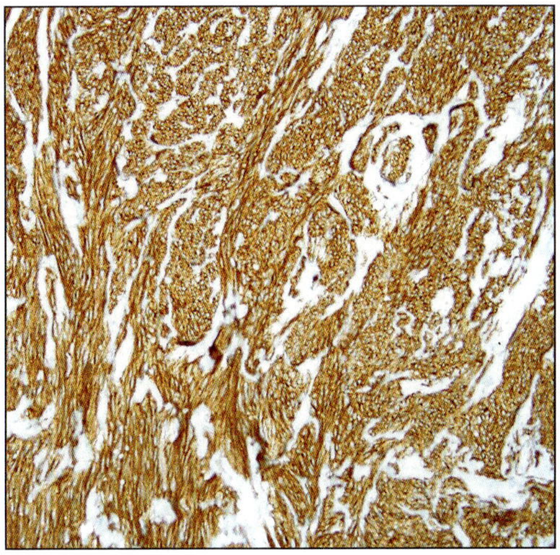

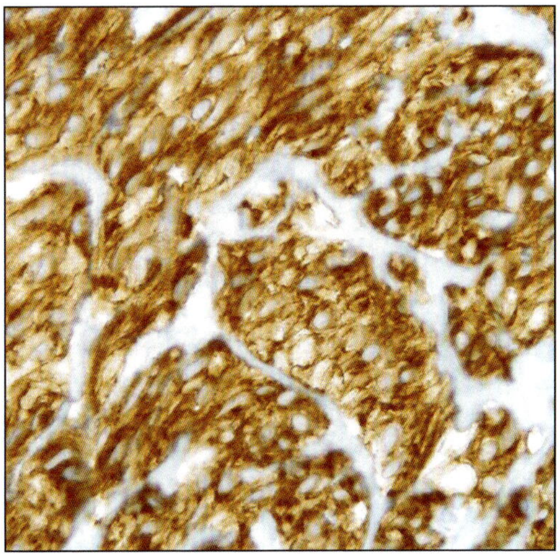

(Left) *CD117 shows strong diffuse labeling in a gastric spindle cell GIST. This is the usual strong staining seen in the majority of such neoplasms. However, similar CD117 expression can be encountered in other tumors.* ***(Right)*** *CD117 shows a higher magnification view of membranous and cytoplasmic labeling in a gastric spindle cell GIST.*

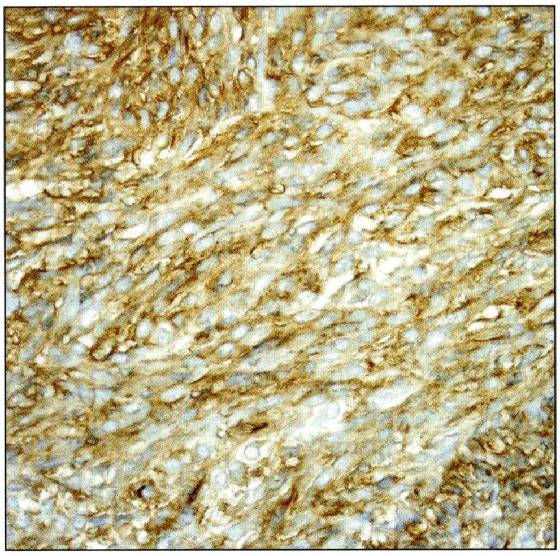

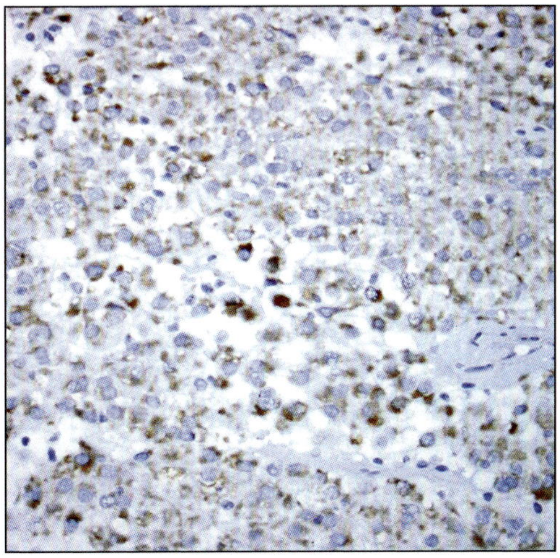

(Left) *CD34 shows cytoplasmic labeling in a gastric spindle cell GIST. Approximately 80% of gastric GISTs express CD34, more than those of the small bowel (~ 60%).* ***(Right)*** *MART-1 shows aberrant labeling in an epithelioid gastric GIST, a common finding that should not be misinterpreted as melanoma. Of course, melanomas can express CD117, so caution must be used in interpreting immunolabeling patterns.*

HAMARTOMATOUS POLYPS OF GI TRACT

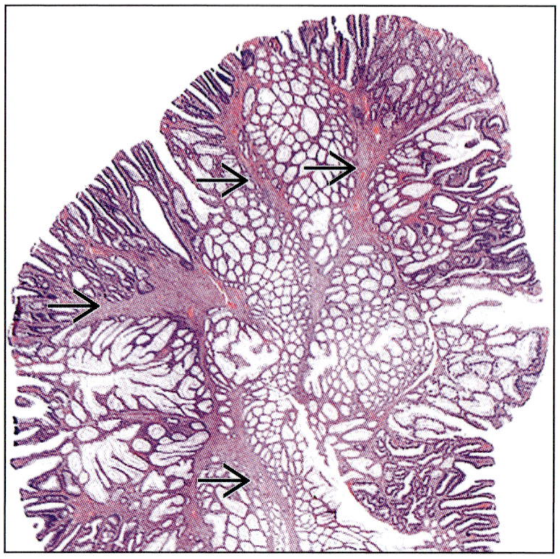

Low-power view of a Peutz-Jeghers polyp shows arborizing smooth muscle bundles →.

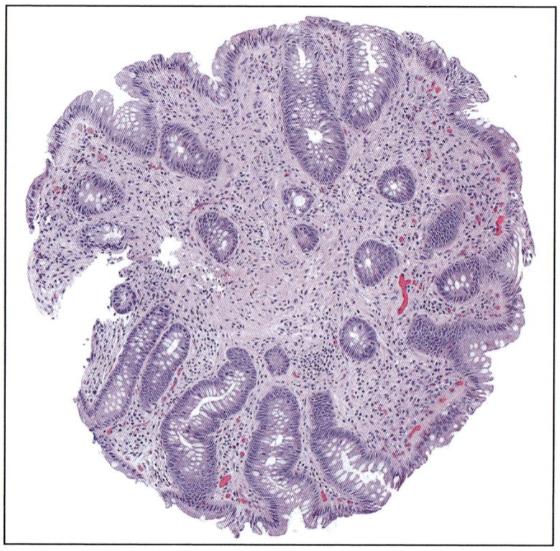

H&E shows a small nondistinctive-appearing hamartomatous polyp from a patient with Cowden syndrome. These polyps often look like healed pseudopolyps or mucosal prolapse-type polyps.

TERMINOLOGY

Definitions

- Nonneoplastic tumor that contains disorganized normal tissues

CLINICAL ISSUES

Presentation

- Hamartomatous polyps may present with hematochezia, anemia, diarrhea, prolapse, abdominal pain, obstruction, or intussusception

MICROSCOPIC PATHOLOGY

Histologic Features

- Cowden/PTEN-hamartoma syndrome polyps
  - Polyps may be numerous; typically small and histologically indistinct
  - Colonic polyps may just look like focal crypt distortion or healed inflammatory pseudopolyps
  - Ganglioneuromas may be seen as well as adenomas
  - Some polyps may resemble juvenile polyps
    - Older literature on juvenile polyps mentions ganglioneuromas, but these likely represented misdiagnosed cases of Cowden/PTEN-hamartoma syndrome
  - May have glycogenic acanthosis in the esophagus
- Juvenile polyps (JP)
  - Polyps may be in stomach, small bowel, and colon
    - Must have > 5 JP in the colon to diagnose syndrome unless positive family history or patient has 1 polyp outside of colon
    - May have isolated colonic JP and not have the syndrome
  - Eroded or ulcerated surface with expanded lamina propria
    - Large pedunculated polyps may have secondary prolapse change that may mimic Peutz-Jeghers polyps (PJP)
  - Cystically dilated glands are histologic hallmark, but often not present in small polyps
  - May have dysplasia or carcinoma arising within polyp
- PJP
  - Polyps can be found in stomach, small bowel, and colon
    - Syndrome can be diagnosed with 2 PJP, but increased cancer risk found in patients with only a single PJP
  - Polyps have arborizing bands of smooth muscle
    - Epithelium is nonneoplastic and has a lobular arrangement around muscle bundles
    - Epithelium may be misplaced within muscle, mimicking invasive carcinoma
  - Small bowel polyps most likely to have characteristic histology
  - Dysplasia is not usually found in PJP
    - Carcinoma thought to arise via a different mechanism (expanded stem cell compartment in nonpolypoid mucosa)

DIFFERENTIAL DIAGNOSIS

Inflammatory Pseudopolyps

- May be indistinguishable from small juvenile polyps (JP)
  - Both may have eroded surface mucosa with hypercellular lamina propria
  - Small JP may not have the cystically dilated glands that are relied on to make diagnosis
- Healed inflammatory polyps are often identical to Cowden polyps (CP)
  - Without appropriate history, CP are extremely difficult to diagnose correctly

HAMARTOMATOUS POLYPS OF GI TRACT

Key Facts

Terminology
- Nonneoplastic tumor that contains disorganized normal tissues

Clinical Issues
- May present with hematochezia, anemia, diarrhea, prolapse, abdominal pain, obstruction, or intussusception

Top Differential Diagnoses
- Inflammatory pseudopolyps may be indistinguishable from small juvenile polyps (JP)
- Healed inflammatory polyps are often identical to CP
- Prominent smooth muscle proliferation of prolapse can mimic a PJP
- Reactive atypia in hamartomatous polyps may mimic adenoma/dysplasia, especially in JP

Polypoid Prolapsing Mucosal Folds (Prolapse-Type Polyps)
- These benign mucosal polyps are often seen at mouth of diverticulum
- Prominent smooth muscle proliferation of prolapse can mimic a PJP
  - May only be able to exclude PJP based on location at mouth of diverticulum
  - Presences of arborizing smooth muscle favors PJP, but may not be present in very small polyps
- Other prolapse phenomena may also mimic PJP

Hyperplastic Polyps (Gastric)
- Based on histology, gastric JP and PJP cannot reliably be differentiated from hyperplastic polyps

Adenoma/Dysplasia
- Reactive atypia in hamartomatous polyps may mimic adenoma/dysplasia, especially in JP
  - JP may have true dysplasia
    - This can be a tricky diagnosis when lesion is eroded/ulcerated

Invasive Adenocarcinoma
- Epithelial misplacement in PJP can mimic invasive adenocarcinoma
  - Misplacement typically lacks desmoplastic stroma

SELECTED REFERENCES

1. Stojcev Z et al: Hamartomatous polyposis syndromes. Hered Cancer Clin Pract. 11(1):4, 2013
2. Latchford AR et al: Juvenile polyposis syndrome: a study of genotype, phenotype, and long-term outcome. Dis Colon Rectum. 55(10):1038-43, 2012
3. Patel SG et al: Familial colon cancer syndromes: an update of a rapidly evolving field. Curr Gastroenterol Rep. 14(5):428-38, 2012
4. Trufant JW et al: Colonic ganglioneuromatous polyposis and metastatic adenocarcinoma in the setting of Cowden syndrome: a case report and literature review. Hum Pathol. 43(4):601-4, 2012
5. Arber N et al: Small bowel polyposis syndromes. Curr Gastroenterol Rep. 13(5):435-41, 2011
6. Latchford AR et al: Gastrointestinal polyps and cancer in Peutz-Jeghers syndrome: clinical aspects. Fam Cancer. 10(3):455-61, 2011
7. van Lier MG et al: High cancer risk and increased mortality in patients with Peutz-Jeghers syndrome. Gut. 60(2):141-7, 2011
8. Lam-Himlin D et al: Morphologic characterization of syndromic gastric polyps. Am J Surg Pathol. 34(11):1656-62, 2010
9. Chen HM et al: Genetics of the hamartomatous polyposis syndromes: a molecular review. Int J Colorectal Dis. 24(8):865-74, 2009
10. Zbuk KM et al: Hamartomatous polyposis syndromes. Nat Clin Pract Gastroenterol Hepatol. 4(9):492-502, 2007

IMAGE GALLERY

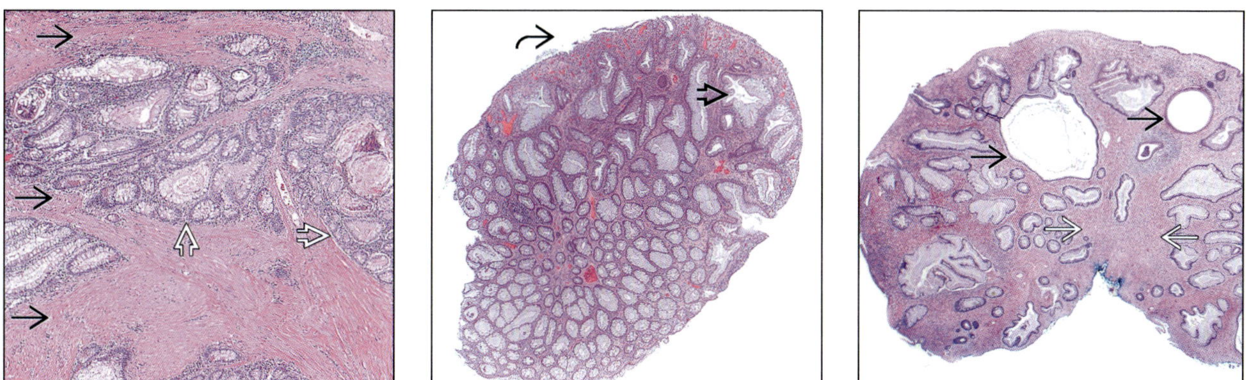

(Left) This hamartomatous polyp has abundant smooth muscle bundles → surrounding benign mucosal islands ⇨. These features are characteristic of Peutz-Jeghers polyps. (Center) This small hamartomatous polyp has an ulcerated surface ↷ with benign dilated glands ⇨ typical of a juvenile polyp. Identical findings could be seen in an inflammatory pseudopolyp. (Right) H&E shows a large juvenile polyp with cystically dilated glands → and an expanded lamina propria ⇨.

SMALL BOWEL ADENOCARCINOMA

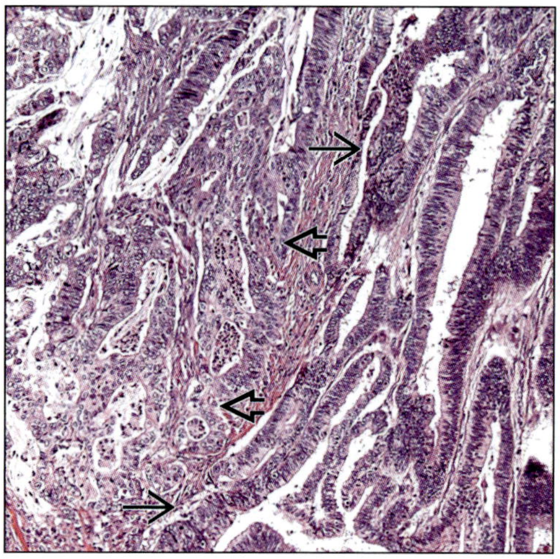

Hematoxylin & eosin shows an adenoma → on the right and an invasive adenocarcinoma ⇨ on the left. Note the presence of a more complex architecture and desmoplastic stroma on the left.

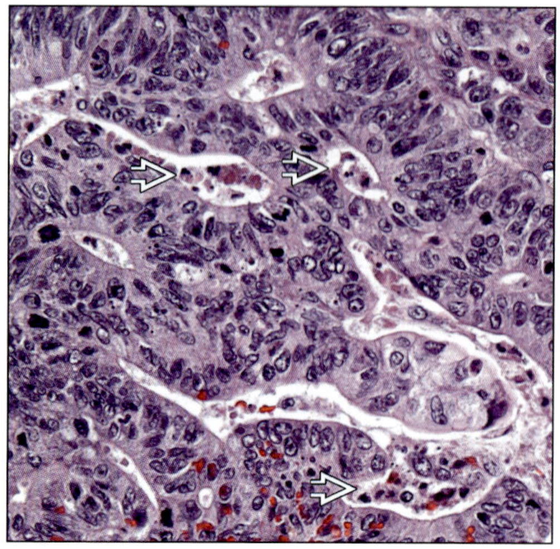

Hematoxylin & eosin shows a high-power view of adenocarcinoma. The overall appearance is very similar to colorectal carcinoma. Note the dirty necrosis ➡.

TERMINOLOGY

Definitions

- Invasive adenocarcinoma arising in small intestine

ETIOLOGY/PATHOGENESIS

Risk Factors

- Crohn disease
- Celiac disease
  - Relative risk ↑ 10-80x
- Polyposis syndromes
  - **Familial adenomatous polyposis (FAP)**
    - Germline mutation in *APC* gene
    - Duodenal and ampullary adenomas
    - Duodenal adenocarcinomas
  - **Lynch syndrome**
    - Most common heritable cause of cancer
    - Small bowel and ampullary carcinomas
  - **Peutz-Jeghers syndrome**
    - Hamartomatous polyposis
    - Small bowel adenocarcinoma cumulative risk: 13%
  - **Neurofibromatosis type 1**
- Uncommon primary tumor, so pathologist should look for 1 of the above mentioned syndromes/diseases when encountered

Molecular Genetic Alterations

- In contrast to colorectal cancer, mutations in *APC* gene are not present
- Mutations in *TP53* and *SMAD4*

CLINICAL ISSUES

Epidemiology

- Incidence
  - ~ 2,400 new cases annually in USA
  - Average age-adjusted annual incidence of 3.9:1,000,000 persons
  - 2.4% of GI tract malignancies
  - M:F = 2:1

Site

- Duodenum (55%)
- Jejunum (18%)
- Ileum (13%)
- Not otherwise specified (14%)

Presentation

- Abdominal pain
- Obstruction
- Anemia
- GI bleeding
- Jaundice, cholestatic
  - Ampullary tumors
- Weight loss

Treatment

- Surgical approaches
  - Resection of primary tumor is mainstay of therapy
    - Segmental small bowel resection with wide excision of mesentery
    - Whipple resection for ampullary/duodenal tumors
- Adjuvant therapy
  - Chemotherapy similar to that given for colorectal cancer
    - Mixed results: Number of patients is too small

Prognosis

- Related to stage of disease
  - Overall 5-year survival: 30.5%
  - Median survival: 19.7 months
- Worse prognosis for duodenal tumors compared to rest of small bowel

SMALL BOWEL ADENOCARCINOMA

Key Facts

Etiology/Pathogenesis

- Uncommon primary tumor, so pathologist should look for 1 of the following diagnoses when encountered: **Crohn disease, celiac disease, polyposis syndromes**

Clinical Issues

- Prognosis related to stage of disease
  - Overall 5-year survival: 30.5%
- ~ 2,400 new cases annually in USA
  - Most found in duodenum: 55%

Microscopic Pathology

- Nearly identical to colorectal carcinoma
- Arises from adenomas or dysplasia (Crohn disease)

Top Differential Diagnoses

- Metastatic adenocarcinoma
- Adenoma with high-grade dysplasia
- Ectopic pancreas
- Endometriosis

DIFFERENTIAL DIAGNOSIS

Metastatic Adenocarcinoma

- Presence of preexisting adenoma or dysplasia suggests small bowel primary
- Pancreatic adenocarcinoma can grow out from ampulla and mimic duodenal/ampullary primary
  - May differentiate similarly to adenoma at surface

Adenoma With High-Grade Dysplasia

- Difficult to differentiate prolapse from invasion around ampulla
  - Desmoplasia is key to diagnosis

Ectopic Pancreas

- Small biopsy specimen that shows only ducts may be misinterpreted as neoplasm

Endometriosis

- Presence of characteristic stroma helps make diagnosis
- Look for ciliated epithelium; argues against neoplasm

DIAGNOSTIC CHECKLIST

Pathologic Interpretation Pearls

- Always look for preexisting conditions/risk factors, such as Crohn disease or polyposis

SELECTED REFERENCES

1. Aparicio T et al: Small bowel adenocarcinoma: Epidemiology, risk factors, diagnosis and treatment. Dig Liver Dis. Epub ahead of print, 2013
2. Chang DK et al: Histomolecular phenotypes and outcome in adenocarcinoma of the ampulla of vater. J Clin Oncol. 31(10):1348-56, 2013
3. Genta RM et al: Advanced precancerous lesions in the small bowel mucosa. Best Pract Res Clin Gastroenterol. 27(2):225-33, 2013
4. Lee HJ et al: Combined loss of E-cadherin and aberrant β-catenin protein expression correlates with a poor prognosis for small intestinal adenocarcinomas. Am J Clin Pathol. 139(2):167-76, 2013
5. Raghav K et al: Small bowel adenocarcinomas-existing evidence and evolving paradigms. Nat Rev Clin Oncol. 10(9):534-44, 2013
6. Wangler MF et al: Unusually early presentation of small-bowel adenocarcinoma in a patient with Peutz-Jeghers syndrome. J Pediatr Hematol Oncol. 35(4):323-8, 2013
7. Hong SH et al: Primary adenocarcinoma of the small intestine: presentation, prognostic factors and clinical outcome. Jpn J Clin Oncol. 39(1):54-61, 2009
8. Hwangbo S et al: Two separated ileal adenocarcinomas in neurofibromatosis type 1. Yonsei Med J. 48(6):1039-42, 2007
9. Green PH et al: Celiac disease and other precursors to small-bowel malignancy. Gastroenterol Clin North Am. 31(2):625-39, 2002
10. Wheeler JM et al: An insight into the genetic pathway of adenocarcinoma of the small intestine. Gut. 50(2):218-23, 2002

IMAGE GALLERY

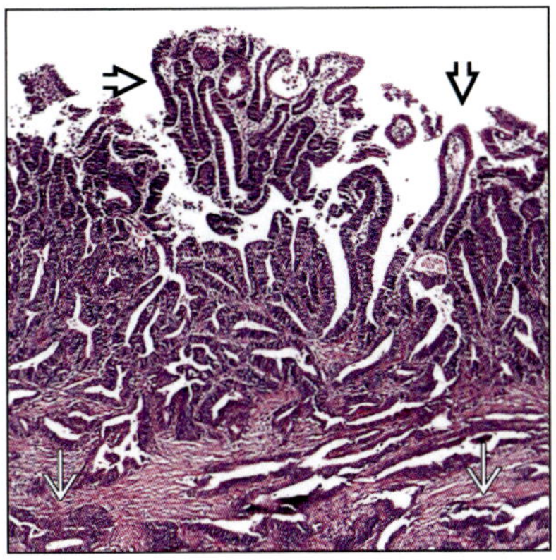

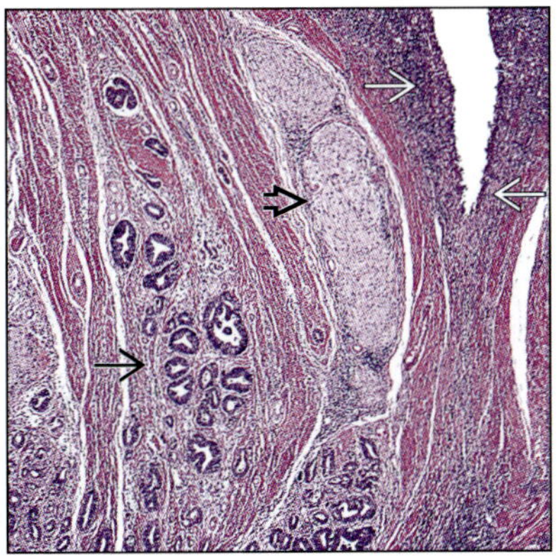

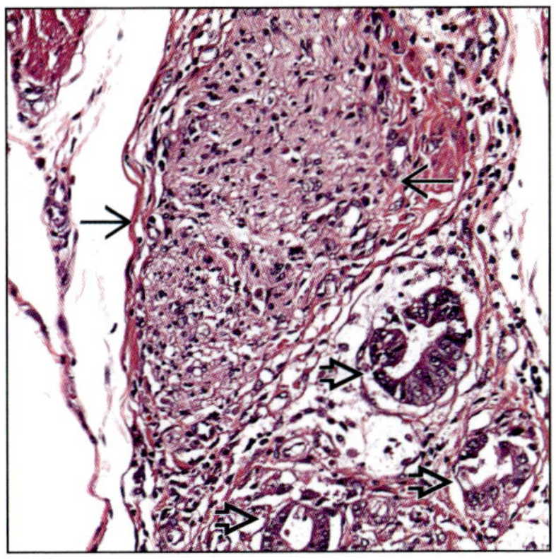

(Left) *Hematoxylin & eosin shows villiform high-grade dysplasia on the surface with invasive adenocarcinoma beneath. This small bowel carcinoma arose in the setting of Crohn disease and dysplasia.* ***(Center)*** *Hematoxylin & eosin shows a low-power view of invasive carcinoma arising in Crohn disease. Note the hypertrophic nerve trunk and fistula tract.* ***(Right)*** *Hematoxylin & eosin shows a higher power view of the hypertrophic nerve and an invasive carcinoma.*

AMPULLARY ADENOCARCINOMA

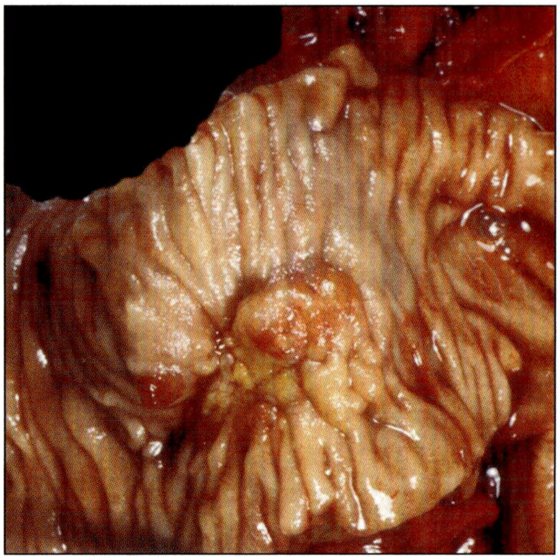

From the luminal aspect of this resection specimen, the ampulla is replaced by a protruding tumor grossly involving the duodenal mucosa of the papilla and periampullary duodenum.

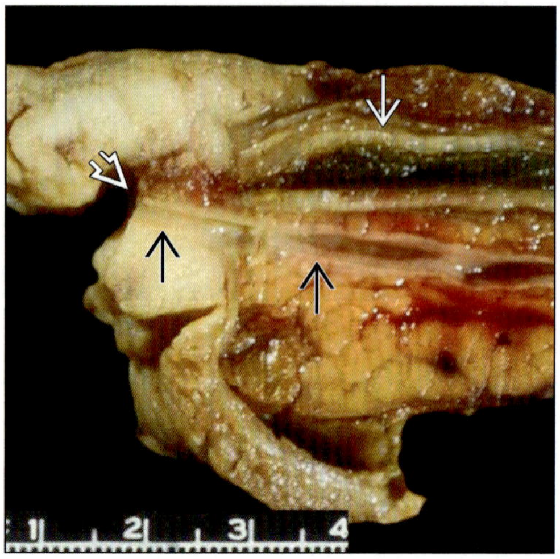

This ampullary adenocarcinoma consists of an exophytic white tumor involving the orifice ➡ of the common bile duct ➡ but not invading the pancreatic duct ⇒.

TERMINOLOGY

Synonyms

- Periampullary adenocarcinoma

Definitions

- Adenocarcinoma arising in ampullary region and periampullary duodenal adenocarcinoma are collectively termed ampullary adenocarcinoma
  - ~ 90% of all carcinomas of region

ETIOLOGY/PATHOGENESIS

Genetics

- Familial adenomatous polyposis
  - Biliary tract adenocarcinoma and dysplasia

CLINICAL ISSUES

Epidemiology

- Incidence
  - Relatively uncommon
    - ~ 0.2% of GI tract malignancies
    - Ampulla is most common site of small bowel adenocarcinoma
- Age
  - Most common in 7th-8th decades of life
  - Patients with familial adenomatous polyposis develop ampullary carcinoma at younger age than patients with sporadic cases
- Gender
  - Slightly more common in men (M:F = 1.48:1)

Presentation

- Jaundice
- Weight loss
- Abdominal pain
- Distended, palpable gallbladder (Courvoisier sign)

Treatment

- Resection (Whipple procedure)
  - Resectability is ~ 60%
- Role of adjuvant chemoradiation therapy (5-FU based) is controversial

Prognosis

- 5-year survival rate after surgical resection is ~ 50%
  - Significantly better than that of pancreatic adenocarcinoma
  - Comparable to that of duodenal adenocarcinoma

MACROSCOPIC FEATURES

General Features

- Variable gross appearance
  - Intraampullary: Arises within ampulla itself
  - Periampullary duodenal: Arises from duodenal mucosa surrounding ampulla
  - Mixed ampullary/duodenal
- Majority arise from preexisting adenomas
- May be exophytic, ulcerated, or mixture of both

Size

- Often small
  - ~ 20% are < 1 cm in diameter, and 75% are < 4 cm

MICROSCOPIC PATHOLOGY

Histologic Features

- Intestinal-type adenocarcinoma
  - Most common type (> 50%)
  - Histologically indistinguishable from tumors of colorectum
- Pancreatobiliary-type adenocarcinoma
  - 2nd most common type
  - Closely resembles primary tumors of pancreas or extrahepatic bile ducts

AMPULLARY ADENOCARCINOMA

Key Facts

Terminology
- Ampullary adenocarcinoma comprises both adenocarcinomas arising in ampullary region and periampullary duodenal adenocarcinomas

Etiology/Pathogenesis
- Familial adenomatous polyposis
  - Biliary tract adenocarcinoma and dysplasia

Clinical Issues
- 5-year survival rate after surgery is ~ 50%

Macroscopic Features
- Tumors may be intraampullary, periampullary duodenal, mixed exophytic, or mixed ulcerated

Microscopic Pathology
- Intestinal type
- Pancreatobiliary type
- Papillary carcinoma (noninvasive)
- Invasive papillary carcinoma
- Mucinous (colloid) carcinoma
- Adenosquamous carcinoma

Ancillary Tests
- Intestinal type is usually positive for CK20 and CDX2; often negative for CK7
- Pancreatobiliary type is usually positive for CK7; often negative for CK20 and CDX2

Diagnostic Checklist
- Intestinal type of histologic differentiation is associated with favorable outcome in comparison to pancreatobiliary type

---

  - High-grade nuclear pleomorphism in presence of architecturally well-formed glands
  - Desmoplastic stroma
  - Perineural invasion is common
- Papillary carcinoma (noninvasive)
  - Exophytic tumor arising in intraampullary mucosa
  - Resembles similar papillary neoplasms of pancreas or bile ducts
  - Does not invade stroma
- Invasive papillary carcinoma
  - < 10% of ampullary adenocarcinomas
  - Complex, branching papillary structures with fibrovascular cores or micropapillae
    - Diagnosis is based on papillary architecture rather than cytologic appearance
- Mucinous (colloid) carcinoma
  - < 10% of ampullary adenocarcinomas
  - Consists predominantly (> 50%) of extracellular mucin pools with floating carcinoma cells
  - Often associated with adenomatous component
- Adenosquamous carcinoma
  - < 3% of ampullary carcinomas
  - Exhibits both glandular and squamous differentiation
  - Squamous component should be significant (> 25%), but focal glandular differentiation is sufficient for diagnosis
- Other rare histologic types
  - Signet ring cell carcinoma
  - Clear cell carcinoma
  - Adenocarcinoma with hepatoid differentiation

ANCILLARY TESTS

Immunohistochemistry
- CEA and CA19-9 positive
- Intestinal type
  - Positive for CK20 and CDX2; often negative for CK7
- Pancreatobiliary type
  - Positive for CK7; often negative for CK20 and CDX2

DIFFERENTIAL DIAGNOSIS

Distal Bile Duct Carcinoma
- Majority exhibit pancreatobiliary-type histology
- Fusiform growth pattern along bile duct

Pancreatic Adenocarcinoma
- Vast majority exhibit pancreatobiliary-type histology
- Pancreatic adenocarcinoma usually arises from main pancreatic duct; ampullary involvement represents peripheral extension
- No associated ampullary adenoma

DIAGNOSTIC CHECKLIST

Clinically Relevant Pathologic Features
- Important to distinguish ampullary from pancreatic or biliary adenocarcinoma because ampullary adenocarcinomas have better prognosis

Pathologic Interpretation Pearls
- Thorough sampling to rule out invasion is warranted in noninvasive papillary carcinomas

SELECTED REFERENCES

1. Bronsert P et al: Intestinal-type of differentiation predicts favourable overall survival: confirmatory clinicopathological analysis of 198 periampullary adenocarcinomas of pancreatic, biliary, ampullary and duodenal origin. BMC Cancer. 13(1):428, 2013
2. Mantas D et al: FAP related periampullary adenocarcinoma. Int J Surg Case Rep. 4(8):684-6, 2013
3. Adsay V et al: Ampullary region carcinomas: definition and site specific classification with delineation of four clinicopathologically and prognostically distinct subsets in an analysis of 249 cases. Am J Surg Pathol. 36(11):1592-608, 2012
4. Schultz NA et al: Frequencies and prognostic role of KRAS and BRAF mutations in patients with localized pancreatic and ampullary adenocarcinomas. Pancreas. 41(5):759-66, 2012

AMPULLARY ADENOCARCINOMA

Microscopic and Immunohistochemical Features

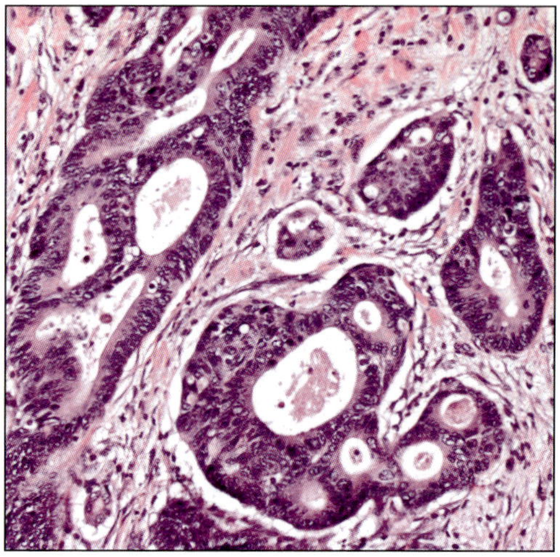
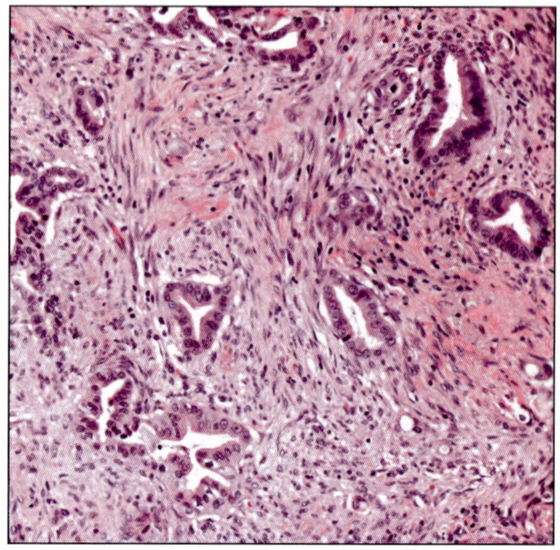

(Left) *In the intestinal type, the tumor consists of columnar cells with stratified, elongated nuclei and a cribriform pattern with luminal necrosis. This type resembles colonic adenocarcinoma.* ***(Right)*** *Pancreatobiliary-type adenocarcinomas consist of well-formed tubules with a single layer of cuboidal to low-columnar cells in a background of prominent desmoplastic stroma.*

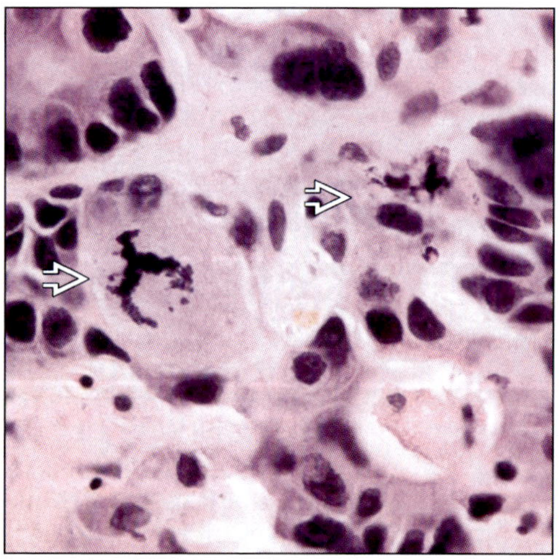
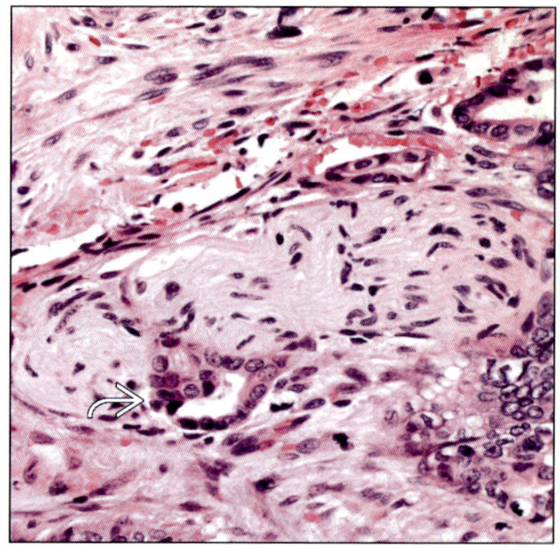

(Left) *Pancreatobiliary-type adenocarcinoma often features nuclear pleomorphism and atypical mitoses within architecturally well-formed glands.* ***(Right)*** *This nerve is partially wrapped by malignant glands. Prominent perineural invasion is a characteristic feature of pancreatobiliary-type ampullary adenocarcinomas.*

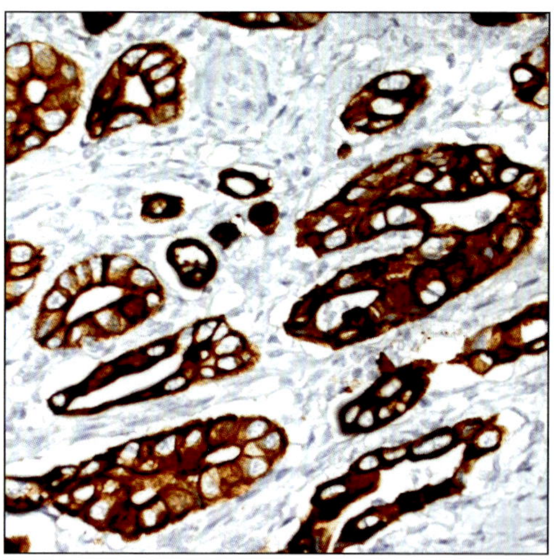
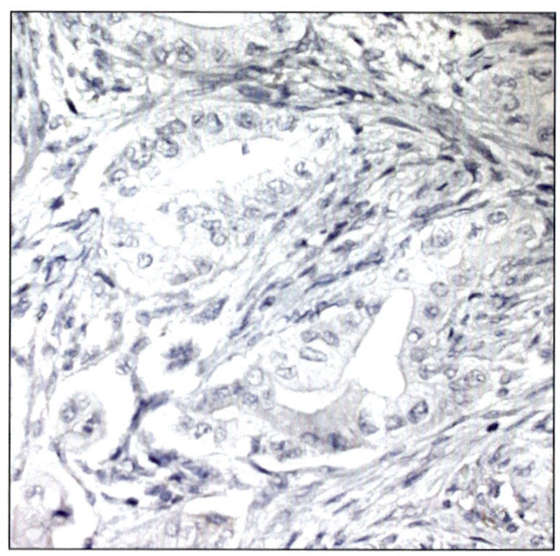

(Left) *This pancreatobiliary-type adenocarcinoma shows infiltrating well-formed glands that strongly express CK7. These tumors also express moderate to intense marking with CEA and CA19-9.* ***(Right)*** *Pancreatobiliary-type ampullary adenocarcinoma demonstrates negative expression of CK20. This type is often negative for CK20 and CDX2. Conversely, intestinal-type adenocarcinoma usually stains positively with CK20 and CDX2 and is negative for CK7.*

Variant Microscopic Features

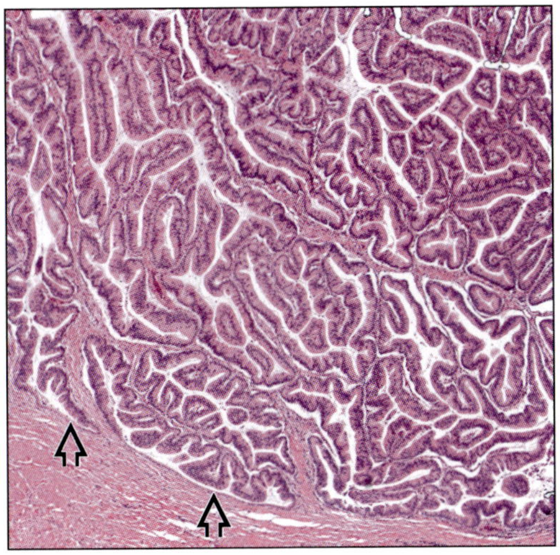

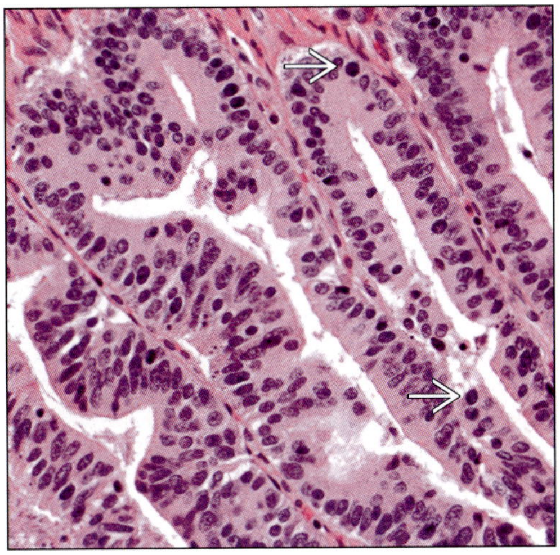

(Left) *Noninvasive papillary carcinomas of the ampulla are exophytic tumors resembling similar papillary neoplasms of the pancreas or bile ducts. They have a pushing border and no submucosal invasion.* ***(Right)*** *In some areas, this noninvasive papillary tumor exhibits enlarged nuclei with nuclear stratification, scattered mitoses, and micropapillary architecture.*

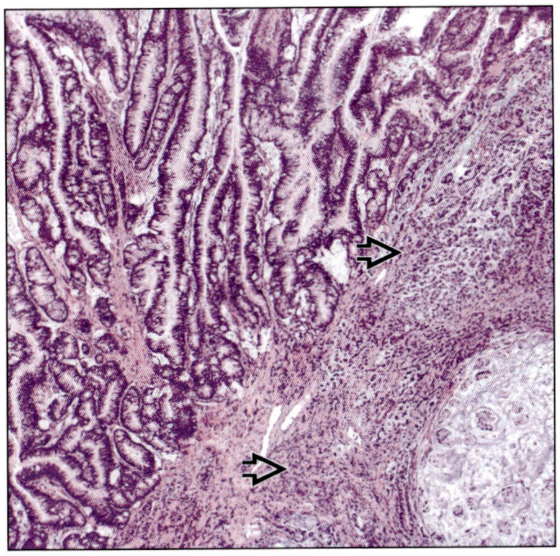

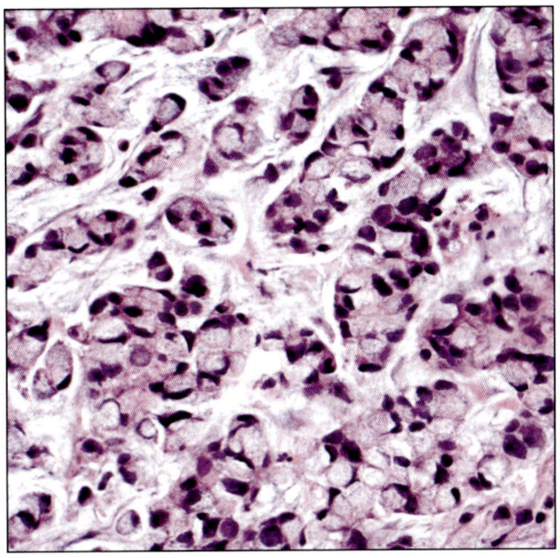

(Left) *This signet ring cell adenocarcinoma is associated with a large tubulovillous adenoma with high-grade dysplasia.* ***(Right)*** *The infiltrating component consists of clusters of single signet ring cells in a background of mucinous or desmoplastic stroma. Although pure signet ring cell carcinoma is rare in the ampulla, the presence of signet ring cells as a minor component is not uncommon.*

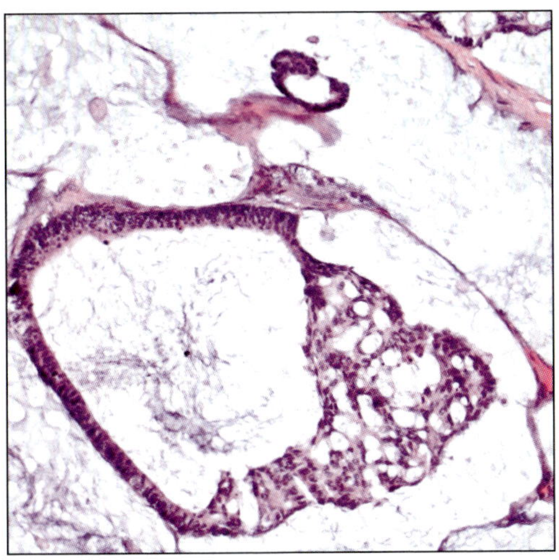

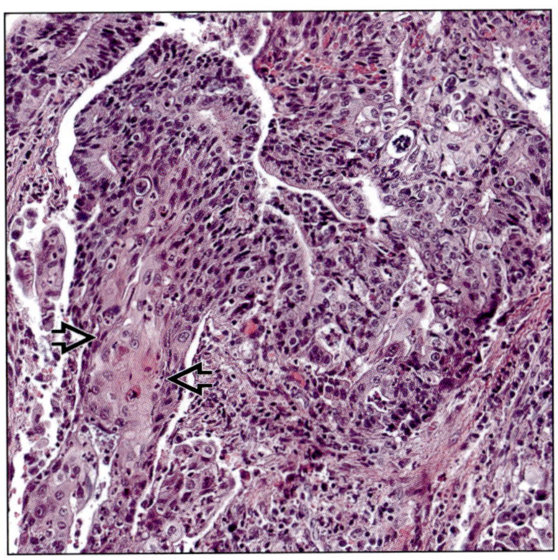

(Left) *This mucinous carcinoma shows a strip of malignant cells and a cluster of malignant cells with a cribriform pattern suspended in extracellular mucin pools.* ***(Right)*** *This adenosquamous carcinoma contains a component of keratinizing squamous cell carcinoma as well as a glandular component. The squamous component should be significant (> 25%) to support the diagnosis of adenosquamous cell carcinoma.*

HEPATOBLASTOMA

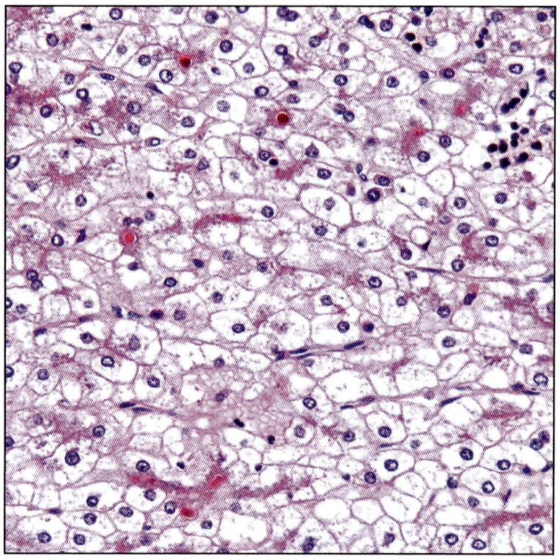

Pure fetal histology consists of uniform polygonal cells that are smaller than normal hepatocytes, have round nuclei, no nucleoli, and clear cytoplasm. This pattern is clinically significant.

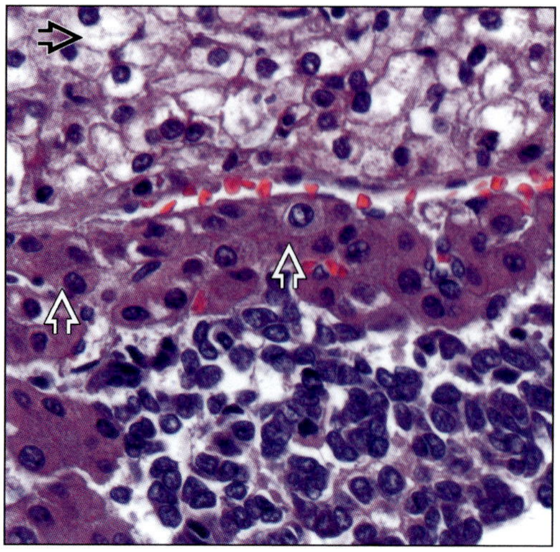

The amount of small undifferentiated cells (bottom right field) should be reported. In contrast, the fetal epithelial cells ➡ above have abundant cytoplasm with variable amounts of glycogen.

TERMINOLOGY

Abbreviations

- Hepatoblastoma (HB)

Definitions

- Predominantly pediatric liver tumor that histologically mimics developing fetal or embryonal liver

ETIOLOGY/PATHOGENESIS

Genetics

- Neoplasm: β-catenin mutation-associated Wnt pathway activation in 70-90%

CLINICAL ISSUES

Epidemiology

- Incidence
  - Constitutes 2.1% of all pediatric cancers among patients between 1 and 19 years of age
  - Increased reporting in low-birth-weight infants but etiology is unknown
- Age
  - Most common malignant liver neoplasm in children
    - 88% in children ≤ 5 years and 3% > 15 years
    - Mean age at diagnosis: 19 months
- Gender
  - Male predominance
    - M:F = 3:2

Site

- 58% involve right lobe
- 27% involve both lobes

Presentation

- Painless abdominal mass
  - Hepatomegaly

Laboratory Tests

- Increased serum α-fetoprotein in 75-96% of patients
  - Often ≥ 100,000 ng/mL
    - Caveat: Neonates < 6 months of age normally have elevated α-fetoprotein
  - Useful marker of response to therapy and recurrence

Treatment

- Surgical resection
  - Only 1/3 to 1/2 have resectable disease at presentation
  - Preoperative chemotherapy converts > 50% of inoperable tumors to resectable tumors
- Orthotopic liver transplant

Children's Oncology Group Staging System (Pretreatment Staging)

- Stage I: Completely resected tumors with negative margins
- Stage II: Grossly resected tumors with residual disease
  - Microscopic positive margin
- Stage III: Unresectable tumors
  - Biopsy diagnosis, partially resected, macroscopic residual tumor, tumor rupture
  - Positive abdominal lymph node
- Stage IV: Tumors with metastasis to lungs, other organs, or sites distant from abdomen

Prognosis

- Tumor stage is key prognostic factor in survival
  - 90% event-free survival with primary complete resection of tumor
  - < 70% event-free survival in those with nonmetastatic, unresectable tumor

Metastasis

- 10-20% of patients have metastases at presentation
- Most frequently spread to lung but can involve bone, brain, eye, or ovaries

HEPATOBLASTOMA

Key Facts

Etiology/Pathogenesis
- Aberrant Wnt/β-catenin activation

Clinical Issues
- Most common malignant liver neoplasm in children
- Typically presents with abdominal mass
- Most patients have increased serum α-fetoprotein
- Key prognostic factor of survival is tumor stage
  - May require preoperative chemotherapy before tumor is resectable

Microscopic Pathology
- Most common component is epithelial subtypes
  - Pure fetal epithelial histology is associated with favorable prognosis
  - Commonly embryonal and fetal epithelial patterns are seen together
  - Macrotrabecular is composed of fetal- or embryonal-type cells in wide trabeculae
  - Any amount of small undifferentiated cells often resembling neuroblasts is associated with poorer prognosis
- Mixed hepatoblastoma (HB) is composed of epithelial and mesenchymal components
  - Mesenchymal component can be immature spindle cells to fibrous tissue
  - Osteoid-like and even teratoid elements can be found

Top Differential Diagnoses
- Normal liver parenchyma; positive nuclear &/or cytoplasmic β-catenin staining in HB
- Hepatocellular carcinoma; presence of both fetal and embryonal cells is diagnostic of HB

- 20-30% survival if there is metastatic disease at presentation

Conditions Associated With HB
- Familial adenomatous polyposis, Beckwith-Wiedemann, Li-Fraumeni, and Simpson-Golabi-Behmel syndromes
- Trisomy 18, glycogen storage disease types I-IV, and hemihypertrophy
- No known histologic features predict syndromic tumors

IMAGE FINDINGS

Radiographic Findings
- Solitary or multifocal mass
  - Heterogeneous and hypervascular
  - Calcification is frequently observed

MACROSCOPIC FEATURES

General Features
- Solitary or multifocal, coarsely lobulated, heterogeneous mass
  - Fetal pattern areas resemble normal liver, light brown and moderately firm
  - Embryonal and small cell patterns are softer, fleshy to gelatinous, gray-tan or pale pink
  - Mesenchymal, osteoid-like areas are firm, fibrous, or calcified
  - Teratoid, melanotic component may be dark brown or black
- Carefully search for vascular invasion

Size
- Large; can be > 15 cm

MICROSCOPIC PATHOLOGY

Histologic Features
- Epithelial patterns
  - Fetal
    - Uniform cells arranged in slender cords (2-3 cells thick) and thin trabeculae
    - Fetal epithelial cells are smaller than normal hepatocytes
    - Central round to oval nuclei, inconspicuous nucleolus, and abundant clear to pink cytoplasm with distinct membrane
    - Alternating light and dark areas based on cytoplasmic glycogen content; may have fat
    - Low mitotic index (≤ 2 mitoses/10 high-power fields)
  - Crowded fetal (fetal with mitoses)
    - Similarities to pure fetal pattern, but cells are closely packed and have higher mitotic count (≥ 2 mitoses/10 high-power fields)
    - Slightly increased nuclear to cytoplasmic ratio, round nuclei, and eosinophilic cytoplasm
    - Intermixed with pure fetal pattern and merged into embryonal pattern; can be difficult to differentiate
  - Embryonal
    - Primitive cells in sheets, pseudorosettes, acini, or tubules
    - Small, angulated nuclei (larger than fetal nuclei) with coarse nuclear chromatin, prominent nucleoli, scant cytoplasm, indistinct membranes
    - Mitotic figures more frequent
  - Small undifferentiated
    - Can be difficult to recognize and diagnose
    - Resembles neuroblast, blastemal cells, or cells found in "small round blue cell" neoplasms
    - Grows in sheets, lacks cohesiveness, and is infiltrative
    - High nuclear to cytoplasmic ratio with almost no cytoplasm, hyperchromatic nuclei, inconspicuous nucleoli

HEPATOBLASTOMA

- Can have rhabdoid-like cells with eccentric cytoplasm
- Variable mitotic rate
  - Extramedullary hematopoiesis occurs in fetal and embryonal patterns
    - Not useful to distinguish these epithelial patterns based on this finding alone
- Mesenchymal component
  - Highly cellular primitive mesenchymal cells (immature spindle cells) with scant cytoplasm and elongated, plump nuclei
  - Collagenous stroma with loose fibrosis &/or mature fibrous tissue
  - Osteoid-like areas
    - Immunoreactive for cytokeratin and epithelial membrane antigen; a metaplastic phenomenon
  - Bone, cartilage, and rhabdomyoblasts
- Teratoid component
  - Primitive neuroglia, ganglion cells, or melanin pigment
  - Can also show bone, cartilage, rhabdomyoblasts, squamous cells, and mucinous glands

Morphologic Classification

- Epithelial HB (majority of HBs)
  - Epithelial patterns can occur alone or in combination with other epithelial patterns
    - Embryonal subtype alone or with fetal component
    - Squamous epithelium and mucinous glands can be part of an epithelial HB
  - Pure fetal histology HB
    - 100% composed of fetal epithelial cells, not crowded fetal
    - Low mitotic index (≤ 2 mitoses/10 high-power fields)
  - Macrotrabecular HB
    - Fetal &/or embryonal cells in wide trabeculae, > 10 cells thick
  - Small undifferentiated or small cell anaplastic HB
    - For a diagnosis of pure small undifferentiated HB, > 70% of tumor must be composed of small undifferentiated cells
    - Any amount of small undifferentiated cells should be reported; provide percentage of small undifferentiated cells
    - May be located toward center of an embryonal region
- Mixed HB
  - Both epithelial and mesenchymal elements
- Mixed HB with teratoid (heterologous) features

Prognostic Factors

- Stage IV associated with uniformly poor prognosis (39% 5-year, event-free survival)
- Histology
  - Pure fetal epithelial HB is associated with excellent prognosis (100% 5-year, event-free survival)
  - Worse prognosis than pure fetal epithelial HB seen in
    - HB with any amount of small cell undifferentiated cells
    - Potentially macrotrabecular HB
- α-fetoprotein < 100 ng/mL confers worse prognosis

ANCILLARY TESTS

Immunohistochemistry

- Nuclear β-catenin staining in epithelial and mesenchymal components (70% of HB)
  - Positive in small undifferentiated cells
- Positive glypican-3 and Hep-Par1 staining in fetal and embryonal epithelial cells
- Positive glutamine synthetase staining in fetal and variably in embryonal cells
- INI1/BAF47 loss in some small undifferentiated cells, especially if rhabdoid phenotype

DIFFERENTIAL DIAGNOSIS

Normal Liver Parenchyma

- Must distinguish fetal epithelial cells of hepatoblastoma from normal hepatocytes, particularly near a margin
  - HB has nuclear &/or cytoplasmic immunoreactivity for β-catenin
  - Fetal cells are smaller than normal hepatocytes

Hepatocellular Carcinoma

- May be indistinguishable from macrotrabecular variant of HB
  - Biphasic pattern with both fetal and embryonal cells points to HB
  - Nuclear β-catenin and glypican-3 are more consistently positive in HB

DIAGNOSTIC CHECKLIST

Clinically Relevant Pathologic Features

- Stage I pure fetal HB cured by surgical resection alone
- Important to report any amount of small undifferentiated cells; confers worse prognosis

SELECTED REFERENCES

1. Spector LG et al: The epidemiology of hepatoblastoma. Pediatr Blood Cancer. 59(5):776-9, 2012
2. Wang LL et al: Effects of neoadjuvant chemotherapy on hepatoblastoma: a morphologic and immunohistochemical study. Am J Surg Pathol. 34(3):287-99, 2010
3. Meyers RL et al: Predictive power of pretreatment prognostic factors in children with hepatoblastoma: a report from the Children's Oncology Group. Pediatr Blood Cancer. 53(6):1016-22, 2009
4. Finegold MJ et al: Protocol for the examination of specimens from pediatric patients with hepatoblastoma. Arch Pathol Lab Med. 131(4):520-9, 2007
5. Rowland JM: Hepatoblastoma: assessment of criteria for histologic classification. Med Pediatr Oncol. 39(5):478-83, 2002
6. Stocker JT: Hepatic tumors in children. Clin Liver Dis. 5(1):259-81, viii-ix, 2001

HEPATOBLASTOMA

Microscopic Features

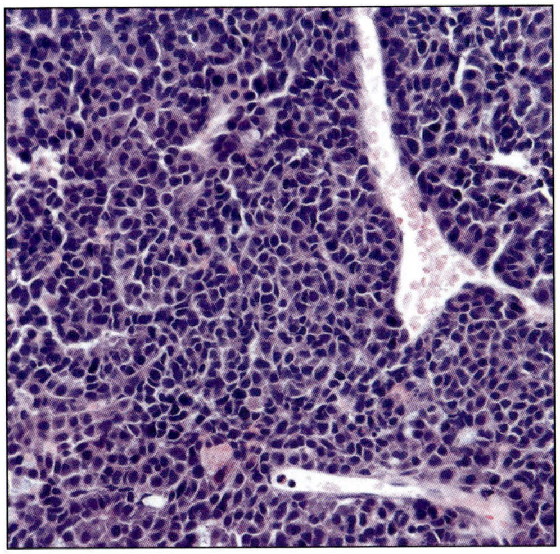

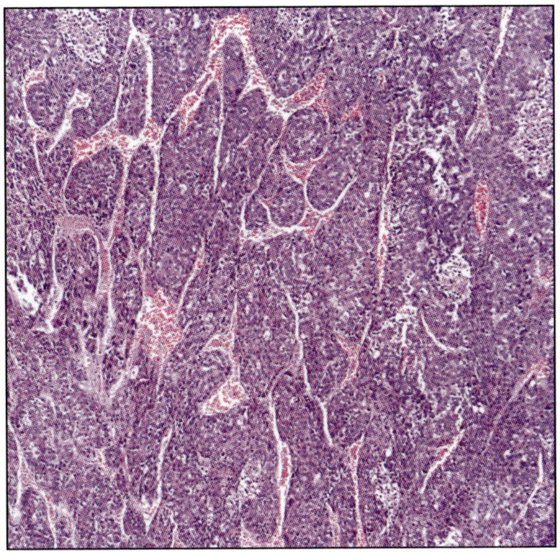

(Left) *Sheets and poorly formed nests of embryonal epithelial cells have angulated nuclei and less cytoplasm than fetal epithelial cells, which can often coexist within the same tumor. Embryonal cells have nuclear or cytoplasmic reactivity to β-catenin and are diffusely positive for glypican-3.* ***(Right)*** *Macrotrabecular HB can mimic hepatocellular carcinoma at low power. Look for mesenchymal components or fetal epithelial pattern to assist in the diagnosis.*

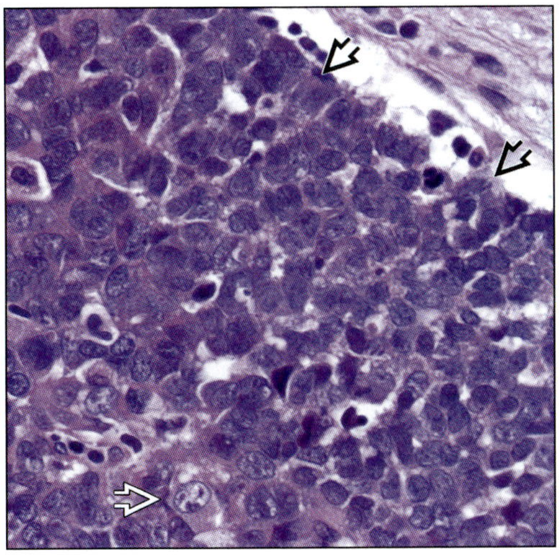

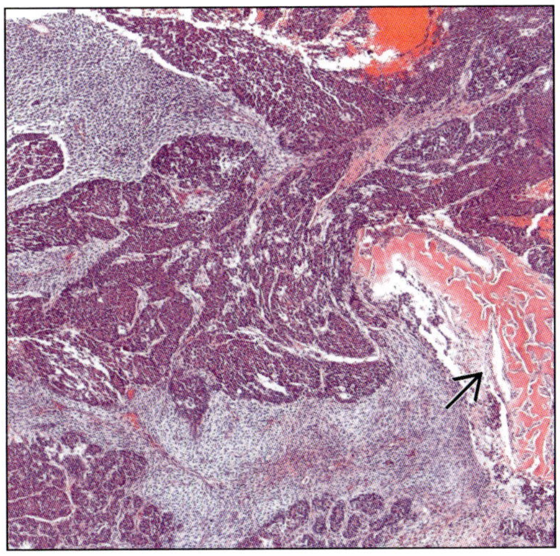

(Left) *This HB shows embryonal epithelial cells merging into a focus of small undifferentiated cells. The latter have even less cytoplasm and are often dyscohesive. These cells look like neuroblasts or blastemal cells but have positive nuclear stain for β-catenin. Even a microscopic focus of small undifferentiated cells confers a poorer prognosis.* ***(Right)*** *This mixed HB has embryonal epithelial cells, spindled mesenchymal component, and a focus of osteoid-like tissue.*

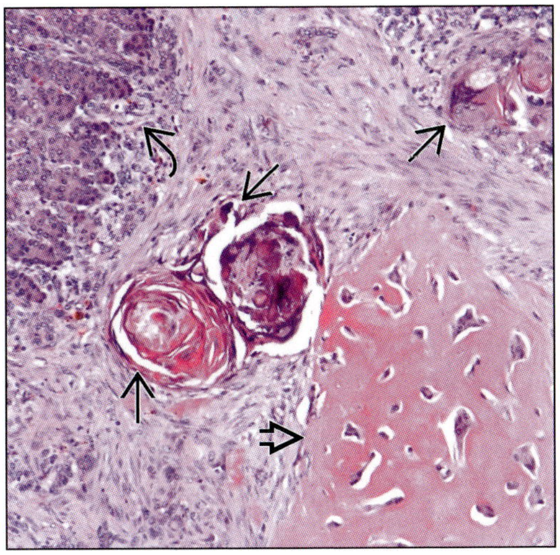

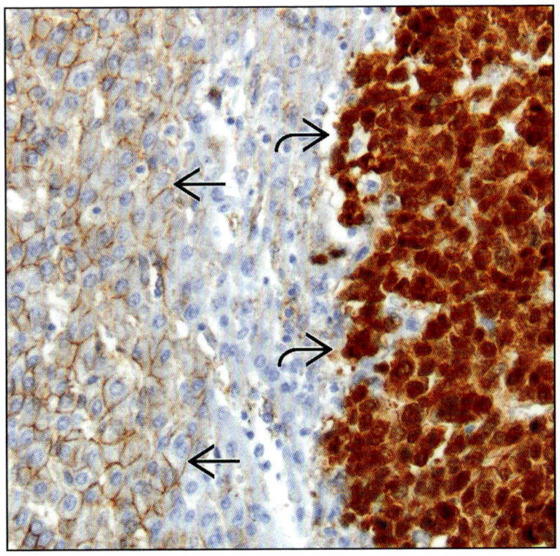

(Left) *This mixed HB has neoplastic epithelial cells in cords, squamoid nests within dense fibrous stroma, and an osteoid-like focus. This is not considered a mixed HB with teratoid features because there is no neural or neuroectodermal differentiation.* ***(Right)*** *Immunohistochemical staining for β-catenin can be useful. The liver parenchyma shows membranous staining of normal hepatocytes whereas the hepatoblastoma shows nuclear staining in neoplastic cells.*

HEPATOCELLULAR CARCINOMA

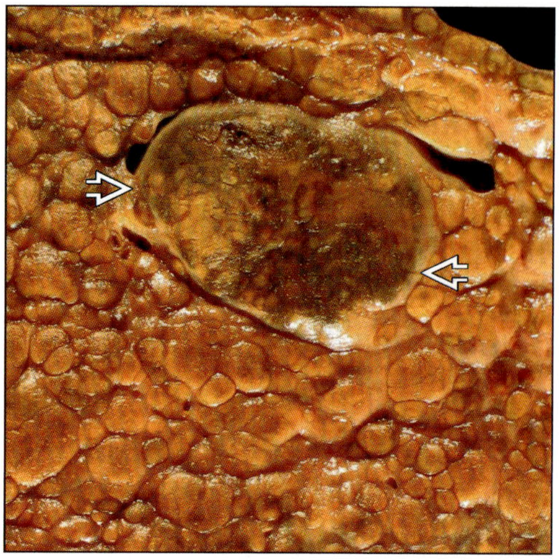

Gross photograph shows a large bile-stained tumor nodule ➡ in a background of cirrhosis. This is a classic presentation of hepatocellular carcinoma.

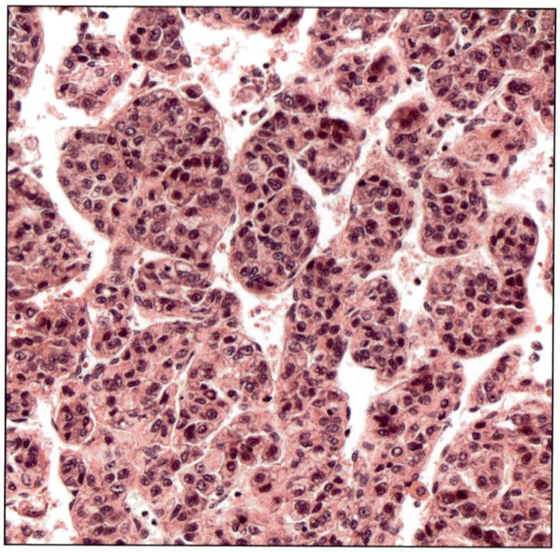

Hepatocellular carcinoma is typically composed of neoplastic cells resembling hepatocytes with a high nuclear to cytoplasmic ratio, which are organized into thick, disordered trabeculae.

TERMINOLOGY

Abbreviations

- Hepatocellular carcinoma (HCC)

Synonyms

- Hepatoma

Definitions

- Primary malignant neoplasm of liver with hepatocytic differentiation

ETIOLOGY/PATHOGENESIS

Developmental Anomaly

- HCC can occur in patients with various congenital anomalies, including Alagille syndrome, ataxia-telangiectasia, Abernethy malformation, and bile salt export protein (BSEP) deficiency

Environmental Exposure

- Aflatoxin B1, a mycotoxin produced by fungi of *Aspergillus* genus that contaminates food, is major cause of HCC in China and southern Africa
- Alcoholic cirrhosis is major cause of HCC in Western populations
- Other exposures linked to HCC include anabolic steroids, Thorotrast, oral contraceptives, and smoking

Infectious Agents

- Chronic viral hepatitis (hepatitis B and hepatitis C) is leading cause of HCC worldwide

Genetic Disorders

- Handful of hepatocellular adenomas and carcinomas reported in familial adenomatous polyposis
  - Increasing rate of hepatoblastomas in male infants

Metabolic

- Various metabolic disorders, including hemochromatosis, tyrosinemia, hypercitrullinemia, α-1-antitrypsin deficiency, and fructosemia, are associated with increased risk of HCC

Cirrhosis

- 70-90% of HCC arises in cirrhosis
- Macronodular cirrhosis is more strongly associated with HCC than is micronodular cirrhosis

Progression of Benign Tumor

- HCC can arise in preexisting hepatocellular adenoma

CLINICAL ISSUES

Epidemiology

- Incidence
  - Varies widely depending on geography in parallel with prevalence of hepatitis B, hepatitis C, and aflatoxin exposure
    - East Asia and southern Africa have highest incidence worldwide, up to 150 per 100,000
    - In USA, annual incidence is ~ 4 per 100,000
- Age
  - Incidence increases with advancing age and then falls off in elderly patients; however, average age varies depending on geography
    - In parts of world with high incidence, average age is 35 years
    - In USA, average age is 60 years
  - Can occur in children, particularly in those with metabolic or genetic disorders
- Gender
  - More common in men

Presentation

- Abdominal pain due to stretching of Glisson capsule
- Malaise, weight loss, hepatomegaly

HEPATOCELLULAR CARCINOMA

Key Facts

Etiology/Pathogenesis
- Chronic viral hepatitis is leading cause of hepatocellular carcinoma (HCC) worldwide
- 70-90% of HCC arises in cirrhosis
- Handful of hepatocellular adenomas and carcinomas reported in familial adenomatous polyposis

Clinical Issues
- In USA, annual incidence is ~ 4 per 100,000
- α-fetoprotein (AFP) is elevated in 70-90% of patients
- In USA, 5-year survival is 30-40% overall, but 75% for tumors < 5 cm

Macroscopic Features
- Typically soft, bile-stained with hemorrhage and necrosis
- Can be solitary tumor, multiple discrete tumors, or small indistinct nodules throughout portion of liver
- Gross venous or bile duct invasion commonly occurs

Microscopic Pathology
- Grows as thickened hepatic plates separated by sinusoids without desmoplastic stroma
- Tumor cells resemble hepatocytes with polygonal shape, round vesicular nuclei, and prominent nucleoli
- Bile pigment in dilated canaliculi is helpful in distinguishing HCC from its mimics

Ancillary Tests
- Positive for Hep-Par1, glypican-3, and CAM5.2 (CK8 and CK18)

- Decompensation of previously stable cirrhotic patient with jaundice and rapidly accumulating ascites
- Fever, leukocytosis, and liver mass mimicking hepatic abscess
- Increasingly, small asymptomatic tumors are being found during surveillance of cirrhotic patients

Laboratory Tests
- α-fetoprotein (AFP) is elevated in 70-90% of patients

Natural History
- Metastasis occurs in 40-60% of patients
  - Most common locations are lymph nodes in porta hepatis, celiac axis, and around pancreas
- HCC has tendency for intravascular spread with involvement of hepatic and portal veins
  - Hematogenous spread most commonly occurs to lungs, but also adrenal glands, bone, stomach, heart, pancreas, kidney, spleen, and ovary
- Tumor seldom breaches Glisson capsule; therefore, dissemination throughout peritoneal cavity is rare

Treatment
- Surgical approaches
  - Resection is possible if sufficient reserve liver function
  - Transplantation is option if patient meets Milan criteria of single tumor < 5 cm, or < 4 tumors, none > 3 cm
- Drugs
  - Sorafenib
    - Tyrosine kinase inhibitor that has proven to be at least somewhat effective in advanced cases
- Ablation therapy
  - Radiofrequency or microwave ablation or direct percutaneous ethanol injections are options for small tumors
  - Angiographic embolization of hepatic artery can infarct tumor and prolong survival

Prognosis
- Better prognosis associated with age < 50 years, female gender, resectable tumor, better differentiated tumor, low mitotic index, absence of vascular invasion, encapsulated tumor, and absence of cirrhosis
- In USA, 5-year survival is 75% for patients with tumors < 5 cm and 30-40% overall

MACROSCOPIC FEATURES

General Features
- Soft tumor that can be bile-stained, with variable hemorrhage and necrosis
- Can be solitary tumor, solitary tumor with satellite nodules, multiple discrete tumors, or multiple small indistinct nodules throughout portion of liver or entire liver
  - Pedunculated tumors are rare, more easily resected, and have better prognosis
  - Encapsulated tumors are rare, usually solitary tumors that arise in cirrhotic livers, and have better prognosis
- Gross venous or bile duct invasion may be seen and should be sought

MICROSCOPIC PATHOLOGY

Histologic Features
- Architectural patterns
  - Trabecular pattern: Tumor cells grow as thickened hepatic plates separated by sinusoids without desmoplastic stroma
  - Pseudoglandular or acinar pattern: Tumor cells grow in solid nests with central degenerative changes
  - Compact pattern: Trabeculae grow compressed together
  - Scirrhous pattern: Resemble trabecular HCC but with abundant stroma
  - Giant cell pattern: Multinucleate giant cells

HEPATOCELLULAR CARCINOMA

- Spindle cell pattern is often referred to as sarcomatoid HCC
- Tumor cell morphology
  - Tumor cells resemble hepatocytes with polygonal shape, round vesicular nuclei, and prominent nucleoli
    - Inclusions can be seen in tumor cells, including Mallory hyaline, hyaline globules, and pale bodies
    - Clear cells may be present and even numerous due to accumulation of glycogen, water, or fat
  - Presence of bile pigment in dilated canaliculi is helpful in distinguishing HCC from its mimics

Cytologic Features

- Neoplastic cells resemble hepatocytes but with enlarged nuclei, nuclear membrane irregularity, coarse chromatin, and prominent macronucleoli
  - May have dispersed cell pattern with numerous stripped, atypical nuclei
- Tumor cells tend to be more monotonous with less anisonucleosis and higher nuclear to cytoplasmic ratio than benign hepatocytes
- Thick, disordered plates or balls of neoplastic cells, focally lined by sinusoidal endothelial cells ("endothelial wrapping")
- Large tissue fragments traversed by blood vessels

Fibrolamellar Variant

- 5% of hepatocellular carcinomas
- Arises in noncirrhotic livers
- Affects both sexes equally, usually < 35 years of age
- Better prognosis than conventional HCC; 5-year survival rate of ~ 50%
- Grossly has lobular appearance with fibrous septa or central stellate scar
- Nests and sheets of large, eosinophilic, polygonal tumor cells with vesicular nuclei and prominent nucleoli separated by fibrous stroma

ANCILLARY TESTS

Histochemistry

- Reticulin
  - Reactivity: Not applicable
  - Staining pattern
    - Diminished or absent in sinusoids; may outline abnormally thick trabeculae as well

Immunohistochemistry

- Positive for Hep-Par1, glypican-3, and CAM5.2 (CK8 and CK18)
- AFP staining is highly specific but insensitive (25%)
- Polyclonal CEA and CD10 demonstrate canalicular pattern
- Sinusoidal capillarization demonstrated with CD34

DIFFERENTIAL DIAGNOSIS

Cholangiocarcinoma

- Mucicarmine (+); expresses CK7, CK19, and CA19-9
- Desmoplastic stroma
- Mixed HCC/cholangiocarcinoma may show features of both

Metastatic Neuroendocrine Tumor

- Prominent collagenous stroma; positive staining for neuroendocrine markers

Metastatic Adenocarcinoma

- Mucicarmine (+); MOC-31(+), keratin profile not limited to 8 and 18

Angiomyolipoma

- Presence of adipose tissue and muscular arteries; HMB-45(+), Hep-Par1(-)

Renal Cell Carcinoma

- History of renal cell carcinoma or renal tumor, no cirrhosis
- Hep-Par1(-), pax-2(+), pax-8(+)

Hepatic Adenoma

- Patient demographics differ; cirrhosis is absent, and trabeculae are at most 2 or 3 cells thick

Regenerative Nodule in Cirrhosis

- Cytologically benign, absence of trabecular or pseudoglandular growth pattern
- Portal tracts present in nodule
- Intact reticulin

Dysplastic Nodule in Cirrhosis

- Cytologic atypia and mild architectural abnormalities
- Contains portal tracts, lacks invasion of portal tracts by tumor
- Intact reticulin

GRADING

Edmondson and Steiner

- Grade I (well differentiated): Small hepatocytic tumor cells arranged as trabeculae
- Grade II (moderately differentiated): Larger tumor cells with abnormal nuclei and eosinophilic cytoplasm; pseudoglandular structures may be seen
- Grade III (poorly differentiated): More frequent tumor giant cells
- Grade IV (undifferentiated): Poorly differentiated tumor cells with hyperchromatic nuclei, little cytoplasm, and loss of trabecular architecture

SELECTED REFERENCES

1. Li M et al: Hepatocelluar carcinoma associated with attenuated familial adenomatous polyposis: a case report and review of the literature. Clin Colorectal Cancer. 11(1):77-81, 2012
2. Stuart KE et al: Hepatocellular carcinoma in the United States. Prognostic features, treatment outcome, and survival. Cancer. 77(11):2217-22, 1996
3. Hurlimann J et al: Immunohistochemistry in the differential diagnosis of liver carcinomas. Am J Surg Pathol. 15(3):280-8, 1991

HEPATOCELLULAR CARCINOMA

Gross and Microscopic Features

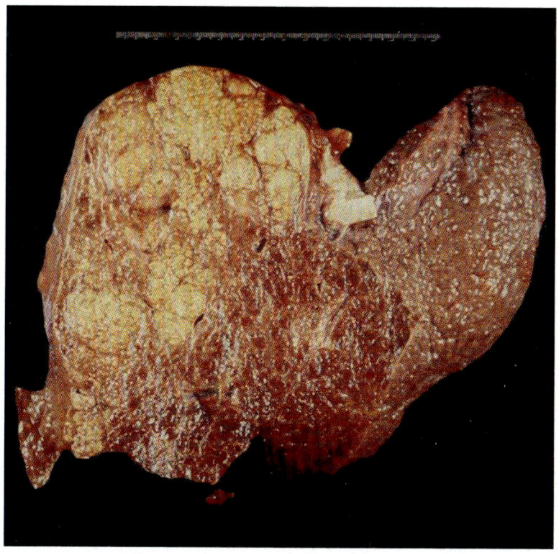

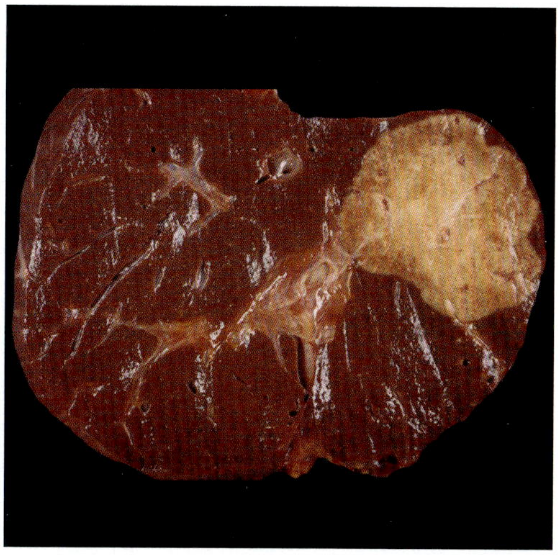

(Left) *This large, multinodular hepatocellular carcinoma (HCC) arises in a background of cirrhosis.* ***(Right)*** *This hepatocellular carcinoma is unifocal, yellow-tan, and well circumscribed. The background liver is not cirrhotic.*

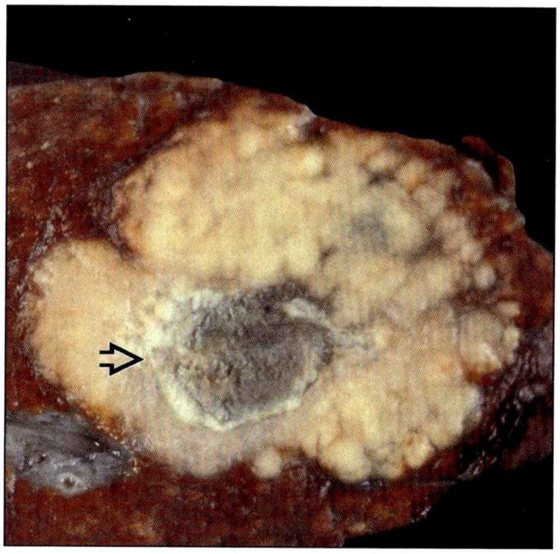

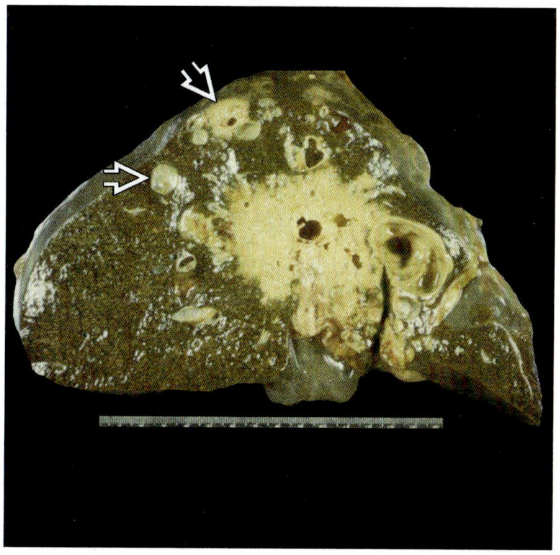

(Left) *This hepatocellular carcinoma arose in a background of hereditary hemochromatosis; note the rust-colored cirrhotic liver in the background. There is also central necrosis ⇨.* ***(Right)*** *This hepatocellular carcinoma is composed of a large central mass with small satellite tumor nodules ➡. There is a background of cirrhosis.*

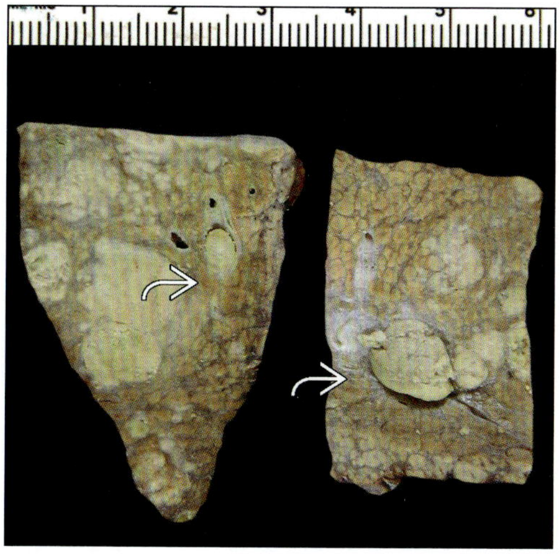

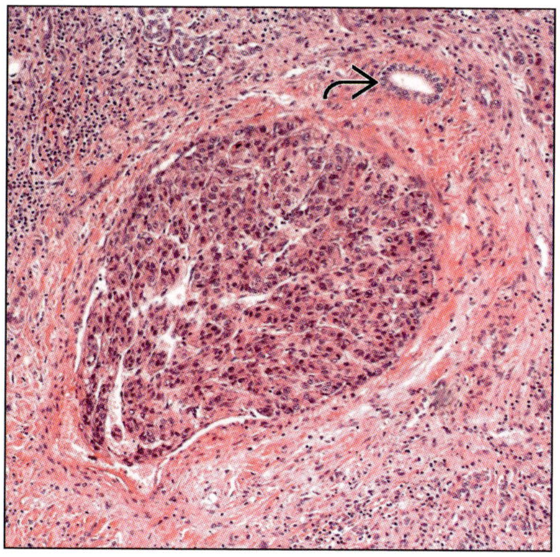

(Left) *This example of the diffuse pattern of HCC shows innumerable small white-tan nodules of a tumor in a background of cirrhosis. Careful inspection shows that 2 of these nodules represent gross venous invasion ↪.* ***(Right)*** *A histologic section of a tumor shows venous invasion by HCC. A portal vein is distended and filled with trabeculae of hyperchromatic neoplastic cells. Note the adjacent accompanying bile duct ↪.*

HEPATOCELLULAR CARCINOMA

Microscopic Features

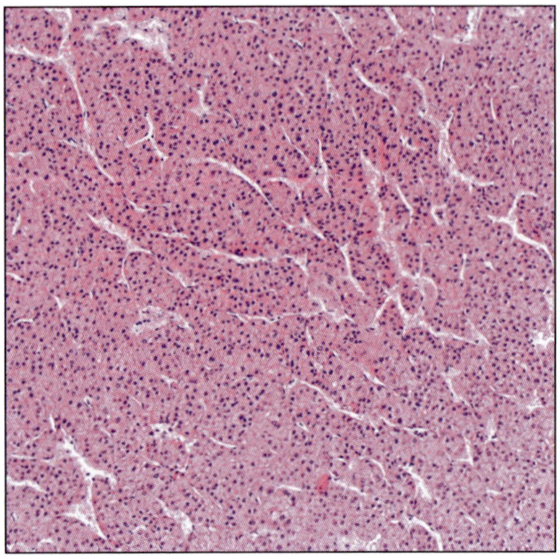
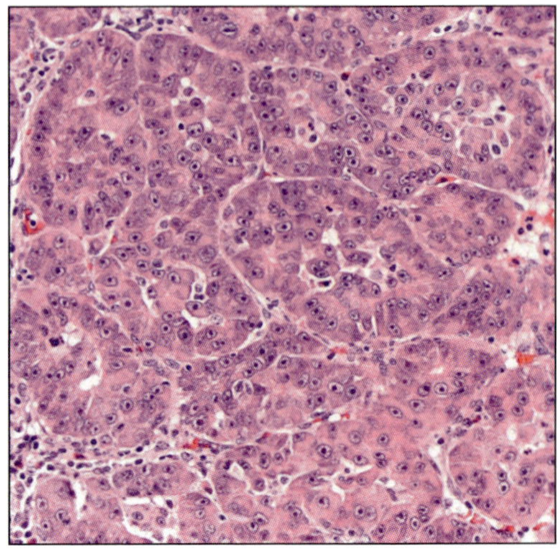

(Left) *The trabecular pattern of hepatocellular carcinoma is characterized by thickened trabeculae separated by sinusoids. In this focus, the trabeculae appear to be ~ 6-8 cells thick.* ***(Right)*** *This hepatocellular carcinoma is growing in a pattern of rounded trabeculae with central degenerative changes.*

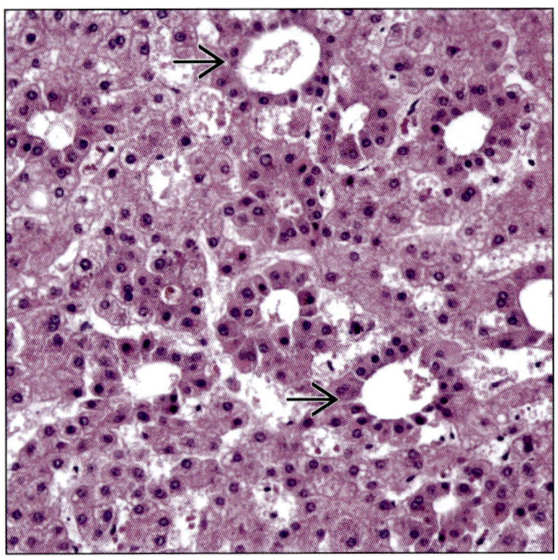
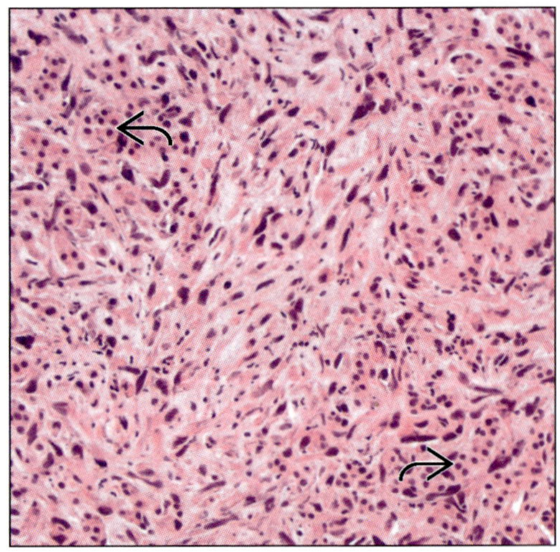

(Left) *In the pseudoglandular pattern of hepatocellular carcinoma, dilated spaces in the centers of trabeculae mimic glands →.* ***(Right)*** *This example of sarcomatoid hepatocellular carcinoma has extensive spindle cell change. Notice the interlacing of spindle cells with more compact epithelioid tumor cells →.*

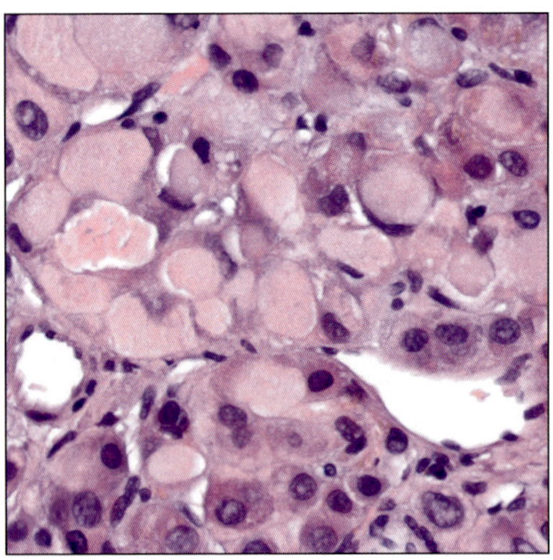
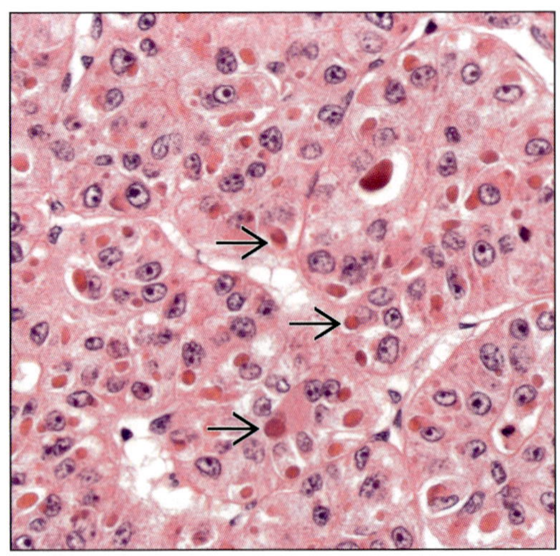

(Left) *These tumor cells in HCC contain pale eosinophilic inclusions (presumably fibrinogen) in the cytoplasm that are known as pale bodies.* ***(Right)*** *Mallory hyaline can be seen in hepatocellular carcinoma. In this tumor, many of the tumor cells contain an oval eosinophilic inclusion →. Although Mallory hyaline in HCC can have the characteristic ropey appearance of alcoholic hyaline, it often is more globular and rounded.*

HEPATOCELLULAR CARCINOMA

Microscopic and Gross Features and Variants

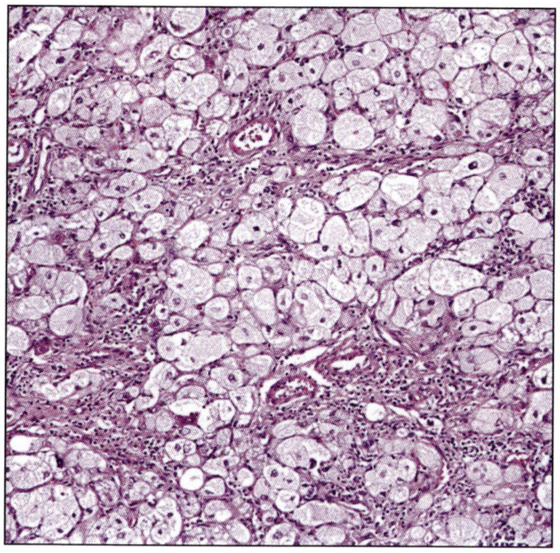

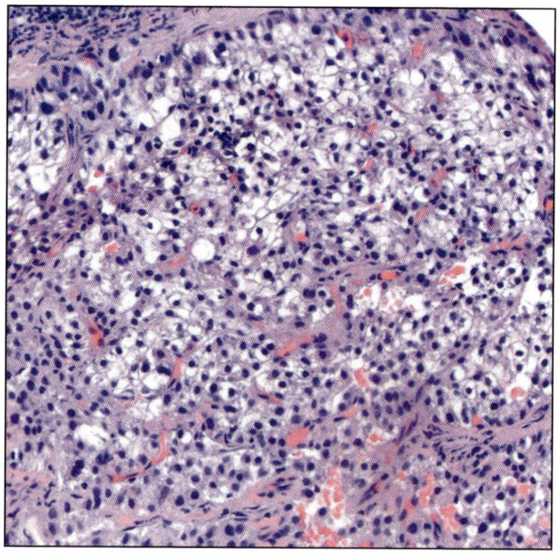

(Left) *The clear cell variant of hepatocellular carcinoma contains tumor cells with abundant glycogen in the cytoplasm, creating a clear appearance reminiscent of clear cell renal cell carcinoma.* ***(Right)*** *Metastatic renal cell carcinoma in the liver is easily mistaken for the clear cell variant of hepatocellular carcinoma. This patient had an identical renal tumor excised a few years prior to the development of this tumor in the liver.*

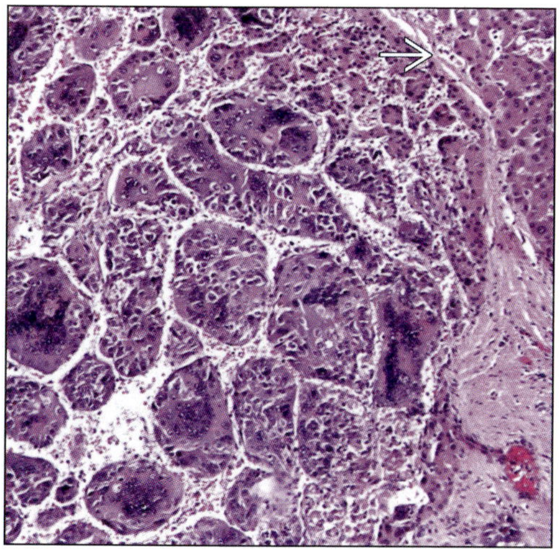

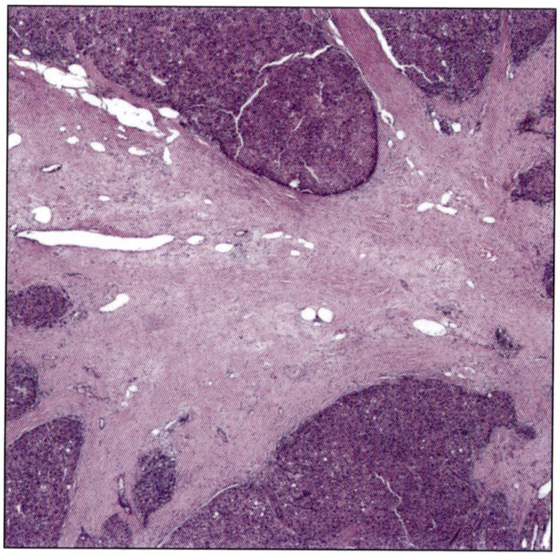

(Left) *This giant cell variant of hepatocellular carcinoma features striking multinucleated tumor giant cells. An area of more typical HCC is present at the periphery of the field ⇒.* ***(Right)*** *The scirrhous pattern of HCC has prominent stroma and may form a large central fibrous scar that can mimic focal nodular hyperplasia or the fibrolamellar variant of HCC. However, the other histologic features of fibrolamellar variant of HCC are absent.*

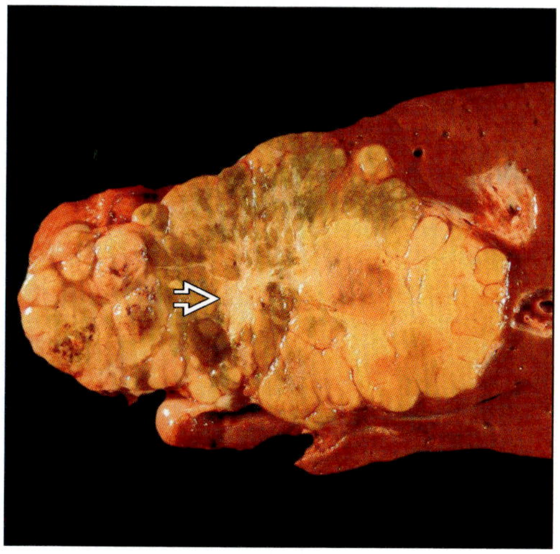

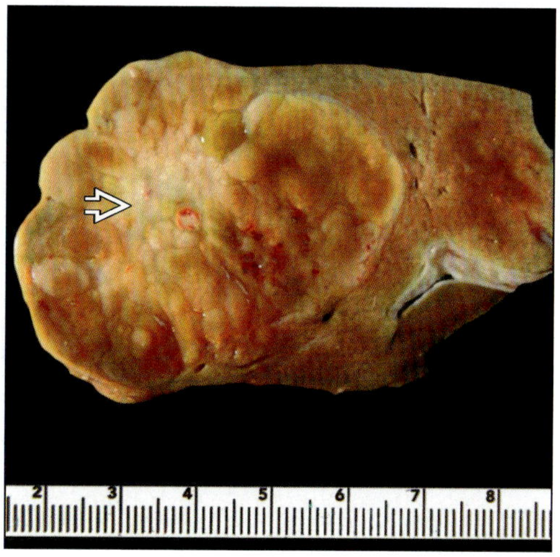

(Left) *The fibrolamellar variant of hepatocellular carcinoma typically has a lobular growth pattern and central scar ⇒. Also note the absence of cirrhosis in the background liver.* ***(Right)*** *Clinically, this fibrolamellar HCC in a young woman was thought to be focal nodular hyperplasia. Note the lobular growth pattern and central scar ⇒, which are typical of both focal nodular hyperplasia and fibrolamellar HCC.*

HEPATOCELLULAR CARCINOMA

Microscopic Features

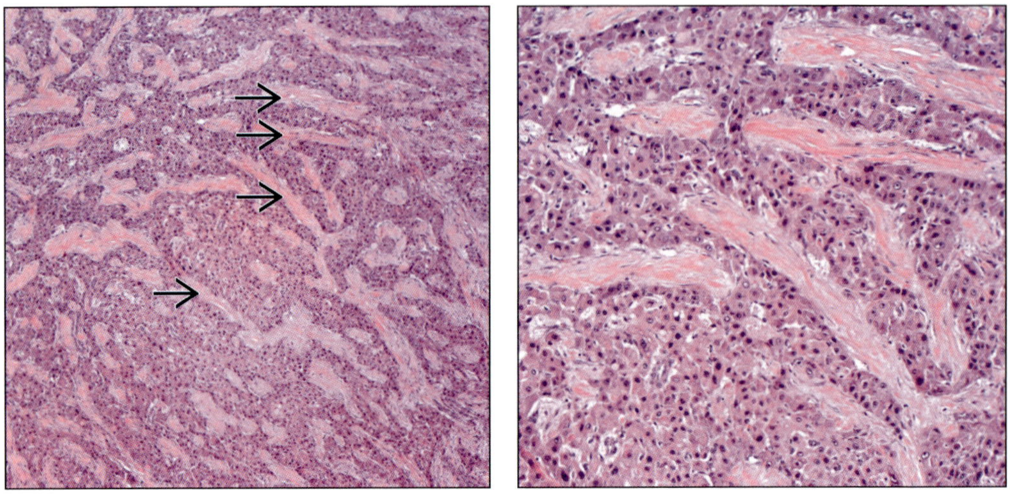

(Left) *Low-power view of fibrolamellar HCC shows cords of neoplastic hepatocytes separated by parallel arrays of collagenous stroma* →. ***(Right)*** *High magnification of fibrolamellar HCC shows fibrous septae composed of parallel collagen fibers separating trabeculae of plump eosinophilic tumor cells.*

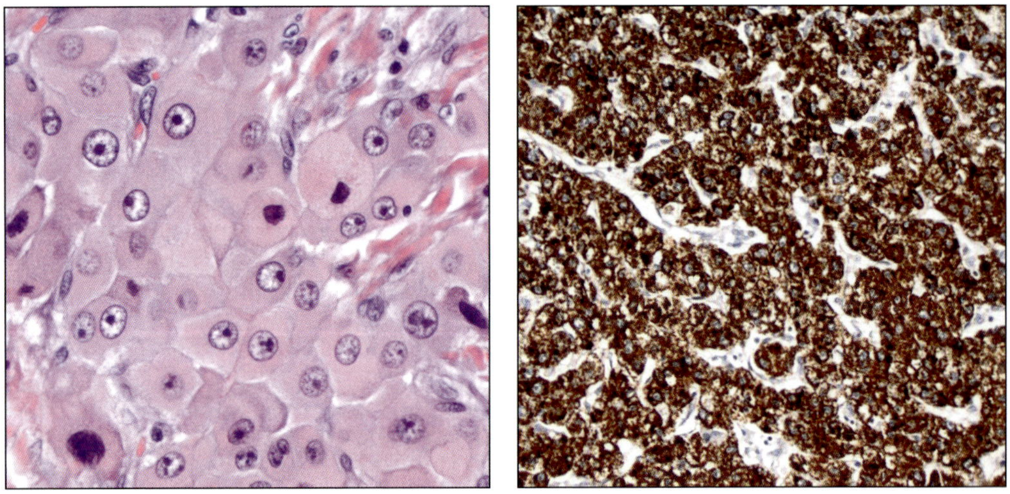

(Left) *In the fibrolamellar variant of HCC, the tumor cells are large, eosinophilic, and polygonal. They have large, vesicular nuclei with prominent nucleoli. The eosinophilic cytoplasm is due to large numbers of mitochondria.* ***(Right)*** *Hep-Par1 immunohistochemical stain in hepatocellular carcinoma shows strong positive cytoplasmic staining.*

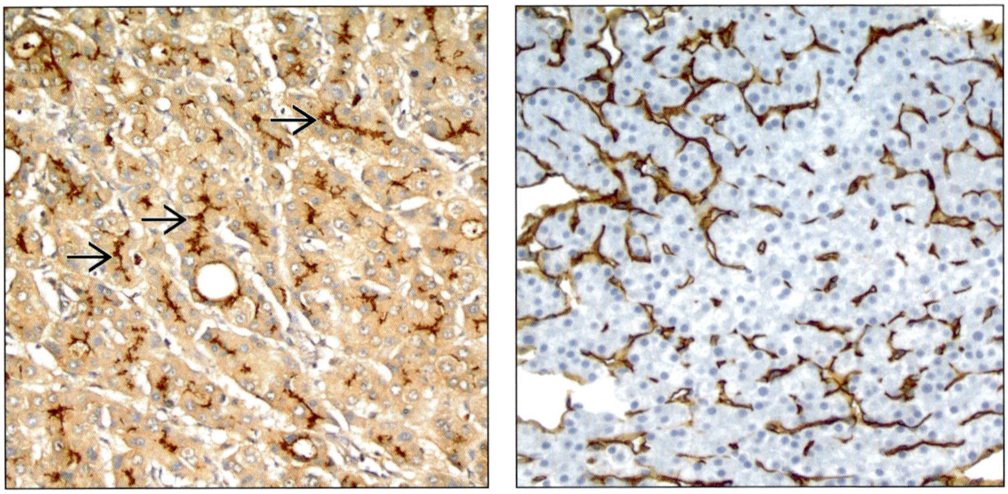

(Left) *Polyclonal CEA immunostain shows staining of bile canaliculi* → *in hepatocellular carcinoma, producing a so-called canalicular pattern. This is in contrast to the pattern typical of ductal adenocarcinoma in which diffuse cytoplasmic staining is seen.* ***(Right)*** *CD34 in hepatocellular carcinoma stains the sinusoidal endothelium. The sinusoids in hepatocellular carcinoma become "capillarized" and thus express antigens normally found in capillary endothelium but not in normal sinusoidal endothelium.*

Microscopic and Cytologic Features

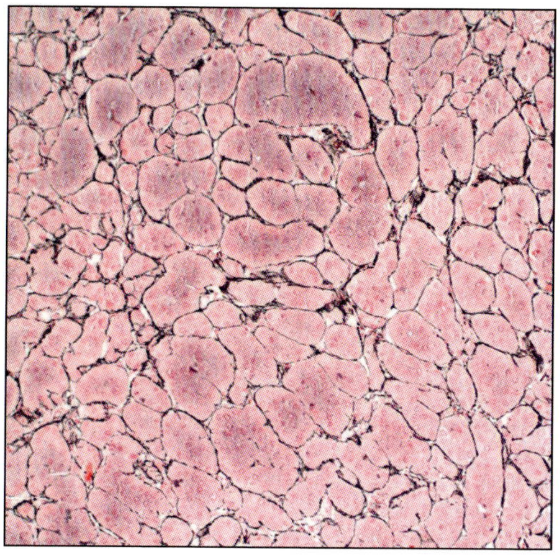

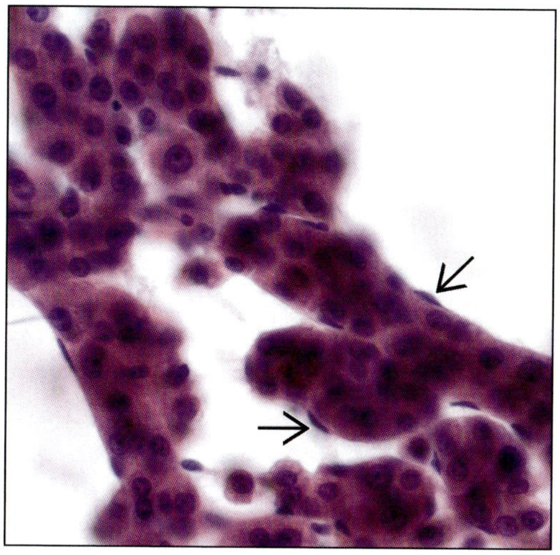

(Left) *Reticulin stain in hepatocellular carcinoma demonstrates an abnormal trabecular growth pattern with thickened, disorganized trabeculae. Reticulin is also frequently reduced in amount or even absent in HCC.* ***(Right)*** *Fine-needle aspiration (FNA) biopsy smear of HCC shows a trabecular growth pattern composed of thick trabeculae of neoplastic hepatocytes. Endothelial wrapping is present at the edges of the tumor* ⇨.

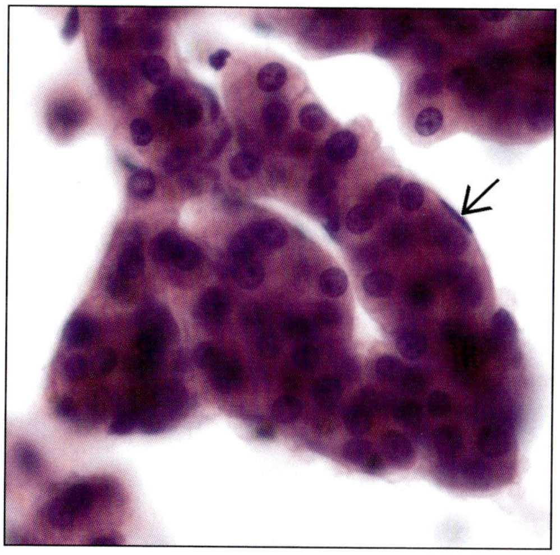

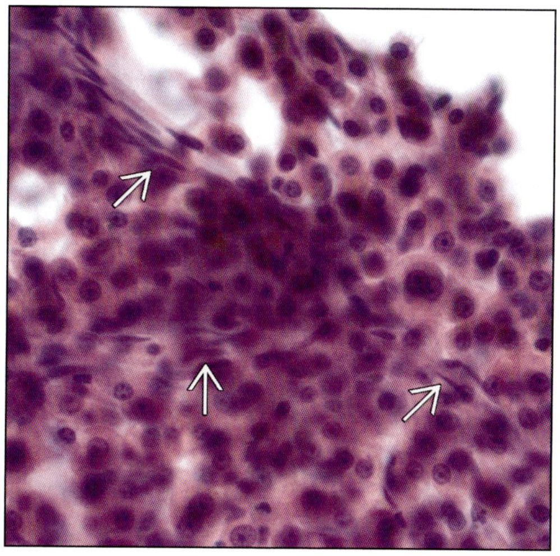

(Left) *Note the smooth contours of this group of HCC cells from an FNA created by endothelial wrapping* ⇨. *Note the increased nuclear density.* ***(Right)*** *This FNA biopsy smear of HCC shows a large cluster of neoplastic hepatocytes with traversing blood vessels* ➡ *typical of this tumor. A similar phenomenon occurs commonly in renal cell carcinoma.*

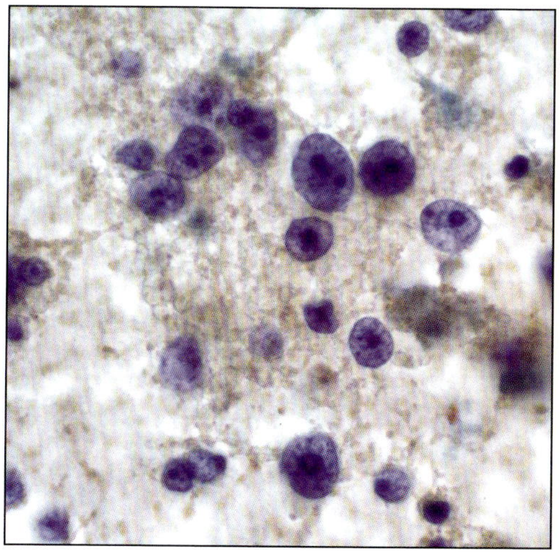

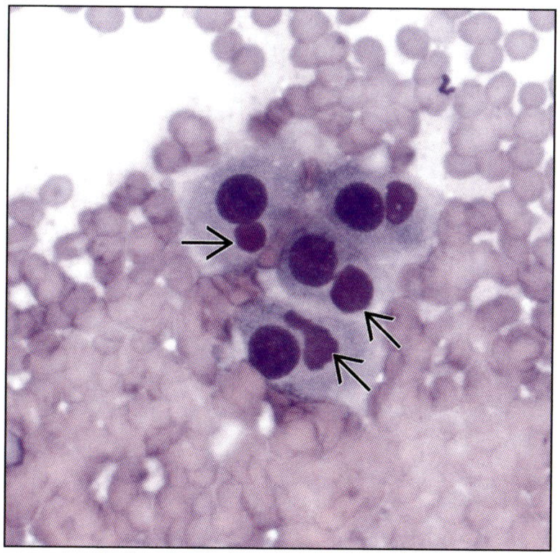

(Left) *This FNA smear of an HCC shows innumerable stripped atypical nuclei scattered throughout the slide. This pattern is not an uncommon one for HCC.* ***(Right)*** *In this air-dried preparation the malignant hepatocytes contain cytoplasmic inclusions, consistent with Mallory hyaline* ⇨. *Note that many of the inclusions appear round or more oval than they do in alcohol-related Mallory hyaline.*

PANCREATIC DUCTAL ADENOCARCINOMA

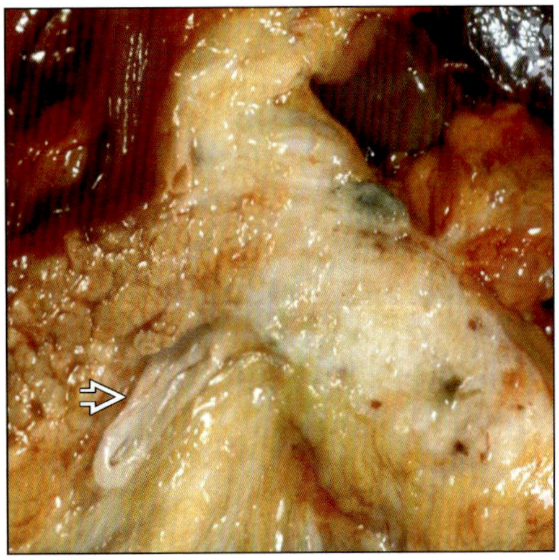

This gross photograph shows the cut surface of a large pancreatic adenocarcinoma. The surface is firm, white, and gritty. Note the dilated pancreatic duct ⇨.

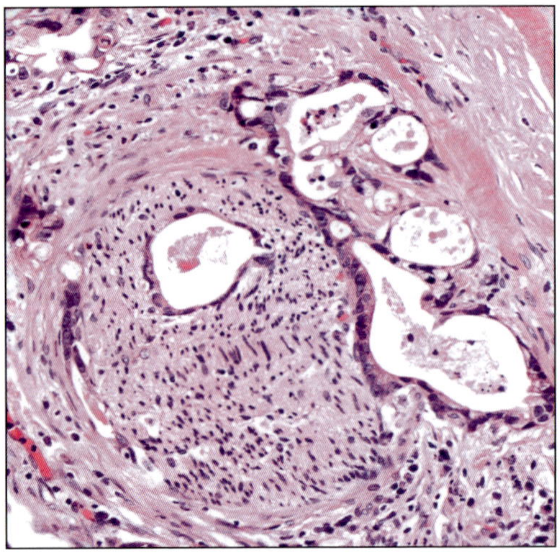

Perineural invasion is a common feature of pancreatic ductal adenocarcinoma.

TERMINOLOGY

Abbreviations

- Pancreatic ductal adenocarcinoma (PDAC)

Synonyms

- Pancreatic adenocarcinoma
- Duct cell adenocarcinoma

Definitions

- Malignant epithelial neoplasm arising in pancreatic ductal system
  - 85-90% of all pancreatic neoplasms
- Predominantly glandular differentiation

ETIOLOGY/PATHOGENESIS

Hereditary Risk Factors

- Family history of pancreatic cancer
- Hereditary pancreatitis
- Peutz-Jeghers syndrome
- Familial atypical multiple mole melanoma syndrome
- *BRCA2* and *BRCA1* mutations

Medical Risk Factors

- Chronic pancreatitis
- Diabetes mellitus
- Previous cholecystectomy or partial gastrectomy

Environmental and Occupational Risk Factors

- Cigarette smoking approximately doubles risk
- Diet high in meat, fat, nitrates, and pork products ↑ risk
- Obesity
- Chemicals (solvents, DDT, gasoline)
- Occupational (coal gas workers, metal working, hide tanning, dry cleaning)

Precursor Lesions

- Pancreatic intraepithelial neoplasia

CLINICAL ISSUES

Epidemiology

- Age
  - Peak incidence in 7th and 8th decades
    - Rare before age 40
- Gender
  - M > F (1.3:1)
- Ethnicity
  - More common in Maoris, native Hawaiians, and African Americans in the United States

Presentation

- Very nonspecific symptoms may result in delay in diagnosis
  - Epigastric pain radiating to the back
  - Weight loss
  - Painless jaundice
  - Signs of biliary obstruction
- Disease associations
  - Trousseau syndrome (migratory thrombophlebitis)
  - Diabetes mellitus
  - Sister Mary Joseph sign (palpable periumbilical nodules)
  - Courvoisier sign (distended, palpable gallbladder)

Treatment

- Resection
  - Only 10-20% of cases are resectable at diagnosis
- Chemotherapy before resection, after resection, or both
  - Gemcitabine seems most promising

Prognosis

- Dismal
  - Overall 5-year survival is < 5%

PANCREATIC DUCTAL ADENOCARCINOMA

Key Facts

Terminology
- Adenocarcinoma arising in pancreatic ductal system
  - Comprises 85-90% of all pancreatic neoplasms

Etiology/Pathogenesis
- Hereditary risk factors
  - Family history of pancreatic cancer
  - Hereditary pancreatitis
  - Peutz-Jeghers syndrome
  - Familial atypical multiple mole melanoma syndrome
  - *BRCA2* and *BRCA1* mutations

Clinical Issues
- Most cases are unresectable at presentation
- Nonspecific symptoms often mean delay in diagnosis

Macroscopic Features
- Majority in head of pancreas
- Poorly defined, firm mass with intense fibrotic reaction
  - Carcinoma may be difficult to distinguish from background pancreatitis

Microscopic Pathology
- Small, haphazardly infiltrating glands embedded in dense desmoplastic stroma
- Many histologic patterns and variants
- Immunopositive for many antigens
  - Cytokeratins 7, 8, 18, 19
  - CEA, CA19-9, CA125, B72.3
  - MUC1, MUC4, MUC5AC, and MUC6 (25%)

IMAGE FINDINGS

General Features
- CT scan is most commonly used radiological method for diagnosis and staging
- Magnetic resonance angiography can be used to examine vascular anatomy and determine resectability
- Endoscopic ultrasound is also very reliable for diagnosis and staging
- ERCP/MRCP help visualize ductal system

MACROSCOPIC FEATURES

General Features
- Majority in head of pancreas
  - Minority in body or tail
  - Minority diffusely involves whole gland
- Solitary (majority) or multifocal
- Firm, solid, poorly defined, white-yellow mass
  - May have cystic degeneration
- Usually intense fibrotic reaction
  - May make carcinoma difficult to distinguish from background pancreatitis
- Pancreatic duct may be dilated
- May cause stenosis of common bile duct
- Tumors often grossly extend beyond pancreas

MICROSCOPIC PATHOLOGY

Histologic Features
- Invasive malignant glands
  - Range from very well-differentiated to very poorly differentiated
  - Glands grow in haphazard fashion and are very infiltrative
- Nuclear features
  - Nuclear crowding and overlapping
  - Nuclei vary in size, shape, and intracellular location from cell to cell within a given neoplastic gland
  - Loss of polarity
  - Irregular chromatin distribution
  - Irregular nuclear contour
- Dense desmoplastic stroma
  - Fibroblasts and other inflammatory cells
  - Neoplastic tumor cells may represent only small component of tumor mass with rest made up of desmoplastic reaction
- Mucin production
- Perineural invasion is very common
  - Present in > 75% of cases
- Angiolymphatic invasion is common
- Tumor may infiltrate larger blood vessels and cause thrombi
- Tumor cells may grow along basement membrane of adjacent intact epithelium, such as in pancreatic ducts (cancerization), bile duct, and duodenum
- Associated pancreatitis is common
  - Parenchymal atrophy
  - Fibrosis
  - Islet cell clustering ("pseudohyperplasia")

ANCILLARY TESTS

Immunohistochemistry
- Positive for cytokeratins 7, 8, 18, 19
- Positive for CEA, CA19-9, CA125, B72.3
- Positive for MUC1, MUC4, MUC5AC, and MUC6 (25%)
- Positive for claudin-4, fascin, mesothelin, PSCA (60%), S100 proteins
- Loss of nuclear expression of p16 (> 90%) and SMAD4 (55%)
- Overexpression of p53 (50-75%)

Histologic Patterns and Variants
- Foamy gland pattern
  - Deceptively bland, benign-appearing cells with microvesicular cytoplasm
  - Mimics pancreatic intraepithelial neoplasm (PanIN), benign glands, or histiocytes
- Clear cell pattern

PANCREATIC DUCTAL ADENOCARCINOMA

  - Clear cytoplasm resembles renal cell carcinoma
  - Common focal finding in conventional ductal adenocarcinoma
- Colloid carcinoma
  - Neoplastic epithelial cells suspended in large pools of extracellular mucin
  - Colloid component must comprise at least 80% of tumor
  - Almost always arises in association with intraductal papillary mucinous neoplasm (IPMN)
- Signet ring cell carcinoma
  - At least 50% of tumor composed of infiltrating, noncohesive cells with intracytoplasmic mucin
- Adenosquamous carcinoma
  - Squamous differentiation in at least 30% of entire lesion
- Large duct adenocarcinoma
  - Composed of large, dilated, invasive glands, often with simple architecture
  - May simulate (dilated) PanIN
- Microadenocarcinoma pattern
  - Small uniform cells arranged in microglandular structures
  - Represents a mixture of ductal adenocarcinoma, endocrine neoplasm, and acinar cell carcinoma
- Medullary carcinoma
  - Poorly differentiated carcinoma with pushing rather than infiltrating borders
  - Associated with microsatellite instability, hereditary nonpolyposis colorectal cancer (HNPCC)
- Undifferentiated carcinoma ± osteoclastic-like giant cells
  - May have giant cell, spindle cell, or glandular component
- Hepatoid carcinoma
  - Significant component demonstrates hepatocellular differentiation
  - Mark with Hep-Par1, CD10, polyclonal CEA, AFP

DIFFERENTIAL DIAGNOSIS

Chronic Pancreatitis

- Often involves younger patients (< 40 years)
- Diffuse scarring of gland without a discrete mass
- Relatively preserved lobular architecture

Normal/Reactive Duct Changes

- Very well-differentiated tumors may mimic normal or reactive pancreatic ducts but can be distinguished by
  - Small glands immediately adjacent to muscular arteries without intervening stroma or acini
  - Incomplete gland formation
  - Disorganized, haphazard growth of neoplastic glands
  - 4x variation in nuclear size within single gland

Ampullary/Periampullary Carcinomas

- Differentiation from PDAC is based on epicenter of mass grossly and presence of precursor lesions

Acinic Cell Carcinoma

- Highly cellular carcinoma with acinar, trabecular, &/or solid patterns
- Eosinophilic granular cytoplasm
- Basally located nuclei with single prominent nucleolus
- Positive for trypsin and chymotrypsin
- Negative for CK7

Neuroendocrine Neoplasms

- Nesting &/or trabecular patterns
- Often have hyalinized stroma
- Uniform nuclei with salt-and-pepper chromatin
- Positive for chromogranin, synaptophysin

DIAGNOSTIC CHECKLIST

Clinically Relevant Pathologic Features

- Perineural or angiolymphatic invasion in retroperitoneal soft tissue margin is underrecognized basis for surgical failure
  - > 1/2 of patients have extrapancreatic nerve involvement in this area
- Lymph node metastases are present at time of surgery in 70-80% of patients

SELECTED REFERENCES

1. Bronsert P et al: Intestinal-type of differentiation predicts favourable overall survival: confirmatory clinicopathological analysis of 198 periampullary adenocarcinomas of pancreatic, biliary, ampullary and duodenal origin. BMC Cancer. 13(1):428, 2013
2. Fendrich V et al: Familial pancreatic cancer-status quo. Int J Colorectal Dis. Epub ahead of print, 2013
3. Maron R et al: Inhibition of pancreatic carcinoma by homo- and heterocombinations of antibodies against EGF-receptor and its kin HER2/ErbB-2. Proc Natl Acad Sci U S A. 110(38):15389-94, 2013
4. Mirzoeva OK et al: Subtype-Specific MEK-PI3 Kinase Feedback as a Therapeutic Target in Pancreatic Adenocarcinoma. Mol Cancer Ther. 12(10):2213-2225, 2013
5. Murphy SJ et al: Genetic Alterations Associated With Progression From Pancreatic Intraepithelial Neoplasia to Invasive Pancreatic Tumor. Gastroenterology. Epub ahead of print, 2013
6. Wang WY et al: A Gene Expression Signature of Epithelial Tubulogenesis and a Role for ASPM in Pancreatic Tumor Progression. Gastroenterology. Epub ahead of print, 2013
7. Xue Y et al: MicroRNAs as diagnostic markers for pancreatic ductal adenocarcinoma and its precursor, pancreatic intraepithelial neoplasm. Cancer Genet. 206(6):217-21, 2013
8. Bartsch DK et al: Familial pancreatic cancer--current knowledge. Nat Rev Gastroenterol Hepatol. 9(8):445-53, 2012
9. Shi C et al: Familial pancreatic cancer. Arch Pathol Lab Med. 133(3):365-74, 2009
10. Hruban RH et al: Pancreatic adenocarcinoma: update on the surgical pathology of carcinomas of ductal origin and PanINs. Mod Pathol. 20 Suppl 1:S61-70, 2007
11. Cubilla A et al: Pancreas cancer. I. Duct adenocarcinoma. A clinical-pathologic study of 380 patients. Pathol Annu. 13 Pt 1:241-89, 1978

PANCREATIC DUCTAL ADENOCARCINOMA

Microscopic Features

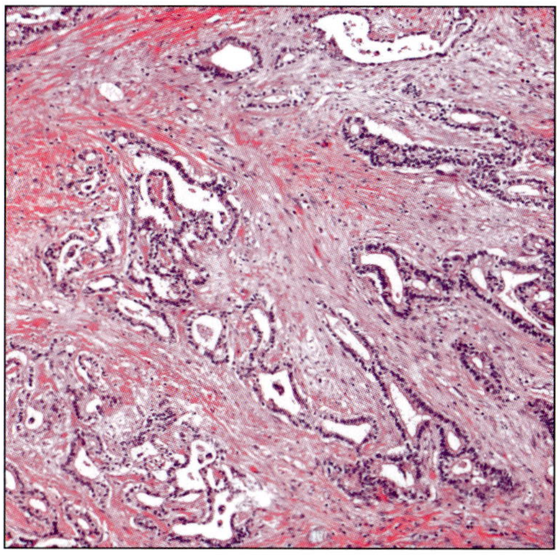

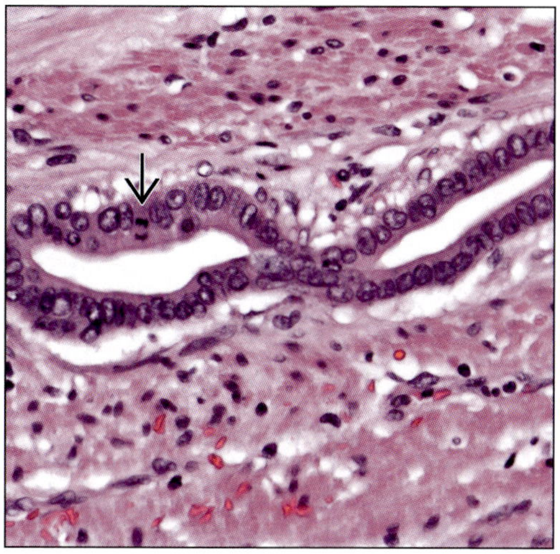

(Left) *Ductal adenocarcinoma typically features small to medium-sized glands with haphazard growth embedded in dense desmoplastic stroma.* ***(Right)*** *Cytologic clues to the diagnosis of well-differentiated pancreatic adenocarcinoma include variation in nuclear size, haphazard arrangement of nuclei, irregular nuclear membranes, and mitoses →.*

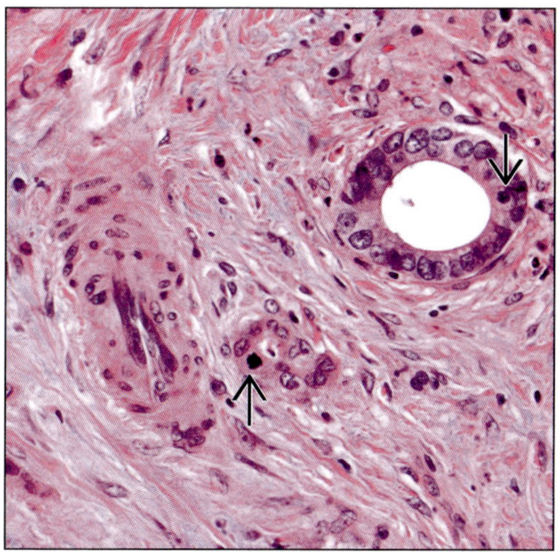

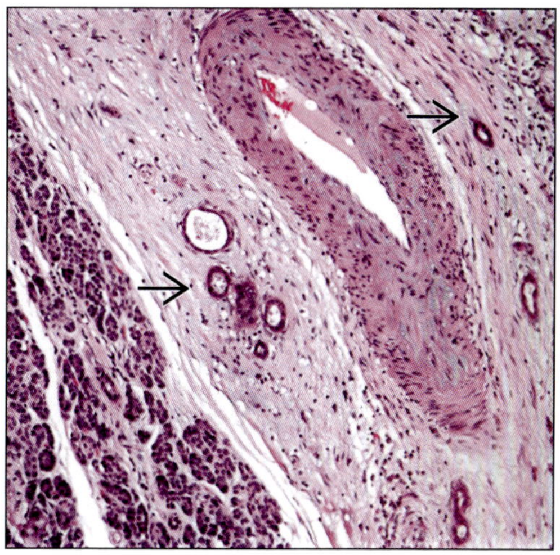

(Left) *Glands directly adjacent to a muscular artery are a clue to malignancy. Note the prominent mitoses → and irregular nuclear membranes in these neoplastic glands.* ***(Right)*** *This photograph shows small infiltrating malignant glands → directly adjacent to a muscular artery without intervening acinar parenchyma. This abnormal growth pattern is a sign of malignancy.*

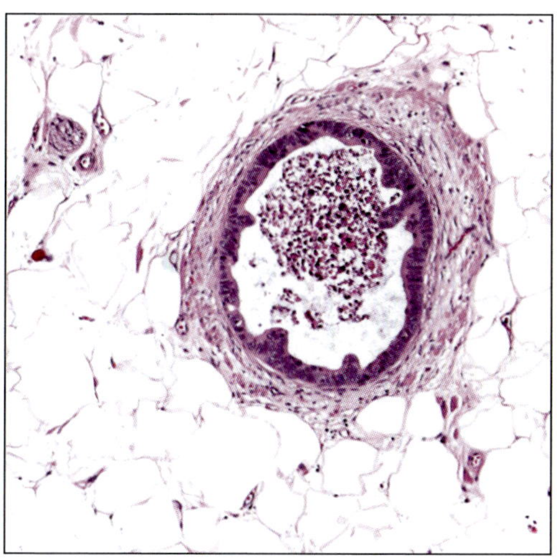

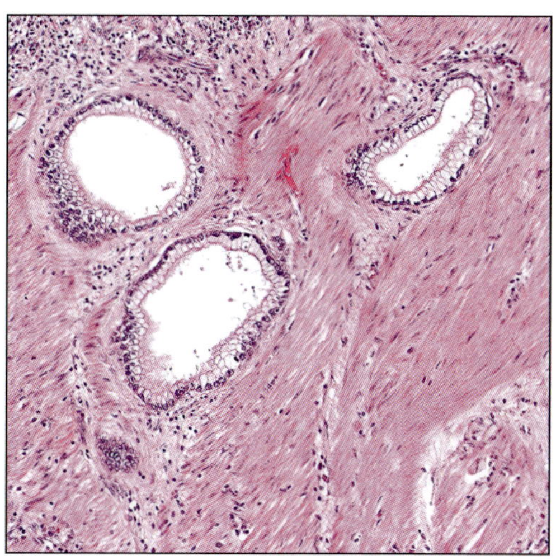

(Left) *This well-differentiated malignant gland is present within the peripancreatic fat.* ***(Right)*** *The foamy gland pattern features well-formed glands with clear foamy cytoplasm. In this case, the tumor infiltrates the muscularis propria of the duodenum.*

PANCREATIC DUCTAL ADENOCARCINOMA

Microscopic Features

(Left) This foamy gland pattern features basally located round nuclei, microvesicular cytoplasm, and distinctive cytoplasmic condensation (brush border-like zone) ➔. The cytology is deceptively bland and mimics pancreatic intraepithelial neoplasm (PanIN) 1A. *(Right)* This high-power photograph of the foamy gland pattern shows a group of cells with microvesicular cytoplasm, raisinoid nuclei, and a low nuclear to cytoplasmic ratio. This pattern may mimic a collection of foamy histiocytes.

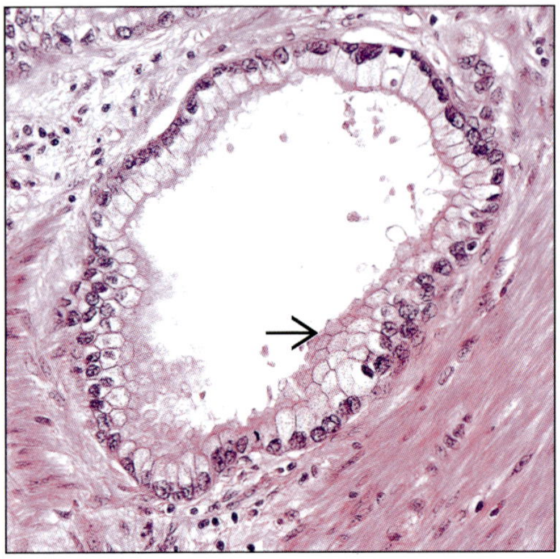

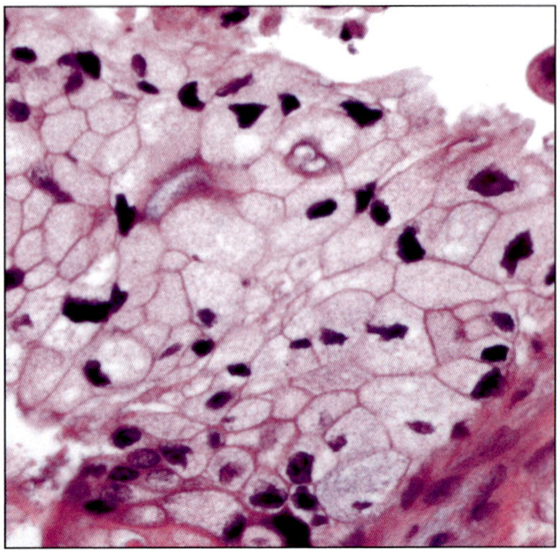

(Left) The mucinous or colloid pattern of pancreatic adenocarcinoma features neoplastic epithelium that is suspended in, or partially lines, large pools of extracellular mucin. *(Right)* A high-power view of the mucinous (colloid) pattern shows detached clusters of malignant cells floating in pools of mucin. Colloid carcinomas are almost always associated with intraductal papillary mucinous neoplasm, especially of the intestinal type.

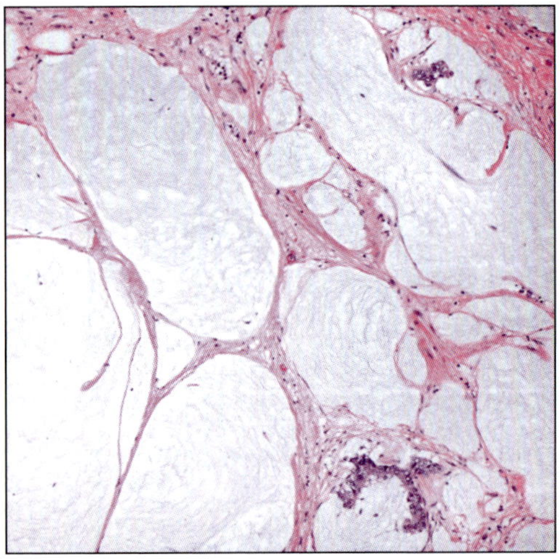

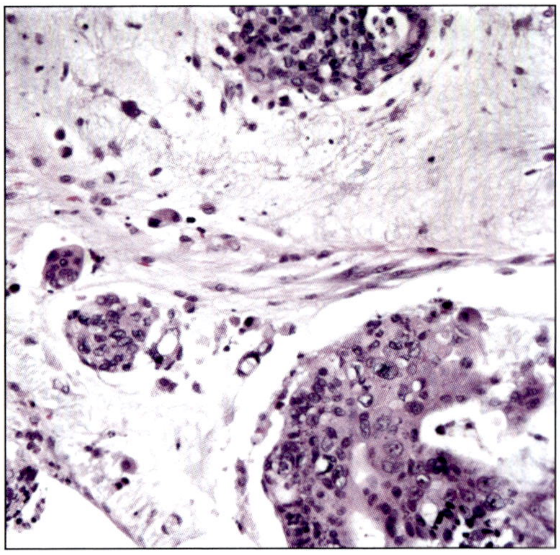

(Left) A large component of the tumor cells have signet ring cell morphology in this signet ring cell variant of pancreatic ductal adenocarcinoma. *(Right)* This example of poorly differentiated adenocarcinoma lacks well-formed glands. The tumor is composed of sheets of poorly differentiated tumor cells as well as single malignant cells. Heterogeneous morphology, encompassing well, moderate, and poor differentiations, is often seen in pancreatic ductal adenocarcinoma.

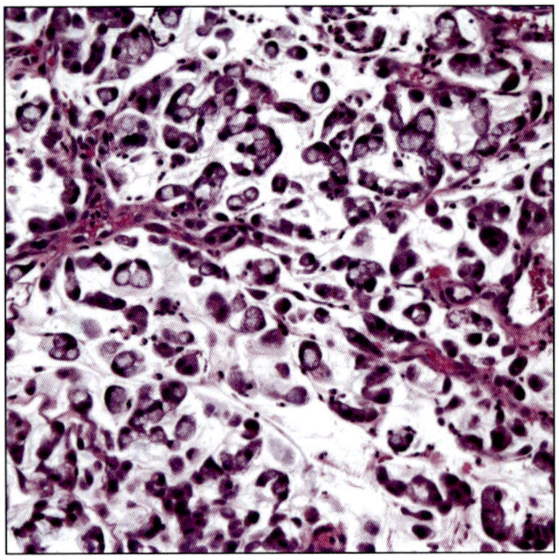

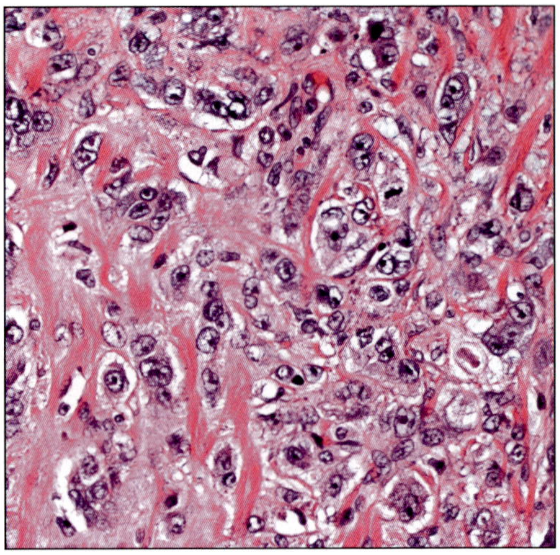

Microscopic Features

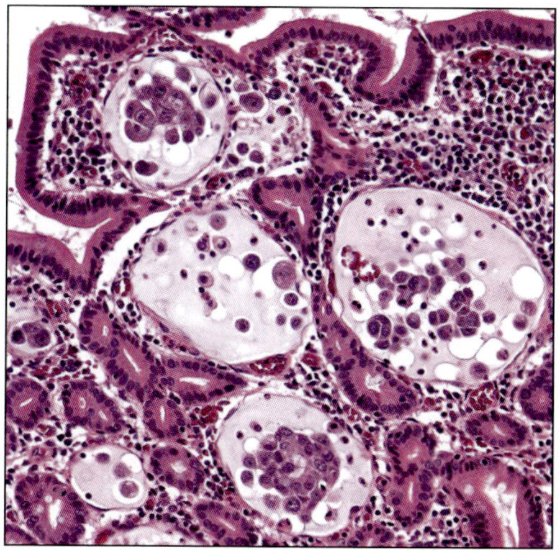

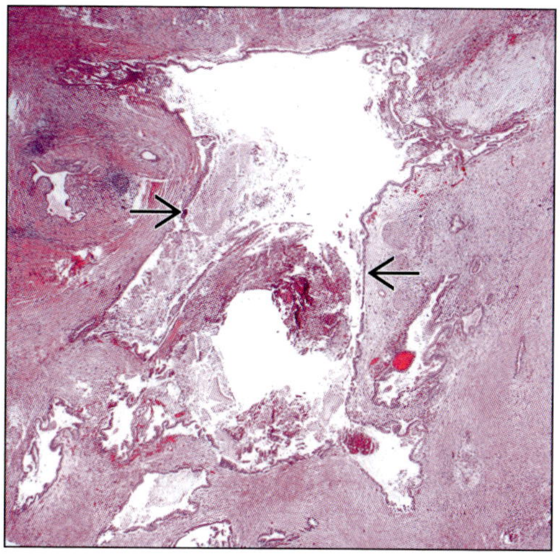

(Left) *This photograph shows extensive involvement of the duodenal lymphovascular spaces by pancreatic ductal adenocarcinoma.* ***(Right)*** *Ductal adenocarcinoma, large duct type, is characterized by cystically dilated neoplastic ducts → that can mimic PanIN or branch-duct intraductal papillary mucinous neoplasm (IPMN). It can be differentiated from the latter based on the absence of low-grade epithelium in the duct lining.*

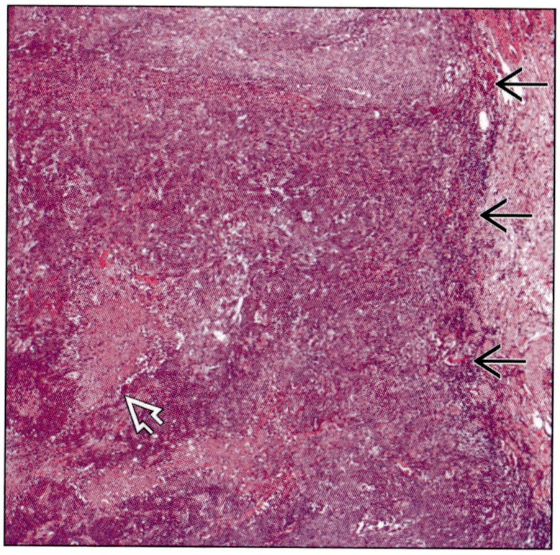

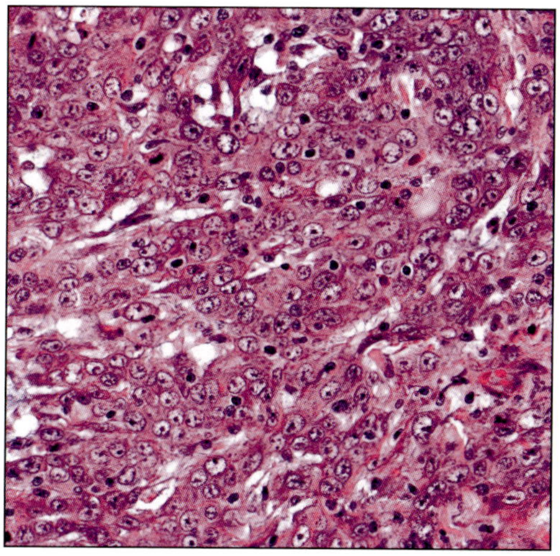

(Left) *This example of the medullary variant of pancreatic ductal carcinoma has well-defined borders → and foci of necrosis ➡.* ***(Right)*** *Medullary pancreatic carcinoma features a syncytial growth pattern containing poorly differentiated cells with scattered tumor-infiltrating lymphocytes.*

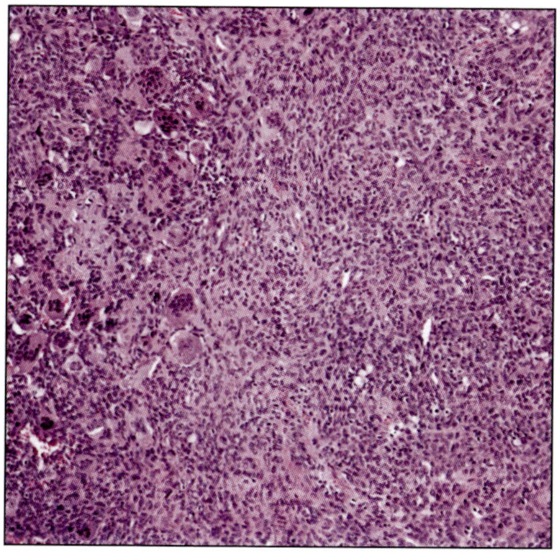

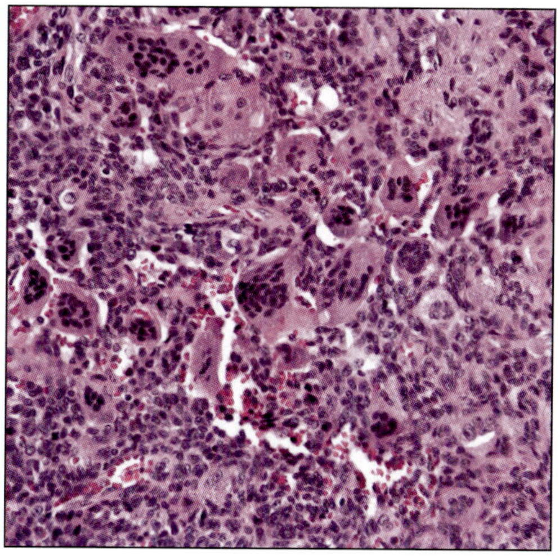

(Left) *This case of undifferentiated pancreatic ductal adenocarcinoma shows clusters of giant cells on the left and a poorly differentiated, spindled pattern on the right. The undifferentiated variant may or may not have giant cells.* ***(Right)*** *This high-power photomicrograph highlights the numerous giant cells in this case of undifferentiated pancreatic ductal adenocarcinoma.*

Genitourinary

Collecting System

Genital Tract

Kidney

BLADDER CARCINOMA

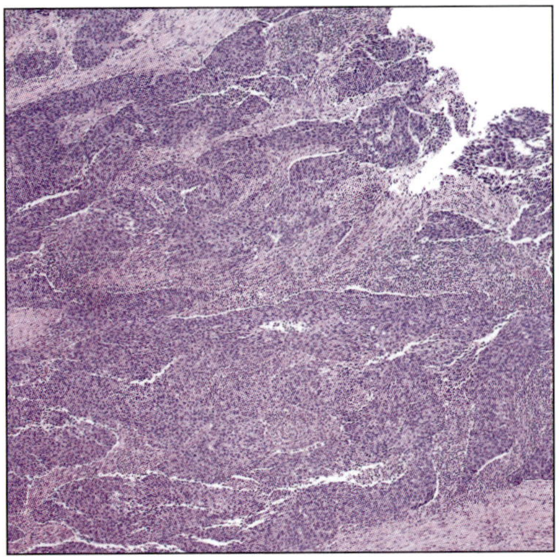

Low-power view shows urothelial carcinoma (UCa) extensively infiltrating the lamina propria. The invasive UCa nests are haphazard and show reactive desmoplastic response in the stroma.

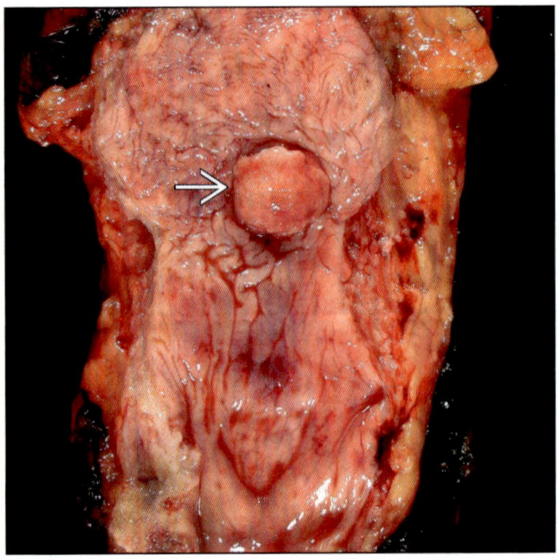

Gross photograph shows a large polypoid mass of UCa ➔ at the posterior bladder wall. Most UCas arise at the trigonal/bladder outlet area.

TERMINOLOGY

Synonyms

- Transitional cell carcinoma

Definitions

- In USA, > 90% of bladder carcinomas are urothelial carcinoma (UCa); < 10% are squamous cell carcinoma, adenocarcinoma, and small cell carcinoma
- Flat urothelial neoplasm
  - **Urothelial dysplasia**
    - Flat growth by urothelial cells thought to be neoplastic but cytologically falls below threshold for carcinoma in situ (CIS)
  - **Urothelial CIS**
    - Flat growth by cytologically malignant urothelial cells that has not invaded through basement membrane
- Papillary urothelial neoplasm
  - Urothelial neoplasm with papillary growth on fibrovascular stalk in exophytic or endophytic manner
  - WHO/ISUP 2004 grading for papillary neoplasm
    - **Urothelial papilloma**
    - **Papillary urothelial neoplasm of low malignant potential (PUNLMP)**
    - **Papillary UCa (PUCa), low grade**
    - **PUCa, high grade**
- Invasive UCa
  - UCa that invades beyond the basement membrane

ETIOLOGY/PATHOGENESIS

Environmental Exposure

- Tobacco smoking with 2.5x higher risk
- Chemicals such as arylamines (e.g., aniline, 2-naphthylamine, benzidine)

Other Possible Risk Factors

- Chronic urinary tract infection, calculi, drugs (e.g., analgesics and cyclophosphamide)
- Schistosomiasis is well-established risk factor for squamous cell carcinoma but may also increase risk for UCa

Model of Bladder Cancer Development and Progression (Dual Track Pathway)

- Alterations in Chr 9 initiating event to either pathway
  - **Hyperplasia/papillary pathway**
    - 70-80% transform to hyperplastic urothelium and progress to low-grade prostate carcinoma (PCa)
    - Linked to mutations in *HRAS* and *FGFR3*
    - Most tumors recur as PUCa, and ~ 15% become invasive UCa by alterations in *P53* and *RB*
  - **Flat pathway**
    - 20-30% transform to CIS/dysplasia
    - Linked to alterations in *P53* and *RB*
    - Most tumors progress to invasive UCa

CLINICAL ISSUES

Epidemiology

- Incidence
  - Bladder cancer is 4th leading cause of cancer morbidity and 8th cause of cancer mortality in USA
- Age
  - Disease of older adults with peak incidence in 70s; rare in individuals younger than 45 years old
  - Urothelial papilloma and PUNLMP relatively more common in patients < 50 years old
- Gender
  - 3-4x more common in men than women
- Ethnicity
  - About 2x more common in whites than blacks

BLADDER CARCINOMA

Key Facts

Clinical Issues

- Bladder cancer is 4th leading cause of cancer morbidity and 8th cause of cancer mortality in USA
- Disease of older adults with peak incidence in 70s; rare in individuals younger than 45 years old
- 3-4x more common in men than women
- About 2x more common in whites than blacks

Microscopic Pathology

- **Urothelial CIS**: Flat urothelial neoplasm with unequivocal high-grade cytology
- **Low-grade PUCa**: Papillae lined by urothelium with mild degree of distortion and low-grade dysplasia
- **High-grade PUCa**: Papillae lined by urothelium with moderate to high-grade cytology
- **Inverted papillary urothelial carcinoma**: Endophytic rounded growth into lamina propria with regular outline and absent stromal reaction
- **Invasive UCa**
  - Irregular jagged nests, single cell infiltration, or tentacular finger-like projections
  - May show ↑ amount of cytoplasm and eosinophilia (squamoid change)
  - Stroma may have desmoplasia, retraction artifact, myxoid change, or pseudosarcomatous stroma
- Variants include UCa with divergent differentiation, nested UCa, micropapillary UCa, plasmacytoid UCa, and lymphoepithelioma-like UCa among others
- Urothelial lineage-associated markers GATA3 and S100P help confirm UCa
- CK7(+), CK20(+/-), HMWCK(+), and p63(+)

Presentation

- Hematuria, dysuria, and frequency
- Advanced disease may present with abdominal pain and weight loss

Natural History

- Most patients present with PUCa before or concurrently with CIS
- Primary (de novo) or isolated CIS without prior or concurrent PUCa rare

Prognosis

- For noninvasive urothelial neoplasm, dependent on grade
  - Urothelial papilloma: 0% recurrence
  - PUNLMP: 25-47% recurrence
  - Low-grade PUCa: 48-71% recurrence, < 5% progression and death
  - High-grade PUCa: 20% progression to invasive UCa
  - CIS: ~ 50% progress to invasive UCa in 5 years
- For invasive UCa, dependent on stage
- Locally advanced disease, even in absence of lymph node metastasis, is associated with poor prognosis
  - Estimated 5-year overall survival rates for pT3aN0, pT3bN0, and pT4aN0 disease are 64%, 49%, and 44%, respectively
- Most variant morphology of UCa presents with higher stage; behavior may be similar to usual UCa when compared stage to stage

MACROSCOPIC FEATURES

General Features

- Most common site is trigone/bladder outlet
- More often multifocal
- Noninvasive PUCa
  - Elevated or papillary lesion, which may increase in size and complexity with increasing grade
  - Inverted growth has more nodular appearance
  - Low or high-grade PUCa can be small or large; grading based on cytology; urothelial papilloma and PUNLMP generally < 2 cm
- CIS
  - Mucosal erythema or discoloration
- Invasive UCa
  - Papillary, polypoid, fungating, or ulcerating solid mass

MICROSCOPIC PATHOLOGY

Histologic Features

- **Urothelial CIS**
  - Unequivocal high-grade cytology
  - Marked nucleomegaly, irregular nuclei, prominent nucleoli, coarse dark chromatin, and abundant mitosis
  - Cellular crowding and loss of polarity
  - Morphologic variations
    - Clinging CIS: Denudation with few residual preserved CIS cells
    - Pagetoid CIS: Individual malignant cells spread in adjacent benign urothelium
    - Undermining CIS: Clusters of malignant cells covered by benign urothelium
    - May extend to involve von Brunn nests or cystitis cystica/glandularis in lamina propria
- **PUNLMP**
  - Papillae lined by thickened urothelium with normal cytology and maintained polarity
  - Papillae with minimal branching
- **Low-grade PUCa**
  - Papillae lined by urothelium with mild degree of architectural distortion and low-grade dysplasia
  - Pleomorphism is random
  - Mitosis may be present at base
- **High-grade PUCa**
  - Papillae lined by urothelium with moderate to high-grade cytology
  - Nucleomegaly, irregular nuclei, prominent nucleoli, and coarse dark chromatin

BLADDER CARCINOMA

- Mitosis may be brisk and seen in all layers
- Papillae exhibit architectural complexities, including branching, confluence, and fusion
- May have epithelial denudation

- **Inverted papillary urothelial carcinoma**
  - Endophytic rounded growth into lamina propria with regular outline and absent stromal reaction
  - Similar to exophytic PUCa, classified as PUNLMP, low or high grade based on cytologic atypia
- **Invasive UCa**
  - Invasive epithelial features
    - Irregular jagged nests, single cell infiltration, or tentacular finger-like projections
    - May show ↑ amount of cytoplasm and eosinophilia (squamoid change) referred to as "paradoxical differentiation"
    - Vast majority of invasive UCa exhibits high-grade cytology, notable exception in some variant morphologies
  - Stromal changes
    - Desmoplasia, retraction artifact, myxoid change, pseudosarcomatous stroma, or no stromal response
- **Variant morphology of UCa**
  - **UCa with divergent differentiation**
    - UCa may exhibit glandular (i.e., adenocarcinoma) or squamous differentiation
    - Squamous differentiation with cell bridges, keratinization, and keratin pearl formation
    - Glandular differentiation includes enteric gland, mucinous gland, or signet ring cell formation
    - Divergent differentiation can be extensive; surface CIS or PUCa that can be focal is clue for diagnosis
  - **Nested UCa**
    - Invasive UCa with deceptively benign appearance growing as infiltrating nests of bland-appearing malignant urothelial cells
    - At the surface, it closely resembles von Brunn nest proliferation
    - Unlike von Brunn nest, nested UCa shows more irregular nests with confluence and back-to-back pattern, and shows at least random pleomorphism
    - Most do not have surface CIS or PUCa component
    - Most present with (at least) muscle-invasive disease
    - Lymphovascular invasion common
  - **Large-nested UCa**
    - Invasive UCa consisting of large nests with pushing borders
    - Nests are typically more apart and connect to surface
    - Cells have low-grade cytology
    - Most have surface CIS or PUCa component
  - **UCa with small tubules**
    - Invasive UCa with predominance of tubular change
    - Similar to nested variant, composed of bland-appearing malignant urothelial cells
    - Nested UCa may have focal tubular change
    - May look like tubular nephrogenic adenoma or Gleason 3 prostatic adenocarcinoma
  - **Microcystic UCa**
    - Invasive UCa with small and large cysts (suggested to be at least 25%)
    - Cysts are lined by transitional or flattened cells and may have eosinophilic luminal secretions
    - Similar to nested variant, composed of bland-appearing malignant cells
    - Does not contain glandular cells
    - May resemble cystitis cystica at surface
  - **Micropapillary UCa**
    - Small nests or micropapillae in retraction-like spaces
    - Resembles micropapillary carcinoma of breast or ovary
    - Most exhibit high-grade cytology
    - Nuclei polarized exterior of nests
    - Multiple nests may be seen inside spaces
    - Surface PUCa may exhibit micropapillations or filiforms in layers of malignant urothelial cells
  - **Plasmacytoid UCa**
    - Invasive UCa characterized by infiltrative dyscohesive cells with eccentric nuclei that resemble plasma cells or poorly differentiated carcinoma
    - Tumor cells express plasma cell-associated marker CD138; a potential pitfall
    - Amount of plasmacytoid morphology varies in published series, although most report it to be at least 30%
    - Invasive tumor cells in single cells, cords (resembling lobular carcinoma), small nests, or solid sheets
    - May form a mass or is widely infiltrative in a linitis plastica-like spread
    - Has propensity to spread or recur in serosal spaces, such as in peritoneum presenting as carcinomatosis
  - **Lymphoepithelioma-like carcinoma**
    - Invasive UCa characterized by syncytium of poorly differentiated UCa in background of dense lymphoplasmacytic infiltrates
    - Resembles undifferentiated nasopharyngeal carcinoma; not EBV related
  - **UCa with rhabdoid features**
    - Exceedingly rare and occurs in association with poorly differentiated UCa
    - Characterized by plump oval to round cells with abundant cytoplasm and intracytoplasmic inclusion displacing nuclei
    - Rhabdoid cells are dyscohesive, infiltrating as single cells, in small nests, or as diffuse sheets
  - **Lipid-rich UCa**
    - Presence of large cells that contain multiple clear vacuoles, which indent nucleus to resemble lipoblasts or signet ring cells
    - Almost always admixed with conventional or other variants of UCa
    - Lipid-rich cells comprise 10-50% of tumor
  - **Clear cell (glycogen-rich) UCa**
    - Tumor cells with clear cytoplasm and may show solid alveolar growth to resemble clear cell renal cell carcinoma
  - **Sarcomatoid UCa/carcinosarcoma**

- UCa containing admixture of epithelial and mesenchymal malignancies by morphology or immunophenotype
- Epithelial component may include invasive UCa, CIS, or PUCa
- Mesenchymal component often malignant spindle cells
- Heterologous malignant mesenchymal elements may be present, such as bone (osteosarcoma), cartilage (chondrosarcoma), or skeletal muscles (rhabdomyosarcoma)

- **UCa with trophoblastic cells**
  - UCa may contain trophoblastic cells with associated production of βHCG, confirmed by immunohistochemistry &/or serum or urine assay
  - ~ 35% of UCa may express βHCG, usually higher grade tumors, with more staining in more undifferentiated or anaplastic cells
  - "Pure" choriocarcinoma may occur rarely in bladder; may arise from urothelial metaplasia
  - Prognosis and treatment response to radiation poorer in UCa with βHCG expression
- **UCa with myxoid stroma and chordoid features**
  - UCa with abundant extracellular mucin in absence of glandular differentiation
  - Tumor cells arranged in microcysts or small cellular aggregates
  - Resembles extraskeletal myxoid chondrosarcoma, chordoma, and myxomatous yolk sac tumor
- **UCa with osteoclast giant cells**
  - Solid growth of mononuclear cells with evenly distributed osteoclast giant cells
  - Mononuclear cells are plump with ovoid to round nuclei with vesicular chromatin, mostly exhibiting mild atypia

ANCILLARY TESTS

Immunohistochemistry

- Urothelial lineage-associated markers GATA3 and S100P help confirm UCa
  - GATA3 is also expressed by breast ductal carcinoma, a subset of cervical carcinomas and paraganglioma
- UCa mostly CK7(+), CK20(+/-), HMCK(+), thrombomodulin (+), and p63(+)
- Uroplakin most specific for urothelial lineage; however suffers from low sensitivity, particularly in higher grade tumors
- Smoothelin shows differential strong expression in muscularis propria vs. muscularis mucosae and can be useful in staging of muscle-invasive disease

DIFFERENTIAL DIAGNOSIS

Poorly Differentiated Prostate Carcinoma

- May be difficult to distinguish from poorly differentiated UCa
- Relatively more monomorphic and does not usually exhibit marked pleomorphism
- May have associated glandular growth of cells with prominent nucleoli
- PSA, PAP, or PSMA (+)
- GATA3, p63, or HMWCK (-)

Gynecologic Carcinomas Involving Bladder

- Cervical squamous carcinoma
  - p63(+) and a subset is GATA3(+)
  - Lacks CIS or PUCa component in bladder surface
- Poorly differentiated uterine carcinomas
  - Often WT1(+), GATA3(-)

Pseudocarcinomatous Hyperplasia

- May simulate invasive UCa
- Often with prior radiotherapy or chemotherapy
- Squamoid changes present and associated with blood vessels and fibrin
- Mucosal hemorrhage common and diffuse radiation-induced atypia present (if patient has history)

Papillary Nephrogenic Adenoma

- May mimic PUCa
- Papillae lined by 1 or few layers of cells and with associated tubular proliferations
- Cells lack atypia and may exhibit hobnailing
- pax-2(+) and GATA3(-), or p63(-)

DIAGNOSTIC CHECKLIST

Clinically Relevant Pathologic Features

- Histologic type, including presence and amount of variant morphology
- Grade, most meaningful in noninvasive UCa
- Stage
  - In transurethral resection (TUR) specimens, diagnosis of high-grade UCa requires reporting of presence or absence of muscularis propria and status of involvement
    - Muscle should be specified if muscularis propria; reporting as "muscle present" is not appropriate
    - Repeat TUR is required if muscularis propria is not present for sampling adequacy
- Margin status in cystectomy

SELECTED REFERENCES

1. Amin MB: Histological variants of urothelial carcinoma: diagnostic, therapeutic and prognostic implications. Mod Pathol. 22 Suppl 2:S96-S118, 2009
2. Zhai QJ et al: Histologic variants of infiltrating urothelial carcinoma. Arch Pathol Lab Med. 131(8):1244-56, 2007
3. McKenney JK et al: The role of immunohistochemistry in the diagnosis of urinary bladder neoplasms. Semin Diagn Pathol. 22(1):69-87, 2005
4. Wu XR: Urothelial tumorigenesis: a tale of divergent pathways. Nat Rev Cancer. 5(9):713-25, 2005
5. Eble JN et al: World Health Organization Classification of Tumours. Pathology & Genetics. Tumours of the Urinary System and Male Genital Organs. Lyon: IARC Press, 2004

BLADDER CARCINOMA

Papillary and Flat Urothelial Neoplasms

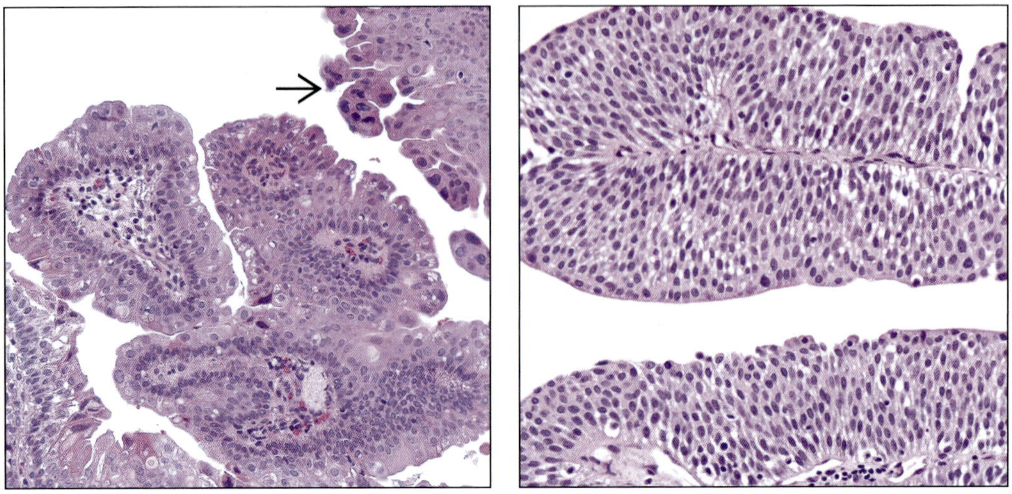

(Left) *Urothelial papilloma shows papillae lined by normal-appearing urothelium, including presence of surface umbrella cells →. The cells lack cellular atypia or mitoses.* ***(Right)*** *PUNLMP, in contrast to urothelial papilloma, shows increased thickness of urothelial cells with bland cytology. Nuclei are oblong, and tumor characteristically exhibits well-maintained cellular polarity from base toward the surface. Papillae with central fibrovascular core are often simple, delicate, and do not exhibit complex branching and fusion.*

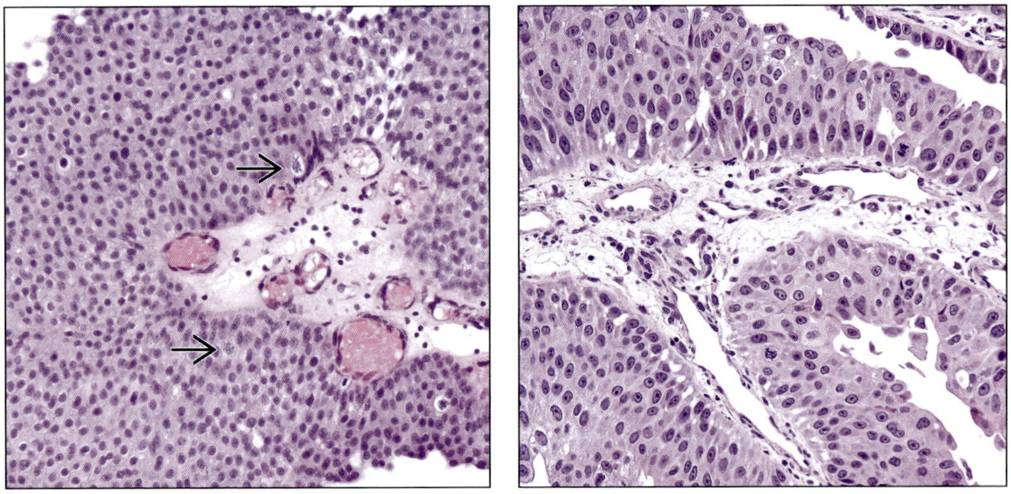

(Left) *Low-grade PUCa shows tumor cells with nuclear rounding and mildly disordered cell polarity. Mitoses can be seen, usually at the base →.* ***(Right)*** *High-grade PUCa shows tumor cells with unequivocal high-grade cytology. The nuclei are enlarged and more rounded and have irregular outlines and marked nucleomegaly. There is loss of the normal perpendicular arrangement of cells toward the surface. Note that grading of papillary neoplasm is based on cytomorphology of neoplastic cells.*

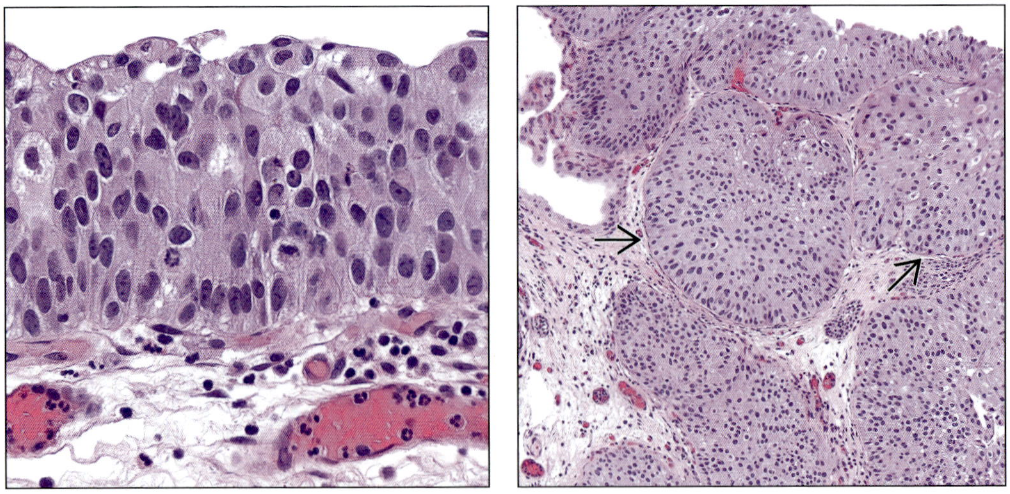

(Left) *UCa in situ shows cellular pleomorphism and presence of enlarged irregular hyperchromatic nuclei. There is such marked disorganization of the neoplastic cells that, in some places, the nuclei overlap. Note presence of prominent nucleoli and abundant mitoses.* ***(Right)*** *UCa in situ from the surface may extend downward to involve von Brunn nests →. Recognition of this extension is important not to overcall as invasion into the lamina propria, particularly in fragmented specimens.*

Invasive Urothelial Carcinoma

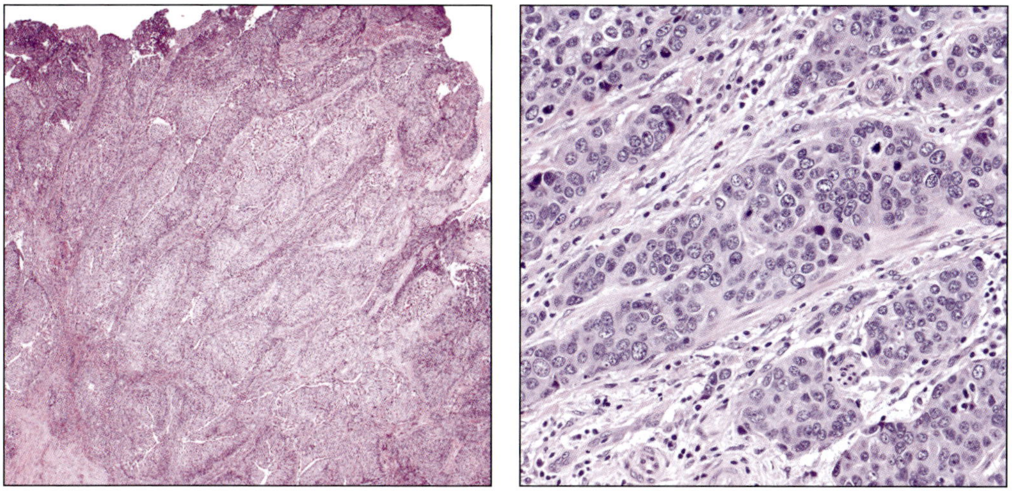

(Left) *Low-power view shows UCa with extensive invasion of the lamina propria. Recognition of the depth of invasion in the bladder wall is important for staging of invasive UCa, including in transurethral resection specimens.* ***(Right)*** *These invasive nests of UCa are irregular, variable in size, jagged, and surrounded by desmoplastic reaction. The neoplastic cells have modest eosinophilic cytoplasm and exhibit pleomorphism, enlarged crowded nuclei, and brisk mitotic activity.*

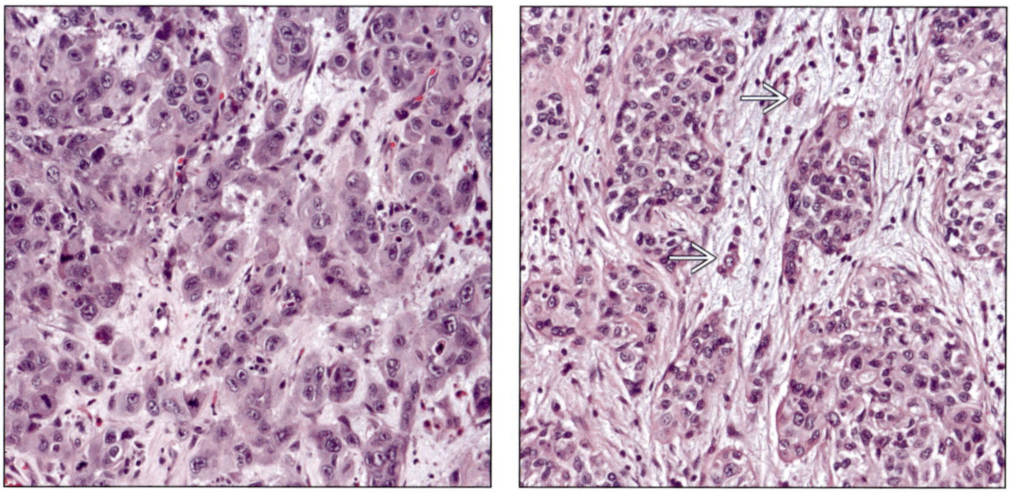

(Left) *Invasive UCa shows some smaller nests and individual infiltrating cells with abundant cytoplasm. This paradoxical differentiation or squamoid change, particularly if appreciated in single cells or small nests, is almost diagnostic for invasion. Note presence of stromal desmoplasia.* ***(Right)*** *Invasive UCa shows infiltrating larger and smaller nests and single cells ➔. The invasive nests dissect in the desmoplastic stroma. Note that some of the cells have relatively more abundant cytoplasm.*

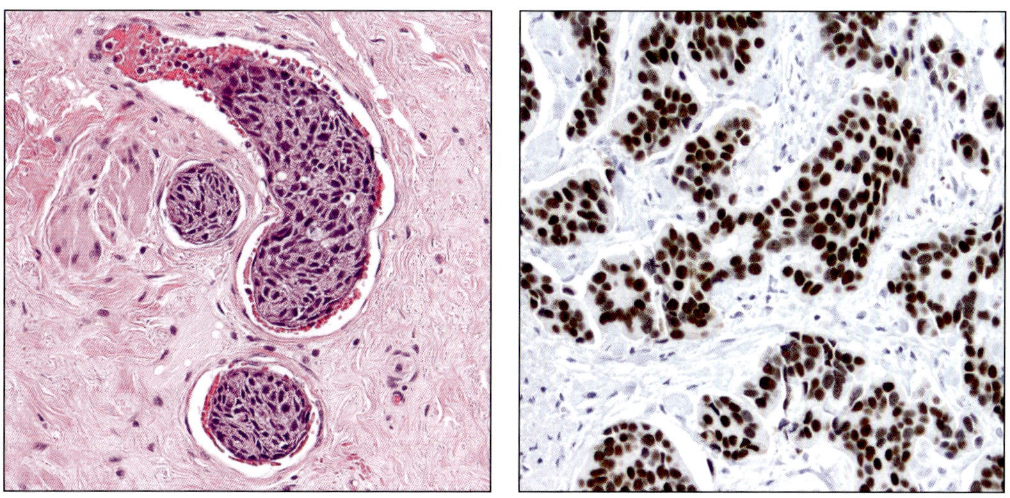

(Left) *UCa exhibits lymphovascular invasion (LVI). The tumor clusters follow the contour of blood vessels. Note presence of admixed hematopoietic cells in the lumen. UCa commonly exhibits retraction artifact and should be distinguished from LVI.* ***(Right)*** *GATA3 shows diffuse nuclear staining of UCa and is useful in distinguishing UCa from nonurothelial tumors in bladder and at metastatic sites. Ductal carcinoma of the breast and some cervical carcinomas may also express GATA3.*

BLADDER CARCINOMA

Staging, Immunohistochemistry, & Variant Morphologies

(Left) *UCa shows invasion into the muscularis propria layer and is considered one of the crossroads for radical management. Identification of the presence of muscularis propria and reporting of status of involvement is warranted for staging adequacy.* ***(Right)*** *Low-power view of invasive UCa shows tumor infiltrating through the muscularis propria layer and into the perivesical soft tissue →. Boundary between muscularis propria and perivesical tissue is often irregular, making staging of microscopic invasion at this site difficult.*

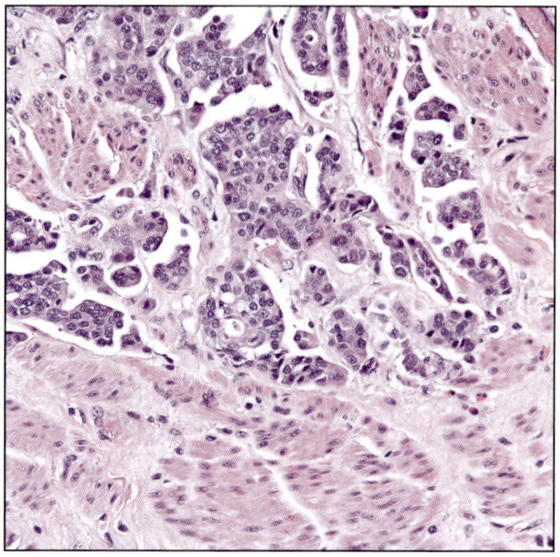

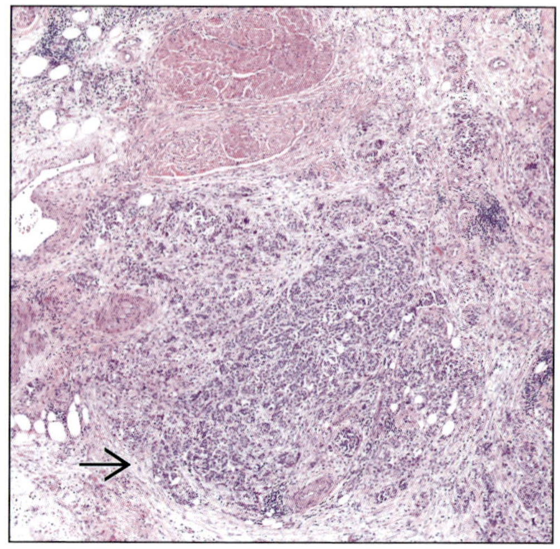

(Left) *CK20 shows diffuse full-thickness staining of urothelium in UCa in situ. In benign and reactive urothelium, CK20 staining is seen only at the surface umbrella cells or is absent. CD44 is often used to complement CK20, which shows full-thickness staining in reactive urothelium and only basal or absent staining in UCa in situ.* ***(Right)*** *p53 shows increased nuclear staining in UCa in situ. Diffuse staining (> 50% positive nuclei) is helpful, but may not always be present, in UCa in situ.*

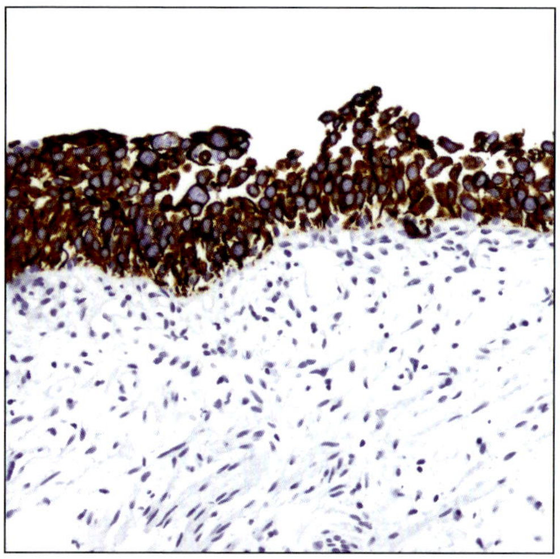

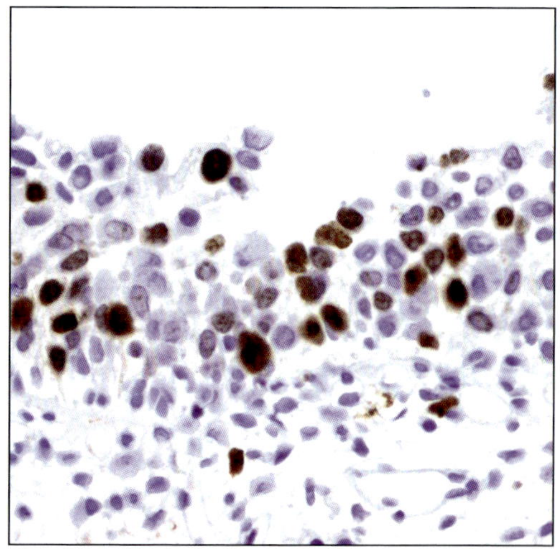

(Left) *Low-power view shows UCa with glandular differentiation. Part of the tumor shows UCa with solid nests of polygonal malignant cells ↗. In addition, there is adenocarcinoma characterized by glandular structures lined by tall columnar cells →.* ***(Right)*** *Low-power view of invasive UCa with squamous differentiation shows prominent keratin production. Search for UCa component, particularly at the surface as in this case, is important to distinguish this tumor from pure squamous cell carcinoma.*

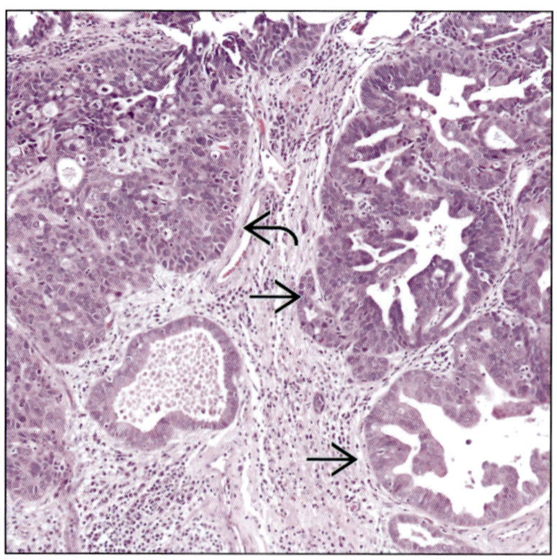

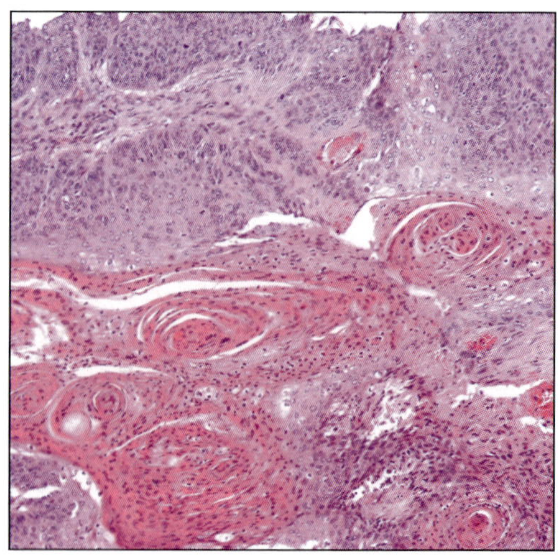

Variant Morphologies

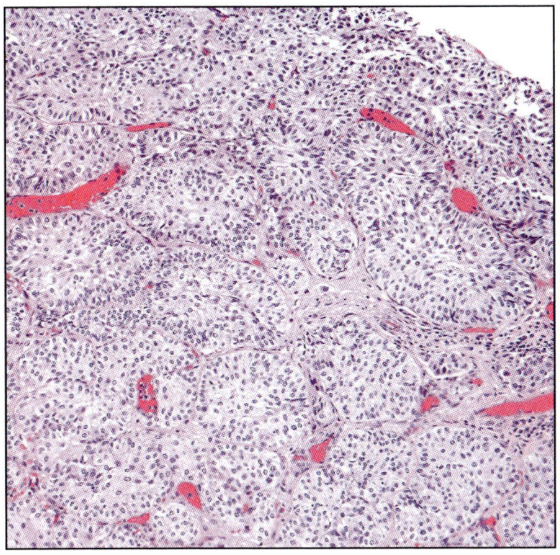

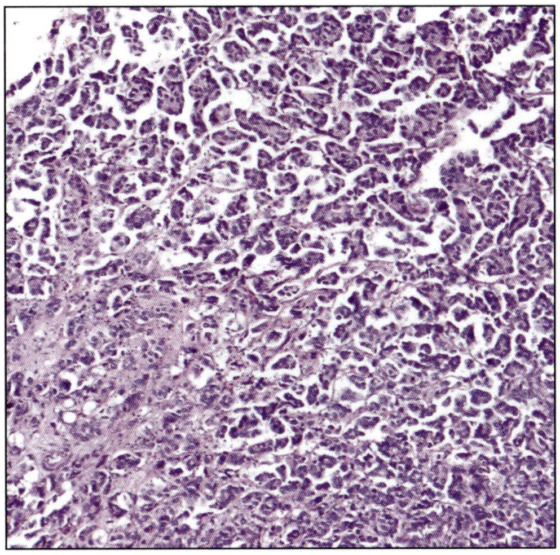

(Left) *Nested UCa shows nests of bland-appearing cells that resemble a von Brunn nest proliferation. Distinction of this variant can be very difficult in superficial biopsy. Compared to von Brunn nests, nested UCa may show more irregular, tightly packed nests with confluence and fusion. Identification of muscularis propria invasion is key in making the diagnosis.* ***(Right)*** *Micropapillary UCa shows small nests of carcinoma cells within lacunar spaces that are often back-to-back.*

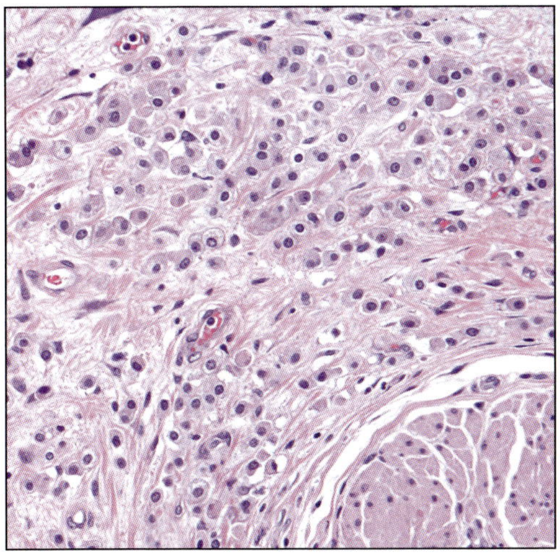

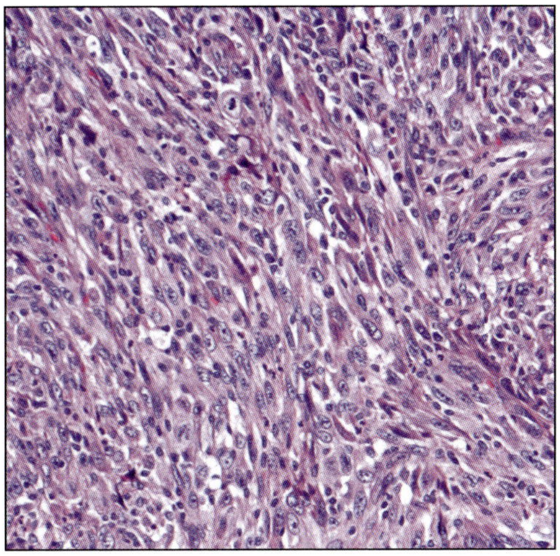

(Left) *Plasmacytoid UCa shows infiltrating dyscohesive individual tumor cell with abundant cytoplasm and off-centric nucleus mimicking plasma cells. Tumor cells may also express plasma-cell-associated marker CD138. This variant usually presents with higher stage and greater proclivity for extension into serosal surfaces.* ***(Right)*** *Sarcomatoid UCa shows presence of high-grade spindle cells. Heterologous elements (e.g., malignant bone, cartilage) may arise from this tumor.*

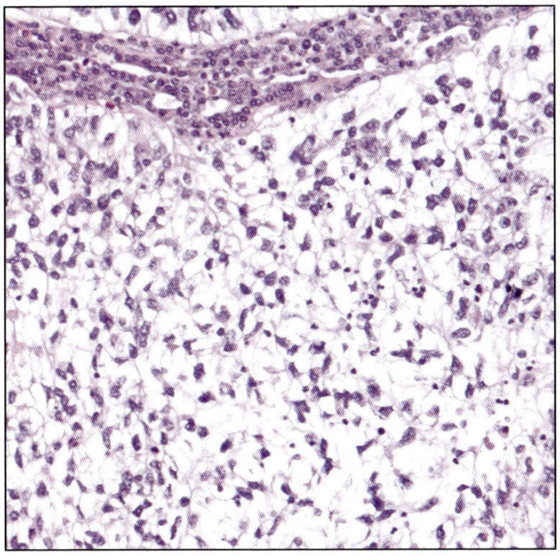

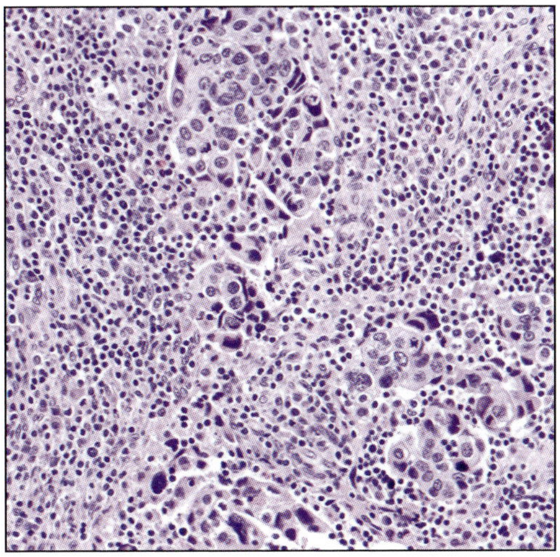

(Left) *Clear cell UCa shows neoplastic cells with clear cytoplasm mimicking clear cell renal cell carcinoma.* ***(Right)*** *Lymphoepithelioma-like carcinoma is characterized by presence of syncytium of poorly differentiated UCa cells in a background of dense lymphoplasmacytic infiltrates resembling undifferentiated carcinoma in nasopharynx. Tumor cells may be masked by the background infiltrates and mimic an inflammatory process. Epithelial markers can highlight the UCa cells.*

URETER UROTHELIAL CARCINOMA

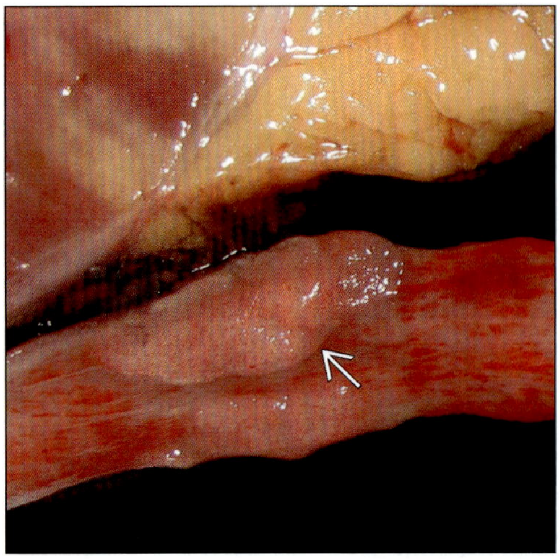

Gross image of a segment of an opened ureter shows an irregular sessile polypoid mass ➔ almost filling the ureteral lumina. Urothelial carcinoma (UCa) is relatively more common at the lower ureter.

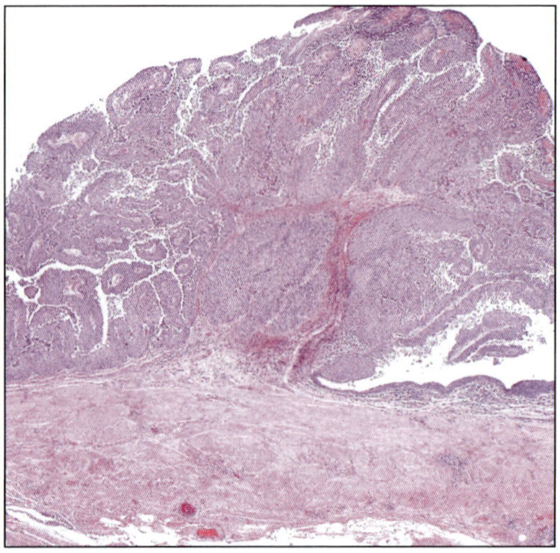

High-grade ureteral UCa shows a complex papillary growth not invading the underlying stroma. Ureteral UCa may exhibit infiltrative or exophytic growths and cause symptoms related to urinary tract obstruction.

TERMINOLOGY

Abbreviations

- Urothelial carcinoma (UCa)

Synonyms

- Ureter transitional cell carcinoma

Definitions

- Carcinoma arising from ureteral urothelium
- Available clinicopathologic data similar with those for renal pelvicaliceal UCa; almost always lumped together in the literature as upper urinary tract cancer

ETIOLOGY/PATHOGENESIS

Risk Factors

- Similar to those in bladder cancer
  - Tobacco, long-term occupational exposure to aromatic carbons and phenacetin

Lynch Syndrome (Hereditary Nonpolyposis Colorectal Cancer Syndrome [HNPCC])

- Autosomal dominant condition with increased risk of cancers of mainly colon, uterus, and upper urinary tract
- Due to inherited mutations in mismatch repair genes, most commonly *MSH2* (~ 90%)
- ~ 6% Lifetime increased risk of upper urinary tract cancer in both ureter and renal pelvis; not established as a risk for bladder UCa
  - Higher incidence of ureter location of UCa in Lynch syndrome at ~ 50%

CLINICAL ISSUES

Epidemiology

- Incidence
  - Rare; estimated that there will be 2,710 new cases and 900 deaths from ureter and other urinary organ cancer in USA in 2013
- Age
  - Range: 40s-90s with peak in 60s-70s; similar to bladder and pelvicaliceal UCa
- Gender
  - More common in men, but lesser gender difference than in bladder UCa

Site

- Distribution of upper urinary tract cancer
  - Renal pelvis 36%, upper ureter 5%, mid ureter 7%, lower ureter 56%, and multifocal 22%

Presentation

- Hematuria, flank pain, irritative voiding symptoms, and weight loss
- May have symptoms related to urinary tract obstruction

Endoscopic Findings

- Papillary, sessile, or infiltrative tumor
- Normal bladder cystoscopy and positive urine cytology suggest upper urinary tract cancer

Treatment

- Surgical approaches
  - Ureterectomy, ± adjuvant therapy depending on stage
- Drugs
  - Unlike in bladder cancer, intraluminal chemotherapy (e.g., BCG, thiotepa) and immunotherapy are sparsely used in ureter cancer and with no guidelines

Prognosis

- Poor survival, similar to pelvicaliceal UCa
- Stage is most important prognostic variable
  - T0: No evidence of primary tumor
  - T1: Tumor invades subepithelial connective tissue

URETER UROTHELIAL CARCINOMA

Key Facts

Etiology/Pathogenesis

- Familial cases: Lynch syndrome or hereditary nonpolyposis colorectal cancer syndrome (HNPCC)
  - ~ 6% lifetime increased risk of upper urinary tract cancer, greater for ureter than renal pelvis

Clinical Issues

- Normal bladder cystoscopy and positive urine cytology suggest upper urinary tract cancer
- Distribution of upper urinary tract cancer
  - Renal pelvis 36%, upper ureter 5%, mid ureter 7%, lower ureter 56%, and multifocal 22%
- Up to ~ 6% will have contralateral ureteral cancer and ~ 17% will have concurrent bladder cancer

Microscopic Pathology

- Classification similar to bladder or pelvicaliceal UCa (WHO, 2004); nonurothelial carcinoma variants rare in ureter

- T2: Tumor invades muscularis propria
- T3: Tumor invades beyond muscularis propria into periureteric fat
- T4: Tumor invades adjacent organ
- N status (N1-N3): Stratified by size of nodal metastasis and number of positive nodes

- UCa in ureter suggested to have worse prognosis than UCa in pelvicaliceal system
  - Some studies, however, showed that after adjustment for tumor stage, location for upper urinary tract cancer is no longer a predictor of cancer-specific survival
- Up to ~ 6% of patients will have contralateral ureteral cancer and ~ 17% will have concurrent bladder cancer

IMAGE FINDINGS

CT Findings

- May present with luminal mass and signs of ureteral obstruction (e.g., hydronephrosis)
- Flat tumors may not be easily discernible, unless there is wall thickening or mass effect

MICROSCOPIC PATHOLOGY

Histologic Features

- Classification similar to bladder or pelvicaliceal UCa (WHO, 2004)
  - Papillary urothelial neoplasms
    - Urothelial papilloma and papillary urothelial neoplasm of unknown malignant potential (PUNLMP) rare in ureter
    - Papillary UCa, low grade
    - Papillary UCa, high grade
  - Flat urothelial neoplasms
    - Urothelial dysplasia
    - UCa in situ
  - Invasive carcinoma, conventional UCa, and variants morphology
  - Squamous cell carcinoma, small cell carcinoma, adenocarcinoma, and sarcomatoid carcinoma rarer in ureter
- Carcinoma may spread/infiltrate through ureteral wall or adventitial tissue without involving overlying ureter mucosa
  - Potential pitfall for false-negative margin, particularly in frozen section ureteral margin

SELECTED REFERENCES

1. Rouprêt M et al: European guidelines on upper tract urothelial carcinomas: 2013 update. Eur Urol. 63(6):1059-71, 2013
2. Cutress ML et al: Long-term endoscopic management of upper tract urothelial carcinoma: 20-year single-centre experience. BJU Int. 110(11):1608-17, 2012
3. Lughezzani G et al: Prognostic factors in upper urinary tract urothelial carcinomas: a comprehensive review of the current literature. Eur Urol. 62(1):100-14, 2012

IMAGE GALLERY

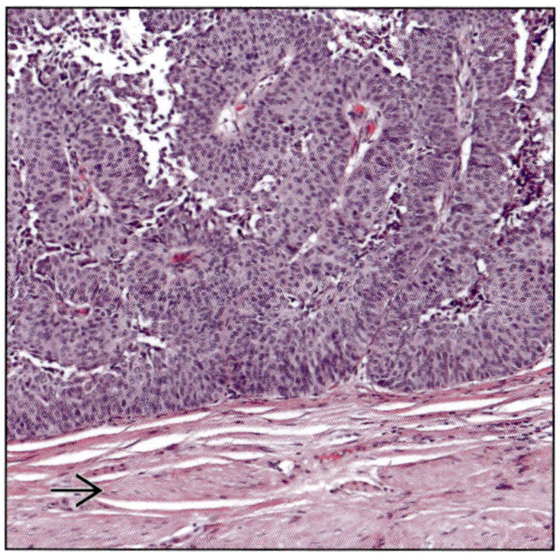
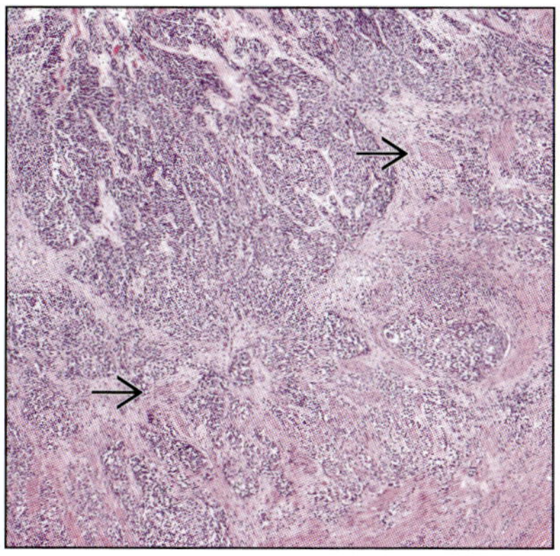
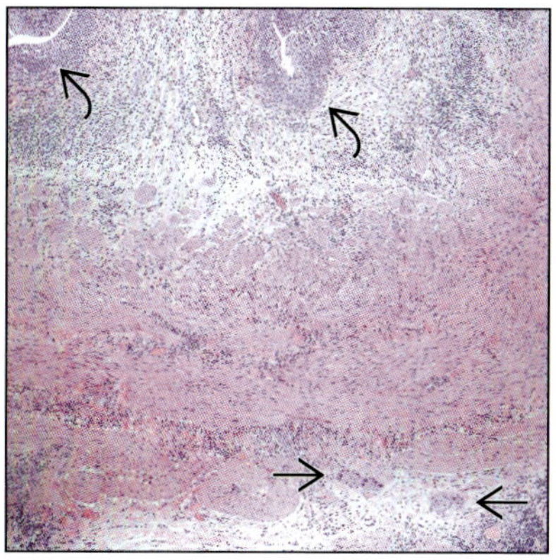

(Left) *Noninvasive high-grade ureteral papillary UCa shows regular boundary with underlying connective tissue. Note the relative closeness of ureteral muscularis propria ⇨ to the surface.* ***(Center)*** *Invasive high-grade ureteral UCa shows infiltration into the ureter muscularis propria ⇨, which has smaller caliber bundles than those in the bladder proper.* ***(Right)*** *Cross section of a ureter shows a benign urothelial mucosa ⇨. However, deep in the wall are infiltrative nests of UCa ⇨, a feature that may present as a pitfall in margin assessment, particularly in frozen sections.*

GERM CELL TUMOR

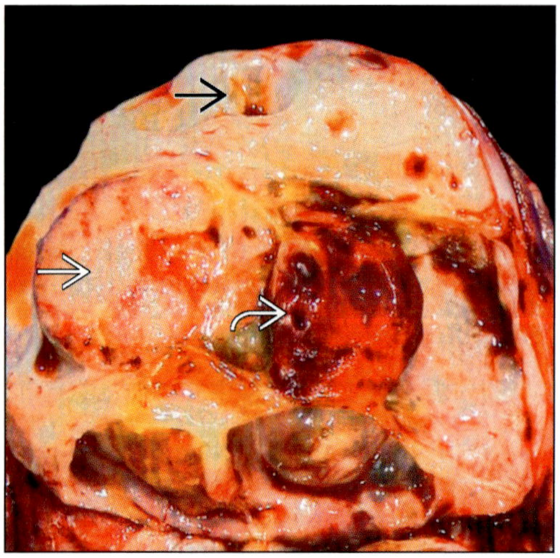

Photo shows MGCT with typical variegation. The cystic mucoid areas represent TT ➔, the tan fleshy area represents seminoma ➔, and hemorrhagic and necrotic areas represent EC ➔. (Courtesy S. Shen, MD.)

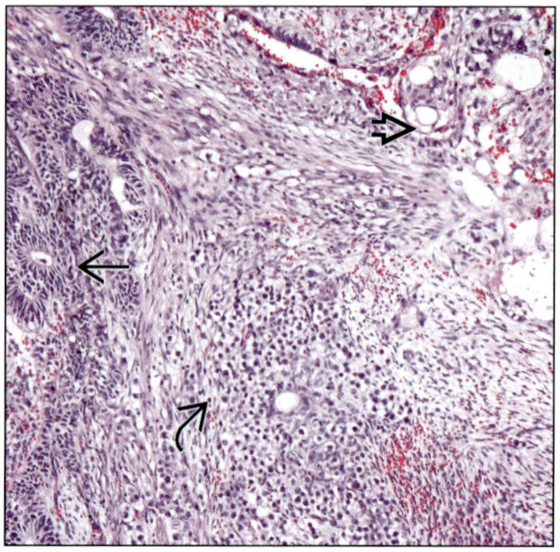

MGCT shows admixture of TT ➔ with primitive neuroepithelium, and YST ➔ with variable patterns, including microcysts and seminoma ➔ with sheets and infiltrates of tumor cells with clear cytoplasm.

TERMINOLOGY

Abbreviations

- Germ cell tumor (GCT)

Definitions

- **GCT**
  - Group of tumors arising from germ cells that are capable of differentiating into embryonic and extraembryonic elements
- Occurrence of testicular GCTs cluster in 3 age groups
  - **Pediatric GCTs**
    - Occur mostly in infants and young children
    - Most are **pure** GCTs and include mostly pure yolk sac tumors (YST) (~ 75% of childhood GCTs) and pure teratomas (TTs)
  - **Postpubertal GCTs**
    - Majority arise in men 20-45 years of age, with peak incidence in 30s
    - GCTs in this age group are **pure** or **mixed**: Pure classical seminoma (CS, ~ 30-45%), pure embryonal carcinoma (EC, < 5%), or mixed germ cell tumor (MGCT, ~ 30-40%)
    - YST, TT, and choriocarcinoma (CC) are more commonly encountered as component of MGCTs; pure form rare in adults
    - Described familial GCT cases are mostly in this age group
  - **Older adult GCTs**
    - Rare; majority are spermatocytic seminoma (SS) in patients with mean age of 53 years
- From clinical standpoint, GCTs are divided into 2 groups
  - **Seminomatous GCT (SGCT)**
    - Only pure CS
  - **Nonseminomatous GCT (NSGCT)**
    - Includes pure and mixed nonseminoma GCTs
  - Compared to NSGCT, SGCT usually arises in patients older by 10 years, is less likely to metastasize, is sensitive to radiotherapy, and responds better to chemotherapy
    - Response of NSGCTs with chemotherapy getting better with platinum-based regimens
- **Intratubular germ cell neoplasia (ITGCN)**
  - Uncommitted neoplastic germ cells proliferating peripherally within seminiferous tubules
  - Considered precursor of most GCTs and common in seminiferous tubules of postpubertal GCTs; **not** seen in pediatric pure YST, pure TT, or SS

ETIOLOGY/PATHOGENESIS

Risk Factors

- Family history, prior history of GCT, contralateral GCT, cryptorchidism, testicular dysgenesis syndrome, undescended testis (cryptorchidism), Klinefelter syndrome

Familial GCT

- ~ 1.5% of testicular GCT (TGCT) patients have positive family history for GCT
- Sons of TGCT-affected individuals: 4-6x ↑ risk
- Siblings of TGCT-affected individuals: 8-10x ↑ risk
- Most affected families have 2 members with TGCT
- However, no high-penetrance cancer susceptibility gene has been described so far
  - Hereditary GCT not yet firmly established

Cytogenetic Changes

- Postpubertal GCTs typically have 1 or more copies of Chr 12p or other forms of Chr 12 abnormalities
  - Most common is isochromosome 12 (i[12p]) seen in ~ 80% of testicular GCTs
- Pediatric GCTs are usually diploid

GERM CELL TUMOR

Key Facts

Terminology

- GCT: Group of tumors arising from germ cells that are capable of differentiating into embryonic and extraembryonic elements
- Pediatric GCTs: Most are pure GCTs and include mostly pure yolk sac tumor (YST) (~ 75% of childhood GCTs) and pure teratoma (TT)
- Postpubertal GCTs: Majority of GCTs arise in men 20-45 years old, with peak incidence in 30s
  - Most are pure classic seminoma (CS) (~ 30-45%), pure embyonal carcinoma (EC) (< 5%), or MGCT (~ 30-40%)
- ITGCN: Considered precursor of most GCTs and common in postpubertal GCTs
- Clinically, GCTs are divided into SGCT and NSGCT with differing behavior and therapy

Etiology/Pathogenesis

- Familial GCTs: ~ 1.5% of TGCT patients have positive family history for GCT
  - Affected individuals' sons have 4-6x higher risk for TGCT, siblings have 8-10x higher risk for TGCT
- Postpubertal GCTs typically have 1 or more copies of Chr 12p or other forms of Chr 12 abnormalities

Microscopic Pathology

- Distinction of CS, EC, YST, TT, CC, SS, and components of MGCT are based mainly on morphologic assessment

Ancillary Tests

- Helpful immunostains: Oct3/4, CD117, CD30, α-fetoprotein, and Glypican-3

CLINICAL ISSUES

Epidemiology

- Age
  - Postpubertal GCTs
    - Nonseminomatous GCT usually occurs in patients aged 25-35 years
    - CS occurs at ages ranging from 35-45 years (10 years older than NSGCT)
- Ethnicity
  - Occurs 5x more often in white men than black men; 3x more often in white men than Asian men

Presentation

- Typically a painless testicular mass
- ~ 10% present due to symptoms from distant metastasis

Laboratory Tests

- α-fetoprotein elevated in YST
- Borderline elevation of β-HCG in GCT with syncytiotrophoblasts and markedly high in CC (usually > 50,000 mIU/mL)
- Serum LDH, α-fetoprotein, and β-HCG levels important in prognosis and are incorporated in AJCC TNM staging

Treatment

- Decision is made based on stage and whether tumor is SGCT or NSGCT
  - SGCT: Radical orchiectomy and surveillance for stage I; radiotherapy, cisplatin-based, or multidrug chemotherapy depending on stage
  - NSGCT: Radical orchiectomy and retroperitoneal lymph node dissection for all stages; additional chemotherapy depending on stage

Prognosis

- Depends on tumor type, stage, and therapy
- In USA, overall survival is good (95%), attributed to advancement in therapy

MACROSCOPIC FEATURES

Classical Seminoma

- Well-circumscribed homogeneous gray-white mass ± lobulations and usually devoid of necrosis or hemorrhages
- May have punctate hemorrhages from syncytiotrophoblasts
- Range: < 1-24 cm; mean: 5 cm

Embryonal Carcinoma

- Usually poorly circumscribed and with variegated irregular surface exhibiting abundant necrosis and hemorrhage
- Tumor usually presents smaller than CS

Yolk Sac Tumor

- Homogeneous gray-white mass with gelatinous surface ± hemorrhage
  - "Pure CS-appearing" tumor in infants and young children

Teratoma

- Often circumscribed solid &/or cystic mass
- Cysts may contain keratinous debris or mucinous fluid
- May have hairs, teeth, bone, or cartilage

Mixed Germ Cell Tumor

- Variegated solid &/or cystic
- Variation depends on components
  - NSGCT components usually associated with necrosis, hemorrhages, and cystic changes

MICROSCOPIC PATHOLOGY

Intratubular Germ Cell Neoplasia

- Large atypical cells with large nucleus, nucleolomegaly, and prominent cytoplasmic membrane within seminiferous tubules usually at periphery

GERM CELL TUMOR

Key Immunohistochemical Reactivity for GCTs and Differential Diagnosis

Antibody	CS	EC	YST	SS	SCT	Melanoma
Oct3/4	+	+	-	-	-	-
CD117	+	-	V	+	-	V
CD30 (BerH2)	-/rare focal + cells	+	-	-	-	-
α-fetoprotein	-	-	+	-	-	-
Glypican-3	-	-	+	-	-	-
PAN-CK (AE1/AE3)	-	+	+	-	-	-

V: Variable; CS: Classical seminoma; EC: Embryonal carcinoma; YST: Yolk sac tumor; SS: Spermatocytic seminoma; SCT: Sertoli cell tumor.

- Seminiferous tubules usually with thickened basement membrane, decreased or absent spermatogenesis, and ITGCN cells admixed with mainly Sertoli cells

Classical Seminoma
- Mainly solid growth but may exhibit interstitial and other rare patterns
- Characteristically shows sheets of tumor cells compartmentalized by thin fibroconnective septae with occasional lymphoplasmacytic infiltrates
- Tumor cells have clear cytoplasm, prominent cytoplasmic border, regular nuclei, and large central nuclei; cells typically do not overlap
- ~ 30% may have granulomas

Embryonal Carcinoma
- Mainly exhibits solid, glandular, or papillary growths
- Characterized by large high-grade pleomorphic cells with indistinct cytoplasmic border, modest amphophilic cytoplasm, large nuclei, and prominent irregular nucleoli; cells usually overlap
- Hemorrhages and necrosis common

Yolk Sac Tumor
- Variable patterns, including reticular (80%, micro- or macrocystic), endodermal sinus pattern (Schiller-Duval bodies), solid, papillary, glandular-alveolar, parietal, enteric, hepatoid, spindled, myxomatous, and mixed
- Bland cells with varied shape; can be cuboidal, columnar, flattened, or spindled
- Clear to eosinophilic cytoplasm, overlapping border, and relatively regular nuclei with no to mild atypia

Teratoma
- **Mature teratoma**
  - Mixture of ectodermal (e.g., epidermis, neuronal tissue), endodermal (e.g., gastrointestinal or respiratory mucosa), and mesodermal (e.g., cartilage, bone) tissues
- **Immature teratoma**
  - Presence of primitive endoderm, neuroectoderm, or mesoderm (undifferentiated spindle cells), including blastemal cells
- May have carcinomatous or sarcomatous transformation

Choriocarcinoma
- Admixture of syncytiotrophoblasts (giant multinucleated cells) and cytotrophoblasts (smaller polygonal cells with prominent membrane and uniform nuclei)
- Hemorrhage is invariably present, forming pseudocystic hemorrhagic nodules
- Lymphovascular invasion is common

Mixed Germ Cell Tumor
- Combination of any CS, EC, YST, TT, or CC in varying proportions
- Most common combinations are EC + TT and EC + CS, but any combination may occur
- Usually exhibits hemorrhages and necrosis
- YST and EC component are often intermingled (e.g., embryoid bodies, diffuse embryonal pattern)

Spermatocytic Seminoma
- Hallmark is presence of 3 distinct cell types
  - Small lymphocyte-like cells: Scant cytoplasm with dark round nuclei
  - Intermediate cells: Most common, with modest cytoplasm and round nuclei with granular chromatin
  - Large cells: Nuclei with filamentous or "spireme" chromatin

ANCILLARY TESTS

Immunohistochemistry
- PLAP: Positive in all GCT
- Important immunostains include Oct3/4, CD117, CD30, α-fetoprotein, and Glypican-3
- Oct 3/4: Positive in ITGCN, CS, and EC
- β-HCG and human placental lactogen: Positive in CC (syncytiotrophoblasts)
- SOX2: Positive in EC
- Inhibin: Negative in GCT and positive in sex cord-stromal tumors

SELECTED REFERENCES

1. Young RH: Testicular tumors--some new and a few perennial problems. Arch Pathol Lab Med. 132(4):548-64, 2008
2. Ulbright TM: Germ cell tumors of the gonads: a selective review emphasizing problems in differential diagnosis, newly appreciated, and controversial issues. Mod Pathol. 18 Suppl 2:S61-79, 2005
3. Ulbright TM: Germ cell neoplasms of the testis. Am J Surg Pathol. 17(11):1075-91, 1993

Microscopic and Gross Features

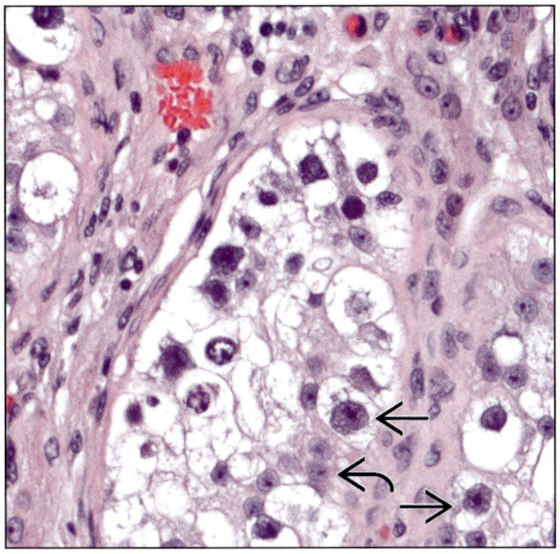

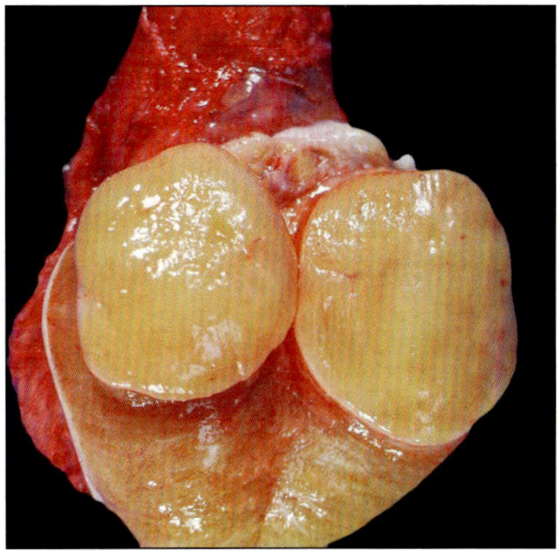

(Left) *ITGCN shows seminiferous tubules with no spermatogenesis and containing large atypical cells with abundant clear cytoplasm, prominent cell border, and large nuclei with nucleolomegaly →. ITGCN cells are more often at the periphery, intermingled with residual Sertoli cells ↩.* ***(Right)*** *This gross photograph shows CS with no necrosis or hemorrhage. The tumor is well-circumscribed, bulging, tan, fleshy, and homogeneous. (Courtesy S. Shen, MD.)*

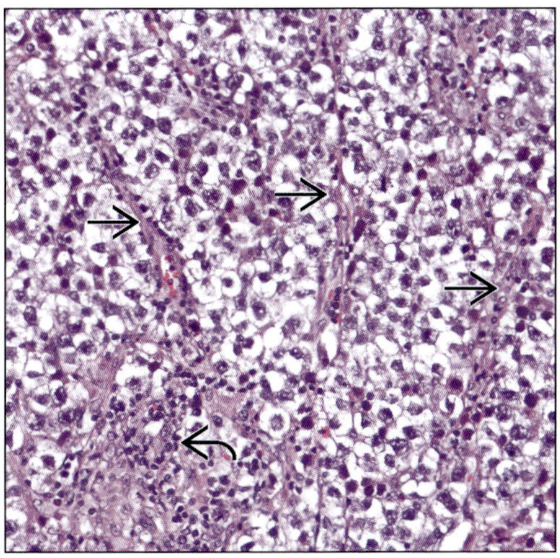

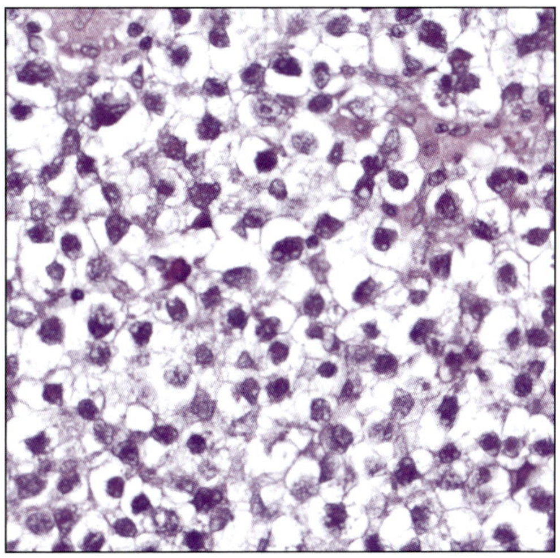

(Left) *Low-power view shows CS characterized by solid growth of clear cells separated by thin fibrovascular septae → and with occasional lymphoplasmacytic infiltrates ↩.* ***(Right)*** *High-power view of CS shows evenly spread clear cells with prominent cytoplasmic border and no significant overlapping. The nuclei are large with variably prominent nucleoli. However, CS may show increased mitosis and nuclear atypia (a.k.a. anaplastic seminoma [not shown]).*

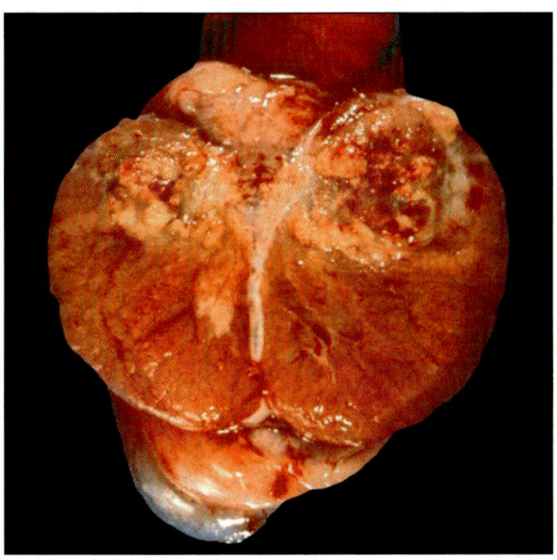

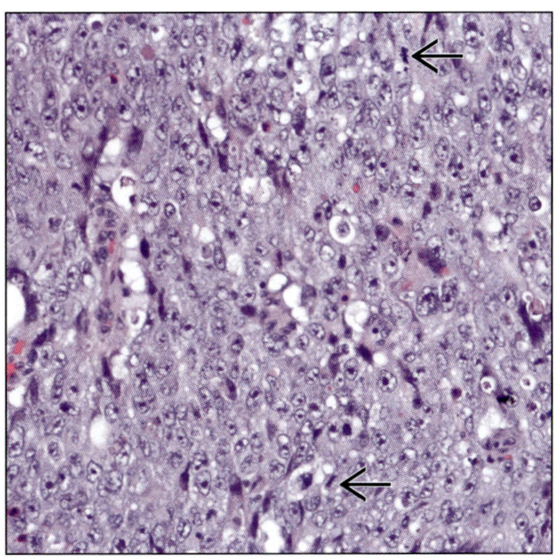

(Left) *EC with a variegated cut surface, hemorrhage, and necrosis is shown. The tumor is poorly circumscribed. The rete testis and spermatic cord are more commonly involved in EC than in seminoma. (Courtesy S. Shen, MD.)* ***(Right)*** *EC shows solid sheet of high-grade pleomorphic cells with overlapping nuclei and brisk mitotic activity →. Solid growth is the most common EC pattern. Morphologic diagnosis of EC is often straightforward due to the presence of these "angry-looking" cells.*

GERM CELL TUMOR

Microscopic and Gross Features

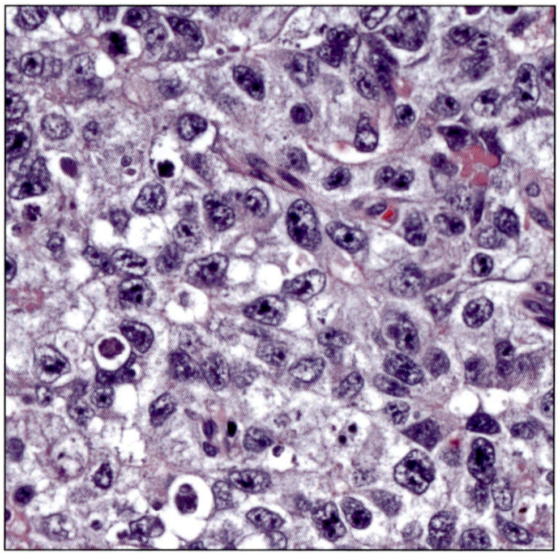

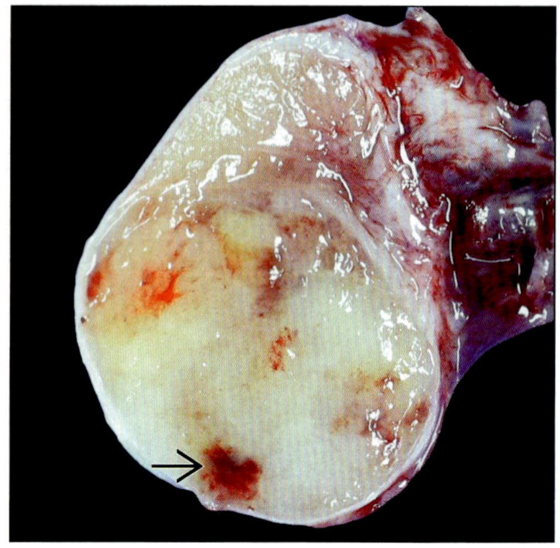

(Left) *High-power view of EC shows the pleomorphic high-grade cells with large variable nuclei, irregular outline, coarse chromatin, and prominent nucleoli. Other than the high-grade nuclei, notable differences from CS are the nuclear overlap and less distinct cell border.* ***(Right)*** *Large YST with relatively homogeneous, white, mucoid cut surface is shown. Focal hemorrhage is present* →*. A gelatinous or myxoid appearance is common in pediatric YSTs that are histologically pure. (Courtesy S. Shen, MD.)*

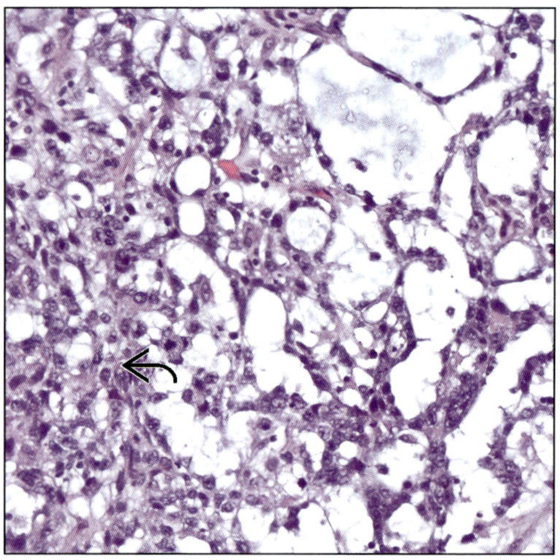

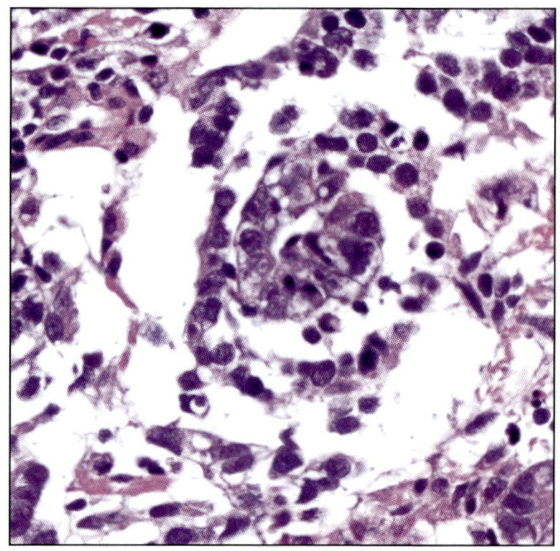

(Left) *Low-power view of YST shows microcysts and focal solid area* ↶*. Microcystic configuration is the most common pattern of YST. The cells vary from cuboidal to flat. YST typically shows variable pattern and cytomorphology.* ***(Right)*** *This image shows a Schiller-Duval body in YST characterized by a central vessel surrounded by a layer of tumor cells and a space created by another layer of tumor cells, giving a glomeruloid appearance. This pattern is the most specific pattern for YST. YST cells are typically bland appearing.*

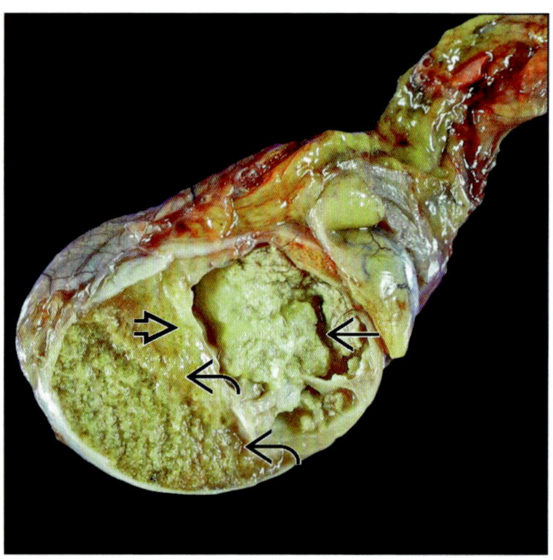

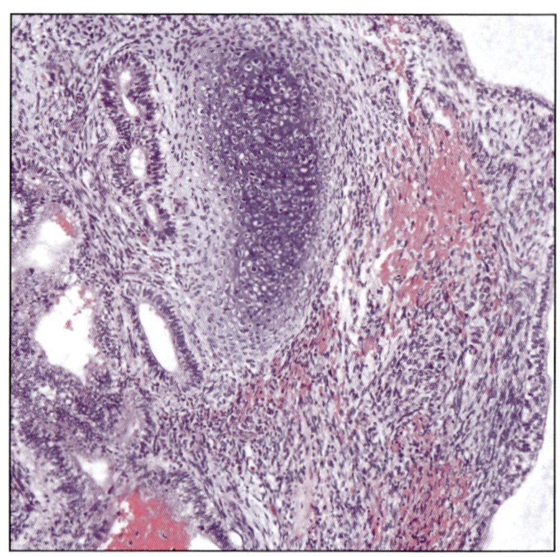

(Left) *This mature TT shows a predominantly cystic mass with chalky keratin debris* →*. Solid mucoid and gelatinous components* ⇨ *are also present and frequently correlate microscopically with immature teratomatous components. Uninvolved testis is pushed to 1 side* ↶*. (Courtesy S. Shen, MD.)* ***(Right)*** *Low-power view shows TT with mature elements, including cartilage, intestinal glands, and spindle cell mesenchymal stroma. In testicular TT, presence of immature elements has no prognostic bearing.*

Microscopic and Immunohistochemical Features

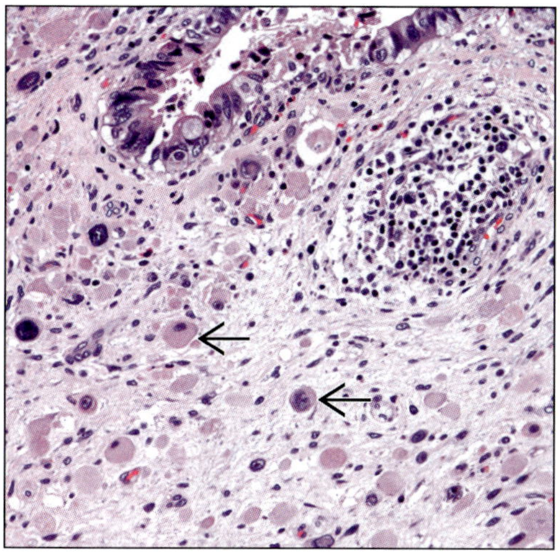
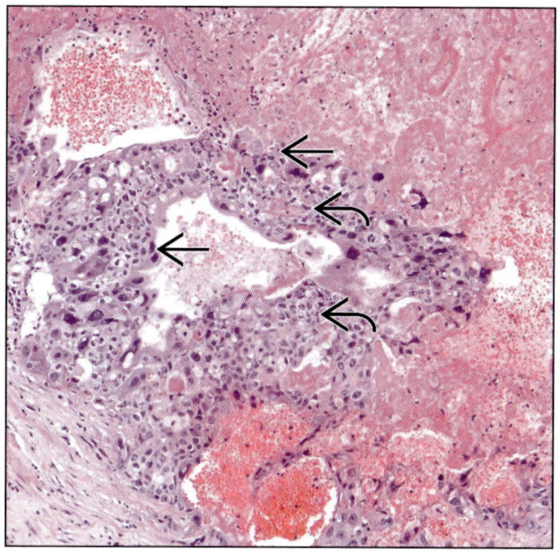

(Left) *Sarcomatous transformation in TT shows rhabdomyoblasts consisting of plump cells with abundant dense eosinophilic cytoplasm and eccentric atypical nuclei →.* ***(Right)*** *CC shows a hemorrhagic cystic nodule with focal proliferation of mononuclear cells (cytotrophoblasts and intermediate trophoblasts) ↪ surrounded or "capped" by syncytiotrophoblasts →. The latter are larger with dense eosinophilic cytoplasm and often multinucleate with smudgy nuclear chromatin.*

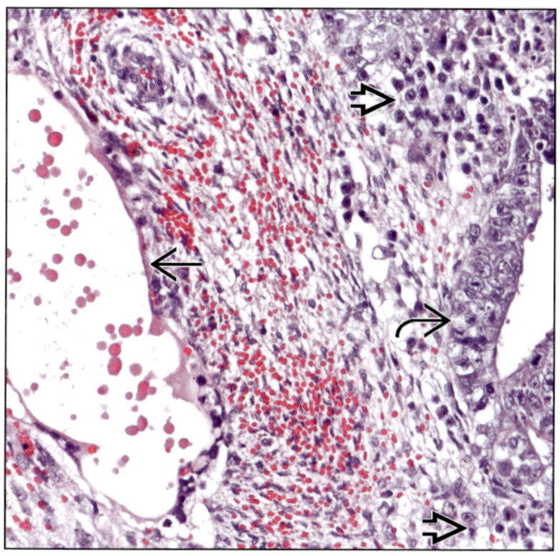
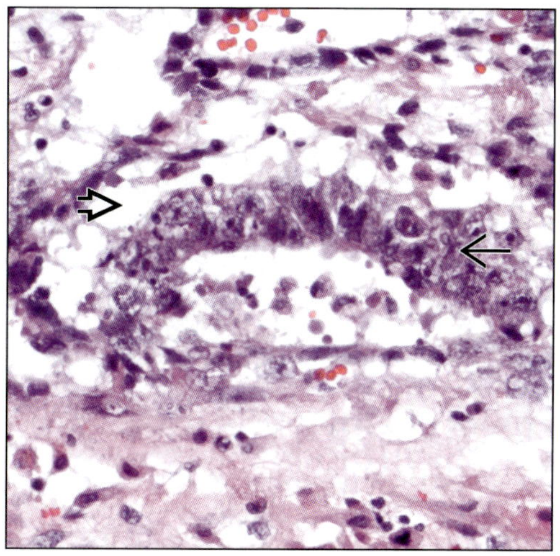

(Left) *MGCT consists of YST with polyvesicular vitelline pattern →, EC consisting of glands ↪ and seminoma with clear cells ⇨. Note the abundant hyaline globules associated with YST. In postpubertal GCTs, YST is almost always seen as a component of MGCT.* ***(Right)*** *This high-power view shows an embryoid body in MGCT consisting of a central embryonic disc → composed of EC cells and surrounded by YST cells creating an amniotic-like cavity ⇨.*

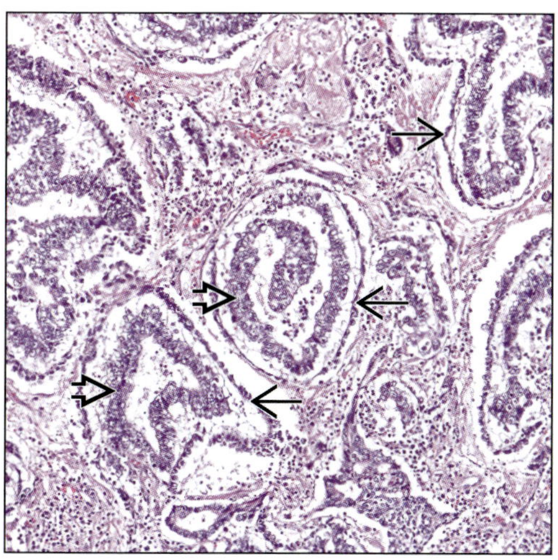
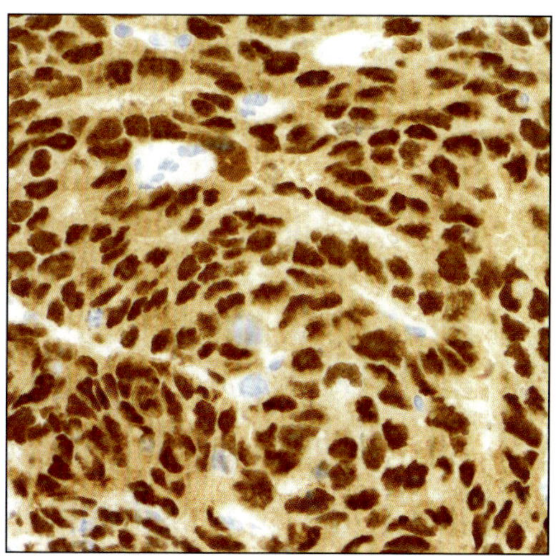

(Left) *Low power of MGCT shows diffuse embryoma pattern characterized by intimate admixture of YST & EC components. YST → is seen wrapping around EC component ⇨.* ***(Right)*** *High-power view shows diffuse nuclear staining of Oct3/4 in EC cells. Oct3/4 is also positive in CS and is not expressed by the other GCTs. This marker is helpful in differentiating EC and CS from other tumors in testis that may exhibit solid growth, such as YST, SS, Sertoli cell tumor, and melanoma.*

PROSTATE CARCINOMA

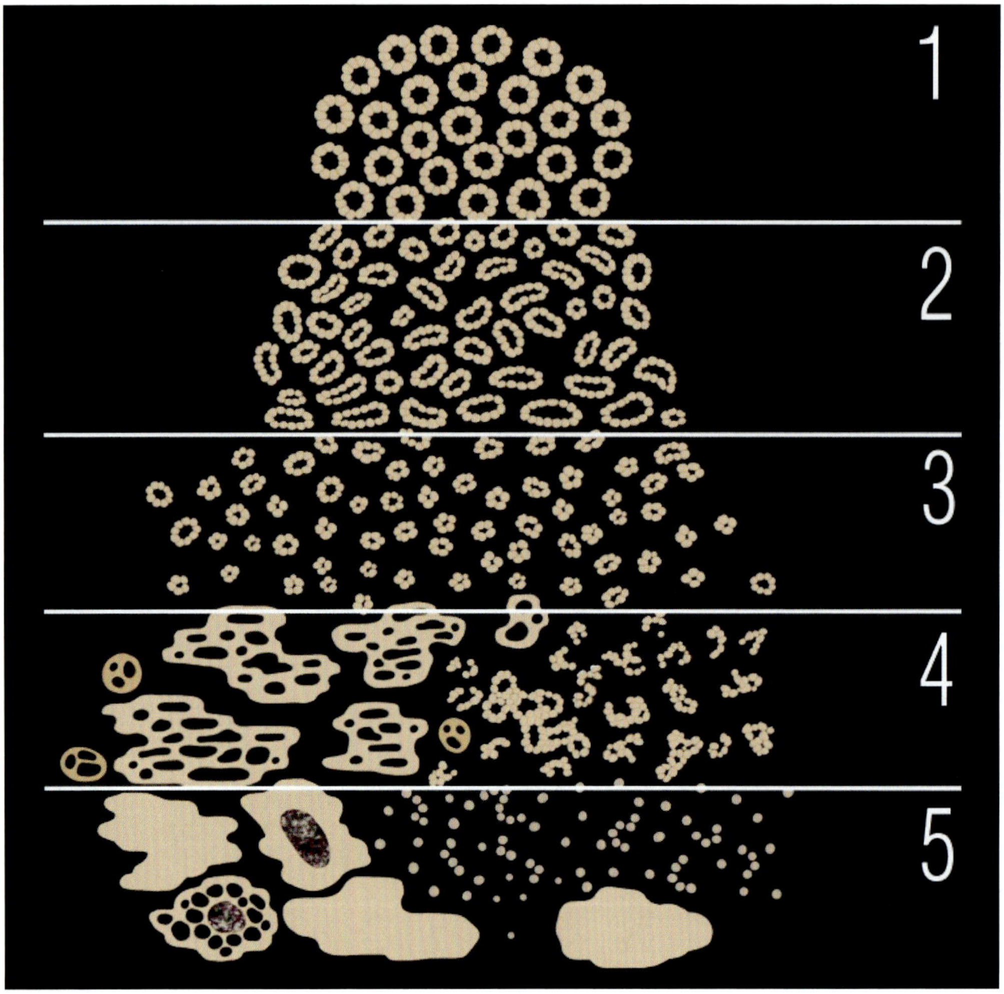

Schematic diagram shows the modified Gleason grading system for PCa. The Gleason score is a powerful prognostic variable in predicting PCa behavior. This grading system is based purely on glandular architectural patterns, divided into 5 histologic categories or grades with decreasing differentiation. First developed in 1966 by Dr. Donald F. Gleason, it underwent refinements in 1974 and 1977 and had its latest modification by ISUP in 2005. This grading scheme is now universally accepted and recognized by the WHO and by the AJCC as the grading system of choice for PCa.

TERMINOLOGY

Abbreviations

- Prostate carcinoma (PCa)

Synonyms

- Prostatic adenocarcinoma

Definitions

- Malignant neoplasm of acinar cell phenotype
- ≥ 95% of prostate carcinomas are **acinar adenocarcinomas**
  - Basis of epidemiologic, pathogenetic, and clinical features of PCas
- < 5% of prostate carcinomas include urothelial carcinoma, small cell carcinoma, carcinoma with squamous differentiation, basal cell/adenoid cystic carcinoma, and sarcomatoid carcinoma

ETIOLOGY/PATHOGENESIS

Molecular Genetics

- *TMPRSS2* and *ETS* gene fusion
  - ~ 50% of PCa patients harbor these recurrent gene fusions
  - ETS family of transcription factors include *ERG*, *ETV1*, *ETV4*, and *ETV5*
  - *TMPRSS2*:*ERG* gene fusion most common (~ 90%)
    - ERG brought under control of androgen-regulated promoter causing protein overexpression
    - In ~ 2/3 of cases, fusion results from deletion
    - Fusion may also occur by more complex rearrangement, such as translocation
    - Associated with blue-tinged mucin, cribriform pattern, intraductal spread, macronucleoli, and signet ring cells
  - Clinical significance not fully understood
- *PTEN* mutation

PROSTATE CARCINOMA

Key Facts

Terminology

- Malignant neoplasm of acinar cell phenotype

Etiology/Pathogenesis

- ~ 50% of PCa harbor *TMPRSS2* and *ETS* gene fusion
- *SPOP* mutation in *TMPRSS2:ETS*-negative PCa
- Compelling evidence suggests familial predisposition to prostate cancer in some cases
  - Implicated genetic factors: *BRCA2*, *ELAC2* on Chr 17p, *RNASEL* on Chr 1q25, *MSR1* on Chr 8p22-23, *NBS1* on Chr 5, and *CHEK2* on Chr 22q

Microscopic Pathology

- Diagnosis based on constellation of architectural, nuclear, cytoplasmic, and intraluminal features
- Crowded uniform glands that infiltrate between preexisting benign glands
  - Small caliber, crowded clusters, rigid or "sharp" lumina, tinctorial staining of cytoplasm distinct from adjacent benign glands
- Nuclear enlargement and hyperchromasia with prominently enlarged &/or multiple and peripherally located nucleoli
- Luminal features, e.g., mucin, amorphous materials, and crystalloids
- Pathognomonic features for malignant glands
  - Glomerulations or collagenous micronodules
- Less differentiated tumors have poorly formed, fused, or large cribriform glands
- Poorly differentiated tumors may grow as infiltrative single cells or solid sheets
- Negative for basal cell markers (e.g., HMWCK, CK5/6, p63); overexpesses AMACR

  - Mutated in 20-40% of PCas, more often in advanced stage
  - Significant co-occurrence with *TMPRSS2:ERG* suggests a late genetic event or "second hit"
- *SPOP* mutation
  - Mutated in 6-13% of PCa
  - Unlike *PTEN*, alterations occur in *TMPRSS2:ERG*(-) PCa, suggesting a different class of PCa
- Other genes and molecular alterations
  - Most common chromosomal alterations in prostate cancer are losses at 1p, 6q, 8p, 10q, 13q, 16q, and 18q, and gains at 1q, 2p, 7, 8q, and Xq
  - Other genes implicated in PCa include tumor suppressor genes *GSTP1, CDKN1B, NKX3-1, KLF6, RB,* and *TP53,* and oncogenes *MYC, BCL2, KIT,* and *STAT5*
  - Mutations in androgen receptor gene may promote cancer growth at lower circulating androgen levels

Hereditary Prostate Cancer

- Compelling evidence suggests familial predisposition to prostate cancer in some cases
  - Hereditary factor difficult to identify because PCa is so common
  - 2x ↑ risk if 1 first-degree relative and 9x ↑ risk if 3 first-degree relatives are diagnosed with prostate cancer
- High-risk alleles identified with either autosomal dominant or X-linked mode of inheritance
- Implicated genetic factors include *BRCA2*, *ELAC2* on Chr 17p, *RNASEL* on Chr 1q25, *MSR1* on Chr 8p22-23, *NBS1* on Chr 5, and *CHEK2* on Chr 22q

Risk Factors

- Older age, black race, and positive family history well established
- Others include red meat diet, obesity, metabolic disease, environmental factors (e.g., exposure to cadmium, pesticides, rubber, textile, and chemicals), and vitamin D deficiency

CLINICAL ISSUES

Epidemiology

- Incidence
  - Most common cause of cancer morbidity and 2nd cause of cancer mortality in men in USA
  - It is estimated that there will be 238,590 new cases of and 29,720 deaths from PCa in the USA in 2013
- Age
  - PCa is a disease of older men and incidence increases dramatically with age
  - Incidence is remarkably low in men < 50 years old; ~ 60% of cases occur in men > 65 years old
  - Diagnosis rate peaks in men 65-74 years old
  - Median age at diagnosis: 67 years old
- Ethnicity
  - Incidence rates highest in higher resource areas, such as USA, Canada, Australia, New Zealand, Western Europe, Scandinavia, and Caribbean
  - In USA, blacks have highest incidence rates, which is ~ 60% higher than in whites
    - Rates are much lower in Asian Americans, Native Americans, and Alaska Natives
  - Mortality rate is also highest in black Americans (54.9 per 100,000 men) and lowest in Asian Americans and Pacific Islanders

Presentation

- Majority of PCa in USA are asymptomatic
  - Tumor detected due to early detection program
- Main indication for needle biopsy are elevated serum PSA level and abnormal digital rectal examination
- When symptomatic, presents with obstructive urinary symptoms, pelvic pain from local extension, and bone-related symptoms from metastasis

Natural History

- Latent form of PCa extremely common; up to 80% of PCa in 9th decade
- Most PCa patients die from other causes, most commonly from cardiovascular disease

PROSTATE CARCINOMA

Prognosis

- Dependent on stage and Gleason grade

MACROSCOPIC FEATURES

General Features

- Unlike most other visceral organ tumors, PCa often has no reliably distinguishable gross mass lesion
  - Grossly evident tumors are usually pT3, ≥ Gleason score (GS) 8, or ≥ 1 cm in size
    - Indurated yellow to yellow-tan homogeneous areas
    - More dense or firmer than surrounding benign spongy parenchyma
  - Typically lack necrosis or hemorrhage
- Tumors usually in posterior or posterolateral aspect (peripheral zone [PZ]) of gland

Site

- 75-80% of PCas arise in PZ, and 15-25% arise in transition zone (TZ)
- Multifocal tumors present in > 50% of PCas

MICROSCOPIC PATHOLOGY

Histologic Features

- Diagnosis based on constellation of architectural, nuclear, cytoplasmic, and intraluminal features
  - Some individual features may also be seen in benign glands
- **Architectural features**
  - Better differentiated tumors consist of compact or loose collections of well-formed glands
    - Small, crowded, uniform glands infiltrate between preexisting benign glands
  - Malignant glands usually differ in appearance from surrounding benign glands
    - Smaller caliber glands
    - Crowded or compact gland clusters
    - Rigid or "sharp" glandular lumina
    - May have periglandular clefts
  - Malignant glands should lack basal cells
  - Less differentiated tumors consist of poorly formed, fused, or large cribriform glands
  - Poorly differentiated tumors may grow as infiltrative single cells or solid sheets
- **Nuclear features**
  - Nuclear enlargement and hyperchromasia
  - Prominently enlarged nucleoli
  - Single or multiple peripherally located nucleoli
  - Parachromatin clearing
  - Mitoses are rare; highly suggestive of malignancy if present
  - Apoptotic bodies (rare)
  - Nuclei commonly uniform, nonpleomorphic
- **Cytoplasmic features**
  - Typically cuboidal to columnar cells with modest cytoplasm
  - Amphophilic, clear or pale granular cytoplasm
  - Taller cells with clear to pale pink cytoplasm and basally located nuclei more common in TZ
- **Intraluminal features**
  - Blue mucin
    - Usually prominent collection of wispy, blue-tinged intracellular mucin
  - Eosinophilic amorphous secretions
    - Granular eosinophilic luminal material
  - Crystalloids
    - Geometric bright eosinophilic rhomboid to prismatic structures with sharp edges, usually associated with eosinophilic amorphous secretions
    - Present in up to 41% of PCas
    - Seen in atypical adenomatous hyperplasia and uncommonly in benign glands
  - Corpora amylacea are extremely rare in PCa, should strongly suggest benign glands
  - Intraluminal necrosis may be present in high-grade tumors, highly indicative of malignancy
- **Pathognomonic features for malignant glands**
  - Glomerulations
    - Cribriform cellular luminal proliferations in otherwise well-formed glands attached to 1 pole
  - Collagenous micronodules (mucinous fibroplasia)
    - Hyalinized eosinophilic material usually associated with abundant intraluminal blue mucin
    - Often imparts an anastomosing epithelial pattern
  - Circumferential perineural or intraneural invasion
    - Gland should completely surround nerve or be seen within nerve
    - Benign glands may focally touch or indent a nerve; very rarely may be intraneural
  - Growth within adipose tissue
    - Intraprostatic fat is exceedingly rare
    - Indicates extraprostatic extension (EPE)

Morphologic Variants and Variations

- **Ductal adenocarcinoma**
  - Large glandular and papillary architecture lined by tall columnar cells, often with pseudostratified growth
  - Often occurs admixed with acinar adenocarcinoma; requires > 80% ductal component for diagnosis
  - ISUP 2005 consensus recommends grading as Gleason grade 4; if necrosis is present, grade 5
- **Atrophic variant**
  - PCa with glands lined by cells with scant cytoplasm, resembling atrophy
  - Infiltrative growth, cytology of malignancy
  - In contrast, benign atrophic glands typically have dense hyperchromatic nuclei and lobular growth
- **Pseudohyperplastic variant**
  - Large or dilated glands, with branching and papillary infolding, resembling hyperplasia
  - Tall columnar cells with abundant pale to slightly granular cytoplasm and basally located nuclei
  - Commonly with luminal eosinophilic amorphous secretions and may have crystalloids
  - Diagnostic malignant nuclear features retained, in contrast to benign hyperplastic glands
- **Foamy gland (xanthomatous) variant**
  - PCa with abundant foamy cytoplasm

  - Malignant nuclear features not always present, as nuclei may be small and pyknotic
  - Presence of infiltrative pattern; may require immunostains
- **Mucinous (colloid) adenocarcinoma**
  - ≥ 25% of resected tumor shows extracellular mucin
  - Intraluminal mucinous material does not qualify, and extraprostatic origin must be excluded
- **Signet ring cell variant**
  - ≥ 25% of resected tumor shows signet ring cell (arbitrary definition)
  - Tumor cells contain optically clear vacuoles displacing nuclei and are widely infiltrative
  - May be mucin-producing PCa (mucinous carcinoma with signet ring cells)
- **PCa with Paneth cell-like differentiation**
  - PCa containing neuroendocrine cells with bright eosinophilic cytoplasmic granules resembling Paneth cells of gastrointestinal tract
- **Other rarer variations**
  - **Lymphoepithelioma-like variant**
    - As in other organs, characterized by syncytial growth amid dense lymphocytic background
  - **Oncocytic variant**
    - PCa with abundant granular eosinophilic cytoplasm and ultrastructurally contains abundant mitochondria
  - **PCa with stratified epithelium (PIN-like)**
    - Glands lined by ≥ 2 layers of malignant cells

Key Elements to Report

- Gleason score
- Tumor quantity
  - Provide length in mm in biopsy
- Extraprostatic extension (EE)
- Margin status
- Perineural invasion
- Lymphovascular invasion
- Seminal vesicle invasion
- In biopsy
  - Atypical small acinar proliferation (ASAP)
  - High-grade prostatic intraepithelial neoplasia

ANCILLARY TESTS

Immunohistochemistry

- PCa should have no basal cells
  - Absent staining for basal cell markers HMWCK, CK5/CK6, or p63
- Overexpress AMACR, in contrast to benign glands
- Prostatic lineage specific marker such as PSA, PAP, and PSMA helpful for diagnosis at metastatic sites

DIFFERENTIAL DIAGNOSIS

General Features

- Given broad morphologic spectrum, differential diagnosis for PCa ranges from innocuous benign normal structures to secondary high-grade cancers
- PCa most often mimicked by benign prostatic glandular lesions; difficulty enhanced in limited samples (e.g., biopsy)
  - Use of ancillary immunohistochemistry helpful in some scenarios
  - Pattern-based approach facilitates work-up and judicious selection of adjuvant stains

GRADING

Gleason Grading System (GS)

- Universally accepted grading system for PCa
- Assessment of gland architecture at low/intermediate magnification: Classified into 5 basic grades
- In resection specimens, GS is sum of primary and secondary Gleason grades
  - Primary grade is most prevalent grade and secondary is 2nd most common grade
- International Society of Urological Pathology (ISUP) 2005 consensus conference proposed several modifications and guidelines
  - In needle biopsies, include tertiary pattern in Gleason score if it is higher than secondary grade
    - Similar rule applies for transurethral resection and enucleation (simple prostatectomy) specimens
    - In high-grade cancers, ignore lower grade if < 5% (e.g., 4 + 4, if pattern 3 is < 5%)
    - For cancers with more than 1 grade, include the higher grade even if it is < 5% (e.g., 3 + 4, even if grade 4 is < 5%)
  - Assign individual GS to all cores as an aggregate if submitted in 1 container; assign GS to each core separately designated (e.g., ink or separately submitted) by urologist
  - In radical prostatectomy, provide GS (primary and secondary grades); separately mention tertiary grade
  - Assign separate GS to dominant tumor(s) for multifocal tumors in radical prostatectomy
  - Individualized Gleason grading approach for some PCa morphologic variants and subtypes
- **Gleason pattern 1**
  - Circumscribed nodule of tightly packed, uniform, round to oval, well-formed glands, with no or minimal infiltration of adjacent parenchyma
  - Using these strict criteria, exceedingly rare and controversial in current practice
    - Most described pre-immunohistochemistry were likely atypical adenomatous hyperplasia
- **Gleason pattern 2**
  - Nodular with minimal peripheral infiltration, less uniform and more loosely arranged glands
  - Also very rare and typically found in TZ
  - Usually incidental with associated higher grades, but occasionally secondary pattern in resection specimens
  - ISUP recommends that GS 3 or 4 should rarely, if ever, be diagnosed in needle biopsy specimens
    - Architecture cannot be assessed in its entirety
    - Poor reproducibility among experts
- **Gleason pattern 3**
  - Most common pattern

PROSTATE CARCINOMA

Differential Diagnosis for Prostate Carcinoma

Histologic Pattern	Prostate Carcinoma	Main Differential Diagnoses
Small glandular proliferation	Glandular Gleason pattern 3	Crowded benign glands, not otherwise specified
	Atrophic pattern	Simple atrophy
	Post-treatment cancer	Outpouching of high-grade PIN
		Partial atrophy
		Postatrophic hyperplasia (PAH)
		Atypical adenomatous hyperplasia (AAH, adenosis)
		Sclerosing adenosis
		Basal cell hyperplasia
		Seminal vesicle epithelium
		Ejaculatory duct
		Cowper glands
		Mesonephric remnants
		Nephrogenic adenoma
		Verumontanum mucosal gland hyperplasia
		Radiation atypia
Atypical large glandular proliferation	Cribriform Gleason patterns 3, 4, and 5	High-grade PIN
	Ductal adenocarcinoma	Urothelial carcinoma involving prostatic ducts and acini
	Pseudohyperplastic pattern	Colorectal carcinoma involving prostate
		Cribriform hyperplasia
		Squamous metaplasia
		Urothelial metaplasia
Infiltrative single cell pattern	Single cell Gleason 5 pattern	Dense inflammation
	Post-treatment carcinoma	Granulomatous prostatitis
		Lymphoma
		Small cell carcinoma
Clear cell pattern	Hypernephroid Gleason pattern 4	Prostatic xanthoma
	Glandular Gleason pattern 3	
Oncocytic pattern	Gleason pattern 4	Paraganglion/paraganglioma
		Carcinoid tumor
Poorly to undifferentiated carcinoma	Solid Gleason pattern 5	Urothelial carcinoma
Spindle cell pattern	Sarcomatoid carcinoma	Pseudosarcomatous myofibroblastic proliferation
		Stromal sarcoma
		Leiomyosarcoma
Small cell pattern	Small cell carcinoma	Lymphoma
		Rhabdomyosarcoma

  - Predominantly well-formed, individual glands that infiltrate between benign ducts and acini
  - Includes smaller but well-formed glands (microacini)
  - Glands typically smaller than in patterns 1 or 2
- **Gleason pattern 4**
  - Most commonly fused, poorly formed glands
    - Tangentially sectioned grade 3 glands may mimic fused pattern 4 glands
  - 2nd most common pattern is cribriform structures with either regular or irregular outlines
  - Uncommon "hypernephroid" pattern, consists of solid sheets of cells with optically clear cytoplasm
- **Gleason pattern 5**
  - Lacks glandular differentiation: Manifests as solid sheets, cords, or single infiltrative tumor cells
  - Also includes solid, cribriform, or papillary structures with central comedo-type necrosis

SELECTED REFERENCES

1. Paner GP et al: Best practice in diagnostic immunohistochemistry: prostate carcinoma and its mimics in needle core biopsies. Arch Pathol Lab Med. 132(9):1388-96, 2008
2. Humphrey PA: Diagnosis of adenocarcinoma in prostate needle biopsy tissue. J Clin Pathol. 60(1):35-42, 2007
3. Epstein JI et al: The 2005 International Society of Urological Pathology (ISUP) Consensus Conference on Gleason Grading of Prostatic Carcinoma. Am J Surg Pathol. 29(9):1228-42, 2005
4. Srigley JR: Benign mimickers of prostatic adenocarcinoma. Mod Pathol. 17(3):328-48, 2004

PROSTATE CARCINOMA

Gross and Microscopic Features

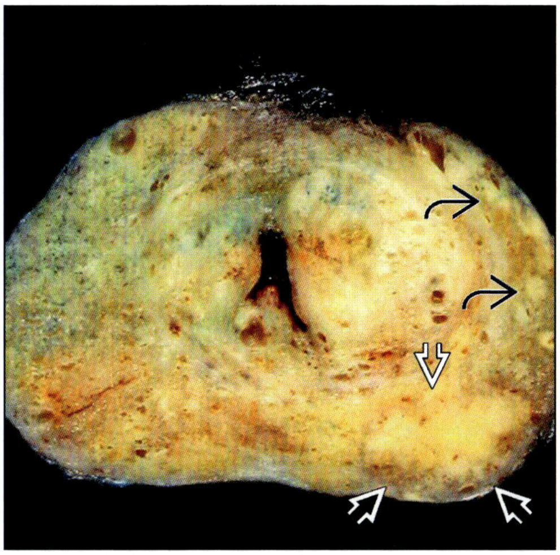

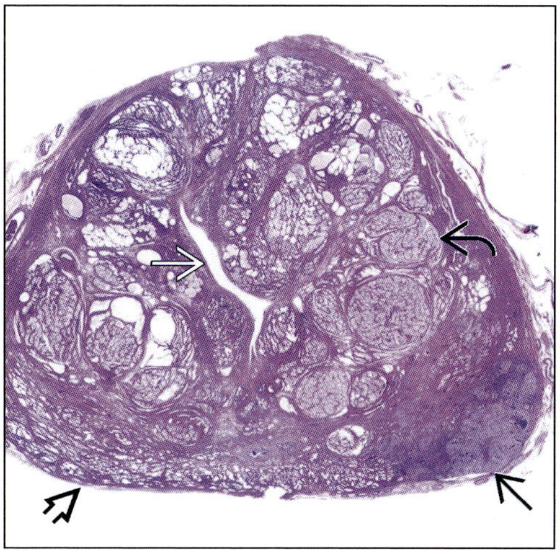

(Left) *This transverse section of prostate shows multifocal PCa predominantly involving the left lobe with a dominant nodule at the posterolateral aspect and additional smaller tumor foci at the lateral aspect of the peripheral zone.* ***(Right)*** *Transverse section of the prostate shows the urethra pushed to the left due to prominent hyperplasia. The peripheral zone shows evidence of prominent atrophy and a carcinoma involving the posterolateral aspect.*

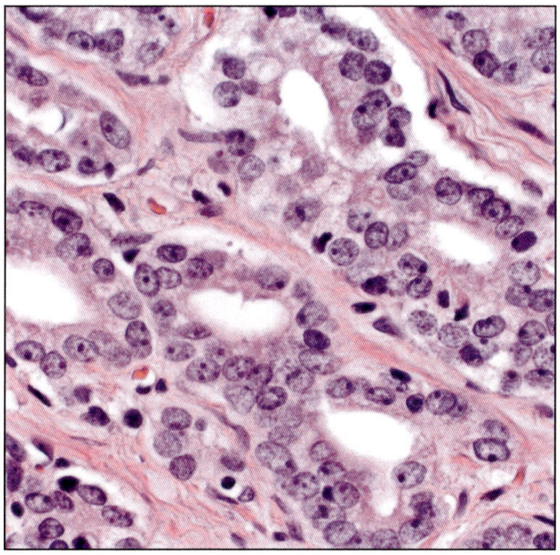

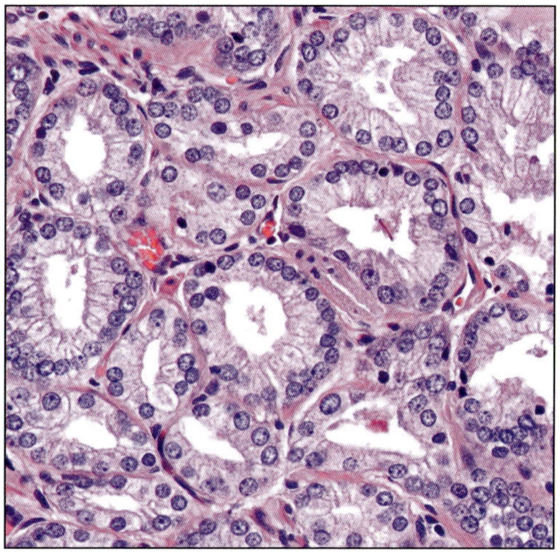

(Left) *Prominent nucleoli, as seen here, are characteristic of PCa, but they are not always required for the diagnosis. In addition, nuclei larger than the adjacent nuclei of benign glands and those with double nucleoli and with parachromatin clearing or mitosis are helpful features.* ***(Right)*** *PCa shows pale granular cytoplasm and monotonous-appearing round nuclei. PCa nuclei are typically homogeneous. Nuclear pleomorphism should suggest the possibility of a nonprostatic lesion.*

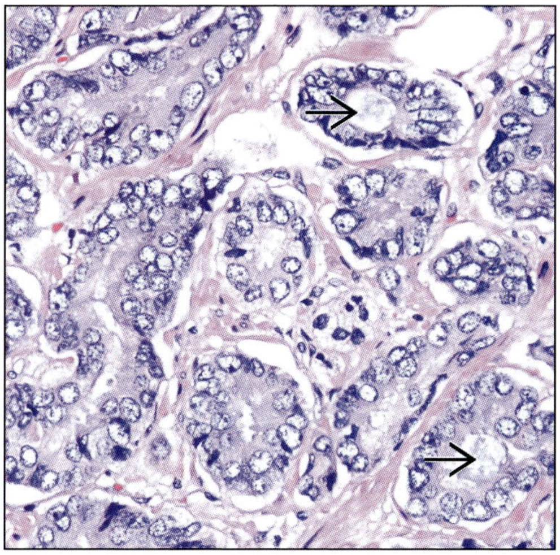

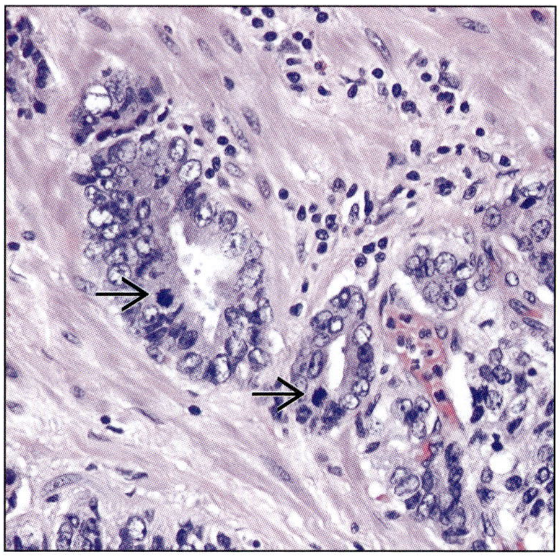

(Left) *PCa glands commonly show parachromatin clearing in the malignant nuclei. These nuclei also show a mild degree of nuclear variability and crowding not typically seen in PCa. PCa nuclei are usually very round and monotonous. Two carcinoma glands contain intraluminal mucin.* ***(Right)*** *PCa shows readily identifiable mitotic figures within the malignant glands. Mitotic figures are very rare in PCa; however, their presence is highly suggestive of adenocarcinoma.*

PROSTATE CARCINOMA

Luminal and Pathognomonic Features

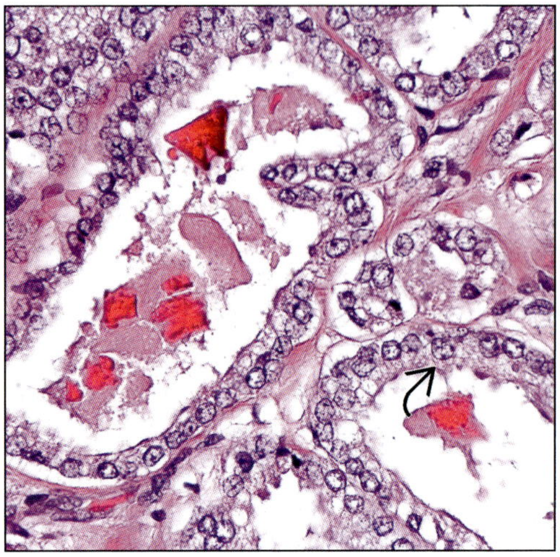
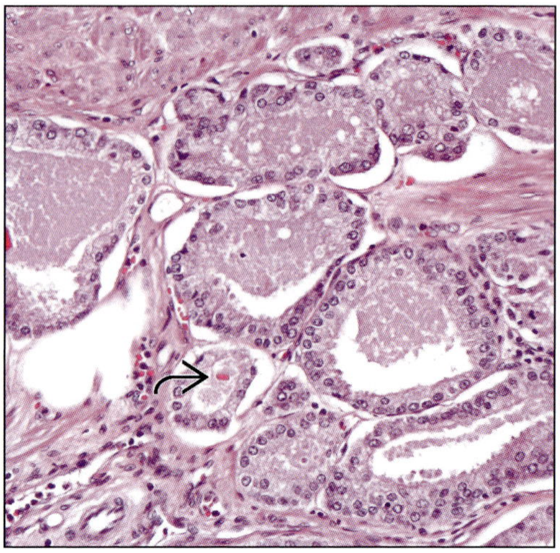

(Left) *H&E shows PCa glands with multiple bright eosinophilic crystalloids in the lumina. The nuclei of these glands are enlarged with prominent nucleoli that are occasionally multiple and peripheral. Crystalloids are common, but not specific, in PCa.* ***(Right)*** *PCa glands contain eosinophilic amorphous secretions in the lumen. Focal crystalloids may be seen admixed with the eosinophilic secretions. Presence of these features warrants close examination of the harboring glands.*

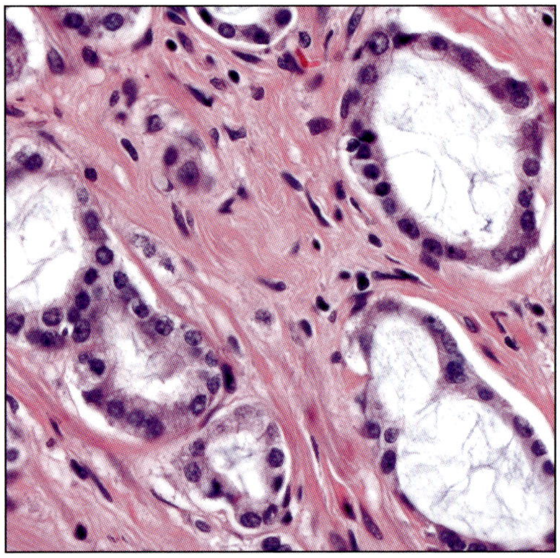
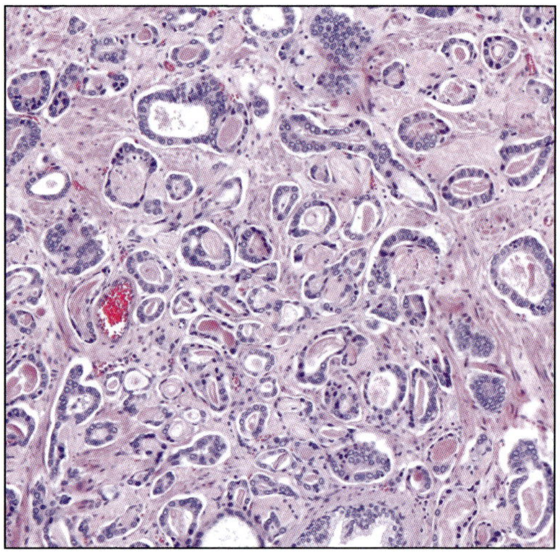

(Left) *PCa glands contain blue mucin in the lumen. Sometimes these mucin may be thin and wispy and may not be easily discernible on scanning magnification.* ***(Right)*** *Collagenous micronodules (mucinous fibroplasia) is a pathognomonic feature of PCa. Early collagenous micronodules consist mostly of mucin with scant fibrous tissue and, with time, the fibrous deposits predominate. Despite the glands assuming a complex architecture because of the collagenous micronodule, these are typically assigned as GS 3 + 3 = 6.*

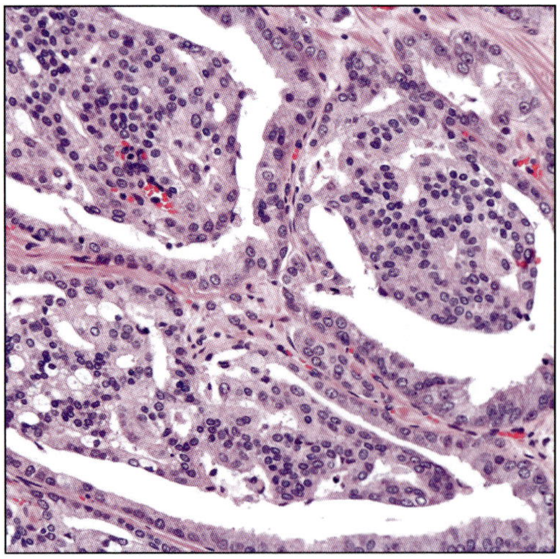
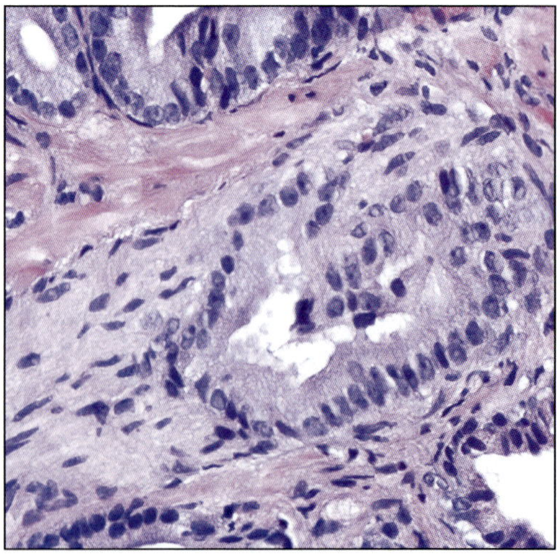

(Left) *H&E shows PCa with glomerulations characterized by intraluminal proliferation of cells that form a cribriform structure attached to 1 pole of the gland. Recent data suggests that glomerulations should be regarded as Gleason grade 4.* ***(Right)*** *High-power view shows PCa gland within a nerve. Intraneural and complete circumferential perineural invasion are pathognomonic features of PCa. Benign glands can be seen adjacent to a nerve and may resemble partial perineural invasion.*

Gleason Grades 2 and 3

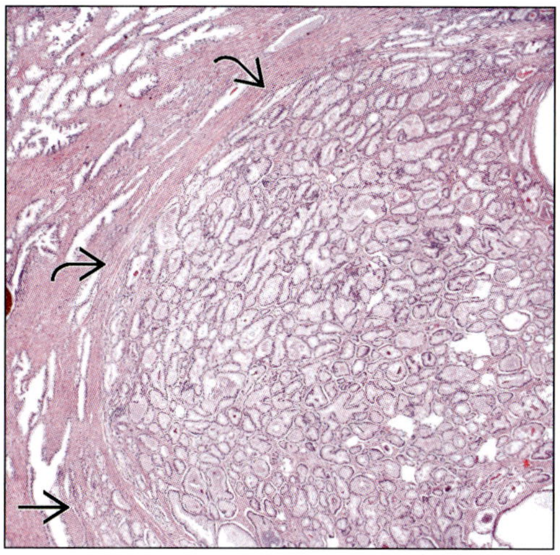

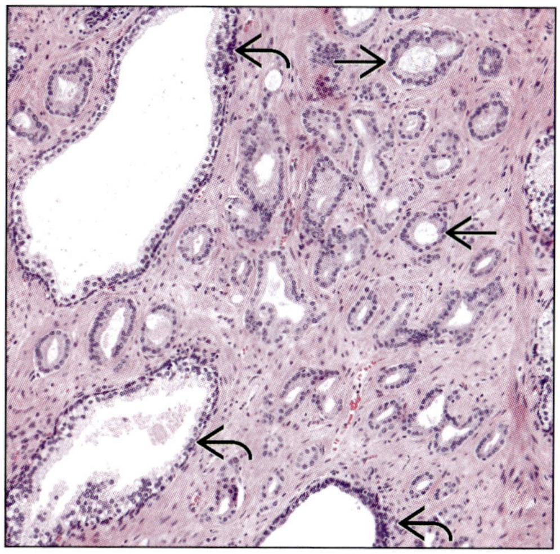

(Left) *This GS 2 + 3 = 5 PCa consists of a circumscribed nodule of slightly irregular medium and large glands (Gleason grade 2)* ↪ *and focally infiltrating glands (Gleason grade 3)* →. ***(Right)*** *Low-power view shows GS 3 + 3 = 6 PCa glands infiltrating between benign glands* ↪. *PCa glands are smaller, haphazardly arranged, have different cytoplasmic tincture and some have rigid lumina* →. *A well-formed gland should have a complete circumference of cells showing central lumina.*

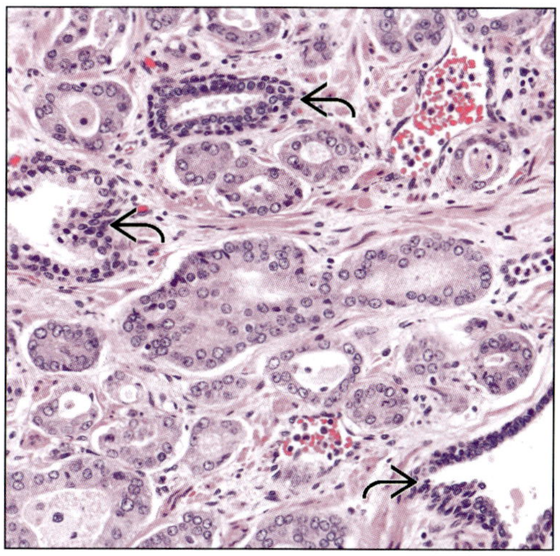

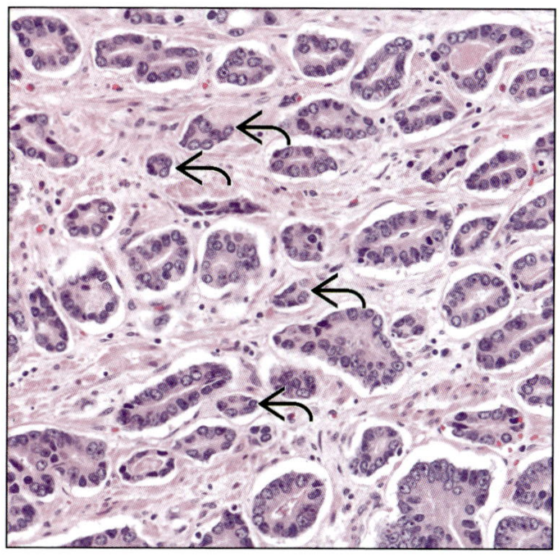

(Left) *These GS 3 + 3 = 6 PCa glands have large nuclei and prominent nucleoli that can be multiple and peripheral. Nuclei of benign glands* ↪ *are smaller and the glands have > 1 layer of cells.* ***(Right)*** *H&E shows GS 3 + 3 = 6 PCa composed of individual infiltrating glands and microacini* ↪. *One has to take into account that not all lumina may be visible on 1 plane of section. Tangentially sectioned glands (vs. ill-formed glands) are suggested by being few in numbers and scattered in between well-formed glands.*

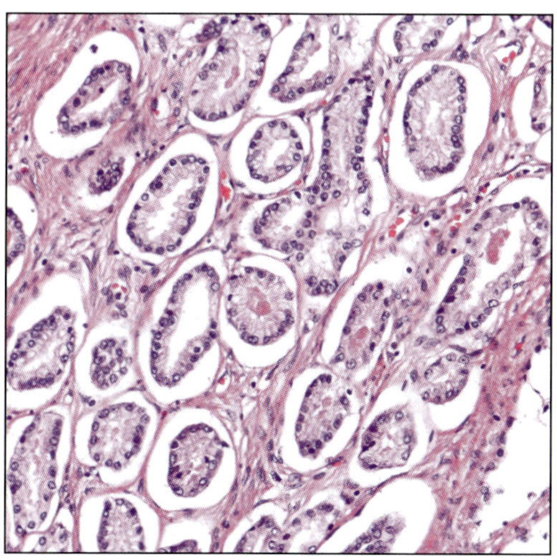

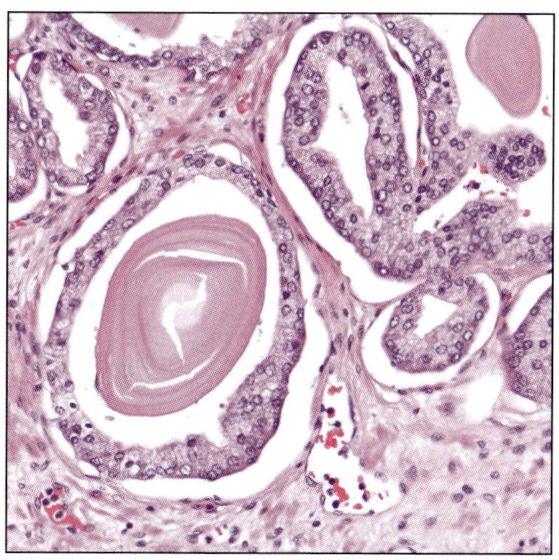

(Left) *This GS 3 + 3 = 6 PCa shows periacini retraction spaces, which is a helpful diagnostic feature. The somewhat linear alignment of the PCa glands is also a helpful hint. These PCa glands consist of columnar cells with basally oriented nuclei. PCa nuclei are relatively homogeneous and very rarely exhibits marked pleomorphism.* ***(Right)*** *High-power view of GS 3 + 3 = 6 PCa shows glands with corpora amylacea. These concretions, while common in benign glands, are rare in PCa.*

PROSTATE CARCINOMA

Gleason Grades 4 and 5

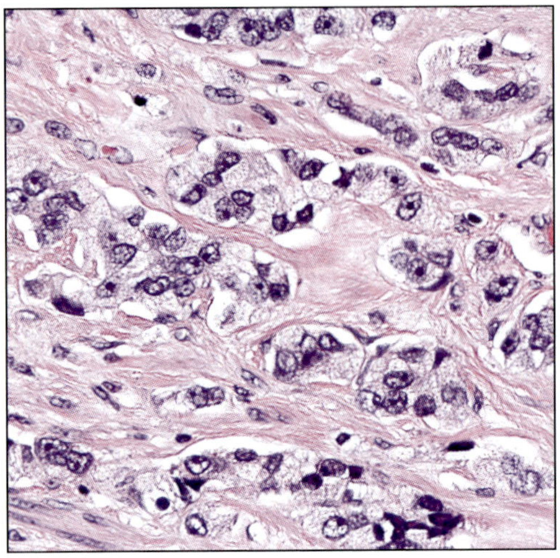
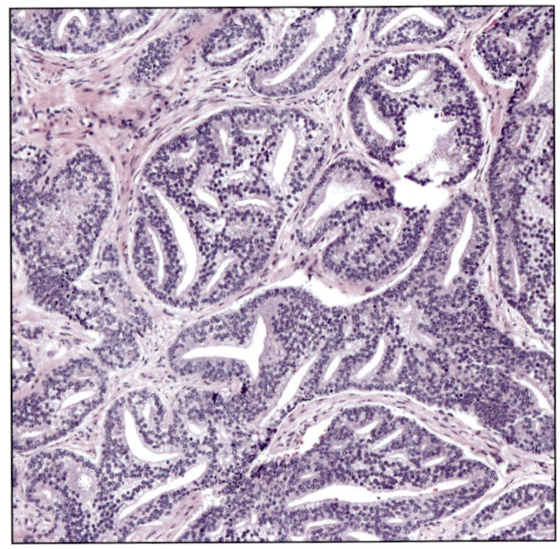

(Left) *High-power view of Gleason grade 4 PCa shows ill-defined glands formed by aggregates of tumor cells that are unable to form a complete circumference and central lumina.* ***(Right)*** *These Gleason grade 4 PCa cribriform glands are larger and central lumina are compartmentalized by multiple cellular bridges. Cribriform PCa gland can be medium or large with an expansile, elongated, or branching shape. Most experts now assign Gleason grade 4 to any cribriform PCa gland that lacks necrosis.*

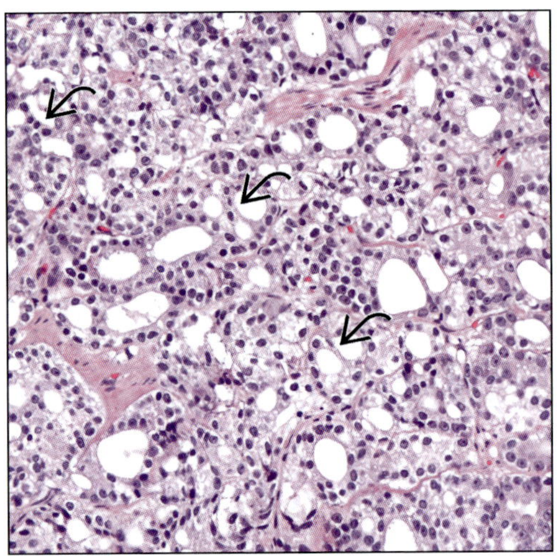
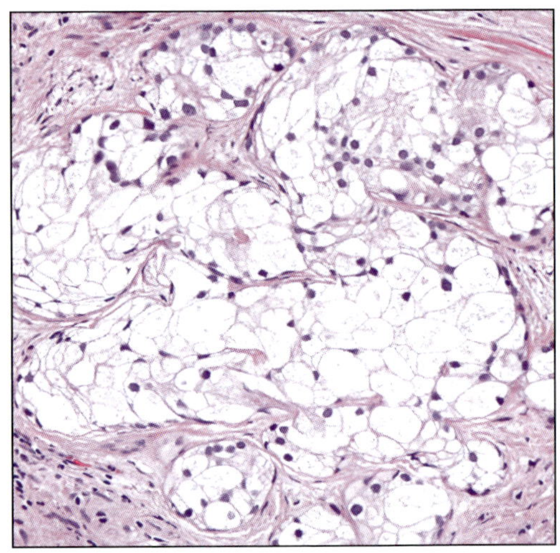

(Left) *This GS 4 + 4 = 8 PCa consists of multiple fused glands. Some lumina are separated by a single layer of cellular bridge that cannot be traced as an exclusive part of 1 gland. In contrast, tightly packed Gleason grade 3 glands can be individually outlined.* ***(Right)*** *H&E shows Gleason grade 4 PCa hypernephroid pattern consisting of solid growth of cells with clear cytoplasm that resemble clear cell RCC. The nuclei are often small and dark with inconspicuous nucleoli.*

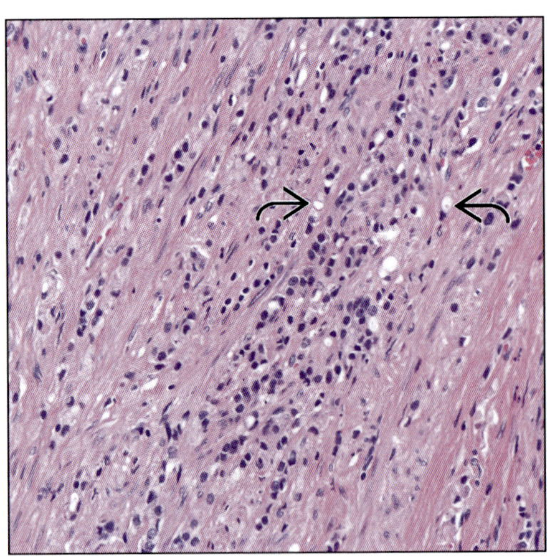
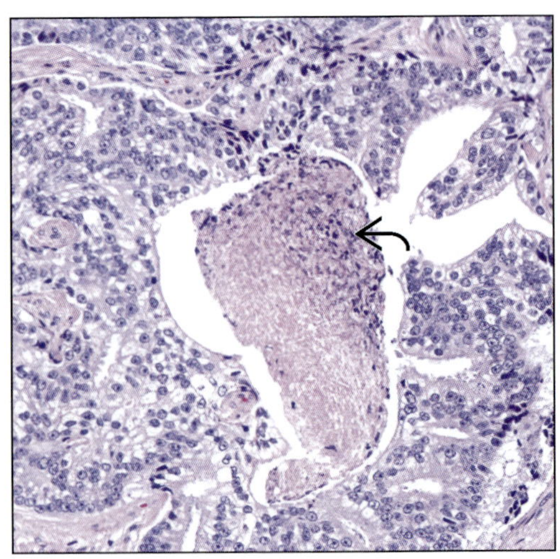

(Left) *H&E shows Gleason grade 5 PCa consisting of cords and single infiltrative tumor cells. These high-grade PCa cells may resemble chronic inflammatory cells. Note that some of the cells exhibit vacuolation.* ***(Right)*** *This large cribriform PCa gland contains luminal necrosis and grading is bumped to Gleason grade 5. The lumen should unequivocally demonstrate necrotic tumor ghost cells. Luminal eosinophilic secretions and inflammatory debris can be mistaken for tumor cell necrosis.*

Gleason Grade 5 and Intraductal Carcinoma

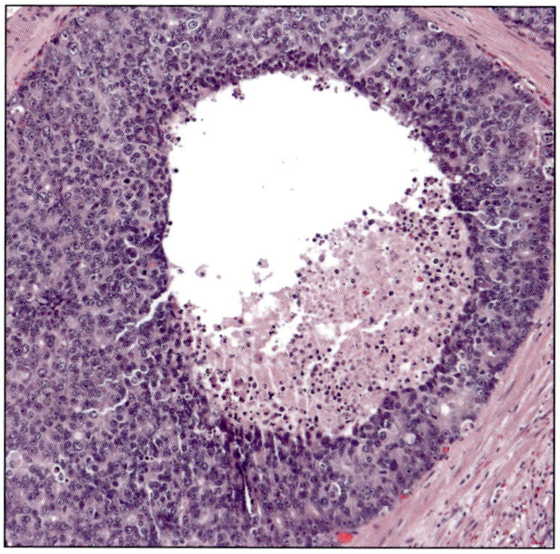

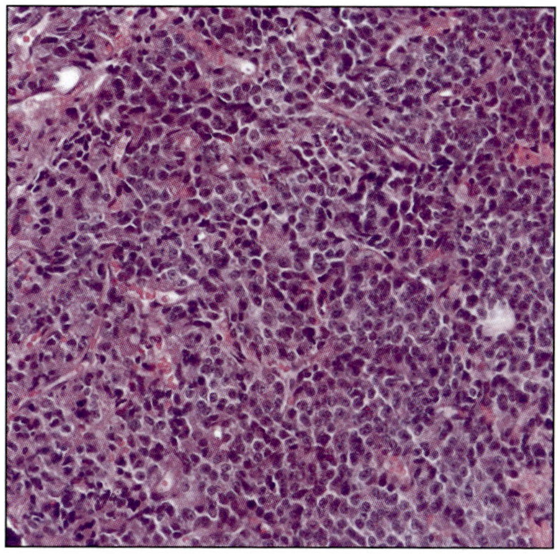

(Left) *This Gleason grade 5 PCa gland shows comedonecrosis. The central lumen contains abundant necrotic tumor cells.* ***(Right)*** *This Gleason grade 5 PCa shows solid growth of poorly differentiated cells. This morphology should be distinguished from a poorly differentiated urothelial carcinoma. Morphologic distinction can be very difficult and often necessitate use of immunostains. Beware that poorly differentiated PCa may exhibit weak or absent PSA expression in up to 13% of cases.*

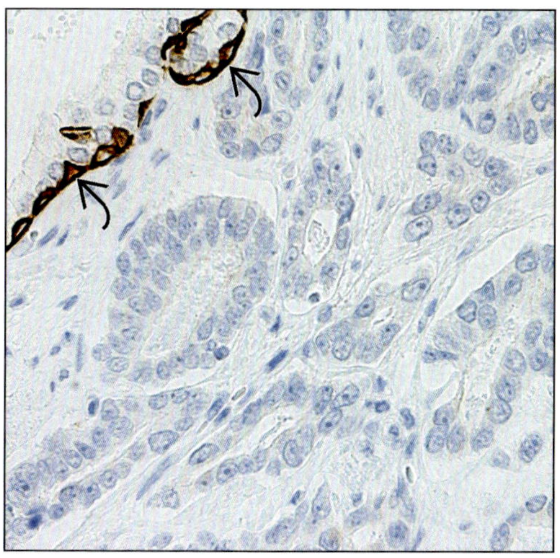

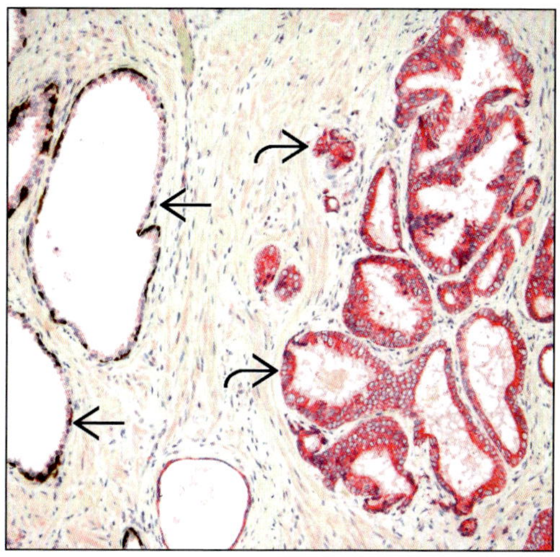

(Left) *HMWCK shows lack of staining in PCa glands. All atypical glands in a suspicious focus should have complete absence of basal cell staining. Adjacent benign gland shows HMWCK staining of the basal cells →.* ***(Right)*** *This cocktail of AMACR (red) and basal cell markers p63 and HMWCK (brown) shows AMACR overexpression and complete absence of basal cell marker immunoreactivity in PCa glands →. Benign glands in contrast show intact basal cells → and no AMACR overexpression.*

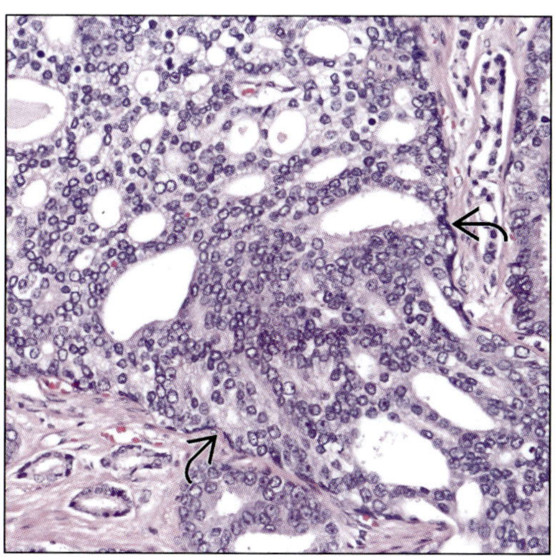

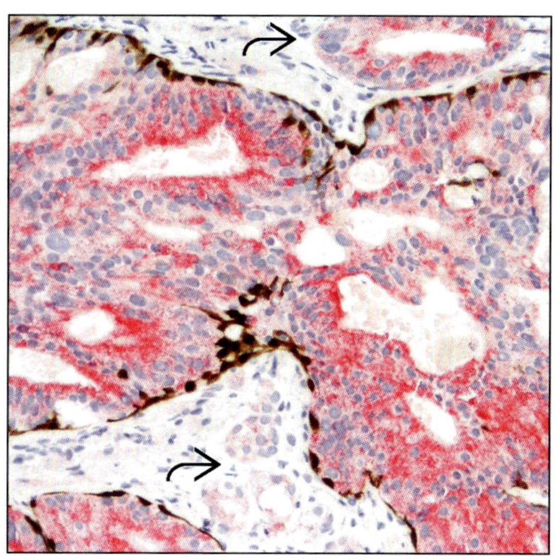

(Left) *H&E shows intraductal carcinoma consisting of large expansile cribriform structures that are composed of cells with large nuclei and prominent nucleoli and has an intact basal cell layer →.* ***(Right)*** *This antibody cocktail of AMACR (red) and basal cell markers p63 and HMWCK (brown) shows AMACR overexpression and basal cell marker staining. Intraductal carcinoma more often coexists with invasive glands → and is considered to be a process succedent to PCa invasion.*

PROSTATE CARCINOMA

Morphologic Variants and Variations

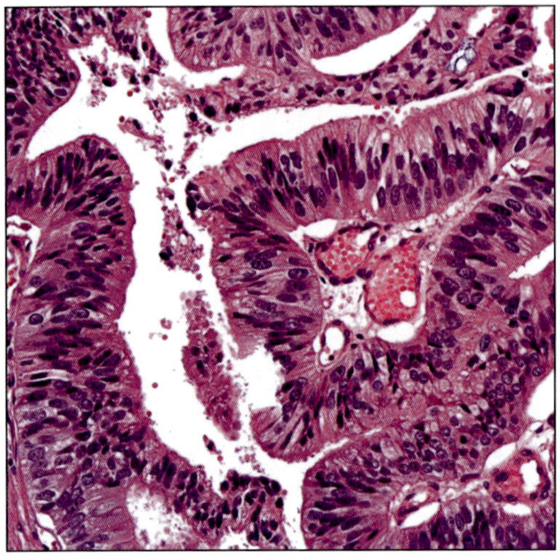

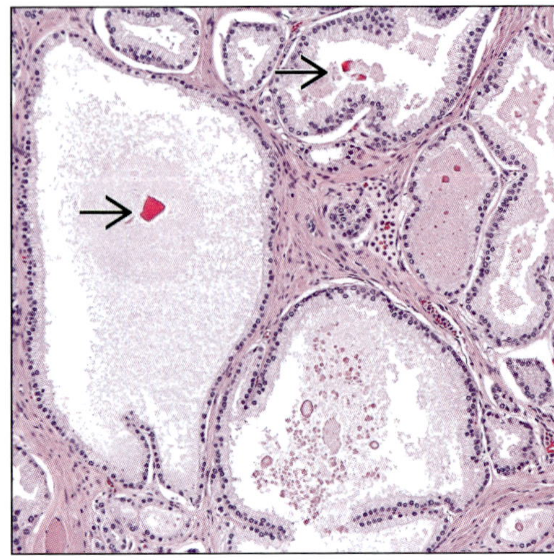

(Left) *Ductal adenocarcinoma shows papillae lined by tall columnar cells with pale cytoplasm and elongated nuclei, exhibiting pseudostratification. Presence of tall columnar cell is a distinguishing feature for this variant.* ***(Right)*** *Pseudohyperplastic PCa shows medium to large dilated glands with papillary infolding, eosinophilic secretions, and few crystalloids →. The cells have abundant cytoplasm and nuclei are usually aligned basally. This variant architecturally resembles benign hyperplasia.*

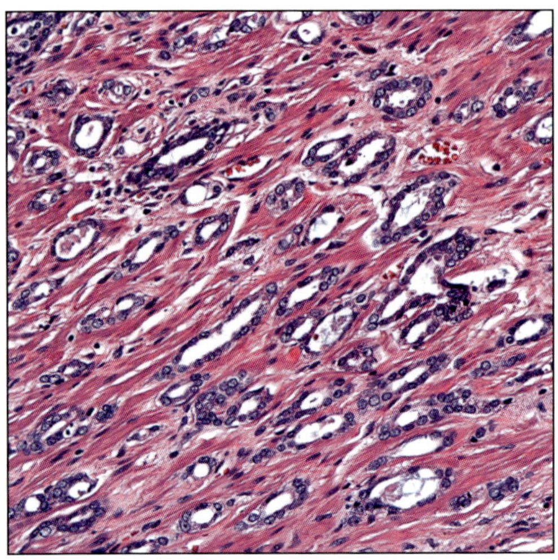

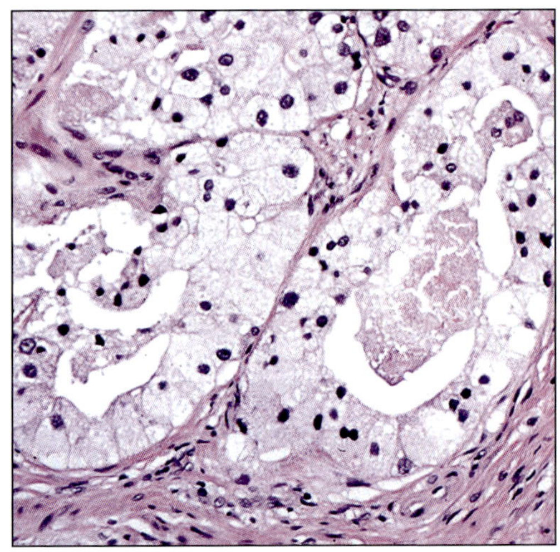

(Left) *Atrophic PCa shows acini lined by cells with attenuated cytoplasm. Features indicative of malignancy include malignant nuclear features (e.g., nucleomegaly, prominent nucleoli), nonlobular growth, luminal features of malignancy, and admixed typical PCa morphology.* ***(Right)*** *Foamy gland PCa shows cells with abundant xanthomatous cytoplasm and small to eosinophilic luminal secretions. Typical malignant nuclear features may not be present, making recognition as PCa difficult.*

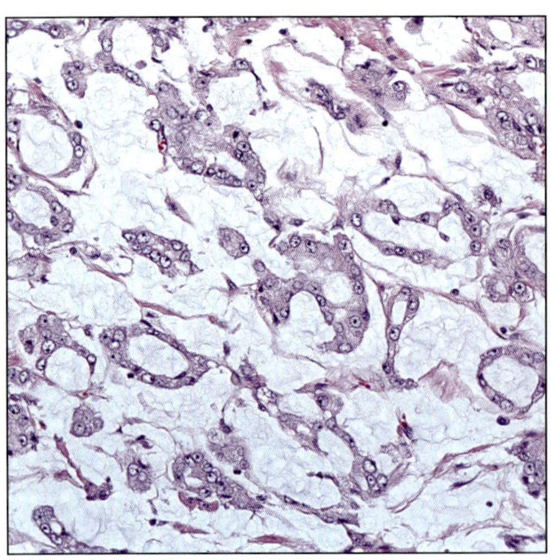

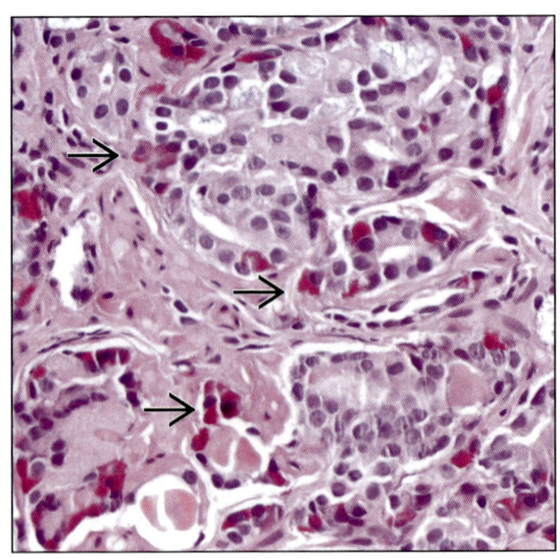

(Left) *Mucinous (colloid) carcinoma is characterized by malignant cells floating in abundant extracellular mucin. This is distinct from the intraluminal mucin seen in more typical forms of PCa. When seen pure in biopsy, confirmation of prostatic origin by immunohistochemistry is necessary.* ***(Right)*** *PCa with Paneth cell-like differentiation shows occasional neuroendocrine cells → with bright eosinophilic cytoplasmic granules resembling Paneth cells of the gastrointestinal tract.*

Differential Diagnosis

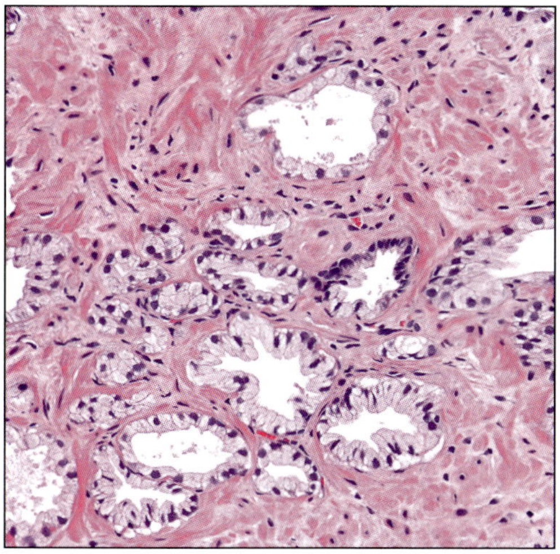
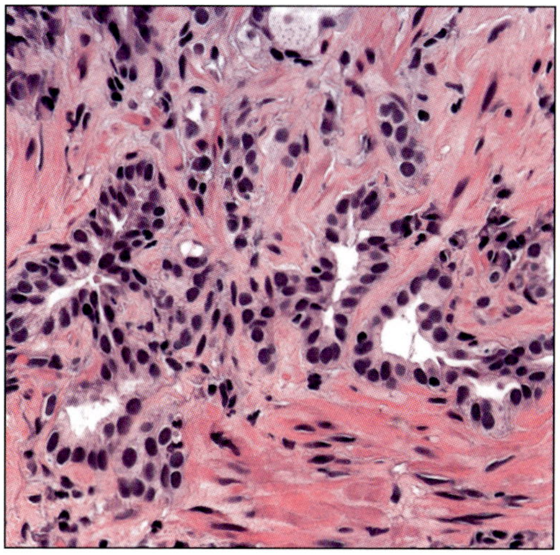

(Left) *H&E shows partial atrophy with relatively ample amount of pale to clear cytoplasm. In contrast to PCa, these glands are somewhat more lobular, more irregular, and lack nuclear and luminal features of malignancy.* **(Right)** *Simple atrophy shows nuclear crowding from loss of cytoplasmic volume. Unlike typical PCa, these atrophic glands are more irregular and angulated. Unlike atrophic PCa, these atrophic glands lack the nuclear and luminal features of malignancy.*

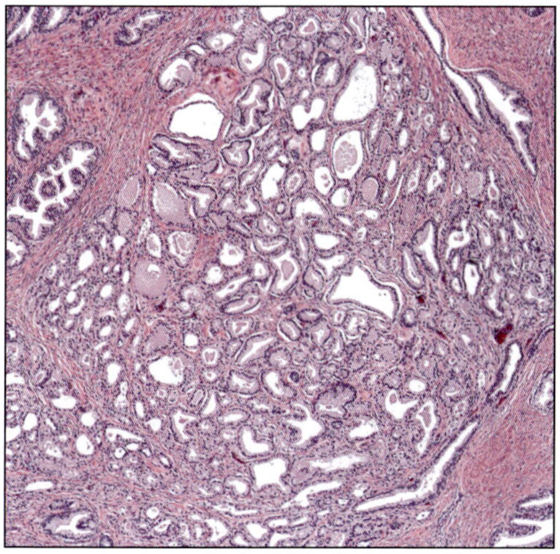
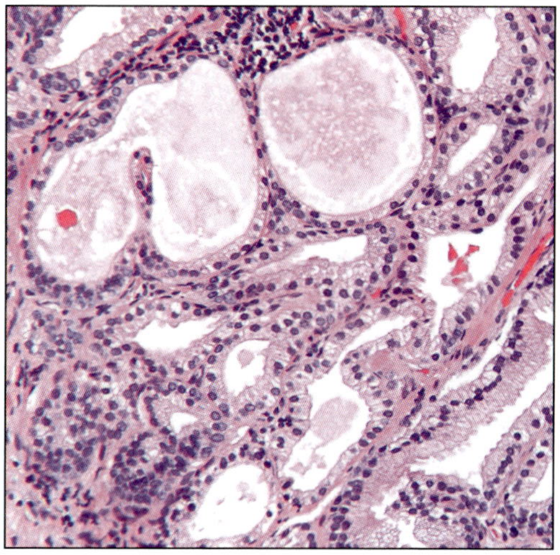

(Left) *Low-power view of AAH shows relatively well-circumscribed proliferation of variably sized acini. The glands at the central aspect are usually larger than in the periphery.* **(Right)** *Intraluminal proteinaceous material and crystalloids may occasionally be seen in AAH. Presence of both of these features in atypical glands compounds the diagnostic difficulty vs. PCa. Immunohistochemistry confirms presence of basal cells in AAH vs. PCa that can be focal or patchy.*

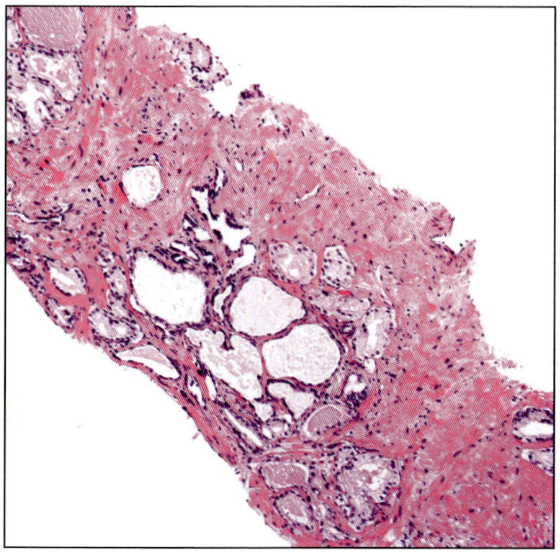
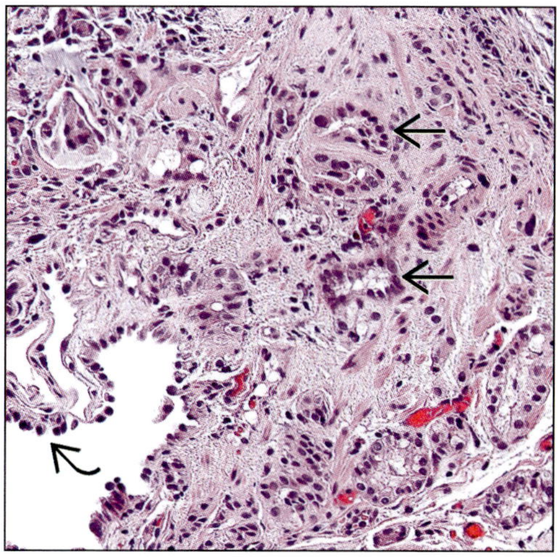

(Left) *PAH encountered in needle biopsy is shown. PAH is 1 of the main differential diagnoses for ASAP in needle biopsy. Diagnosis is relatively less challenging if the entire architecture is appreciated as in this case.* **(Right)** *Nephrogenic adenoma from the prostatic urethra may be sampled in needle biopsy and its tubules ➔ may mimic PCa. Distinction is confounded by the similar positivity for AMACR. Attention to single layer of hobnail cells at the surface ➚ similar to those in tubules is helpful.*

TESTICULAR SERTOLI CELL NEOPLASMS

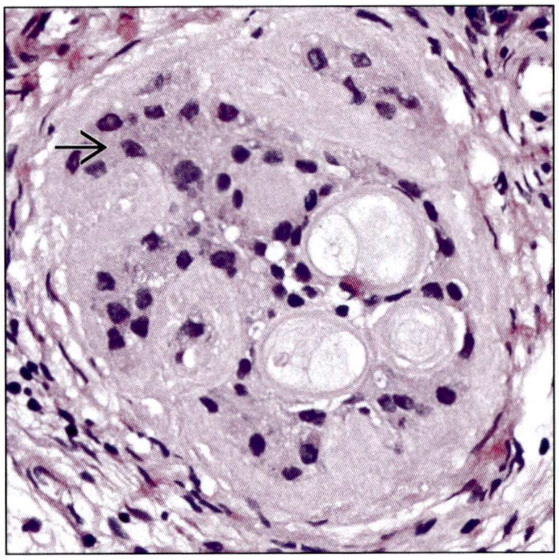

High-power view shows an intratubular large cell hyalinizing Sertoli cell neoplasia (ILCHSCN) in a Peutz-Jeghers syndrome testis, composed of large Sertoli cells ➔ admixed with basement membrane material.

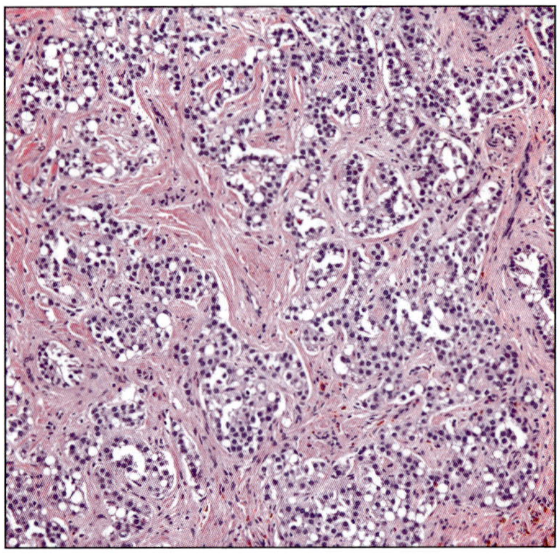

Intermediate-power view shows Sertoli cell tumor (SCT) with small nested cords and tubular growths in a fibrous stroma. SCT grows in variable architectural patterns, with tubule formation being the most common.

TERMINOLOGY

Definitions

- Group of testicular neoplasms with Sertoli cell differentiation linked to syndromes such as Carney complex and Peutz-Jeghers syndrome
  - **Intratubular large cell hyalinizing Sertoli cell neoplasia (ILCHSCN)**: Intraseminiferous tubular neoplasia of large Sertoli cells admixed with globular basement membrane deposits
    - Subset may progress to invasive Sertoli cell tumor (SCT) or large cell calcifying SCT (LCCSCT)
  - **SCT**: Sex cord-stromal tumor exhibiting variable patterns and hallmark tubular growth
  - **LCCSCT**: Variant of SCT composed of large epithelioid cells with abundant eosinophilic cytoplasm and peculiar calcifications
- Most ILCHSCN described in Peutz-Jeghers syndrome
- Vast majority of SCT and ~ 60% of LCCSCT encountered as sporadic tumors
  - ~ 40% of LCCSCT linked to syndromes

ETIOLOGY/PATHOGENESIS

Syndromes/Familial Sertoli Cell Neoplasms

- **Peutz-Jeghers syndrome**
  - Mainly caused by mutations in *STK11/LKB1*
  - Autosomal dominant disorder characterized by multiple hamartomatous polyps and mucocutaneous pigmentations with higher risk for multiple visceral organ cancers (lifetime risk of 37-93%)
  - ILCHSCN, LCCSCT, and SCT described in patients with this syndrome
- **Carney complex**
  - Autosomal dominant multiple neoplasia syndrome
  - Caused by mutations in *PRKAR1A* (45-80%)
  - LCCSCT is a component of this complex

CLINICAL ISSUES

Epidemiology

- Incidence
  - SCT and LCCSCT are rare tumors
- Age
  - **SCT**: ~ 30% occur in 1st decade of life
  - **LCCSCT**: Mostly prepubertal boys to young adult men; mean: ~ 30 years
  - **ILCHSCN**: < 15 years of age; mean: 6.8 years

Presentation

- ILCHSCN may exhibit testicular enlargement but no discrete mass
- SCT and LCCSCT may present as painless testicular mass or enlargement
  - LCCSCT has higher chance for bilaterality, particularly in Carney syndrome
- Hormone-related symptoms, such as gynecomastia (most common), precocious puberty, or advanced skeletal maturation
- Discovery of testicular tumors from other syndromic manifestations
  - Peutz-Jeghers syndrome
    - Mucocutaneous pigmentations, bowel obstruction, or intussusception from multiple gastrointestinal polyps
  - Carney complex
    - Spotty pigmentation of skin, cardiac or cutaneous myxomas, endocrinopathy, schwannomas
- Testicular ultrasound of LCCSCT will show characteristic Christmas tree-like appearance

Laboratory Tests

- High serum estradiol levels
- Serum α-fetoprotein and β-HCG levels not elevated

Prognosis

- **ILCHSCN**: Benign course, but a subset may transform to invasive SCT or LCCSCT

TESTICULAR SERTOLI CELL NEOPLASMS

Key Facts

Terminology
- Group of testicular neoplasms with Sertoli cell differentiation linked to syndromes such as Carney complex and Peutz-Jeghers syndrome
- Most ILCHSCN described in Peutz-Jeghers syndrome
- Most SCT and ~ 60% of LCCSCT are sporadic

Clinical Issues
- **ILCHSCN**: Benign course, but a subset may transform to invasive SCT or LCCSCT
- **SCT**: Majority benign; ~ 10% are malignant and may metastasize
- **LCCSCT**: Majority benign; ~ 20% malignant

Microscopic Pathology
- **ILCHSCN**: Seminiferous tubules with thickened basement membrane
  - Expanded by large Sertoli cells with pale to eosinophilic cytoplasm and globular, eosinophilic basement membrane deposits
- **SCT**: Hallmark tubular growth of regular cuboidal or columnar cells with pale to pink cytoplasm that may be vacuolated
- **LCCSCT**: Large polygonal cells with abundant eosinophilic ground-glass cytoplasm associated with hallmark irregular or psammomatous calcifications

Ancillary Tests
- Inhibin (+), PLAP and OCT3/OCT4 (-)

Top Differential Diagnoses
- Leydig cell tumor
- Granulosa cell tumor
- Adenomatoid tumor

- **SCT**: Majority benign; ~ 10% are malignant and may metastasize
- **LCCSCT**: Majority benign; ~ 20% malignant

MACROSCOPIC FEATURES

General Features
- **ILCHSCN**: Either testicular enlargement with no visible lesion or small ill-defined white lesions
- **SCT**: Small (mean: 3.5 cm), well-circumscribed, homogeneous gray-white to yellow mass
- **LCCSCT**: Usually small (< 4 cm), well-circumscribed, homogeneous gray-white to yellow mass with calcifications

MICROSCOPIC PATHOLOGY

Histologic Features
- **ILCHSCN**: Expanded seminiferous tubules with thickened peritubular basement membrane
  - Tubules filled with large Sertoli cells with abundant pale to eosinophilic cytoplasm and globular, eosinophilic basement membrane deposits
- **SCT**: Tubular (hallmark), microcystic, cords, and nests or solid growths
  - Nodular pattern on low-power view often separated by fibrous or acellular stroma
  - Tubules may be solid, hollow, or dilated
  - Regular cuboidal or columnar cells with bland round nuclei, occasional nucleoli, and pale to pink cytoplasm that may be vacuolated
  - Usually paucicellular, hyalinized, or fibrous stroma
- **LCCSCT**: Nest, cords, and trabecular or focal tubular growth
  - Large polygonal cells with abundant eosinophilic "ground-glass" cytoplasm, nuclei with vesicular chromatin and variably prominent nucleoli
  - Hallmark calcifications that may be large, irregular, wavy, laminated, or psammomatous
  - Myxoid or fibromyxoid stroma

ANCILLARY TESTS

Immunohistochemistry
- Inhibin (+), PLAP and OCT3/OCT4 (-)

DIFFERENTIAL DIAGNOSIS

Leydig Cell Tumor
- Differential diagnosis for SCT and LCCSCT
- Mainly solid growth of large round or polygonal cells with abundant eosinophilic cytoplasm

Granulosa Cell Tumor (GCT)
- Differential diagnosis for SCT
- Mainly microfollicular pattern and formation of Call-Exner bodies (eosinophilic material surrounded by palisading granulosa cells)

Adenomatoid Tumor
- Differential diagnosis for SCT and LCCSCT
- Located in testicular adnexa
- Composed of gland-like or irregular spaces lined by cuboidal to flat bland cells
- Calretinin (+) and WT1(+)

SELECTED REFERENCES

1. Gourgari E et al: Large-cell calcifying Sertoli cell tumors of the testes in pediatrics. Curr Opin Pediatr. 24(4):518-22, 2012
2. Ulbright TM et al: Intratubular large cell hyalinizing sertoli cell neoplasia of the testis: a report of 8 cases of a distinctive lesion of the Peutz-Jeghers syndrome. Am J Surg Pathol. 31(6):827-35, 2007
3. Young RH: Sex cord-stromal tumors of the ovary and testis: their similarities and differences with consideration of selected problems. Mod Pathol. 18 Suppl 2:S81-98, 2005

TESTICULAR SERTOLI CELL NEOPLASMS

Microscopic Features

__(Left)__ SCT shows cords and tubules composed of polygonal cells with modest light eosinophilic cytoplasm and regular nuclei in a fibrous background. Note presence of cytoplasmic vacuolations →, which is common in SCT. __(Right)__ SCT is characterized by tubular formations that can be solid →, hollow ⇒, or dilated ↗. Dilated tubules are occasionally lined by more flattened cells and may ramify to resemble rete testis (retiform pattern). Note the presence of light eosinophilic secretions in tubular lumina.

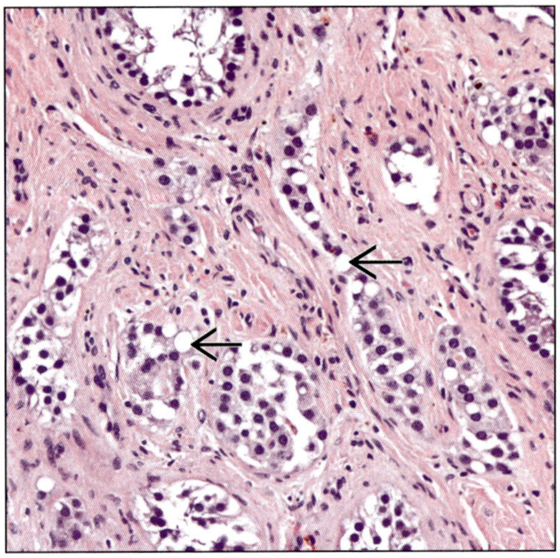

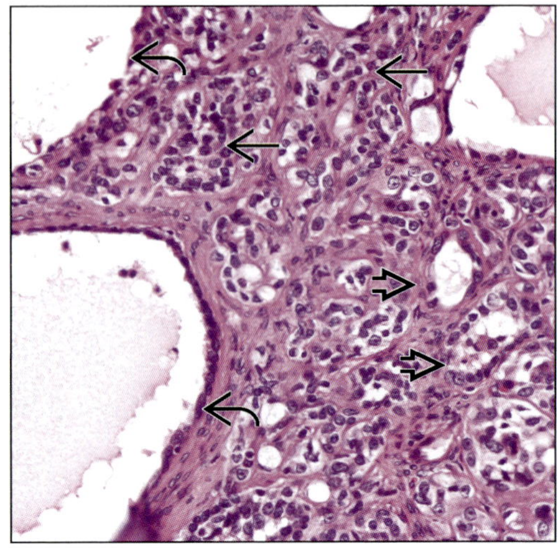

__(Left)__ High-power view shows SCT composed of polygonal cells with a modest amount of pale to light eosinophilic cytoplasm. Some of the tumor cells are also vacuolated. The nuclei usually do not exhibit prominent nucleoli, and mitosis is rare in > 80% of cases, particularly in the well-differentiated (tubule-forming) tumors. __(Right)__ H&E shows SCT exhibiting a more solid growth. The tumor cells have abundant lipid-filled cytoplasmic vacuoles. Some of the vacuoles are multiple and large, which indents the nuclei.

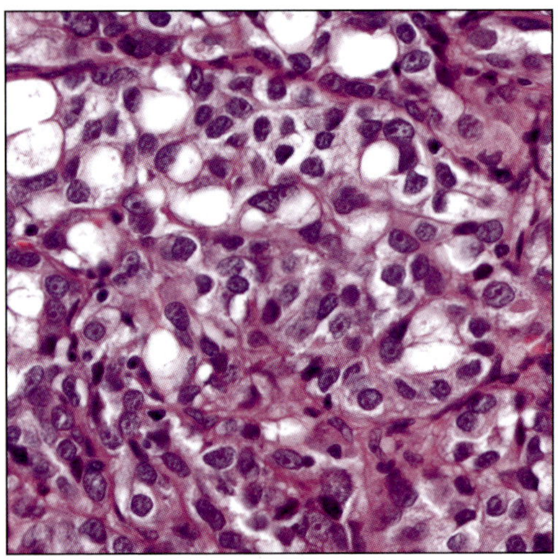

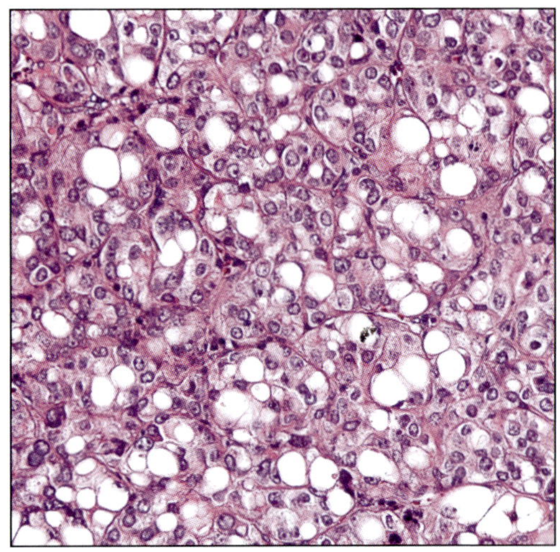

__(Left)__ A well-circumscribed LCCSCT is demarcated from the adjacent testis ⇒ by a thick fibrous capsule. The tumor is composed of cords and nests of tumor cells with hyalinized or myxoid stroma. (Courtesy S. Shen, MD, PhD.) __(Right)__ LCCSCT shows small nests and solid tubules of large polygonal cells with abundant eosinophilic cytoplasm in a myxoid stroma. Presence of calcifications → is a hallmark for LCCSCT and can be marked. These calcifications may make the tumor notably gritty on sectioning.

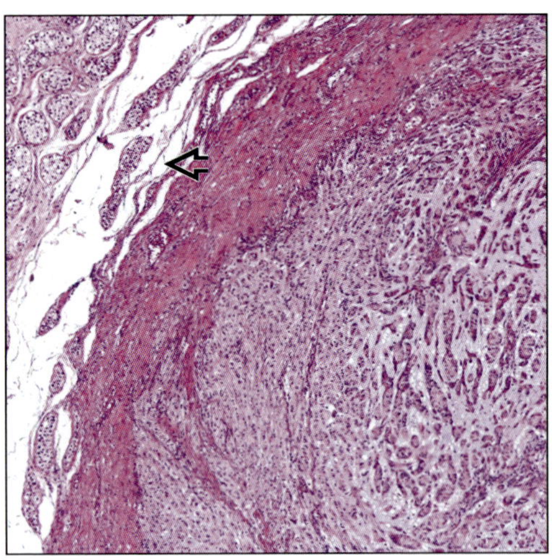

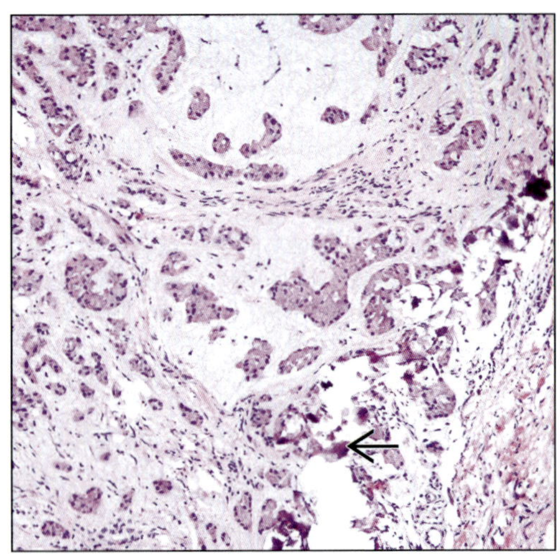

Microscopic Features and Differential Diagnosis

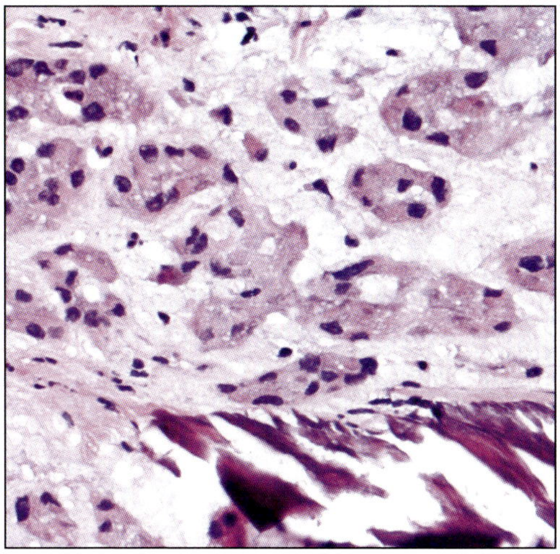

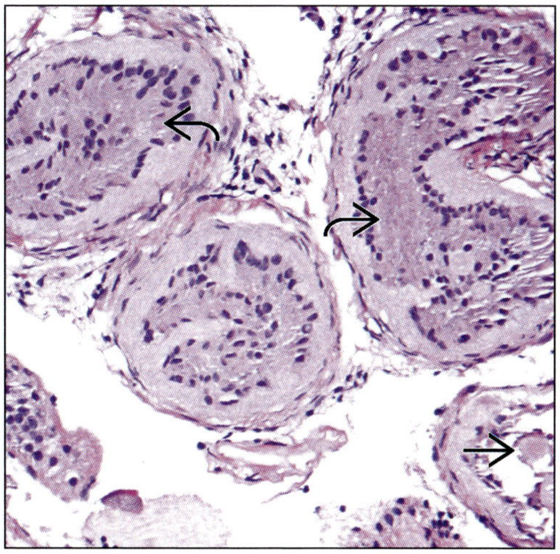

(Left) *High-power view of LCCSCT shows the characteristic large polygonal pink cells with bland nuclei. Note the dense calcifications and scattered neutrophils.* **(Right)** *H&E shows ILCHSCN composed of intratubular proliferations of large Sertoli cells and with dense eosinophilic basement membrane deposits. The deposits are denser at the peritubular area and may also form globules ⇒. The Sertoli cells ↗ have abundant eosinophilic cytoplasm, which can be fibrillary.*

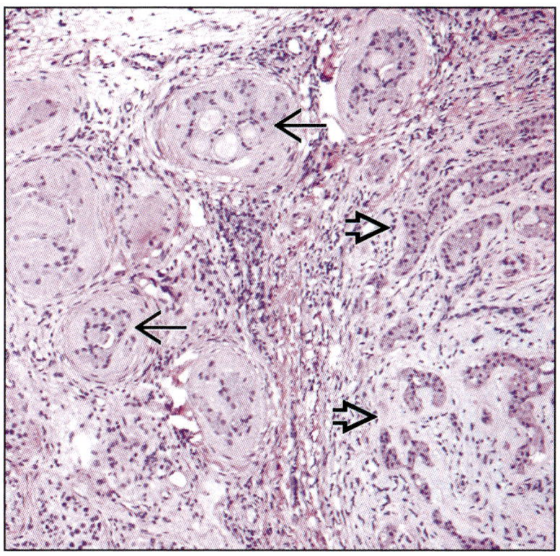

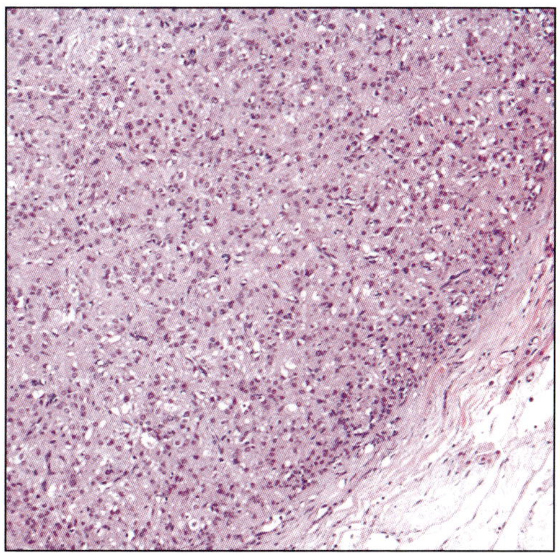

(Left) *Low-power view shows an ILCHSCN ⇒ adjacent to LCCSCT ⇨. ILCHSCN is an intratubular process that does not form a mass lesion. A subset of ILCHSCN may become invasive to form LCCSCT or SCT.* **(Right)** *Low-power view shows Leydig cell tumor with solid growth of polygonal cells with abundant eosinophilic cytoplasm. The tumor may also exhibit tubular or insular growths. The tumor cells are typically uniform with round to ovoid nuclei. Unlike LCCSCT, calcification is not a feature.*

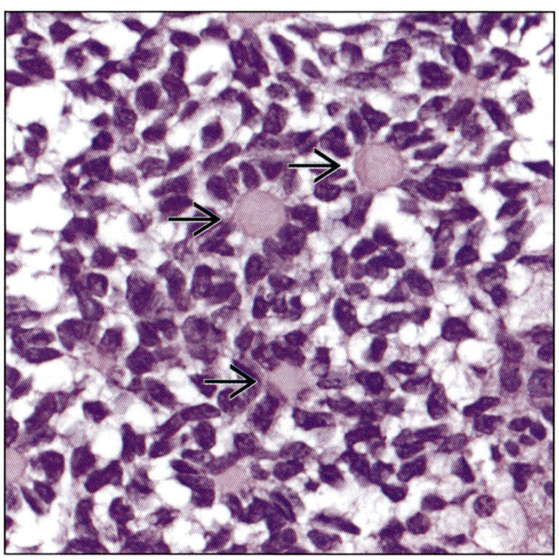

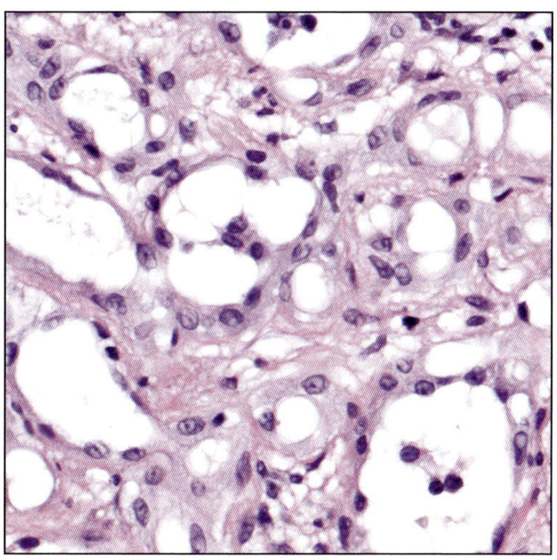

(Left) *A GCT shows typical Call-Exner bodies ⇒ characterized by central eosinophilic material and palisading tumor cells, resulting in a rosette appearance. The tumor cells have scant cytoplasm. (Courtesy S. Shen, MD, PhD.)* **(Right)** *Adenomatoid tumor shows variably sized tubules of cuboidal and flattened cells, and some may resemble vessels or signet ring cells. Unlike SCT, adenomatoid tumor is located in the testicular adnexa and expresses WT1 and calretinin.*

ANGIOMYOLIPOMA

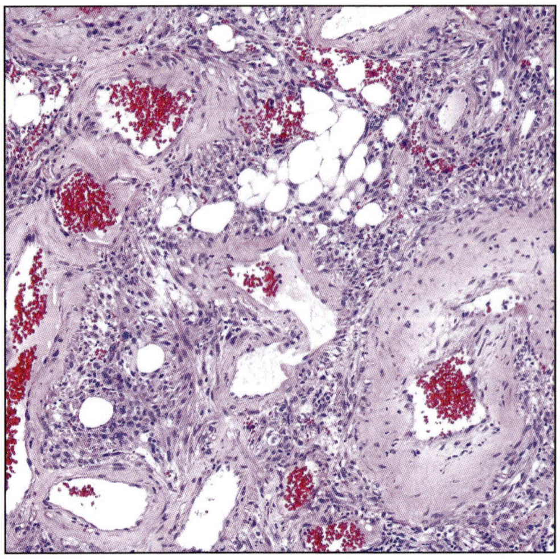

C-AML shows triphasic morphology composed of dysmorphic blood vessels, spindle cells, and fat. Proportion of these components vary so that 1 may predominate (e.g., leiomyomatous or lipoma-like AML).

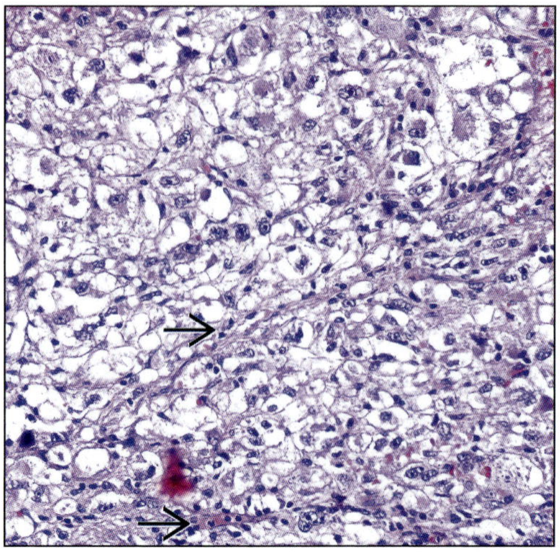

E-AML shows carcinoma-like growth with epithelioid cells containing clear to granular cytoplasm separated by thin vasculatures ➔ and with pleomorphic nuclei, which may resemble high-grade clear cell RCC.

TERMINOLOGY

Abbreviations

- Angiomyolipoma (AML)

Synonyms

- Classic AML (C-AML): Renal PEComa, triphasic AML

Definitions

- **C-AML**
  - Renal mesenchymal neoplasm putatively derived from perivascular epithelioid cells (PECs) with typical triphasic components of dysmorphic blood vessels, fat, and spindle cells
- **Epithelioid AML (E-AML)**
  - Renal mesenchymal neoplasm putatively derived from PECs consisting mainly of polygonal cells
- C-AML and E-AML are closely related to a family of PEC-derived visceral and soft tissue tumors
  - e.g., PEComas, lymphangiomyomatosis, "sugar" tumor of lung, and cardiac rhabdomyomas
- C-AML and E-AML often a spectrum

ETIOLOGY/PATHOGENESIS

Sporadic AML

- > 90% of C-AML and ~ 75% of E-AML are sporadic

Tuberous Sclerosis (TS)-Associated AML

- Genetic alterations in *TSC1* or hamartin (Chr 9q34) and *TSC2* or tuberin (Chr 16p13.3)
- Up to 75% of TS patients will develop AML
- Association of E-AML (~ 25%) to TS stronger

CLINICAL ISSUES

Epidemiology

- Incidence
  - Uncommon, encountered in < 0.2% of population
- Age
  - 14-88 years old; median: 50 years
  - Younger for TS-associated AML (mean: 26 years)
  - E-AML younger than C-AML (mean: 39 vs. 52 years)
- Gender
  - Higher female incidence shown by most studies
    - C-AML: M:F = 1:1-4 and E-AML: M:F = 1:1-6.5

Presentation

- ~ 50% are incidental finding
- ~ 2/3 show signs of bleeding (e.g., hematuria, retroperitoneal hemorrhage) and ~ 1/5 has flank pain

Natural History

- TS-associated AML presents earlier, larger, multifocal or bilateral, and more symptomatic than sporadic AML

Treatment

- Conservative surgery for C-AML, such as partial nephrectomy, enucleation, or embolization
- Expectant management suggested for radiographically typical AML
  - Surgical intervention for suspicion of malignancy, large size, hemorrhage, and intractable pain

Prognosis

- Contemporary studies with C-AML shows benign outcome; retroperitoneal hemorrhage can be fatal
- E-AML has malignancy potential with reported metastasis and deaths
  - Recurrence and metastasis varied from 5-49%
  - Reported mortality rates of 10-33%
  - Differences in aggressiveness influenced by varying diagnostic criteria and types of cases

MACROSCOPIC FEATURES

General Features

- Solitary in 60% and multifocal in 40%

ANGIOMYOLIPOMA

Key Facts

Terminology
- **C-AML**: Renal mesenchymal neoplasm putatively derived from PECs with typical triphasic components of dysmorphic blood vessels, fat, and spindle cells
- **E-AML**: Renal mesenchymal neoplasm putatively derived from PECs consisting of polygonal cells

Etiology/Pathogenesis
- > 90% of C-AML and ~ 75% of E-AML are sporadic
- Up to 75% of TS patients will develop AML
- Association of E-AML (~25%) to TS stronger

Clinical Issues
- Age: 14-88 years old; median: 50 years
- Younger for TS-associated AML (mean: 26 years)
- TS-associated AML presents earlier, larger, multifocal or bilateral, and more symptomatic

Microscopic Pathology
- **C-AML:** Usually triphasic pattern of dysmorphic vessels, fat, and spindle cells in 85% of cases
- In 15%, fat or spindle cells may predominate (comprises 95% of tumor)
- **E-AML:** Carcinoma-like or diffuse mixed epithelioid and plump spindle cell growths
- Nuclei tend to be pleomorphic with brisk mitosis
- Larger pleomorphic multinucleated cells present

Ancillary Tests
- Melanocytic markers (+); epithelial markers (-)

Top Differential Diagnoses
- C-AML: Sarcomatoid RCC or urothelial carcinoma, liposarcoma and smooth muscle tumors
- E-AML: RCC

- Up to 100% of familial AMLs are multifocal/bilateral

Size
- E-AML larger than C-AML
  - C-AML range from 1-30 cm; mean: 8.6 cm
  - E-AML range from 0.2-35 cm; mean: 5.6 cm
- Familial larger than sporadic AMLs (mean: 13 vs. 5 cm)

Gross Appearance
- C-AML
  - Unencapsulated and may bulge or extend to extrarenal fat (not a sign of malignancy)
  - Variable appearance depending on predominance of fat (lipoma-like) or spindle cells (leiomyoma-like)
- E-AML
  - Unencapsulated and may extend outside of kidney
  - More solid with variable amount of hemorrhage, necrosis, or cystic degeneration

MICROSCOPIC PATHOLOGY

Histologic Features
- **C-AML**
  - Usually triphasic pattern of dysmorphic vessels, fat, and spindle cells in up to 85% of cases
  - In 15%, fat or spindle cells may predominate (comprises 95% of tumor)
  - Vessels are ectatic, hyalinized with eccentric lumen
  - Spindle cells have granular cytoplasm, bland nuclei, rare mitosis, and appear to radiate from vessels
  - Fat cells are mature and may have nuclear atypia
  - Rarely, may have epithelial cysts lined by cuboidal or hobnail cells (AML with epithelial cells)
- **E-AML**
  - **Carcinoma-like growth**
    - Cohesive nests, broad alveoli or sheets compartmentalized by vascular septae
  - **Diffuse epithelioid and plump spindle cell growth**
  - Cells have pale to granular eosinophilic cytoplasm
  - Nuclei tend to be atypical or pleomorphic
  - Brisk mitosis (> 5 per HPF) with atypical forms
  - Larger pleomorphic multinucleated cells present
  - Hemorrhages, necrosis, vascular invasion, and extrarenal extension not uncommon

ANCILLARY TESTS

Immunohistochemistry
- Melanocytic markers (HMB-45, MART-1, tyrosinase) (+); rare cells (+) in fat-predominant AML
- Epithelial markers (-); spindle cells actin (+)

DIFFERENTIAL DIAGNOSIS

C-AML
- Sarcomatoid spindle RCC or urothelial carcinoma
  - High grade, keratin (+), and melanocytic markers (-)
- Liposarcoma
  - Lacks dysmorphic vessels and MDM2 or CDK4 (+)
- Smooth muscle tumors (leiomyoma or leiomyosarcoma)
  - So-called "capsuloma" likely fat-poor AML (HMB-45[+])
  - No dysmorphic vessels and melanocytic markers (-)

E-AML
- RCC
  - Clear cell RCC CAIX(+); melanocytic markers (-)

SELECTED REFERENCES

1. He W et al: Epithelioid angiomyolipoma of the kidney: pathological features and clinical outcome in a series of consecutively resected tumors. Mod Pathol. Epub ahead of print, 2013
2. Nese N et al: Pure epithelioid PEComas (so-called epithelioid angiomyolipoma) of the kidney: A clinicopathologic study of 41 cases: detailed assessment of morphology and risk stratification. Am J Surg Pathol. 35(2):161-76, 2011

ANGIOMYOLIPOMA

Gross and Microscopic Features

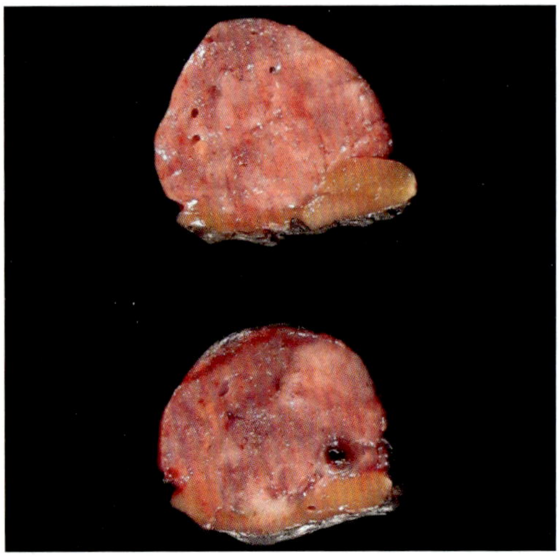

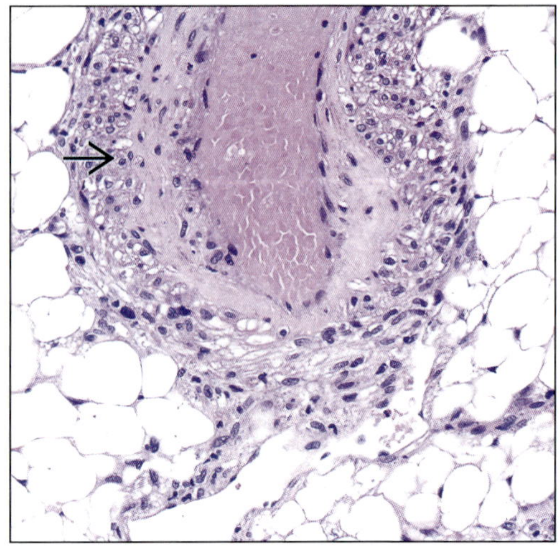

(Left) *Gross photograph of partial nephrectomy for C-AML shows variegated appearance because of varying admixture of spindle cells, fat, and vessels. This tumor protrudes into the perinephric fat, which is not uncommon for AML.* ***(Right)*** *Blood vessels in C-AML are abnormal (ectatic, thickened, and hyalinized). The epithelioid and spindle cells appear to arise from around the vessels or from perivascular epithelioid cells* →*. Spindle cells merge with the fat component, which exhibits some atypia.*

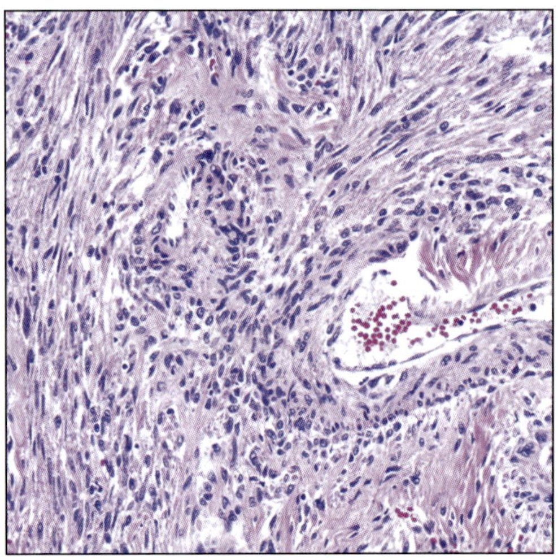

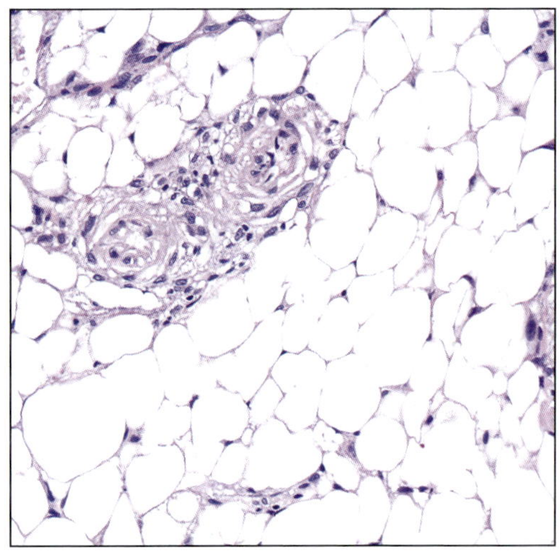

(Left) *C-AML shows predominance of spindle cells (leiomyomatous AML). Tumor cells can be seen originating from around the vessels. In areas with prominent spindle cells, the tumor may have a hemangiopericytoma-like appearance.* ***(Right)*** *C-AML shows predominance of fat (lipoma-like AML) that may exhibit atypia. Careful search for abnormal vessels with spindle or epithelioid cells, as shown in this image, should be made. Lipoma-like AML may resemble a well-differentiated liposarcoma from the retroperitoneum.*

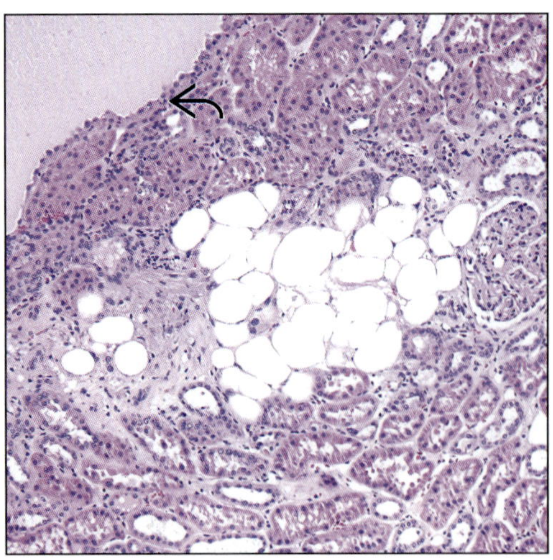

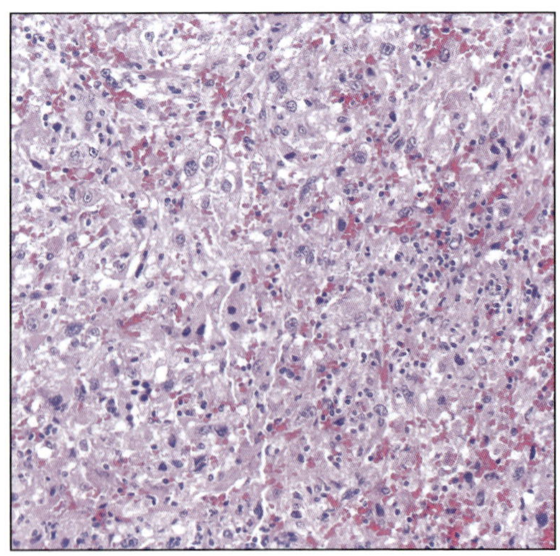

(Left) *Tuberous sclerosis patients may exhibit multiple and bilateral AMLs. As shown in this image, AML can be seen microscopically, incidentally in resected kidneys. Renal cysts* ↗ *are also common in tuberous sclerosis patients.* ***(Right)*** *E-AML shows diffuse epithelioid and plump spindle cell growth. Tumor cells show granular eosinophilic cytoplasm, and the nuclei exhibit some degree of pleomorphism. E-AML more often shows less prominent vascularity and rare fat cells. E-AML may resemble RCC.*

Microscopic Features and Differential Diagnosis

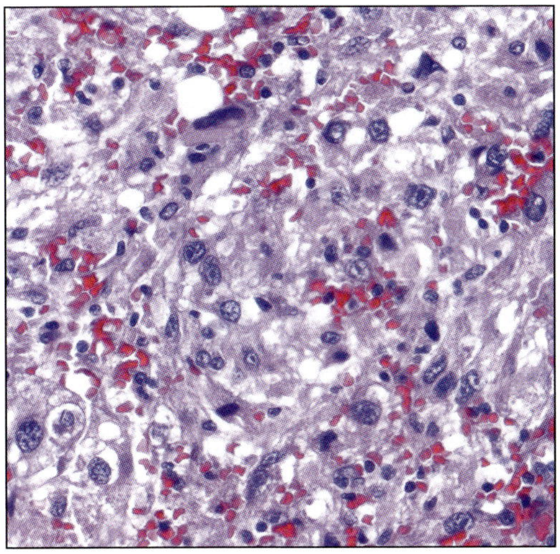

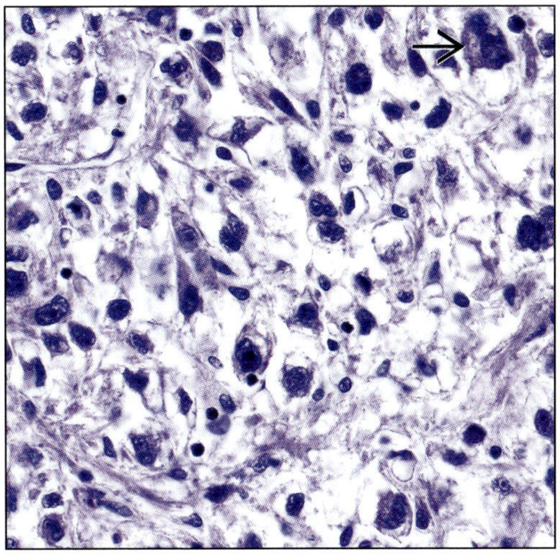

(Left) E-AML shows admixture of epithelioid and spindle cells with granular eosinophilic cytoplasm. The nuclei are more variable with obvious nuclear atypia. ***(Right)*** E-AML shows marked pleomorphism including multinucleation ➙. This degree of nuclear atypia is greater than in usual clear cell RCC, which is the main differential diagnosis. This feature should raise suspicion for E-AML. Admixture of spindle cells and, occasionally, focal areas of abnormal vessels and fat may help in diagnosis.

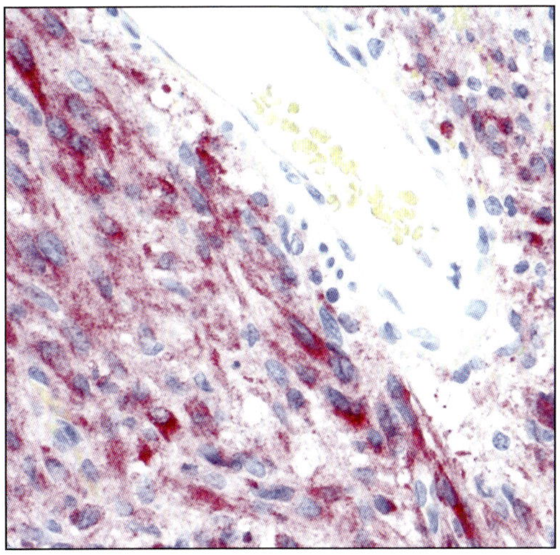

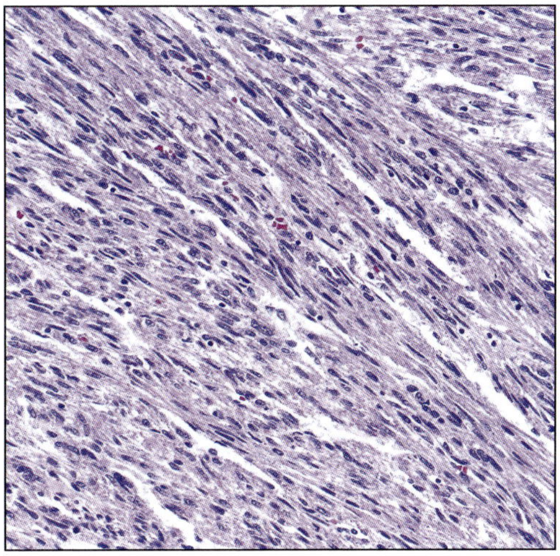

(Left) *MART-1 immunostain shows diffuse cytoplasmic immunoreactivity of the spindle cell component of C-AML. Other melanoma markers, such as HMB-45 and MITF are positive in AML.* ***(Right)*** *C-AML shows predominant spindle cells with absence of fat (leiomyomatous AML). Spindle cells may exhibit fascicular growth with elongated nuclei. These spindle cells are positive for smooth muscle markers. Most experts believe that the so-called capsulomas are likely fat-poor AMLs.*

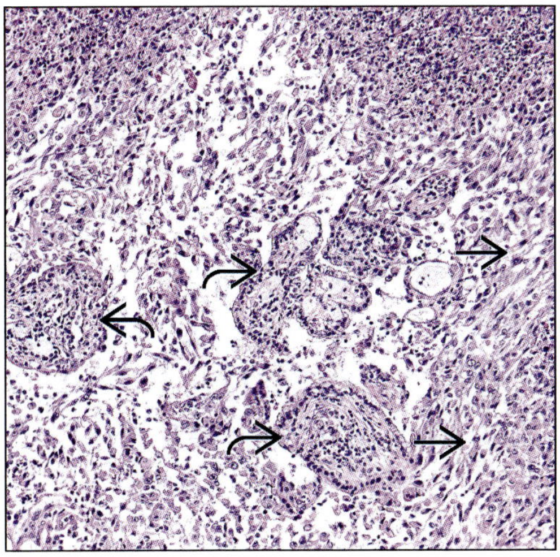

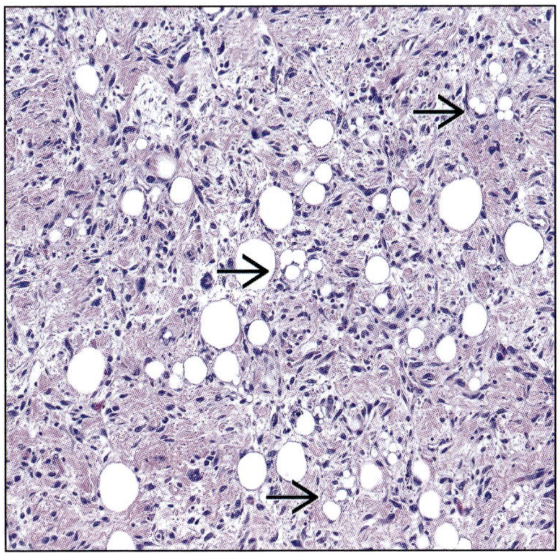

(Left) *Sarcomatoid RCC contains spindle cells ➙ mimicking C-AML. Sarcomatoid spindle cells are high grade and may have brisk mitosis. Search, including by additional sampling, for differentiated area (in this case papillary RCC ↗), may aid in diagnosis.* ***(Right)*** *Dedifferentiated liposarcoma contains an admixture of fat and spindle cells resembling E-AML. Lipoblasts ➙, which show nuclear indentation by fat vacuoles and high-grade spindle cells, are helpful in diagnosis.*

CLEAR CELL RENAL CELL CARCINOMA

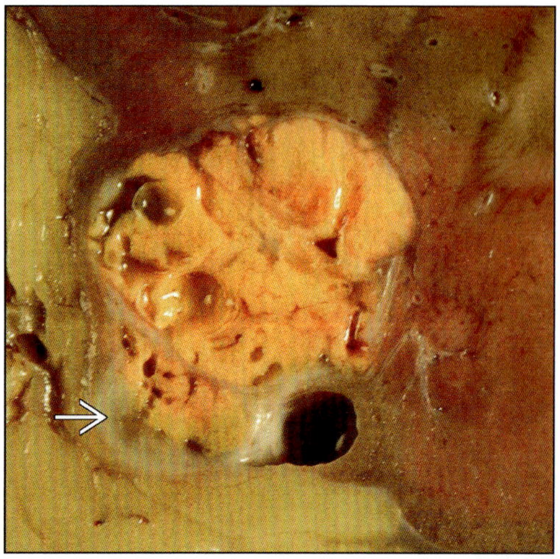

CCRCC shows typical golden-yellow cut surface due to abundant lipid content. This tumor pushes into the renal sinus fat ➔ and should be sampled thoroughly to search for possible invasion (pT3a).

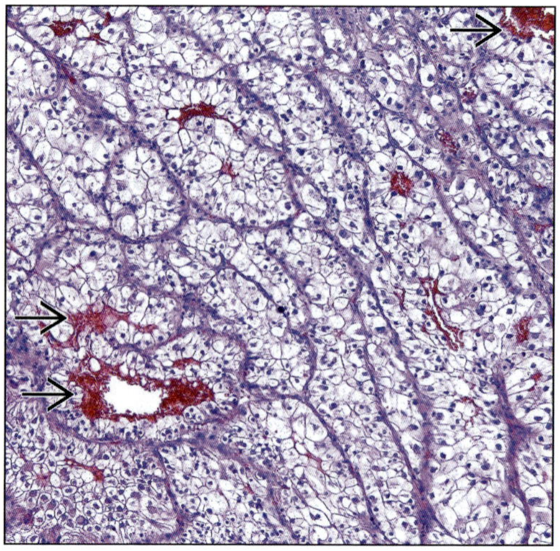

CCRCC consists of optically clear cells arranged in solid alveolar nests surrounded by intricate vascular meshwork imparting a "chicken-wire" appearance. Occasionally, hemorrhage ➔ may occur within nests.

TERMINOLOGY

Abbreviations

- Clear cell renal cell carcinoma (CCRCC)

Synonyms

- Conventional RCC

Definitions

- Malignant renal epithelial neoplasm composed of cells with optically clear cytoplasm in solid alveolar growth

ETIOLOGY/PATHOGENESIS

Sporadic CCRCC

- Vast majority of CCRCC are sporadic tumors
- Up to 90% have somatic inactivation of *VHL* at Chr 3p25-26 by mutation, loss, or DNA methylation
  - Leads to nondegradation of hypoxia-induced factor (HIF); usually degraded by *VHL* gene products
- Inactivating mutation of *PBRM1* on Chr 3p21; 2nd most frequently mutated gene in CCRCC (~ 40%)

Familial CCRCC

- Familial predisposition for CCRCC and no identifiable genetic factor; diagnosis of exclusion
- Usually older onset and presents with solitary CCRCC, similar to sporadic CCRCC
- **von Hippel-Lindau (VHL) disease**
  - Virtually all patients have inactivation of *VHL*
  - CCRCC seen in up to 45% of VHL patients
  - Frequently multifocal and bilateral CRCCs
  - Multiple renal cysts and small "clear cell tumorlets" involved the renal parenchyma
  - At risk of developing up to 600 tumors per kidney
- **Constitutional chromosome 3 translocation**
  - Rare hereditary predisposition for bilateral and multifocal CCRCC due to Chr 3 translocation
- CCRCC may occur in a subset of patients with Birt-Hogg-Dubé syndrome and tuberous sclerosis complex

CLINICAL ISSUES

Epidemiology

- Incidence
  - Most common renal epithelial neoplasm (~ 75%)
- Age
  - 21-89 years (mean: 61)
  - Younger in VHL patients (16-67 years, mean: 39)
- Gender
  - M:F = 1.1:1

Presentation

- Mostly encountered as incidental radiologic findings
- Classic triad of abdominal mass, flank pain, and hematuria seen in only ~ 25% of patients
- In VHL, discovered due to extrarenal symptoms

Treatment

- Surgical approaches
  - Nephrectomy; partial is preferred, particularly if tumor is < 4 cm and not involving hilum
    - Robotic-assisted procedure gaining popularity
  - In VHL patients, conservative surgery performed if tumor reaches 3 cm in size
- Drugs
  - For advanced-stage CCRCC; resistant to chemotherapy
  - Tyrosine kinase inhibitor as 1st option
  - Immunotherapy (IL-2) considered 1 of standards but its use is limited by side effects
  - Therapies targeting HIF or mammalian target of rapamycin (mTOR) pathways show promise

Prognosis

- 5-year disease-specific survival: 76%; poorer behavior compared to papillary RCC and chromophobe RCC

CLEAR CELL RENAL CELL CARCINOMA

Key Facts

Terminology
- Renal epithelial neoplasm composed of cells with optically clear cytoplasm in solid alveolar growth

Etiology/Pathogenesis
- Mostly sporadic; up to 90% have somatic inactivation of *VHL* at Chr 3p25-26
- *PBRM1* on Chr 3p21 2nd frequently mutated gene
- Encountered in VHL, constitutional chromosome 3 translocation, familial CCRCC, and subset of Birt-Hogg-Dubé syndrome and tuberous sclerosis patients

Clinical Issues
- Most common renal epithelial neoplasm (~ 75%)
- 21-89 years (mean: 61); younger in VHL patients
- 5-year disease-specific survival: 76%; poorer behavior than papillary RCC and chromophobe RCC

Macroscopic Features
- Usually well circumscribed with golden-yellow cut surface due to lipid content

Microscopic Pathology
- Solid alveoli/nests separated by meshwork of delicate vessels forming characteristic "chicken-wire" pattern
- Occasionally, hemorrhage occurs within alveoli/nests, forming "blood lakes"
- Tumor cells typically have optically clear cytoplasm due to intracellular glycogen and lipid
- Occasionally, cells have eosinophilic granular cytoplasm; usually have higher grade nuclei
- CAIX diffusely (+), CD10(+), RCC(+), pax-2(+), and pax-8(+)

MACROSCOPIC FEATURES

General Features
- Usually well circumscribed; can be cystic
- Golden-yellow cut surface due to lipid content
- May show hemorrhages, necrosis, or cystic change
- Sarcomatoid change is firm white-tan and infiltrative

Size
- 1.3-15 cm (mean: 6.2)

MICROSCOPIC PATHOLOGY

Histologic Features
- Solid alveoli/nests separated by meshwork of delicate vessels forming characteristic "chicken-wire" pattern
- Occasionally, hemorrhage occurs within alveoli/nests, forming "blood lakes"
- Tumor cells typically have optically clear cytoplasm due to intracellular glycogen and lipid
- Occasionally, cells have eosinophilic granular cytoplasm; usually have higher grade nuclei
- True papillae, if present, should be focal; breakdown of alveoli/nests may form pseudopapillae

ANCILLARY TESTS

Immunohistochemistry
- CAIX diffusely (+), CD10(+), RCC(+), pax-2(+) and, pax-8(+)
- CD117(-), ksp-cadherin (-), CK7(-), AMACR(-), and GATA3(-)

DIFFERENTIAL DIAGNOSIS

Chromophobe RCC
- CCRCC with clear and eosinophilic cells mimic classic and eosinophilic chromophobe RCC, respectively
- With prominent cytoplasmic membrane, perinuclear halo, wrinkled nuclei, and common binucleation
- CD117(+), ksp-cadherin (+), CK7(+), and CAIX(-)

MITF/TFE Translocation Carcinomas
- Usually younger patients with higher stage disease
- **TFE3 carcinomas**: Prominent papillae, occasional psammoma calcifications, and clear cells with voluminous cytoplasm
- **TFEB carcinomas**: Biphasic with nests of larger clear cells and central smaller cells clustered around nodules of hyaline materials
- Epithelial markers focally (+) or (-), TFE3(+) or TFEB(+)

Clear Cell Papillary RCC
- Common in end-stage kidneys and often partly cystic
- Papillary and solid growths containing clear cells with low-grade nuclei aligned away from basal aspect
- CAIX(+), CK7(+) and AMACR(-)

Epithelioid Angiomyolipoma
- Higher grade, abundant mitosis, admixed plump spindle cells, and giant pleomorphic cells
- Epithelial markers (-) and melanocytic markers (+) (e.g., HMB45, MITF, and MART-1)

SELECTED REFERENCES

1. Li L et al: New insights into the biology of renal cell carcinoma. Hematol Oncol Clin North Am. 25(4):667-86, 2011
2. Valera VA et al: Misdiagnosis of clear cell renal cell carcinoma. Nat Rev Urol. 8(6):321-33, 2011
3. Verine J et al: Hereditary renal cancer syndromes: an update of a systematic review. Eur Urol. 58(5):701-10, 2010
4. Amin MB et al: Prognostic impact of histologic subtyping of adult renal epithelial neoplasms: an experience of 405 cases. Am J Surg Pathol. 26(3):281-91, 2002

CLEAR CELL RENAL CELL CARCINOMA

Microscopic Features

(Left) *CCRCC shows abundant hemorrhage within the central aspects of alveolar nests, creating multiple "blood lakes."* ***(Right)*** *CCRCC is typically composed of tumor cells with optically clear cytoplasm due to abundant glycogen and fat content that are not preserved with processing. Few nuclei show prominent nucleoli → visible on low-power view, consistent with Fuhrman nuclear grade (FNG) 3. Most of the nuclei are small without nucleoli, consistent with FNG 1. Grading is based on the highest nuclear grade present.*

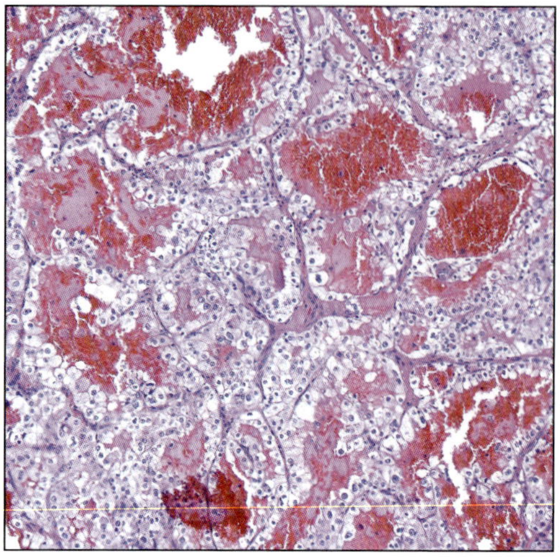

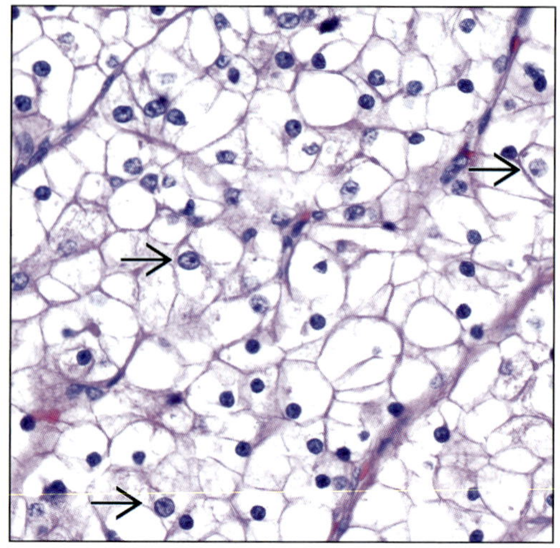

(Left) *CCRCC shows FNG 4 nuclei characterized by marked pleomorphism and multinucleation. The high-grade nuclei increase the chance for recurrence and metastasis.* ***(Right)*** *CCRCC with eosinophilic cytoplasm retains the basic architecture of intricate vessels and solid alveolar nests. Cells in CCRCC with eosinophilic cytoplasm usually have higher grade nuclei. This tumor may resemble other renal tumors with eosinophilic cytoplasm; the intricate vasculature is a helpful distinguishing feature.*

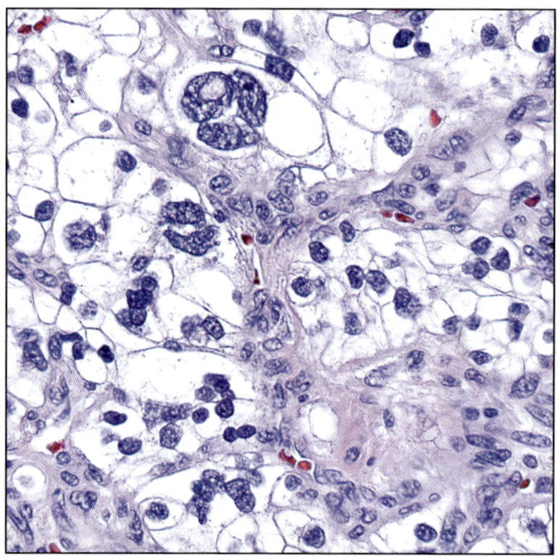

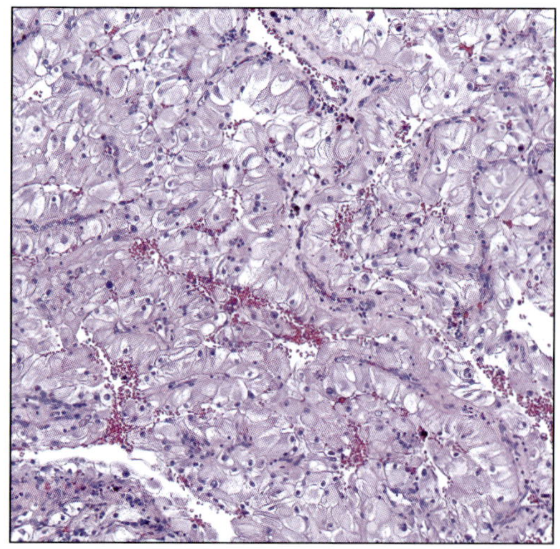

(Left) *VHL patients' kidneys harbor multiple microscopic "clear cell tumorlets," seen here between normal renal tubules. The cytology of these cells is similar to that of CCRCC. It is debatable whether to consider these microscopic clear cell foci as CCRCC.* ***(Right)*** *A VHL patient's kidney shows microcysts →. These small cysts are lined by 1 or few layers of clear cells with low-grade nuclei. Management of VHL patients requires regular surveillance and intervention for renal masses that reach 3 cm in size.*

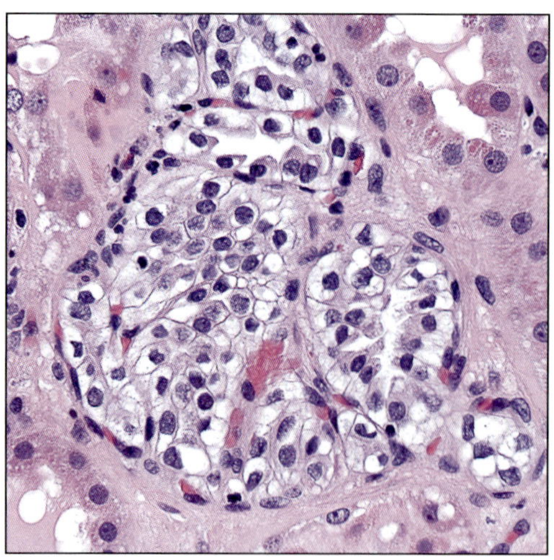

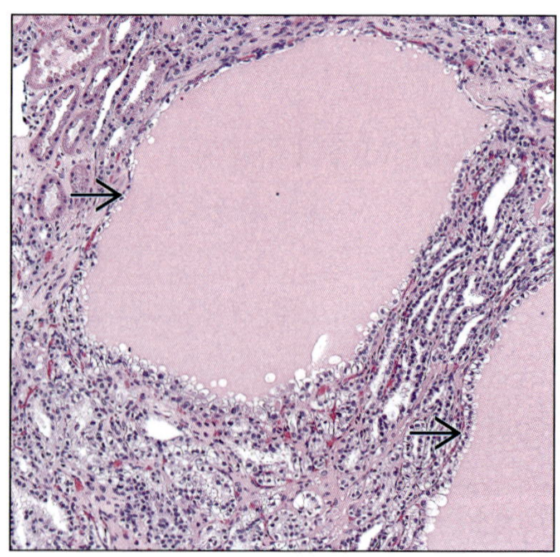

Immunohistochemistry and Differential Diagnosis

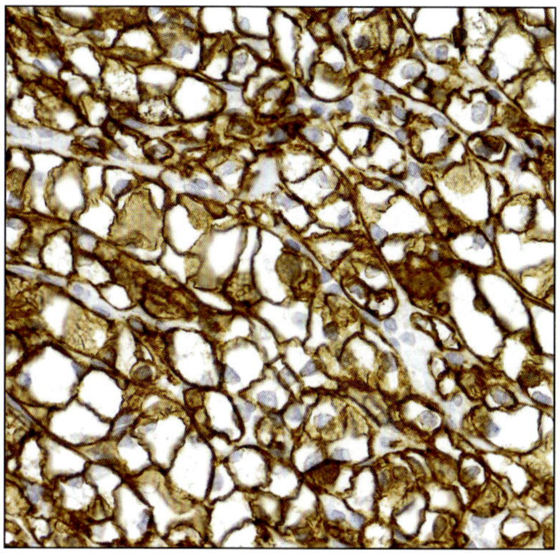
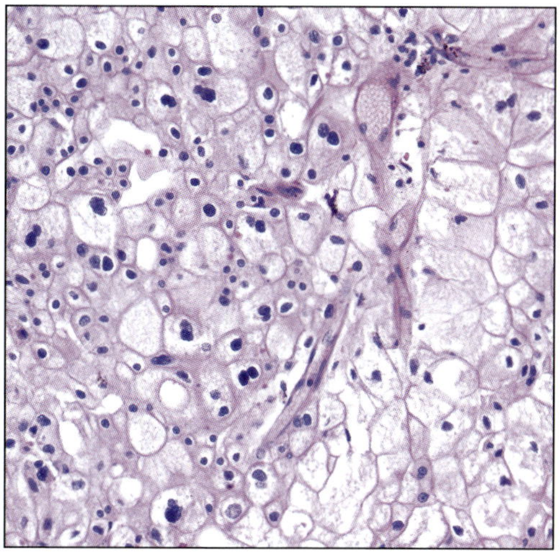

(Left) *CCRCC typically shows strong diffuse membranous staining with CAIX, a helpful marker in the differential diagnosis from most other renal tumors with pale or clear cytoplasm.* ***(Right)*** *Chromophobe RCC shows tumor cells with flocculent cytoplasm, prominent cell membrane (plant cell-like), perinuclear halo, koilocytoid nuclear atypia, and common binucleation. Unlike CCRCC, this tumor is diffusely CD117 and ksp-cadherin positive and CAIX negative.*

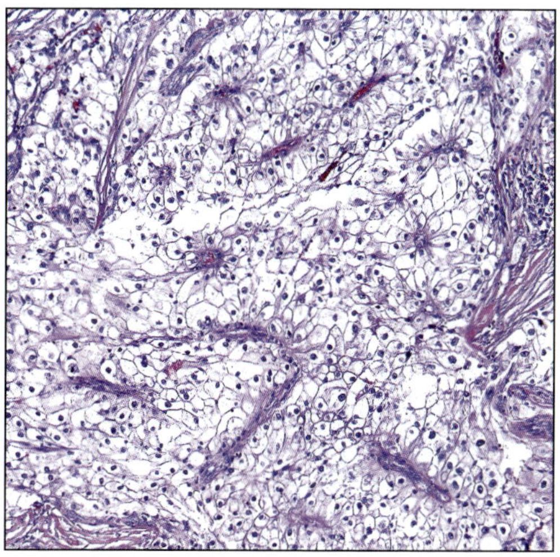
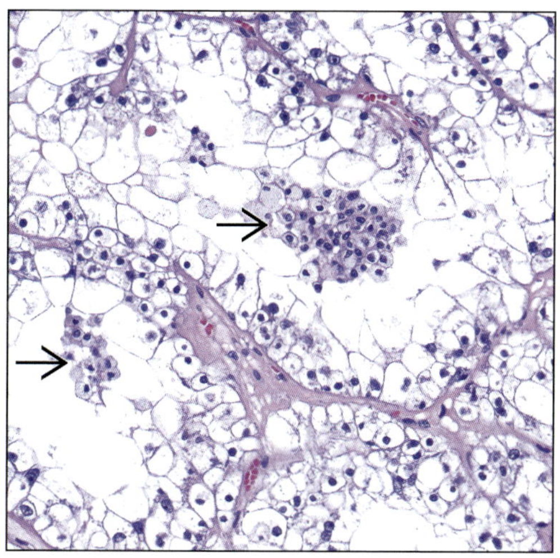

(Left) *TFE3 translocation carcinoma shows clear cells with abundant or voluminous cytoplasm. This tumor is more common in younger individuals and presents with higher stage. Diagnoses can be confirmed by TFE3 positivity.* ***(Right)*** *TFEB carcinoma shows dual population of cells consisting of larger clear cells arranged in nests surrounded by thin vessels and with central collections of smaller cells ➔. This tumor occurs in younger individuals and can be confirmed by TFEB positivity.*

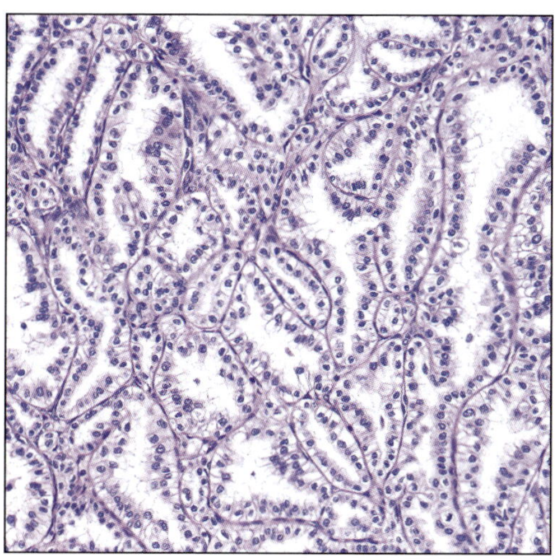
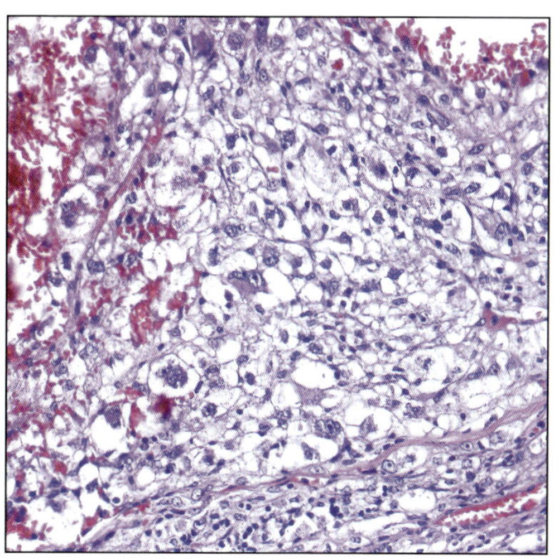

(Left) *Clear cell papillary RCC may show solid areas that may resemble CCRCC. However, clear cell papillary RCC shows tubules lined by clear cells with low-grade nuclei lined at the luminal aspect. This tumor is also CAIX(+), but unlike CCRCC, it is CK7(+).* ***(Right)*** *Epithelioid AML may exhibit a carcinoma-like growth and resemble CCRCC. Epithelioid AML usually shows nuclear pleomorphism with multinucleation and abundant mitosis. This tumor is pankeratin (-) and HMB45(+), unlike CCRCC.*

PAPILLARY RENAL CELL CARCINOMA

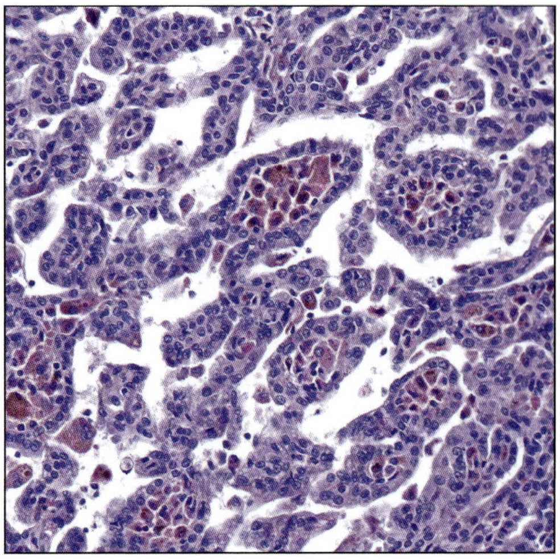

PRCC type 1 shows papillae lined by small cuboidal cells with amphophilic cytoplasm and low-grade nuclei. Papillae contain hemosiderin-laden histiocytes from an old hemorrhage, which is common in PRCC.

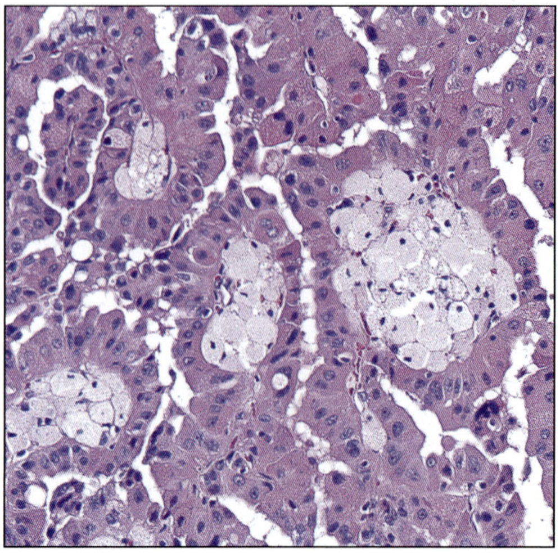

PRCC type 2 shows papillae lined by cells with abundant eosinophilic cytoplasm and nuclei with prominent nucleoli. Type 2 cells usually have higher grade nuclei. Foamy histiocytes are common in papillary cores.

TERMINOLOGY

Abbreviations

- Papillary renal cell carcinoma (PRCC)

Synonyms

- Chromophil renal cell carcinoma

Definitions

- Renal epithelial neoplasm predominantly exhibiting papillary or tubulopapillary architectures
- Published cut-off for papillae varies from 50-75%

ETIOLOGY/PATHOGENESIS

Sporadic PRCC

- Vast majority of PRCC are sporadic tumors
- Majority show Chr +7, +17, and -Y

Hereditary PRCC Syndrome

- Autosomal dominant; characterized by multiple type 1 PRCCs related to a germline *MET* mutation
- No associated extrarenal manifestations, unlike other renal tumor syndromes

Hereditary Leiomyomatosis and Renal Cell Cancer (HLRCC) Syndrome

- Some renal tumors previously classified as PRCC type 2
  - Subsequently, renal tumors were identified to have unique features absent in PRCC (i.e., large inclusion-like nucleolus and perinucleolar clearing)

CLINICAL ISSUES

Epidemiology

- Incidence
  - ~10-15% of renal tumors; 2nd most common type
- Age
  - 22-83 years (mean: 62 years)
- Gender
  - More common in men (M:F = 1.8:1)

Presentation

- Majority of tumors detected incidentally
- Hematuria, flank pain, and abdominal mass

Treatment

- Nephrectomy, partial preferred if tumor is < 4 cm and does not involve the hilum

Prognosis

- 5-year survival rate is 82-90%; better than clear cell RCC but poorer than chromophobe RCC
- Worse prognosis suggested for PRCC type 2 vs. type 1

MACROSCOPIC FEATURES

General Features

- Well circumscribed with fibrous pseudocapsule
- Multifocal in ~ 40%; highest for sporadic renal tumors
- Homogeneous tan to brown or variegated cut surface
  - Hemorrhage is common and produces red to dark brown discoloration
  - Collections of histiocytes cause yellowish streaks
- Sarcomatoid change: Firm white tan with infiltration

Size

- Range: 1.8-18 cm (mean: 6.7 cm)

MICROSCOPIC PATHOLOGY

Histologic Features

- Distinct papillary architectures with fibrovascular cores, usually with foamy histiocytes within the stalk
- Tubulopapillary pattern common; ~ 50% with tubules

PAPILLARY RENAL CELL CARCINOMA

Key Facts

Terminology
- Renal epithelial neoplasm predominantly exhibiting papillary or tubulopapillary architectures

Etiology/Pathogenesis
- Vast majority of PRCCs are sporadic tumors
- Majority of PRCCs show Chr +7, +17, and -Y
- Hereditary PRCC syndrome is characterized by development of multiple type 1 PRCCs related to a germline *MET* mutation

Clinical Issues
- ~ 10-15% of renal tumors; 2nd most common type
- 5-year survival rate is 82-90%; better than clear cell RCC but poorer than chromophobe RCC
- Worse prognosis suggested for PRCC type 2 vs. type 1

Macroscopic Features
- Well circumscribed with fibrous pseudocapsule
- ~ 40% multifocal; highest for sporadic renal tumors
- Hemorrhage is common

Microscopic Pathology
- Distinct papillary architectures with fibrovascular cores, usually with foamy histiocytes within the stalk
- Tubulopapillary pattern common; ~ 50% with tubules
- **PRCC type 1**: Smaller cells with few or modest amphophilic or basophilic cytoplasm, usually with low-grade nuclei
- **PRCC type 2**: Larger cells with abundant eosinophilic cytoplasm, usually with higher grade nuclei

Ancillary Tests
- AMACR(+), CK7(+), and EMA(+)

- Tubules may have intratubular cell proliferation (glomeruloid pattern)
- Tubular pattern may predominate and can be compacted ("solid variant")
- Typing based on cell types
  - **PRCC type 1**: Smaller cells with few or modest amphophilic or basophilic cytoplasm, usually with low-grade nuclei
  - **PRCC type 2**: Larger cells with abundant eosinophilic cytoplasm, usually with higher grade nuclei
  - **PRCC mixed types 1 and 2**: Mixture of cells seen in up to 24% of cases
- Psammomatous calcifications are occasionally present
- Hemorrhages, hemosiderin pigment deposits, necrosis, and cystic change are occasionally present

Grading
- Fuhrman grading system not applicable
- Grading based on nucleolar prominence proposed

ANCILLARY TESTS

Immunohistochemistry
- AMACR(+), CK7(+), and EMA(+)

DIFFERENTIAL DIAGNOSIS

Mucinous Tubular and Spindle Cell Carcinoma
- May resemble sarcomatoid PRCC type 1; also expresses AMACR, CK7, and EMA
- Contains mucinous stroma; can be abundant
- Spindle cells are low grade
- Cytogenetically does not harbor Chr +7, +17, and -Y

Collecting Duct Carcinoma
- May exhibit papillae (focal) and CK7 positivity
- Multinodular and infiltrative, centered at medulla
- High-grade cells, some have hobnail appearance
- Admixed invasive glands (adenocarcinoma) with marked stromal desmoplasia

Metanephric Adenoma
- Exhibits papillae, glomeruloid structures, and psammoma calcifications
- Tumor cells have scant cytoplasm with uniformly low-grade nuclei (primitive-appearing cells)
- WT1(+), CD57(+), and AMACR(-)

Clear Cell Papillary RCC
- Papillae lined by low-grade clear cells with nuclei aligned away from cell base
- Cystic component common; often in end-stage kidneys
- CK7(+), CAIX(+), and AMACR(-)

MiTF/TFE Family Translocation Carcinomas
- Usually in pediatric or young adult patients
- Papillae contain prominent clear cell component, sometimes with voluminous cytoplasm
- Epithelial marker is focally (+) or (-) and TFE3(+)

SELECTED REFERENCES

1. Sika-Paotonu D et al: Nucleolar grade but not Fuhrman grade is applicable to papillary renal cell carcinoma. Am J Surg Pathol. 30(9):1091-6, 2006
2. Lefèvre M et al: Adult papillary renal tumor with oncocytic cells: clinicopathologic, immunohistochemical, and cytogenetic features of 10 cases. Am J Surg Pathol. 29(12):1576-81, 2005
3. Delahunt B et al: Morphologic typing of papillary renal cell carcinoma: comparison of growth kinetics and patient survival in 66 cases. Hum Pathol. 32(6):590-5, 2001
4. Amin MB et al: Papillary (chromophil) renal cell carcinoma: histomorphologic characteristics and evaluation of conventional pathologic prognostic parameters in 62 cases. Am J Surg Pathol. 21(6):621-35, 1997
5. Renshaw AA et al: Solid variants of papillary (chromophil) renal cell carcinoma: clinicopathologic and genetic features. Am J Surg Pathol. 21(10):1203-9, 1997

PAPILLARY RENAL CELL CARCINOMA

Gross and Microscopic Features

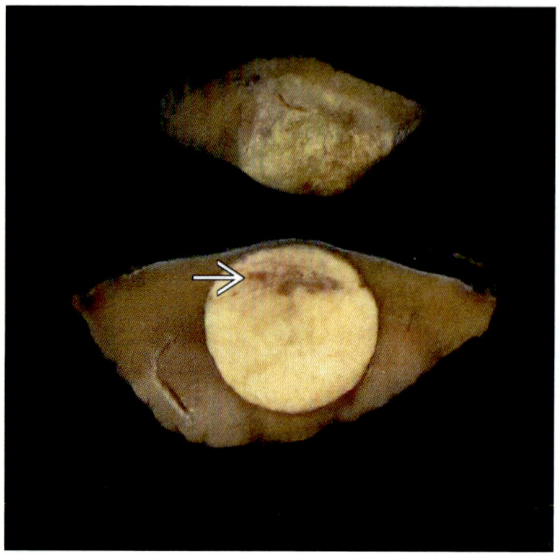
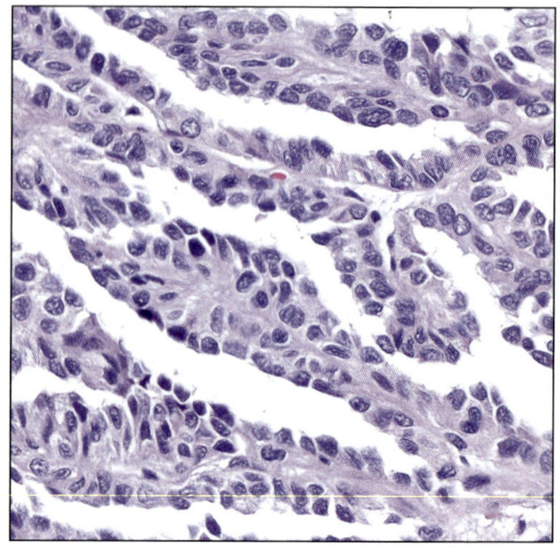

(Left) *PRCC shows a well-circumscribed tumor with solid, light-tan cut surface. Tumor may show pseudocapsule. Red-brown* ➔ *and yellow discoloration from hemorrhages and histiocytic infiltrates, respectively, are common in PRCC.* ***(Right)*** *PRCC type 1 is lined by cells with scant cytoplasm and low-grade nuclei imparting a basophilic appearance. PRCC type 1 papillae are usually lined by 1 layer or a few layers of cells with minimal stratification. PRCC type 1 cells resemble those in most papillary adenomas.*

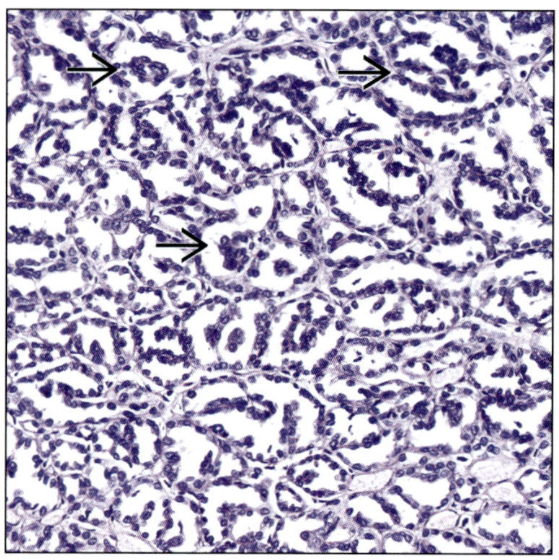
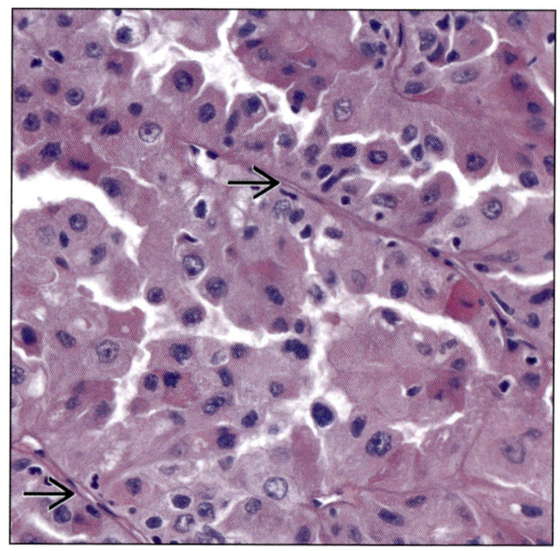

(Left) *PRCC type 1 with predominant tubular growth imparts a solid appearance. Some tubules have glomeruloid pattern* ➔ *due to intratubular cellular proliferation. About 50% of PRCCs have tubular growth, and occasionally, it is predominate, as in this tumor.* ***(Right)*** *High-power view of PRCC type 2 shows cells with larger nuclei and occasional prominent nucleoli than in type 1. PRCC type 2 exhibits relatively more frequent cellular stratification. Papillary cores* ➔ *are thin and contain delicate vasculature.*

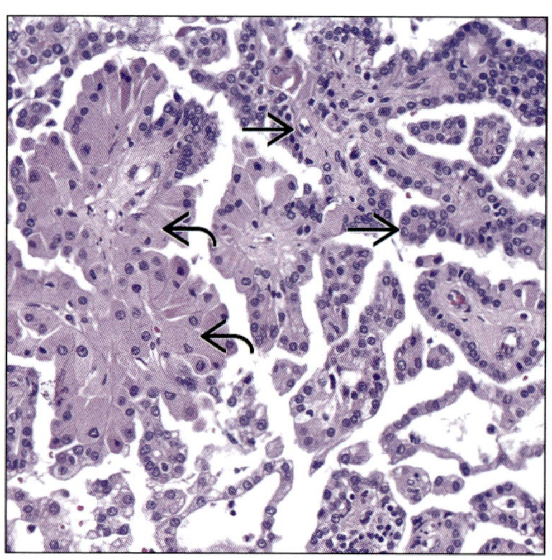
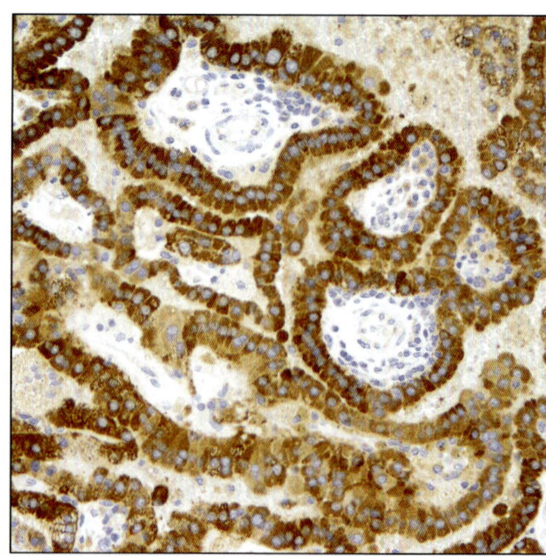

(Left) *PRCC shows mixed small cuboidal cells (type 1)* ➔ *and large eosinophilic cells (type 2)* ↩. *Admixture of these cells are encountered in ~ 1/4 of PRCC. PRCC type 2 is considered to have worse prognosis than type 1. Behavior of mixed PRCC types 1 and 2 is unclear.* ***(Right)*** *PRCC shows strong diffuse cytoplasmic immunoreactivity to AMACR. This immunostain is expressed in > 95% of PRCC and helps to distinguish it from most other renal tumors with papillary growth. PRCC and papillary adenoma are positive with AMACR.*

Differential Diagnosis

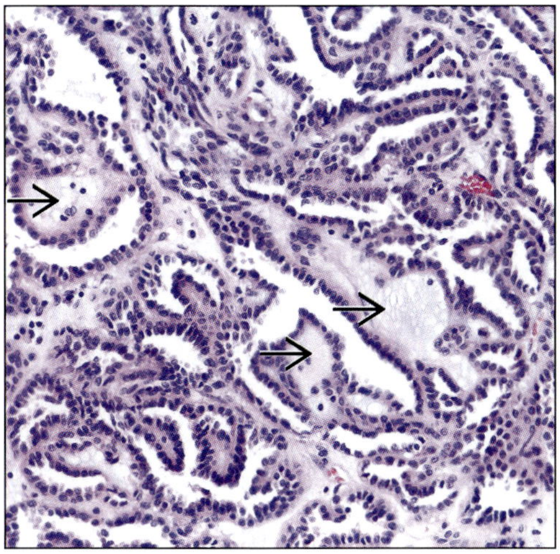
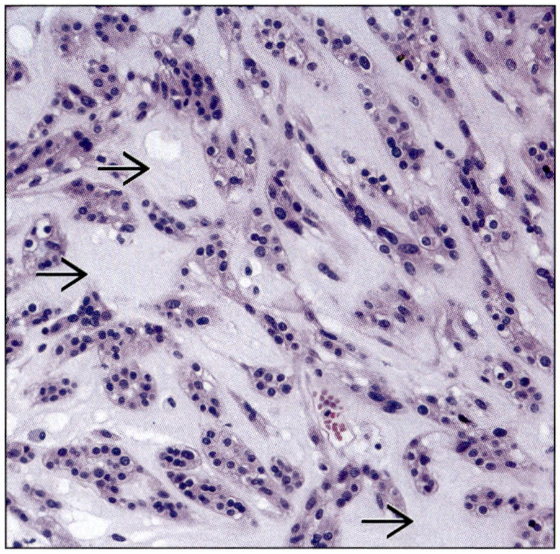

(Left) *Mucinous tubular and spindle cell carcinoma may exhibit focal papillation and resemble PRCC type 1. This tumor, however, exhibits prominent basophilic mucin → in stroma.* ***(Right)*** *Mucinous tubular and spindle cell carcinoma also contains elongated tubular and spindle cells and may mimic a PRCC type 1 with sarcomatoid change. Unlike PRCC, this tumor contains abundant mucin in stroma →, and the cells have bland-appearing nuclei unlike in sarcomatoid spindle cells, which are high grade.*

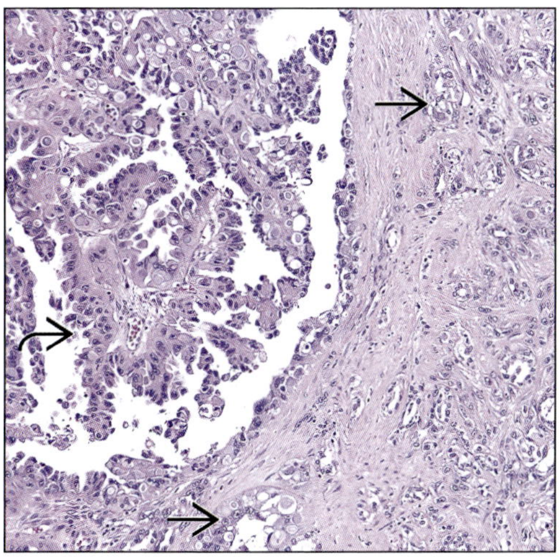
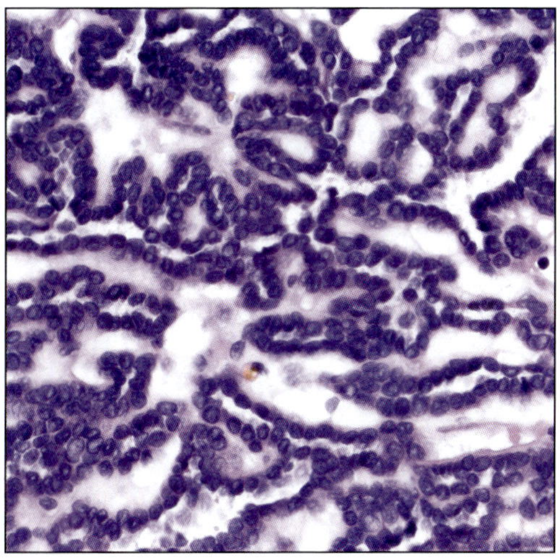

(Left) *Collecting duct carcinoma may exhibit papillary growth and mimic PRCC. Unlike PRCC, this tumor shows higher grade cells with hobnailing ↷. Furthermore, collecting duct carcinoma also exhibits an infiltrative gland component →.* ***(Right)*** *Metanephric adenoma shows papillary, tubulopapillary, and glomeruloid growth similar to PRCC. However, tumor cells have minimal cytoplasm (resembling primitive metanephric cells) and intervening paucicellular stroma.*

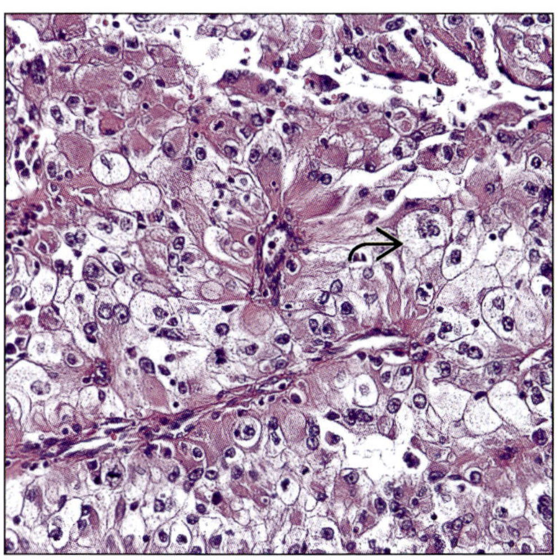
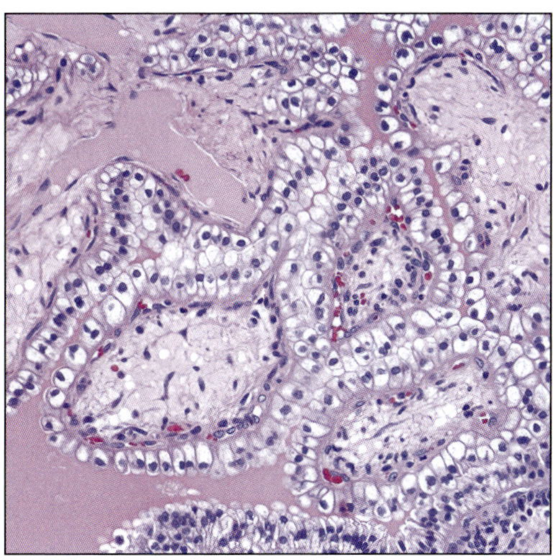

(Left) *TFE3 translocation carcinomas may exhibit papillary growth. The tumor contains high-grade clear cells that may have abundant (voluminous) cytoplasm ↷. Translocation carcinoma is often seen in young adults and pediatric patients.* ***(Right)*** *Clear cell papillary RCC is characterized by papillae lined by clear cells with low-grade nuclei linearly placed away from the basal aspect of the cells. Cystic change is usual, and this tumor is more common in end-stage kidneys but may occur sporadically.*

RENAL ONCOCYTOMA, CHROMOPHOBE, AND HYBRID ONCOCYTIC TUMORS

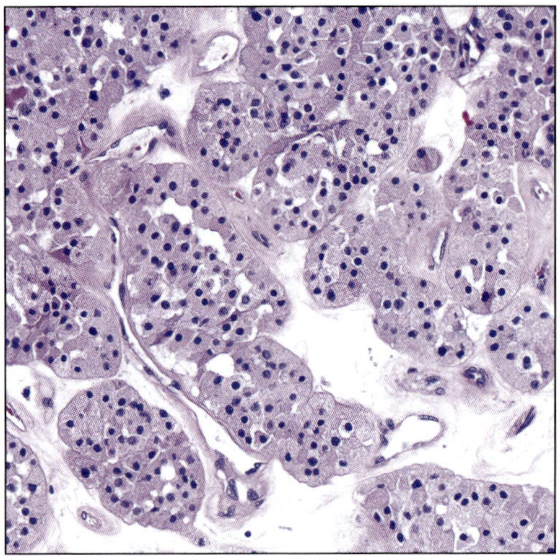

RO is characterized by tumor cells with eosinophilic granular cytoplasm in small nested growth and with round regular nuclei. Broad solid alveolar growth and high-grade irregular nuclei are not permissible in RO.

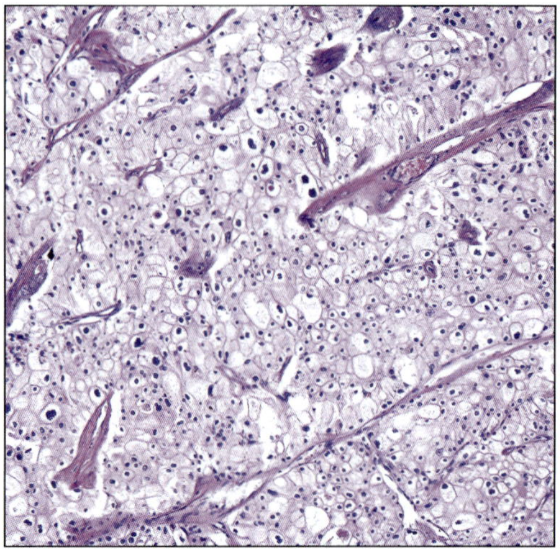

Classic CHRCC shows broad solid alveolar growth and tumor cells with pale or flocculent cytoplasm, prominent cell membrane (plant cell-like), perinuclear halo, koilocytoid nuclear atypia, and binucleation.

TERMINOLOGY

Abbreviations

- Renal oncocytoma (RO)
- Chromophobe renal cell carcinoma (CHRCC)
- Hybrid oncocytic tumor (HOT)

Definitions

- **RO**
  - Benign renal epithelial neoplasm characterized by eosinophilic cells, uniform nuclei, and small nests
- **Renal oncocytosis**
  - Kidney involved by innumerable oncocytic nodules
- **CHRCC**
  - Malignant renal epithelial neoplasm characterized by prominent cytoplasmic membrane, flocculent cells, perinuclear clearing, and koilocytoid nuclei
- **HOT**
  - Tumor with mixed RO and CHRCC cells

ETIOLOGY/PATHOGENESIS

Sporadic Tumors

- Vast majority of RO and CHRCC are sporadic
- Cytogenetics
  - RO: Loss of Chr 1 and Y and 11q23 alteration
  - CHRCC: Multiple loss (Chr 1, 6, 10, 13, 17, 21 & Y)
- Nonfamilial HOT uncommon and oncocytosis rare

Birt-Hogg-Dubé (BHD) Syndrome

- Autosomal dominant characterized by tumors of hair follicles, pneumothorax, and renal tumors
- Alteration of folliculin (*FLCN*) at Chr 17p11.2
- 15-30% develop renal tumors with higher proclivity for HOT (50%), CHRCC (34%), and oncocytosis (58%)

Familial Oncocytomas

- Chr 1 loss; has fewer chromosomal instabilities
- RO often bilateral &/or multifocal

Succinate Dehydrogenase B-Deficient Tumors

- Association with RO initially reported; recent studies show different tumors from RO and common RCCs

CLINICAL ISSUES

Epidemiology

- Incidence
  - RO accounts for 6% of all renal tumors
  - CHRCC 3rd most common renal tumor (~ 5%)
- Age
  - RO: 32-89 years (mean: 67); CHRCC: 27-82 (mean: 59)
  - BHD renal tumors affect younger patients (37-67 years, mean: 51)
- Gender
  - RO: M:F = 3.1:1; CHRCC: M:F = 1.1:1
  - Oncocytosis: M:F = 1:2.5; BHD renal tumors: M:F = 5:1

Presentation

- Mostly incidental (66-83%)
- Hematuria, flank pain, and abdominal mass

Prognosis

- RO: Benign tumor, no potential for metastasis
- CHRCC: 5- and 10-year survival > 90%

MACROSCOPIC FEATURES

General Features

- Familial tumors have higher tendency for multifocality and bilaterality
  - BHD tumors are 73% multifocal and 62% bilateral, and 57% have associated renal oncocytosis
  - Familial oncocytomas are 67% bilateral

RENAL ONCOCYTOMA, CHROMOPHOBE, AND HYBRID ONCOCYTIC TUMORS

Key Facts

Terminology
- **RO**: Benign renal epithelial neoplasm characterized by eosinophilic cells, uniform nuclei, and small nests
- **Renal oncocytosis**: Kidney involved by innumerable oncocytic nodules
- **CHRCC**: Renal epithelial neoplasm characterized by prominent cytoplasmic membrane, flocculent cells, perinuclear clearing, and koilocytoid nuclei
- **HOT**: Tumor with mixed RO and CHRCC cells

Etiology/Pathogenesis
- BHD patients' renal tumors have higher proclivity for HOT (50%), CHRCC (34%), and oncocytosis (58%)

Clinical Issues
- BHD renal tumors: Younger (37-67 years; mean: 51)
- RO: Benign tumor & CHRCC: > 90% 5-year survival

Macroscopic Features
- Multifocality/bilaterality common in familial tumors

Microscopic Pathology
- **RO**: Small nests, tubulocystic with hyalinized stroma, and cells have eosinophilic granular cytoplasm, uniform nuclei, and occasional prominent nucleoli
- **CHRCC, classic type**: Small/large solid nests and cells with pale cytoplasm, distinct cell membrane, perinuclear halo, binucleation, round to irregular (koilocytoid) nuclei with occasional large nucleoli
- **CHRCC, eosinophilic type**: More dense eosinophilic granular cytoplasm
- **CHRCC, mixed type**: Mixed pale and eosinophilic cells; pale cells usually at periphery
- RO and CHRCC: CD117(+) and ksp-cadherin (+)

RO
- Well circumscribed, homogeneous, mahogany brown, with central scarring in ~ 50%; few may have focal perinephric fat extension (not a sign of malignancy)

Oncocytosis
- Dominant nodules range from 2-10.5 cm, with multiple microscopic to small nodules
- Gross features depend on type (RO, CHRCC, or HOT)

CHRCC
- Well circumscribed with central scarring in ~ 20%
- **Classic type**: Beige or light yellow
- **Eosinophilic type**: Mahogany brown (resemble RO)
- Sarcomatoid change: Firm, white-tan with infiltration

MICROSCOPIC PATHOLOGY

Histologic Features
- **RO**
  - Small nests, tubulocystic with hyalinized stroma
  - Large nests or diffuse pattern not permissible; "compact small nests" of RO may appear solid
  - Cells have eosinophilic granular cytoplasm, uniform nuclei and occasional prominent nucleoli
  - Some may have degenerate-appearing nuclei and smaller cells with less cytoplasm (oncoblasts)
  - Mitosis rare; high-grade nuclei **not** allowed
- **Oncocytosis**
  - Dominant/larger tumors are RO, CHRCC, or HOT
  - Smaller nodules from microscopic collections of few tumor cells to macroscopic visible lesions
    - Most have cells like RO, few like CHRCC or HOT
    - May percolate between tubules and glomeruli as irregular solid clusters or form tubules and cysts
- **CHRCC**
  - **Classic type**
    - Small/large solid nests; rare microcysts or tubules
    - Cells with flocculent pale cytoplasm and distinct cytoplasmic membrane (plant cell-like)
    - Perinuclear halo; round to irregular wrinkled dark nuclei (koilocytoid) with occasional large nucleoli
    - Binucleation common; may have large degenerative nuclei (like in RO)
  - **Eosinophilic type**
    - More dense eosinophilic granular cytoplasm
  - **Mixed type** (mixed pale and eosinophilic cells)
    - Pale cells usually at periphery of solid nests
- **HOT**
  - Mixture of RO-like and CHRCC-like cells/areas
  - RO-like with high-grade nuclei excluded (categorized as unclassified RCC)

ANCILLARY TESTS

Immunohistochemistry
- RO and CHRCC: CD117(+) and ksp-cadherin (+)
- RO: CK7(-) or focal (+); classic CHRCC: CK7(+); eosinophilic CHRCC: CK7(+) or focal (+)

Electron Microscopy
- Abundant mitochondria; microvesicles in CHRCC

DIFFERENTIAL DIAGNOSIS

Clear Cell RCC With Eosinophilic Cytoplasm
- Solid alveolar nests with "chicken-wire" vasculatures
- May have higher grade nuclei than RO (> Fuhrman nuclear grade 2 [FNG2])
- CAIX diffusely (+); CD117/ksp-cadherin (-)

SELECTED REFERENCES

1. Tickoo SK et al: Renal oncocytosis: a morphologic study of fourteen cases. Am J Surg Pathol. 23(9):1094-101, 1999
2. Amin MB et al: Renal oncocytoma: a reappraisal of morphologic features with clinicopathologic findings in 80 cases. Am J Surg Pathol. 21(1):1-12, 1997

RENAL ONCOCYTOMA, CHROMOPHOBE, AND HYBRID ONCOCYTIC TUMORS

Gross and Microscopic Features

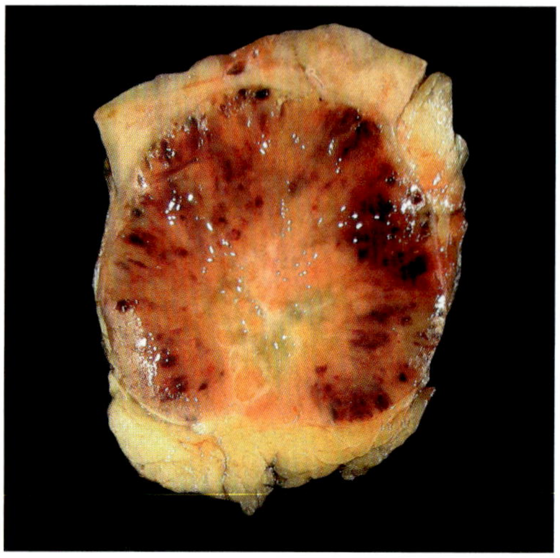
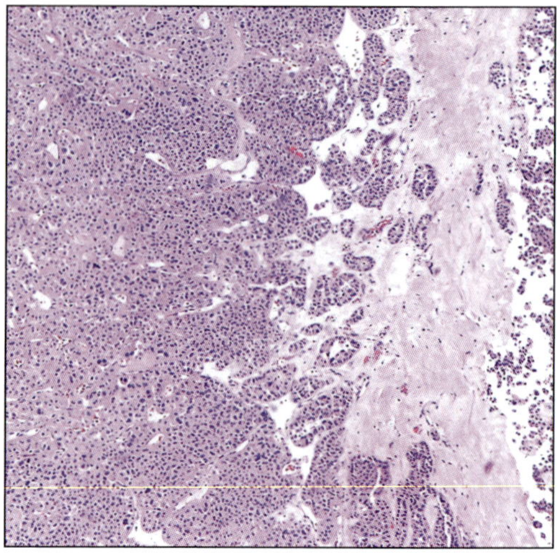

(Left) *Gross photograph of RO shows typical central scar seen in ~ 50% of cases. This finding, however, is not specific and can be seen in ~ 20% of CHRCC, particularly in eosinophilic type. Both RO and eosinophilic CHRCC show mahogany brown appearance.* ***(Right)*** *Low-power view of RO shows nested growth that is more compact at periphery and loose toward the center (central scarring). This RO exhibits random degenerate nuclear atypia, appreciable even on low-power view, which is not uncommon in RO.*

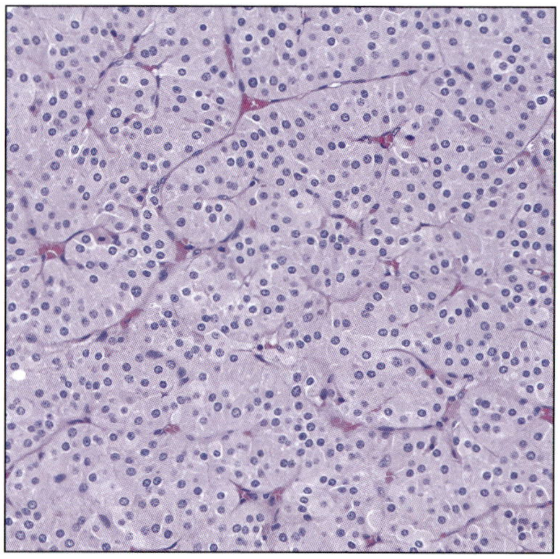
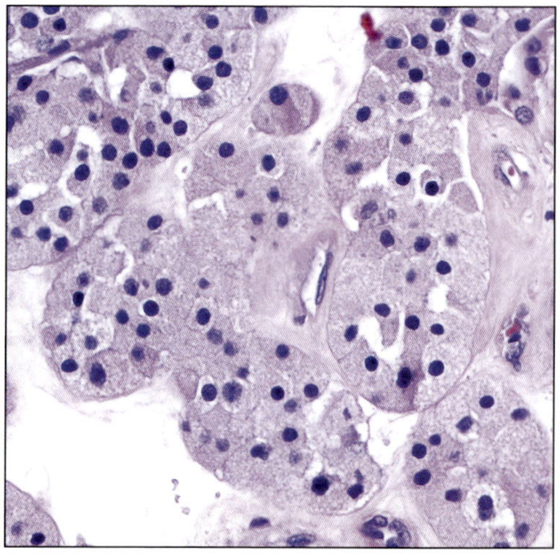

(Left) *RO typically exhibits small nested growth. Diffuse solid or broad large alveolar growths should be excluded in RO. More compact growth of small nests, as seen in this image, may impart a diffuse or solid growth, and should be examined closely for outline of tight small nests of RO.* ***(Right)*** *RO shows round relatively regular nuclei. Presence of marked nuclear irregularity or atypia should prompt consideration of a diagnosis of RCC. Cytoplasm is eosinophilic and granular due to abundance of mitochondria.*

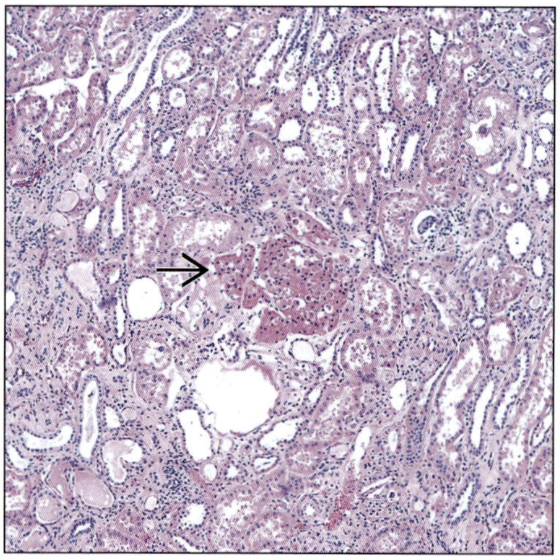
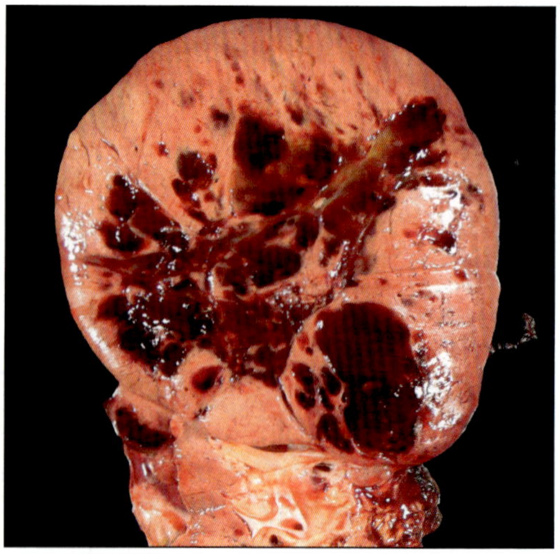

(Left) *Renal oncocytosis shows innumerable oncocytic nodules in the kidney. Some may be small and microscopic, as seen in this image ⇒. This minute oncocytic nodule is composed of low-grade cells with abundant eosinophilic cytoplasm and percolates between renal tubules.* ***(Right)*** *Gross photograph of CHRCC, eosinophilic type, shows well-circumscribed tumor with mahogany brown appearance similar to RO. Considerable overlap from gross to microscopic exists between RO and CHRCC, eosinophilic type.*

Microscopic Features and Differential Diagnosis

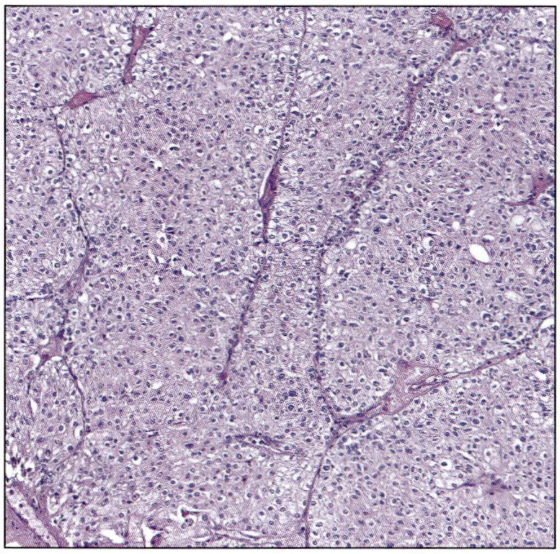
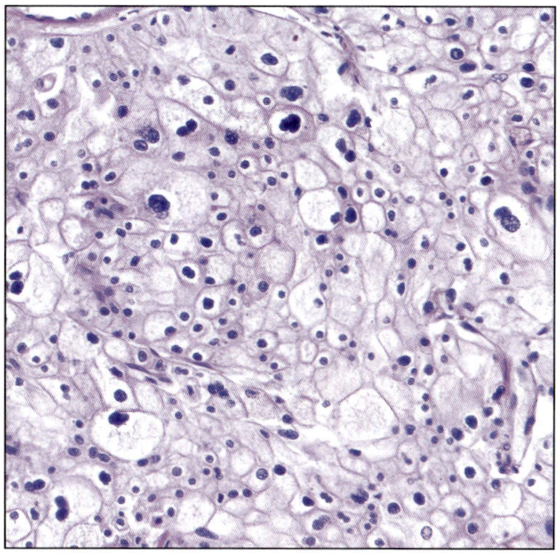

(Left) *Low-power view of CHRCC, classic type, shows the typical broad solid alveolar growth. There is paucity of vessels within the broad alveolar area, unlike in clear cell RCC.* ***(Right)*** *CHRCC, classic type, shows tumor cells with pale or flocculent cytoplasm and prominent cytoplasmic membrane imparting a plant cell-like appearance. Nuclei of CHRCC are innately atypical or pleomorphic despite its being a low-grade tumor. Thus, Fuhrman nuclear grading is not applicable in CHRCC.*

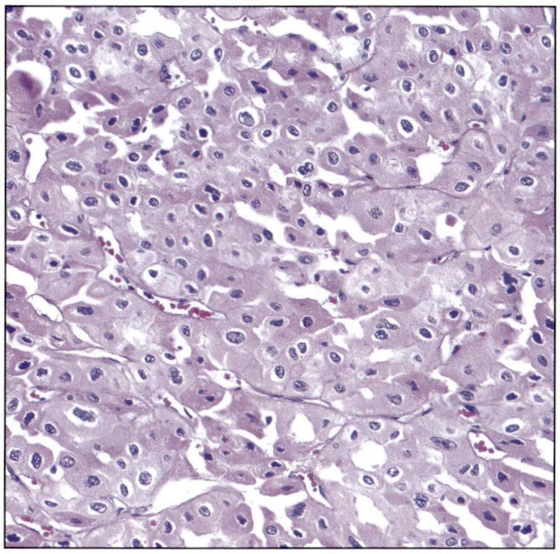
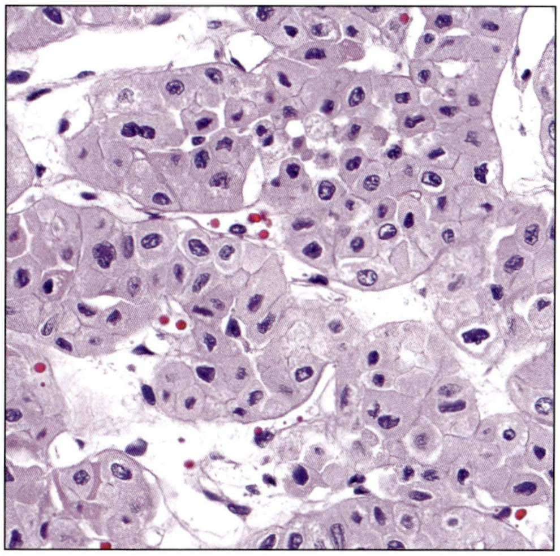

(Left) *CHRCC, eosinophilic type, demonstrates cells with abundant eosinophilic cytoplasm similar to RO. Unlike RO, nuclei exhibit koilocytoid atypia, perinuclear halo, and more frequent binucleation.* ***(Right)*** *CHRCC, eosinophilic type, may exhibit small nested growth similar to RO. Diagnosis can be made by nuclear features. Currently, there are no reliable immunohistochemical stains to distinguish these 2 tumors, and distinction is mainly morphologic.*

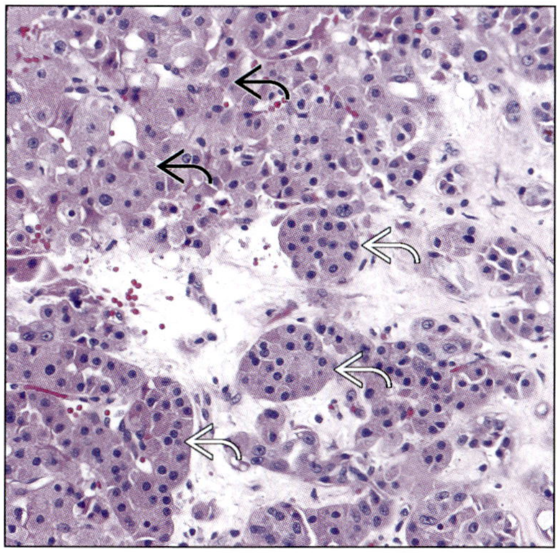
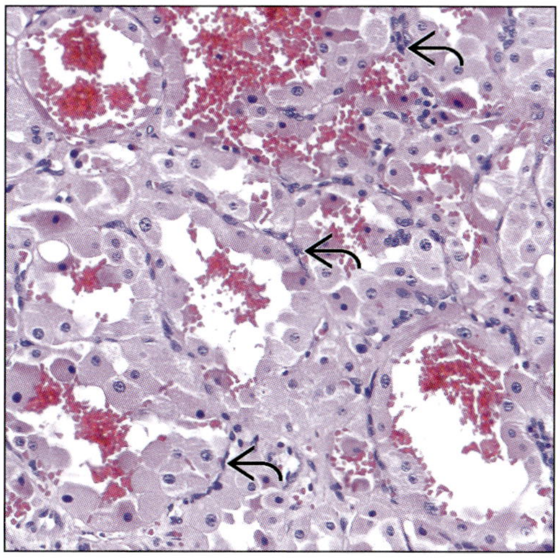

(Left) *HOT shows area of cells with more diffuse growth and relatively variable nuclei, consistent with CHRCC, and another area of cells in smaller nests with more uniform nuclei, consistent with RO. HOT is more frequently encountered in BHD and renal oncocytosis.* ***(Right)*** *Clear cell RCC with eosinophilic cytoplasm may resemble RO and CHRCC, eosinophilic type. Presence of "chicken-wire" vasculatures and nested growth are helpful futures for diagnosis of clear cell RCC.*

RENAL UROTHELIAL CARCINOMA

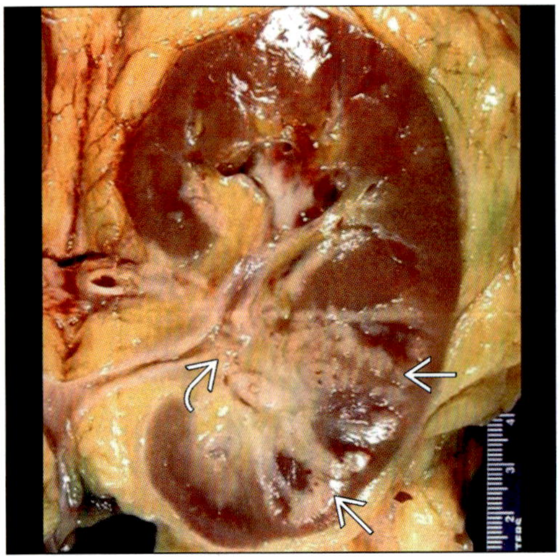

Bivalved resected kidney (coronal plane) shows a urothelial carcinoma (UcA) along the lower pole collecting system ➔ and is invading into the renal parenchyma ➔ with no extension into perinephric fat.

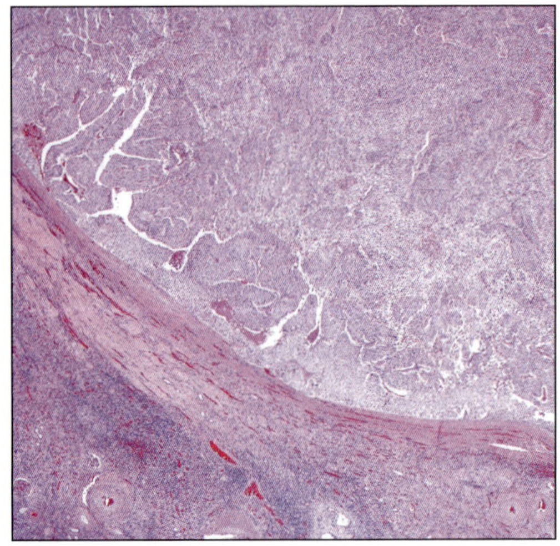

Low-power view shows a papillary UcA involving and filling the renal pelvis lumen. Despite its size, this tumor does not show invasion into the underlying structures, evident by the regular smooth boundary.

TERMINOLOGY

Abbreviations

- Urothelial carcinoma (UcA)

Synonyms

- Renal transitional cell carcinoma, pelvicaliceal UcA

Definitions

- Carcinoma arising from pelvicaliceal urothelium

ETIOLOGY/PATHOGENESIS

Risk Factors

- Similar to bladder cancer
  - Tobacco exposure increases risk by 2.5-7x
  - Long exposure to aromatic amines (e.g., benzidine, β-naphthalene) ↑ risk by 8.3x
    - ~ 7 years of exposure, with latency of ~ 20 years to develop upper tract UcA

Familial Renal UcA

- **Lynch syndrome**, a.k.a. hereditary nonpolyposis colorectal cancer (HNPCC) syndrome
  - Autosomal dominant condition with increase risk for cancer of colon (most common: 63%), uterus (9%), upper urinary tract, stomach, ovary, biliary tract, pancreas, and brain
  - Lifetime risk of cancer up to 80% by age 70 years
  - Associated with inherited mutations in DNA mismatch repair genes
    - Most commonly with *MSH2* (~ 90%), but also observed in small numbers of *MLH1*, *MSH6*, *PMS2*, and EpCAM (*TACSTD1*)
  - ~ 6% Lifetime risk for upper urinary tract UcA
    - 22x higher risk than general population
    - Younger median age of onset (56 years, or 10-15 years younger than sporadic cases)
    - More likely to have bilateral disease than sporadic cases
    - Risk is higher for ureter than renal pelvis UcA; risk for bladder UcA not established
    - UcAs have more potential for high grade than in general population
  - Suspect hereditary upper tract UcA if
    - Patient < 60 years old
    - History of HNPCC-associated cancer
    - First-degree relative < 50 years of age with HNPCC-associated cancer
    - 2 first-degree relatives with HNPCC-associated cancer
  - Suspected patients should undergo DNA testing for confirmation

CLINICAL ISSUES

Epidemiology

- Incidence
  - Upper tract UcA accounts for ~ 5-10% of all UcA
  - Annual incidence of 2 new cases per 100,000 in Western countries
- Age
  - Range: 40s to 90s; median: 69 years (similar to bladder UcA)
- Gender
  - M:F = 2:1

Presentation

- Gross or microscopic hematuria (70-80%)
- Flank pain (20-40%)
- Lumbar mass (10-20%)
- Systemic symptoms, such as anorexia, weight loss, malaise, fatigue, fever, night sweats, or cough for metastasis
- ~ 17% have concurrent bladder cancer

RENAL UROTHELIAL CARCINOMA

Key Facts

Etiology/Pathogenesis

- Familial cases: Lynch syndrome (a.k.a. HNPCC)
  - Associated with inherited mutations in DNA mismatch repair genes, most commonly with *MSH2* (~ 90%), but also observed in small numbers of *MLH1*, *MSH6*, *PMS2*, and EpCAM (*TACSTD1*)
  - ~ 6% lifetime risk for upper urinary tract UcA
  - 22x higher risk than general population

Clinical Issues

- Upper tract UcA accounts for ~ 5-10% of all UcA
- Mostly present with gross or microscopic hematuria (70-80%)
- ~ 17% has concurrent bladder cancer
- In up to ~ 25% of ureteroscopic biopsy, diagnosis cannot be made due to inadequate sampling

Macroscopic Features

- Papillary or polypoid mass involving or filling pelvicalyceal space
- Infiltrative mass may extensively involve kidney and mimic primary high-grade renal carcinoma

Microscopic Pathology

- Histologic classification similar to bladder UcA (WHO, 2004)
- Higher percentage of non-UcA and variant morphology (25%) than bladder
- Other morphologies may occur, e.g., small cell, micropapillary, plasmacytoid, lymphoepithelioma-like, and sarcomatoid carcinomas
- Intratubular growth by UcA (pTis) should not be interpreted as renal parenchymal invasion (pT3)

Endoscopic Findings

- Papillary or sessile mass; may fill renal pelvic cavity
- In up to ~ 25% of ureteroscopic biopsies, diagnosis cannot be made due to inadequate sampling
  - Potential pitfall in diagnosis

Treatment

- Surgical approaches
  - Radical nephroureterectomy (RNU) with excision of bladder cuff is gold standard therapy
    - Indicated for suspicion of infiltrating UcA on imaging, high-grade UcA, multifocality and noninvasive but > 2 cm tumor size

Prognosis

- Dependent on stage (most consistent on multivariate analyses)
  - 5-year specific survival is < 50% for pT2/pT3 and < 10% for pT4
- Other important prognostic factors
  - Grade, tumor size, multifocality, lymphovascular invasion, hydronephrosis, and positive margin after RNU
  - Associated with poor prognosis are advanced age, ECOG performance status ≥ 1, body mass index ≥ 30, systemic symptoms, and previous/synchronous bladder cancer
- Recurrence in bladder occurs in 22-47%
- Recurrence in contralateral upper tract occurs in 2-6%

MACROSCOPIC FEATURES

General Features

- Papillary or polypoid mass involving or filling pelvicalyceal space
- Infiltrative mass may extensively involve renal parenchyma and mimic primary high-grade renal carcinoma

MICROSCOPIC PATHOLOGY

Histologic Features

- Classification similar to bladder UcA (WHO, 2004)
  - Papillary urothelial neoplasms
    - **Urothelial papilloma** and **papillary UcA of unknown malignant potential (PUNLMP)** rare in renal pelvis
    - **Papillary UcA, low grade**
    - **Papillary UcA, high grade**
  - Flat urothelial neoplasms
    - **Urothelial dysplasia**
    - **UcA in situ**
  - **Invasive carcinoma, conventional UcA and variants**
    - Higher percentage of non-UcA and variant morphology (25%) than bladder
  - Most common variants: Squamous cell carcinoma (9.9%) and carcinomas with glandular differentiation (4.4%)
  - Other morphologies may occur, e.g., small cell, micropapillary, plasmacytoid, lymphoepithelioma-like, and sarcomatoid carcinomas
- Intratubular growth by UcA (pTis) should not be interpreted as renal parenchymal invasion (pT3)
- Involvement of renal parenchyma by UcA shows infiltrative, irregular nests in contrast to well-circumscribed mass common among renal cell carcinoma subtypes
- Inverted growth of UcA suggested to be associated with Lynch syndrome

SELECTED REFERENCES

1. Rouprêt M et al: European guidelines on upper tract urothelial carcinomas: 2013 update. Eur Urol. 63(6):1059-71, 2013
2. Crockett DG et al: Upper urinary tract carcinoma in Lynch syndrome cases. J Urol. 185(5):1627-30, 2011

RENAL UROTHELIAL CARCINOMA

Gross and Microscopic Features

*(**Left**) Gross image shows a UcA ⇨ involving the inferior pelvicaliceal system. At the upper aspect, the tumor shows a relatively regular and distinct boundary ⇨ whereas at the inferior aspect, there is focal infiltration of the renal parenchyma ↪. Distinction between renal UcA and primary renal cell carcinoma can often be made by gross examination alone. (**Right**) Low-power view shows a renal pelvis low-grade papillary UcA. It is not uncommon to see large papillary UcA with low-grade cytology in the renal pelvis.*

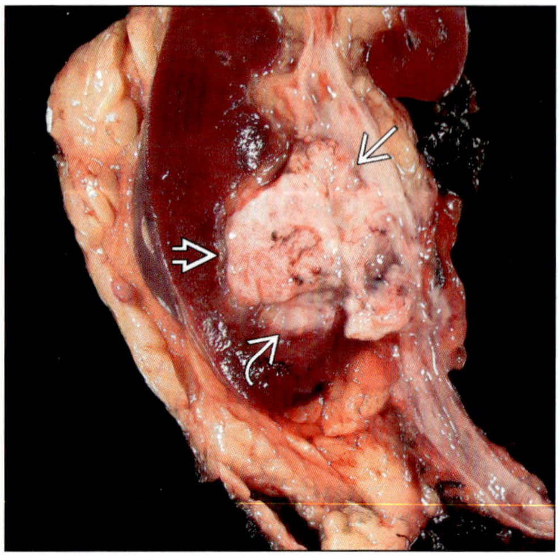

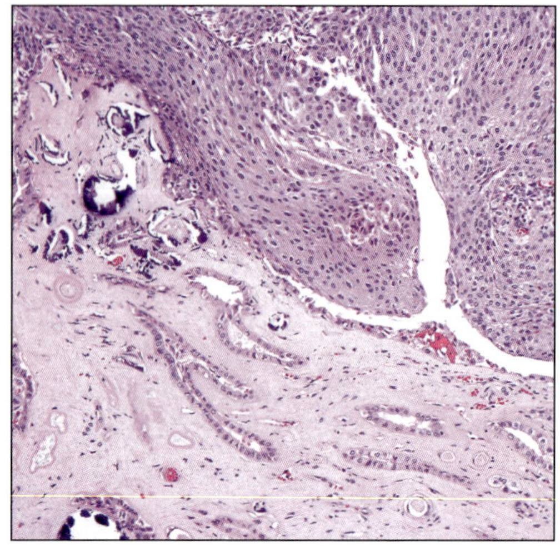

*(**Left**) This renal pelvis low-grade papillary UcA shows similar histology to low-grade UcA elsewhere in the GU tract. The tumor cells exhibit mild nuclear atypia with oval nuclei, vesicular chromatin, and mild cellular disorganization. (**Right**) Low-power view shows a high-grade papillary UcA with necrosis → in the renal pelvis and extending into the ureteropelvic portion. Note the adjacent peripelvic fat ⇨; infiltration of tumor into this fat is staged similar to renal parenchymal invasion.*

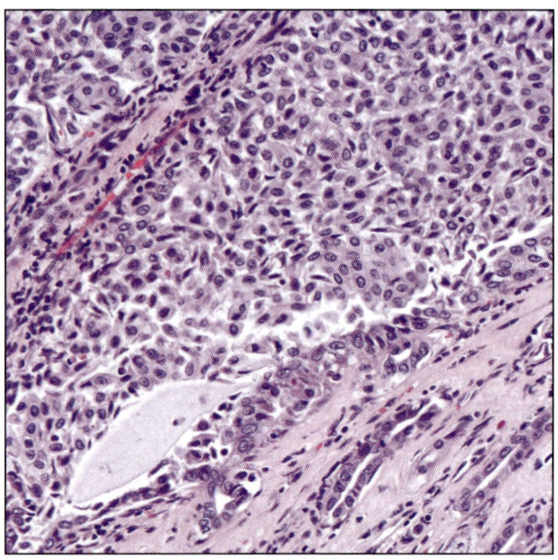

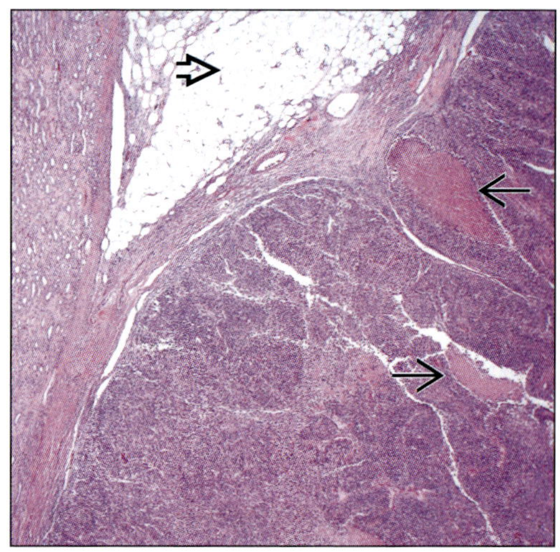

*(**Left**) Low-power view shows a high-grade noninvasive papillary UcA in the renal pelvis with delicate exophytic papillae containing fibrovascular cores. Similar to UcA elsewhere, grading of renal UcA is based entirely on cytomorphological features. (**Right**) High-grade papillary UcA shows fused papillae containing disorganized, large pleomorphic cells with nuclear rounding and frequent overlap. Nuclear chromatin is dense and mitosis is frequent →. No invasion is present in this tumor.*

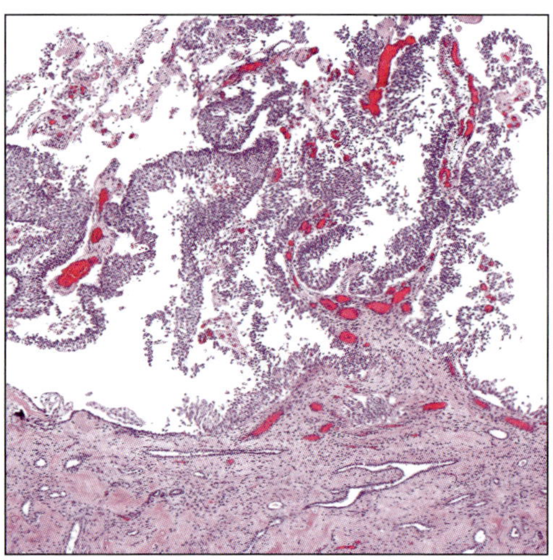

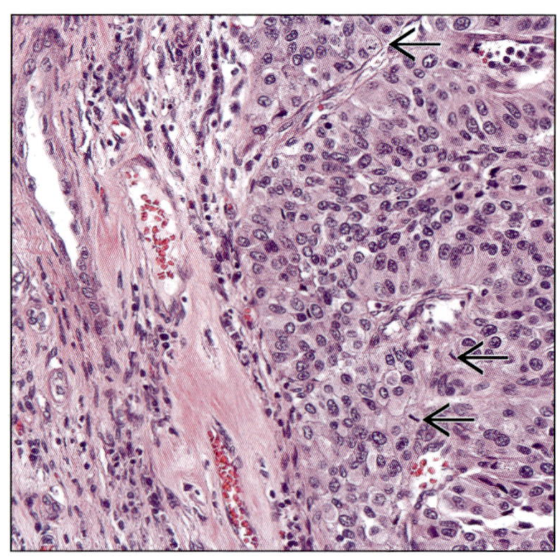

Microscopic and Immunohistochemical Features

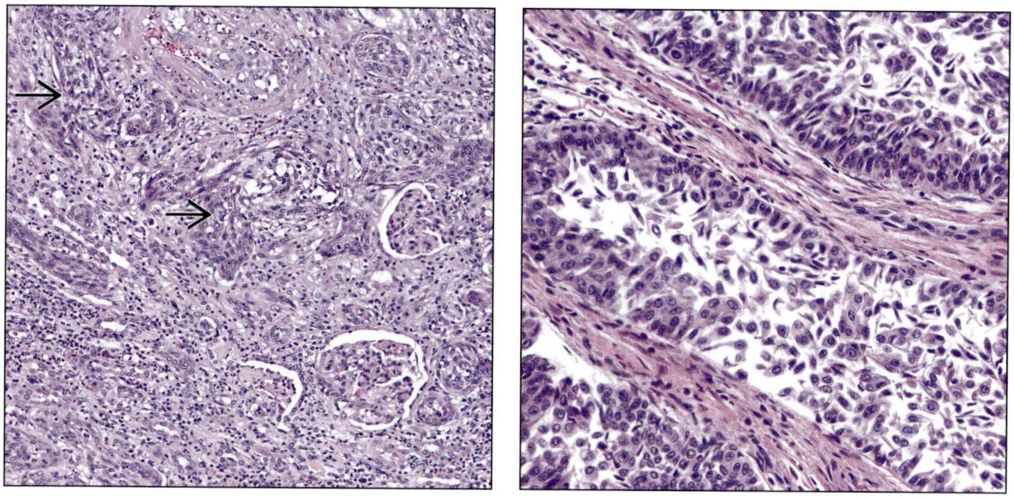

(Left) *Invasive UcA to renal parenchyma is seen infiltrating between glomeruli. There are irregular nests and small cell clusters* → *in a desmoplastic background.* **(Right)** *This noninvasive papillary UcA exhibits an endophytic growth characterized by a smooth, regular outline and no desmoplastic response. Inverted growth is suggested to be a feature of renal UcA in Lynch syndrome. Note the artifactual dyscohesion, which is not uncommon in nephrectomy specimens for UcA.*

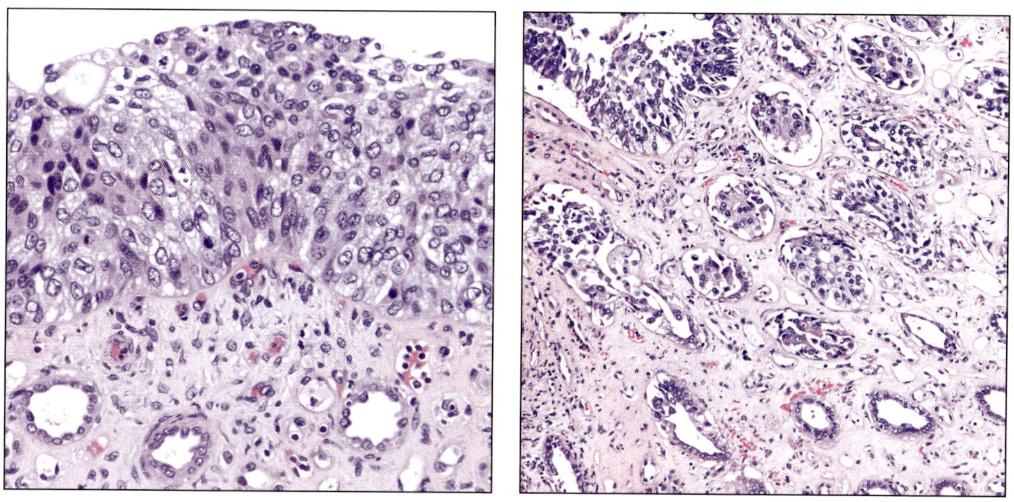

(Left) *H&E shows UcA in situ involving the renal pelvis urothelium. There is cellular disorganization with nuclear pleomorphism and hyperchromaticity.* **(Right)** *Low-power view shows UcA in situ in the renal pelvis urothelium with extension within the collecting ducts. Note the outline of the tumor nests follows the contour of the native tubules with no desmoplastic reaction. This growth remains noninvasive (pTis) and should not be overstaged as renal parenchymal invasion (pT3).*

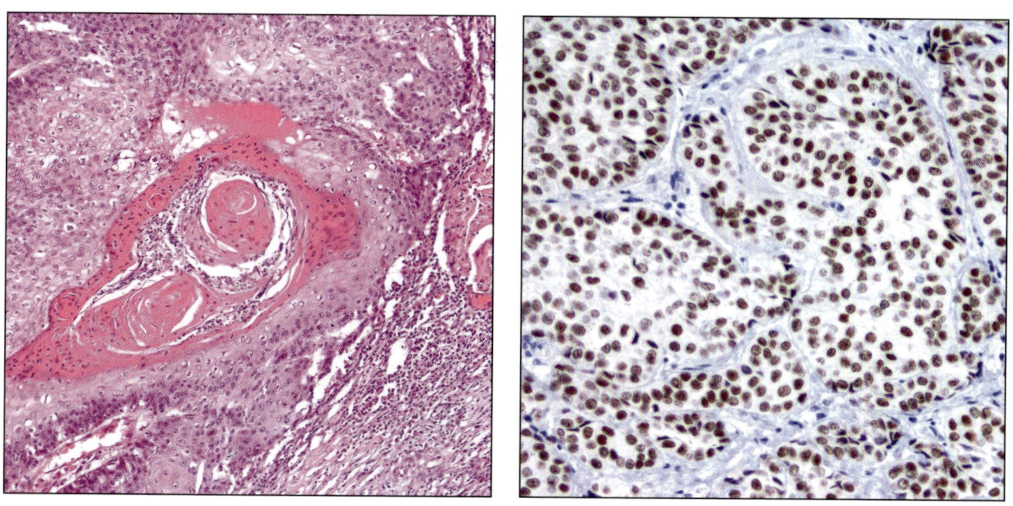

(Left) *Low-power view shows a high-grade UcA with squamous differentiation exhibiting abundant keratinization. In terms of proportion, variant morphology of UcA is more frequent (~ 25%) in the renal pelvis than in the bladder.* **(Right)** *GATA3 shows diffuse nuclear staining in this invasive renal UcA. GATA3 can be helpful in the distinction of UcA from renal carcinoma. Distinction between renal UcA and renal carcinoma has important prognostic and therapeutic implications.*

WILMS TUMOR

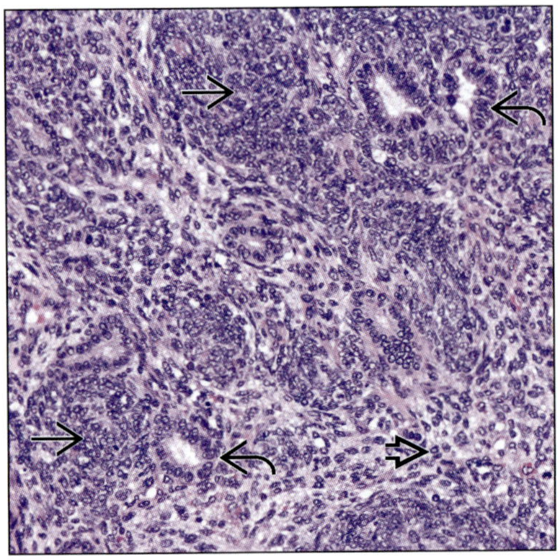

H&E shows Wilms tumor (WT) with classic triphasic histology consisting of undifferentiated blastemal cells ➔, epithelial cells (tubules) ➔, and stromal cells ➔. Proportion of these 3 components in the tumor may vary.

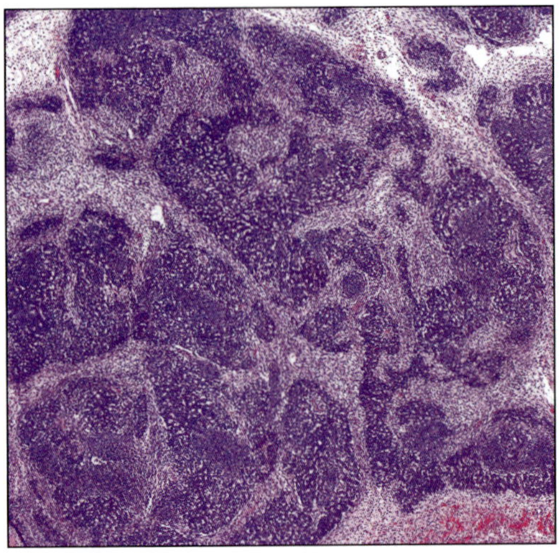

Low-power view shows large nests of blastemal cells with serpentine growth. These are tightly packed undifferentiated cells with high nuclear to cytoplasmic ratio giving the appearance of small round blue cells.

TERMINOLOGY

Abbreviations

- Wilms tumor (WT)

Synonyms

- Nephroblastoma

Definitions

- Malignant immature tumor of nephrogenic blastemal cell origin that may differentiate into epithelial or mesenchymal cells, recapitulating renal embryogenesis

ETIOLOGY/PATHOGENESIS

Gene Alterations in WT

- *WT1*
  - Encodes a 55 kDa zinc finger transcription factor containing 4 carboxy-terminal zinc finger domains that mediate DNA binding
  - Localized at Chr 11p13
  - Transcript critical in early and late stages of genitourinary development
  - Mutations in *WT1* common in sporadic WT and germline mutation consistently present in WT1-associated syndromes
- *CTNNB1*
  - Encodes an 88 kDa β-catenin protein
  - Functions as oncogene located at Chr 3p21
  - β-catenin is a main effector in Wnt/β-catenin signaling pathway
  - Mutations in *CTNNB1* seen in ~ 15% of WT and majority are 3 nucleotide deletions or missense mutations that delete or mutate Ser45
- *WTX*
  - a.k.a. *FAM123B* or *AMER1*, which contributes to stabilization of β-catenin
  - Functions as tumor suppressor gene located at Chr Xq11.1
  - Altered in 7-29% of WT, with most (~ 2/3) carrying deletion of the entire *WTX*
- *IGF2*
  - Encodes an embryonic growth factor located at Chr 11p15
  - Loss of imprinting (LOI) occur in ~ 50% of WT, resulting in aberrant inactivation of *IGF2*
  - LOI found more often in perilobar nephrogenic rests (vs. *WT1* mutations, which tend to be associated with intralobar nephrogenic rests)
- *P53*
  - Tumor suppressor gene located at Chr 17p13.1 and is the most frequently mutated gene in human cancers
  - Altered in ~ 5% of WT by missense mutation
  - Associated with diffusely anaplastic WT (AWT), detected in ~ 75% of cases

Loss of Heterozygosity (LOH) in WT

- LOH at Chr 1p and 16q are shown to be adverse prognostic factors in favorable histology Wilms tumor (FHWT)
  - Testing has sensitivity of 8% and specificity of 96%
  - Presence in FHWT requires more aggressive chemotherapy
  - Current Children Oncology Group (COG) guideline recommends LOH studies for Chr 1p and 16q in FHWT

Other Significant Gene Abnormalities

- Loss of Chr 4q and 14 q specific for AWT
- Gain of Chr 1q and *MYCN*, and loss of Chr 16q, common in AWT and FHWT

Sporadic WT (SWT)

- Mutations in *WT1* occur in 15-20% of SWT

Familial WT (FWT)

- *WT1* **not** considered the predisposition gene in most FWT families

WILMS TUMOR

Key Facts

Terminology
- Malignant immature tumor of nephrogenic blastemal cell origin that may differentiate into epithelial or mesenchymal cells, recapitulating renal embryogenesis

Etiology/Pathogenesis
- Genes altered in Wilms tumor (WT) include *WT1*, *CTNNB1*, *WTX*, *IGF2*, and *P53*
- Mutations in *WT1* occur in 15-20% of SWT
- *WT1* considered **not** the predisposition gene in most FWT families
- WT cases grouped into
  - **SWT**, comprising up to 99% of cases
  - **FWT**, comprising ~ 1- 2% of cases
  - **WT-associated syndromes**, which include *WT1*-associated and overgrowth syndromes

Clinical Issues
- Most common renal tumor of pediatric age group, accounting for 95% of tumors
- Peak incidence at 2-3 years of age
- Clinical outcomes excellent for both COG and SIOP therapies with > 90% overall survival

Microscopic Pathology
- Classic histology of WT is a triphasic pattern composed of undifferentiated **blastemal cells**, **epithelial cells**, and **stromal cells**
- Diffuse anaplasia considered a poor prognostic factor

Ancillary Tests
- WT1(+) in blastemal and epithelial but not stromal elements

- 2 FWT genes mapped
  - *FWT1* at Chr 17q12-q21
  - *FWT2* at Chr 19q13.4
  - Specific genes in these 2 regions have not yet been identified
  - Lack of linkage in some families to *FWT1* and *FWT2* suggests the existence of at least 1 additional FWT gene

WT-Associated Syndromes
- ↑ risk for WT in syndromic settings
- *WT1*-associated syndromes (WTS)
  - **WAGR syndrome**
    - Caused by microdeletions at Chr 11p13 that encompass *WT1* and *PAX6*
  - **Denys-Drash syndrome**
    - Caused by point mutation in zinc finger region of *WT1* at Chr 11p13
  - **Frasier syndrome**
    - Caused by point mutation in *WT1* intron 9 donor splice site at Chr 11p13
- **Overgrowth syndromes (OGS)**
  - **Beckwith-Wiedemann syndrome**
    - Most caused by altered expression of imprinted genes (*KCNQ1OT1, CDKN1C, LIT1* or *H19*, and *IGF2*) located at Chr 11p15.5
  - **Simpson-Golabi-Behmel syndrome**
    - Majority (70%) caused by mutations or deletions of glypican-3 (*GPC3*) at Chr Xq26
  - **Isolated (idiopathic) hemihypertrophy**
    - Abnormality in Chr 11p15 in 20-35% of cases
  - **Perlman syndrome**
    - Unknown cause; *GPC3* mutation suggested

CLINICAL ISSUES

Epidemiology
- Incidence
  - 5th most common pediatric malignancy accounting for 6% of all pediatric renal cancers
    - Estimated incidence of 7 in 1 million children < 16 years of age
    - ~ 650 new cases diagnosed in USA per year
  - Most common renal tumor of pediatric age group accounting for 95% of tumors
  - SWT comprises up to 99% of cases
  - FWT comprises ~ 1-2% of cases
  - Syndrome diagnosis seen in up to 17% of WT patients and OGS seen in ~ 4% of WT patients
- Age
  - Peak incidence at 2-3 years of age
  - ~ 75% occur in children < 5 years of age
- Gender
  - Similar incidence in male and female

Presentation
- Most commonly asymptomatic abdominal mass detected by relatives
- Abdominal pain
- Hematuria seen in ~ 20-30% of cases
- Hypertension from renin overactivity seen in ~ 25% of cases
- Subcapsular hemorrhage of tumor may cause rapidly enlarging abdominal mass, anemia, pain, and fever

Treatment
- Surgical approaches
  - Surgeon has to completely remove the tumor without spillage and adequately assess extent of spread
- Treatment approach differs for COG (includes National Wilms Tumor Study [NWTS]) followed mostly in USA, and the Société Internationale d'Oncologie Pédiatrique (SIOP) followed mostly in Europe
  - COG advocates resection 1st, followed by further therapy depending on stage and histology (i.e., favorable or unfavorable)
  - SIOP advocate neoadjuvant therapy followed by resection, and further therapy depends on stage, histology, and treatment response

WILMS TUMOR

Prognosis

- Clinical outcomes excellent for both COG and SIOP therapies with > 90% overall survival
- Most common site for metastasis is lungs

MACROSCOPIC FEATURES

General Features

- Most are unilateral and unifocal tumors

MICROSCOPIC PATHOLOGY

Histologic Features

- Classic histology of WT is a triphasic pattern composed of undifferentiated blastemal cells, epithelial cells, and stromal cells
- Some WTs may have predominance of 2 or 1 components or may only have 2 (biphasic) or 1 (uniphasic) component
- **Blastemal cells**
  - Tightly packed primitive cells with high nuclear to cytoplasmic ratio (round blue cells)
  - Nuclei have evenly spread chromatin and with indistinct nucleoli
  - Mitotically active and may show nuclear molding
  - Grow in small or large solid nests that can be serpiginous and infiltrative
- **Epithelial components**
  - Variable, includes solid or hollow primitive or mature tubules, glomeruloid structures, and papillae
  - Rarely, focal mucinous cells and squamous cells may be present
- **Stromal components**
  - Spindle cells that are commonly nondescript or with fibroblastic, smooth muscle, or skeletal differentiation
  - Often have myxoid background that resembles embryonic mesenchyme
  - Rarely, cartilage, bone, adipocytes, or neural elements
- **Anaplasia**
  - Criteria for diagnosis (all 3 are nuclear features)
    - Markedly enlarged nuclei (at least 3x size of adjacent nuclei)
    - Nuclear hyperchromasia
    - Multipolar mitotic figure
  - Present in 5% of WT; more common in older children
  - Focal anaplasia
    - Clearly defined focus of anaplasia, without presence of anaplasia elsewhere
    - May have > 1 focus, but should be completely surrounded on all sides by nonanaplastic foci
    - Not considered a poor prognostic factor (i.e., considered favorable histology)
  - Diffuse anaplasia
    - Presence of anaplasia beyond above criteria for focal anaplasia
    - Considered a poor prognostic factor (unfavorable histology by COG)
    - Stage IA WT has 69% 10-year relapse-free survival vs. 91% for FWT
  - Correlates with p53 expression
- **Teratoid WT**
  - Presence of extensive heterologous differentiation in WT, such as mucinous glands, cartilages, skeletal muscles
- **Tumor necrosis**
  - Necrotic WT with < 1/3 viable area is considered completely necrotic; low-risk tumor (by SIOP)

ANCILLARY TESTS

Immunohistochemistry

- WT1(+) in blastemal and epithelial but not stromal elements
- pax-2 or pax-8(+)
- Cytokeratin (+) in epithelial components
- CK7 and CD57 may be positive in epithelial components
- Desmin and CD56 may be positive in blastemal component

DIFFERENTIAL DIAGNOSIS

Small Round Blue Cell Tumors

- Pediatric tumors in this morphologic group may occur in or at vicinity of kidney
  - Neuroblastoma, rhabdomyosarcoma, acute lymphoblastic lymphoma, poorly differentiated synovial sarcoma, and primitive neuroectodermal tumor (PNET)
  - Distinction can often be made with the use of ancillary immunohistochemistry

Immature Teratoma

- May resemble teratoid WT
- More organoid structural differentiation (vs. haphazard elements in teratoid WT)

Metanephric Adenoma

- Primitive cells with high nuclear:cytoplasmic ratio arranged in papillae, tubules, or glomeruloid structures
- May have stromal elements (metanephric adenofibroma)
- Positive for WT1, similar to WT
- Unlike WT, nuclei are bland and mitosis is rare and more common in adults

Papillary Renal Cell Carcinoma

- Papillary and glomeruloid structures of type 1 tumors may resemble epithelial component of WT
- AMACR(+), CK7(+), and WT1(-) unlike WT
- More common in older patients (peak: 60s-70s)

Clear Cell Sarcoma of Kidney

- Similar age group to WT and may resemble blastemal-predominant WT
- Tumor cells with clearing and percolated by "chicken-wire" vasculatures
- CD99(+) and WT1(-), unlike WT

WT Staging System (COG)

Stage	Tumor Extent	Findings	Frequency
I	**Tumor limited to kidney and completely excised**	Tumor confined to kidney	40-45%
		Renal capsule is intact or tumor not ruptured	
		No invasion of lymphatic or veins of renal sinus	
		Resection margin free of tumor	
II	**Tumor extends beyond the kidney, but completely excised**	Tumor with regional or local extension	20%
		Tumor penetrates capsule or perirenal tissue	
		Tumor invades lymphatics or veins outside of kidney	
		Resection margin free of tumor	
III	**Residual nonhematogenous tumor confined to abdomen**	Positive lymph node involvement	20-25%
		Spillage from rupture before or during surgery	
		Peritoneal implants	
		Gross residual tumor in abdomen	
		Microscopic or gross positive resection margin	
		Previous biopsy	
IV	**Hematogenous metastasis**	Tumor deposits beyond stage III (i.e., lungs, liver, brain, or bone or distant lymph nodes)	10%
V	**Bilateral renal involvement**	Each side substages separately (e.g., stage V, substage II [right], substage I [left])	5%

Classification of WT After Neoadjuvant Therapy (SIOP)

Risk Level	Tumor Histology
Low-risk tumors	Cystic partially differentiated WT
	Completely necrotic WT
Intermediate-risk tumors	WT, epithelial type
	WT, stromal type
	WT, mixed type
	WT, regressive type
	WT, focal anaplasia
High-risk tumors	WT, blastemal type
	WT, diffuse anaplasia

Histological Criteria for WT Subtyping After Chemotherapy by SIOP

Tumor Type	Chemotherapy-Induced Changes (%)	% Epithelium	% Stroma	% Blastema
Completely necrotic	100	0	0	0
Regressive	> 66	0-33	0-33	0-33
Mixed	< 66	0-65	0-65	0-65
Epithelial	< 66	66-100	0-33	0-10
Stromal	< 66	0-33	66-100	0-10
Blastemal	< 66	0-33	0-33	66-100

SELECTED REFERENCES

1. Davidoff AM: Wilms tumor. Adv Pediatr. 59(1):247-67, 2012
2. Hamilton TE et al: Wilms tumor: recent advances in clinical care and biology. Semin Pediatr Surg. 21(1):15-20, 2012
3. Huff V: Wilms' tumours: about tumour suppressor genes, an oncogene and a chameleon gene. Nat Rev Cancer. 11(2):111-21, 2011
4. Md Zin R et al: Pathology, genetics and cytogenetics of Wilms' tumour. Pathology. 43(4):302-12, 2011
5. Vujanić GM et al: The pathology of Wilms' tumour (nephroblastoma): the International Society of Paediatric Oncology approach. J Clin Pathol. 63(2):102-9, 2010

WILMS TUMOR

Microscopic Features

(Left) *Low-power view shows WT, which typically has a well-defined border → from the normal kidney parenchyma. WT with predominance of blastemal cells may exhibit more infiltrative growth with irregular boundary.* ***(Right)*** *H&E shows WT with epithelial structures → amidst blastemal and stromal cells. The epithelial component is most often in the form of tubules, and may also form papillae or glomeruloid bodies. Mixed-type WT is considered an intermediate-risk tumor by SIOP working classification.*

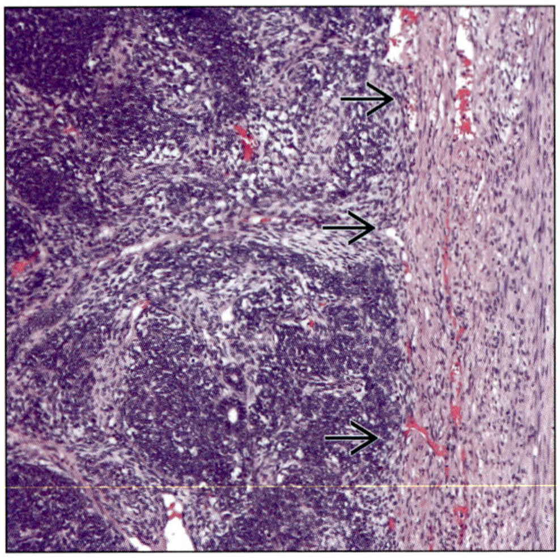

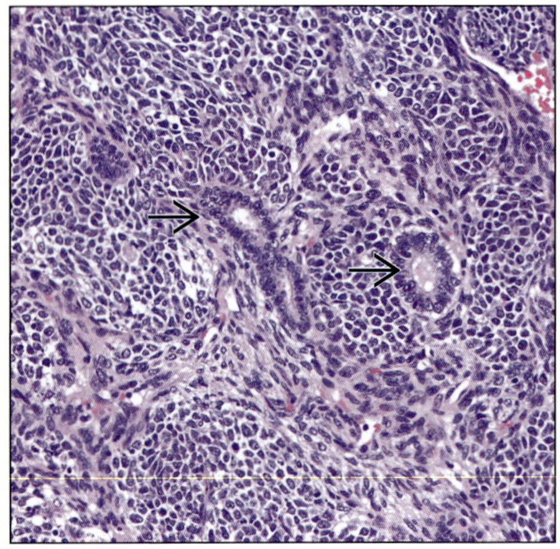

(Left) *H&E shows epithelial component of WT with rosette-like structures or solid tubulopapillary formations. These structures contain cells with relatively regular hyperchromatic nuclei. Anaplasia is usually not appreciated in the epithelial component of WT.* ***(Right)*** *H&E shows well-differentiated hollow tubular epithelial structures in WT. Note the presence of abundant mitosis. Increased mitotic activity (excluding multipolar mitosis) is not considered a poor prognostic factor in WT.*

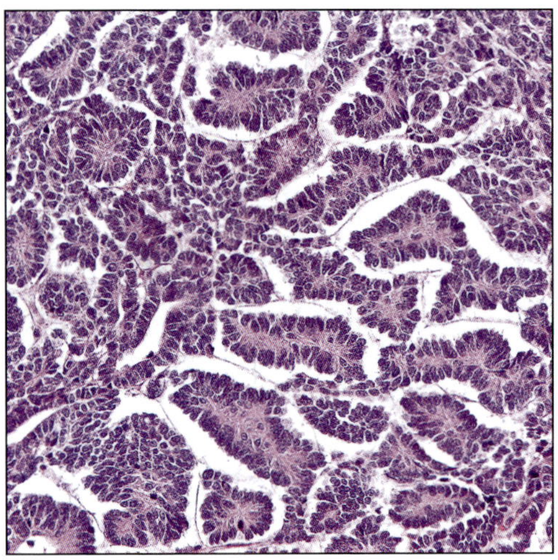

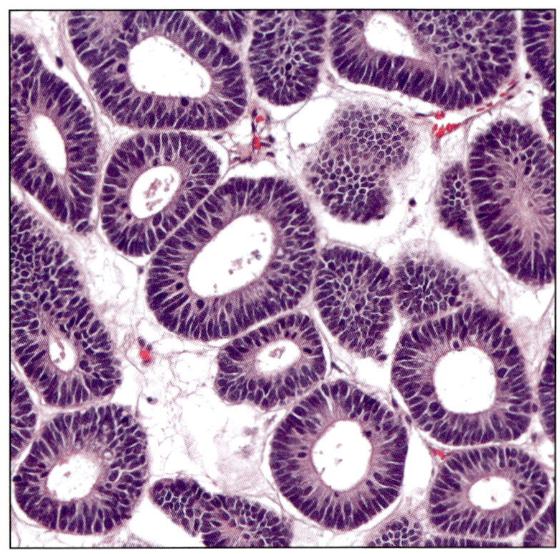

(Left) *WT shows presence of primitive glomeruloid structures consisting of large tubules with intraluminal papillary growths → in a background of spindle cells in myxoid stroma ⇨. A nest of blastemal cells ↗ is present nearby.* ***(Right)*** *H&E shows WT with large solid nests of blastemal cells partly showing peripheral cellular palisading. These immature undifferentiated cells may predominate in WT (blastemal-type WT), which is considered a high-risk tumor by the SIOP working classification.*

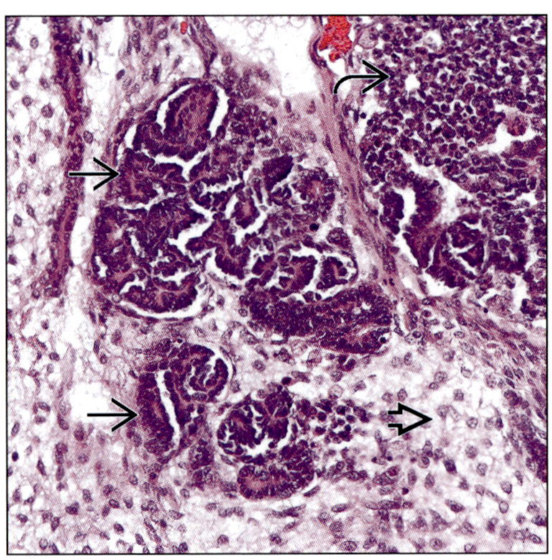

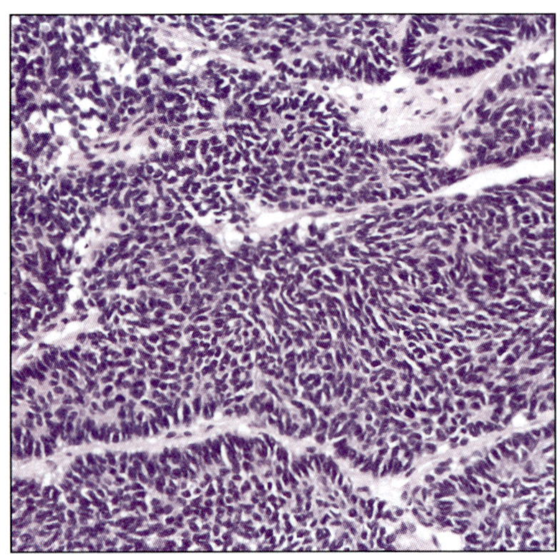

Microscopic Features

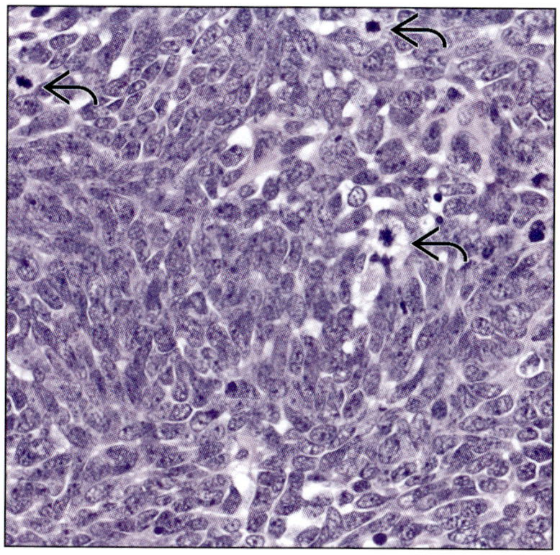

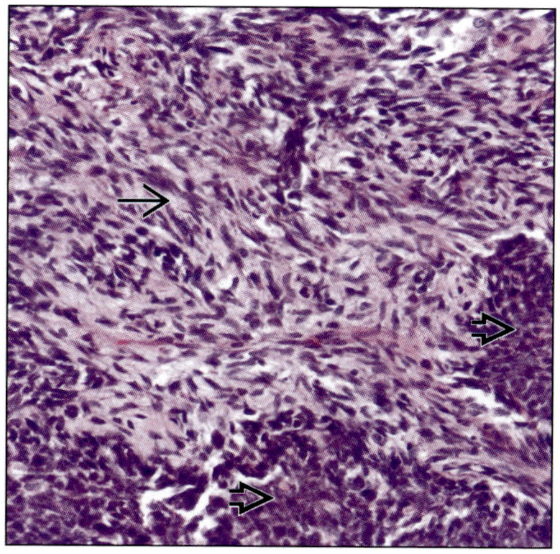

(Left) *High-power view shows blastemal cells of WT. These cells typically have large overlapping nuclei, scant cytoplasm, and evenly distributed chromatin. Note the abundant mitoses. Blastemal cells of WT resemble other small round blue cell tumors that may occur in the kidney or extrarenal sites.* ***(Right)*** *H&E shows stromal cells and blastemal cells in WT. Stromal cells are often nondescript spindle cells. Sometimes these cells exhibit smooth muscle or skeletal muscle differentiation.*

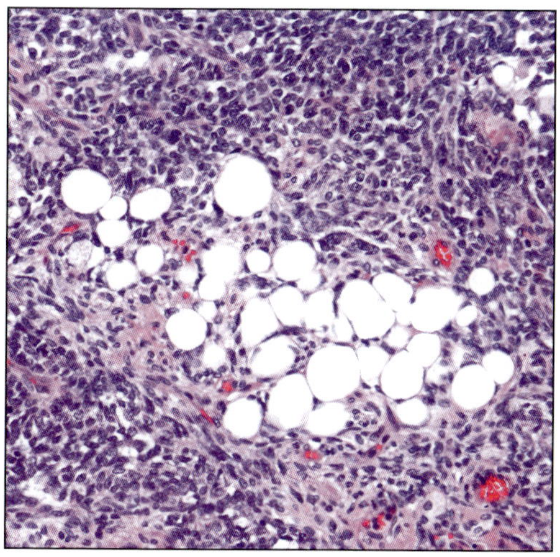

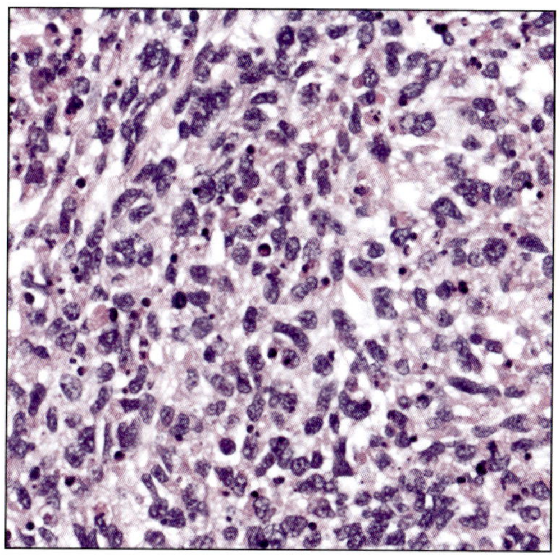

(Left) *H&E shows WT with presence of a cluster of adipocytes in the stromal component. These fat cells exhibit atypia, including variability in size and multivacoulations. Rarely, the stromal component of WT may also contain other heterologous elements, such as cartilage, bone, or glial tissues (not shown).* ***(Right)*** *H&E shows WT with rhabdomyoblastic differentiation. The cells are focally spindled and some show dense eosinophilic cytoplasm with eccentric nuclei.*

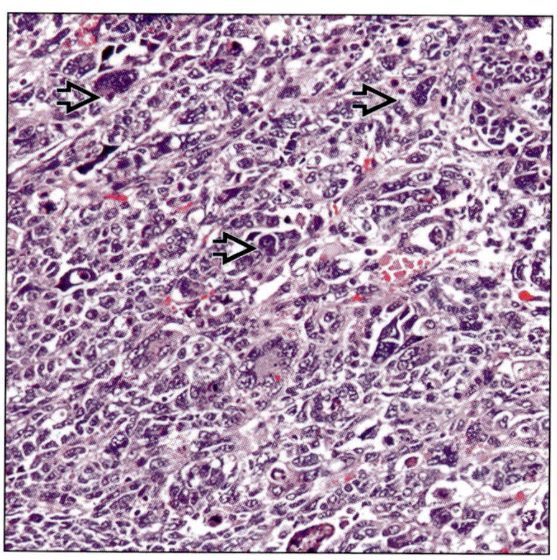

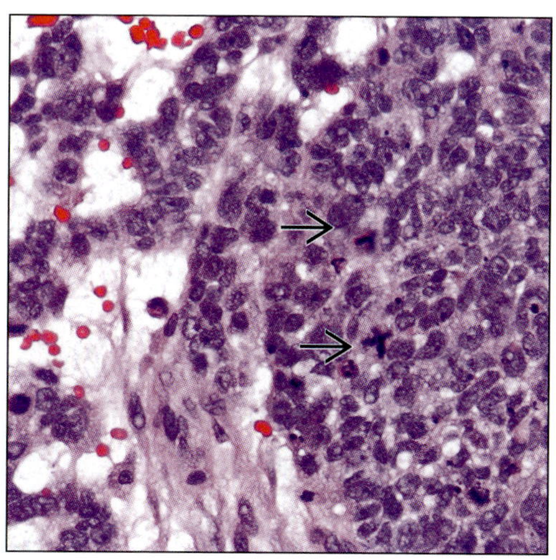

(Left) *H&E shows WT with anaplasia, which is considered an unfavorable histology when diffuse. Features of anaplasia include markedly enlarged nuclei (3x in size compared to the rest of the tumor cells), hyperchromasia, and multipolar mitotic figures. (Courtesy S. Tickoo, MD.)* ***(Right)*** *Multipolar mitotic figures are considered a diagnostic feature of anaplasia in WT. Only diffuse, and not focal, anaplasia is used in making therapeutic decisions in WT. (Courtesy S. Tickoo, MD.)*

WILMS TUMOR

Staging and Immunohistochemistry

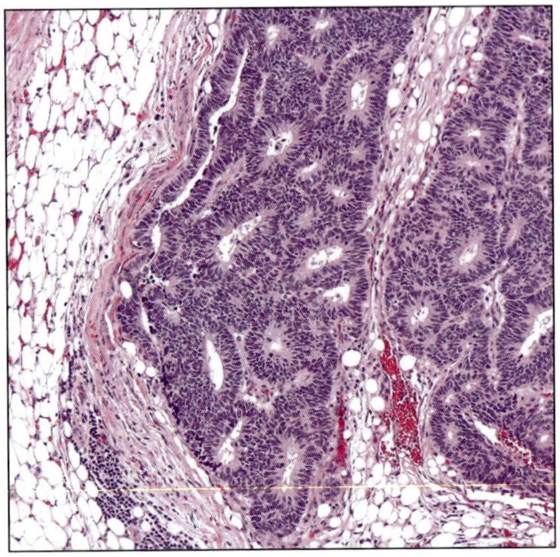

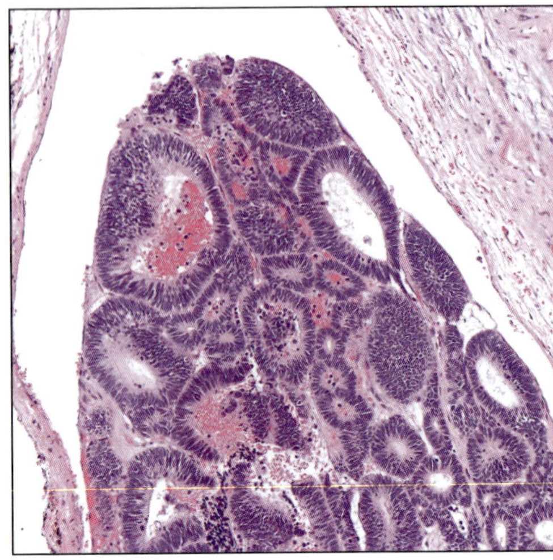

*(**Left**) Section shows WT involving the perinephric fat. This tumor is classified as stage II due to local extension of WT outside of the kidney with complete tumor resection (negative margin). (**Right**) Section shows WT seen within a large vessel. Note that the tumor follows the vessel contour. Involvement of a vessel in the renal sinus in a completely resected WT results in this tumor being classified as stage II. Stage and histology after resection are important pathologic variables that dictate subsequent therapy of WT.*

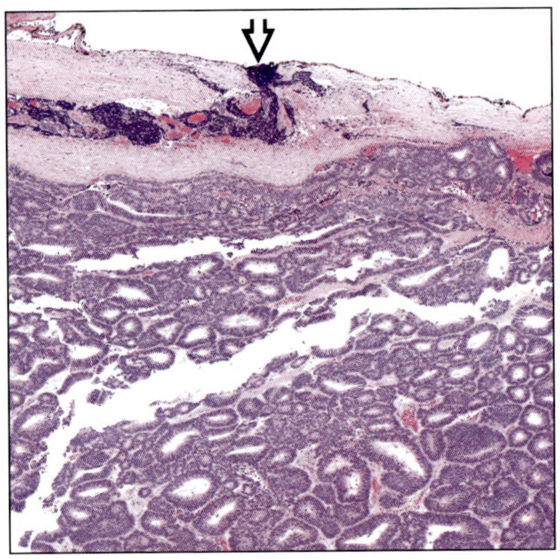

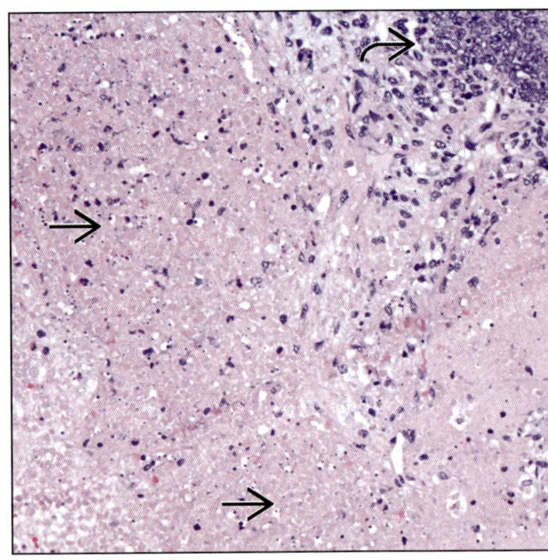

*(**Left**) Section shows WT with capsular rupture demonstrated by a tumor cell involving the inked capsule ⇒, which results in residual tumor in the abdomen. Tumor spillage of any degree before or during surgery is considered a stage III tumor. (**Right**) This WT shows abundant necrosis → characterized by presence of tumor ghost cells (coagulative type necrosis). Note the focal viable cluster of blastemal cells ↪. Completely necrotic WT after chemotherapy is considered a low-risk tumor (by SIOP).*

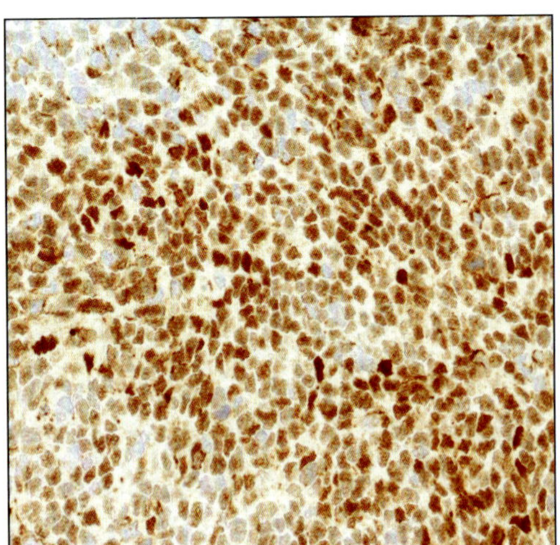

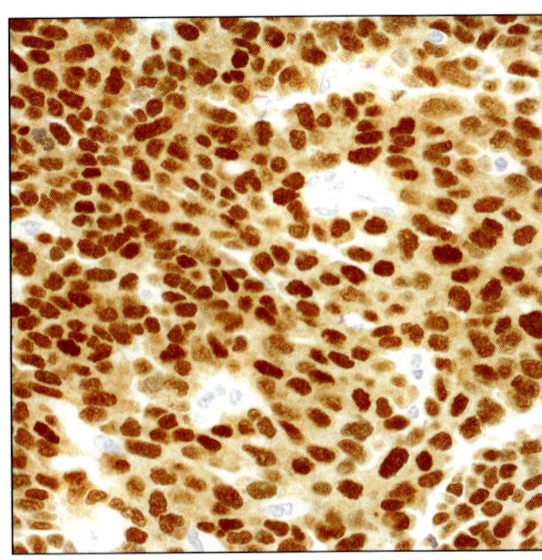

*(**Left**) WT1 shows diffuse nuclear positivity in WT. Blastemal and epithelial cells, and not the stromal cells, are usually positive for WT1 protein. Beware that metanephric adenoma may also be positive for WT1. (**Right**) pax-8 shows diffuse nuclear positivity in WT (pax-8 is nephric-lineage transcription factor crucial for kidney organogenesis). Expression of this protein is helpful in distinguishing WT from other nonrenal tumor mimics, particularly most other small round blue cell tumors.*

Differential Diagnosis

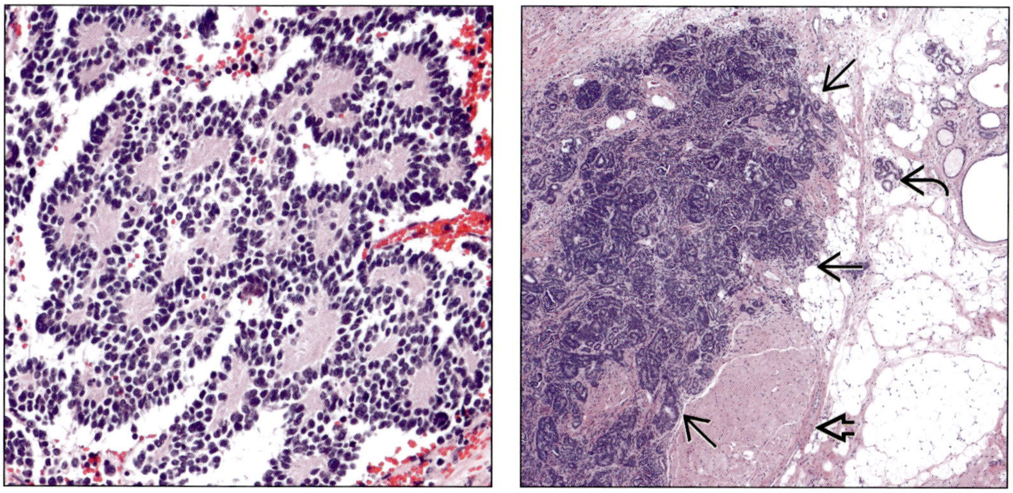

(Left) *H&E shows neuroblastoma with rosette formations, which have central neurophil surrounded by neuroblastic tumor cells (Homer Wright rosettes). This is in contrast to pseudorosettes, which have a central blood vessel. Unlike WT, neuroblastoma may exhibit cytoplasmic, and not nuclear, WT1 positivity.* **(Right)** *Low-power view shows teratoma giving rise to WT →. Adjacent to WT are well-differentiated glands (including intestinal type glands ↪), fat cells and skeletal muscles ⇨.*

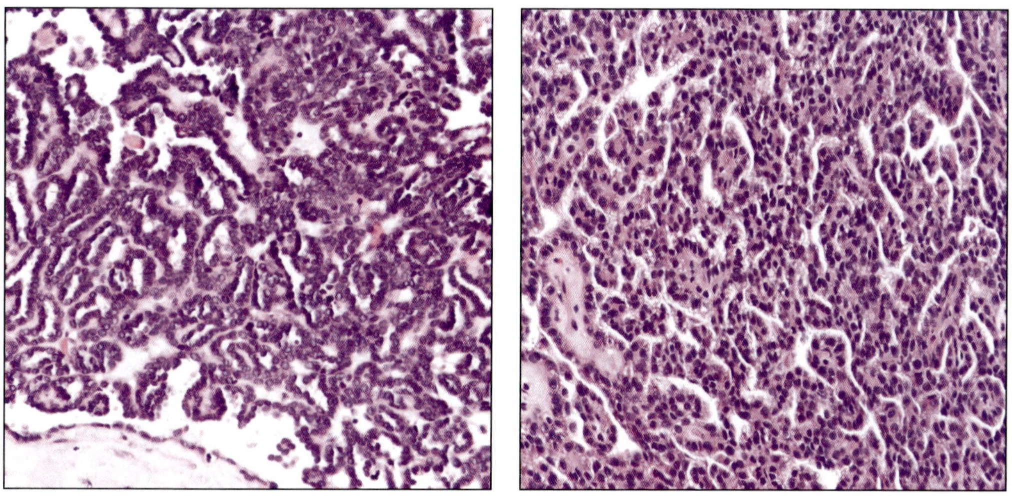

(Left) *Metanephric adenoma shows tubulopapillary and glomeruloid growths of primitive-appearing cells with high nuclear to cytoplasmic ratio. Similar to WT, these tumor cells are positive for nuclear WT1. Unlike epithelial-predominant WT, the nuclei are more regular and lack mitotic figures.* **(Right)** *Papillary renal cell carcinoma type 1 shows papillae lined by cells with amphophilic cytoplasm. These tumors occur mostly in adults and are racemase (+) and WT1(-).*

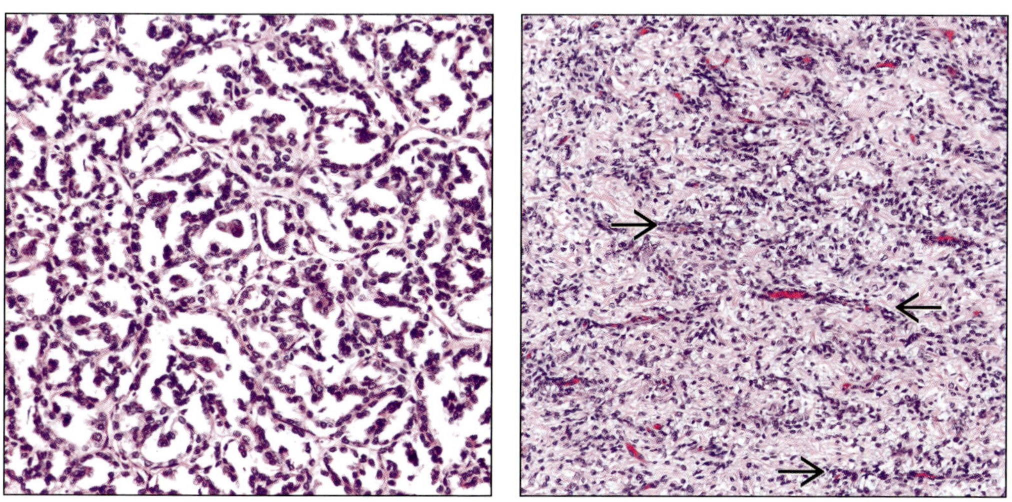

(Left) *H&E shows "solid" variant of papillary renal cell carcinoma type 1 consisting of diffuse glomeruloid growth and may resemble epithelial-predominant WT.* **(Right)** *Clear cell sarcoma of the kidney may resemble blastemal or stromal component of WT. Clear cell sarcoma typically shows polygonal tumor cells with cytoplasmic clearing from mucopolysaccharide material and with presence of arborizing vasculatures →. Unlike WT, clear cell sarcoma is negative for nuclear WT1.*

Gynecology

CERVICAL CARCINOMA

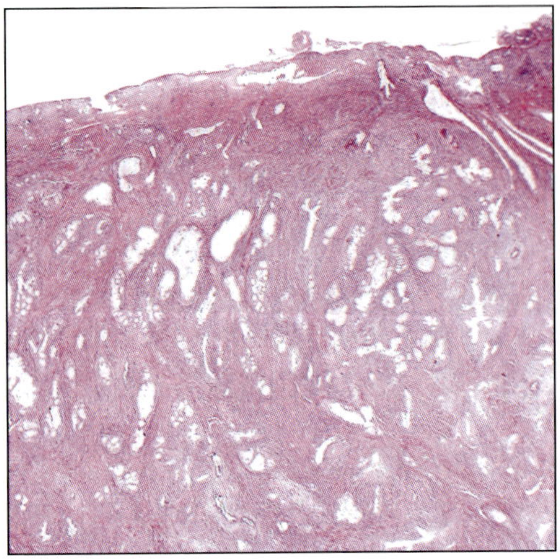

Minimal deviation adenocarcinoma shows deeply infiltrating mucinous glands.

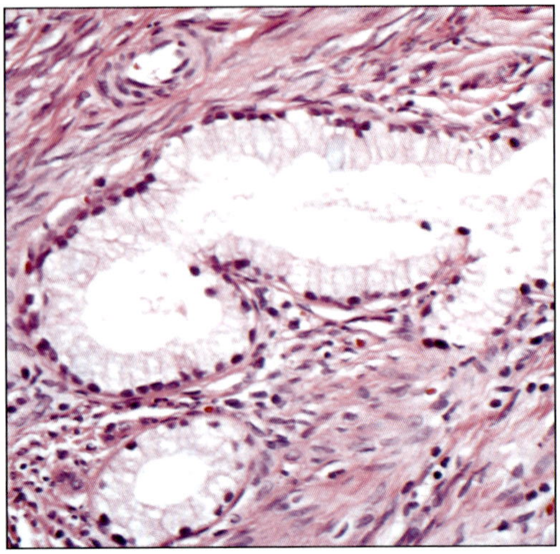

Minimal deviation adenocarcinoma is composed of glands lined by tall columnar cells with abundant apical mucin and bland nuclei.

TERMINOLOGY

Synonyms

- Minimal deviation adenocarcinoma (MDA) is also known as adenoma malignum

Definitions

- Cervical carcinoma
  - Includes multiple types of epithelial tumors
  - Most common are squamous cell carcinomas and adenocarcinomas
  - MDA is a rare subtype of cervical adenocarcinoma
    - Can be subdivided in mucinous and endometrioid types
    - Particularly associated with Peutz-Jeghers syndrome (PJS)
- PJS
  - Autosomal dominant disorder
  - Caused by mutations of *LKB1* (*STK11*) gene
  - Mucocutaneous pigmentation
  - Hamartomatous gastrointestinal polyps
  - Increased cancer risk in multiple sites, including gastrointestinal, pancreas, breast, thyroid, lung, testis, and gynecologic
  - Gynecologic tumors
    - Cervix: Minimal deviation adenocarcinoma
    - Ovary: Sex cord-stromal tumor with annular tubules (SCTATs)

ETIOLOGY/PATHOGENESIS

Peutz-Jeghers Syndrome

- Caused by germline mutations of *LKB1* (*STK11*) gene
- *LKB1* is a serine-threonine kinase that functions as a tumor suppressor gene
  - *LKB1* regulates mTOR pathway and plays a role in the control of cell proliferation
- 25% of cases are de novo

Minimal Deviation Adenocarcinoma

- Comprises 1-3% of cervical adenocarcinomas
- 10% of MDAs (specifically the mucinous subtype) are associated with PJS
- Not associated with human papillomavirus (HPV) infection, unlike the majority of cervical adenocarcinomas

CLINICAL ISSUES

Presentation

- Most patients with MDA present with cervical discharge
- Vaginal bleeding is 2nd most common presentation
- Upon exam, a bulky cervix can be detected in most patients

Treatment

- Surgery is most important modality of treatment
- Chemotherapy and radiation are also employed

Prognosis

- Late detection in most cases leads to poor prognosis
- 1 study (Kuragaki et al) suggests that MDA with *LKB1* mutations have worse prognosis than MDA without mutations

MACROSCOPIC FEATURES

Minimal Deviation Adenocarcinoma

- Barrel-shaped cervix
- Usually no discrete lesion
- Firm, expanded endocervical wall

MICROSCOPIC PATHOLOGY

Histologic Features

- Minimal deviation mucinous adenocarcinoma

Key Facts

Etiology/Pathogenesis

- Peutz-Jeghers syndrome
  - Caused by mutations of *LKB1* (*STK11*) gene
  - Cervix: Minimal deviation adenocarcinoma
  - Ovary: Sex cord-stromal tumor with annular tubules (SCTATs)
- 10% of MDAs (specifically the mucinous subtype) are associated with Peutz-Jeghers syndrome

Microscopic Pathology

- Minimal deviation mucinous adenocarcinoma
- Irregularly shaped glands that deeply infiltrate cervical wall
- Deceptively bland nuclear features

- Irregularly shaped glands that deeply infiltrate cervical wall
- Minimal or no stromal reaction
- Glands are lined by columnar cells with basal nuclei and abundant apical mucin
- Deceptively bland nuclear features, most cases have focal nuclear atypia
- Low mitotic rate
- Diagnosis on cervical biopsies is usually not possible as diagnosis relies primarily on identification of deeply infiltrative glands
- Conization is usually diagnostic

Cytologic Features

- Cytologic examination has low detection rate for MDA as cells show minimal cytologic atypia

ANCILLARY TESTS

Immunohistochemistry

- Minimal deviation mucinous adenocarcinoma
  - Practically all cases positive for HIK1083, a marker for gastric mucin
  - Vimentin and CEA positive in most cases, similar to usual-type cervical adenocarcinomas
  - Most cases are negative for CA125, unlike usual-type cervical adenocarcinomas
- Immunoexpression of proliferation markers (Ki-67 and PCNA) tends to be moderate to high (> 50% of cells), unlike well-differentiated usual-type adenocarcinomas that have low proliferation index
- p53 overexpression is seen in some cases

SELECTED REFERENCES

1. Kwon SY et al: Minimal deviation adenocarcinoma of the cervix and tumorlets of sex-cord stromal tumor with annular tubules of the ovary in Peutz-Jeghers syndrome. J Gynecol Oncol. 24(1):92-5, 2013
2. Takatsu A et al: Clonality analysis suggests that STK11 gene mutations are involved in progression of lobular endocervical glandular hyperplasia (LEGH) to minimal deviation adenocarcinoma (MDA). Virchows Arch. 462(6):645-51, 2013
3. Zhu L et al: A clinicopathological and immunohistochemical study of minimal deviation adenocarcinoma of the uterine cervix. Med Hypotheses. 80(5):643-8, 2013
4. Li G et al: Minimal deviation adenocarcinoma of the uterine cervix. Int J Gynaecol Obstet. 110(2):89-92, 2010
5. Kuragaki C et al: Mutations in the STK11 gene characterize minimal deviation adenocarcinoma of the uterine cervix. Lab Invest. 83(1):35-45, 2003

IMAGE GALLERY

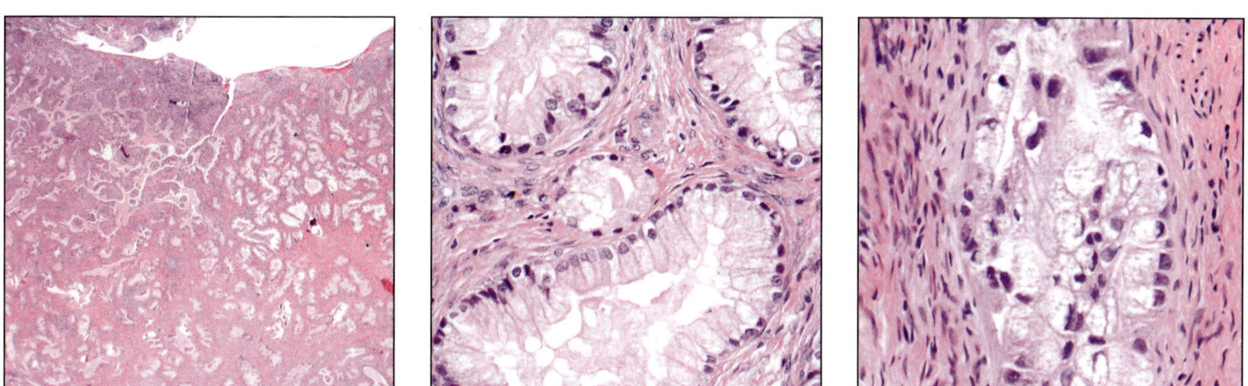

(Left) *Low-power view of minimal deviation adenocarcinoma shows infiltrative glands with irregular outlines.* ***(Center)*** *Minimal deviation adenocarcinoma is composed of glands lined by tall mucinous cells with abundant apical mucin and small, bland, basally located nuclei.* ***(Right)*** *Diligent search commonly leads to the identification of atypical nuclei focally within the tumor. Nuclei are enlarged, hyperchromatic, and irregular.*

ENDOMETRIAL CARCINOMA

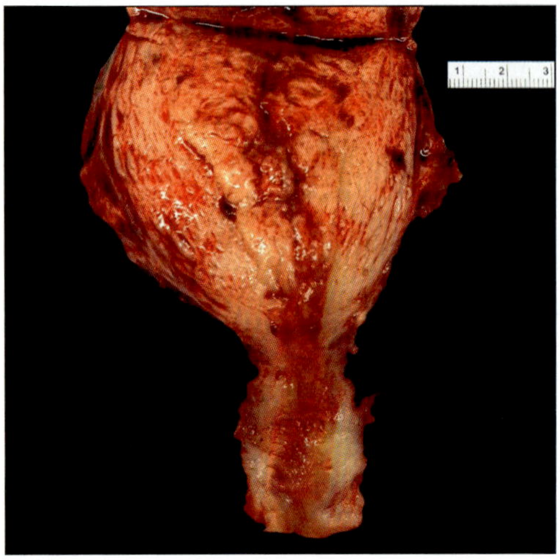

Gross photograph of an endometrial adenocarcinoma, endometrioid type, shows a sessile polypoid lesion involving most of the endometrial cavity.

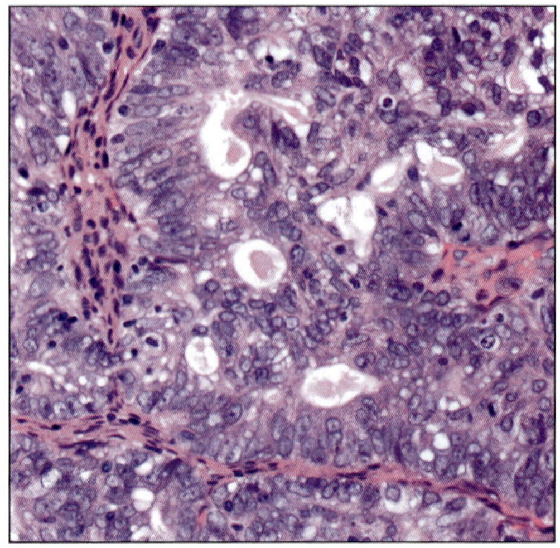

Endometrial adenocarcinoma, endometrioid type, shows cribriforming glands lined by columnar cells, similar to normal endometrial glands.

TERMINOLOGY

Synonyms

- Endometrial adenocarcinoma

Definitions

- Endometrial malignant neoplasms that comprise multiple subtypes
  - Endometrioid adenocarcinoma
  - Serous adenocarcinoma
  - Clear cell adenocarcinoma
  - Malignant mixed müllerian tumor (also known as carcinosarcoma)

ETIOLOGY/PATHOGENESIS

Genetic Predisposition

- Syndromic
  - **Lynch syndrome (LS)**
    - Autosomal dominant
    - Multiple-cancer disorder caused by germline mutations of mismatch repair genes *MLH1*, *MSH2*, *MSH6*, and *PMS2*
    - DNA mismatch repair genes excise errors occurring during DNA replication
    - Less common causes for LS are *EPCAM* deletions and germline *MLH1* promoter hypermethylation
  - **PTEN-hamartoma tumor syndrome (PHTS) (a.k.a. Cowden syndrome [CS]) or PHTS/CS**
    - Autosomal dominant
    - Germline-inactivating mutations of *PTEN* tumor suppression gene
  - **Peutz-Jeghers syndrome (PJS)**
    - Autosomal dominant
    - Mutations in the serine/threonine kinase 11 (*STK11*) gene, also known as *LKB1* gene

Sporadic

- **Endometrioid adenocarcinoma**
  - Unopposed estrogen stimulation due to anovulation, exogenous estrogen, or obesity
- **Nonendometrioid adenocarcinoma**
  - *TP53* mutations in majority of cases
  - May be related to aging and radiation

CLINICAL ISSUES

Epidemiology

- **LS**
  - Accounts for 2-3% of all endometrial cancers and 10% of endometrial cancers diagnosed before age 50
  - In women, lifetime risk for endometrial cancer (~ 60%) is slightly higher than for colorectal cancer (~ 54%)
  - Risk of endometrial cancer development varies with genetic alteration
    - 21-57% for *MLH1* and *MSH2*
    - 17-26% for *MSH6*
    - 15% for *PMS2*
  - Ratio of endometrial to colon cancer is higher for *MSH6*
- **PHTS/CS**
  - Lifetime risk for endometrial cancer has been estimated to range from 5-42%, although it is not well defined
  - Recent study showed that *PTEN*-related endometrial cancer risk begins at age 25 and rises to 30% by age 60
- **PJS**
  - Estimated 9% risk of endometrial cancer by age 65

Presentation

- **LS**
  - Increased risk for cancer of gastrointestinal tract, endometrium, ovaries, pancreatobiliary, urinary tract, brain, and skin
  - Patients with synchronous colorectal and endometrial cancer should be investigated for LS

ENDOMETRIAL CARCINOMA

Key Facts

Etiology/Pathogenesis

- **Lynch syndrome**
  - Multiple-cancer disorder caused by germline mutations of mismatch repair genes *MLH1*, *MSH2*, *MSH6*, and *PMS2*
- **PTEN-hamartoma tumor syndrome (a.k.a. Cowden syndrome)**
  - Germline-inactivating mutations of *PTEN* tumor suppression gene
- **Peutz-Jeghers syndrome**
  - Mutations in serine/threonine kinase *STK11* gene

Clinical Issues

- **Lynch syndrome**
  - Increased risk for cancer of gastrointestinal tract, endometrium, ovaries, pancreatobiliary, urinary tract, brain, and skin
  - Women with synchronous endometrial and ovarian endometrioid adenocarcinomas are more likely to have Lynch syndrome
  - Lifetime risk for endometrial cancer is slightly higher than for colorectal cancer

Ancillary Tests

- **Lynch syndrome**
  - Mismatch repair protein immunohistochemical expression using antibodies against MLH1, MSH2, MSH6, and PMS2
  - *MLH1* promoter hypermethylation
  - Microsatellite instability (MSI)
  - Germline testing

- Women with synchronous endometrial and ovarian endometrioid adenocarcinomas are more likely to have LS
- Carcinomas of lower uterine segment appear to be more frequent in LS than in general population
- Mean age at diagnosis of nonendometrioid tumors is lower in LS vs. sporadic cases

- **PHTS/CS**
  - Multiple-cancer syndrome with hamartomatous growth in many organs
  - Hamartomas of the skin, mucous membranes, breast, thyroid, and endometrium
  - Cancers of the thyroid, breast, endometrium, colorectum and kidney; also melanoma
  - Frequent and multiple uterine leiomyomas
- **PJS**
  - Hamartomatous gastrointestinal polyps and mucocutaneous pigmentation
  - Increased risk for multiple cancers including gastrointestinal, pancreatic, ovarian, cervical, and uterine

Treatment

- Most experts recommend hysterectomy and bilateral salpingo-oophorectomy after childbearing is complete for patients with LS
- No specific recommendations have been defined for PHTS/CS and PJS

Prognosis

- Does not seem to differ for endometrial carcinomas arising in familial or sporadic settings

Surveillance

- Transvaginal ultrasound and endometrial sampling after age 30 is recommended for patients with familial cancer syndromes with increased risk for endometrial cancer

MACROSCOPIC FEATURES

General Features

- Synchronous endometrial and ovarian endometrioid adenocarcinomas
- Carcinomas of lower uterine segment

MICROSCOPIC PATHOLOGY

Histologic Features

- **LS**
  - Both endometrioid and nonendometrioid histology
  - Higher incidence of high-grade nonendometrioid types than among general population, particularly with *MSH2* mutations
  - As in colorectal cancer, tumor-infiltrating lymphocytes and peritumoral lymphocytes in endometrial carcinoma appear to be predictors of microsatellite instability (MSI)
  - Undifferentiated tumor histology, unlike colon cancer, has not been consistently associated with LS
- **PHTS/CS and PJS**
  - Data regarding histologic subtypes in PHTS/CS and PJS are limited

Cytologic Features

- Cytopathologic examination is rarely employed for diagnosis of endometrial carcinoma
- Detached tumor cells can be identified in cervical cytology and peritoneal fluid in some cases

ANCILLARY TESTS

Immunohistochemistry

- **LS**
  - Mismatch repair protein immunohistochemistry using antibodies against MLH1, MSH2, MSH6, and PMS2
  - Loss of nuclear staining is considered abnormal

ENDOMETRIAL CARCINOMA

- Background nonneoplastic cells, particularly lymphocytes, are good internal positive controls
- Concurrent loss of MLH1 and PMS2 expression indicates *MLH1* gene abnormalities
  - When *PMS2* mutations are present, only PMS2 expression is lost
- Concurrent loss of MSH2 and MSH6 expression indicates *MSH2* gene abnormalities
  - When *MSH6* mutations are present, only MSH6 expression is lost
- Immunohistochemical results are used to triage cases for germline testing
- Screening test of choice in endometrial carcinoma as a significant proportion of LS-associated endometrial carcinomas are microsatellite low or microsatellite stable by MSI testing, particularly when *MSH6* is mutated

Molecular Genetics

- LS
  - *MLH1* promoter hypermethylation
    - Methylation of *MLH1* promoter is a sporadic cause of loss of MLH1 protein expression
    - When *MLH1* promoter is methylated, there is no indication for germline testing
    - Performed in DNA extracted from paraffin-embedded tissues
  - MSI
    - Hallmark of defective mismatch repair
    - Can result from sporadic or germline loss of mismatch repair protein function
    - DNA is extracted from both tumor and nonneoplastic tissue
    - Normal tissue can be extracted from paraffin-embedded tissue or peripheral blood lymphocytes
    - Significant proportion of LS-associated endometrial carcinomas are microsatellite low or microsatellite stable by MSI testing, particularly when *MSH6* is mutated
    - Less reliable as LS screening test in endometrial carcinoma compared to colorectal cancer
  - Germline testing
    - Mutational analysis by DNA sequencing of *MLH1*, *MSH2*, *MSH6*, and *PMS2*
    - Performed in DNA extracted from peripheral blood lymphocytes
- PHTS/CS
  - Germline testing
    - *PTEN* sequencing analysis, large deletion/duplication analysis
    - Performed in DNA extracted from peripheral blood lymphocytes
- PJS
  - Germline testing
    - *STK11* gene sequencing analysis, large deletion/duplication analysis
    - Performed in DNA extracted from peripheral blood lymphocytes

DIFFERENTIAL DIAGNOSIS

Lynch Syndrome

- Guidelines for identifying LS in women with gynecologic cancers are less defined than for colorectal cancer
- Endometrial carcinoma may be 1st malignancy diagnosed in women with LS
- Women with endometrial carcinoma before age 50 have a higher likelihood of having LS, but the tumor may develop later in life
- Patients with synchronous endometrioid uterine and ovarian adenocarcinomas are at increased risk for LS and should be screened by immunohistochemistry &/or MSI
- Patients with synchronous endometrial carcinoma and colorectal cancer should be screened by immunohistochemistry &/or MSI

PTEN-Hamartoma Tumor Syndrome and Peutz-Jeghers Syndrome

- Differential between sporadic and familial endometrial carcinoma in these syndromes relies primarily on nongynecologic manifestations and genetic testing

SELECTED REFERENCES

1. Miesfeldt S et al: Management of genetic syndromes predisposing to gynecologic cancers. Curr Treat Options Oncol. 14(1):34-50, 2013
2. Ballinger LL: Hereditary gynecologic cancers: risk assessment, counseling, testing and management. Obstet Gynecol Clin North Am. 39(2):165-81, 2012
3. Daniels MS: Genetic testing by cancer site: uterus. Cancer J. 18(4):338-42, 2012
4. Tan MH et al: Lifetime cancer risks in individuals with germline PTEN mutations. Clin Cancer Res. 18(2):400-7, 2012
5. Resnick KE et al: Current and emerging trends in Lynch syndrome identification in women with endometrial cancer. Gynecol Oncol. 114(1):128-34, 2009
6. Walsh MD et al: Molecular, pathologic, and clinical features of early-onset endometrial cancer: identifying presumptive Lynch syndrome patients. Clin Cancer Res. 14(6):1692-700, 2008
7. Broaddus RR et al: Pathologic features of endometrial carcinoma associated with HNPCC: a comparison with sporadic endometrial carcinoma. Cancer. 106(1):87-94, 2006
8. Soliman PT et al: Women with synchronous primary cancers of the endometrium and ovary: do they have Lynch syndrome? J Clin Oncol. 23(36):9344-50, 2005
9. Giardiello FM et al: Very high risk of cancer in familial Peutz-Jeghers syndrome. Gastroenterology. 119(6):1447-53, 2000

Microscopic Features and Ancillary Techniques

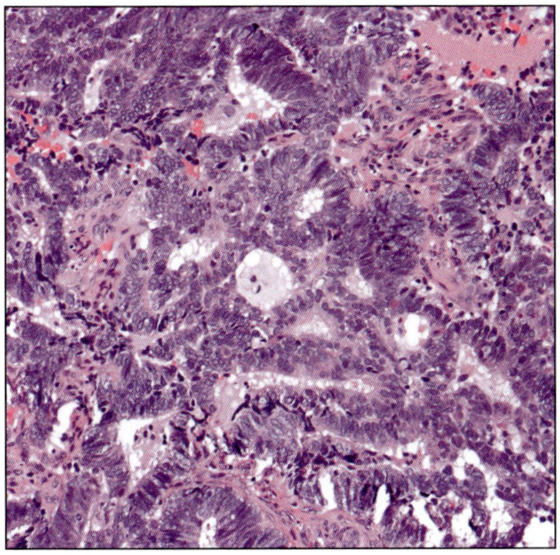
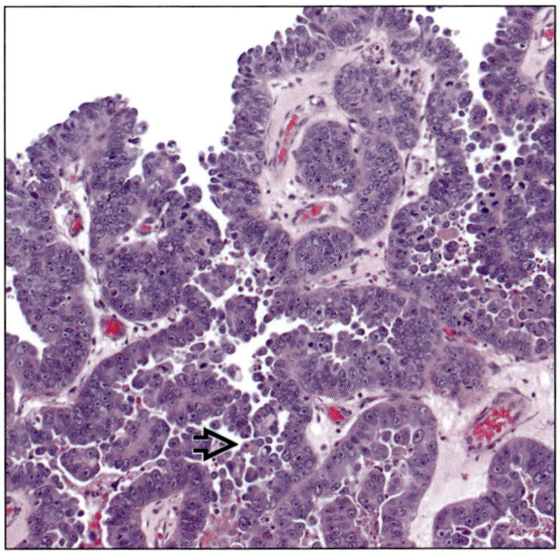

(Left) *Endometrioid adenocarcinoma shows back-to-back glands lined by pseudostratified columnar cells with nuclear atypia. Despite the high frequency of nonendometrioid adenocarcinomas in Lynch syndrome, endometrioid adenocarcinomas are most common in absolute numbers.* ***(Right)*** *Serous adenocarcinoma is composed of broad papillae with cellular budding into intervening spaces ⇨. The cells are markedly atypical with pleomorphic nuclei and prominent nucleoli.*

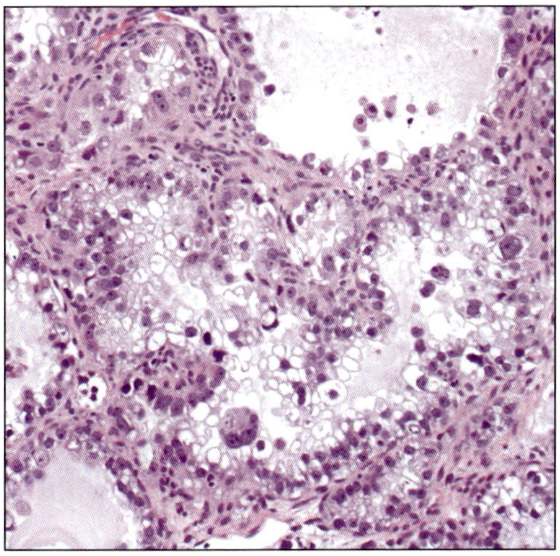
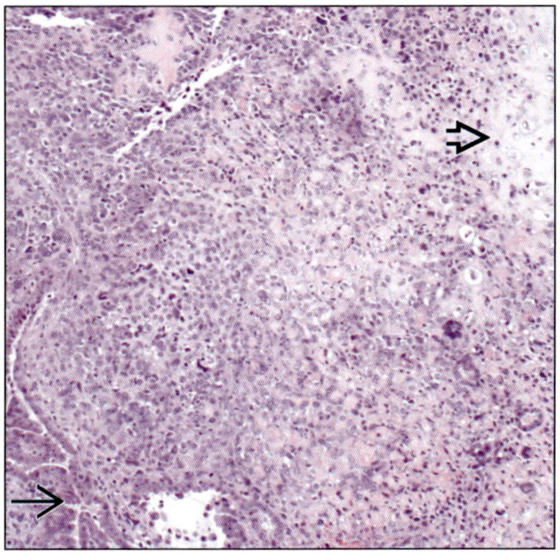

(Left) *Clear cell adenocarcinoma shows tubulopapillary growth of polygonal cells with abundant clear cytoplasm and markedly pleomorphic nuclei. Typical of this tumor are nuclei polarized toward the lumen, known as hobnailing.* ***(Right)*** *Carcinosarcoma consists of an admixture of carcinomatous gland-forming → and sarcomatous chondroid ⇨ components.*

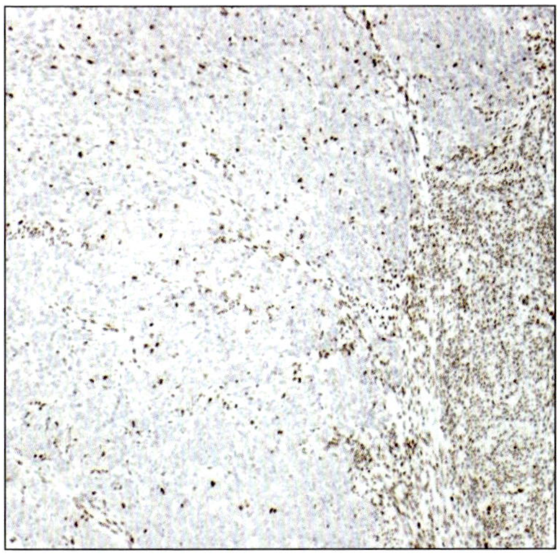
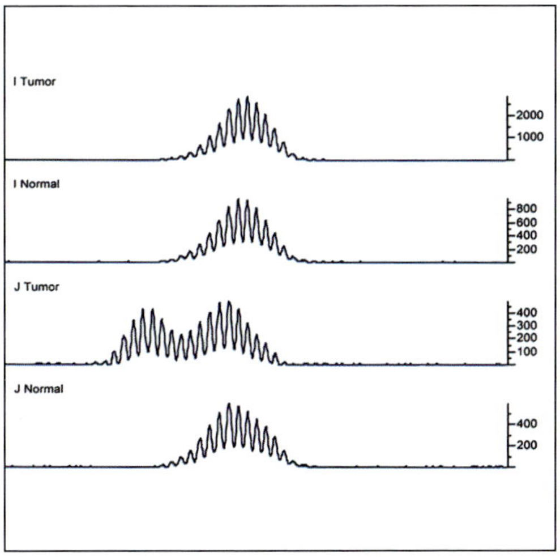

(Left) *Immunohistochemistry for MSH2 is shown in an endometrioid adenocarcinoma in a patient with Lynch syndrome and germline MSH2 gene mutation. Tumor cell nuclei are negative, and infiltrating lymphocytes serve as an internal positive control.* ***(Right)*** *Microsatellite instability testing using a mononucleotide marker (BAT26) shows that the top tumor sample is microsatellite stable whereas the bottom tumor sample is microsatellite unstable.*

FALLOPIAN TUBE CARCINOMA

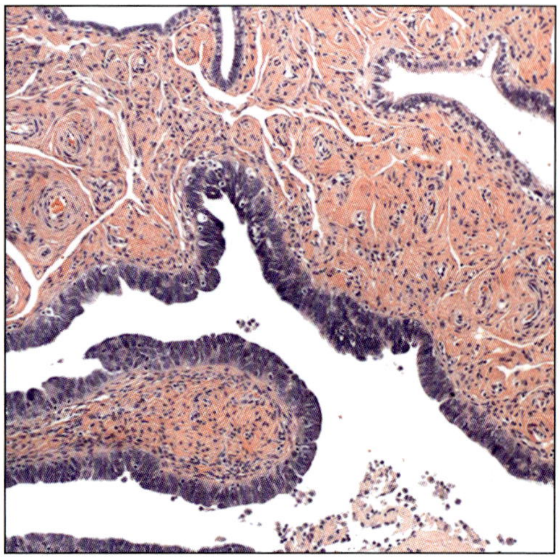

Serous intraepithelial carcinoma shows cellular stratification. Compare with the background normal tubal epithelium.

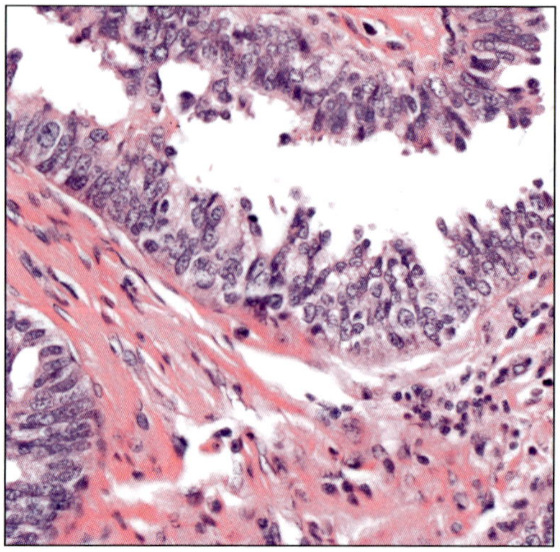

Serous intraepithelial carcinoma shows high nuclear:cytoplasmic ratio and pleomorphic nuclei.

TERMINOLOGY

Abbreviations

- Hereditary breast and ovarian cancer (HBOC)

ETIOLOGY/PATHOGENESIS

Hereditary Breast and Ovarian Cancer

- Caused by germline *BRCA1* and *BRCA2* mutations with increased risk for breast and gynecologic cancers, including ovary, fallopian tube, and peritoneum
- Germline mutations in other genes, such as genes involved in the Fanconi anemia-BRCA pathway, might be related to the development of fallopian tube cancer, but data is limited
- p53 signatures are believed to be precursor lesion for development of serous tubal intraepithelial carcinomas (STIC), which, in turn, represent in situ stage of invasive serous carcinoma

CLINICAL ISSUES

Epidemiology

- Up to 30% of women with unselected fallopian tube carcinoma were found to have germline *BRCA1* and *BRCA2* mutations in a recent study
- In situ tubal carcinoma can be detected before age 40 whereas most invasive tubal carcinomas occur in 50s and 60s
- Patients with fallopian tube carcinoma diagnosed before age 60, of Jewish decent, and with personal or familial history of breast or ovarian cancer are at increased risk of harboring *BRCA1* or *BRCA2* mutations

Presentation

- Most tubal carcinomas diagnosed in HBOC patients are detected at early stages at risk-reducing bilateral salpingo-oophorectomy (RRSO)
- Based on molecular genetic studies, a significant proportion of serous carcinomas involving the ovary and peritoneum are believed to arise from the fallopian tube epithelium

Treatment

- RRSO is recommended between ages 35 and 40, after childbearing is complete
- Oral contraceptives decrease the risk of cancer development
- Hormone replacement therapy has been shown to increase the risk of fallopian tube cancer
- *BRCA1*- and *BRCA2*-related tumors have better response to platinum-based chemotherapy and increased sensitivity to poly ADP-ribose polymerase (PARP) inhibitors compared to sporadic carcinomas

Prognosis

- As for ovarian carcinomas, HBOC tubal carcinomas have a better prognosis than the sporadic counterpart

MACROSCOPIC FEATURES

Gross Findings

- Most RRSO specimens do not have a visible gross lesion
- Majority of both in situ and invasive tubal carcinomas in RRSO specimens are found in the distal fimbria
- Sectioning and extensively examining the fimbriated end (SEE-FIM) protocol describes how to submit fallopian tubes to optimize detection of microscopic carcinomas
  - Fimbriated end is amputated and longitudinally sectioned at 2-3 mm intervals

FALLOPIAN TUBE CARCINOMA

Key Facts

Etiology/Pathogenesis

- Germline *BRCA1* and *BRCA2* mutations with increased risk for breast and gynecologic cancers

Clinical Issues

- Most tubal carcinomas are detected at early stages at risk-reducing bilateral salpingo-oophorectomy (RRSO)

Microscopic Pathology

- Invasive or in situ tubal carcinoma is detected in ~ 5-7% of RRSO specimens
- Majority are serous tubal intraepithelial carcinomas (STIC)

Ancillary Tests

- p53 and Ki-67 (MIB-1) can be performed to confirm diagnosis of STIC

- Remainder fallopian tube is transversely sectioned at 2-3 mm intervals
- Bilateral fallopian tubes received as part of RRSO specimen should be fixed in formalin prior to sectioning

MICROSCOPIC PATHOLOGY

Histologic Features

- Invasive or in situ tubal carcinoma is detected in ~ 5-7% of RRSO specimens
- Majority are STIC
  - Characterized by marked cytologic atypia when compared with the background tubal epithelium
  - Cellular stratification and pseudostratification
  - Disorganization and loss of polarity
  - High nuclear:cytoplasmic ratio and loss of cilia
  - Nuclear enlargement and chromatin irregularities
- Most invasive tumors are high-grade serous carcinomas
- Some carcinomas show undifferentiated or endometrioid histology
- Frozen section examination of RRSO specimen is not recommended unless a grossly visible suspicious lesion, such as a solid nodule, is present

ANCILLARY TESTS

Immunohistochemistry

- p53 and Ki-67 (MIB-1) can be performed to confirm diagnosis of STIC
  - Microscopic foci of morphologically atypical tubal epithelium is expected to show strong and diffuse immunostaining for both p53 and Ki-67 to be diagnostic of STIC
- p53 signature
  - Defined as strong and diffuse p53 immunoreaction in 12 or more consecutive tubal lining epithelial cells
  - To be considered a p53 signature, the focus in question should **not** demonstrate cytologic atypia
  - p53 signatures have been shown to harbor *TP53* mutations by molecular genetic studies
  - Not recommended for diagnostic reporting

Molecular Genetics

- DNA sequencing for germline mutations in *BRCA1* and *BRCA2* genes
- Consider BRCA1 and BRCA2 mutational analysis in all patients diagnosed with fallopian tube carcinoma

SELECTED REFERENCES

1. Mingels MJ et al: Tubal epithelial lesions in salpingo-oophorectomy specimens of BRCA-mutation carriers and controls. Gynecol Oncol. 127(1):88-93, 2012

IMAGE GALLERY

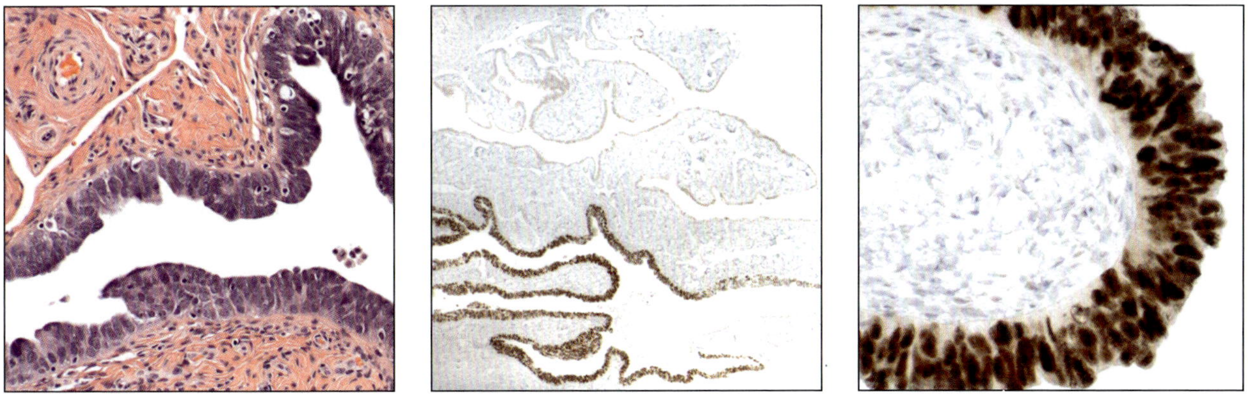

(Left) *Serous intraepithelial carcinoma shows stratification, loss of polarity, and lack of cilia. The cells have high nuclear:cytoplasmic ratio, nuclear enlargement, and chromatin irregularities.* ***(Center)*** *p53 immunostain is positive in serous intraepithelial carcinoma and negative in the background benign epithelium.* ***(Right)*** *p53 immunostain in serous intraepithelial carcinoma shows diffuse and strong nuclear staining.*

OVARIAN CARCINOMA

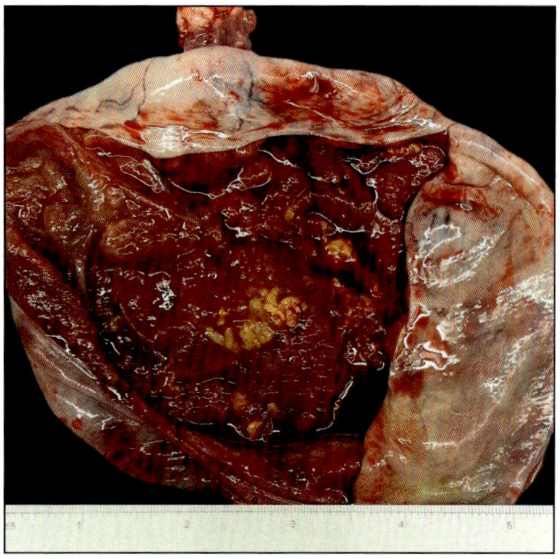

Gross photo shows an ovarian serous carcinoma forming a solid cystic mass.

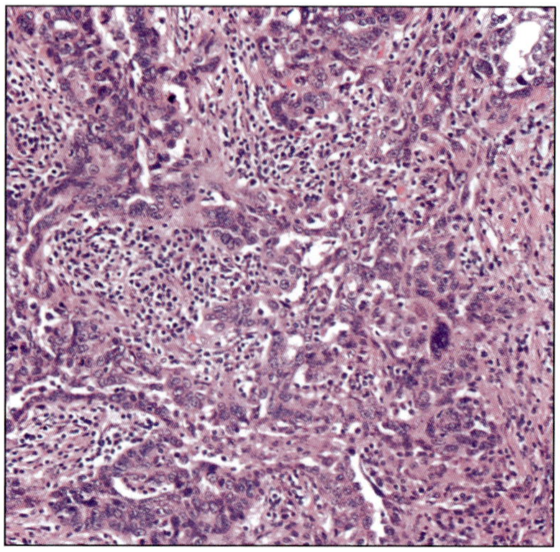

High-grade serous carcinoma forms cleft-like spaces lined by large epithelial cells with marked nuclear atypia.

TERMINOLOGY

Definitions

- **Hereditary breast and ovarian cancer**
  - Germline *BRCA1* and *BRCA2* mutations with ↑ risk for breast and gynecologic cancers
- **Lynch syndrome**
  - Germline mismatch repair gene mutations leading to increased cancer risk, including colorectal and gynecologic
- **Peutz-Jeghers syndrome**
  - Germline *STK11* mutations with increased risk of multiple cancers, such as gastrointestinal, pancreatic, and gynecologic

ETIOLOGY/PATHOGENESIS

Hereditary Breast and Ovarian Cancer (HBOC)

- Autosomal dominant
- Germline *BRCA1* and *BRCA2* mutations
- *BRCA1* and *BRCA2* genes repair DNA damage through homologous recombination

Lynch Syndrome (LS)

- Autosomal dominant
- Germline mutations of *MLH1*, *MSH2*, *MSH6*, and *PMS2* genes
- DNA mismatch repair genes that excise errors occurring during DNA replication

Peutz-Jeghers Syndrome (PJS)

- Autosomal dominant
- Mutations in serine threonine kinase 11 (*STK11*) gene

Germline Mutations of Genes in Fanconi Anemia (FA)-BRCA Pathway

- *RAD51C*, *RAD51D*, *BRIP1*, among others
- Monoallelic germline mutations of these genes have been identified in highly penetrant breast and ovarian cancer families lacking *BRCA1/BRCA2* mutations
- FA-BRCA pathway plays a role in homologous recombination, which mends double-stranded DNA breaks

CLINICAL ISSUES

Epidemiology

- ~ 1 in 4 women with ovarian cancer has hereditary gene mutation related to cancer development
- **Hereditary breast and ovarian cancer**
  - Account for majority of hereditary ovarian cancers
  - 13-15% of women with invasive ovarian cancer harbor germline mutations of *BRCA1* or *BRCA2* genes
  - Proportion of ovarian cancer that is hereditary varies with prevalence of founder mutations in each population
  - In women of Ashkenazi decent, 35-40% of ovarian carcinomas are associated with *BRCA1* or *BRCA2* mutations
  - Lifetime risk for ovarian cancer
    - 35-60% for *BRCA1*
    - 12-25% for *BRCA2*
  - Average age of ovarian cancer onset
    - 50 years for *BRCA1* mutation
    - 60 years for *BRCA2* mutation
    - 63 years in general population
  - Women with very early onset ovarian cancer (< 40 years old) are less likely to harbor *BRCA1/BRCA2* mutations, unlike breast cancer
- **Lynch syndrome**
  - Approximately 2-4% of ovarian cancers are believed to be associated with Lynch syndrome
  - Lifetime risk for ovarian cancer is estimated at 4-11%

OVARIAN CARCINOMA

Key Facts

Clinical Issues

- ~ 1 in 4 women with ovarian cancer has hereditary gene mutation related to cancer development
- **Hereditary breast and ovarian cancer**
  - 13-15% of women with invasive ovarian cancer harbor germline mutations of *BRCA1* or *BRCA2* genes
  - Lifetime risk for ovarian cancer: 35-60% for *BRCA1*, 12-25% for *BRCA2*
- **Lynch syndrome**
  - ~ 2-4% of ovarian cancers are believed to be associated with Lynch syndrome
  - Lifetime risk for ovarian cancer is estimated at 4-11%
- **Peutz-Jeghers syndrome**
  - Estimated 10x increased cancer incidence compared to general population

Microscopic Pathology

- **Hereditary breast and ovarian cancer**
  - Characteristically epithelial tumors
  - Most are high-grade serous carcinomas
  - Borderline tumors and mucinous carcinomas are uncommon
- **Lynch syndrome**
  - Characteristically epithelial invasive tumors
- **Peutz-Jeghers syndrome**
  - Patients are particularly at risk for sex cord-stromal tumors with annular tubules (SCTATs)
  - Up to 35% of women with SCTATs are found to have PJS

  - Mean age at diagnosis of ovarian cancer is 42 years with 1/3 of patients < 40 years old
- **Peutz-Jeghers syndrome**
  - Estimated 10x ↑ cancer incidence compared to general population
  - 1/2 of patients with ovarian tumors present at ≤ 22 years old

Presentation

- **Hereditary breast and ovarian cancer**
  - Patients are at risk for developing ovarian, fallopian tube, and primary peritoneal carcinomas
- **Lynch syndrome**
  - Cancers of gastrointestinal tract, endometrium, ovaries, hepatobiliary, urinary tract, brain, and skin
  - Women with synchronous endometrial and ovarian endometrioid adenocarcinomas are more likely to have Lynch syndrome
- **Peutz-Jeghers syndrome**
  - Hamartomatous gastrointestinal polyps and mucocutaneous pigmentation
  - Increased risk for multiple cancers including colon, pancreas, ovary, cervix, and uterus
  - Ovarian sex cord-stromal tumors may lead to precocious puberty and infertility

Treatment

- **Hereditary breast and ovarian cancer**
  - Risk-reducing bilateral salpingo-oophorectomy (RRSO) in ages 35-40, after childbearing is complete
  - RRSO has been shown to ↓ pelvic cancer risk by 80-95%
  - After RRSO, patients still have estimated 4% risk of primary peritoneal cancer development
  - Oral contraceptives have been shown to reduce ovarian cancer risk by 50% in patients choosing nonsurgical approach
  - *BRCA1/BRCA2*-related ovarian cancers have better response to platinum-based agents compared to nonmutation carriers
  - Increased sensitivity to poly ADP-ribose polymerase (PARP) inhibitors compared to sporadic carcinomas
- **Lynch syndrome**
  - Hysterectomy and bilateral salpingo-oophorectomy recommended after childbearing is complete
- **Peutz-Jeghers syndrome**
  - Tumors arising in PJS setting are treated in same manner as sporadic ovarian tumors of same histologic subtype

Prognosis

- **Hereditary breast and ovarian cancer**
  - *BRCA1/BRCA2*-related ovarian cancers have better prognosis than nonmutation carriers
- **Lynch syndrome and Peutz-Jeghers syndrome**
  - Apparently, there are no prognostic differences between sporadic and hereditary ovarian tumors associated with these syndromes

Surveillance

- **Hereditary breast and ovarian cancer**
  - Transvaginal ultrasound and CA-125 are recommended every 6 months starting at age 30 or 5-10 years before earliest age at onset of ovarian cancer in patient's family
- **Lynch syndrome**
  - No specific recommendations have been outlined for ovarian cancer
- **Peutz-Jeghers syndrome**
  - Annual transvaginal ultrasound starting at age 18-20

MACROSCOPIC FEATURES

Hereditary Breast and Ovarian Cancer

- 2.5-17% of patients undergoing RRSO have occult ovarian, fallopian tube, or peritoneal carcinoma upon pathologic examination
- Extensive sampling of RRSO specimens should be performed including histopathologic examination of entire ovaries and fallopian tubes
- Ovaries should be transversely sectioned in 5 mm intervals along greater axis and all cross sections submitted

OVARIAN CARCINOMA

MICROSCOPIC PATHOLOGY

Histologic Features

- **Hereditary breast and ovarian cancer**
  - Characteristically epithelial tumors
  - Most are high-grade serous carcinomas
  - Solid pseudoendometrioid and transitional patterns, increased mitosis, and tumor-infiltrating lymphocytes may be associated with BRCA-related tumors but data is limited
  - Borderline tumors and mucinous carcinomas are uncommon
  - Ovaries and fallopian tubes should be scrutinized for occult microscopic carcinoma
- **Lynch syndrome**
  - Characteristically epithelial invasive tumors
  - Histologic subtypes include serous, endometrioid, mucinous, and clear cell
  - Higher proportion of endometrioid subtype than nonmutation carriers
- **Peutz-Jeghers syndrome**
  - Patients are particularly at risk for sex cord-stromal tumors with annular tubules (SCTATs)
  - SCTATs in PJS tend to be small, calcified, multifocal, and bilateral
  - Up to 35% of women with SCTATs are found to have PJS
  - Other histologic types have been described in PJS including granulosa cell tumors, Brenner tumors, dysgerminomas, and Sertoli cell tumors

ANCILLARY TESTS

Immunohistochemistry and Molecular Genetics

- **Hereditary breast and ovarian cancer**
  - DNA sequencing for germline mutations in *BRCA1* and *BRCA2* genes
  - Current testing is limited by gene patents to a single company (Myriad Genetics)
  - Commercially available test includes sequencing of all coding exons and exon-intron boundaries as well as testing for common gene rearrangements
  - Current sensitivity for *BRCA1* and *BRCA2* gene analysis is 90%
- **Lynch syndrome**
  - Experience with interpreting testing for somatic alterations by microsatellite instability (MSI) analysis and immunohistochemistry in ovarian cancer is limited compared with colorectal and endometrial cancers
  - Paraffin-embedded tissue can be evaluated for immunohistochemistry for mismatch repair proteins
    - MLH1
    - MSH2
    - MSH6
    - PMS2
  - *MLH1* promoter hypermethylation
  - Germline mutation testing
    - DNA sequencing of *MLH1*, *MSH2*, *MSH6*, and *PMS2*
    - Performed on DNA extracted from peripheral blood lymphocytes
- **Peutz-Jeghers syndrome**
  - Testing for germline alterations of *STK11* gene
  - *STK11* alterations are found in 50-90% of individuals with a clinical diagnosis of PJS
  - Majority of mutations are missense or truncating but up to 30% are large deletions
  - Optimal testing includes both DNA sequencing and analysis for large deletions/duplications
  - Performed on DNA extracted from peripheral blood lymphocytes

DIFFERENTIAL DIAGNOSIS

Hereditary Breast and Ovarian Cancer

- Women with breast and ovarian cancer should undergo genetic counseling and genetic testing for HBOC if indicated

Lynch Syndrome

- Guidelines for identifying LS in women with gynecologic cancers are less defined than for colorectal cancer
- Patients with synchronous endometrioid uterine and ovarian adenocarcinomas are at increased risk for LS and should be screened by immunohistochemistry &/ or MSI analysis

SELECTED REFERENCES

1. Ballinger LL: Hereditary gynecologic cancers: risk assessment, counseling, testing and management. Obstet Gynecol Clin North Am. 39(2):165-81, 2012
2. Pennington KP et al: Hereditary ovarian cancer: beyond the usual suspects. Gynecol Oncol. 124(2):347-53, 2012
3. Soslow RA et al: Morphologic patterns associated with BRCA1 and BRCA2 genotype in ovarian carcinoma. Mod Pathol. 25(4):625-36, 2012
4. Weissman SM et al: Genetic testing by cancer site: ovary. Cancer J. 18(4):320-7, 2012
5. Soliman PT et al: Women with synchronous primary cancers of the endometrium and ovary: do they have Lynch syndrome? J Clin Oncol. 23(36):9344-50, 2005
6. Giardiello FM et al: Very high risk of cancer in familial Peutz-Jeghers syndrome. Gastroenterology. 119(6):1447-53, 2000

Microscopic Features

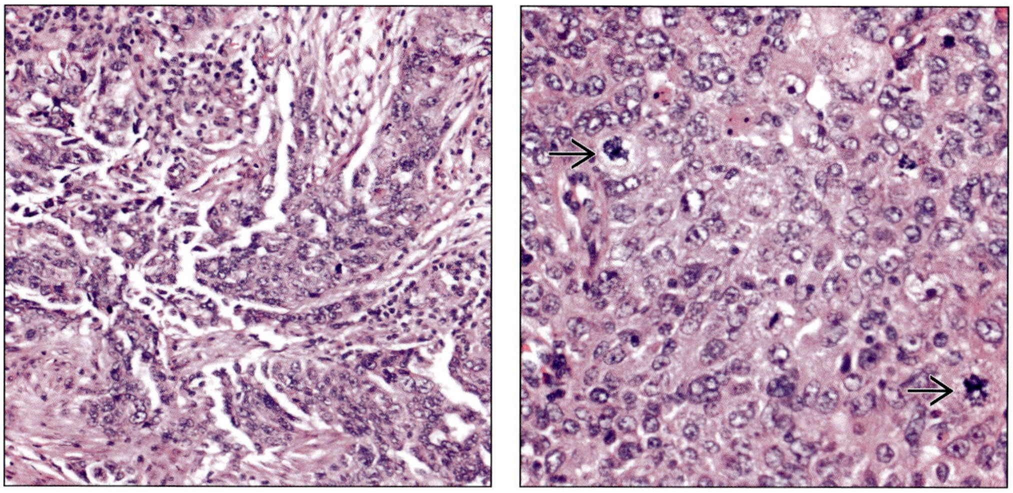

(Left) *Solid pseudoendometrioid and transitional patterns, increased mitosis, and tumor-infiltrating lymphocytes may be associated with BRCA-related tumors. High-grade serous carcinomas are the prototypical ovarian tumors in hereditary breast and ovarian cancer.* ***(Right)*** *Solid areas of high-grade serous carcinoma show marked nuclear pleomorphism with numerous mitotic figures* →.

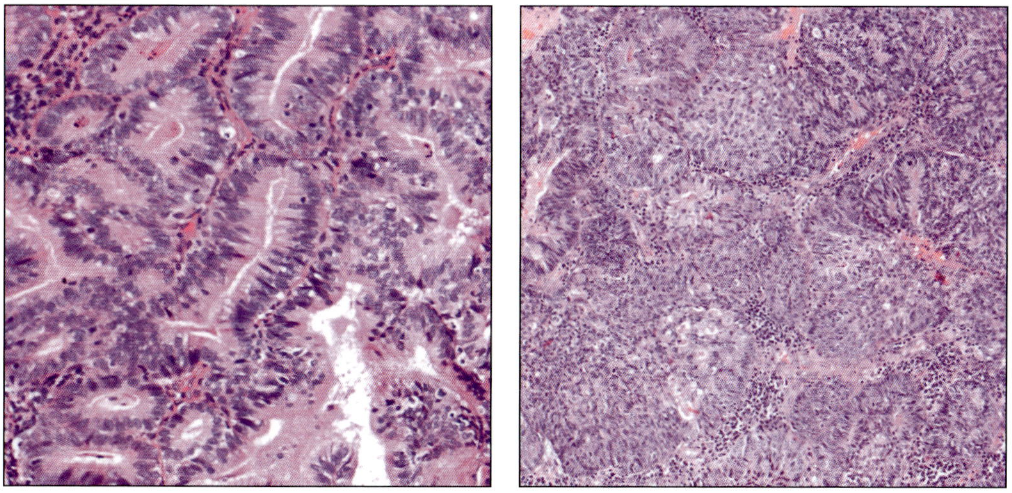

(Left) *Endometrioid adenocarcinoma, FIGO grade 1, is characterized by confluent growth of glands lined by pseudostratified epithelium. Histologic subtypes of tumors that are seen in Lynch syndrome include serous, endometrioid, mucinous, and clear cell.* ***(Right)*** *FIGO grade 2 endometrioid adenocarcinoma is composed of both glandular and solid areas. Ovarian endometrioid adenocarcinomas occur frequently in patients with Lynch syndrome.*

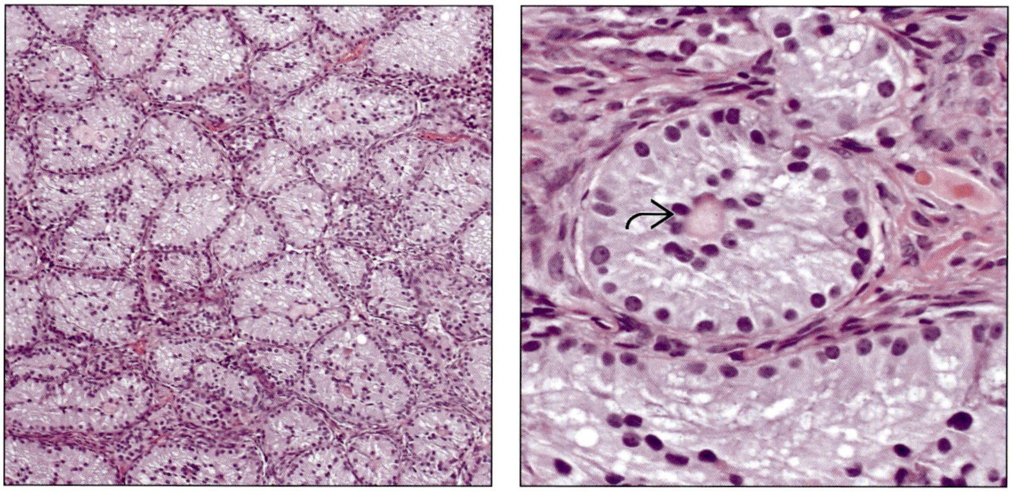

(Left) *Sex cord-stromal tumor with annular tubules (SCTATs) occur in Peutz-Jeghers syndrome. Up to 35% of women with SCTATs are found to have Peutz-Jeghers syndrome.* ***(Right)*** *Sex cord-stromal tumor with annular tubules consist of pale Sertoli cells arranged around hyaline bodies* ↷. *SCTATs in Peutz-Jeghers syndrome tend to be small, calcified, multifocal, and bilateral.*

Nervous System

ASTROCYTOMA

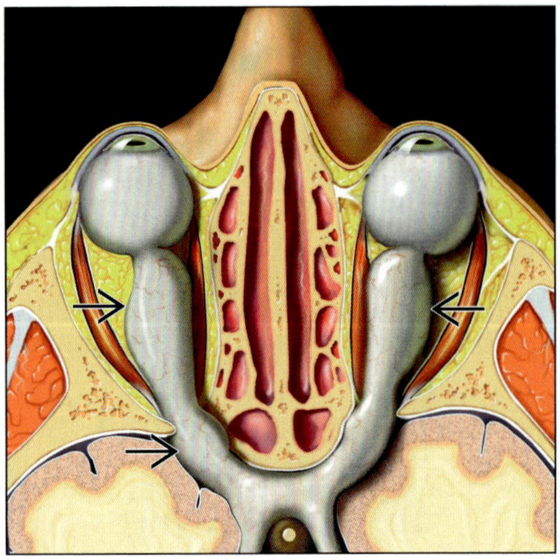

Optic nerve gliomas are characterized by fusiform expansions of the optic nerve. When bilateral &/or multiple ⇒, they are essentially pathognomonic for neurofibromatosis (NF1) syndrome.

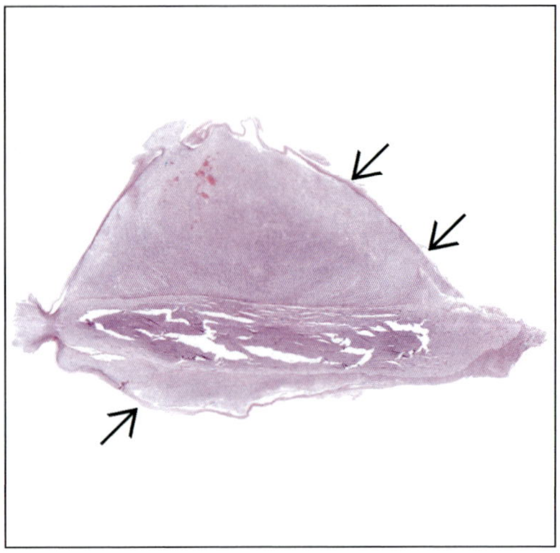

Almost all optic nerve gliomas in NF1 patients are pilocytic astrocytomas. The tumors involve the substance of the optic nerve proper, but also frequently extend into the leptomeninges ⇒.

TERMINOLOGY

Abbreviations

- Neurofibromatosis type 1 (NF1)
- Tuberous sclerosis complex (TSC)
- Subependymal giant cell astrocytoma (SEGA)

Definitions

- Astrocytomas represent primary CNS neoplasms demonstrating a phenotype similar to astrocytic glia

ETIOLOGY/PATHOGENESIS

Neurofibromatosis Type 1

- Results from germline inactivation of *NF1* gene encoding for neurofibromin
- Pilocytic astrocytoma most frequent primary CNS tumor arising in neurofibromatosis type 1
- Diffuse gliomas grades II-IV may also develop, particularly after childhood years
- Subset of astrocytomas, particularly low grade, remain difficult to precisely classify using current WHO guidelines

Neurofibromatosis Type 2

- Results from germline inactivation of *NF2* gene encoding for merlin
- Main glioma in NF2 is ependymoma, but astrocytomas may also rarely develop

Noonan Syndrome

- Combines facial features and cardiac abnormalities; associated with mutations in genes encoding for components of RAS signaling pathway
  - Mutation in *PTPN11* most frequent (50%) but also caused by mutations in *KRAS*, *SOS1*, *RAF1*, and *NF1*
- May develop low-grade astrocytomas and glioneuronal tumors

Turcot Syndrome

- Defined as concomitant brain tumors in setting of familial colon cancer
- Germline heterozygous mutations in mismatch repair genes (*MLH1, MSH2, MSH6, PMS1, PMS2*) associated with Turcot syndrome and glioma development (Turcot type 1)
- Germline mutations in *APC* associated with medulloblastoma/PNET (Turcot type 2)

Constitutional Mismatch Repair-Deficiency Syndrome

- Homozygous or compound heterozygous mutations in mismatch repair genes
- Multiple cancers, including gliomas, colon cancer
- May be associated with clinical features of NF1 (e.g., café au lait spots)

Li-Fraumeni Syndrome

- Associated with germline *TP53* mutations
- Multiple cancers, including sarcomas, breast cancer, leukemias, adrenocortical carcinomas, choroid plexus tumors, and gliomas

Tuberous Sclerosis Complex

- Results from germline mutations in *TSC1* or *TSC2* genes
- Subependymal giant cell astrocytoma (SEGA) is a low-grade astrocytoma that develops almost exclusively in TSC

Melanoma Astrocytoma Syndrome

- Associated with germline mutations of chromosome region 9p21 (involving the *CDKN2A* gene or the *P14* (*ARF*) specific exon 1-β)
- Cutaneous melanoma and high-grade astrocytomas (glioblastomas) in family members

ASTROCYTOMA

Key Facts

Terminology

- Astrocytomas represent primary CNS neoplasms demonstrating a phenotype similar to astrocytic glia

Microscopic Pathology

- Pilocytic astrocytoma (WHO grade I)
  - Classic biphasic pattern with alternating compact ("piloid") and loose (microcyst-rich) areas
  - When affecting optic nerve, involves substance of nerve and extends into subarachnoid space
- Subependymal giant cell astrocytoma (SEGA) (WHO grade I)
  - Large eosinophilic cells with macronucleoli
- Low-grade astrocytomas, subtype indeterminate
  - Subset of NF1 gliomas difficult to classify; may have features of both pilocytic and diffuse astrocytomas
- Diffuse astrocytoma (WHO grade II)
  - Hypercellularity and atypia when compared to nonneoplastic brain
- Anaplastic astrocytoma (WHO grade III)
  - Increased cellularity compared to grade II and evident mitotic activity
- Glioblastoma (WHO grade IV)
  - Infiltrating astrocytoma with mitotic activity + necrosis &/or microvascular proliferation

Ancillary Tests

- GFAP(+), OLIG2(+), S100(+)
- NFP stains entrapped axons in diffuse astrocytomas; pilocytic astrocytomas more circumscribed
- Expression of neuronal markers (synaptophysin, neurofilament protein) frequent in SEGA
- Ki-67 labeling index generally increases with grade

CLINICAL ISSUES

Presentation

- Gradual visual loss main symptom in NF1 patients with optic nerve gliomas
- Seizures may be initial presentation in cortically based tumors
- Signs of increased intracranial pressure (headaches, nausea/vomiting) in posterior fossa or intraventricular tumors (e.g., SEGA)

Treatment

- Optic nerve gliomas (pilocytic astrocytomas) in NF1 children are usually observed without treatment
- Diffuse astrocytomas in NF1 may require additional treatment, although irradiation is avoided as much as possible
- High-grade astrocytomas (WHO grades III-IV) require treatment after surgery, usually irradiation + chemotherapy
- SEGAs in TSC respond to mTOR pathway inhibitors

Prognosis

- Prognosis of astrocytic neoplasms depends strongly on grade (WHO grades I-IV) and molecular alterations
- Pilocytic astrocytomas in NF1 may behave in a favorable fashion, particularly when involving optic pathways
  - May stabilize or even regress in absence of treatment
  - Pilocytic astrocytomas with anaplasia demonstrate variable outcome
    - Aggressive behavior in a subset of cases, although not as predictably poor as infiltrating high-grade astrocytomas
- High-grade astrocytomas in NF1 associated with poor outcome similar to sporadic tumors
- High-grade astrocytomas in Turcot may have a better outcome compared to sporadic tumors

IMAGE FINDINGS

MR Findings

- Pilocytic astrocytoma
  - Well demarcated, contrast enhancement, often cyst with enhancing mural nodule configuration
  - Predilection for optic nerve/pathways in young NF1 patients
  - Fusiform expansion of optic nerve
  - Bilateral optic nerve glioma almost pathognomonic for NF1
  - May also arise in brainstem, cerebellum, cerebral hemispheres, and spinal cord
- Diffusely infiltrating astrocytomas
  - Occur throughout neural axis in sporadic and syndrome associated settings
  - Diffuse astrocytomas (WHO grade II) form ill-defined, T2-hyperintense masses lacking contrast enhancement
  - Anaplastic astrocytomas may show variable contrast enhancement
  - Glioblastomas almost always enhance, and may show ring enhancement reflecting central necrosis
- SEGA
  - Arises in lateral ventricles near foramen of Monro
  - Additional CNS manifestations of tuberous sclerosis, e.g., subependymal nodules, cortical tubers, may be present
  - Presence of contrast enhancement and size distinguishes it from subependymal nodules

MICROSCOPIC PATHOLOGY

Histologic Features

- Pilocytic astrocytoma (WHO grade I)
  - Classic biphasic pattern with alternating compact ("piloid") and loose (microcyst-rich) areas
  - Rosenthal fibers and eosinophilic granular bodies characteristic

ASTROCYTOMA

- May contain hyalinized &/or glomeruloid microvasculature
- Mitotic activity rare to absent
- When affecting optic nerve, involves substance of nerve and extends into subarachnoid space
- Pilomyxoid variant, characterized by monomorphous cells, myxoid background, and perivascular pseudorosettes, is associated with more aggressive clinical behavior

- Pilocytic astrocytoma with anaplastic features
  - Previously defined as pilocytic astrocytomas with brisk mitotic activity (≥ 4-5/10 HPF), hypercellularity, and atypia ± necrosis
  - No WHO grade assignment yet
  - Associated NF1 syndrome in 24%
- SEGA (WHO grade I)
  - Large eosinophilic cells with macronucleoli
  - Vague fascicular formation, occasional perivascular pseudorosettes and microcalcifications
  - Frequent mast cells
  - Mitotic figures and necrosis rare to absent
- Pleomorphic xanthoastrocytoma (WHO grade II)
  - Circumscribed astrocytoma containing pleomorphic cells, xanthic change, fascicular architecture, and eosinophilic granular bodies
  - Rare reports in NF1 patients, including curious occurrence in 2 NF1 siblings
- Low-grade astrocytoma, subtype indeterminate
  - Subset of NF1-associated astrocytoma remains difficult to classify
  - May have features of both pilocytic and diffuse astrocytomas
  - A subset demonstrates increased cytoplasmic size and macronucleoli
    - May demonstrate partial neuronal differentiation by immunohistochemistry &/or electron microscopy
- Glioneuronal tumors
  - Dysembryoplastic neuroepithelial tumor (DNT)
    - Cortical-based, multinodular, usually sporadic low-grade neoplasm strongly associated with chronic seizures
    - Bland, round oligodendroglial-like cells, specific glioneuronal element between nodules
    - Microcysts, "floating" neurons in mucin pools
    - Occasionally occurs in NF1 patients
  - Ganglioglioma
    - Biphasic neoplasm with neoplastic glial and neuronal components
    - Neoplastic ganglion cells with atypia, binucleation
    - Glial component may be pilocytic or diffuse
  - Rosette forming glioneuronal tumor
    - Characterized by a component of small, uniform neurocytes and distinctive small, synaptophysin-positive neurocytic rosettes
    - Variable glial component resembling pilocytic astrocytoma
    - DNT-like areas may be present
    - Predilection for the 4th ventricle
    - Most often sporadic but reported in NF1 and Noonan patients
- Diffuse astrocytoma (WHO grade II)
  - Hypercellularity and atypia when compared to nonneoplastic brain
  - Underlying axons &/or neurons evident on H&E or highlighted by immunohistochemistry
  - Absent to very rare mitotic activity
- Anaplastic astrocytoma (WHO grade III)
  - Increased cellularity compared to grade II and evident mitotic activity
- Glioblastoma (WHO grade IV)
  - Infiltrating astrocytoma with mitotic activity + necrosis &/or microvascular proliferation
  - Presence of a sarcomatous component (i.e., gliosarcoma) previously described in NF1 and Turcot syndrome
  - Component of bizarre multinucleated giant cells described in several cases of Turcot syndrome
  - Other variants reported in NF1 include giant cell and adenoid

ANCILLARY TESTS

Immunohistochemistry

- GFAP(+), OLIG2(+), S100(+)
- Neurofilament protein highlights entrapped axons in diffusely infiltrating astrocytomas; pilocytic astrocytomas are more circumscribed
- Strong nuclear p53 immunostaining frequent in diffuse astrocytomas
- Mutant IDH-1 (R132H) protein usually absent in NF1-associated infiltrating gliomas compared with sporadic counterparts
- Expression of neuronal markers (synaptophysin, neurofilament protein) frequent in SEGA
- Ki-67 labeling index generally increases with grade
- Markers of mTOR pathway activation frequently immunopositive in SEGA as well as NF1-associated pilocytic and indeterminate astrocytomas

In Situ Hybridization

- *BRAF* duplications present in majority of sporadic pilocytic astrocytomas, but only rarely in NF1-associated cases
- *CDKN2A* and 10q deletions, as well as *NF1* inactivation frequent in NF1-associated high-grade astrocytomas

Molecular Genetics

- Homozygous *NF1* gene inactivation is a feature of NF1-associated neoplasms including gliomas
  - Leads to RAS and mTOR pathway activation
  - Partial (heterozygous) *NF1* loss in nonneoplastic stromal and hematopoietic cells (e.g., microglia) required for optic glioma development in model systems
- *CDKN2A* homozygous deletions (~ 50%) and *TP53* mutations (~ 35%) represent important somatic genetic events in sporadic glioblastoma
- *NF1* gene point mutations/deletions also occur in a subset (< 20%) of sporadic primary glioblastoma
- Astrocytomas developing in Li-Fraumeni patients with germine *TP53* mutations may develop secondary *IDH1* mutation (R132C rather than R132H)

Gene Expression Profiling

- Gene expression profiles separate NF1-associated and sporadic pilocytic astrocytomas despite histologic similarities
- Gene expression profiles of SEGA include up-regulation of genes involved in tumorigenesis and downregulation of developmental genes, probably mediated by increased mTOR activity

DIFFERENTIAL DIAGNOSIS

Gliosis

- Piloid gliosis is main nonneoplastic entity in differential diagnosis with pilocytic astrocytoma
  - Lacks biphasic architecture, microcysts, and eosinophilic granular bodies
  - Seen around slow-growing tumors in hypothalamic region, posterior fossa, and spinal cord
  - Also a feature of spinal cord cavities (syrinx)
- Glial hyperplasia variably occurs in association with NF1
  - Glial clusters and perineuronal satellitosis described as nonneoplastic features of NF1 brains
  - Lacks hypercellularity, proliferation, and atypia of infiltrating glioma
  - Immunohistochemical stains (p53, Ki-67) may be helpful in distinction

Malignant Peripheral Nerve Sheath Tumor (MPNST)/Sarcoma

- Associated malignancies in NF1 (MPNST and sarcoma) and Li-Fraumeni (sarcoma)
- May involve CNS by direct extension from intracranial primaries or metastases from distant sites
- Difficult to differentiate from gliosarcoma with a predominant sarcomatous component
- Identification of a malignant, GFAP(+), reticulin-poor glial component required for diagnosis of gliosarcoma

Metastatic Carcinoma

- Must be considered, particularly in Turcot syndrome
- Cytokeratin (CAM5.2) positive, GFAP negative

Metastatic Melanoma

- May be difficult to distinguish from high-grade glioma
- Expression of specific melanocytic markers (e.g., Melan-A, HMB-45, tyrosinase) in addition to S100; GFAP negative

DIAGNOSTIC CHECKLIST

Clinically Relevant Pathologic Features

- Gliomas of optic nerve in NF1 patients are almost always pilocytic astrocytomas
- NF1 patients may also develop unclassifiable and higher grade gliomas, particularly after the childhood years

Pathologic Interpretation Pearls

- Think of SEGA and TSC when large cells with ample cytoplasm and macronucleoli are encountered in a mass from the lateral ventricle

SELECTED REFERENCES

1. Neal MT et al: Pleomorphic xanthoastrocytoma in two siblings with neurofibromatosis type 1 (NF-1). Clin Neuropathol. 31(1):54-6, 2012
2. Karafin M et al: Rosette forming glioneuronal tumor in association with Noonan syndrome: pathobiological implications. Clin Neuropathol. 30(6):297-300, 2011
3. Jentoft M et al: Phenotypic variations in NF1-associated low grade astrocytomas: possible role for increased mTOR activation in a subset. Int J Clin Exp Pathol. 4(1):43-57, 2010
4. Kyritsis AP et al: Inherited predisposition to glioma. Neuro Oncol. 12(1):104-13, 2010
5. Lusis EA et al: Glioblastomas with giant cell and sarcomatous features in patients with Turcot syndrome type 1: a clinicopathological study of 3 cases. Neurosurgery. 67(3):811-7; discussion 817, 2010
6. Rodriguez FJ et al: Anaplasia in pilocytic astrocytoma predicts aggressive behavior. Am J Surg Pathol. 34(2):147-60, 2010
7. Tyburczy ME et al: Novel proteins regulated by mTOR in subependymal giant cell astrocytomas of patients with tuberous sclerosis complex and new therapeutic implications. Am J Pathol. 176(4):1878-90, 2010
8. Reuss D et al: Hereditary tumor syndromes and gliomas. Recent Results Cancer Res. 171:83-102, 2009
9. Watanabe T et al: Selective acquisition of IDH1 R132C mutations in astrocytomas associated with Li-Fraumeni syndrome. Acta Neuropathol. 117(6):653-6, 2009
10. Rodriguez FJ et al: Gliomas in neurofibromatosis type 1: a clinicopathologic study of 100 patients. J Neuropathol Exp Neurol. 67(3):240-9, 2008
11. Wimmer K et al: Constitutional mismatch repair-deficiency syndrome: have we so far seen only the tip of an iceberg? Hum Genet. 124(2):105-22, 2008
12. Yokota O et al: Glial clusters and perineuronal glial satellitosis in the basal ganglia of neurofibromatosis type 1. Acta Neuropathol. 116(1):57-66, 2008
13. Poley JW et al: Biallelic germline mutations of mismatch-repair genes: a possible cause for multiple pediatric malignancies. Cancer. 109(11):2349-56, 2007
14. Gutmann DH et al: Molecular analysis of astrocytomas presenting after age 10 in individuals with NF1. Neurology. 61(10):1397-400, 2003
15. Kluwe L et al: Loss of NF1 alleles distinguish sporadic from NF1-associated pilocytic astrocytomas. J Neuropathol Exp Neurol. 60(9):917-20, 2001
16. Tachibana I et al: Investigation of germline PTEN, p53, p16(INK4A)/p14(ARF), and CDK4 alterations in familial glioma. Am J Med Genet. 92(2):136-41, 2000
17. Kleihues P et al: Tumors associated with p53 germline mutations: a synopsis of 91 families. Am J Pathol. 150(1):1-13, 1997
18. Lopes MB et al: Immunohistochemical characterization of subependymal giant cell astrocytomas. Acta Neuropathol. 91(4):368-75, 1996

ASTROCYTOMA

Low-Grade Astrocytomas

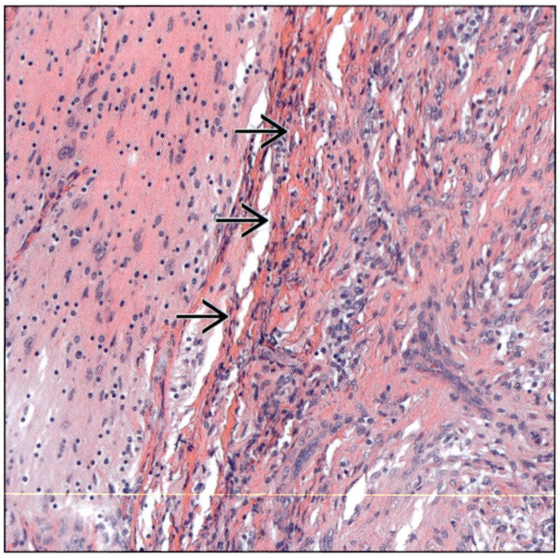
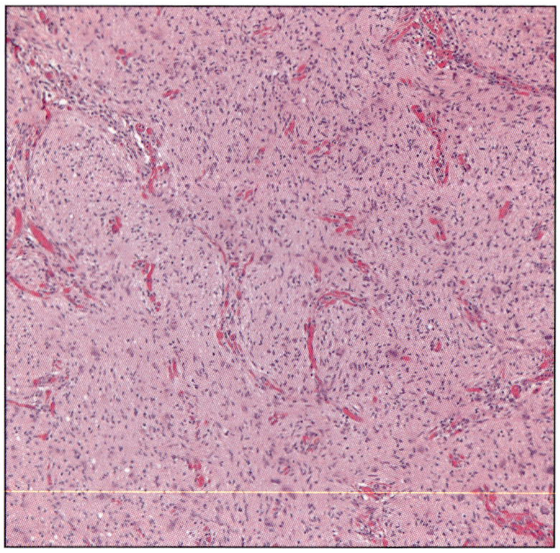

(Left) *Pilocytic astrocytomas of the optic nerve frequently extend into the leptomeninges →, although this finding should not be interpreted as reflecting more aggressive biology.* ***(Right)*** *Pilocytic astrocytomas of the optic nerve may demonstrate infiltrative behavior, which is identifiable in cross sections as increased cellularity of optic nerve fascicles. As in other anatomic sites, infiltration in pilocytic astrocytoma is not necessarily associated with more aggressive behavior.*

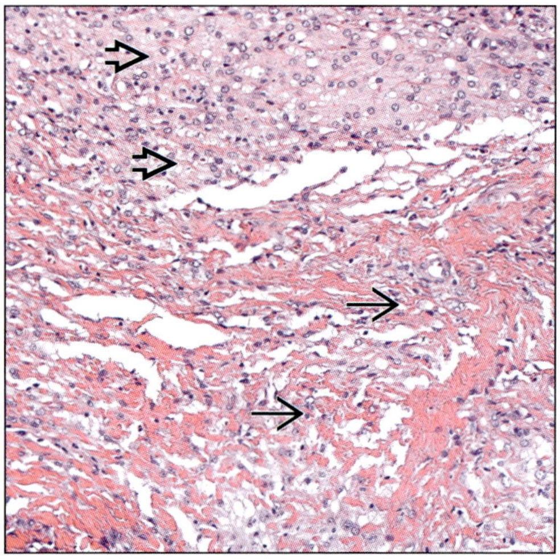
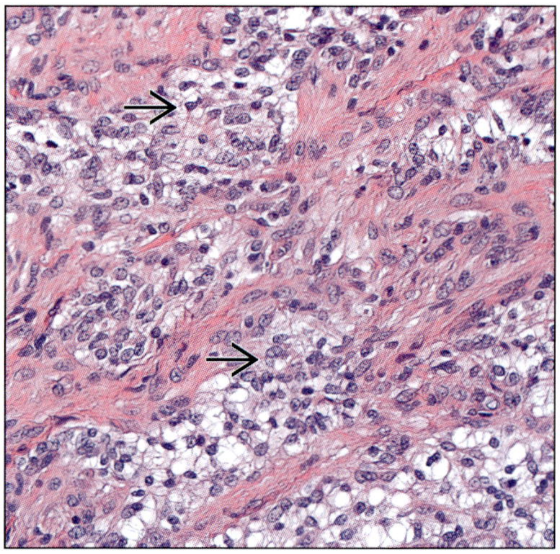

(Left) *Optic nerve gliomas in NF1 patients may be hypercellular ⇨, and on occasion may be associated with underlying, reactive meningothelial hyperplasia →. It is important to not mistake the latter for meningioma in small, nonrepresentative biopsies.* ***(Right)*** *Hypercellular pilocytic astrocytoma of the optic nerve forms bland, ill-formed nests →. Despite the increase in cellularity, almost no mitotic activity was present in this relatively large specimen.*

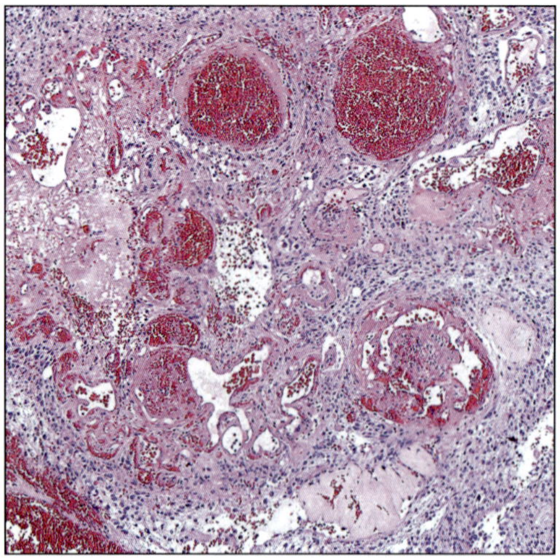
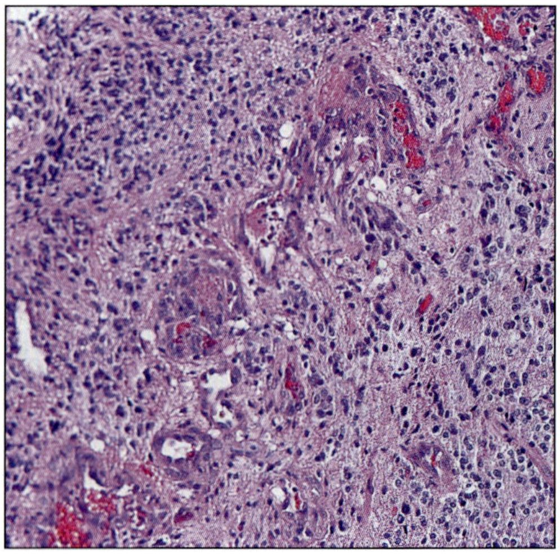

(Left) *NF1-associated pilocytic astrocytomas have similar histologic features as their sporadic counterparts, including frequent enlarged vessels with degenerative changes (e.g., mural hyalinization).* ***(Right)*** *Microvascular glomeruloid changes are often encountered in pilocytic astrocytomas. They are still compatible with WHO grade I CNS neoplasms despite their similarity to the florid microvascular proliferation typical of high-grade gliomas, particularly glioblastoma.*

Low-Grade Astrocytomas

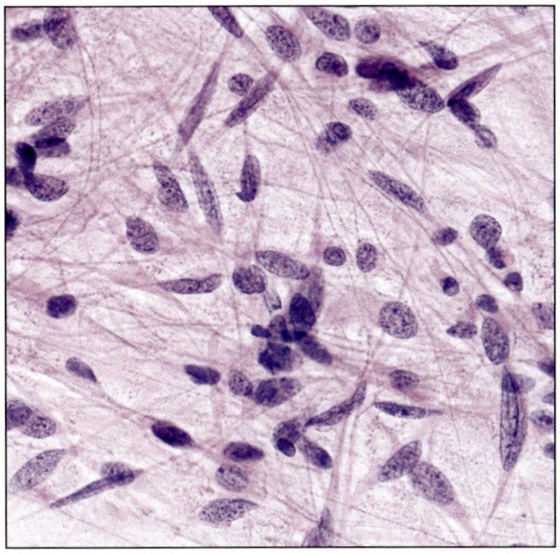

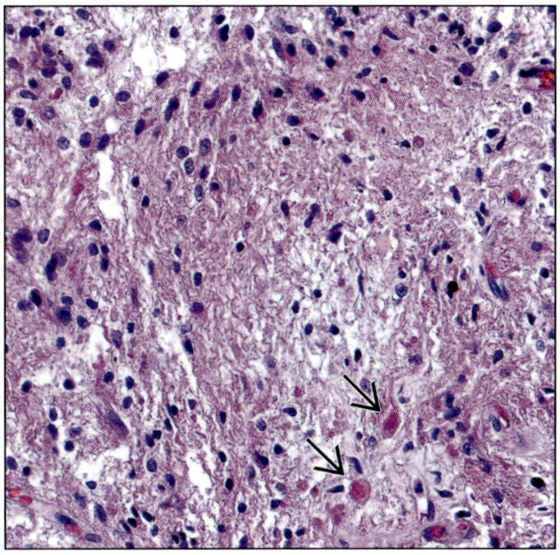

(Left) *The cytologic features of pilocytic astrocytomas are best appreciated in smear preparations, which include bright, bipolar eosinophilic processes and delicate oval nuclei.* ***(Right)*** *The most characteristic architectural feature of NF1-associated or sporadic pilocytic astrocytoma is the compact piloid areas where Rosenthal fibers ➔ are relatively easy to find. The main differential diagnosis is with piloid gliosis, which may develop around a variety of slow-growing neoplasms.*

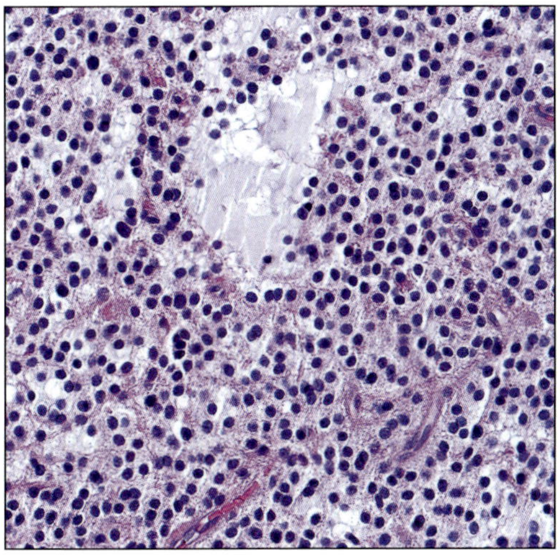

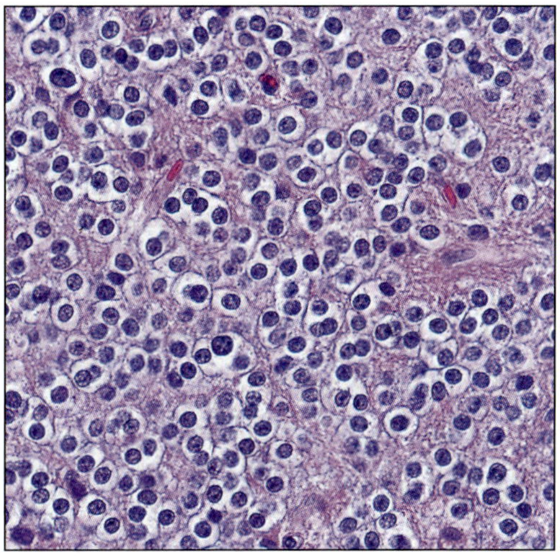

(Left) *Loose-textured areas rich in microcysts represent the other component of pilocytic astrocytomas.* ***(Right)*** *Monotonous, oligodendroglioma-like cells are a conspicuous feature of this cerebellar NF1-associated pilocytic astrocytoma. Oligodendroglioma-like areas often occur in pilocytic astrocytomas. Clues to the correct diagnosis in this case included the presence of focal piloid architecture elsewhere, cerebellar location, and characteristic imaging findings.*

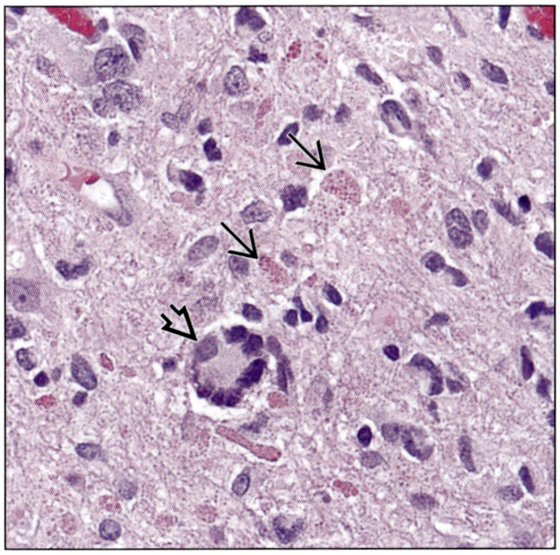

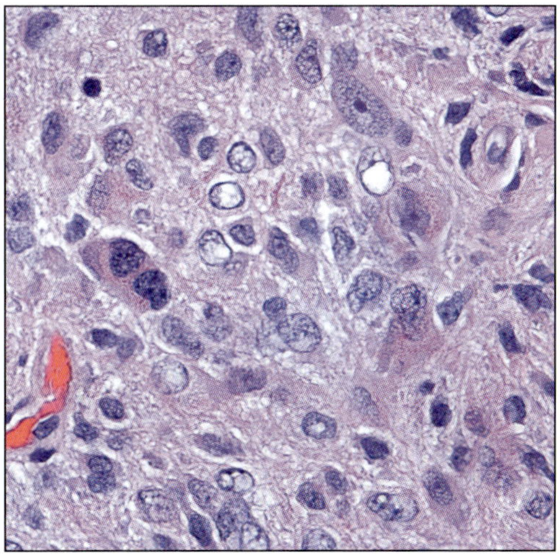

(Left) *Eosinophilic granular bodies (EGBs) ➔ are also frequent, but not specific, acellular components of pilocytic astrocytoma. EGBs are typical of circumscribed, low-grade glial or glioneuronal neoplasms and are almost never encountered in diffuse gliomas. Multinucleated giant cells ➲ are also often present in pilocytic astrocytomas.* ***(Right)*** *Some NF1-associated pilocytic astrocytomas may contain hypercellular pleomorphic areas and rare mitoses.*

Low-Grade Astrocytomas

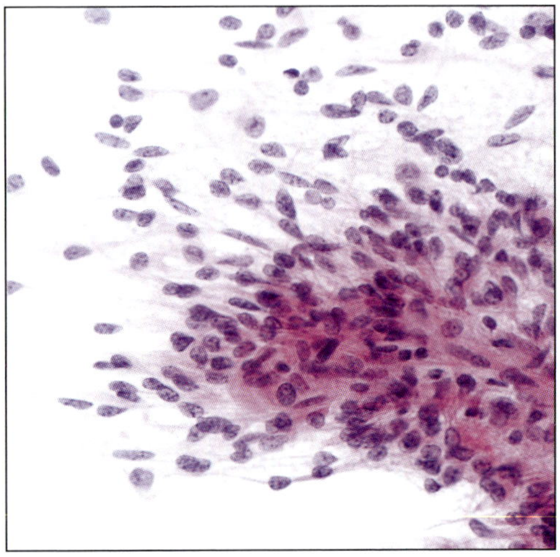

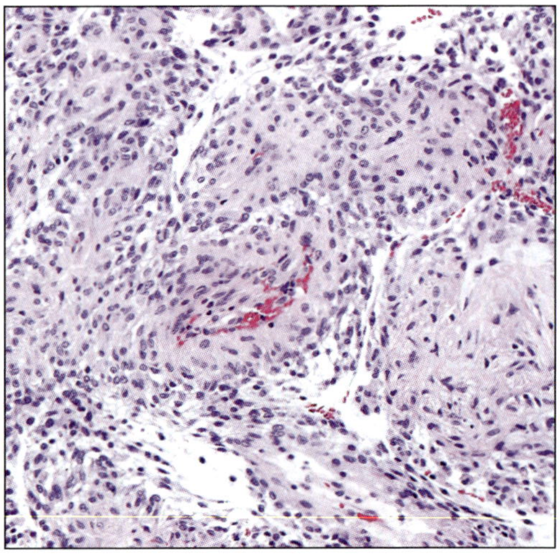

(Left) *The whole spectrum of pilocytic astrocytoma variants may occur in NF1 patients, including the WHO grade II pilomyxoid variant. In cytologic preparations, these tumors contain oval, monotonous cells in tight association with intratumoral vessels.* ***(Right)*** *Compared to conventional pilocytic astrocytomas, the pilomyxoid variant exhibits more monotonous cytologic and architectural features. A myxoid stroma and perivascular arrangement of cells are typical. EGBs are rare to absent.*

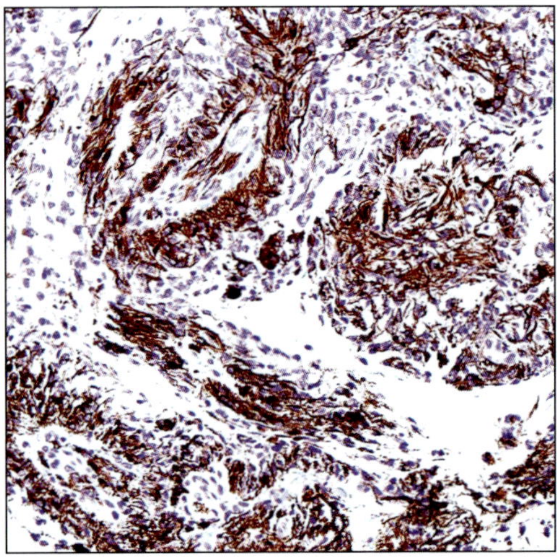

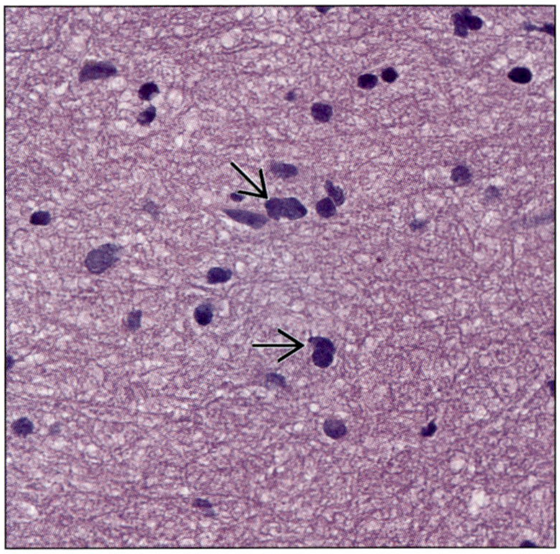

(Left) *GFAP expression is a feature of all pilocytic astrocytomas. In the pilomyxoid astrocytoma variant, it particularly stains around vessels, highlighting the characteristic perivascular processes.* ***(Right)*** *NF1 patients may develop other astrocytomas, including diffuse astrocytoma (grade II). These tumors contain hyperchromatic, "naked" nuclei with irregular nuclei membranes ➔ infiltrating underlying CNS parenchyma.*

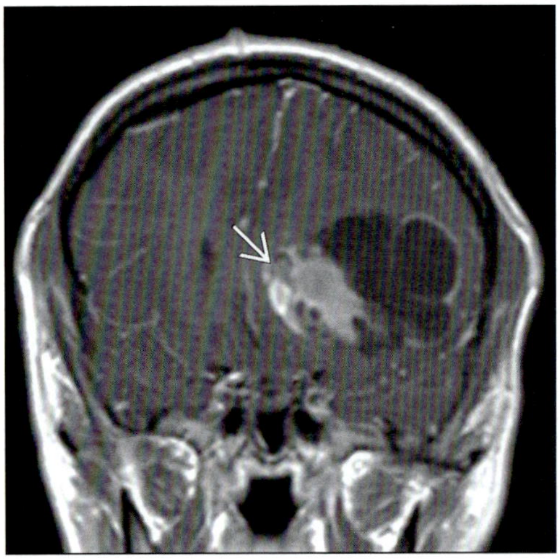

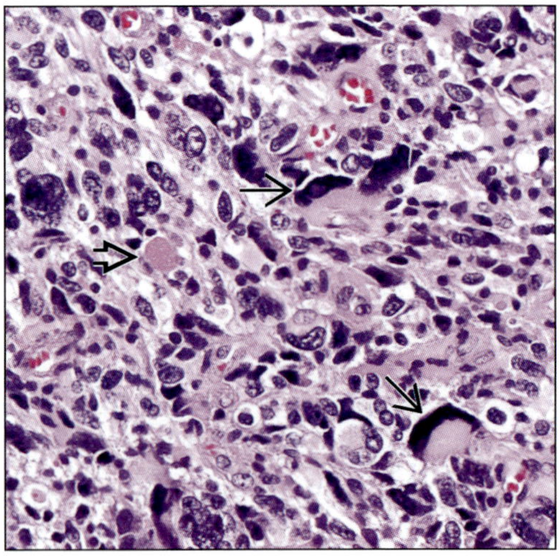

(Left) *Post-contrast MR T1-weighted image shows a cyst with an enhancing mural nodule ➔ in an NF1 patient. Histologically, this tumor was a pleomorphic xanthoastrocytoma, a glioma subtype that may develop in NF1 patients on rare occasions.* ***(Right)*** *This NF1-associated plemorphic xanthoastrocytoma contains large pleomorphic cells ➔ and scattered eosinophilic granular bodies ⇨, hallmarks of this glioma subtype.*

Low-Grade Astrocytomas, Indeterminate

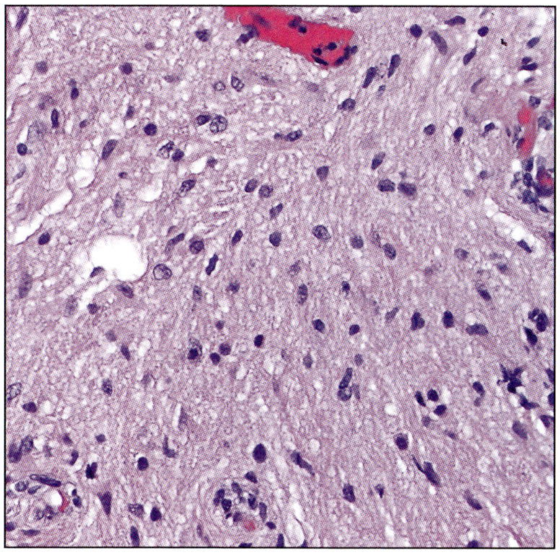

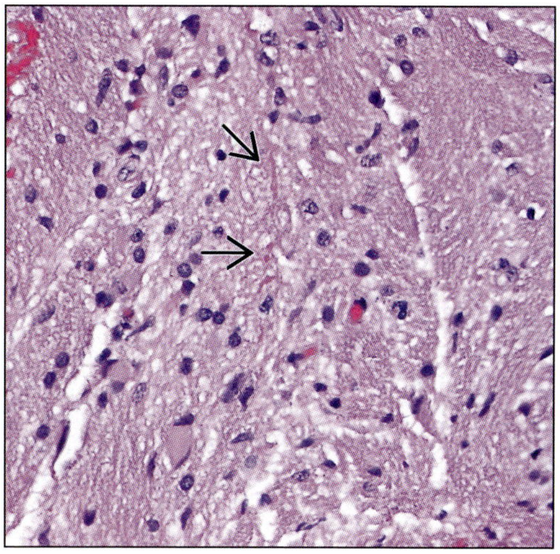

(Left) *Although most low-grade astrocytomas in NF1 patients are pilocytic, a subset represent classification challenges. In this example, there is tissue infiltration, but also cytoplasmic eosinophilia and focal compact architecture elsewhere.* ***(Right)*** *In this NF1-associated low-grade astrocytoma, there is conspicuous parenchymal infiltration. However, bright eosinophilic cytoplasmic processes raise at least the possibility of pilocytic astrocytoma ⇒. Rosenthal fibers are absent.*

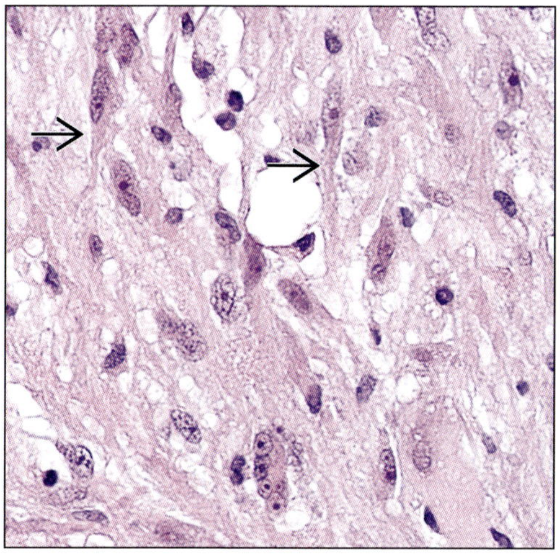

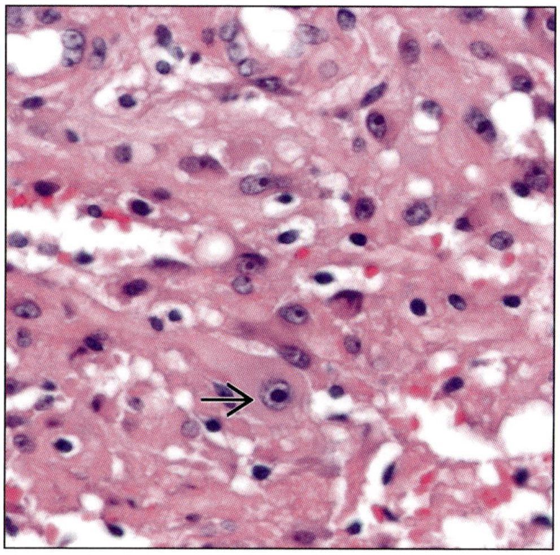

(Left) *Some low-grade astrocytomas in NF1 patients demonstrate architectural features of pilocytic astrocytoma, but additionally may show unusual cytologic features, including plump cytoplasmic processes ⇒ and macronucleoli.* ***(Right)*** *Conspicuous macronucleoli ⇒ represent an eye-catching feature of some NF1-associated low-grade astrocytomas. Although they may be reminiscent of ganglion cells, the eosinophilic cytoplasm and cell processes suggest glial differentiation.*

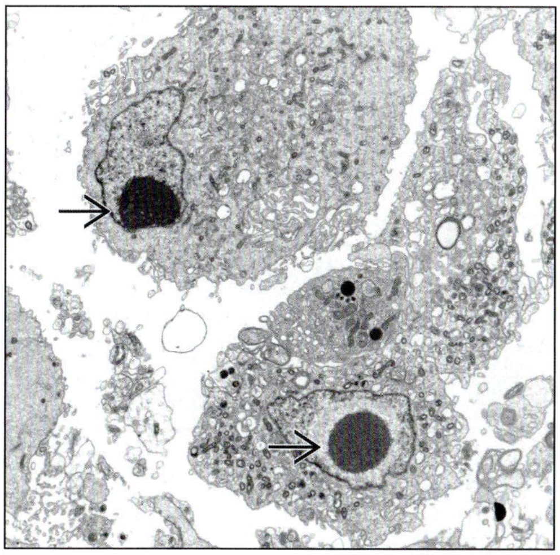

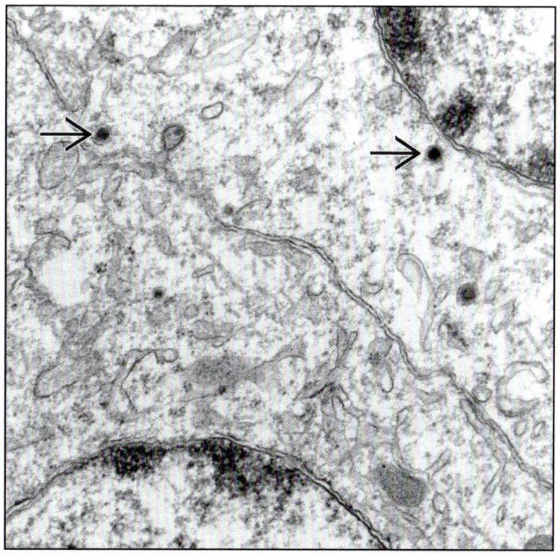

(Left) *Macronucleoli represent a remarkable ultrastructural feature ⇒ of this low-grade indeterminate astrocytoma from a NF1 patient.* ***(Right)*** *A subset of low-grade NF1-associated astrocytomas in addition to immunohistochemical and ultrastructural features of glial differentiation may contain neurosecretory granules ⇒, as well as other ultrastructural evidence of neuronal differentiation.*

Pilocytic Astrocytoma With Anaplasia

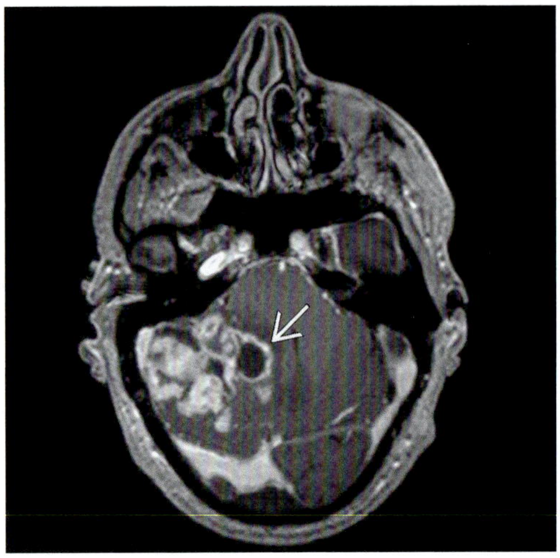

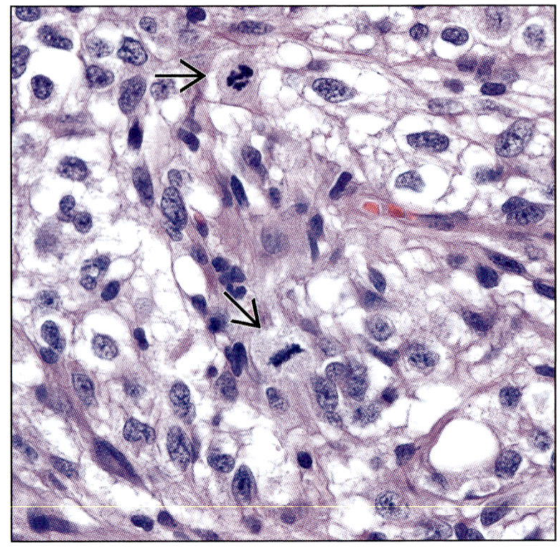

***(Left)** A small subset of pilocytic astrocytomas, including those originating in NF1 patients, may develop clinical &/or histologic malignant/anaplastic features. In this cerebellar pilocytic astrocytoma, a more ominous biology is anticipated by large size, rapid progression, multinodularity, and heterogeneous enhancement* ➡*. **(Right)** Brisk mitotic activity present throughout the specimen* → *is the main histologic feature of pilocytic astrocytomas that develop anaplastic features.*

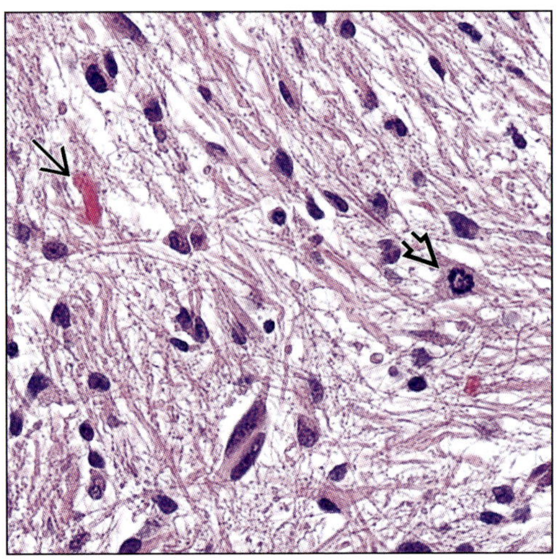

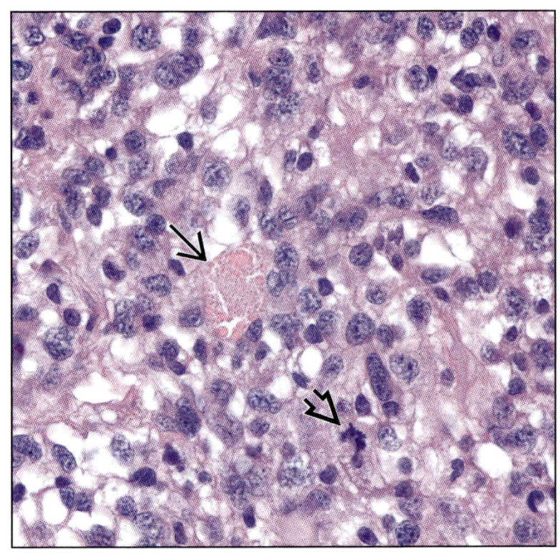

***(Left)** By definition, pilocytic astrocytomas with anaplasia must contain recognizable morphologic attributes of pilocytic astrocytoma, e.g., piloid cytoplasmic processes and Rosenthal fibers* →*. Anaplastic features are ascribed by the presence of concurrent brisk mitotic activity* ⇨*. **(Right)** In this NF1-associated pilocytic astrocytoma with anaplastic features, there are concurrent features of pilocytic astrocytoma (granular bodies* →*) and anaplasia (frequent mitoses* ⇨*).*

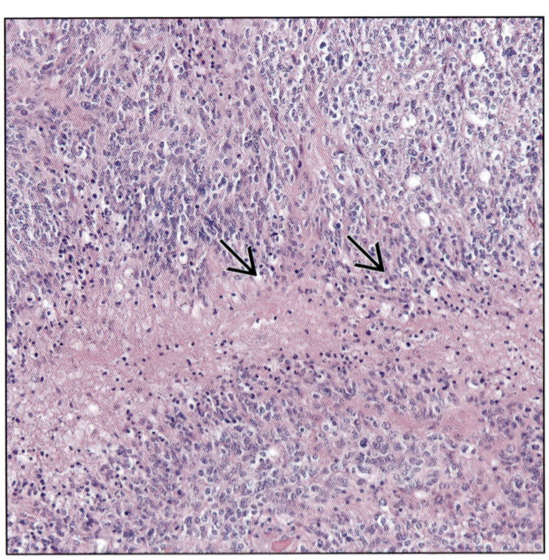

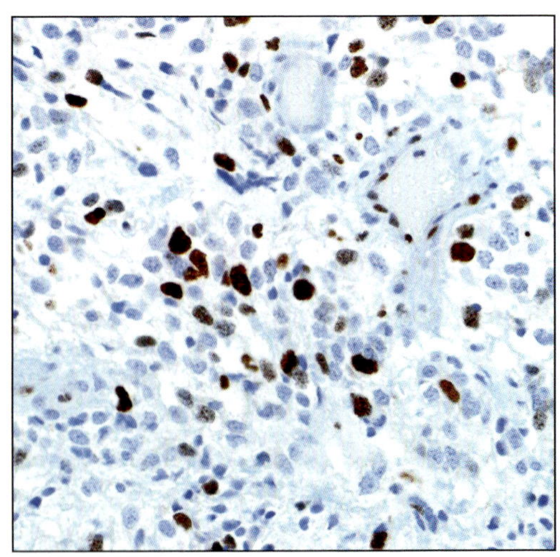

***(Left)** A subset of pilocytic astrocytomas with anaplasia contain areas of necrosis, including pseudopalisading* →*. The presence of necrosis in addition to brisk mitotic activity is associated with a greater potential for aggressive behavior in these tumors. **(Right)** An elevated Ki-67 labeling index in pilocytic astrocytomas with anaplasia confirms the proliferative activity that is characteristic of these tumors, whether sporadic or NF1 associated.*

Glioneuronal Tumors

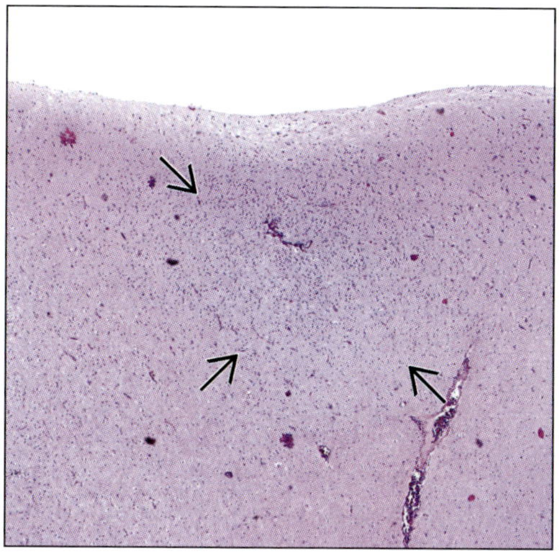

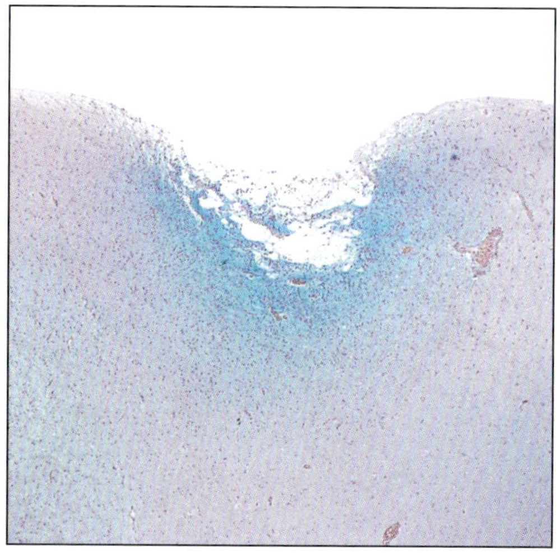

(Left) *Low-grade glioneuronal tumors also develop in NF1 patients, albeit at a lower frequency. Diagnosis of dysembryoplastic neuroepithelial tumor (DNT) was made in this example based on bland, intracortical nodules →. Intact specimens that preserve the lesion's architecture are optimal.* ***(Right)*** *Intracortical nodules of dysembryoplastic neuroepithelial tumor are acid mucopolysaccharide rich and are particularly highlighted by the Alcian blue special stain.*

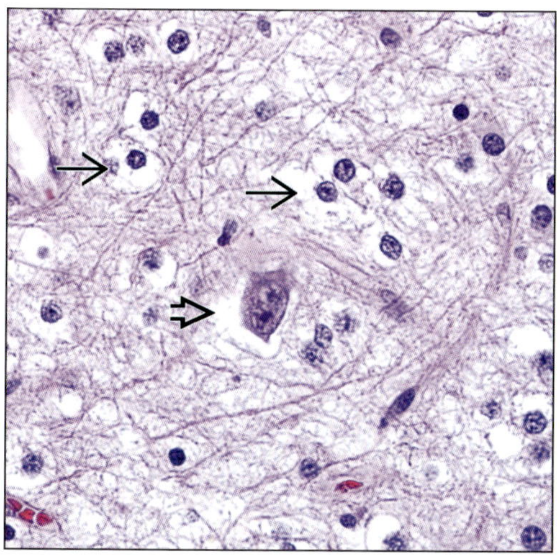

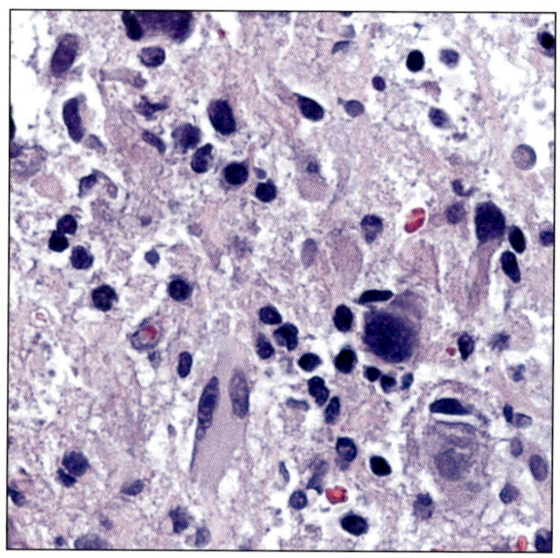

(Left) *DNT is composed of bland, round, monotonous cells similar to those present in oligodendroglioma →. In contrast to oligodendrogliomas, intralesional neurons in DNT are often found in mucoid pools ("floating neurons"), lacking perineuronal satellitosis →.* ***(Right)*** *Gangliogliomas represent glioneuronal tumors that also may arise in the setting of NF1. In addition to a glial component, they contain neoplastic ganglion cells.*

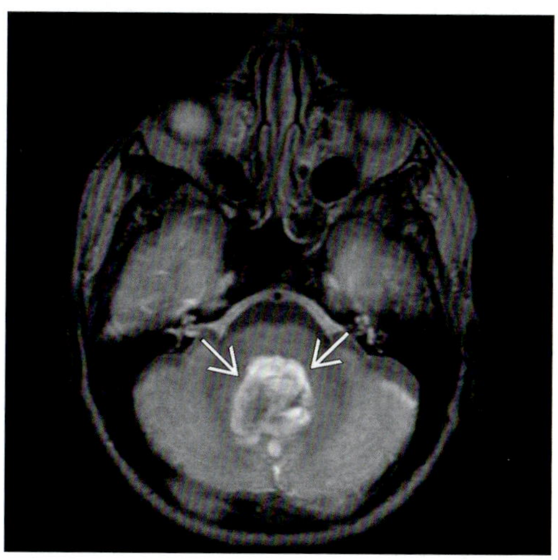

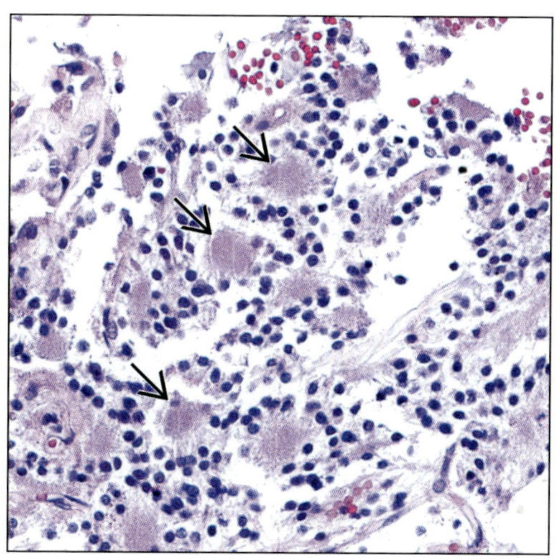

(Left) *Rosette-forming glioneuronal tumor is a distinctive neoplasm that may occasionally occur in the setting of inherited genetic syndromes, as in this patient with Noonan syndrome. This neoplasm has a distinctive predilection for the 4th ventricle region →.* ***(Right)*** *The most distinctive feature of rosette-forming glioneuronal tumor is the presence of small rosettes with an eosinophilic fibrillar core surrounded by bland neurocytes →. This example developed in a Noonan patient.*

ASTROCYTOMA

Subependymal Giant Cell Astrocytoma

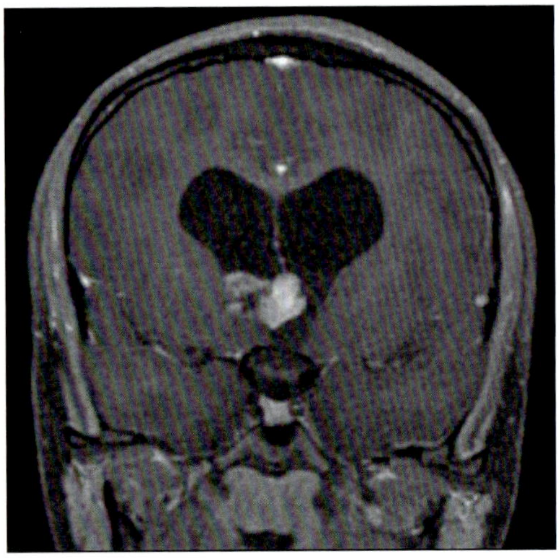

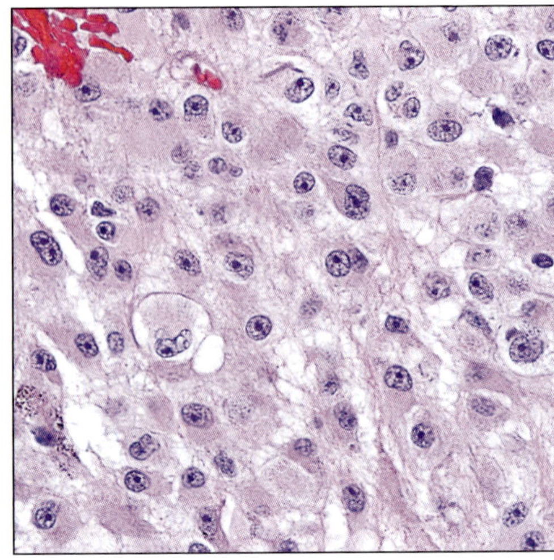

(Left) *Subependymal giant cell astrocytomas (SEGAs) appear as well-demarcated, contrast-enhancing lesions on post-contrast T1-weighted MR images. They arise in the lateral ventricle, almost always near the foramen of Monro.* ***(Right)*** *The neoplastic cells in SEGA contain abundant eosinophilic cytoplasm, as well as large nuclei with prominent nucleoli. These tumors are low grade, and mitotic activity is scant or altogether absent. Necrosis is also rare in these tumors.*

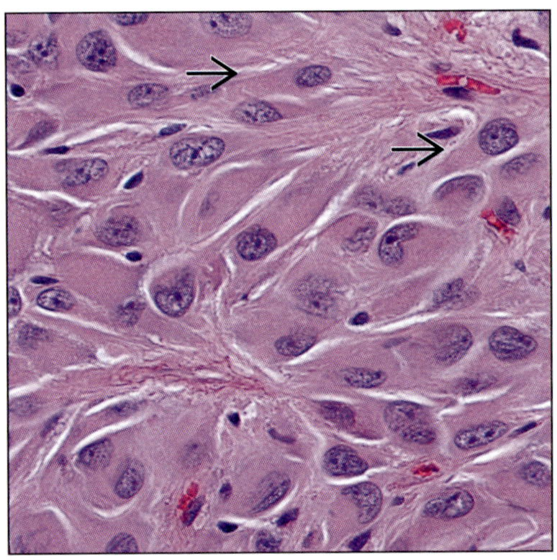

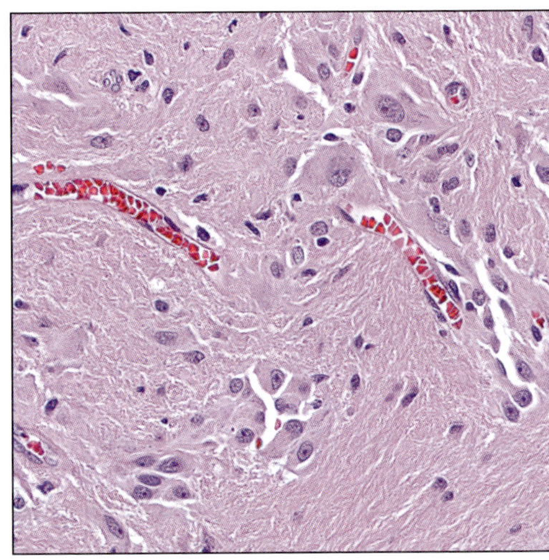

(Left) *Dense cytoplasmic eosinophilia is a prominent feature of some SEGAs. A subset of the cells may also have more fusiform contours →, and even be arranged in vague fascicles. The presence of large nuclei with macronucleoli raises the possibility of a neuronal tumor, and in fact these neoplasms show immunohistochemical and ultrastructural evidence of neuronal differentiation, at least in part.* ***(Right)*** *Nests embedded in fibrillary stroma may be identified in areas of most SEGAs.*

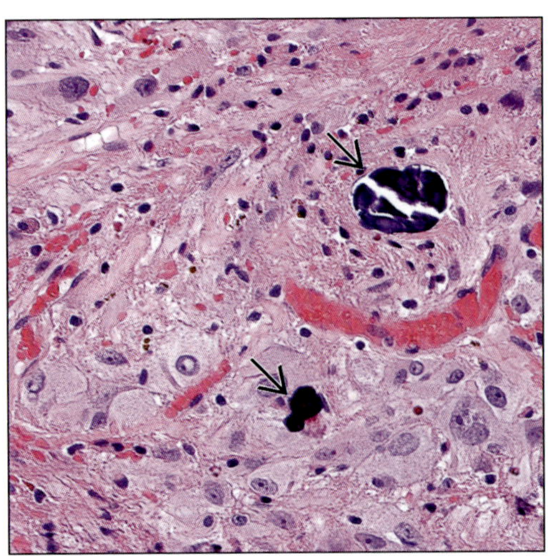

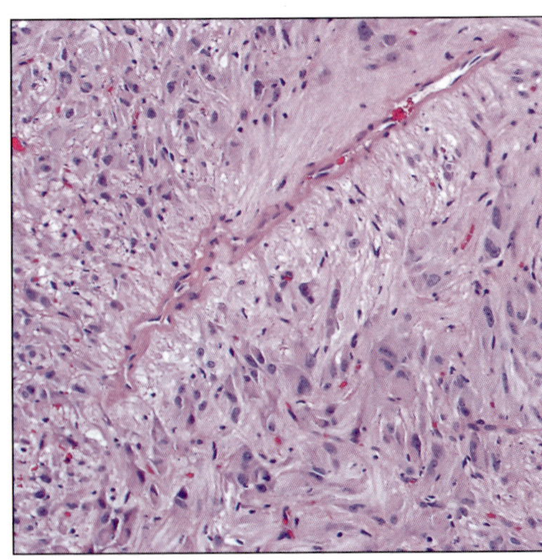

(Left) *Foci of microcalcification → may be present in a subset of SEGAs. The large cells with ample cytology suggest the diagnosis, particularly when encountering an intraventricular neoplasm located near the foramen of Monro.* ***(Right)*** *Perivascular, fibrillar neoplastic cell processes may be present in SEGA. Given its uniform intraventricular location, ependymoma represents the main diagnostic consideration. However, the cells of SEGA are larger and the immunophenotype is distinct.*

Subependymal Giant Cell Astrocytoma

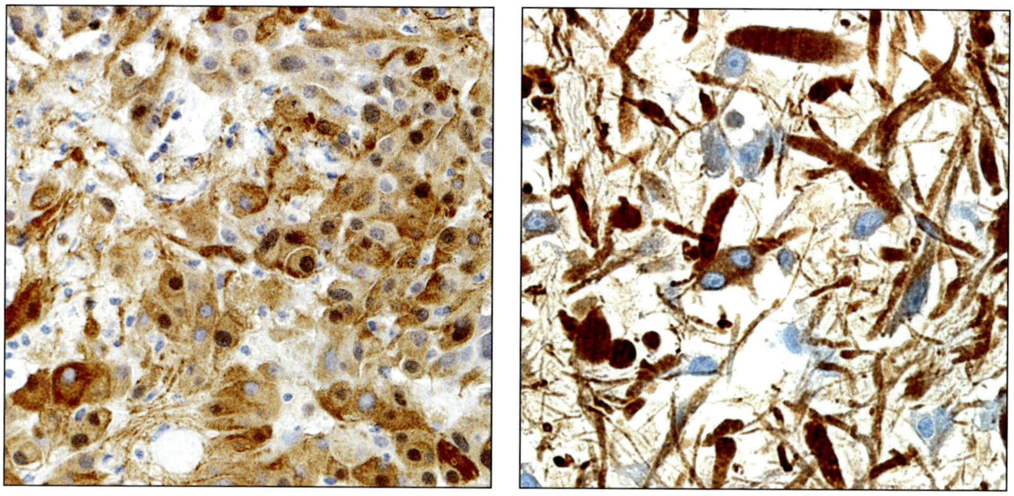

(Left) *Strong, uniform immunoreactivity for S100 is an almost universal feature of SEGA, including cytoplasmic and nuclear labeling. S100 is a sensitive (although not entirely specific) marker for glial differentiation in primary neoplasms of the central nervous system.* ***(Right)*** *GFAP expression is also frequent in SEGA and highlights perinuclear cytoplasm as well as cell processes. The presence of GFAP expression confirms that these neoplasms are indeed glial.*

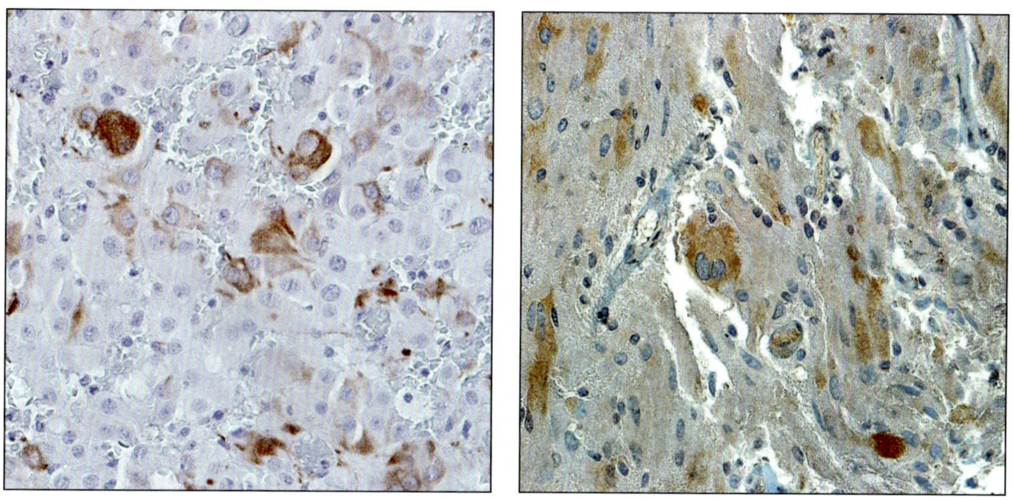

(Left) *Immunohistochemical stain for GFAP is frequent in SEGA, although it is variable. In some cases, such as this example, convincing expression may be limited to a minority of neoplastic cells, in contrast to most diffuse astrocytomas.* ***(Right)*** *In addition to expressing glial markers, SEGA frequently demonstrates immunohistochemical evidence of neuronal differentiation, such as synaptophysin expression. This suggests a mixed glioneuronal phenotype.*

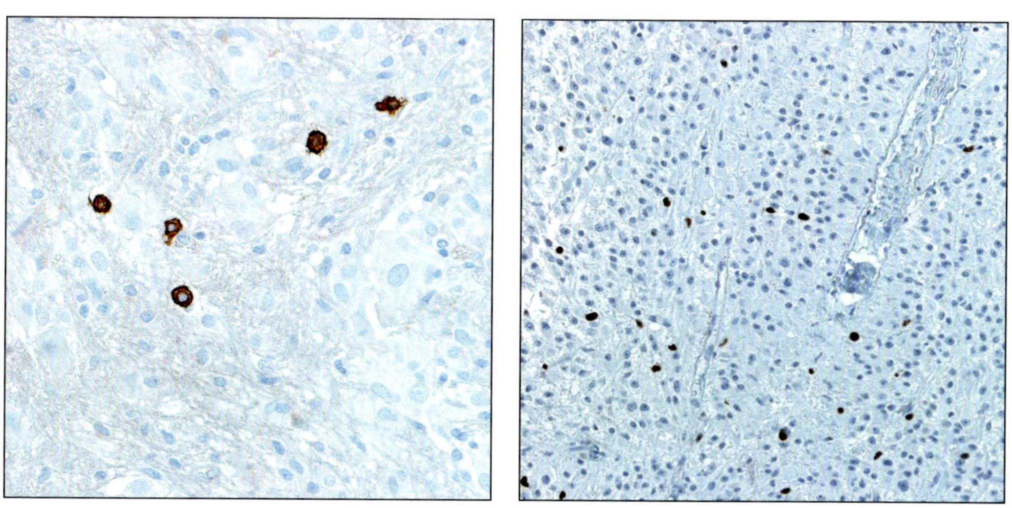

(Left) *SEGA is one CNS tumor type that frequently contains a component of mast cells. Mast cells may be recognized by strong CD117 (KIT) expression.* ***(Right)*** *General low proliferative activity is an important feature of SEGA. Mitotic activity is always difficult to find in these tumors, and the Ki-67 labeling index is very low, as demonstrated by this particular example. This explains in part its slow progression, even in subtotally resected cases.*

High-Grade Astrocytomas

(Left) High-grade astrocytomas may also develop in NF1 patients, particularly after the childhood years. These tumors may arise anywhere in the neural axis and demonstrate aggressive imaging features, including heterogeneous contrast enhancement ➡. *(Right)* Astrocytic neoplasm in an NF1 patient demonstrates hypercellularity, nuclear hyperchromasia, glial processes, and frequent mitotic figures ➡, consistent with at least an anaplastic astrocytoma.

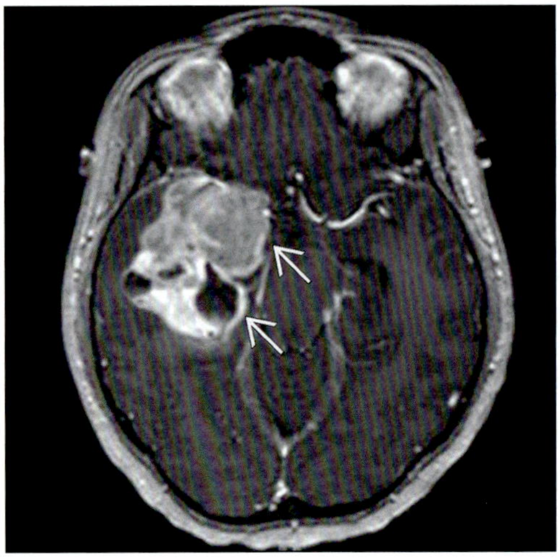

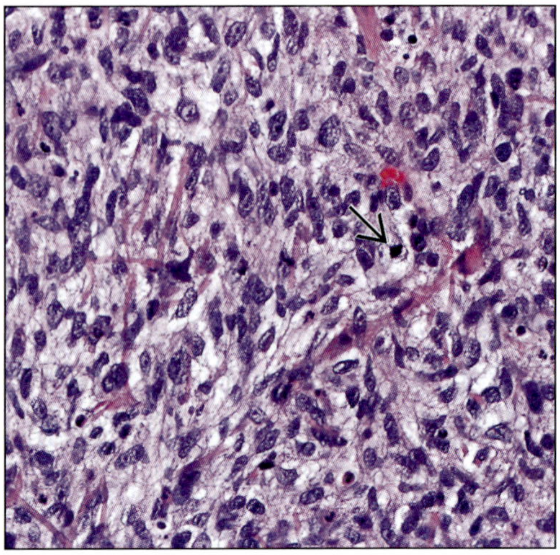

(Left) This patient with a family and personal history of cutaneous melanoma developed a large ring-enhancing mass ➡ that histologically proved to be a glioblastoma. *(Right)* Pseudopallisading necrosis is a frequent feature in high-grade brain parenchymal neoplasms, particularly glioblastoma. This example developed in a patient with a personal and family history of cutaneous melanoma. This combination of tumors is sometimes associated with germline CDKN2A gene mutations.

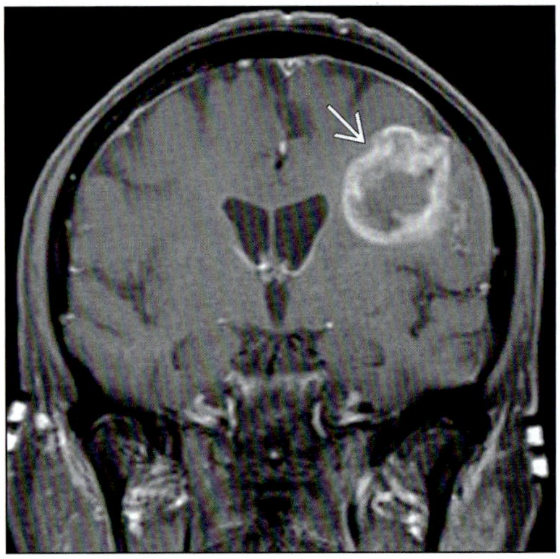

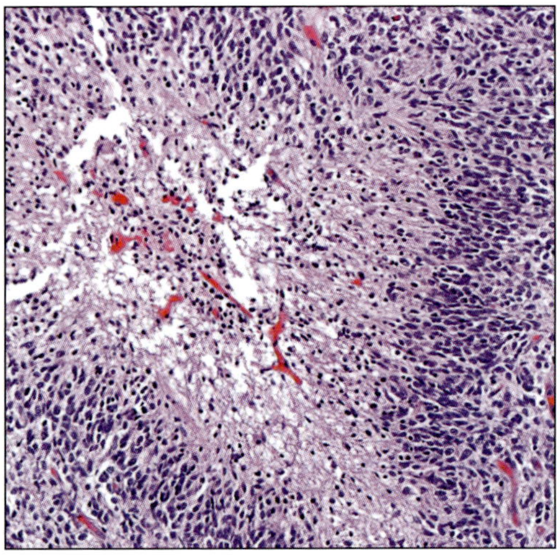

(Left) High-grade astrocytomas may develop in constitutional mismatch repair-deficiency syndrome. This patient had clinical features of NF1 but also microsatellite unstable colorectal cancer and lymphoma. A tripolar mitotic figure is evident ➡, as well as entrapped neurons ⇨. *(Right)* This NF1-associated giant cell glioblastoma is characterized by large multinucleated glial cells. Multinucleated giant cells have also been described in glioblastomas associated with Turcot syndrome.

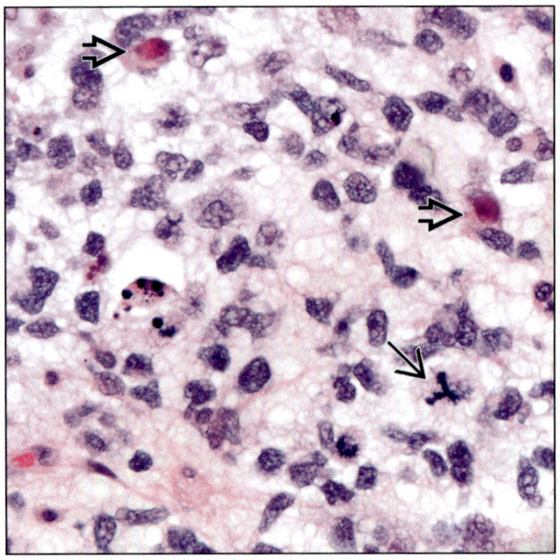

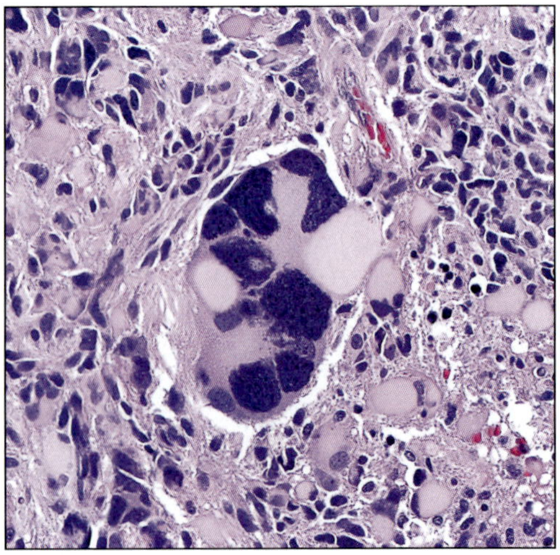

High-Grade Astrocytomas

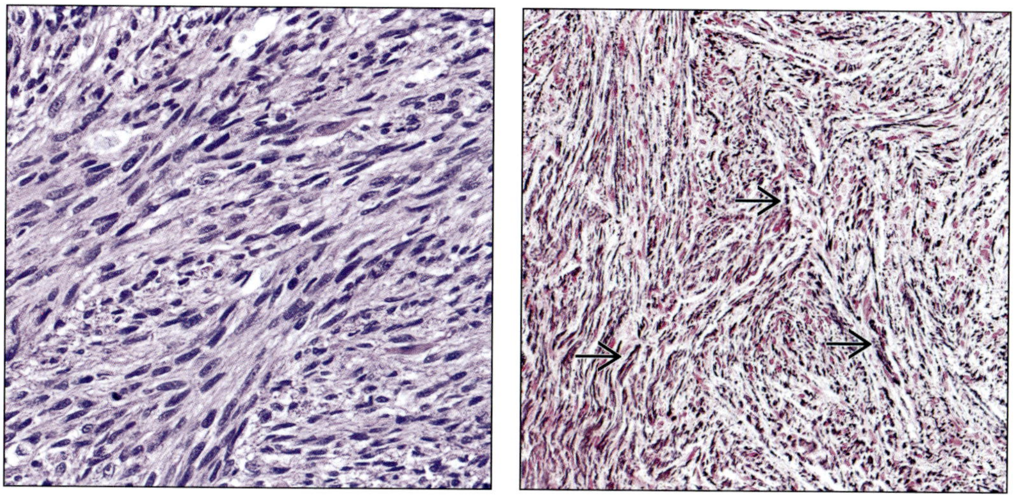

(Left) *Gliosarcoma in an NF1 patient contains a malignant spindle cell/ mesenchymal component arranged in well-formed fascicles, a morphology that corresponds to fibrosarcoma.* ***(Right)*** *Reticulin shows a prominent pericellular pattern of staining in the malignant mesenchymal component of gliosarcoma* ⇒*. In addition, loss of GFAP expression in the sarcomatous component is another feature that may be demonstrated by immunohistochemistry, and required for the diagnosis.*

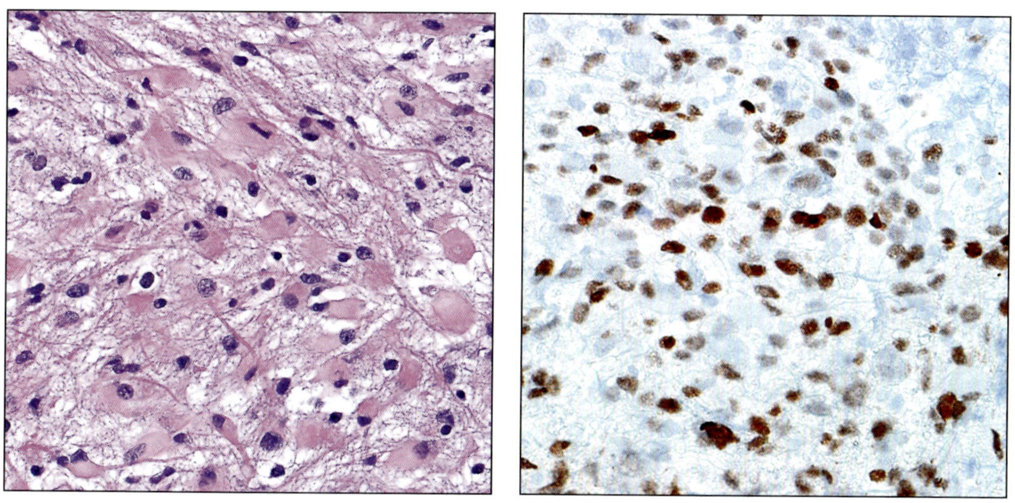

(Left) *This anaplastic astrocytoma developed in a patient with Li-Fraumeni syndrome. High-grade astrocytomas are also a feature of Li-Fraumeni syndrome, characterized by germline mutations in the tumor suppressor gene TP53.* ***(Right)*** *A gemistocytic astrocytoma developing in a patient with Li-Fraumeni syndrome shows strong p53 labeling. Strong, uniform p53 immunostaining in most tumor cells is a frequently used, albeit imperfect surrogate for TP53 mutations.*

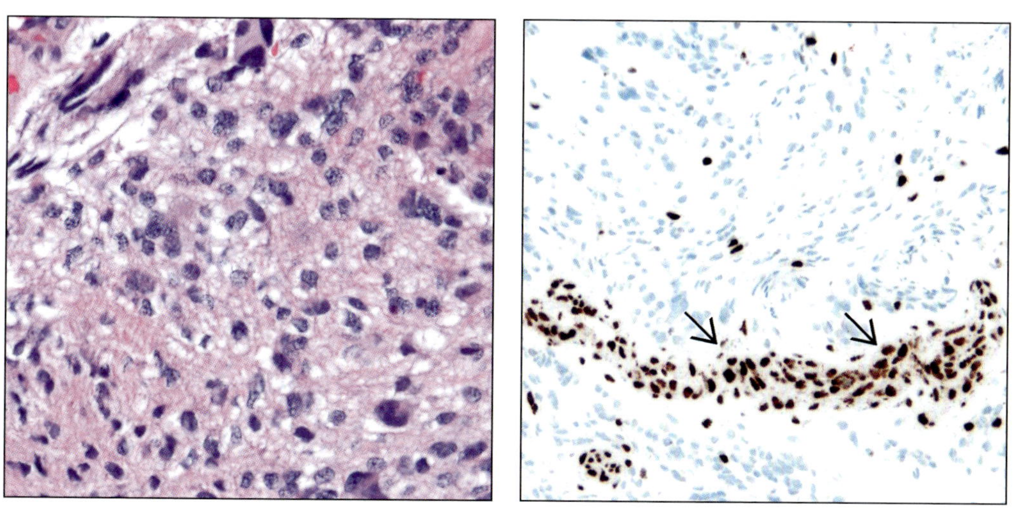

(Left) *This tumor developed in a patient with Turcot type 1 syndrome, associated with deficiency in mismatch repair enzymes. Mitotic activity was identifiable elsewhere, supporting a high-grade astrocytoma.* ***(Right)*** *This high-grade astrocytoma developing in a patient with Turcot type 1 syndrome demonstrates MSH6 loss by IHC in tumor cells, but not in vessels or other nonneoplastic elements* ⇒*. MSH2 was also lost (not shown). (Courtesy C. Giannini, MD.)*

CHOROID PLEXUS TUMORS

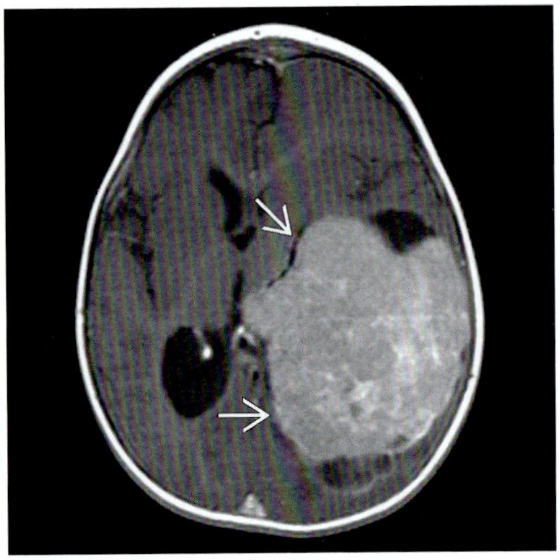

Choroid plexus carcinomas are malignant neoplasms that almost always develop in young children and demonstrate variable contrast enhancement ➡. (Courtesy T. Vanegas, MD.)

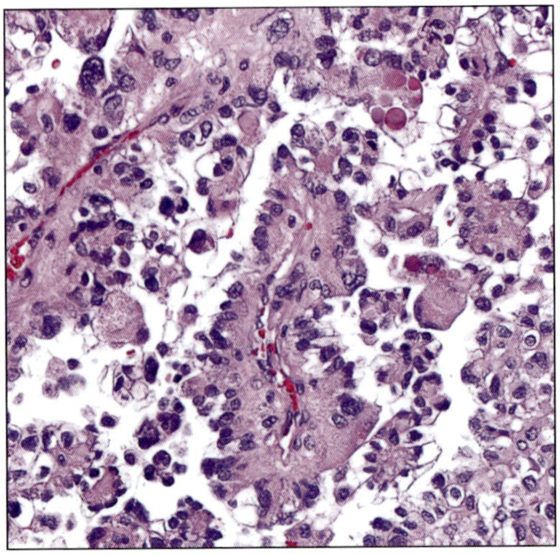

Choroid plexus carcinomas usually have a papillary architecture and variable pleomorphism. This young patient developed a rhabdomyosarcoma, which strongly suggests Li-Fraumeni syndrome.

TERMINOLOGY

Definitions

- Spectrum of neoplasms arising in ventricular locations and with anatomic, morphologic, and immunophenotypic similarities with choroid plexus

ETIOLOGY/PATHOGENESIS

Sporadic Tumors

- Most choroid plexus tumors are sporadic, but choroid plexus carcinomas are strongly associated with germline *TP53* mutations

Li-Fraumeni Syndrome

- Tumor predisposition syndrome most commonly secondary to germline *TP53* mutations
- Most CNS neoplasms in Li-Fraumeni patients are astrocytomas (~ 60%)
- Also develop medulloblastomas and choroid plexus tumors (carcinomas > papillomas)

Rhabdoid Predisposition Syndrome

- Choroid plexus carcinomas reported in some patients, but there is morphologic and immunophenotypic overlap with atypical teratoid/rhabdoid tumors (AT/RT)

Aicardi Syndrome

- X-linked dominant **sporadic** syndrome occurring almost exclusively in females
- Agenesis of corpus callosum, chorioretinal lacunae, and infantile spasms
- Associated with choroid plexus papillomas and cysts

CLINICAL ISSUES

Epidemiology

- Incidence
  - Rare brain tumors overall (< 1%)
  - Relatively high proportion of brain tumors in infants

Presentation

- Symptoms attributable to hydrocephalus and increased intracranial pressure

Prognosis

- Varies from excellent (choroid plexus papilloma) to poor (choroid plexus carcinoma)

MICROSCOPIC PATHOLOGY

Histologic Features

- Choroid plexus papilloma
  - Papillary architecture with fibrovascular cores lined by cuboidal to columnar epithelium
  - Pleomorphism, sheet-like growth, and necrosis are rare but may be present in isolation
  - Mitotic activity rare to absent
- Atypical choroid plexus papilloma
  - Mitotic activity ≥ 2 per 10 high-power fields
  - ↑ cellularity, nuclear pleomorphism, sheet-like growth, and necrosis may be present but not required for diagnosis
- Choroid plexus carcinoma
  - Overtly malignant histology
  - Brisk mitotic activity
  - Hypercellularity, pleomorphism, solid growth, and necrosis common
  - Brain invasion may be present

CHOROID PLEXUS TUMORS

Key Facts

Terminology
- Spectrum of neoplasms arising in ventricular locations and with anatomic, morphologic, and immunophenotypic similarities with choroid plexus

Etiology/Pathogenesis
- Most are sporadic
  - Choroid plexus carcinomas are strongly associated with germline *TP53* mutations
- Li-Fraumeni syndrome: Most CNS neoplasms are astrocytomas, but some are also choroid plexus tumors (carcinoma > papilloma)
- Rhabdoid predisposition syndrome: Reported cases of choroid plexus carcinoma may in fact be atypical teratoid/rhabdoid tumors (AT/RT)
- Aicardi syndrome: Associated with choroid plexus papillomas and cysts

Microscopic Pathology
- Papilloma: Papillary architecture with fibrovascular cores lined by cuboidal to columnar epithelium; mitotic activity rare to absent
- Atypical papilloma: Mitotic activity ≥ 2 per 10 high-power fields
- Carcinoma: Overtly malignant histology, brisk mitotic activity

Ancillary Tests
- *TP53* alterations associated with poorer prognosis in choroid plexus tumors in some studies
- Notch pathway activation induces choroid plexus tumors in mice and is present in a subset of human choroid plexus tumors

ANCILLARY TESTS

Immunohistochemistry
- Cytokeratin and podoplanin expressed by choroid plexus tumors
- S100 protein and transthyretin also frequently expressed
- GFAP expression in a subset
- Frequent p53 immunopositivity in carcinomas
- Kir7.1 and stanniocalcin-1 expression in nonneoplastic choroid plexus and most choroid plexus tumors

Molecular Genetics
- *TP53* alterations associated with poorer prognosis in choroid plexus tumors in some studies
- Notch pathway activation induces choroid plexus tumors in mice and is present in a subset of human choroid plexus tumors

DIFFERENTIAL DIAGNOSIS

Normal Choroid Plexus
- Cobblestone appearance, less cellularity than papilloma, microcalcifications

Cribriform Neuroepithelial Tumor
- Very rare low-grade intraventricular neoplasm with cribriform/trabecular architecture
- Surface EMA staining, INI1 loss

Ependymoma
- May have a papillary pattern (papillary or myxopapillary ependymoma)
- Prominent pseudorosettes, true rosettes
- Dot-like or surface EMA immunopositivity

Papillary Tumor of Pineal Region
- Similar morphologic and immunophenotypic features
- Pineal gland location not a feature of choroid plexus tumors
- Lacks Kir7.1 and stanniocalcin-1 positivity

Atypical Teratoid/Rhabdoid Tumor
- May have morphologic and immunophenotypic overlap with choroid plexus carcinoma
- INI1 protein loss

Metastatic Carcinoma
- Usually not an issue in children but main consideration in adult patients

GRADING

WHO Grades I-III
- Papilloma (WHO grade I), atypical papilloma (WHO grade II), and carcinoma (WHO grade III)

SELECTED REFERENCES

1. Gozali AE et al: Choroid plexus tumors; management, outcome, and association with the Li-Fraumeni syndrome: the Children's Hospital Los Angeles (CHLA) experience, 1991-2010. Pediatr Blood Cancer. 58(6):905-9, 2012
2. Schittenhelm J et al: Atypical teratoid/rhabdoid tumors may show morphological and immunohistochemical features seen in choroid plexus tumors. Neuropathology. 31(5):461-7, 2011
3. Tabori U et al: TP53 alterations determine clinical subgroups and survival of patients with choroid plexus tumors. J Clin Oncol. 28(12):1995-2001, 2010
4. Gonzalez KD et al: Beyond Li Fraumeni Syndrome: clinical characteristics of families with p53 germline mutations. J Clin Oncol. 27(8):1250-6, 2009
5. Frye RE et al: Choroid plexus papilloma expansion over 7 years in Aicardi syndrome. J Child Neurol. 22(4):484-7, 2007
6. Dang L et al: Notch3 signaling initiates choroid plexus tumor formation. Oncogene. 25(3):487-91, 2006
7. Hasselblatt M et al: Identification of novel diagnostic markers for choroid plexus tumors: a microarray-based approach. Am J Surg Pathol. 30(1):66-74, 2006
8. Jeibmann A et al: Prognostic implications of atypical histologic features in choroid plexus papilloma. J Neuropathol Exp Neurol. 65(11):1069-73, 2006

CHOROID PLEXUS TUMORS

Imaging and Microscopic Features

(Left) *Choroid plexus neoplasms almost always arise within the ventricular system. This sagittal T1-weighted MR image shows a choroid plexus papilloma involving the 4th ventricle, a common location in adults ➔.* ***(Right)*** *Choroid plexus tumors encompass a spectrum ranging from benign (grade I) to malignant (grade III). This grade I choroid plexus papilloma contains numerous papillae lined by cuboidal to columnar cells.*

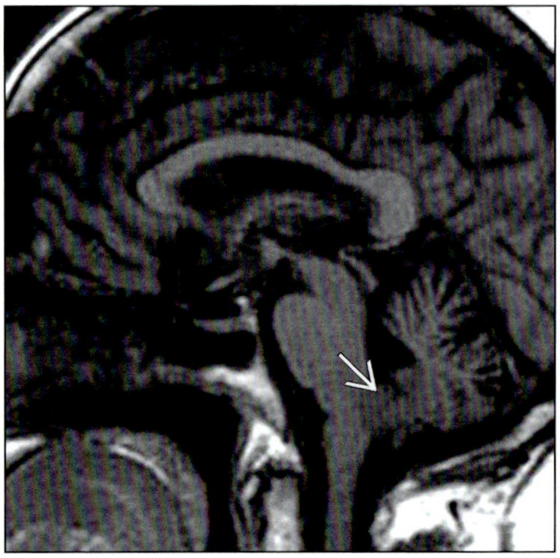

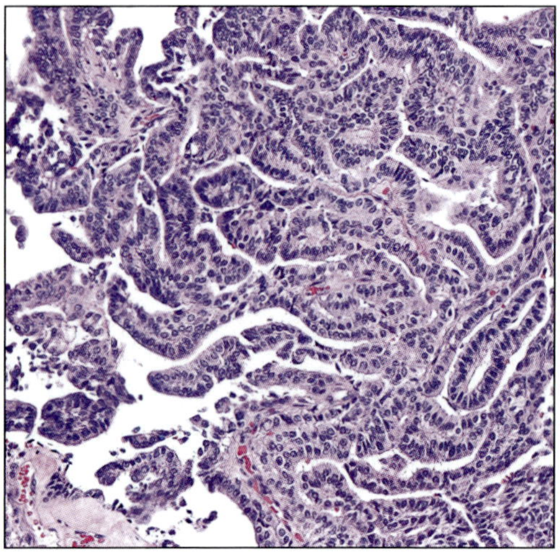

(Left) *Distinctive fibrovascular cores are hallmarks of choroid plexus tumors ➔. This choroid plexus papilloma has bland cytology and lacks mitotic activity and necrosis, which is consistent with a grade I neoplasm.* ***(Right)*** *This choroid plexus tumor has a more solid pattern of growth, which may be a feature of a subset of tumors. Mitotic activity is not subtle ➔, which is consistent with an atypical choroid plexus papilloma, indicating a WHO grade II.*

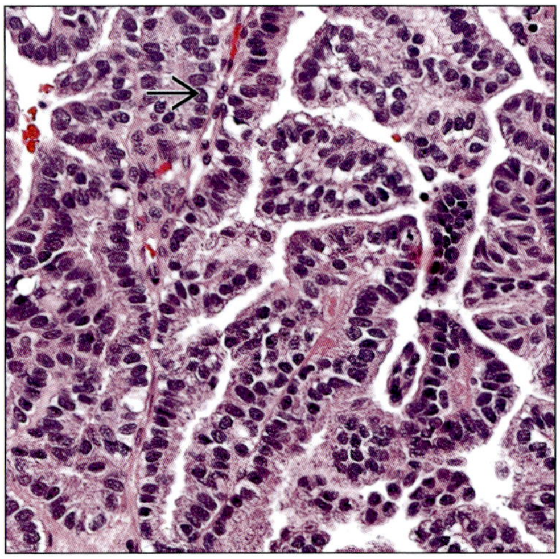

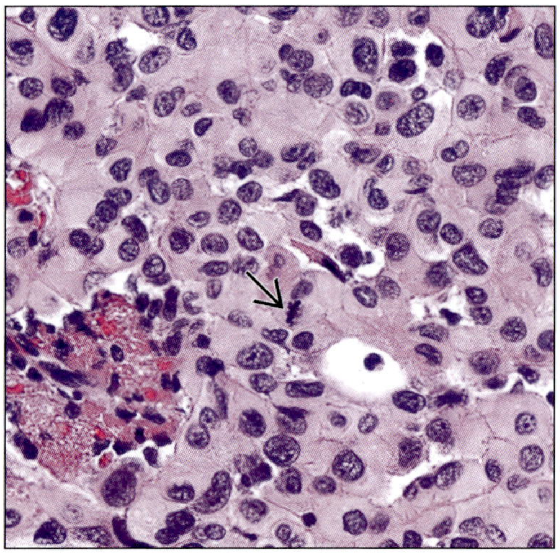

(Left) *Keratin expression is a universal feature of choroid plexus neoplasms. Strong labeling with cytokeratin CAM5.2 is strongly supportive of the diagnosis in the right context.* ***(Right)*** *Choroid plexus tumors may also express a variety of markers. This example expresses S100, with a nuclear and cytoplasmic pattern.*

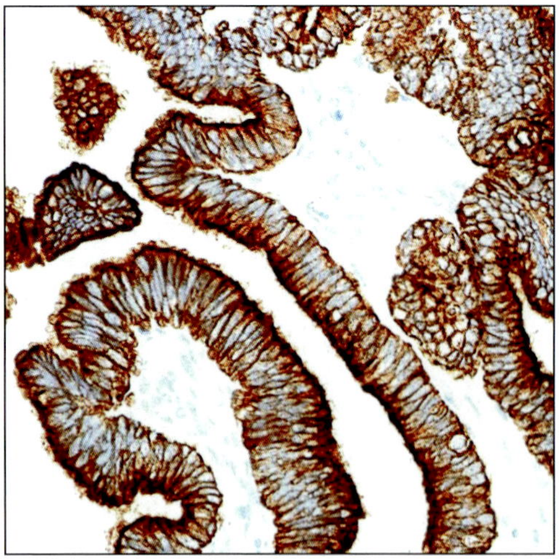

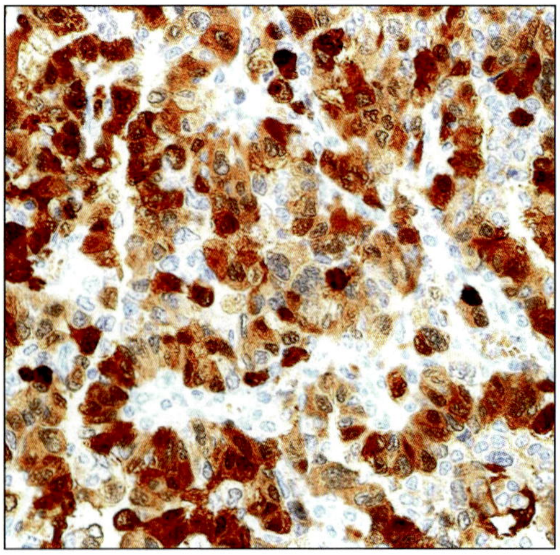

Diagrammatic and Microscopic Features

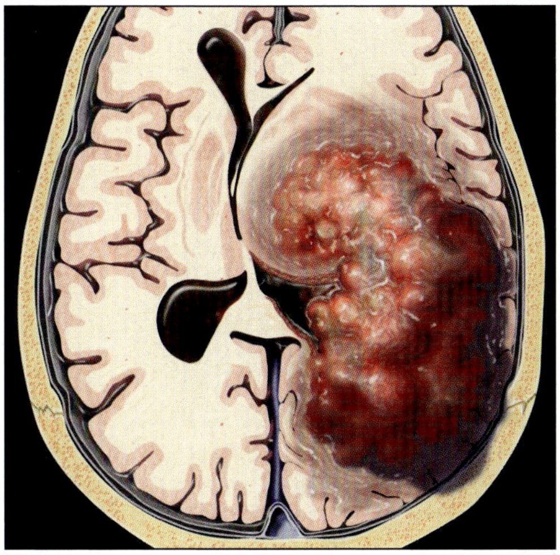

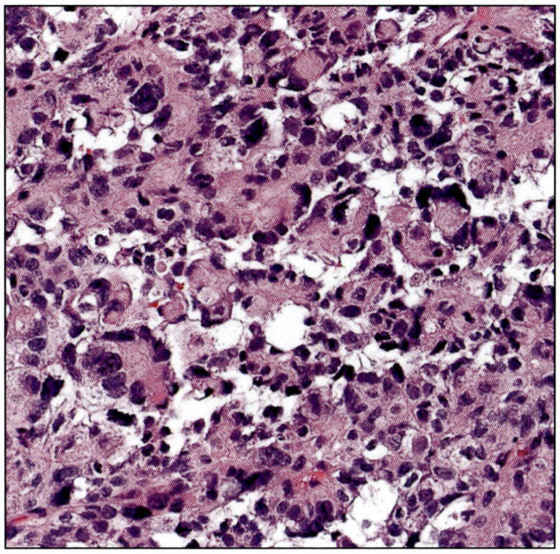

(Left) *Choroid plexus carcinomas are highly malignant neoplasms and may form huge, fleshy masses with associated edema and mass effect.* ***(Right)*** *Many choroid plexus carcinomas demonstrate cytologic features of malignancy, particularly nuclear enlargement, hyperchromasia, and pleomorphism. In this example, a papillary architecture is still evident.*

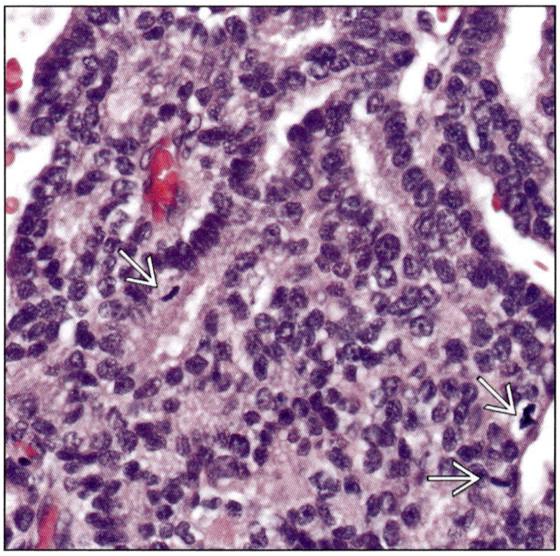

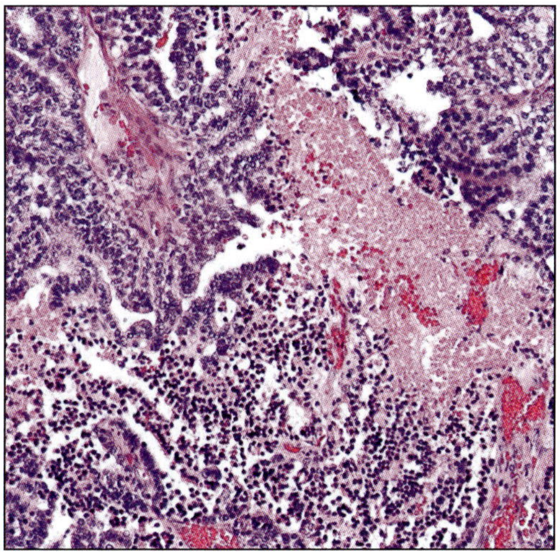

(Left) *A subset of choroid plexus papillomas may contain minimal atypia and are well differentiated at the architectural level. However, the presence of brisk mitotic activity* ➔ *in a choroid plexus neoplasm is very worrisome and consistent with a carcinoma.* ***(Right)*** *Sheets of coagulative necrosis are not uncommon in choroid plexus carcinomas. In combination with brisk mitotic activity, it strongly supports the diagnosis.*

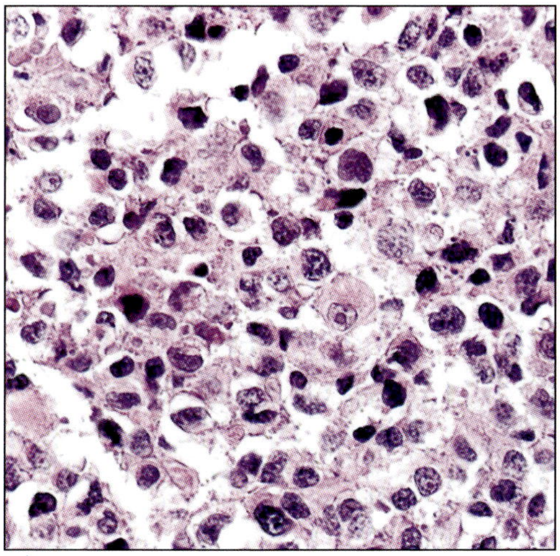

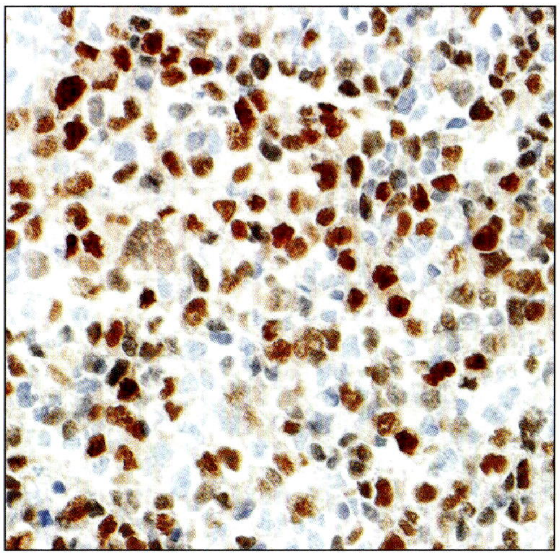

(Left) *This tumor developed in a young patient after treatment for a choroid plexus carcinoma and had morphologic and immunophenotypic features of rhabdomyosarcoma. The combination of choroid plexus carcinoma and sarcoma in a young patient is strongly suggestive of a tumor predisposition syndrome, particularly Li-Fraumeni.* ***(Right)*** *Strong nuclear myogenin labeling confirmed the diagnosis of rhabdomyosarcoma in this young patient treated for choroid plexus carcinoma.*

EPENDYMOMA

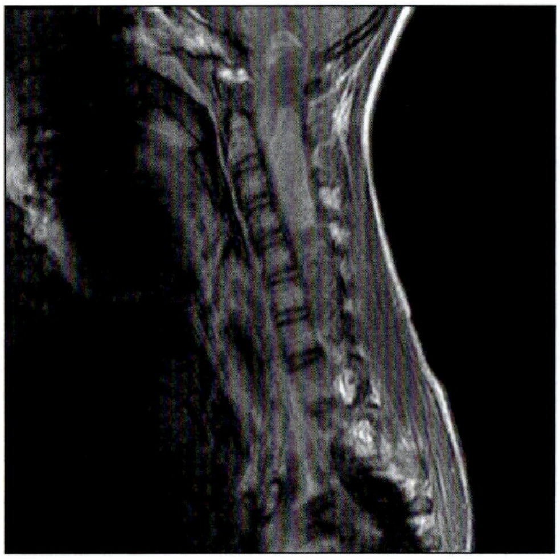

As this T1-weighted MR shows, ependymomas in NF2 patients have a predilection for the cervical cord. Ependymomas form well-circumscribed masses, and most demonstrate contrast enhancement.

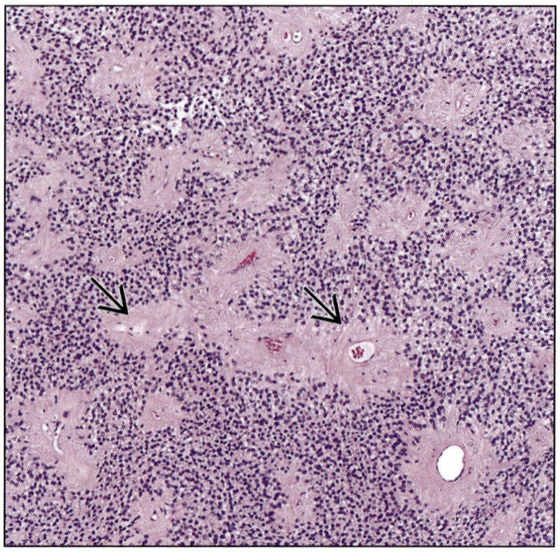

Among the main architectural features of ependymomas at low power are perivascular pseudorosettes, which impart an anuclear area around intratumoral vessels ⇒.

TERMINOLOGY

Definitions

- Circumscribed CNS neoplasm with dual glial and epithelial differentiation, properties resembling ependymal lining of ventricular system/central spinal cord canal

CLINICAL ISSUES

Site

- May arise anywhere in neuraxis
  - Predilection for spinal cord (adults) and posterior fossa/supratentorial compartment (children)
- Most frequent primary spinal cord neoplasm in adults
- Predilection for cervical cord/cervicomedullary junction in patients with neurofibromatosis type 2 (NF2)

Presentation

- Present in ~ 1/3 to 1/2 of NF2 patients on imaging
- NF2-ependymomas (when present) are multiple in most patients (58%)
- Majority of NF2 patients are asymptomatic

Treatment

- Clinical follow-up is indicated for asymptomatic tumors in NF2
- Goal of surgery is complete surgical resection if feasible

Prognosis

- Most NF2-associated ependymomas are indolent
  - Progression occurs in only a minority of patients

IMAGE FINDINGS

MR Findings

- Well-circumscribed neoplasms
- ↑ T2 signal, homogeneous contrast enhancement
- Heterogeneous enhancement in necrotic tumors
- Associated cyst/spinal cord syrinx may be present
- Leptomeningeal dissemination in a subset of cases (intracranial tumors)

MICROSCOPIC PATHOLOGY

Histologic Features

- Subtypes include cellular, myxopapillary, papillary, clear cell, tanycytic, giant cell, and anaplastic
- Most histologic subtypes have been reported in NF2 patients, including myxopapillary, tanycytic, and anaplastic
- Perivascular pseudorosettes present in majority of ependymomas to variable extent
  - Glial processes surrounding vessels create an anuclear zone
  - More accentuated in ependymomas but may be present to a lesser extent in astrocytic and neuronal neoplasms
- True ependymal rosettes
  - Well-defined lumina resembling ependymal linings
  - When large, known as ependymal canals
  - May be minute and recognized by EMA immunohistochemistry (dot-like pattern) or electron microscopy
  - Less frequent than pseudorosettes but essentially diagnostic in right context
- Usually sharp interface with CNS parenchyma
  - Gliosis with Rosenthal fibers may be present
  - Infiltration is rare but may be found in supratentorial/recurrent &/or anaplastic tumors

EPENDYMOMA

Key Facts

Terminology
- Circumscribed CNS neoplasm with dual glial and epithelial differentiation, properties resembling the ependymal lining of the ventricular system/central spinal cord canal

Clinical Issues
- Ependymomas may arise anywhere in the neuraxis
- Most frequent primary spinal cord neoplasm
- Predilection for cervical cord/cervicomedullary junction in NF2 patients
- NF2 ependymomas (when present) are multiple in most patients (58%)
- Majority of NF2 patients are asymptomatic
- Most NF2-associated ependymomas are indolent

Microscopic Pathology
- Most histologic subtypes have been reported in NF2 patients, including myxopapillary, tanycytic, and anaplastic
- Perivascular pseudorosettes are present in majority of ependymomas to variable extent
- True ependymal rosettes
- Usually sharp interface with CNS parenchyma

Ancillary Tests
- Molecular genetics
  - Alterations in the *NF2* gene in 76% of NF2-associated spinal ependymomas
  - Most mutations truncating (nonsense or frameshift)

Cytologic Features
- Uniform, bland oval cells with relatively short processes
- Aggregation/clinging of cells around vessels (pseudorosettes) is characteristic

ANCILLARY TESTS

Molecular Genetics
- Alterations in *NF2* gene in 76% of NF2-associated spinal ependymomas
  - Most mutations truncating (nonsense or frameshift)

Gene Expression Profiling
- Relevant subtypes cluster acording to anatomic site and clinical behavior

DIFFERENTIAL DIAGNOSIS

Schwannoma
- May coexist with ependymoma and meningioma in NF2 patients, usually extramedullary
- S100(+) but EMA(-)

Meningioma
- May coexist with schwannoma and ependymoma in NF2 patients
- Extramedullary location
- Membranous (rather than dot-like) EMA expression, GFAP negative

Astrocytoma
- May also develop in NF2 patients
- Most intramedullary tumors in NF2 are ependymomas
  - Strong index of suspicion, even in the absence of overt ependymal features

Paraganglioma
- Clinical and histologic overlap with myxopapillary ependymoma in the filum terminale
- Strong synaptophysin and chromogranin positivity

Metastatic Carcinoma
- Rare in the spinal cord proper
- Increased pleomorphism, strong cytokeratin expression

GRADING

WHO Grades I-III
- Myxopapillary (WHO grade I), conventional (WHO grade II), anaplastic (WHO grade III)
- Criteria for anaplasia: Brisk mitotic activity, often with microvascular proliferation and pseudopalisading necrosis
- Adverse histologic factors may depend on anatomic site and be less significant in spinal cord tumors

SELECTED REFERENCES

1. Raghunathan A et al: Histological Predictors of Outcome in Ependymoma are Dependent on Anatomic Site Within the Central Nervous System. Brain Pathol. 23(5):584-94, 2013
2. Hagel C et al: Clinical presentation, immunohistochemistry and electron microscopy indicate neurofibromatosis type 2-associated gliomas to be spinal ependymomas. Neuropathology. 32(6):611-6, 2012
3. Plotkin SR et al: Spinal ependymomas in neurofibromatosis type 2: a retrospective analysis of 55 patients. J Neurosurg Spine. 14(4):543-7, 2011
4. Tihan T et al: The prognostic value of histological grading of posterior fossa ependymomas in children: a Children's Oncology Group study and a review of prognostic factors. Mod Pathol. 21(2):165-77, 2008
5. Ebert C et al: Molecular genetic analysis of ependymal tumors. NF2 mutations and chromosome 22q loss occur preferentially in intramedullary spinal ependymomas. Am J Pathol. 155(2):627-32, 1999

EPENDYMOMA

Diagrammatic and Microscopic Features

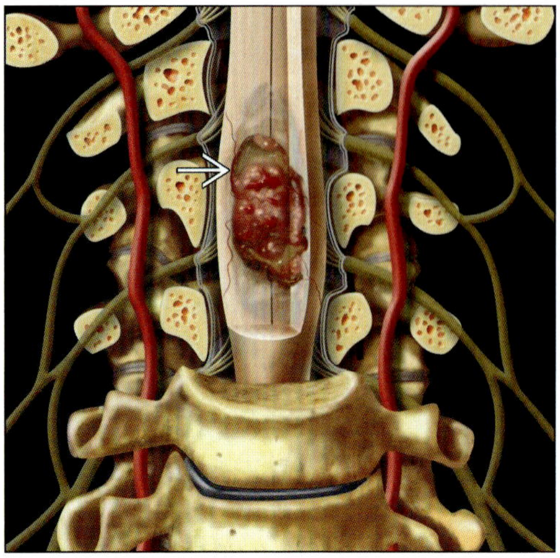

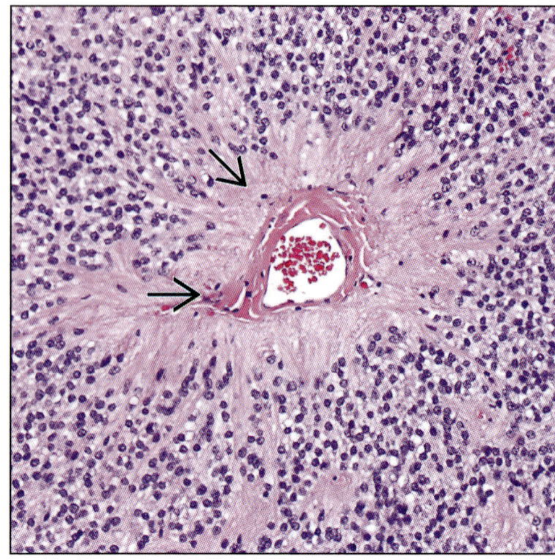

(Left) *Ependymomas are well-circumscribed neoplasms that may develop anywhere along the neural axis but with a predilection for the spinal cord, particularly in adults and patients with NF2. Associated cystic changes are not uncommon* →. ***(Right)*** *Perivascular pseudorosettes are frequent in ependymomas. They are composed of anuclear perivascular zones containing numerous neoplastic glial cell processes* →.

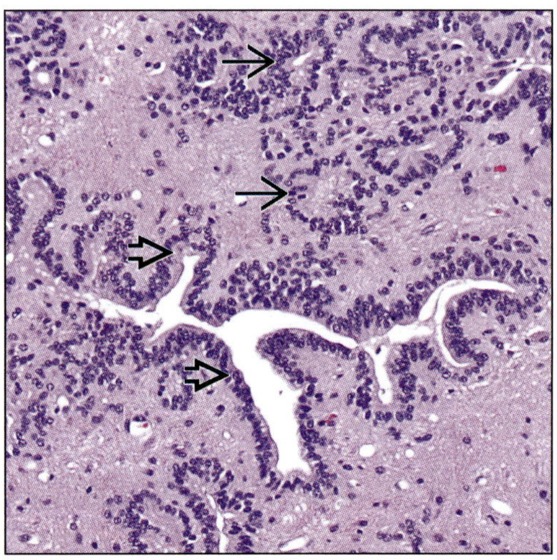

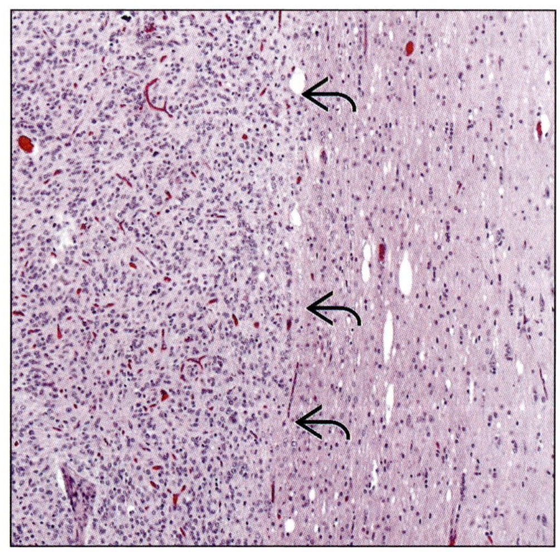

(Left) *A more specific histologic feature of ependymoma is the presence of well-developed epithelial surfaces resembling the lining of the ventricular system and central canal of the cord. These surfaces may be conspicuous in some tumors and include ependymal rosettes* → *as well as larger elongated ependymal canals* →. ***(Right)*** *Among primary CNS neoplasms, ependymomas tend to be the most well circumscribed, and a sharp interface with brain parenchyma is seen in most cases* →.

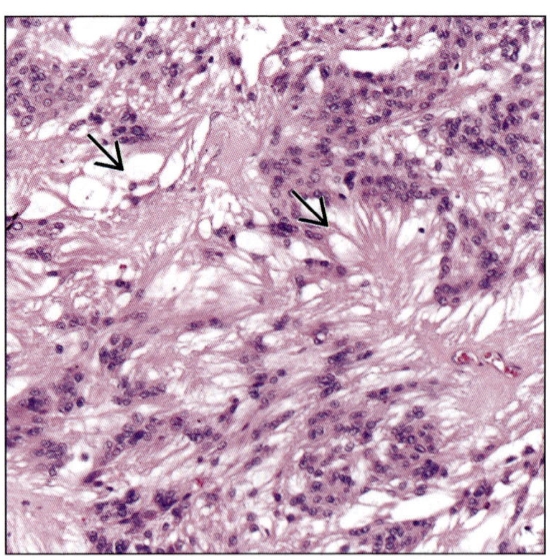

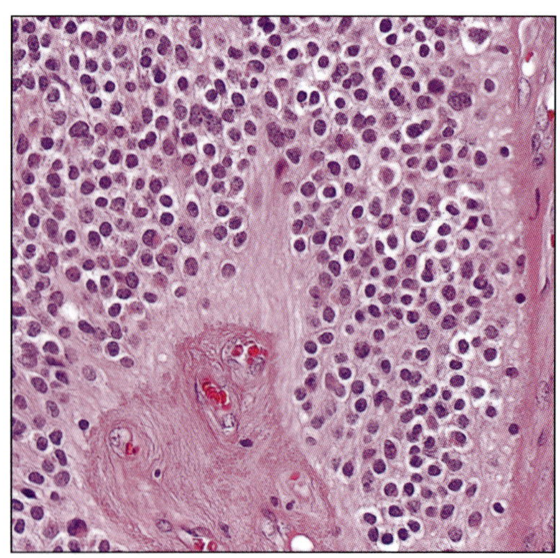

(Left) *Myxopapillary ependymoma is a distinctive subtype containing myxoid cuffs in pseudorosettes and stroma* →. *These tumors have a predilection for the distal cord/filum terminale region and are assigned a grade I under the current WHO classification.* ***(Right)*** *Clear cell ependymoma is an ependymoma subtype characterized by the presence of round/oval nuclei and cytoplasmic clearing. The latter property raises the differential with oligodendroglial and neurocytic tumors.*

EPENDYMOMA

Microscopic Features

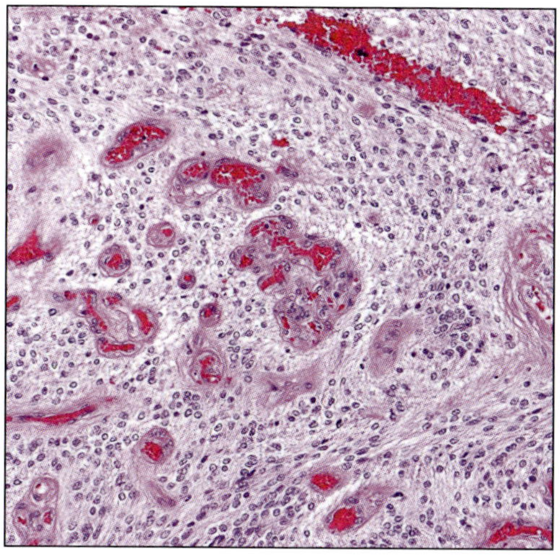

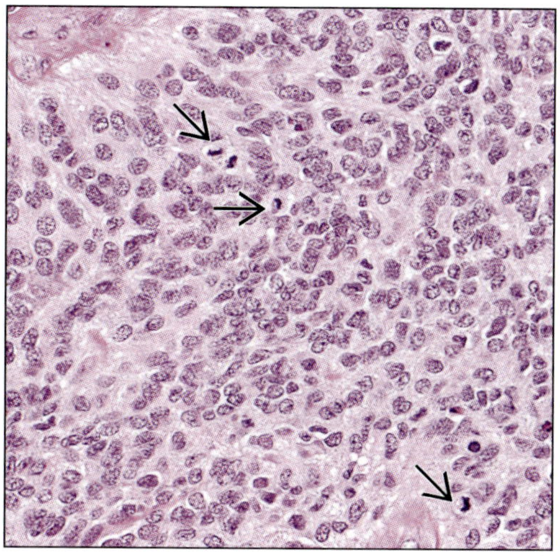

(Left) *Microvascular proliferation is a worrisome feature in ependymomas and usually 1 of the histologic properties ascribed to the anaplastic subtype (WHO grade III).* ***(Right)*** *The hallmark of anaplastic ependymoma is the presence of brisk mitotic activity. This particular example has at least 3 mitoses ⇒ in a single high-power field.*

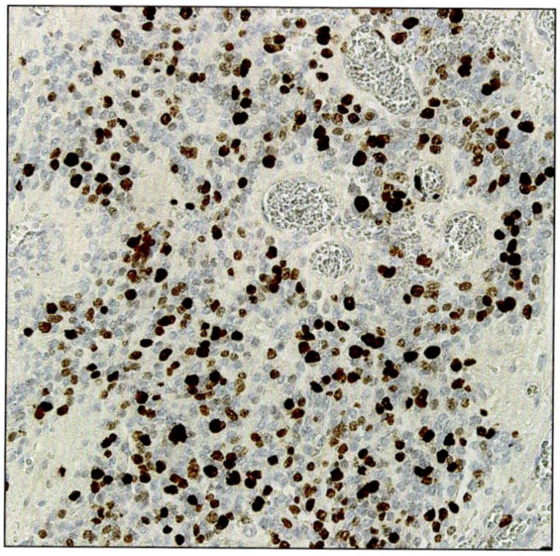

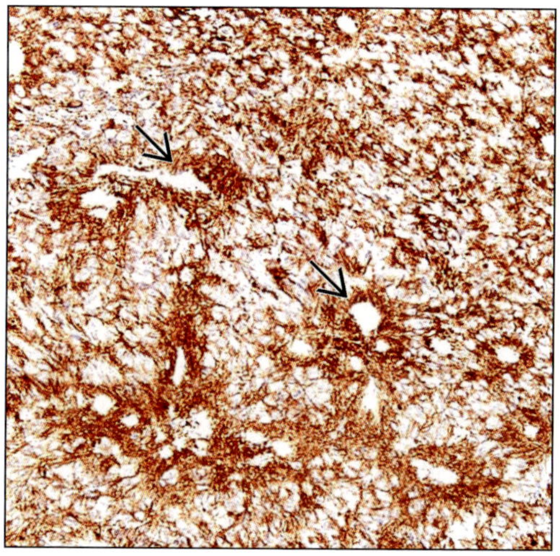

(Left) *The Ki-67 labeling index is very high in this ependymoma, consistent with its anaplastic histologic features.* ***(Right)*** *GFAP expression is variable in ependymomas but usually accentuated around vessels, highlighting perivascular pseudorosettes ⇒. This pattern of staining is not surprising since pseudorosettes are rich in GFAP-containing glial processes.*

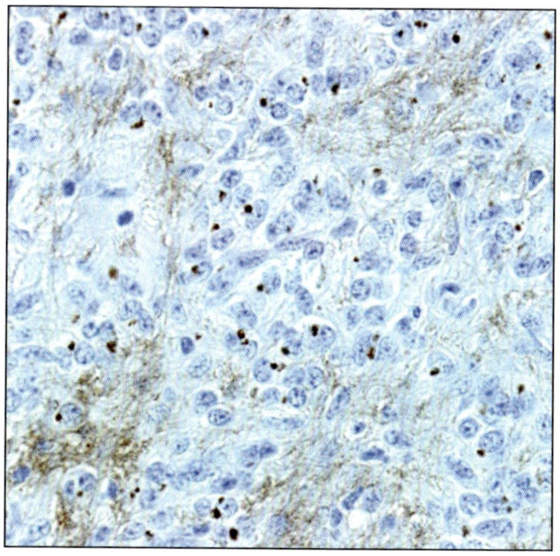

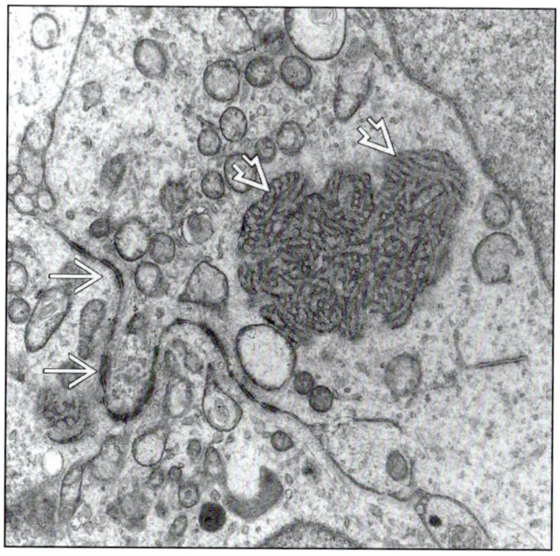

(Left) *A useful immunohistochemical marker in the evaluation of ependymoma is epithelial membrane antigen, which stains with a characteristic paranuclear/intercellular dot-like pattern. This pattern of staining is attributed to microlumina rich in microvilli, which may be demonstrated by electron microscopy.* ***(Right)*** *Electron microscopy is still a useful ancillary technique in the diagnosis of ependymoma. Features include well-formed intercellular junctions ➡ and microlumina ➡.*

MEDULLOBLASTOMA/CNS-PNET

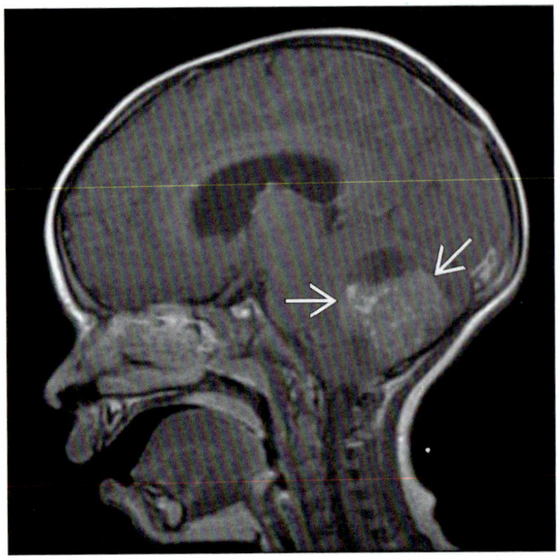

Medulloblastomas form heterogeneous masses in the cerebellum with variable contrast enhancement on post-contrast T1-weighted MR images ➡. Nodularity may be present.

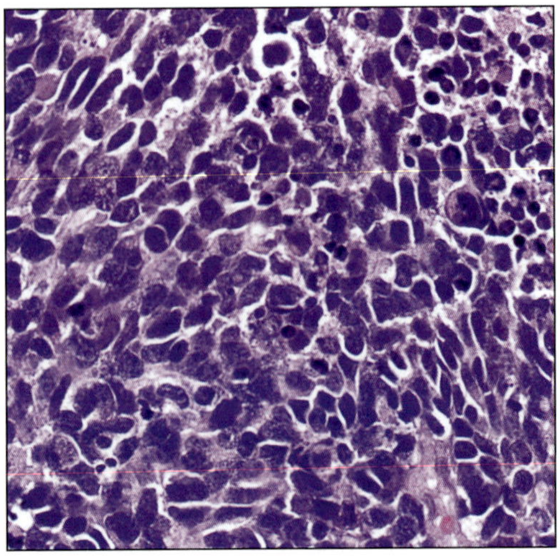

Most medulloblastomas arise sporadically. A subset develop in the setting of tumor-predisposing syndromes. This tumor developed in a patient with Li-Fraumeni syndrome, characterized by germline TP53 mutations.

TERMINOLOGY

Abbreviations

- Central nervous system primitive neuroectodermal tumor (CNS-PNET)

Definitions

- Malignant embryonal neoplasms with predominant neuronal differentiation arising in CNS parenchyma (CNS-PNET) or cerebellum/4th ventricle region (medulloblastoma)
- Unrelated to peripheral PNET/Ewing sarcoma
- WHO grade IV

ETIOLOGY/PATHOGENESIS

Sporadic Tumors

- Vast majority of medulloblastomas and CNS-PNET develop sporadically without a family history
- Frequency of cancer predisposing syndrome higher in very young patients (< 3 years)

Gorlin Syndrome/Nevoid Basal Cell Carcinoma Syndrome

- Caused by germline mutations in *PTCH1* (most frequent), *PTCH2*, or *SUFU*, resulting in activation of sonic hedgehog signaling pathway
- Patients develop numerous basal cell carcinomas, ovarian fibromas, and nonneoplastic manifestations (odontogenic keratocysts, calcification of the falx cerebri, skeletal abnormalities)
- Cancer predisposing syndrome most strongly associated with medulloblastoma (~ 6% of medulloblastoma patients)

Turcot Syndrome Type 2

- Caused by germline mutations in *APC* leading to activation of WNT signaling pathway
- Patients may develop medulloblastomas and CNS-PNET

Hereditary Retinoblastoma

- Patients may develop embryonal tumors involving CNS in addition to retinoblastoma (i.e., trilateral retinoblastoma)
- Usually midline, ~ 80% centered in pineal gland (pineoblastoma)
- Remainder mostly in suprasellar region

Li-Fraumeni Syndrome

- Autosomal dominant syndrome characterized by germline *TP53* mutations
- Leads to development of a variety of neoplasms, including sarcomas, adrenocortical carcinomas, and brain tumors
- Astrocytomas and choroid plexus carcinomas more typical of syndrome, but medulloblastomas may also develop

CLINICAL ISSUES

Epidemiology

- Age
  - Predominantly childhood neoplasms
    - ~ 20-30% of medulloblastoma develop in adults (usually 2nd-3rd decades)

Site

- Medulloblastoma
  - By definition, involves posterior fossa
    - Cerebellar vermis, cerebellar hemispheres > 4th ventricle
- CNS-PNET
  - Cerebral hemispheres most frequently affected
  - Often near cerebral ventricles
  - Occasionally suprasellar region, brainstem, spinal cord

MEDULLOBLASTOMA/CNS-PNET

Key Facts

Terminology

- Malignant embryonal neoplasms with predominant neuronal differentiation arising in CNS parenchyma (central nervous system primitive neuroectodermal tumor [CNS-PNET]) or cerebellum/4th ventricle region (medulloblastoma)

Etiology/Pathogenesis

- Tumor predisposition syndromes associated with medulloblastoma/CNS-PNET include Gorlin syndrome, Turcot syndrome type 2, hereditary retinoblastoma, Li-Fraumeni syndrome
- Majority of medulloblastomas and CNS-PNETs develop sporadically without a family history

Microscopic Pathology

- Desmoplastic/nodular: Pale nodules reflective of neuronal differentiation, and proliferative reticulin-rich internodular areas; frequent in Gorlin syndrome
- Classic: Prototypical embryonal round blue cell tumor
- Anaplastic/large cell: Characterized by nuclear enlargement (anaplastic) or large nuclei with macronucleoli (large); histologic marker of poor prognosis
- CNS-PNET subtypes include cerebral neuroblastoma, ganglioneuroblastoma, medulloepithelioma, ependymoblastoma, ETANTR, undifferentiated, and nodular
- Molecular subtypes of medulloblastoma and CNS-PNET separated based on gene expression profiles

Presentation

- Medulloblastoma
  - Ataxia, nausea, vomiting, headache
- CNS-PNET
  - Symptoms secondary to mass effect, hydrocephalus

Treatment

- Craniospinal irradiation and chemotherapy

Prognosis

- Aggressive neoplasms with propensity for CSF dissemination
- Potentially curable tumors with aggressive therapy (unlike high-grade astrocytomas)
- Prognosis better for medulloblastoma than CNS-PNET

IMAGE FINDINGS

MR Findings

- Relatively well-circumscribed tumors
- Variable enhancement
- Spinal MR usually performed to assess for CSF dissemination

MICROSCOPIC PATHOLOGY

Histologic Features

- Medulloblastoma
  - Hypercellular neoplasm composed of cells with high nuclear:cytoplasmic ratios
  - Pathologic subtypes
    - Desmoplastic/nodular: Characterized by pale nodules reflective of neuronal differentiation, and proliferative reticulin-rich internodular areas; frequent in Gorlin syndrome
    - Medulloblastoma with extensive nodularity: May reside in desmoplastic nodular spectrum; affects young children and is associated with better prognosis; a significant proportion associated with Gorlin syndrome
    - Classic: Prototypical embryonal round blue cell tumor; most frequent medulloblastoma subtype
    - Anaplastic/large cell: Characterized by nuclear enlargement (anaplastic) or large nuclei with macronucleoli (large); histologic marker of poor prognosis
- CNS-PNET
  - Heterogeneous group of neoplasms
    - Hypercellular neoplasms with increased mitotic activity
    - Relatively circumscribed neoplasms, but may infiltrate CNS parenchyma
    - Variable extent of neuronal and glial differentiation
  - Histologic subtypes
    - Cerebral neuroblastoma, ganglioneuroblastoma, medulloepithelioma, ependymoblastoma, embryonal tumor with abundant neuropil and true rosettes (ETANTR), undifferentiated, and nodular

ANCILLARY TESTS

Immunohistochemistry

- Synaptophysin expression present in almost all medulloblastomas/CNS-PNET, although extent of staining variable
- Other markers of neuronal differentiation (e.g., neurofilament protein, chromogranin, NeuN) may also be positive, but less consistent
- GFAP may also be expressed
  - Usually around vessels or nodules in desmoplastic/nodular medulloblastoma variant

Gene Expression Profiling

- 4 distinct molecular subgroups of medulloblastoma recognized
  - *WNT* subgroup
    - Least frequent subgroup (~ 10%) but excellent prognosis (long term survival rates > 90%)
    - Classic histology in almost all

MEDULLOBLASTOMA/CNS-PNET

- β-catenin mutations, monosomy 6; nuclear β-catenin immunolocalization
- Sonic hedgehog (*SHH*) subgroup
  - Frequent in young children and adults, desmoplastic/nodular histology in a proportion (but not all)
  - Intermediate prognosis
  - 9q deletions, *PTCH1/SMO/SUFU* mutations, *GLI2* amplifications; SFRP1, YAP1 and GAB1 detectable by immunohistochemistry
  - *SHH* medulloblastomas with *TP53* mutations have a high frequency of **germline** *TP53* mutations
- Group 3
  - Poor prognosis; mostly classic histology, but relatively high frequency of anaplastic/large cell histology
  - *MYC* amplification; NPR3 expression
- Group 4
  - Most frequent subgroup (~ 35%), intermediate prognosis
  - Isochromosome 17q frequent
- Medulloblastoma subgroups may currently be separated using special platforms in formalin-fixed paraffin-embedded tissues
- PNET is a more heterogeneous group, but distinct from medulloblastoma
  - 3 molecular subgroups of CNS-PNET also characterized by gene expression
    - Group 1 (primitive neural): Worst prognosis; *LIN28* positive
    - Group 2 (oligo-neural): Intermediate prognosis; *OLIG2* positive
    - Group 3 (mesenchymal): Better prognosis; *LIN28*/*OLIG2* negative

DIFFERENTIAL DIAGNOSIS

Neurocytic Tumors

- Central neurocytoma (intraventricular), extraventricular neurocytoma (hemispheric), and cerebellar liponeurocytoma
- Better differentiated, low proliferation
  - Mitoses rare, low Ki-67 labeling index
- Synaptophysin positive (as medulloblastoma/PNET) but also frequently NeuN positive

Lymphoma

- Primary CNS lymphoma almost always large B cell
  - Usually afflicts elderly patients or develops in setting of immunosuppression
  - LCA(+), CD20(+)
- Secondary CNS involvement by lymphoma usually superficial (leptomeninges)

Glial Neoplasms

- May arise at any age and any location in the neuraxis
- Poorly differentiated astrocytomas may be difficult to separate from CNS-PNET
- High-grade oligodendrogliomas may resemble PNET and express neuronal markers
  - Mutant *IDH1*(+), *OLIG2*(+), 1p19q codeleted
- In adults, high-grade gliomas may develop a PNET component
  - Usually high grade (III-IV)
  - Infiltrating glial and PNET components distinct
- Anaplastic ependymoma: EMA(+), perivascular pseudorosettes, true ependymal rosettes

Atypical Teratoid Rhabdoid Tumor

- Component of rhabdoid predisposition syndrome
- May contain a predominant undifferentiated round blue cell component, particularly in very young patients
- Polyphenotypic pattern by immunohistochemistry (EMA, GFAP, SMA, and CK [+])
- INI1 loss in neoplastic cells

Metastasis

- Metastatic embryonal tumors
  - Retinoblastoma, neuroblastoma
- Small cell carcinoma
  - Should be considered in adults

Pineoblastoma

- Embryonal tumor that by definition arises in pineal gland region
- Often grouped with CNS-PNET category, but more properly designated a pineal parenchymal tumor
- May arise in setting of hereditary retinoblastoma (trilateral retinoblastoma)

Olfactory Neuroblastoma (Esthesioneuroblastoma)

- Tumor of adults, cribriform plate involvement

SELECTED REFERENCES

1. Zhukova N et al: Subgroup-specific prognostic implications of TP53 mutation in medulloblastoma. J Clin Oncol. 31(23):2927-35, 2013
2. Northcott PA et al: Rapid, reliable, and reproducible molecular sub-grouping of clinical medulloblastoma samples. Acta Neuropathol. 123(4):615-26, 2012
3. Picard D et al: Markers of survival and metastatic potential in childhood CNS primitive neuro-ectodermal brain tumours: an integrative genomic analysis. Lancet Oncol. 13(8):838-48, 2012
4. Taylor MD et al: Molecular subgroups of medulloblastoma: the current consensus. Acta Neuropathol. 123(4):465-72, 2012
5. Ellison DW et al: Medulloblastoma: clinicopathological correlates of SHH, WNT, and non-SHH/WNT molecular subgroups. Acta Neuropathol. 121(3):381-96, 2011
6. Garrè ML et al: Medulloblastoma variants: age-dependent occurrence and relation to Gorlin syndrome--a new clinical perspective. Clin Cancer Res. 15(7):2463-71, 2009
7. Rieber J et al: Novel oncogene amplifications in tumors from a family with Li-Fraumeni syndrome. Genes Chromosomes Cancer. 48(7):558-68, 2009
8. Amlashi SF et al: Nevoid basal cell carcinoma syndrome: relation with desmoplastic medulloblastoma in infancy. A population-based study and review of the literature. Cancer. 98(3):618-24, 2003
9. Eberhart CG et al: Histopathologic grading of medulloblastomas: a Pediatric Oncology Group study. Cancer. 94(2):552-60, 2002

MEDULLOBLASTOMA/CNS-PNET

Diagrammatic, Gross, and Microscopic Features

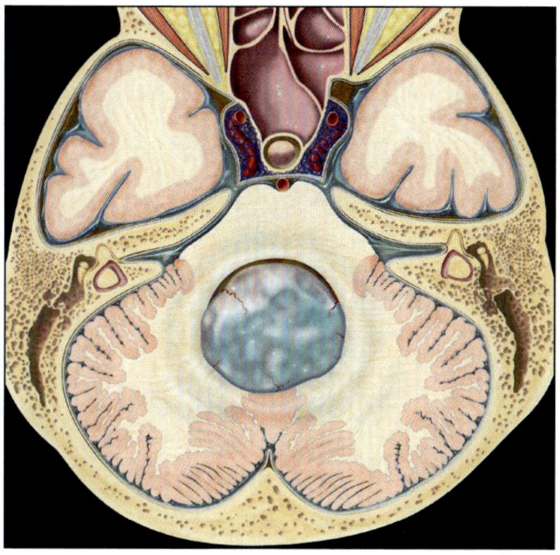

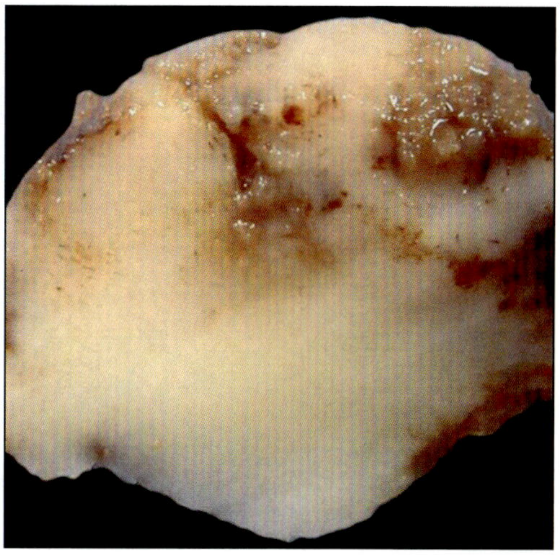

(Left) *Medulloblastomas generally form well-circumscribed masses that, by definition, are centered in the cerebellum/4th ventricle region. Although they may appear well circumscribed, they have a propensity for CSF dissemination. Therefore, not only intracranial imaging but also spinal imaging is recommended for appropriate evaluation.* ***(Right)*** *Medulloblastomas are highly cellular neoplasms and may demonstrate a gray-white appearance on gross cut surface examination.*

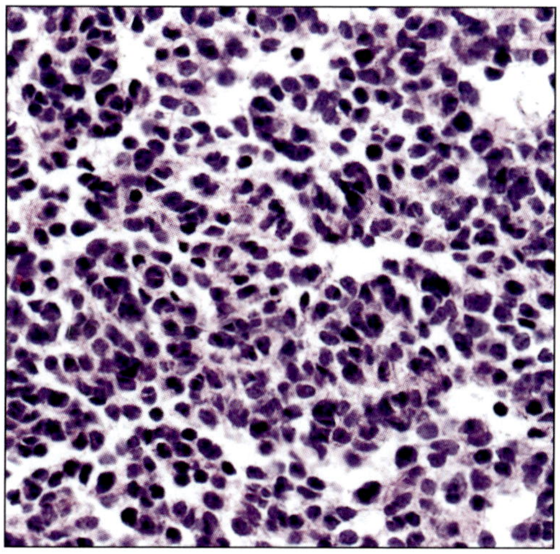

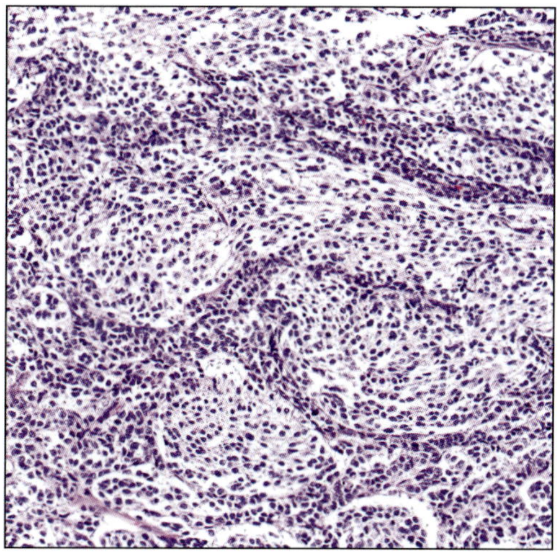

(Left) *Classic medulloblastoma represents the main histologic subtype, characterized by sheets of packed round cells with apoptotic bodies and mitotic activity. Nuclear size varies from small to moderate.* ***(Right)*** *Desmoplastic/nodular medulloblastoma is characterized by pale nodules alternating with a proliferative desmoplastic cellular infiltrate. Molecularly, they demonstrate sonic hedgehog activation and are overrepresented in Gorlin syndrome.*

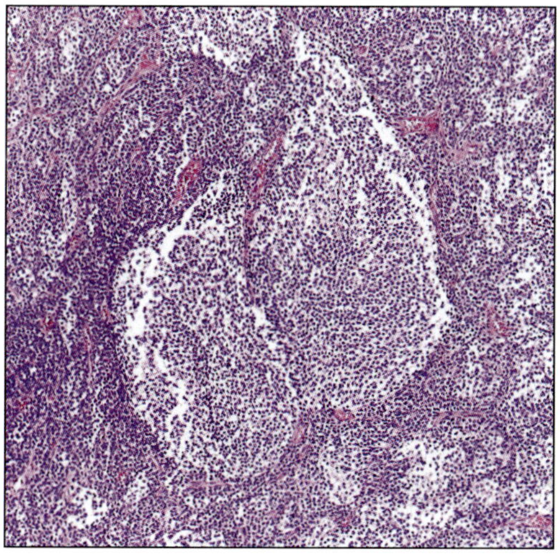

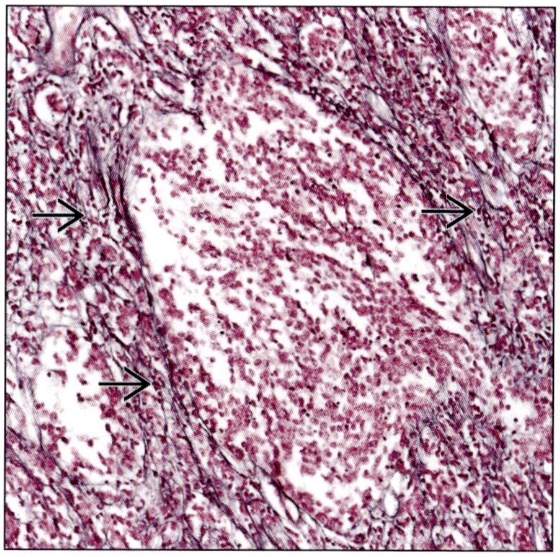

(Left) *Nodules in the desmoplastic/nodular medulloblastoma variant are characterized by variable sizes and shapes. They may be ill defined or well circumscribed, appearing as an area of pallor as shown here. They reflect neuronal differentiation in any embryonal tumor.* ***(Right)*** *The nodules of the desmoplastic/nodular variant of medulloblastoma are reticulin poor, which contrasts with the dense pericellular reticulin of internodular areas ➙.*

Microscopic Features

(Left) *The anaplastic variant of medulloblastoma is defined mainly on the basis of nuclear enlargement. Cell-to-cell wrapping →, apoptotic bodies, and increased mitotic activity are frequent.* ***(Right)*** *The large cell variant is a unique variant of medulloblastoma recognized on the basis of cytologic features. The cells are large, round, and contain a prominent nucleoli. Areas of anaplastic and large cell medulloblastoma may coexist.*

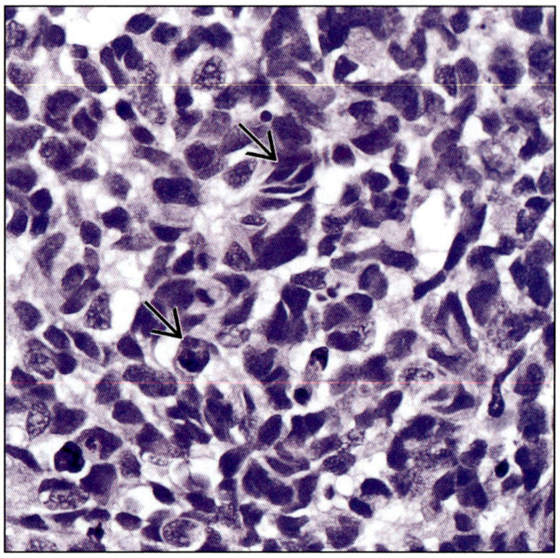

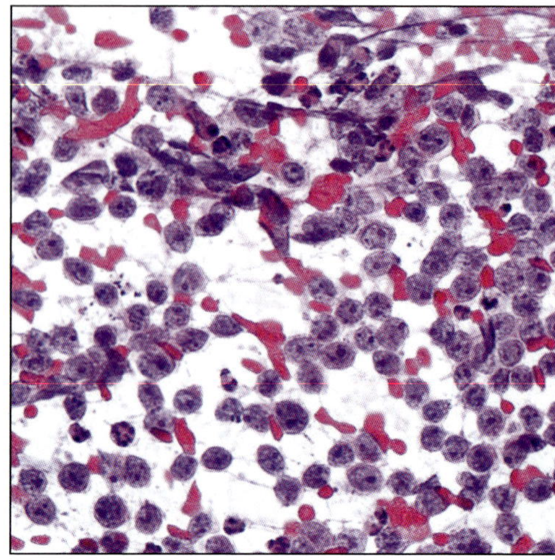

(Left) *Synaptophysin expression is frequent in medulloblastomas and CNS-PNET. Strong expression is evident in this example, but it varies from strong to weak.* ***(Right)*** *GFAP expression may also be present in medulloblastomas and CNS-PNET, although to a limited extent. Labeling tends to be more frequent and stronger around intratumoral vessels →. GFAP expression is also frequent around the nodules of the nodular/desmoplastic variant of medulloblastoma.*

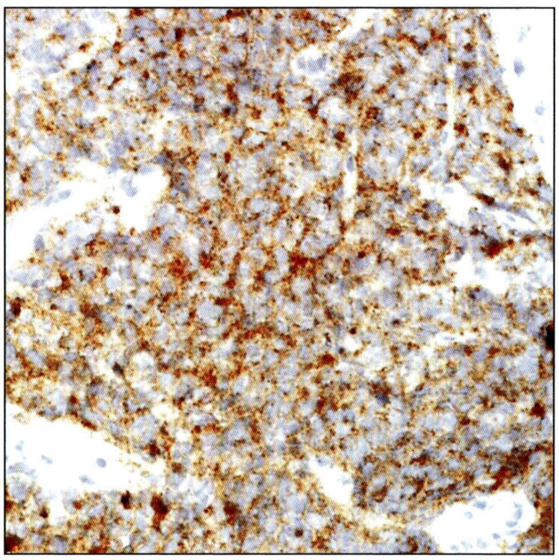

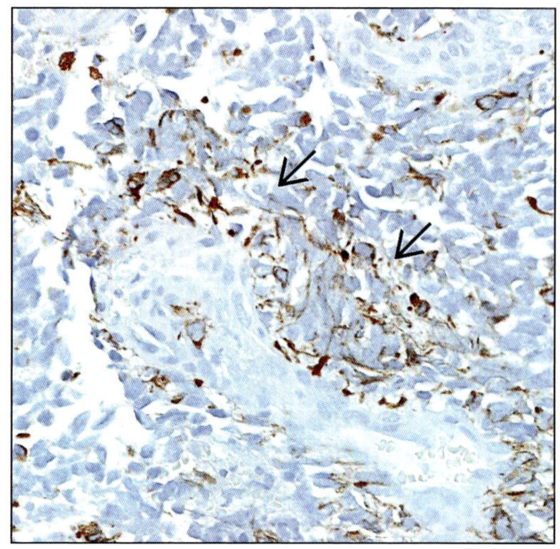

(Left) *Immunohistochemical staining for β-catenin demonstrates a membranous/cytoplasmic pattern in most medulloblastomas. When nuclear staining, it identifies the diagnostically favorable WNT subgroup.* ***(Right)*** *Nuclear INI1 labeling is a feature of all medulloblastomas. INI1 loss by neoplastic cells characterizes atypical teratoid rhabdoid tumor, which is an important entity in the differential diagnosis, particularly of the anaplastic/large cell variant.*

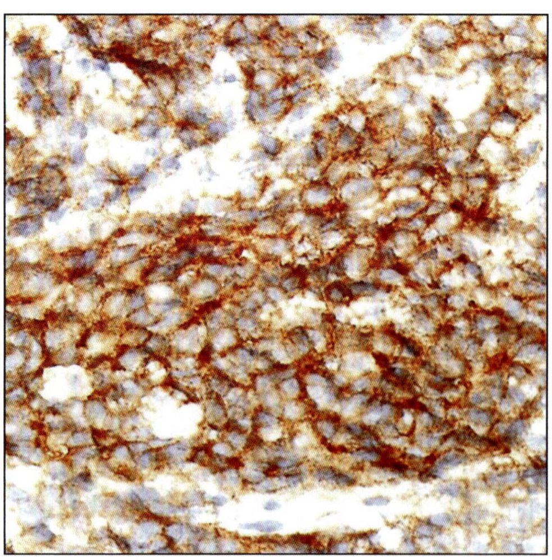

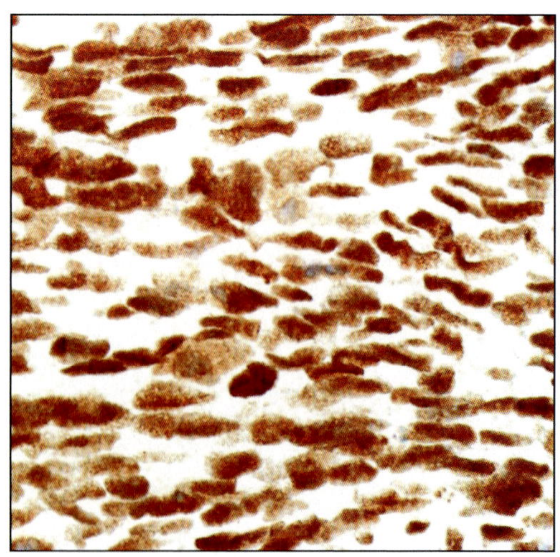

Imaging and Microscopic Features

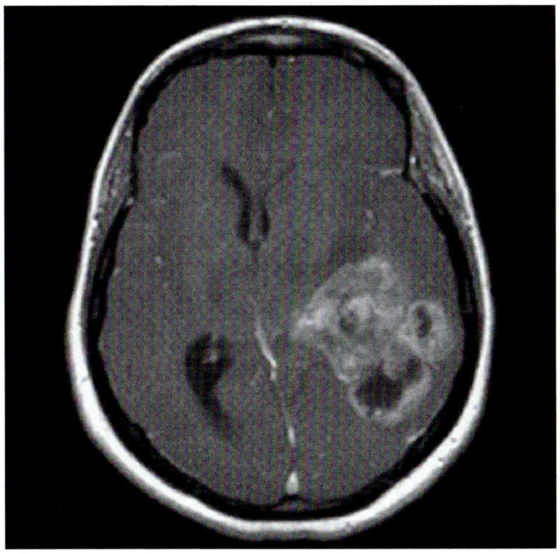
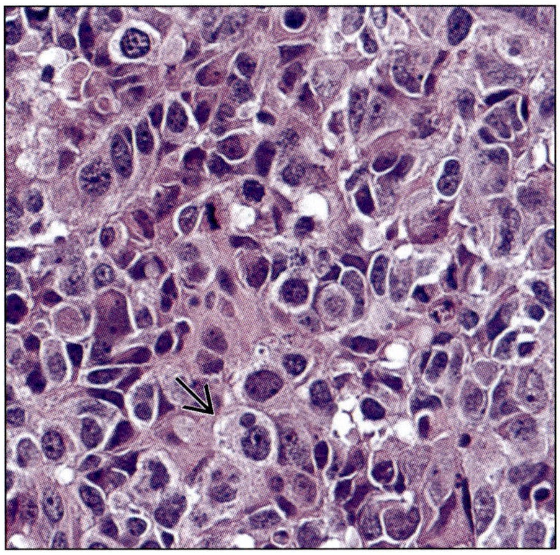

(Left) *CNS-PNETs represent malignant embryonal neoplasms usually developing in the supratentorial compartment. This example developed in a patient with familial adenomatous polyposis (i.e., Turcot type 2 syndrome).* ***(Right)*** *Supratentorial PNETs can arise in familial adenomatous polyposis (FAP) syndrome. This example has considerable nuclear variability and large cells with a ganglioid appearance ⇒.*

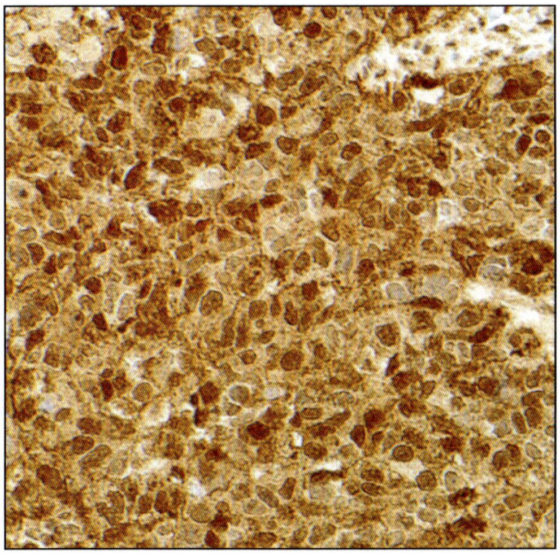
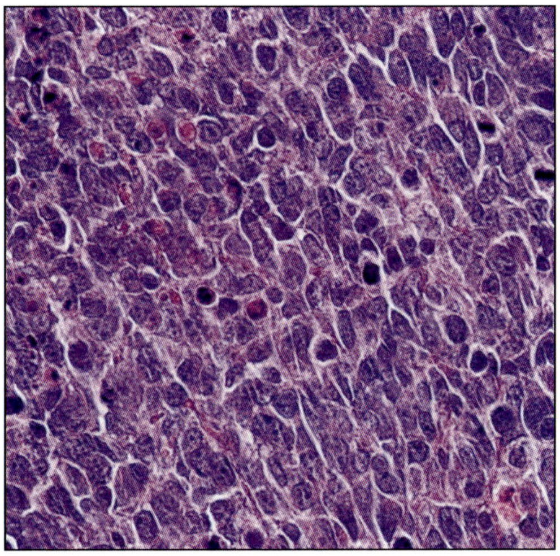

(Left) *Nuclear β-catenin staining (seen in this CNS-PNET in a patient with FAP), reflects activation of the WNT signaling pathway; this pathway is also operational in a subset of medulloblastomas.* ***(Right)*** *CNS-PNET are highly cellular neoplasms composed of sheets of cells with high nuclear:cytoplasmic ratios, frequent apoptotic bodies, and mitotic activity. They are analogous to medulloblastoma, although they are distinct at the molecular level.*

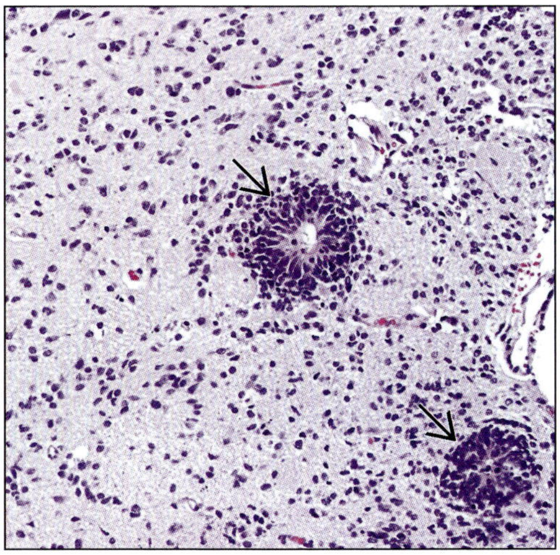
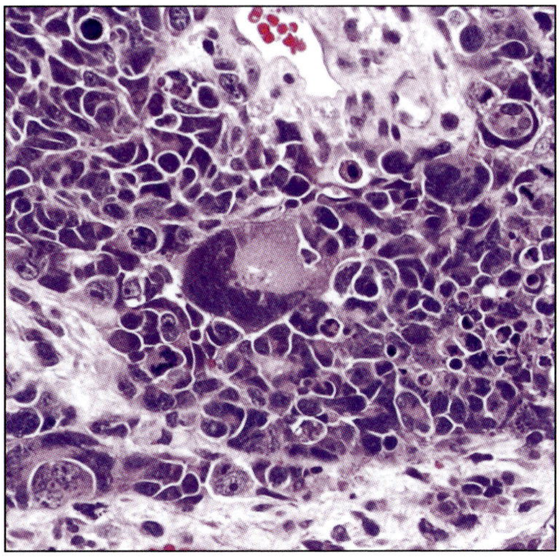

(Left) *Distinctive subtypes of CNS-PNET include the embryonal tumor with abundant neuropil and true rosettes (ETANTR), which, as the name implies, contains large areas of neuropil as well as distinctive rosettes with central lumina ⇒.* ***(Right)*** *A PNET component may be part, and a dominant feature, of high-grade gliomas with PNET components. Careful histologic and immunohistochemical analysis must be pursued in those tumors to identify the glial component.*

MENINGIOMA

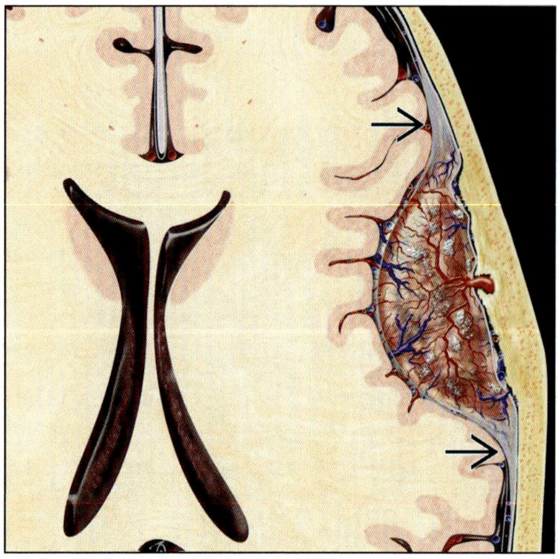

Meningiomas are usually well-circumscribed neoplasms that arise in relation to the dura ⇒. They are well vascularized, which explains the typical contrast enhancement in imaging studies.

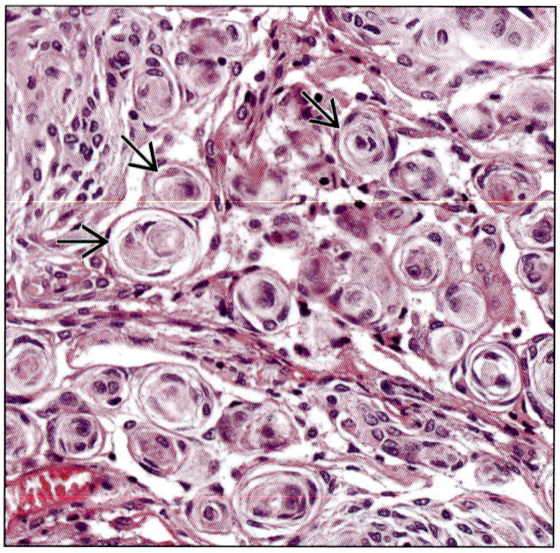

The prototypical histologic meningioma subtype is the meningotheliomatous, characterized by cohesive nests and indistinct cell borders. Whorls are conspicuous in this neurofibromatosis type 2-associated example ⇒.

TERMINOLOGY

Definitions

- Neoplasm with differentiation along meningothelial (arachnoid) cell types, usually associated with dura

ETIOLOGY/PATHOGENESIS

Neurofibromatosis Type 2 (NF2)

- *NF2* gene frequently inactivated in meningioma
- Multiple meningiomas represent a frequent component of NF2 syndrome

Schwannomatosis With Multiple Meningiomas

- Most schwannomatosis patients develop schwannomas only
- Rare families described with multiple schwannomas and meningiomas and with *SMARCB1* germline mutations
  - Meningiomas predominantly intracranial and located in falx cerebri

Familial Multiple Meningioma Disease

- Most meningiomas arise sporadically; familial in 1-5%, multiple in < 10%
- May occur in a subset of families lacking other tumor types (e.g., schwannomas)
- Germline mutation in *SUFU* (negative regulatior of Hh signaling) with loss of heterozygosity identified in 1 family with multiple meningiomas
- Subset of familial multiple spinal meningiomas associated with heterozygous *SMARCE1* inactivating mutations and clear cell histology

MICROSCOPIC PATHOLOGY

Histologic Features

- Frequent features include cohesive nests of cells with indistinct borders, nuclear grooves/inclusions, whorls, and psammoma bodies (i.e., concentric calcifications)
- Subtypes include meningothelial, fibrous (fibroblastic), transitional, psammomatous, angiomatous, microcystic, secretory, lymphoplasmacytic-rich, chordoid (WHO grade II), clear cell (WHO grade II), rhabdoid (WHO grade III), and papillary (WHO grade III)
- NF2-associated meningiomas histologically similar to sporadic counterparts
- May be associated with meningioangiomatosis in either sporadic or NF2-associated cases

ANCILLARY TESTS

Cytogenetics

- Chromosome 22 loss most frequent alteration (~ 2/3 of cases)
  - Most frequent in fibroblastic, transitional, and psammomatous subtypes
- Losses of 1p, 6q, 10, 14q, &/or 18q associated with atypical or anaplastic subtypes
- Gains of 1q, 9q, 12q, 15q, 17q, &/or 20q also associated with atypical or anaplastic subtypes

Molecular Genetics

- Inactivating mutations in *NF2* present in ~ 1/2 of meningiomas
- Oncogenic mutations in *AKT1* and *SMO* present in a meningioma subset associated with activation of PI3K and sonic hedgehog pathways
- Combined *TRAF7* and *KLF4* mutations characterize secretory meningioma and are mutually exclusive with *NF2* mutations

MENINGIOMA

Key Facts

Etiology/Pathogenesis

- *NF2* gene frequently inactivated in meningioma
- Multiple meningiomas represent a frequent component of the NF2 syndrome
- Rare families described with multiple schwannomas and meningiomas and with *SMARCB1* germline mutations
- May occur in a subset of families lacking other tumor types (e.g., schwannomas)
- Subset of familial multiple spinal meningiomas associated with heterozygous *SMARCE1* inactivating mutations and clear cell histology

Ancillary Tests

- Inactivating mutations in *NF2* present in ~ 1/2 of meningiomas
- Oncogenic mutations in *AKT1* and *SMO* present in a meningioma subset associated with activation of PI3K and sonic hedgehog pathways
- Combined *TRAF7* and *KLF4* mutations characterize secretory meningioma and are mutually exclusive with *NF2* mutations

Top Differential Diagnoses

- Meningothelial hyperplasia
- Schwannoma
- Glioblastoma/gliosarcoma
- Metastatic carcinoma
- Mesenchymal neoplasms
  - Solitary fibrous tumor/hemangiopericytoma, dural sarcoma

DIFFERENTIAL DIAGNOSIS

Meningothelial Hyperplasia

- Reactive proliferation associated with a variety of superficial CNS insults (hemorrhage, inflammation, neoplasms)
- Limited in size

Schwannoma

- Important differential with fibrous meningioma and predilection for cerebellopontine angle
- Smears poorly; S100(+), EMA(-)

Mesenchymal Neoplasms

- Solitary fibrous tumor more differentiated, ropy collagen; hemangiopericytoma, increased cellularity and more aggressive clinical behavior
  - CD34(+), EMA(-)
- Dural sarcomas usually high grade, overtly malignant with high cellularity, fascicular pattern of growth, brisk mitotic activity

Glioblastoma/Gliosarcoma

- Superficial high-grade gliomas may extend to dura
- GFAP(+), usually EMA(-)

Metastatic Carcinoma

- Cytokeratin (+) whereas meningiomas are usually cytokeratin (-)

GRADING

WHO Grade I

- Low proliferative activity (< 4 mitoses per 10 high-power fields) and lack of brain invasion

WHO Grade II

- Increased mitotic activity (≥ 4 per 10 high-power fields) **or** ≥ 3 of the following: Hypercellularity, sheet-like growth, macronucleoli, small cell change, necrosis (in the absence of embolization) **or** brain invasion **or** chordoid/clear cell histologic subtypes

WHO Grade III

- ≥ 20 mitoses per 10 high-power fields **or** histologic malignancy (i.e., resembling carcinoma or sarcoma) **or** rhabdoid/papillary histologic subtypes

SELECTED REFERENCES

1. Brastianos PK et al: Genomic sequencing of meningiomas identifies oncogenic SMO and AKT1 mutations. Nat Genet. 45(3):285-9, 2013
2. Clark VE et al: Genomic analysis of non-NF2 meningiomas reveals mutations in TRAF7, KLF4, AKT1, and SMO. Science. 339(6123):1077-80, 2013
3. Reuss DE et al: Secretory meningiomas are defined by combined KLF4 K409Q and TRAF7 mutations. Acta Neuropathol. 125(3):351-8, 2013
4. Smith MJ et al: Loss-of-function mutations in SMARCE1 cause an inherited disorder of multiple spinal meningiomas. Nat Genet. 45(3):295-8, 2013
5. Aavikko M et al: Loss of SUFU function in familial multiple meningioma. Am J Hum Genet. 91(3):520-6, 2012
6. van den Munckhof P et al: Germline SMARCB1 mutation predisposes to multiple meningiomas and schwannomas with preferential location of cranial meningiomas at the falx cerebri. Neurogenetics. 13(1):1-7, 2012
7. Christiaans I et al: Germline SMARCB1 mutation and somatic NF2 mutations in familial multiple meningiomas. J Med Genet. 48(2):93-7, 2011
8. Bacci C et al: Schwannomatosis associated with multiple meningiomas due to a familial SMARCB1 mutation. Neurogenetics. 11(1):73-80, 2010
9. Stemmer-Rachamimov AO et al: Meningioangiomatosis is associated with neurofibromatosis 2 but not with somatic alterations of the NF2 gene. J Neuropathol Exp Neurol. 56(5):485-9, 1997
10. Wellenreuther R et al: Analysis of the neurofibromatosis 2 gene reveals molecular variants of meningioma. Am J Pathol. 146(4):827-32, 1995

MENINGIOMA

Imaging and Microscopic Features

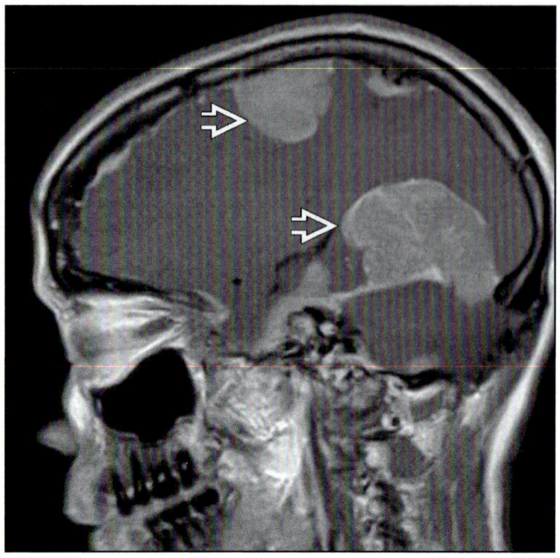

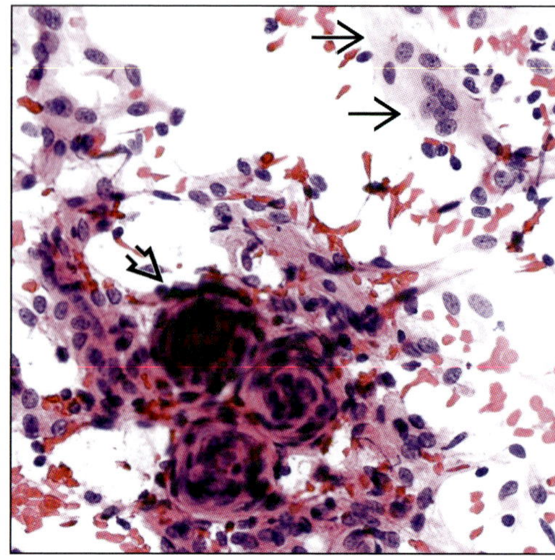

(Left) *Meningiomas are the 2nd most common neoplasms in NF2 patients. They are usually dura-based, multiple in these patients, and demonstrate strong, homogeneous contrast enhancement after administration of gadolinium in T1-weighted MR sequences ⇨.* ***(Right)*** *Diagnostic properties of meningioma are usually evident on smear preparations, including flat cells → and whorls with psammoma bodies ⇨.*

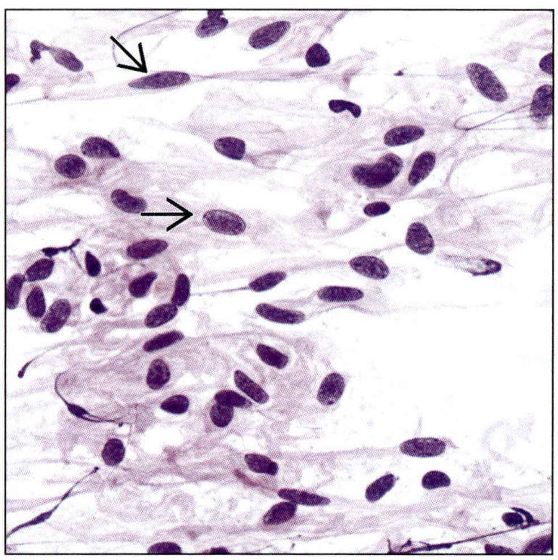

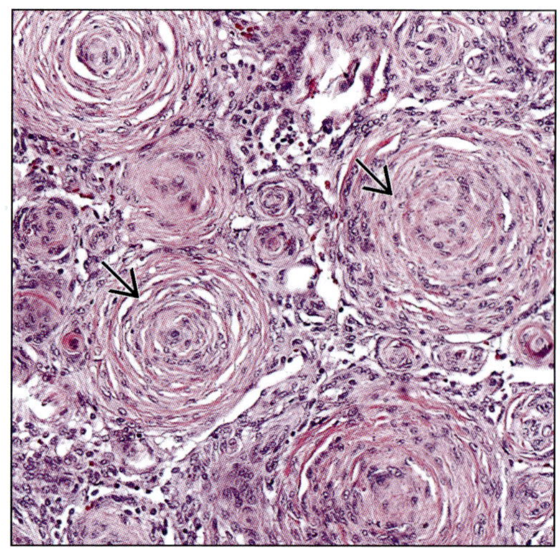

(Left) *Meningiomas are usually characterized by bland, flat cells with oval nuclei in smear preparations. In this specific example arising in a woman with NF2, Barr bodies are present →. Barr bodies, representing the inactive X chromosome, are a cytologic feature supporting the female sex and often seen in meningiomas.* ***(Right)*** *The presence of whorls is 1 of the architectural hallmarks of meningioma. Numerous whorls are present in this meningioma arising in a patient with NF2 →.*

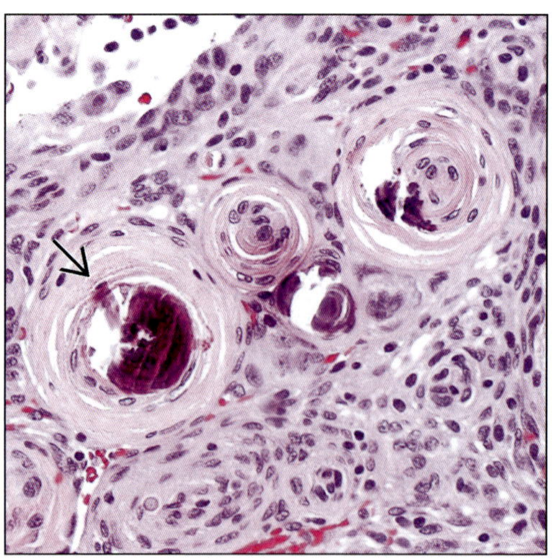

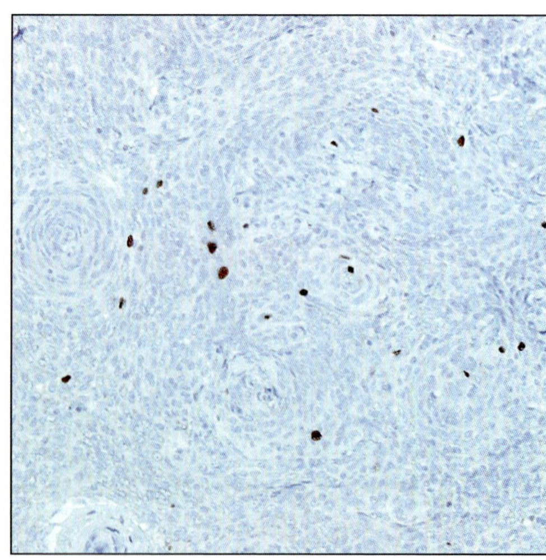

(Left) *Psammoma bodies → represent peculiar calcifications with concentric arrangements occurring in the center of meningioma whorls. When numerous and occupying every field, the diagnosis of psammomatous meningioma may be appropriate.* ***(Right)*** *Most meningiomas are WHO grade I and demonstrate low proliferative rates. Ki-67/MIB1, which labels cells that are actively in the cell cycle, stains only rare nuclei in these tumors.*

Microscopic Features

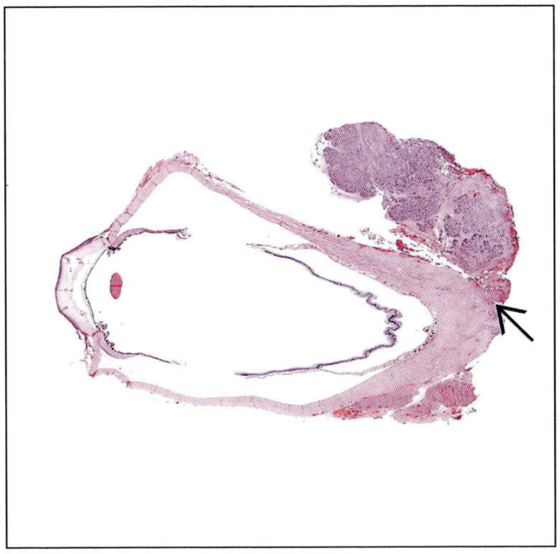

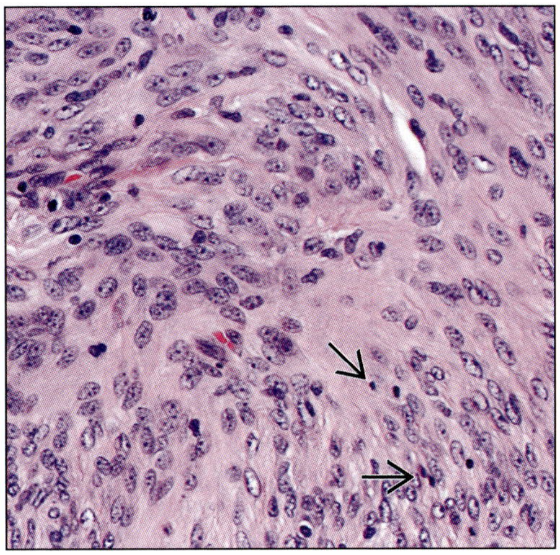

(Left) *Meningiomas in NF2 patients are usually multiple and may arise in any anatomic site, including the orbit. Many intraorbital meningiomas develop in close relation to the optic nerve sheath* →. ***(Right)*** *Increased mitotic activity may occur in a subset of meningiomas and represents an important criterion for grading. In this atypical meningioma (WHO grade II), mitotic activity is not subtle* → *and exceeds 4 mitotic figures per 10 high-power fields.*

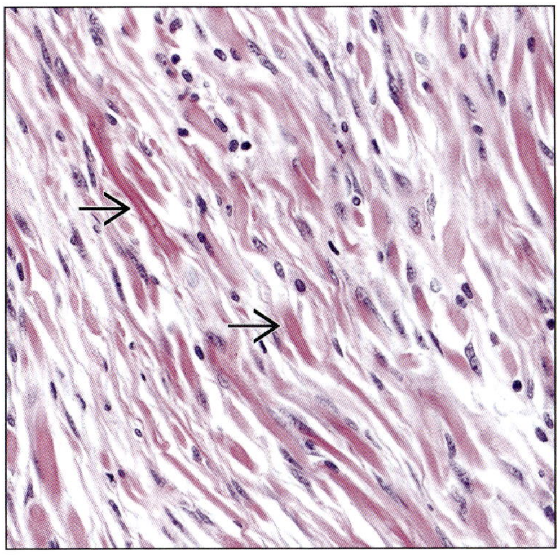

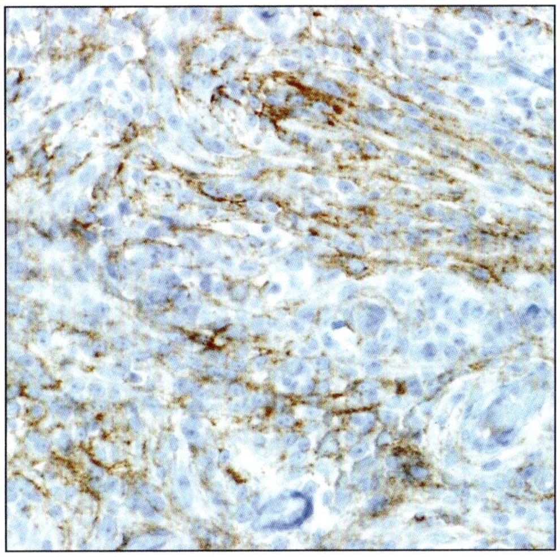

(Left) *The fibrous meningioma subtype is characterized by the presence of spindle cells. Bright, eosinophilic collagen bundles may be present* →*, which raises the differential diagnosis to a variety of mesenchymal neoplasms, particularly solitary fibrous tumor.* ***(Right)*** *Most meningiomas, regardless of the subtype, express EMA, although the immunoreactivity is variable and usually not to the extent of epithelium. A linear/membranous pattern is common.*

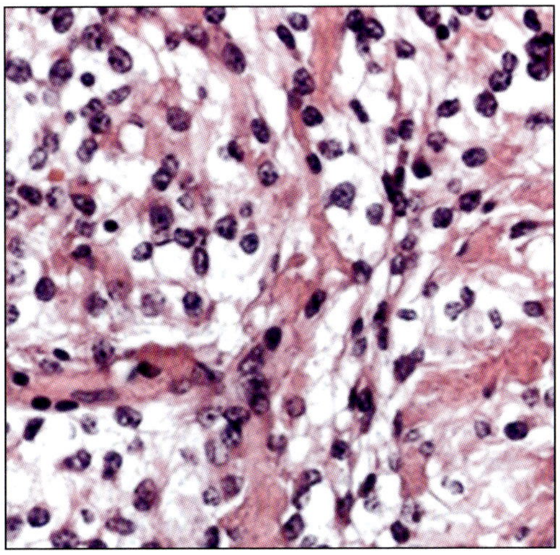

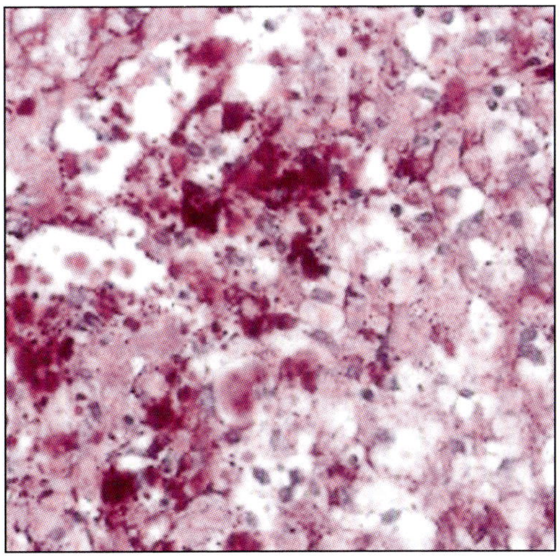

(Left) *Clear cell meningioma is a unique subtype with more aggressive behavior. This tumor arose in a patient with a germline heterozygous SMARCE1 mutation, a recently recognized familial meningioma syndrome. These patients are predisposed to the development of clear cell meningiomas. (Courtesy D.G. Evans, MD.)* ***(Right)*** *Meningiomas associated with SMARCE1 mutations are of the clear cell type. PAS highlights glycogen. (Courtesy D. G. Evans, MD.)*

PINEOBLASTOMA

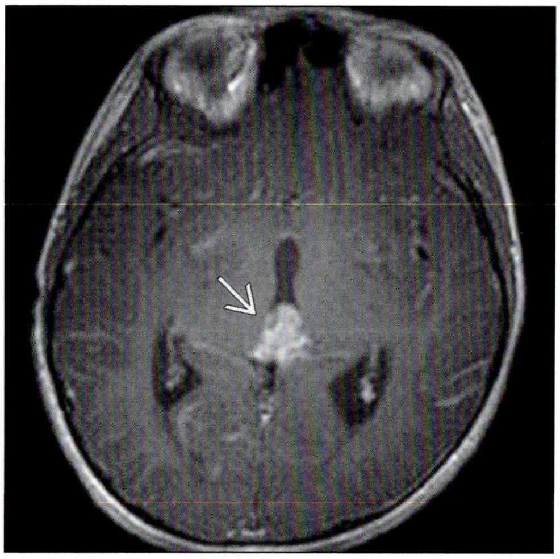

Pineoblastomas are malignant neoplasms presenting as contrast-enhancing masses in the pineal region ➡. Associated hydrocephalus is a frequent finding.

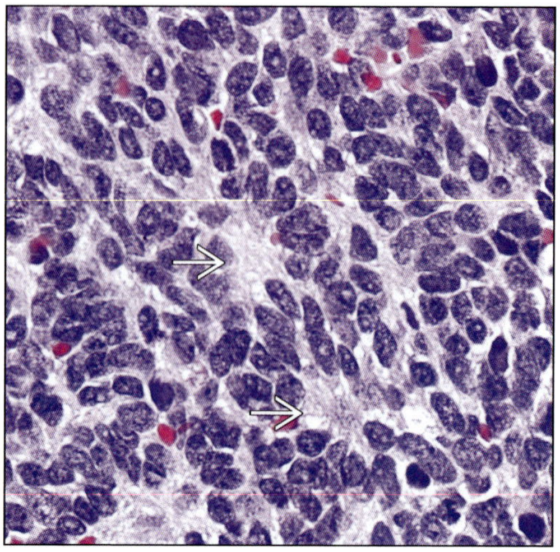

Pineoblastomas are hypercellular, round blue cell tumors. Neuronal differentiation is reflected in the form of small Homer Wright rosettes ➡.

TERMINOLOGY

Definitions

- Malignant, high-grade embryonal neoplasm centered in pineal region

ETIOLOGY/PATHOGENESIS

Syndrome Association

- Most pineoblastomas arise sporadically without syndrome association
- May arise in patients with *RB1* germline mutations
- Also may develop in setting of Turcot type 2 (familial adenomatous polyposis) with associated *APC* mutations
- Rare report of pineoblastoma developing in a patient with germline *DICER1* mutation and subsequent loss of heterozygosity

Trilateral Retinoblastoma Syndrome

- Bilateral retinoblastoma + intracranial/midline embryonal tumor, *RB1* germline mutation
- Occurs in < 1% of patients with retinoblastoma
- Intracranial tumor frequently (~ 80%) in pineal region = pineoblastoma ("3rd eye")
- 1 report of trilateral retinoblastoma in Peutz-Jeghers syndrome patient with germline *LKB1/STK11* mutation

CLINICAL ISSUES

Epidemiology

- ~ 40% of pineal parenchymal tumors, ~ 20% of nonmedulloblastoma primitive neuroectodermal tumors (PNET) affecting CNS
- More common in children < 3 years of age

Presentation

- Pineal region mass with associated hydrocephalus, tectal plate compression, paralysis of vertical gaze

Prognosis

- Related to age (worse in young children)
- Poor in patients with trilateral retinoblastoma syndrome

IMAGE FINDINGS

MR Findings

- Heterogeneous enhancing mass

CT Findings

- Calcifications rare to absent

MICROSCOPIC PATHOLOGY

Histologic Features

- Sheets of tightly packed round cells with brisk mitotic activity, similar to other embryonal neoplasms
- Lack of pineocytomatous rosettes
- Homer Wright rosettes → acellular synaptophysin positive cores; Flexner-Wintersteiner rosettes → contain a central lumen, consistent with retinoblastic differentiation

ANCILLARY TESTS

Immunohistochemistry

- Expresses same neuronal antigens as other PNETs and pineal parenchymal tumors express (e.g., synaptophysin)
  - GFAP usually negative (highlights entrapped astrocytes)
- High Ki-67 labeling index

PINEOBLASTOMA

Key Facts

Terminology
- Malignant, high-grade embryonal neoplasm centered in pineal region

Etiology/Pathogenesis
- May arise in patients with *RB1* germline mutations
- Trilateral retinoblastoma: Bilateral retinoblastoma + intracranial/midline embryonal tumor
  - Intracranial tumor frequently (80%) in pineal region = pineoblastoma ("3rd eye")

Clinical Issues
- ~ 40% of pineal parenchymal tumors

Microscopic Pathology
- Sheets of tightly packed round cells with brisk mitotic activity, similar to other embryonal neoplasms

Ancillary Tests
- Expresses same neuronal antigens that other PNETs and pineal parenchymal tumors express

Molecular Genetics
- Genomic imbalance lower in pineoblastomas compared with other CNS-PNET in single nucleotide polymorphism (SNP) array studies
  - Copy number gains in gene regions of *PCDHGA3* (5q31.3) and *FAM129A* (1q25)
  - Copy number losses in gene region of *OR4C12* (11p11.12)
- Cytogenetic alterations in *RB1* and *TP53* mutations are not a feature of sporadic pineoblastoma

DIFFERENTIAL DIAGNOSIS

Pineal Parenchymal Tumors
- Pineocytoma (WHO grade I) and pineal parenchymal tumor of intermediate differentiation (WHO grades II-III)
- Grading systems complex but based on mitotic activity and extent of differentiation (i.e., neurofilament protein expression)

Medulloblastoma/CNS-PNET
- Similar histology but distinct anatomic location and molecular features

Papillary Tumor of Pineal Region
- Epithelial morphology and keratin expression (CAM 5.2)

Germ Cell Tumors
- Mainly germinoma, but other patterns also possible
- Immunoreactivity for germ cell markers (PLAP, OCT4, SALL4, AFP)

Metastatic Carcinoma
- Important consideration in adults
- Expression of epithelial markers (keratin, EMA)

SELECTED REFERENCES

1. Raizis AM et al: Trilateral retinoblastoma in a patient with Peutz-Jeghers syndrome. Am J Med Genet A. 161A(5):1096-100, 2013
2. Sabbaghian N et al: Germline DICER1 mutation and associated loss of heterozygosity in a pineoblastoma. J Med Genet. 49(7):417-9, 2012
3. Miller S et al: Genome-wide molecular characterization of central nervous system primitive neuroectodermal tumor and pineoblastoma. Neuro Oncol. 13(8):866-79, 2011
4. Antoneli CB et al: Trilateral retinoblastoma. Pediatr Blood Cancer. 48(3):306-10, 2007
5. Gadish T et al: Pinealoblastoma in a patient with familial adenomatous polyposis: variant of Turcot syndrome type 2? Report of a case and review of the literature. Dis Colon Rectum. 48(12):2343-6, 2005
6. Li MH et al: Molecular genetics of supratentorial primitive neuroectodermal tumors and pineoblastoma. Neurosurg Focus. 19(5):E3, 2005
7. Jouvet A et al: Pineal parenchymal tumors: a correlation of histological features with prognosis in 66 cases. Brain Pathol. 10(1):49-60, 2000

IMAGE GALLERY

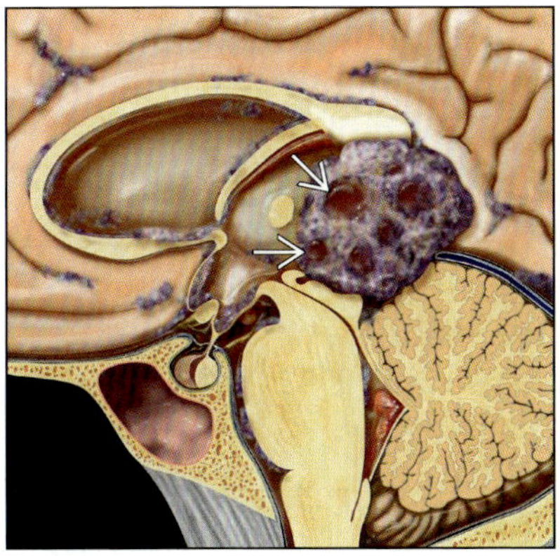
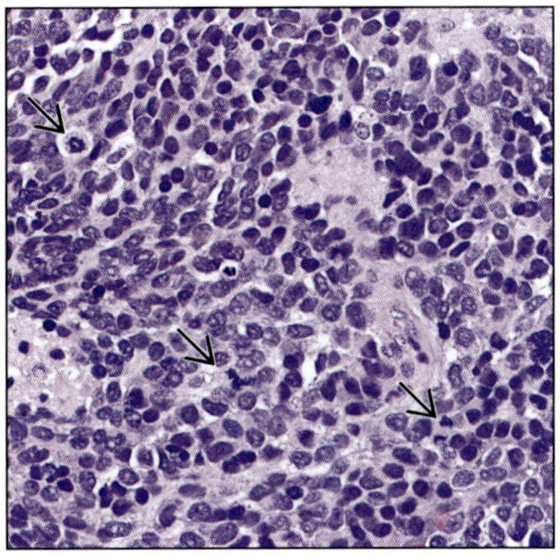
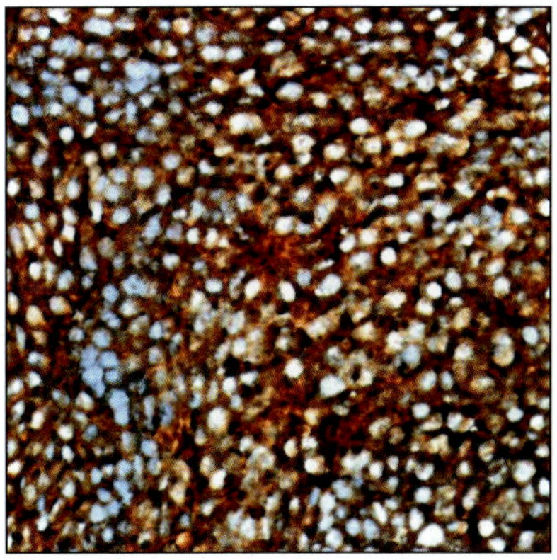

(Left) *Pineoblastomas may present as large masses with an epicenter in the pineal region and associated areas of heterogeneity* ➡*.* ***(Center)*** *Brisk mitotic activity* ➡ *is an important histologic property of pineoblastoma that distinguishes it from other, better differentiated pineal parenchymal tumors. Necrosis may also be present.* ***(Right)*** *All pineal parenchymal tumors are characterized by the expression of neuronal markers, particularly synaptophysin.*

RETINOBLASTOMA

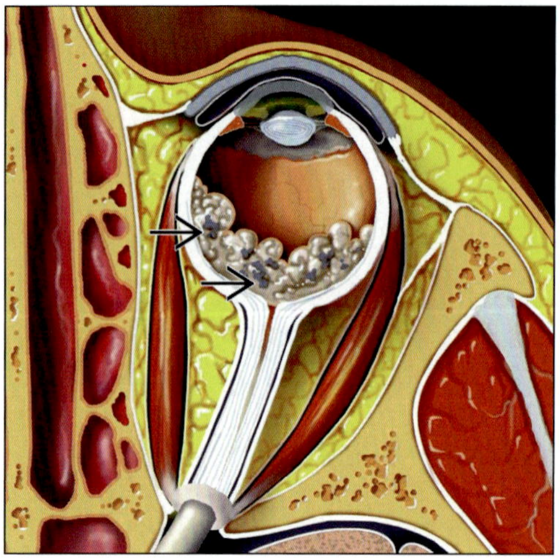

Retinoblastoma may have lobulated contours and extend through the limiting membrane into the vitreous. Punctate calcifications ➔ are characteristic.

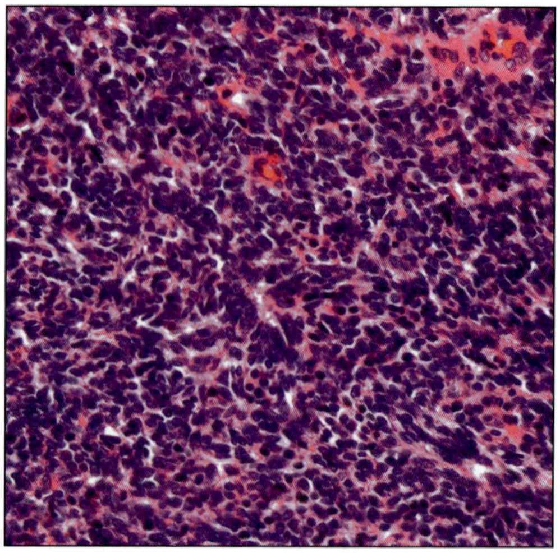

Retinoblastoma is a cellular malignant neoplasm composed of cells with high nuclear:cytoplasmic ratios, forming sheets.

TERMINOLOGY

Abbreviations

- Retinoblastoma (RB)

Definitions

- Malignant embryonal neoplasm centered in the retina and demonstrating variable photoreceptor differentiation

ETIOLOGY/PATHOGENESIS

Developmental Anomaly

- Loss or inactivation of both alleles of retinoblastoma gene (*RB1*)
  - Located at 13q14
  - Tumor suppressor gene
- Knudson "2-hit" hypothesis
  - RB results from 2 independent mutations
    - 1st mutation may be either somatic (sporadic) or germinal (inherited)
    - 2nd mutation is sporadic

CLINICAL ISSUES

Epidemiology

- Incidence
  - Most common intraocular malignancy in children
- Age
  - Average age at diagnosis is 18-24 months
  - Younger in bilateral/familial cases
- Gender
  - No predilection
- Ethnicity
  - No predilection

Site

- Sporadic RB is usually unilateral
- Inherited RB is often bilateral
  - May include pineal tumor (so-called trilateral RB)
  - Quadrilateral RB is very rare and includes bilateral RB plus pineal and suprasellar tumors

Presentation

- Leukocoria (white pupil)
  - Frequently noticed in photographs
- Strabismus
- Decreased visual acuity
- Glaucoma
- Red, painful eye
- Up to 40% have genetic predisposition
  - 5-10% have family history of RB
  - Remainder are new germline mutations

Treatment

- Depends on tumor size, intraocular location, and histopathologic risk factors

Prognosis

- If untreated, invariably fatal
- Poor prognosis if direct scleral invasion or invasion of optic nerve
- 90% cure rate if noninvasive
- 2nd cancers common in patients with *RB1* mutations
  - Incidence is higher in inherited RB
  - Osteosarcoma, soft tissue sarcoma, melanoma, Hodgkin lymphoma, breast carcinoma

IMAGE FINDINGS

General Features

- Calcified intraocular mass
- Diagnosis often made by imaging only

RETINOBLASTOMA

Key Facts

Etiology/Pathogenesis

- Loss or inactivation of both alleles of retinoblastoma gene (*RB1* gene)
  - Knudson "2-hit" hypothesis

Clinical Issues

- Most common intraocular malignancy in children
- Average age at diagnosis: 18-24 months
- Up to 40% have genetic predisposition
- 2nd cancers common in patients with *RB1* mutations
  - Osteosarcoma, soft tissue sarcoma, melanoma, Hodgkin lymphoma, breast carcinoma
- Leukocoria is most common clinical presentation

Image Findings

- Calcified intraocular mass
- Diagnosis often made by imaging only

Microscopic Pathology

- Small round blue cell tumor
- Variable appearance based on degree of differentiation
  - Flexner-Wintersteiner rosettes have central lumen
  - Fleurette shows photoreceptor differentiation
- Ischemic necrosis common
- Calcifications common

Top Differential Diagnoses

- Primitive neuroectodermal tumor (PNET)
- Leukemia/lymphoma
- Astrocytoma
- Medulloepithelioma

MACROSCOPIC FEATURES

General Features

- Creamy white appearance, calcifications and necrosis
- Growth patterns
  - Endophytic: Growth inward toward vitreous cavity
  - Exophytic: Growth outward toward subretinal space and choroid
    - Detaches retina; still may fill vitreous cavity
  - Diffusely infiltrating: Thickens retina

MICROSCOPIC PATHOLOGY

Histologic Features

- Small round blue cell tumor
- Flexner-Wintersteiner rosettes
  - Tumor cells surround central lumen that contains acid mucopolysaccharide
  - Tumor nuclei are placed away from central lumen
- Homer Wright rosettes
  - Lack well-defined lumen
- Fleurette
  - Photoreceptor differentiation (well-differentiated RB, "retinocytoma" when completely made of fleurettes)
  - Pattern resembles a fleur-de-lis
- Ischemic necrosis common
  - Surrounds perivascular tumor cells
- Calcifications common
- May invade optic nerve and extend to brain or CSF
- High-risk characteristics include anterior chamber involvement, massive posterior uveal invasion, postlaminar optic nerve invasion, and posterior uveal + optic nerve invasion

DIFFERENTIAL DIAGNOSIS

Primitive Neuroectodermal Tumor (PNET)

- If in eye, would be considered metastatic/secondary extension

Leukemia/Lymphoma

- Immunohistochemical stains for lymphoid markers helpful

Astrocytoma

- Small round blue cell pattern generally not seen in astrocytoma; GFAP(+)

Medulloepithelioma

- Larger rosettes, tubular architecture
- May be benign or malignant; teratoid (i.e., containing heteroplastic elements) or nonteratoid

SELECTED REFERENCES

1. Kaliki S et al: High-risk retinoblastoma based on international classification of retinoblastoma: analysis of 519 enucleated eyes. Ophthalmology. 120(5):997-1003, 2013
2. Kashyap S et al: Clinical predictors of high risk histopathology in retinoblastoma. Pediatr Blood Cancer. 58(3):356-61, 2012
3. Gao YJ et al: Clinical characteristics and treatment outcome of children with intraocular retinoblastoma: a report from a Chinese cooperative group. Pediatr Blood Cancer. 57(7):1113-6, 2011
4. Palamar M et al: Evolution in regression patterns following chemoreduction for retinoblastoma. Arch Ophthalmol. 129(6):727-30, 2011
5. Serrano C et al: Low penetrance hereditary retinoblastoma in a family: what should we consider in the genetic counselling process and follow up? Fam Cancer. 10(3):617-21, 2011
6. Ghosh S et al: Diagnostic accuracy in retinoblastoma. J Indian Med Assoc. 108(8):509, 512-3, 2010
7. Sastre X et al: Proceedings of the consensus meetings from the International Retinoblastoma Staging Working Group on the pathology guidelines for the examination of enucleated eyes and evaluation of prognostic risk factors in retinoblastoma. Arch Pathol Lab Med. 133(8):1199-202, 2009

RETINOBLASTOMA

Clinical and Other Features

(Left) *Leukocoria, or white pupil, is a common presentation of retinoblastoma. This is frequently noticed in photographs. (Courtesy D. Shatzkes, MD.)* ***(Right)*** *Retinoblastoma forms variably sized masses on funduscopic examination. Tumors → are usually white and fluffy. The optic nerve ➡ and macula ⇨ are uninvolved. (Courtesy D. Dries, MD.)*

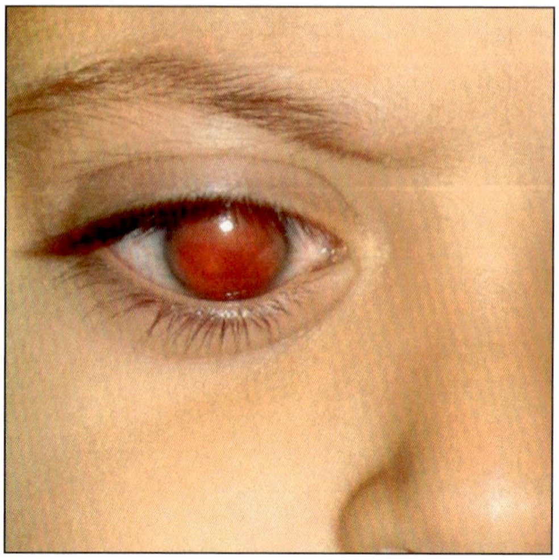

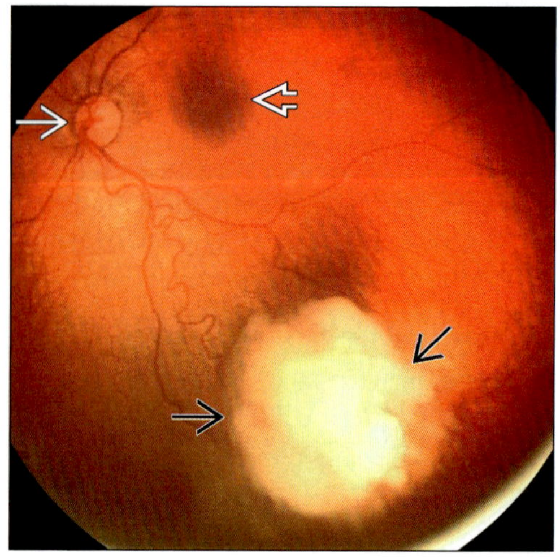

(Left) *Gross pathology shows the macroscopic appearance of the eye after exenteration. Retinoblastoma is a calcified mass that fills the vitreous cavity. (Courtesy B. Ey, MD.)* ***(Right)*** *Retinoblastomas may form large intraocular masses, which block the normal retinal light reflex. Necrosis is a frequent finding and may be identified on low magnification →.*

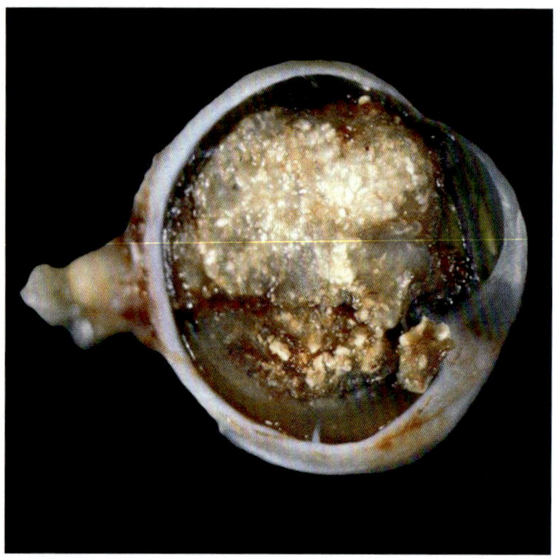

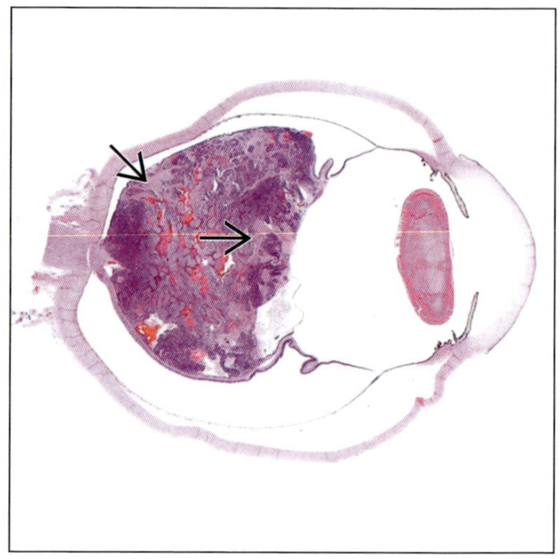

(Left) *Axial CT shows a large, lobulated, partially calcified left intraocular mass ➡, typical of retinoblastoma.* ***(Right)*** *Knudsen "2-hit" hypothesis refers to the sequence in which both copies of a tumor suppressor gene must be mutated for a tumor to develop. The 1st hit may be either inherited (germline, bottom) or sporadic (somatic, top). The 2nd hit is always sporadic (red chromosome contains a mutant copy of a tumor suppressor gene).*

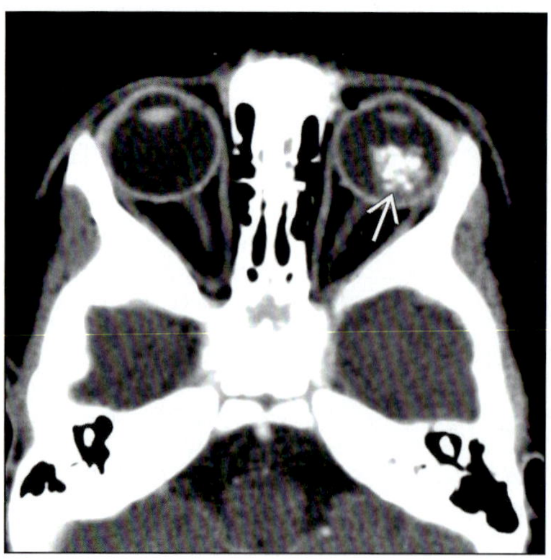

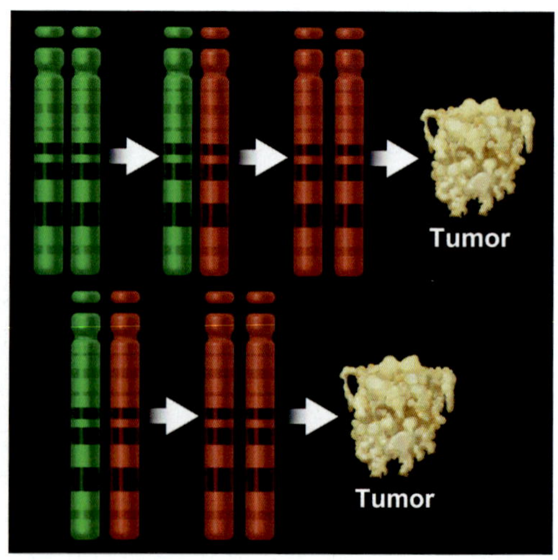

RETINOBLASTOMA

Microscopic Features

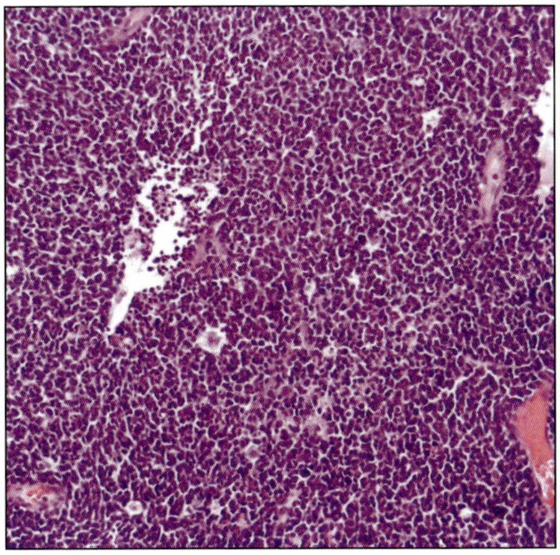
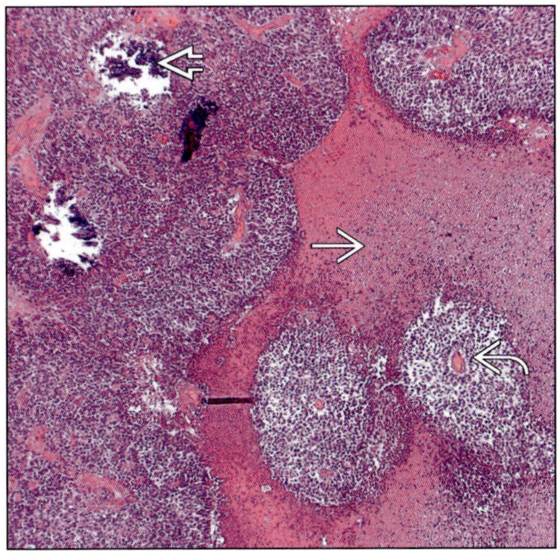

(Left) *Sheets of small round blue cells make up this poorly differentiated retinoblastoma. This field could be mistaken for PNET if the location was not known.* **(Right)** *Necrosis → and calcifications → are very common in retinoblastoma. The necrosis is often seen around vascular spaces →, as the tumor outgrows its blood supply. Calcifications are an important marker in radiologic studies.*

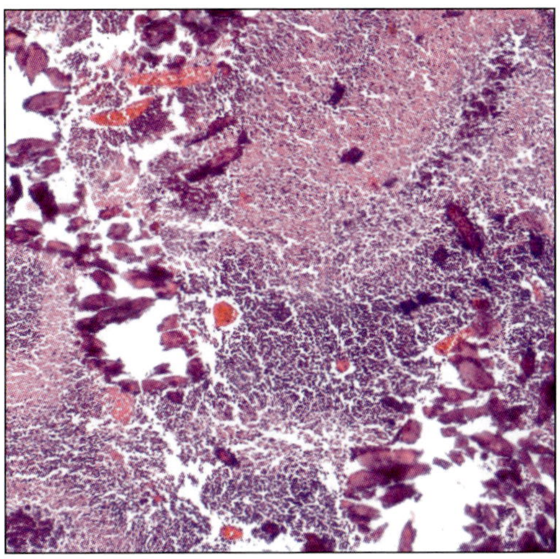
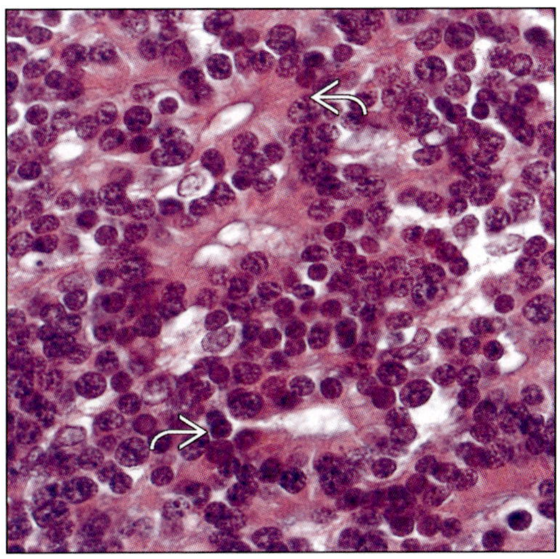

(Left) *Calcifications may be prominent in some examples and are a useful diagnostic finding in x-ray-based imaging studies.* **(Right)** *Flexner-Wintersteiner rosettes → are seen in moderately differentiated retinoblastomas. They have central lumina filled with mucopolysaccharide, and the surrounding tumor cells have their nuclei located away from the lumina.*

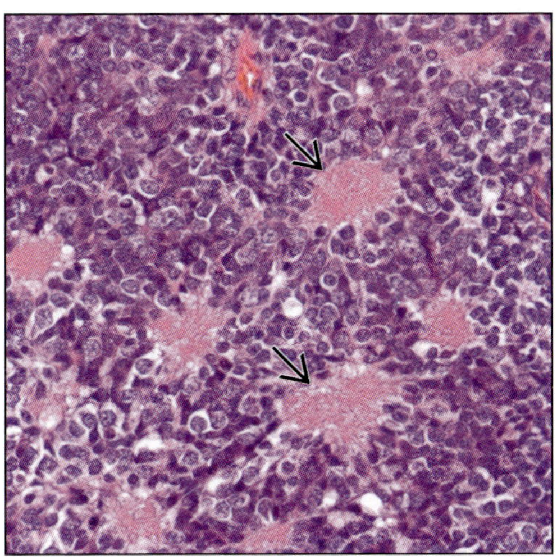
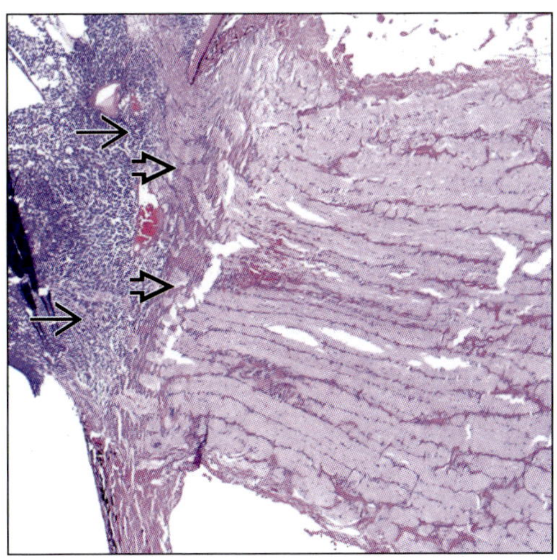

(Left) *Homer Wright rosettes are less specific structures characterized by an anuclear center lacking lumina →. They may be encountered in a variety of tumor types.* **(Right)** *Invasion of the optic nerve → is a negative prognostic factor in retinoblastoma and must be carefully evaluated in all specimens. Extent of invasion is important and the lamina cribrosa represents an important landmark →. Invasion beyond the lamina cribrosa is associated with an ominous prognosis.*

Pulmonary

ADENOCARCINOMA, LUNG

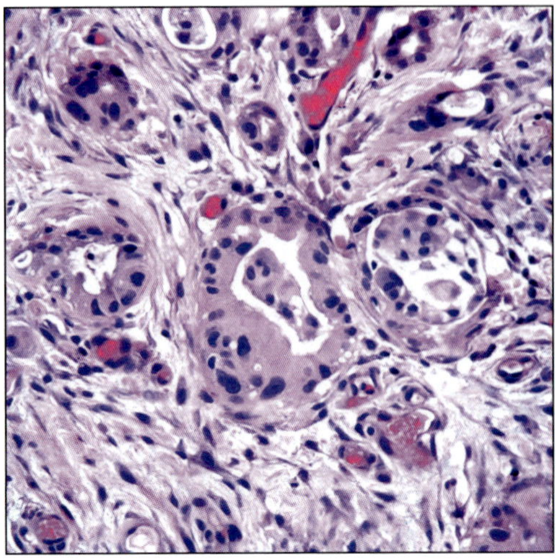

High-power view shows a well-differentiated adenocarcinoma with an acinar growth pattern. The glands are irregular with nuclear atypia and scattered mitotic figures.

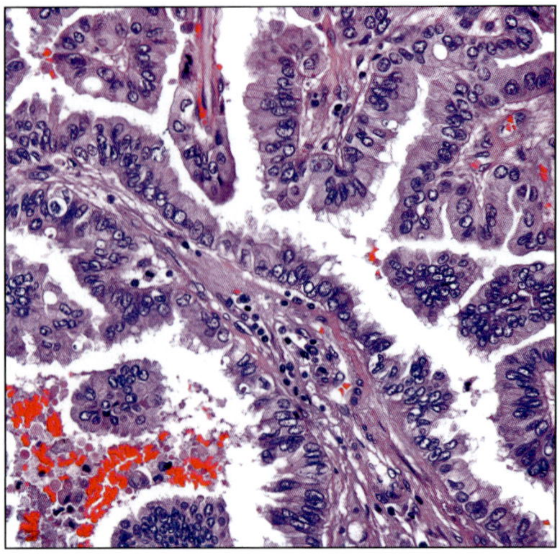

High-power view shows a true papillary carcinoma of the lung. Note the presence of true papillae. The nuclear characteristics of this tumor may mimic those seen in thyroid carcinomas.

TERMINOLOGY

Definitions

- Malignant epithelial neoplasm with glandular differentiation

ETIOLOGY/PATHOGENESIS

Environmental Exposure

- Close association with tobacco use

Association With Familial Syndromes

- Lung adenocarcinoma shows increased frequency and occurs at a younger age than the general population in Bloom Syndrome, hereditary retinoblastoma, and *BRCA2*

Etiology

- Tumor probably originates from endobronchial glands

CLINICAL ISSUES

Epidemiology

- Incidence
  - In past decade, adenocarcinomas have become more prevalent than any other non-small cell carcinoma
  - Currently is most common non-small cell carcinoma
- Age
  - Although more common in adults, adenocarcinomas also occur in younger individuals
  - Adenocarcinomas are more common in 6th and 7th decades of life

Presentation

- Cough
- Weight loss
- Difficulty breathing
- Chest pain
- Cushing syndrome
- Superior vena cava syndrome
- Pancoast syndrome
- Hemoptysis

Treatment

- Surgical approaches
  - Segmentectomy, lobectomy, pneumonectomy
- Adjuvant therapy
  - Chemotherapy, radiation therapy, or both
  - Cases positive for epidermal growth factor receptor (*EGFR*) mutation may receive targeted treatment

Prognosis

- Depends on stage at time of diagnosis
- Patients with carcinomas positive for *EGFR* mutation may have better prognosis
- It is also possible that tumors with better differentiated histology have more favorable outcome
- It may also be related to other pulmonary function factors as well as other medical conditions

MACROSCOPIC FEATURES

General Features

- Peripheral or central tumors
  - Tumors may show necrosis &/or hemorrhage
  - Homogeneous tan surface
  - Well-circumscribed but not encapsulated

Sections to Be Submitted

- Tumor in relation to pleural surface
  - Pleural involvement crucial for staging tumors < 3 cm in size

Size

- Varying size from 0.6 cm to > 10 cm

ADENOCARCINOMA, LUNG

Key Facts

Terminology
- Malignant epithelial neoplasm with glandular differentiation

Etiology/Pathogenesis
- Close association with tobacco smoking
- Lung adenocarcinoma shows increased frequency and occurs at a younger age than general population in
  - Bloom syndrome
  - *BRCA2*
  - Hereditary retinoblastoma

Macroscopic Features
- Peripheral or central tumors
- Varying size from 0.6 cm to > 10 cm

Microscopic Pathology
- Acinar
- Solid
- Papillary
- Micropapillary
- Mixed

Ancillary Tests
- EGFR by FISH
- Analysis of exons 18, 19, 20, and 21

Top Differential Diagnoses
- Adenocarcinoma from extrathoracic origin
- Atypical adenomatous hyperplasia (AAH)
- Adenoid cystic carcinoma (ACC)
- Fetal adenocarcinoma (monophasic pulmonary blastoma)
- Papillary carcinoma of thyroid origin

MICROSCOPIC PATHOLOGY

Histologic Features
- Malignant glandular component

Predominant Pattern/Injury Type
- Acinar
- Solid
- Papillary
- Mixed
- Micropapillary

Predominant Cell/Compartment Type
- Epithelial

True Papillary Carcinoma
- Should be composed of at least 75% true papillae with fibrovascular cores
- This particular pattern is believed to be more aggressive
- Lymph node metastases in this pattern are commonly seen
- TTF-1(+) and thyroglobulin (-)

Papillary Carcinoma with Morular Component
- Similar criteria to true papillary carcinoma
- Presence of morular component in alveolar spaces
- Morules are of different sizes and always in intraalveolar location
- TTF-1(+) and thyroglobulin (-)

Micropapillary Carcinoma
- Composed of small micropapillae without fibrovascular cords
- This pattern is often seen in combination with true papillary carcinoma
- TTF-1(+) and thyroglobulin (-)

Hepatoid Adenocarcinoma
- Composed of cords of neoplastic cells resembling hepatic parenchyma
- This pattern is commonly placed among large cell carcinomas of lung
- TTF-1 may show focal positive staining

Warthin-Like Adenocarcinoma
- Prominent lymphoid component similar to tumors in salivary gland
- Some cases of mucoepidermoid carcinoma may also display similar features
- Glandular proliferation with cells producing mucin embedded in inflammatory background
- TTF-1 may show positive staining

Adenomatoid Tumor-Like Adenocarcinoma
- Bland appearance similar to true adenomatoid tumor
- In some cases, can be confused with so-called alveolar adenoma
- TTF-1 and keratin 7 positive

ANCILLARY TESTS

Histochemistry
- Mucicarmine
  - Reactivity: Positive
  - Staining pattern
    - Cytoplasmic
- PAS-diastase
  - Reactivity: Positive
  - Staining pattern
    - Cytoplasmic

EGFR by Fluorescent In Situ Hybridization (FISH)
- Analysis of exons 18, 19, 20, and 21

DIFFERENTIAL DIAGNOSIS

Adenocarcinoma From Extrathoracic Origin
- Immunohistochemistry positive for TTF-1; keratin 7 would favor lung origin in vast majority of cases

ADENOCARCINOMA, LUNG

Immunohistochemistry

Antibody	Reactivity	Staining Pattern	Comment
CEA-M	Positive	Cytoplasmic	
TTF-1	Positive	Nuclear	Often negative in mucinous tumors
CD15	Positive	Cytoplasmic	Often negative in poorly differentiated tumors
MOC-31	Positive	Cytoplasmic	Some mesotheliomas may show focal positive staining
CK-PAN	Positive	Cytoplasmic	
CK7	Positive	Cytoplasmic	
Surfactant	Positive	Cytoplasmic	Negative in many cases of primary lung origin
CDX-2	Positive		
EpCAM/BER-EP4/ CD326	Positive	Cell membrane	Some mesotheliomas are positive
NAPSIN-A	Positive	Cell membrane	Positive in most well-differentiated tumors
PRP	Negative		
Mammaglobin	Negative		
ERP	Negative		Some lung adenocarcinomas may be positive
CK20	Negative		Some lung adenocarcinomas may show weak positive staining

Atypical Adenomatous Hyperplasia (AAH)

- Lesion ≤ 0.5 cm in diameter
- Shares similar histological features with bronchioloavelolar carcinoma (BAC)

Adenoid Cystic Carcinoma (ACC)

- Shows characteristic double layer-forming glands
- Immunohistochemical studies show myoepithelial differentiation

Fetal Adenocarcinoma (Monophasic Pulmonary Blastoma)

- Presence of morules and embryonic-type glandular structures
- Presence of cytoplasmic mucin content in favor of adenocarcinoma

Papillary Carcinoma of Thyroid Origin

- Histologically, tumors with papillary pattern may show similar histological features
- Positive TTF-1 and negative staining for thyroglobulin favors primary lung cancer

DIAGNOSTIC CHECKLIST

Pathologic Interpretation Pearls

- Size of lesion separates carcinoma from AAH
- Cases designated as AAH are < 5 mm in diameter

GRADING

Low Grade

- Well-differentiated adenocarcinoma composed of easily identifiable glandular structures and arranged in back-to-back arrangement
- Absence of necrosis, increased mitotic activity, and nuclear atypia
- Glandular tumoral structures may be separated by extensive areas of collagenization

Intermediate Grade

- Moderately differentiated adenocarcinoma composed of identifiable glands
- Tumor may show more nuclear atypia and mitotic activity
- Glandular structures may show more disarray

High Grade

- Poorly differentiated adenocarcinoma may show solid areas with ↑ mitotic activity and nuclear atypia
- Necrosis and hemorrhage may be present

SELECTED REFERENCES

1. Planck M et al: Identification of Transcriptional Subgroups in EGFR-Mutated and EGFR/KRAS Wild-Type Lung Adenocarcinoma Reveals Gene Signatures Associated with Patient Outcome. Clin Cancer Res. 19(18):5116-26, 2013
2. Weissferdt A et al: Well-differentiated adenocarcinoma-bronchioloalveolar carcinoma-in situ adenocarcinoma: a conundrum. Adv Anat Pathol. 20(5):347-51, 2013
3. Yoshida T et al: Solid predominant histology predicts EGFR tyrosine kinase inhibitor response in patients with EGFR mutation-positive lung adenocarcinoma. J Cancer Res Clin Oncol. 139(10):1691-700, 2013
4. Wahbah M et al: Changing trends in the distribution of the histologic types of lung cancer: a review of 4,439 cases. Ann Diagn Pathol. 11(2):89-96, 2007
5. Moran CA: Pulmonary adenocarcinoma: the expanding spectrum of histologic variants. Arch Pathol Lab Med. 130(7):958-62, 2006
6. Prudkin L et al: Epidermal growth factor receptor abnormalities in lung cancer. Pathogenetic and clinical implications. Ann Diagn Pathol. 10(5):306-15, 2006
7. Moran CA et al: Papillary lung carcinoma with prominent "morular" component. Am J Clin Pathol. 122(1):106-9, 2004
8. Amin MB et al: Micropapillary component in lung adenocarcinoma: a distinctive histologic feature with possible prognostic significance. Am J Surg Pathol. 26(3):358-64, 2002

Microscopic Features

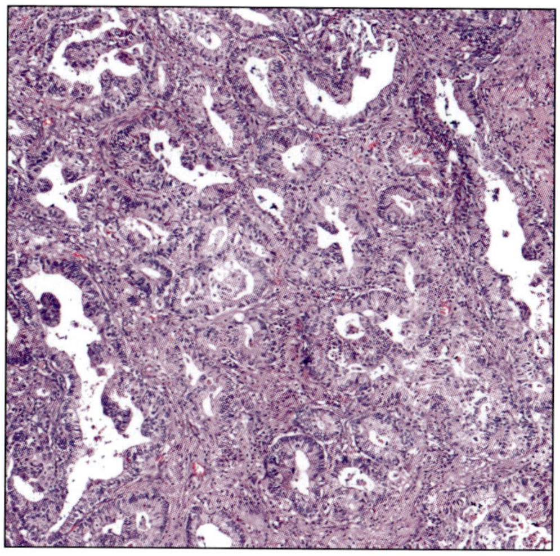

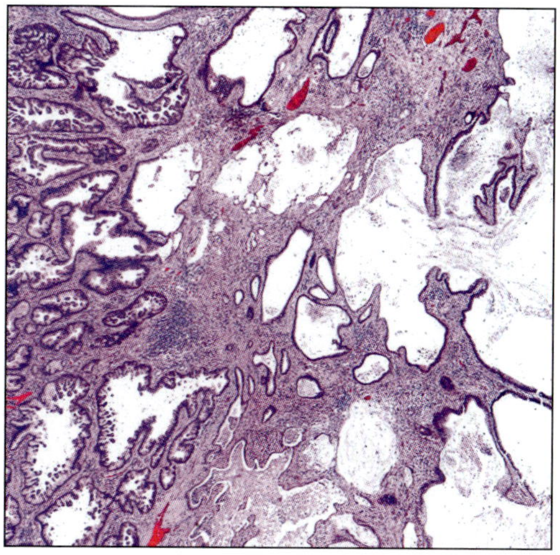

(Left) *Adenocarcinoma shows an acinar pattern of growth. The neoplastic glandular proliferation is composed of glands of different sizes in a back-to-back arrangement.* ***(Right)*** *Adenocarcinoma in which a nonmucinous component merges with a mucinous component shows cystic changes whereas the nonmucinous component reveals a more acinar component.*

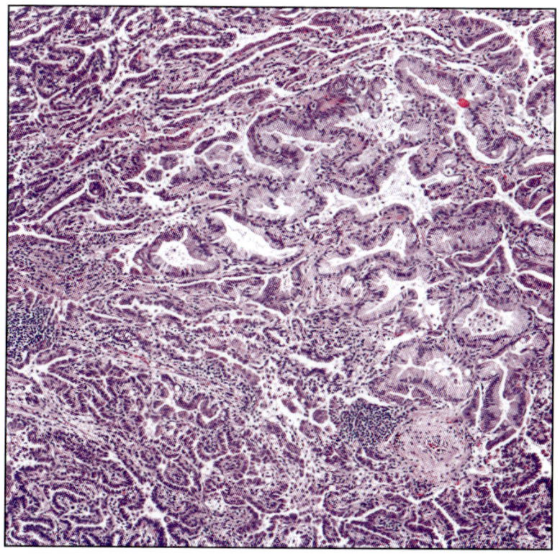

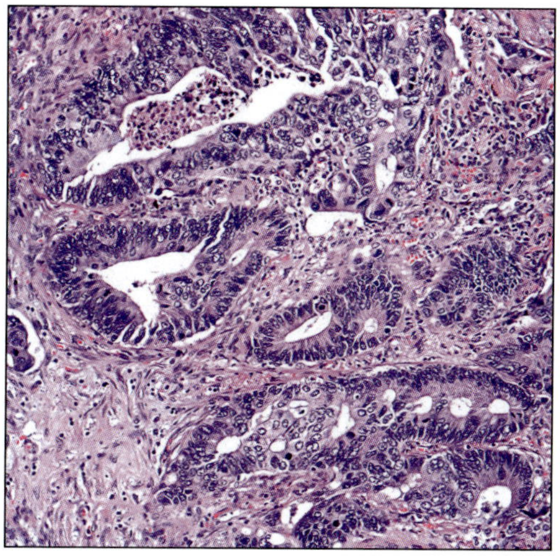

(Left) *Adenocarcinoma shows predominantly a nonmucinous type of glandular epithelium. In focal areas, a nonmucinous type of proliferation merges with glands composed of a mucinous type of epithelium. This component may be subtle.* ***(Right)*** *High-power view shows a moderately differentiated adenocarcinoma revealing glandular structures with nuclear atypia and mitotic activity. The glands have a vague enteric type of differentiation, mimicking a metastasis from colon.*

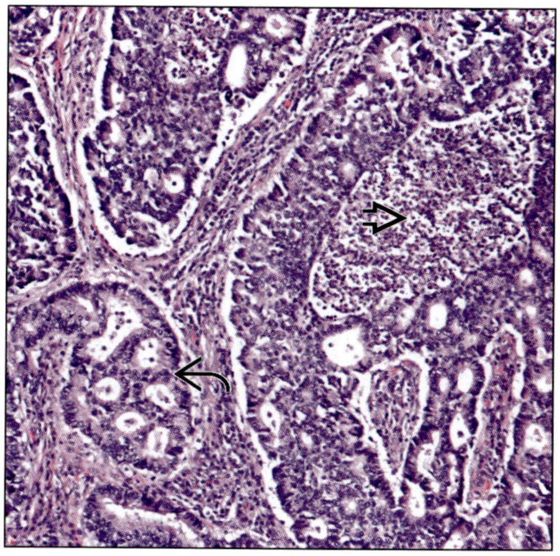

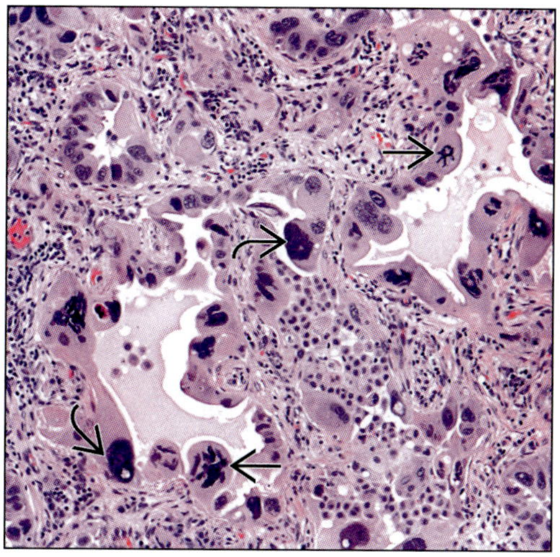

(Left) *Adenocarcinoma is shown with comedo-like necrosis ⇨ and with an acinar pattern ↶ that demonstrates a vague neuroendocrine morphology whereas in some areas it shows conventional glandular differentiation.* ***(Right)*** *Adenocarcinoma with the presence of numerous multinucleated giant cells ↷ is seen in this photomicrograph. Note the presence of atypical bizarre mitotic figures →.*

ADENOCARCINOMA, LUNG

Microscopic Features

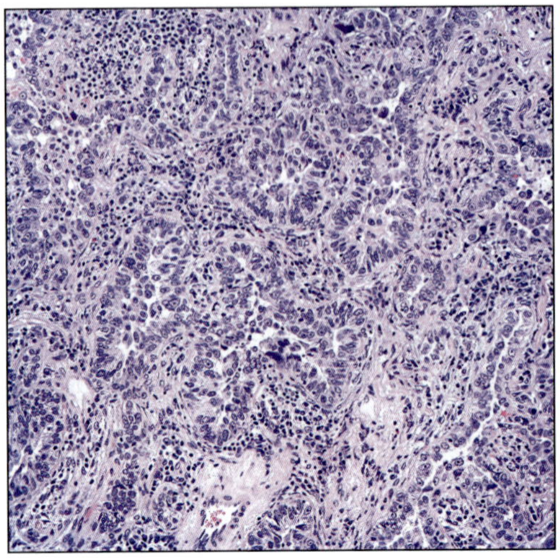

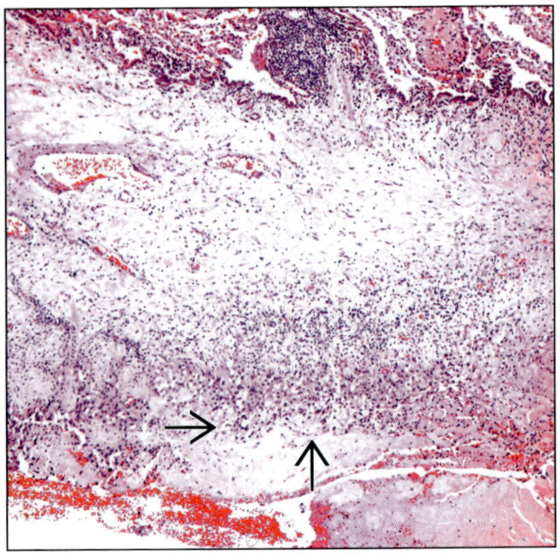

(Left) *Moderately differentiated adenocarcinoma displays easily recognizable glandular structures of different sizes. The glands are separated by an inflammatory reaction. Some of the glands are collapsed and show more nuclear atypia.* ***(Right)*** *Adenocarcinoma → involves the pleural surface. This particular feature is highly important in tumors < 3 cm in which pleural involvement will upgrade the pathologic staging of the tumor to a higher level (T2).*

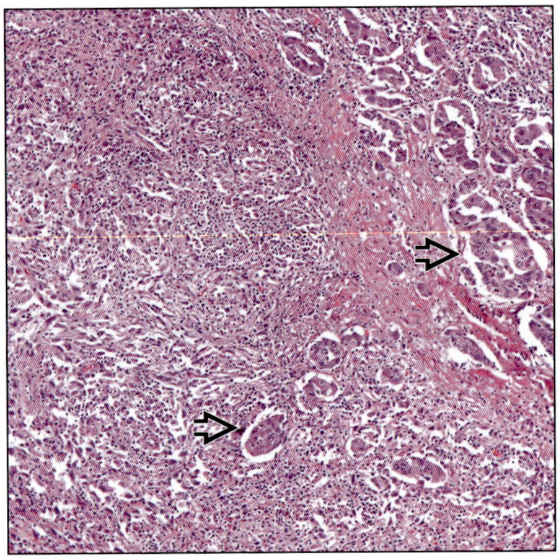

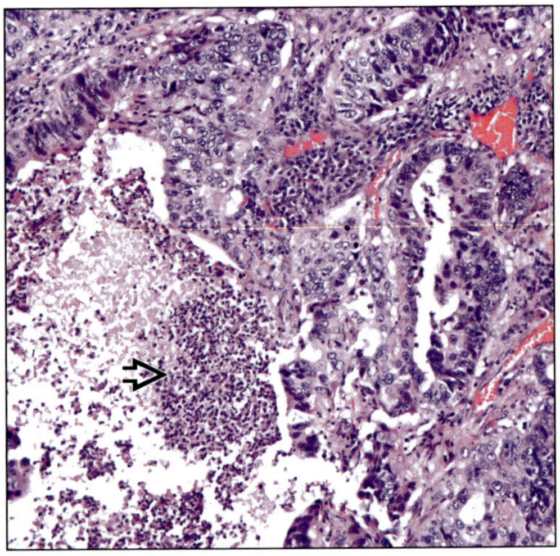

(Left) *This poorly differentiated adenocarcinoma of lung has only focal areas with glandular differentiation ⇨. Most of the tumor has a predominantly solid growth pattern.* ***(Right)*** *Adenocarcinoma with prominent inflammatory changes ⇨ is seen in this photomicrograph. These changes may be very extensive or may form abscess areas within the tumor.*

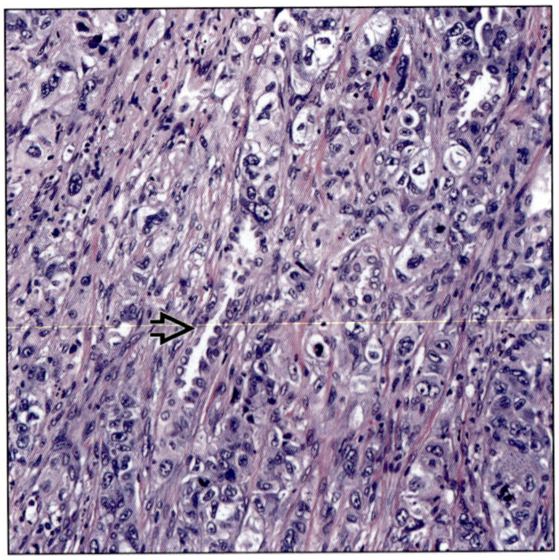

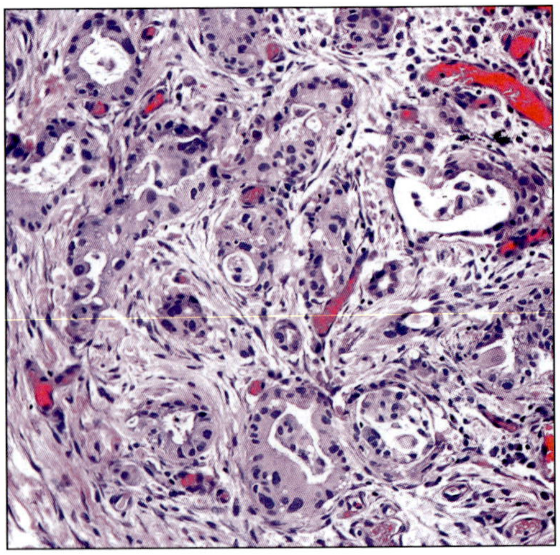

(Left) *Intermediate-power view of a poorly differentiated adenocarcinoma with vague glandular formation ⇨ is shown. The presence of glandular differentiation in some poorly differentiated adenocarcinomas may be focal.* ***(Right)*** *Well-differentiated adenocarcinoma with an acinar growth pattern is composed of small glandular proliferation of different sizes. The glands are arranged in a haphazard pattern with fibrotic and inflammatory reaction.*

Microscopic Features

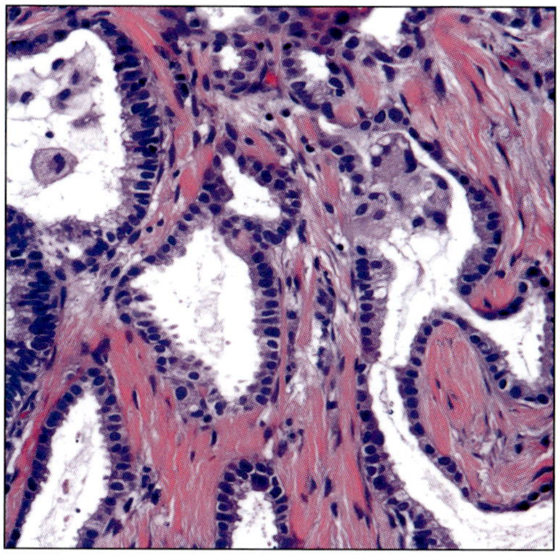

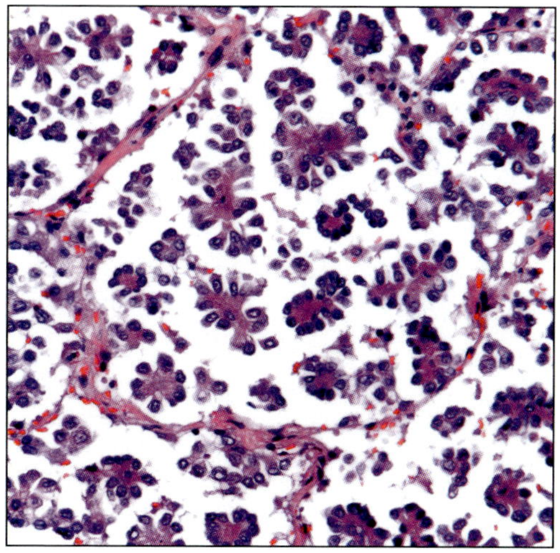

(Left) *High-power view of a well-differentiated adenocarcinoma is composed of malignant glands with low cuboidal epithelium.* ***(Right)*** *High-power view shows a micropapillary adenocarcinoma of the lung. Note that the micropapillae filling the alveolar spaces are devoid of fibrovascular cord, contrary to true papillae.*

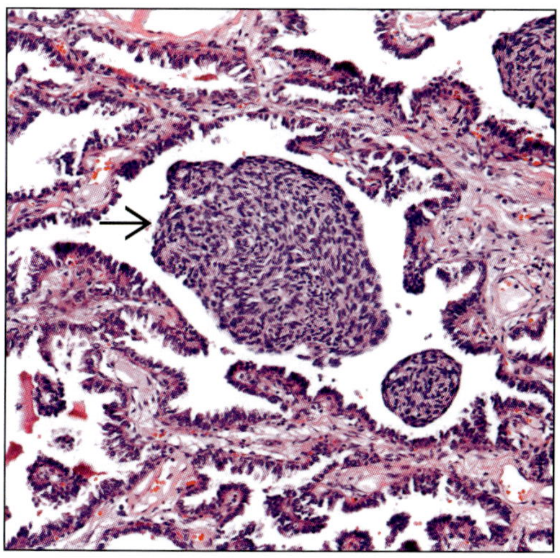

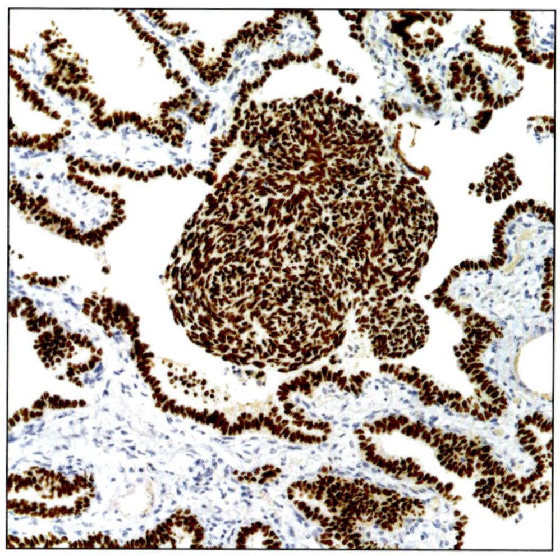

(Left) *High-magnification view shows a papillary adenocarcinoma with morular component. Note the presence of the morules* → *within the alveolar spaces, in contrast to those seen in monophasic blastomas, which are in the interstitium at the base of the glands.* ***(Right)*** *Immunohistochemical stain for TTF-1 with strong nuclear staining in the morular component of the tumor is shown. Note that adjacent neoplastic glands are also positive.*

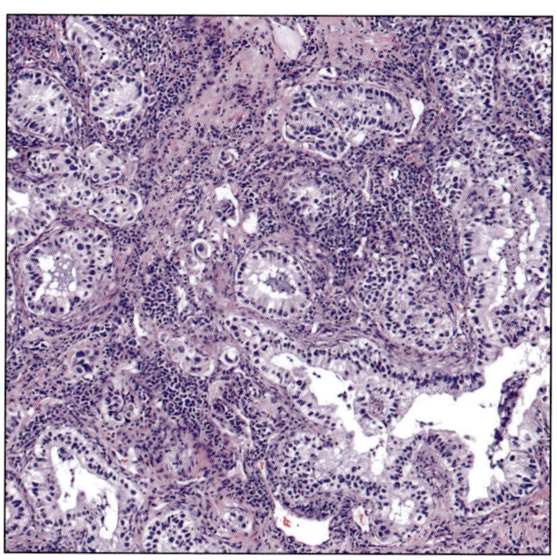

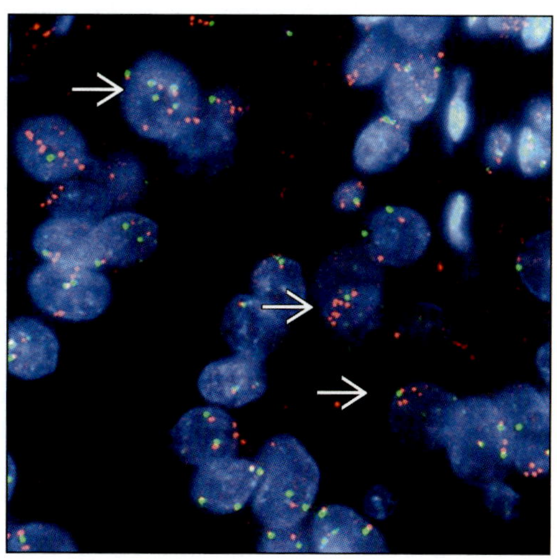

(Left) *Moderately differentiated adenocarcinoma shows the malignant glandular proliferation admixed with areas of fibrosis and inflammatory reaction.* ***(Right)*** *FISH shows gene amplification of the characteristic EGFR mutation* → *in a pulmonary adenocarcinoma.*

ADENOCARCINOMA WITH LEPIDIC (BRONCHIOLOALVEOLAR) PREDOMINANT PATTERN

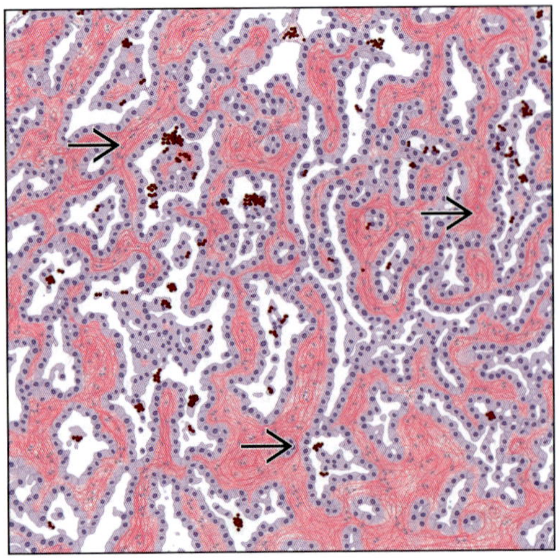

Illustration of adenocarcinoma with a lepidic predominant pattern shows growth of neoplastic cells along alveolar structures without evidence of stromal ⇒, vascular, or pleural invasion.

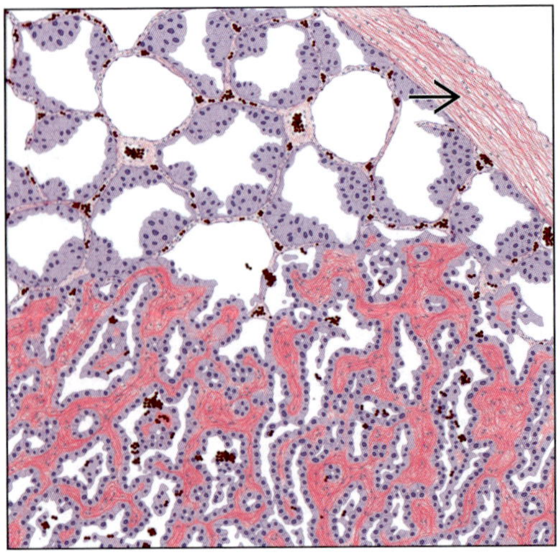

Illustration of an adenocarcinoma with a lepidic predominant pattern highlights the absence of pleural involvement by the tumor ⇒. This is an important criterion for the diagnosis of BAC.

TERMINOLOGY

Abbreviations

- Adenocarcinoma with a lepidic predominant pattern (BAC)

Synonyms

- Adenocarcinoma in situ
- Minimally invasive adenocarcinoma
- Adenocarcinoma with a bronchioloalveolar carcinoma pattern

Definitions

- Lesion with relatively bland cytologic features that arises in periphery of lung and spreads along walls of distal air spaces
- A bronchioloalveolar carcinoma pattern of adenocarcinoma shows growth of neoplastic cells along preexisting alveolar structures (lepidic growth)
  - In situ adenocarcinoma
  - No evidence of stromal, vascular, or pleural invasion

ETIOLOGY/PATHOGENESIS

Environmental Exposure

- Adenocarcinoma with a lepidic (bronchioloalveolar) predominant pattern appears not to be associated with tobacco use

Association With Familial Syndromes

- BAC associated with familial tumor syndromes is rare
- Risk of developing lung cancer is increased in
  - Li-Fraumeni syndrome, as compared with general population
  - Peutz-Jeghers syndrome, with a cumulative cancer risk of 15% by age 60
  - Xeroderma pigmentosum

CLINICAL ISSUES

Epidemiology

- Incidence of true BAC is not high and may represent less than 10% of all lung carcinomas
- Tumor can occur at any age

Presentation

- Cough
- Chest pain
- Shortness of breath

Treatment

- Surgical approaches
  - Wedge resection, lobectomy, or pneumonectomy

Prognosis

- As currently defined, patients with BAC tumors ≤ 2 cm are expected to do well

MACROSCOPIC FEATURES

General Features

- Localized tumor mass
- Multinodular pattern: Extensive areas of lung parenchyma are involved in miliary fashion
- Diffuse pattern: No distinct tumor mass or nodule is present

MICROSCOPIC PATHOLOGY

Histologic Features

- Conventional type
  - Tumor cells are small and dark with hyperchromatic nuclei and scant cytoplasm
  - Tumor cells display prominent hobnail appearance and are devoid of nucleoli or mitotic figures

ADENOCARCINOMA WITH LEPIDIC (BRONCHIOLOALVEOLAR) PREDOMINANT PATTERN

Key Facts

Terminology
- Adenocarcinoma with a lepidic (bronchioloalveolar) predominant pattern
  - Adenocarcinoma with no evidence of stromal, vascular, or pleural invasion
  - In situ adenocarcinoma

Etiology/Pathogenesis
- Adenocarcinoma with a lepidic pattern appears not to be associated with tobacco smoking
- Risk of developing lung cancer is increased in
  - Li-Fraumeni syndrome as compared with general population
  - Peutz-Jeghers syndrome, with a cumulative cancer risk of 15% by age 60

Macroscopic Features
- Multinodular pattern: Extensive areas of lung parenchyma are involved in miliary fashion
- Diffuse pattern: No distinct tumor mass or nodule

Top Differential Diagnoses
- Atypical adenomatous hyperplasia (AAH)
  - Tumor nodule of < 0.5 cm in greatest dimension
- Metastatic adenocarcinoma
  - Immunohistochemical studies may be helpful in determining primary site
- Invasive adenocarcinoma
  - Adenocarcinoma with a lepidic pattern is a tumor with no lymphatic, pleural, or interstitial invasion
  - To rule out invasion, entire specimen has to be examined

Immunohistochemistry

Antibody	Reactivity	Staining Pattern	Comment
KERATIN-LMW	Positive	Cytoplasmic	
CEA-M	Positive	Cytoplasmic	Helpful in both mucinous and nonmucinous tumors
CK7	Positive	Cytoplasmic	
TTF-1	Positive	Nuclear	In some mucinous cases, stain may be negative
NAPSIN-A	Positive		
CK20	Negative		May show focal positive staining in tumor cells in some cases
CDX-2	Negative		May show focal positive staining in tumor cells in some mucinous tumors
GCDFP-15	Negative		

- Mucinous adenocarcinoma in situ is by definition a low-grade adenocarcinoma
  - Tumor cells are tall, columnar, and contain abundant mucinous cytoplasm

DIFFERENTIAL DIAGNOSIS

Atypical Adenomatous Hyperplasia
- Tumor nodule < 0.5 cm in greatest dimension
- Histology very similar to BAC

Metastatic Adenocarcinoma
- Past or present history of adenocarcinoma outside of thoracic cavity
- Immunohistochemical studies may be helpful in determining primary site

Pulmonary Invasive Adenocarcinoma
- BAC lacks presence of vascular, lymphatic, pleural, or interstitial involvement by tumor cells

DIAGNOSTIC CHECKLIST

Clinically Relevant Pathologic Features
- Noninvasive pattern
- Diagnosis of BAC cannot be achieved in biopsy specimens
- Histopathological examination of entire tumor is required for diagnosis of BAC
- Lymph node sampling is required to properly rule out metastatic disease

Pathologic Interpretation Pearls
- Alveolar wall lined by neoplastic cells
- Absence of pleural invasion
- Absence of interstitial invasion

SELECTED REFERENCES

1. Travis WD et al: New pathologic classification of lung cancer: relevance for clinical practice and clinical trials. J Clin Oncol. 31(8):992-1001, 2013
2. Weissferdt A et al: Well-differentiated adenocarcinoma-bronchioloalveolar carcinoma-in situ adenocarcinoma: a conundrum. Adv Anat Pathol. 20(5):347-51, 2013
3. Travis WD et al: Tumours of the lung, pleura, thymus, and heart. Pathology & Genetics: World Health Organization (WHO). Lyon: IARC Press. 38, 2004
4. Colby TV et al: Tumors of the lower respiratory tract. Atlas of Tumor Pathology: Armed Forces Institute of Pathology (AFIP). (13):203, 1995
5. Liebow AA: Bronchiolo-alveolar carcinoma. Adv Intern Med. 10:329-58, 1960

ADENOCARCINOMA WITH LEPIDIC (BRONCHIOLOALVEOLAR) PREDOMINANT PATTERN

Gross and Microscopic Features

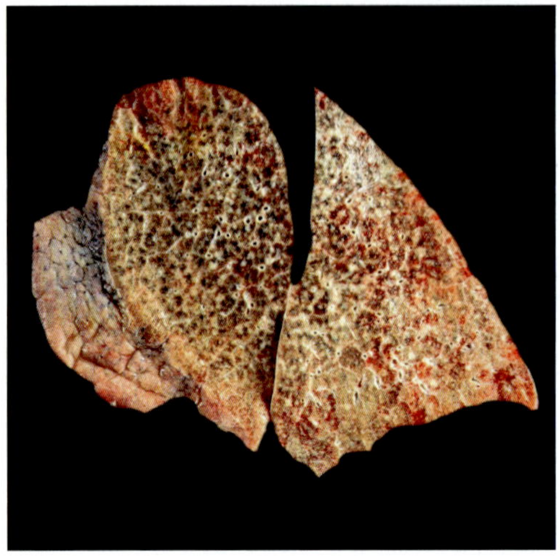
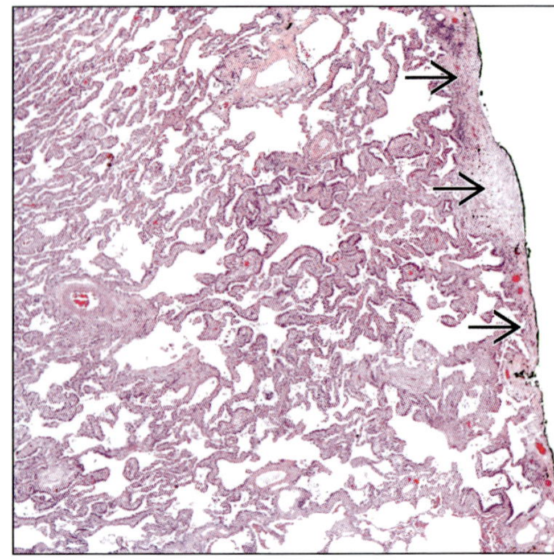

(Left) *Gross photograph shows multiple small pulmonary nodules of different sizes. This represents the multinodular pattern of bronchioloalveolar cell carcinoma.* ***(Right)*** *Nodular (nonmucinous) pattern of adenocarcinoma with a lepidic predominant pattern is shown. The tumor is in a subpleural location without pleural [→] or interstitial involvement.*

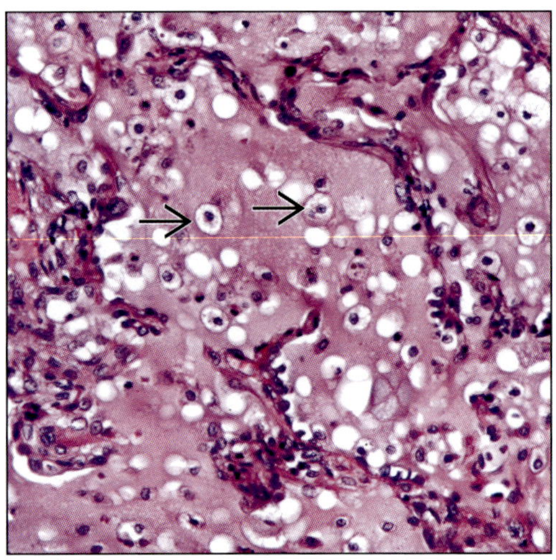
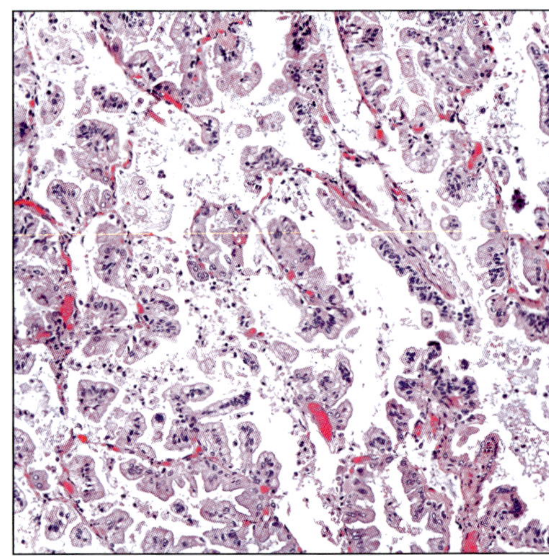

(Left) *H&E shows adjacent areas of normal lung parenchyma in a pneumonic type of adenocarcinoma with a lepidic predominant pattern. The alveoli are filled with fluid and numerous floating macrophages [→].* ***(Right)*** *This photomicrograph shows a characteristic adenocarcinoma with a lepidic predominant pattern. Note the absence of tumor infiltrating the interstitium. However, absence of pleural invasion must also be excluded for this diagnosis.*

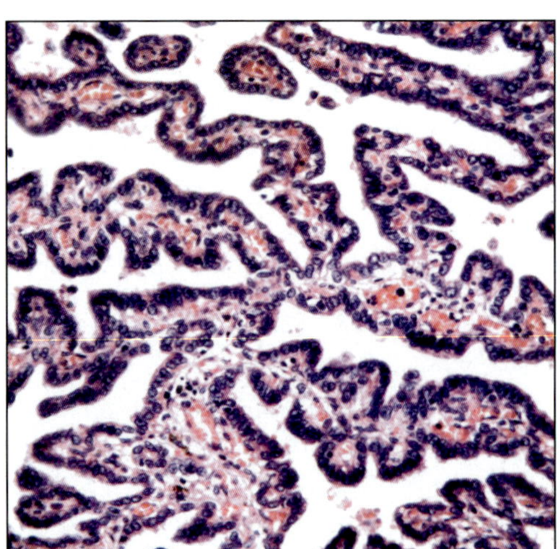
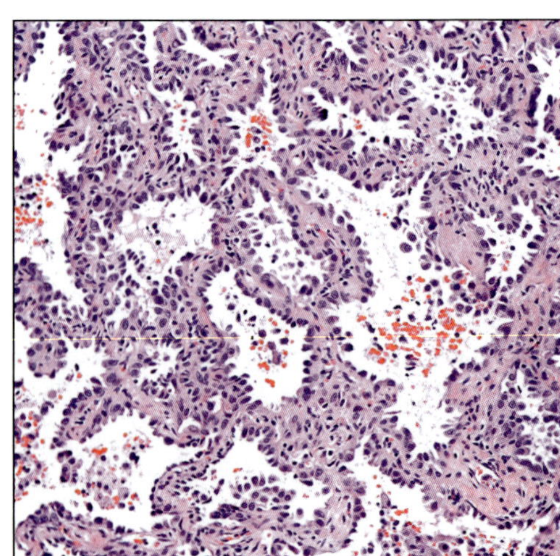

(Left) *Adenocarcinoma with a lepidic predominant pattern is seen composed of cellular proliferation lining the alveolar walls. The cells are low to flat cuboidal with pyknotic nuclei and an absence of mitotic activity or nuclear atypia. Note the lack of interstitial involvement.* ***(Right)*** *Adenocarcinoma with a lepidic predominant pattern is shown, in which the alveolar walls are lined by cells displaying more nuclear atypia. However, the tumor cells do not show mitotic activity.*

ADENOCARCINOMA WITH LEPIDIC (BRONCHIOLOALVEOLAR) PREDOMINANT PATTERN

Microscopic Features

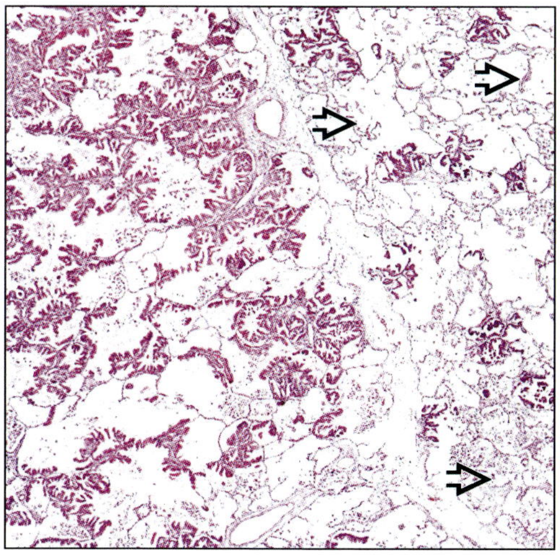

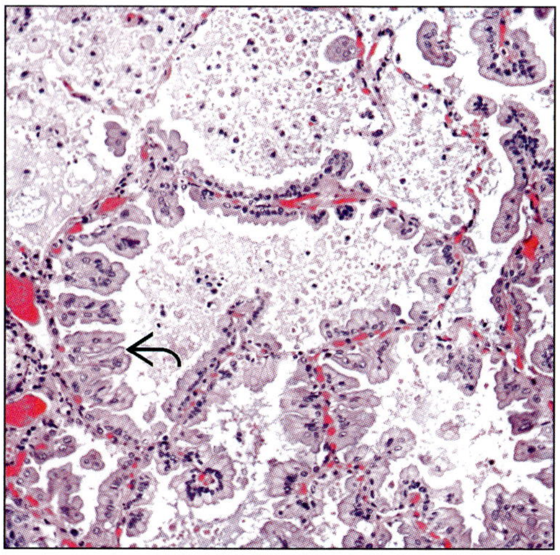

***(Left)** Predominantly alveolar pattern in adenocarcinoma is shown, in which malignant cells line the alveolar walls. Also note the presence of areas of normal lung parenchyma. **(Right)** Bronchioloalveolar cell carcinoma pattern shows a classical pattern of the lepidic growth. Note the presence of neoplastic cells lining the alveolar wall. Still, one is able to follow the "normal" architecture of the lung parenchyma.*

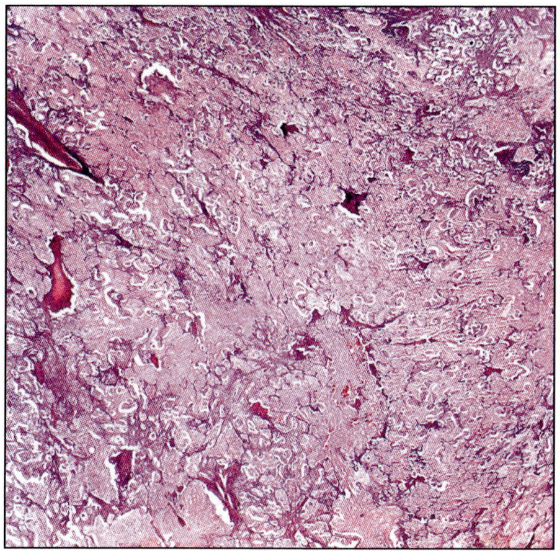

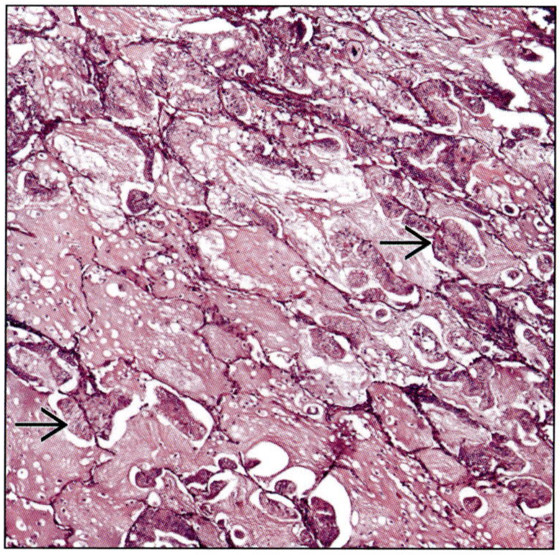

***(Left)** Low power view of this adenocarcinoma shows extensive areas of lung parenchyma replaced with proteinaceous fluid filling the alveolar spaces. This pattern represents the so-called pneumonic pattern of adenocarcinoma. **(Right)** Pneumonic pattern of adenocarcinoma in which the alveoli are filled with edematous fluid is shown here with only focal areas of alveoli replaced by mucinous epithelium.*

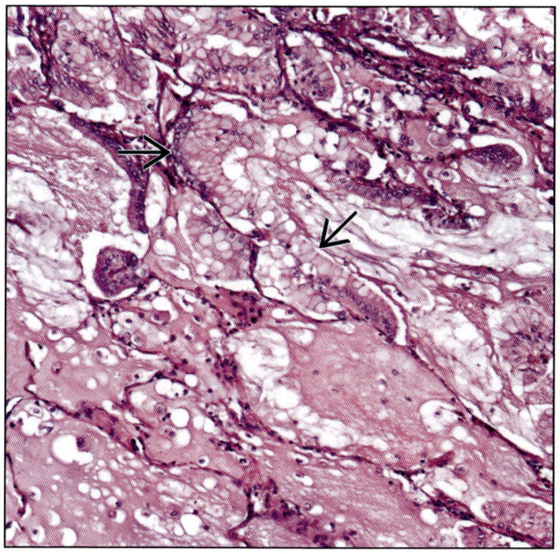

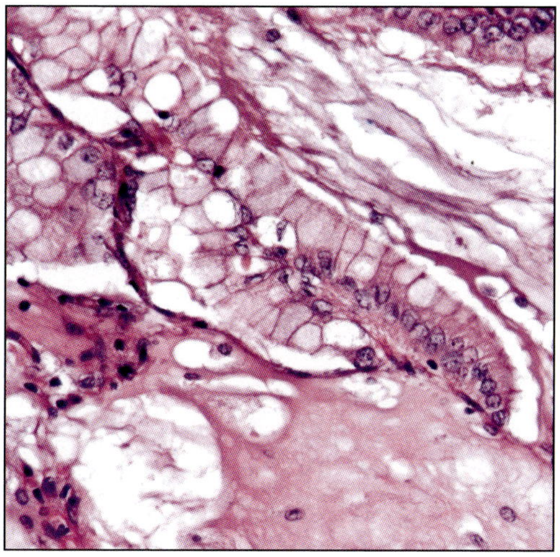

***(Left)** Closer view shows the pneumonic variant of adenocarcinoma with a lepidic predominant pattern. Note the presence of mucinous epithelium replacing the alveolar lining. **(Right)** Mucinous type of epithelium replaces the alveolar lining. The mucinous epithelium is composed of columnar cells with nuclei displaced toward the base. No cellular atypia or mitotic activity is present.*

LYMPHANGIOLEIOMYOMATOSIS

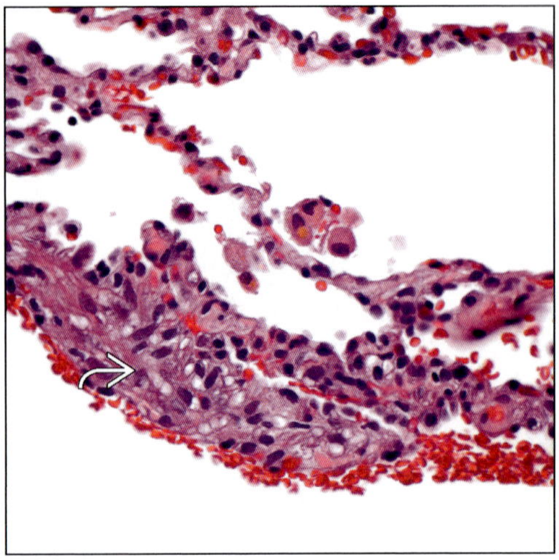

High-power view of the smooth muscle proliferation ➡ in lymphangioleiomyomatosis (LAM) is shown. Distinguishing between sporadic and tuberous sclerosis-associated LAM may not be possible on histologic grounds.

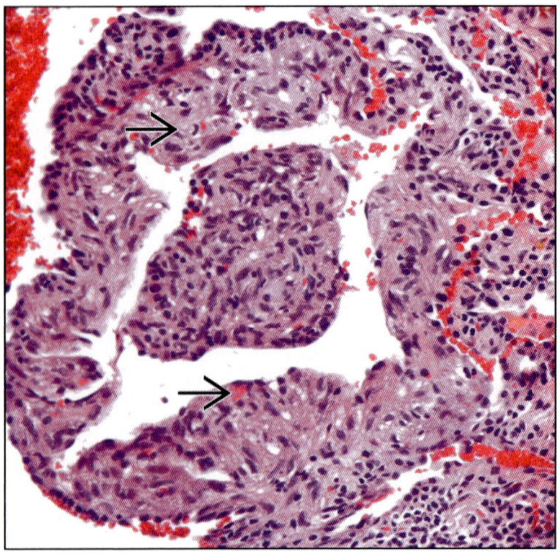

High-power magnification of LAM shows the classical presence of smooth muscle proliferation. The muscle proliferation is obvious and has obliterated the normal alveolar lining ➡.

TERMINOLOGY

Abbreviations

- Lymphangioleiomyomatosis (LAM)

Synonyms

- Lymphangiomyomatosis

Definitions

- Nonneoplastic lung condition characterized by presence of immature muscle proliferation

ETIOLOGY/PATHOGENESIS

Etiology

- Unknown
- May share similar genetic relationship with tuberous sclerosis complex

CLINICAL ISSUES

Epidemiology

- Incidence
  - LAM occurs in ~ 2 cases per million patients
  - May be underreported
- Age
  - More common in premenopausal women
  - Rarely described in children
- Gender
  - Commonly affects women

Presentation

- Cough
- Shortness of breath
- Chylous effusion
- Pneumothorax
- Hemoptysis

Treatment

- No specific treatment
- Possible treatments
  - Hormonal manipulation
  - Oophorectomy
  - Lung transplantation

Prognosis

- Predominantly cystic lesions may have poor prognosis
- 85% survival at 5 years
- 70% survival at 10 years

IMAGE FINDINGS

General Features

- Bilateral multiple nodular and cystic changes in lung parenchyma
- Unilateral involvement is also possible

MACROSCOPIC FEATURES

General Features

- Multiple cysts with honeycomb appearance

MICROSCOPIC PATHOLOGY

Histologic Features

- Cystic changes
- Hemorrhage
- Spindle cell proliferation
  - In alveolar walls
  - Lining cystic structures
  - With focal clear cell change
  - Lacking atypia or mitotic activity
- Adjacent lung parenchyma may show type II pneumocyte hyperplasia

LYMPHANGIOLEIOMYOMATOSIS

Key Facts

Etiology/Pathogenesis
- Unknown etiology
- Occurs in ~ 6% of tuberous sclerosis patients
- May share similar genetic relationship with tuberous sclerosis complex

Clinical Issues
- Incidence
  - More common in premenopausal women
  - Rarely described in children

Microscopic Pathology
- Cystic changes with smooth muscle proliferation
- Spindle cell proliferation lining cystic structures
  - In alveolar walls
  - With focal clear cell change
  - Lacking atypia or mitotic activity

Ancillary Tests
- Spindle cells are positive for SMA, HMB-45, and ER/PR

Top Differential Diagnoses
- Tuberous sclerosis
  - Distinction between sporadic and familial LAM may not be possible on histologic grounds
  - Associated with numerous tumors, hamartomas, and cysts
- Leiomyoma
  - Usually forms a solid tumor mass
- Leiomyosarcoma
  - LAM lacks atypia or mitotic activity

Immunohistochemistry

Antibody	Reactivity	Staining Pattern	Comment
Actin-sm	Positive	Cytoplasmic	In muscle component
Desmin	Positive	Cytoplasmic	In muscle component
HMB-45	Positive	Cytoplasmic	More often in clear cells
IGF-1	Positive	Cytoplasmic	
MMP-1	Positive	Cytoplasmic	
ER	Positive	Nuclear	May be focal
PR	Positive	Nuclear	May be focal
S100	Negative		
CK-PAN	Negative		Positive in alveolar cell and entrapped lung

ANCILLARY TESTS

Immunohistochemistry
- Spindle cells are positive for SMA, HMB-45, and for ER/PR

DIFFERENTIAL DIAGNOSIS

Tuberous Sclerosis
- Tuberous sclerosis-associated LAM has similar features to sporadic tumors
  - Such distinction may not be possible on histologic grounds alone
- It is important to obtain a clinical history of tuberous sclerosis

Leiomyoma
- Usually forms a tumor mass
- Unusual for leiomyoma to present with prominent cystic changes

Leiomyosarcoma
- LAM lacks atypia or mitotic activity

SELECTED REFERENCES

1. Badri KR et al: Exonic mutations of TSC2/TSC1 are common but not seen in all sporadic pulmonary lymphangioleiomyomatosis. Am J Respir Crit Care Med. 187(6):663-5, 2013
2. Bissler JJ et al: Everolimus for angiomyolipoma associated with tuberous sclerosis complex or sporadic lymphangioleiomyomatosis (EXIST-2): a multicentre, randomised, double-blind, placebo-controlled trial. Lancet. 381(9869):817-24, 2013
3. Cudzilo CJ et al: Lymphangioleiomyomatosis screening in women with tuberous sclerosis. Chest. 144(2):578-85, 2013
4. Mavroudi M et al: Lymphangioleiomyomatosis: current and future. J Thorac Dis. 5(1):74-9, 2013
5. Wataya-Kaneda M et al: Trends in the prevalence of tuberous sclerosis complex manifestations: an epidemiological study of 166 Japanese patients. PLoS One. 8(5):e63910, 2013
6. Henske EP et al: Lymphangioleiomyomatosis - a wolf in sheep's clothing. J Clin Invest. 122(11):3807-16, 2012
7. Maruyama H et al: Multifocal micronodular pneumocyte hyperplasia and lymphangioleiomyomatosis in tuberous sclerosis with a TSC2 gene. Mod Pathol. 14(6):609-14, 2001
8. Capron F et al: Pulmonary lymphangioleiomyomatosis and Bourneville's tuberous sclerosis with pulmonary involvement: the same disease? Cancer. 52(5):851-5, 1983

LYMPHANGIOLEIOMYOMATOSIS

Microscopic Features

(Left) *Low-power view of lung parenchyma in LAM shows little change at this magnification. However, note the presence of cysts and the thickening of some of those cysts' walls →.* ***(Right)*** *Higher magnification shows alternating normal alveolar structures ⇨ and other cystic structures lined by smooth muscle proliferation → in pulmonary lymphangioleiomyomatosis.*

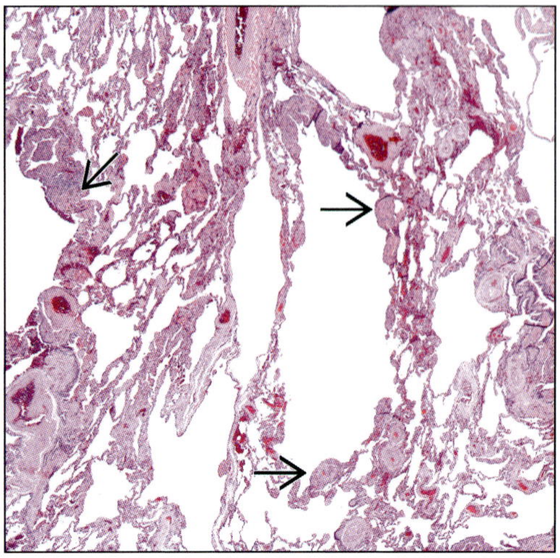
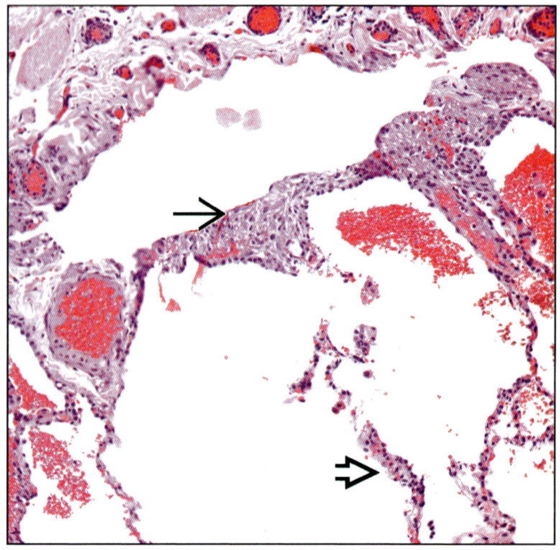

(Left) *LAM shows areas of nonneoplastic vascular proliferation →; some of the vessels contain fresh blood. Note the presence of muscle proliferation adjacent to the dilated vascular structures ↪.* ***(Right)*** *This LAM shows a very subtle area of muscle proliferation ↪ adjacent to an alveolar space ⇨. In some cases, the presence of muscle may be only focal and can easily be missed in a cursory review.*

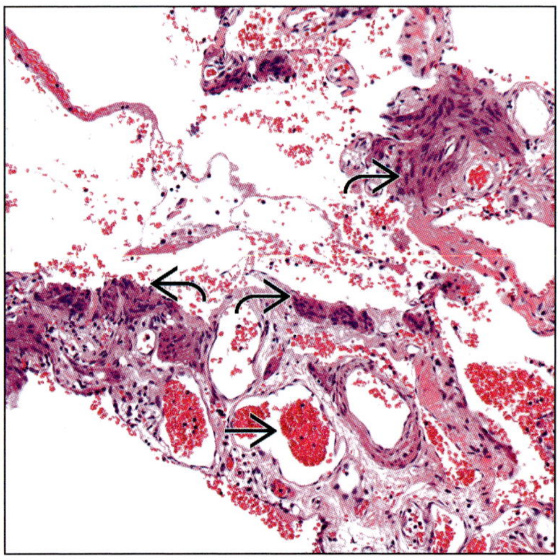
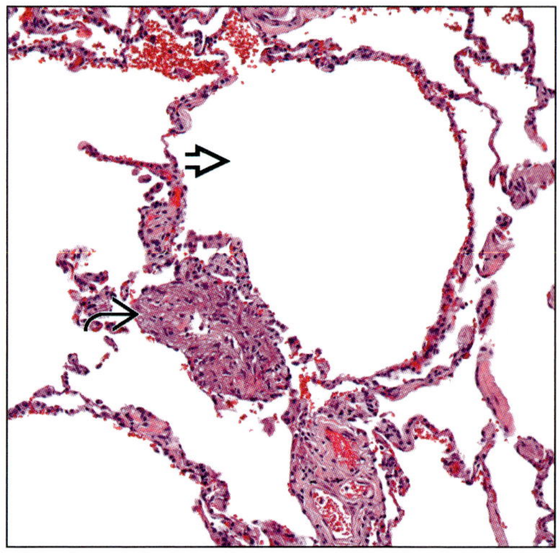

(Left) *An unusual feature that may be seen in some cases of LAM is the presence of pneumocyte hyperplasia ↪. Such change may be in the form of small nodules that can raise the possibility of a malignant epithelial neoplasm.* ***(Right)*** *Low-power view of LAM shows 2 focal areas of muscle proliferation ↪. Note that the rest of the pulmonary parenchyma appears to be within normal limits.*

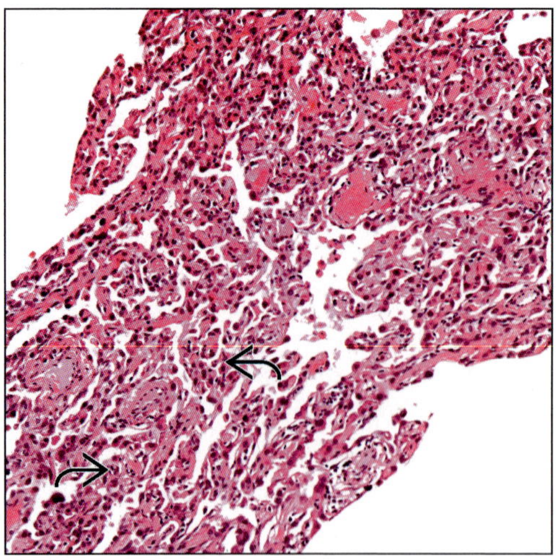
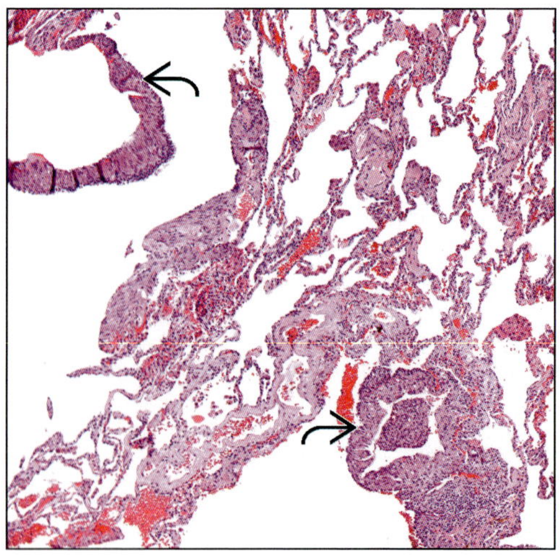

Microscopic Features

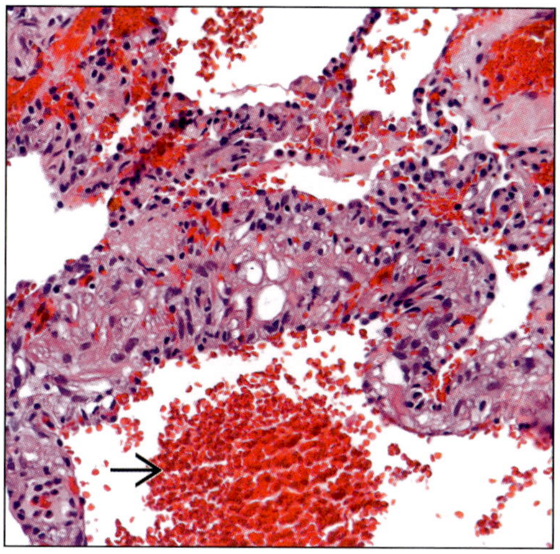
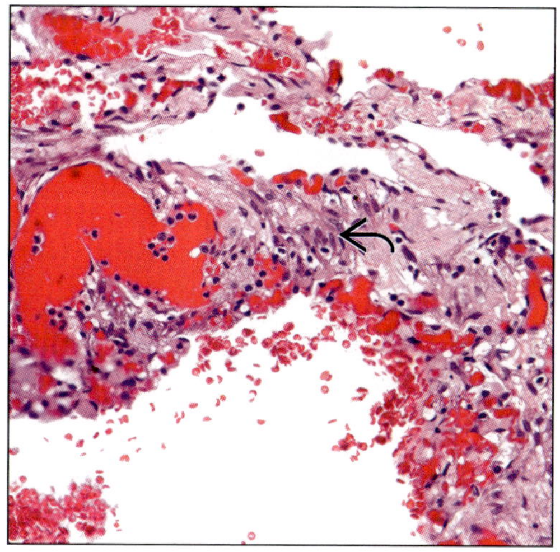

(Left) *This LAM shows areas of congestion and hemorrhage with the presence of fresh blood* →. *However, note that the alveolar wall has been replaced by a muscle proliferation, which also shows some clear cell changes. Due to the areas of hemorrhage and congestion, these areas can be missed.* ***(Right)*** *Hemorrhage and congestion in LAM can at times be very marked, and areas of muscle proliferation can be difficult to find. Muscle proliferation* ↷ *can be easily missed.*

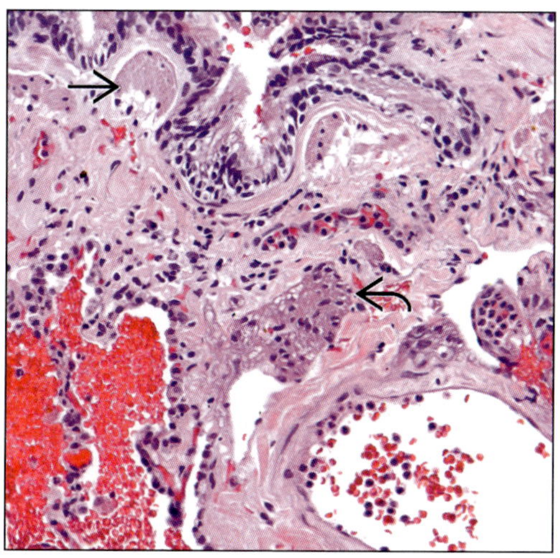
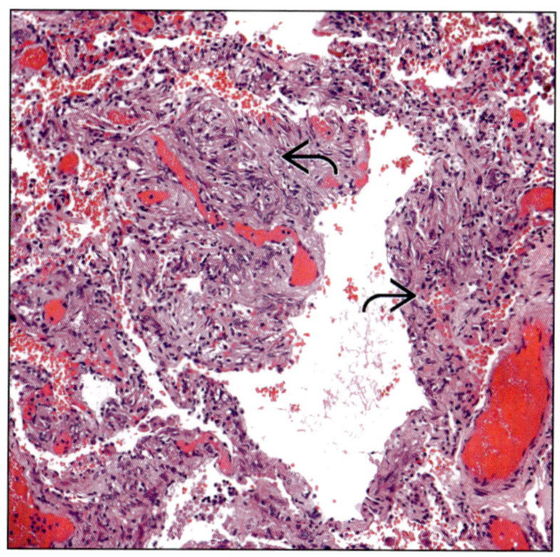

(Left) *The presence of muscle proliferation must be separated from the normal muscle layers that surround normal airway structures. Note the difference between the muscle of LAM* ↷ *and the normal muscular layer around the airway* →. ***(Right)*** *In some cases of LAM, the muscle proliferation can be marked and can actually mimic a smooth muscle tumor. The muscle proliferation* ↷ *in this case is extensive, destroying normal lung architecture.*

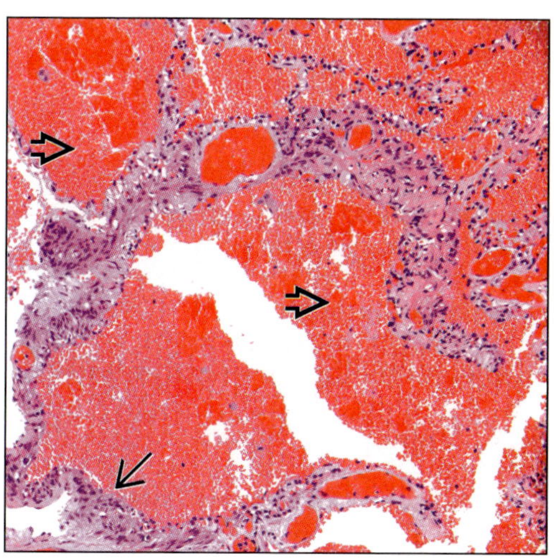
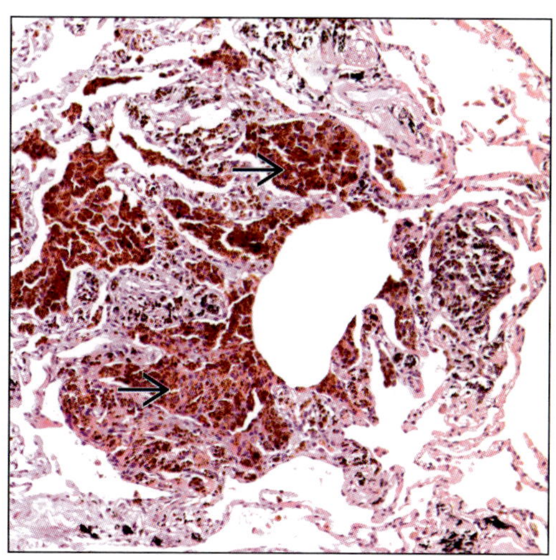

(Left) *Despite the presence of dilated alveolar spaces filled with fresh blood* ⇨, *smooth muscle proliferation* → *is still visible.* ***(Right)*** *One additional feature that may be seen in most of the cases of LAM is the presence of hemosiderin-laden macrophages* → *filling alveolar spaces, as shown here.*

NEUROENDOCRINE CARCINOMA, LUNG

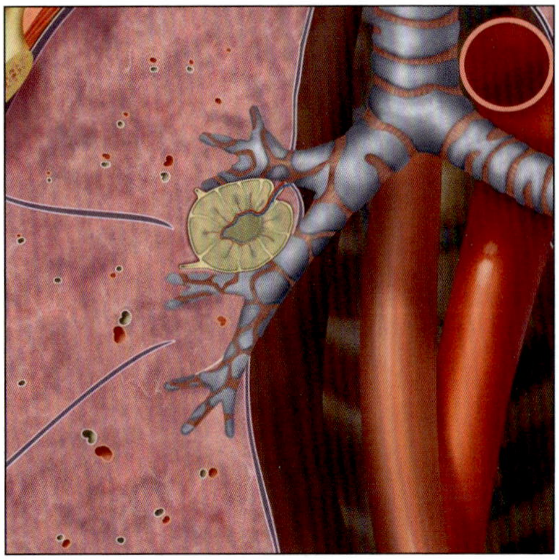

Graphic of a neuroendocrine carcinoma of the lung shows 1 of the usual locations of these tumors. The tumors are usually endobronchial and obstruct the bronchial lumen.

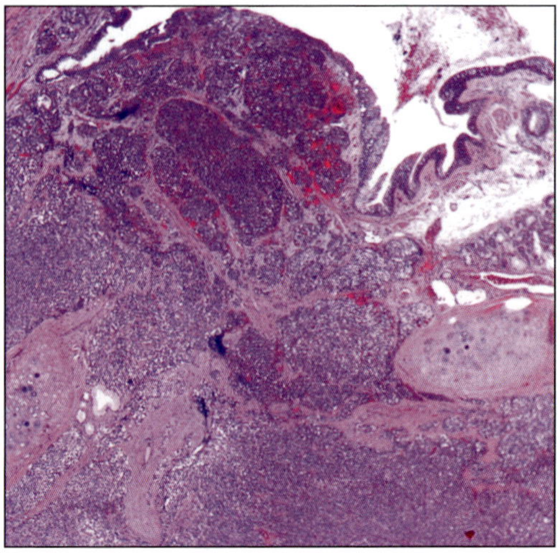

Low-power view of a low-grade endobronchial neuroendocrine carcinoma (carcinoid tumor) shows organized pattern of growth.

TERMINOLOGY

Synonyms

- Carcinoid tumor, atypical carcinoid, small cell carcinoma, large cell carcinoma

Definitions

- Spectrum of neoplasms ranging from low- to high-grade malignancy showing neuroendocrine differentiation

ETIOLOGY/PATHOGENESIS

Etiology

- Tumor is thought to be derived from Kulchitsky cells
- Patients with hereditary retinoblastoma syndrome have an increased risk of developing neuroendocrine lung tumors

CLINICAL ISSUES

Presentation

- Incidental finding
- Paraneoplastic syndromes
- Chest pain, cough, dyspnea, or hemoptysis

Treatment

- Surgical approaches
  - Low- and intermediate-grade tumor
- Adjuvant therapy
  - High-grade tumors

Prognosis

- Low-grade neoplasms
  - Survival rate at 5 years: > 75%
- Intermediate-grade neoplasms
  - Survival rate at 5 years: ~ 50%
- High-grade neoplasms
  - Survival rate at 5 years: May be < 5%

MACROSCOPIC FEATURES

General Features

- Endobronchial or intraparenchymal tumor
- High-grade tumor may show extensive areas of necrosis

Size

- 0.5 to > 10 cm in diameter

MICROSCOPIC PATHOLOGY

Histologic Features

- Low-grade tumors
  - < 3 mitotic figures per 10 high-power field (HPF)
  - Necrosis is absent
- Intermediate-grade tumors
  - 3-10 mitotic figures per 10 HPF
  - Comedo-like necrosis
- High-grade tumors
  - > 10 mitotic figures per 10 HPF
  - Necrosis is present
- Large cell neuroendocrine carcinoma requires neuroendocrine pattern and positive staining with neuroendocrine markers (chromogranin-A, synaptophysin, CD56)
  - Cells with prominent nucleoli
  - Neuroendocrine markers must be positive
  - Electron microscopic studies show neurosecretory granules
  - Comedo-like necrosis
- Small cell carcinoma
  - Miotic figures > 10 per 10 HPF applies only to resected specimens
  - Neuroendocrine markers are not required for diagnosis

NEUROENDOCRINE CARCINOMA, LUNG

Key Facts

Terminology
- Spectrum of neoplasms ranging from low- to high-grade malignancy

Etiology/Pathogenesis
- Patients with hereditary retinoblastoma syndrome have an increased risk of developing neuroendocrine lung tumors

Clinical Issues
- Paraneoplastic syndromes

Macroscopic Features
- Endobronchial or intraparenchymal tumor
- 0.5 to > 10 cm in diameter

Microscopic Pathology
- Neuroendocrine pattern, mitotic activity, necrosis
- Low-grade tumors: < 2 mitotic figures per 10 HPF; absence of necrosis
- Intermediate-grade tumor: 3-10 mitotic figures per 10 HPF; comedo-like necrosis
- High-grade tumors: > 10 mitotic figures per 10 HPF; necrosis is present
- Large cell neuroendocrine carcinoma requires neuroendocrine pattern and positive staining with neuroendocrine markers (chromogranin-A, synaptophysin, CD56)
- In small cell carcinoma, mitotic count of > 10 per 10 HPF applies only to resected specimens, not biopsy material

Ancillary Tests
- Chromogranin-A, CD56, synaptophysin

Predominant Pattern/Injury Type
- Nesting
- Diffuse
- Mucinous
- Glandular

Predominant Cell/Compartment Type
- Oncocytic
- Spindle
- Melanocytic
- Epithelial, neuroendocrine
- Clear

DIFFERENTIAL DIAGNOSIS

Low-Grade Neuroendocrine Carcinoma
- < 3 mitotic figures and absence of necrosis
- Well-organized growth pattern

Intermediate-Grade Neuroendocrine Carcinoma
- Mitotic activity from 3-9 per 10 HPF and necrosis
- Often a combination of well-organized nested pattern and diffuse pattern of growth

High-Grade Neuroendocrine Carcinoma
- > 10 mitotic figures per 10 HPF, necrosis &/or hemorrhage (in resected specimens)
- Positive neuroendocrine markers (synaptophysin, chromogranin-B, &/or CD56) in cases of large cell neuroendocrine carcinoma
- In cases of small cell carcinoma, neuroendocrine markers may be negative

Carcinoid Tumorlet
- These tumors are usually < 5 mm in diameter
- Tumorlets and carcinoid tumors share same immunophenotype

Metastatic Neuroendocrine Carcinoma of Extrathoracic Origin
- Clinical history of previous tumor is of utmost importance
- Immunohistochemical study for TTF-1 may be helpful

Pulmonary Paraganglioma
- Paragangliomas and neuroendocrine tumors show positive staining for neuroendocrine markers
- Usually negative for keratin
- Generally do not show mitotic activity
- Usually show cells with macronuclei

Large Cell Carcinoma
- Must show neuroendocrine pattern and positive neuroendocrine markers

Large Cell Carcinoma With Neuroendocrine Differentiation
- Histology is that of conventional non-small cell carcinoma with positive neuroendocrine markers

Large Cell Carcinoma With Neuroendocrine Pattern
- Tumors show neuroendocrine histologic pattern but negative staining for neuroendocrine markers

DIAGNOSTIC CHECKLIST

Clinically Relevant Pathologic Features
- Mitotic rate

Pathologic Interpretation Pearls
- Neuroendocrine pattern
- Rosettes
- Necrosis
- Mitotic activity
- Positive neuroendocrine markers in large cell neuroendocrine carcinoma

NEUROENDOCRINE CARCINOMA, LUNG

Immunohistochemistry

Antibody	Reactivity	Staining Pattern	Comment
Chromogranin-A	Positive	Cytoplasmic	Strongly positive but not global
Synaptophysin	Positive	Cytoplasmic	Diffuse positive staining
CD56	Positive	Cytoplasmic	Diffuse staining
KERATIN-LMW	Positive	Cytoplasmic	Diffuse staining
TTF-1	Positive	Nuclear	In most cases
CD57	Positive	Cytoplasmic	In some cases
Bombesin	Positive	Cytoplasmic	In some cases
LEU-7	Positive	Cytoplasmic	In some cases
CK7	Positive	Cytoplasmic	Diffuse positive staining
CDX-2	Negative		

Molecular Features of Neuroendocrine Carcinomas

Gene Alterations	Result
RB gene; hereditary retinoblastoma syndrome	Well-differentiated and moderately differentiated carcinomas
11q deletion	Well-differentiated and moderately differentiated carcinomas
10q and 13q losses	Well-differentiated and moderately differentiated carcinomas
3q gain	Small cell carcinoma
10q-, 16q-, and 17p deletions	High-grade neuroendocrine carcinomas
LOH at 3p14.2-p21.3	More common in moderately differentiated carcinomas

GRADING

Low-Grade Neuroendocrine Carcinoma (Carcinoid Tumor)

- Tumors with < 3 mitoses per 10 HPF and no necrosis

Intermediate-Grade Neuroendocrine Carcinoma (Atypical Carcinoid)

- Tumors with ≥ 3 but > 10 per 10 HPF and necrosis

High-Grade Neuroendocrine Carcinoma

- Small cell carcinoma
- Large cell neuroendocrine carcinoma
  - For large cell neuroendocrine carcinoma, neuroendocrine markers must be positive

SELECTED REFERENCES

1. Allan B et al: Malignant neuroendocrine tumors: incidence and outcomes in pediatric patients. Eur J Pediatr Surg. 23(5):394-9, 2013
2. den Bakker MA et al: Neuroendocrine tumours--challenges in the diagnosis and classification of pulmonary neuroendocrine tumours. J Clin Pathol. 66(10):862-9, 2013
3. Grand B et al: High grade neuroendocrine lung tumors: Pathological characteristics, surgical management and prognostic implications. Lung Cancer. 81(3):404-9, 2013
4. Kalemkerian GP et al: Small cell lung cancer. J Natl Compr Canc Netw. 11(1):78-98, 2013
5. Kinoshita T et al: The differences of biological behavior based on the clinicopathological data between resectable large-cell neuroendocrine carcinoma and small-cell lung carcinoma. Clin Lung Cancer. 14(5):535-40, 2013
6. Nakamura H et al: Aberrant anaplastic lymphoma kinase expression in high-grade pulmonary neuroendocrine carcinoma. J Clin Pathol. 66(8):705-7, 2013
7. Alì G et al: Expression of p-AKT and p-mTOR in a large series of bronchopulmonary neuroendocrine tumors. Exp Ther Med. 2(5):787-792, 2011
8. Iyoda A et al: Expression profiling and identification of potential molecular targets for therapy in pulmonary large-cell neuroendocrine carcinoma. Exp Ther Med. 2(6):1041-1045, 2011
9. Moran CA et al: Neuroendocrine carcinomas of the lung: a critical analysis. Am J Clin Pathol. 131(2):206-21, 2009
10. Dörffel Y et al: Neuroendocrine tumors: characterization with contrast-enhanced ultrasonography. Ultraschall Med. 29(5):506-14, 2008
11. García-Yuste M et al: Neuroendocrine tumors of the lung. Curr Opin Oncol. 20(2):148-54, 2008
12. Gustafsson BI et al: Bronchopulmonary neuroendocrine tumors. Cancer. 113(1):5-21, 2008
13. Yao JC et al: One hundred years after "carcinoid": epidemiology of and prognostic factors for neuroendocrine tumors in 35,825 cases in the United States. J Clin Oncol. 26(18):3063-72, 2008
14. Moran CA et al: Neuroendocrine carcinomas (carcinoid, atypical carcinoid, small cell carcinoma, and large cell neuroendocrine carcinoma): current concepts. Hematol Oncol Clin North Am. 21(3):395-407; vii, 2007
15. Cerilli LA et al: Neuroendocrine neoplasms of the lung. Am J Clin Pathol. 116 Suppl:S65-96, 2001

Low-Grade NE Carcinoma (Carcinoid Tumor)

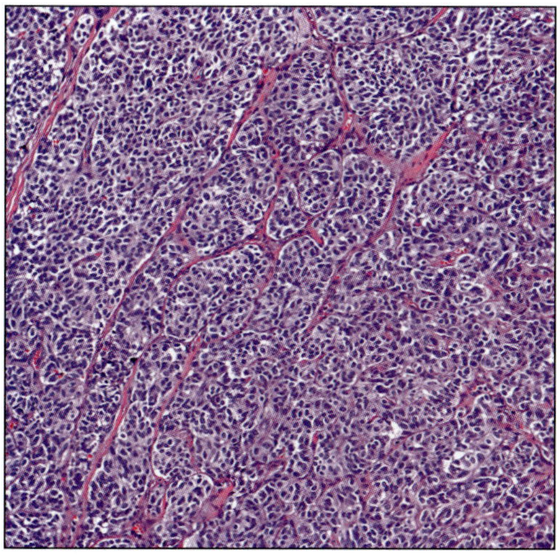
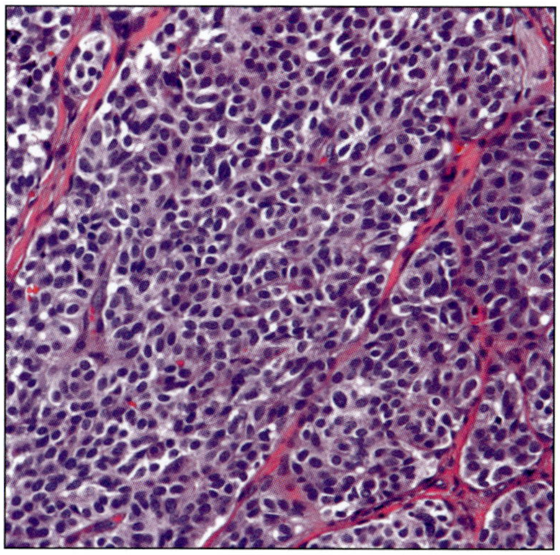

(Left) *H&E shows the nesting pattern in a low-grade neuroendocrine carcinoma. Note the well-organized growth and delicate bands of fibroconnective tissue separating the nests of tumor cells.* ***(Right)*** *Homogeneous cellular proliferation without nuclear atypia, necrosis, or hemorrhage is shown. Notice the well-organized pattern of growth, which is 1 important parameter in low-grade neuroendocrine lung tumors.*

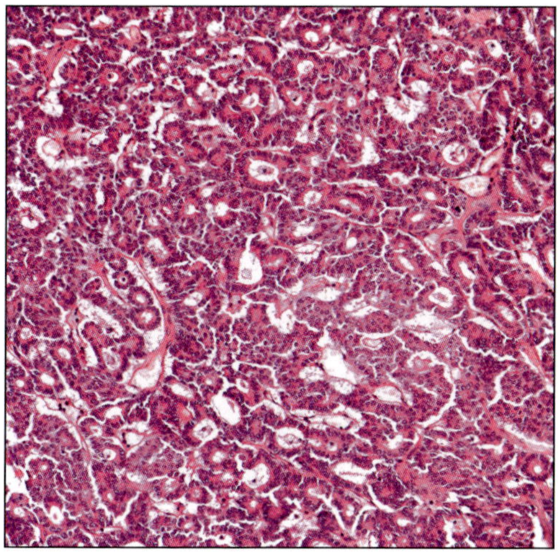
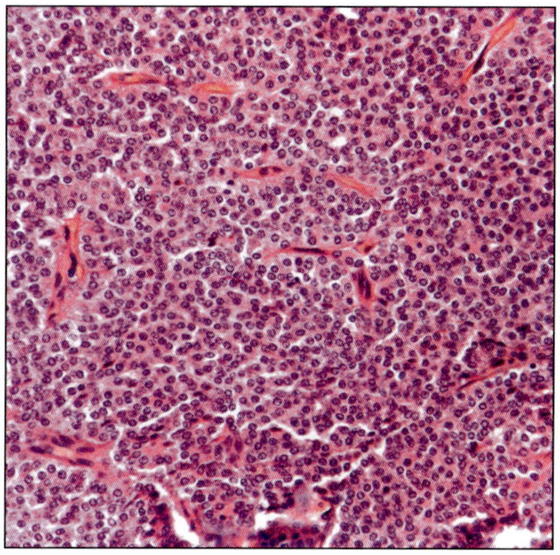

(Left) *Tubular (glandular) pattern of a low-grade neuroendocrine carcinoma is shown. This glandular pattern at low-power view may mimic adenocarcinoma.* ***(Right)*** *Sheets of cells with a homogeneous pattern are shown in a low-grade neuroendocrine carcinoma. Note the absence of necrosis &/or hemorrhage. These features are highly important in low-grade tumors in helping to separate them from higher grade tumors.*

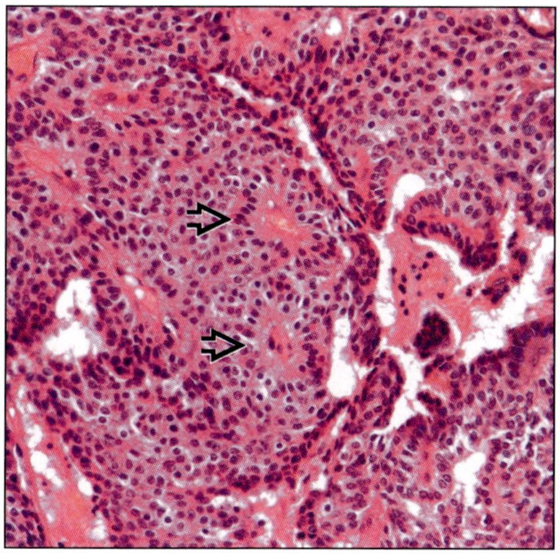
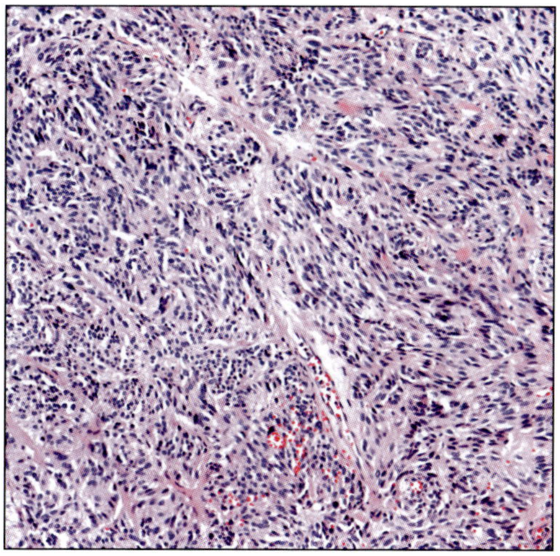

(Left) *H&E shows rosettes* ⇨ *in a well-differentiated neuroendocrine carcinoma. Also important to note is the absence of mitotic activity &/or necrosis.* ***(Right)*** *Low-grade neuroendocrine carcinoma with prominent spindle cell growth pattern is shown. The tumor does not show necrosis, hemorrhage, or mitotic activity, which are not features of low-grade tumors.*

Low-Grade NE Carcinoma (Carcinoid Tumor)

*(**Left**) Well-differentiated neuroendocrine carcinoma shows glands composed of rather small cells without mitotic activity. This pseudoglandular architecture may be erroneously interpreted as adenocarcinoma. Thus, a careful cytological examination of the neoplastic cells is important. (**Right**) H&E shows glandular pattern of low-grade neuroendocrine carcinoma. This complex architecture may mimic a well-differentiated adenocarcinoma.*

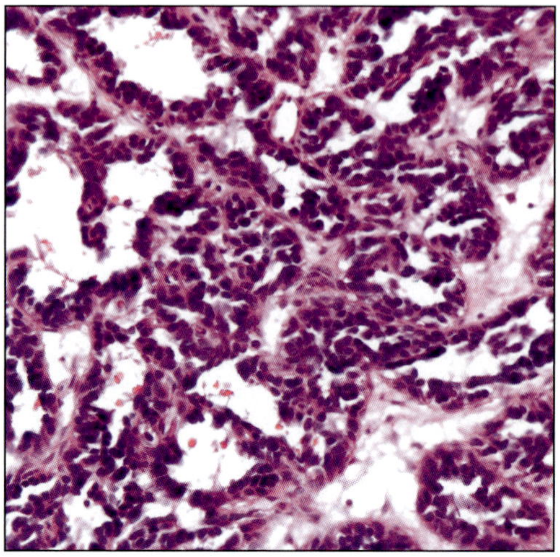

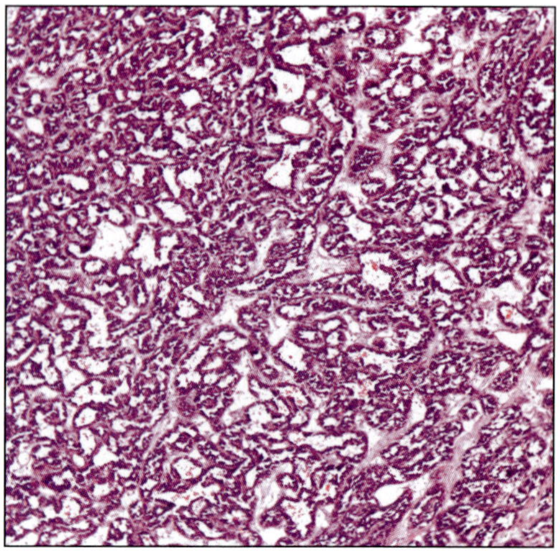

*(**Left**) Well-differentiated neuroendocrine carcinoma shows subtle nesting pattern with spindle cell proliferation. This architectural pattern may be misinterpreted as sarcoma or other neoplasms of neuroectodermal origin, such as melanomas. (**Right**) Spindle cells without nuclear atypia or mitotic activity are shown. The pattern of growth mimics a neural neoplasm. A spindle cell pattern may also be seen in higher grade tumors.*

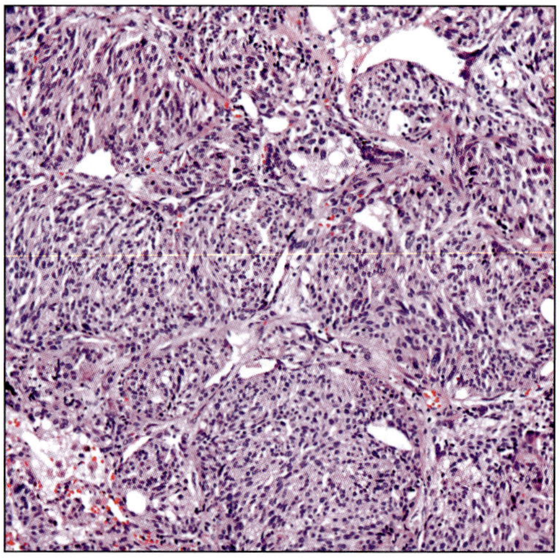

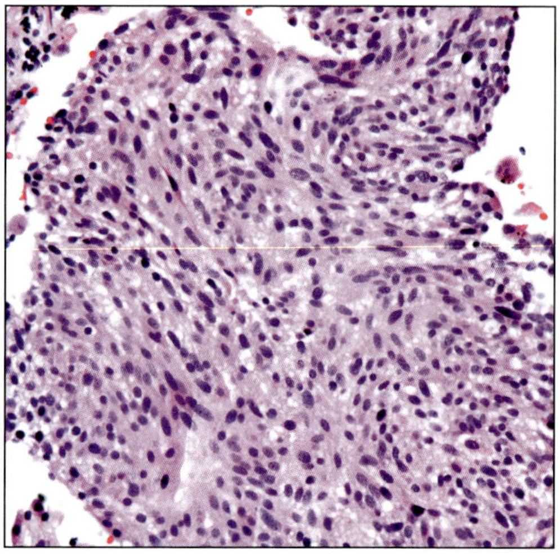

*(**Left**) Low-grade neuroendocrine carcinoma is shown with areas of metaplastic bone formation. Bone formation in neuroendocrine carcinomas is rare. This metaplastic change is rarely extensive. (**Right**) Closer view of the metaplastic bone formation in neuroendocrine carcinoma shows pseudoglandular arrangement of the neoplastic neuroendocrine cells.*

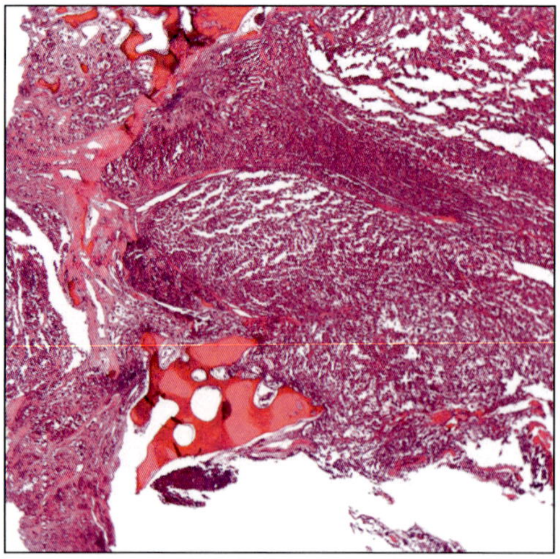

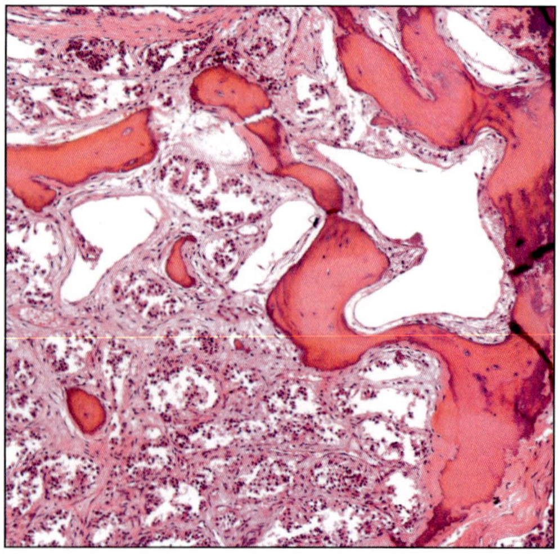

Intermediate-Grade NE Carcinoma (Atypical Carcinoid)

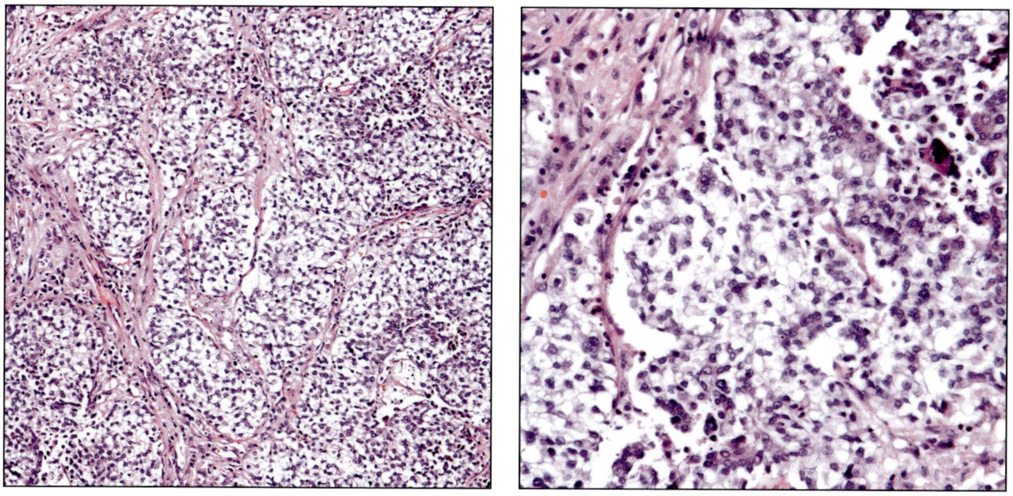

(Left) *Atypical carcinoid (AC) shows the characteristic nesting growth pattern of neuroendocrine carcinoma; however, the neoplastic cellular proliferation is composed of clear cells. The presence of extensive areas of clear cell change in neuroendocrine carcinomas is rare.* ***(Right)*** *Closer view shows neuroendocrine cellular proliferation composed predominantly of clear cells with small round and homogeneous nuclei. Nucleoli are inconspicuous.*

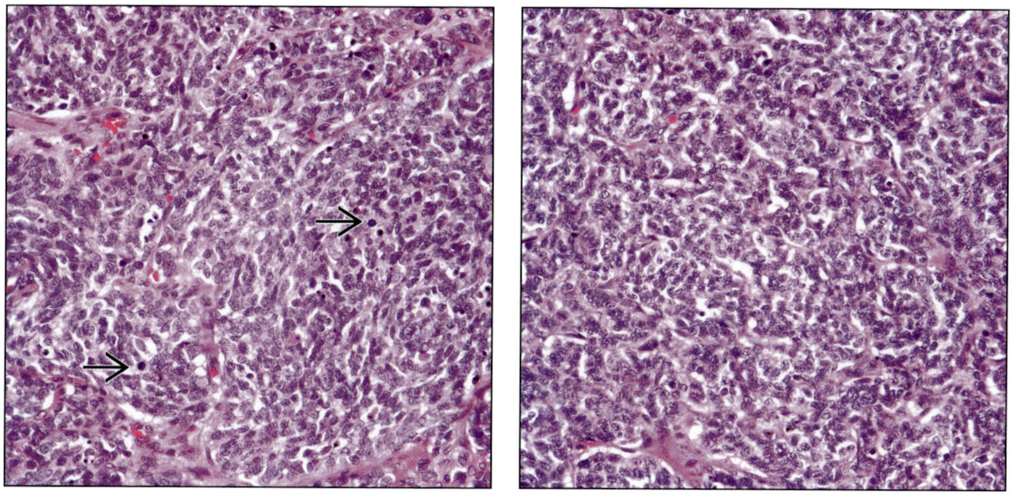

(Left) *H&E shows spindle cell neuroendocrine carcinoma with easily identifiable mitotic figures* →. *The mitotic count in neuroendocrine carcinoma is the most important feature in the classification of these tumors.* ***(Right)*** *Sheets of neoplastic cells are shown in a disorganized pattern of growth. Nuclear atypia is evident and should prompt the search for mitotic activity.*

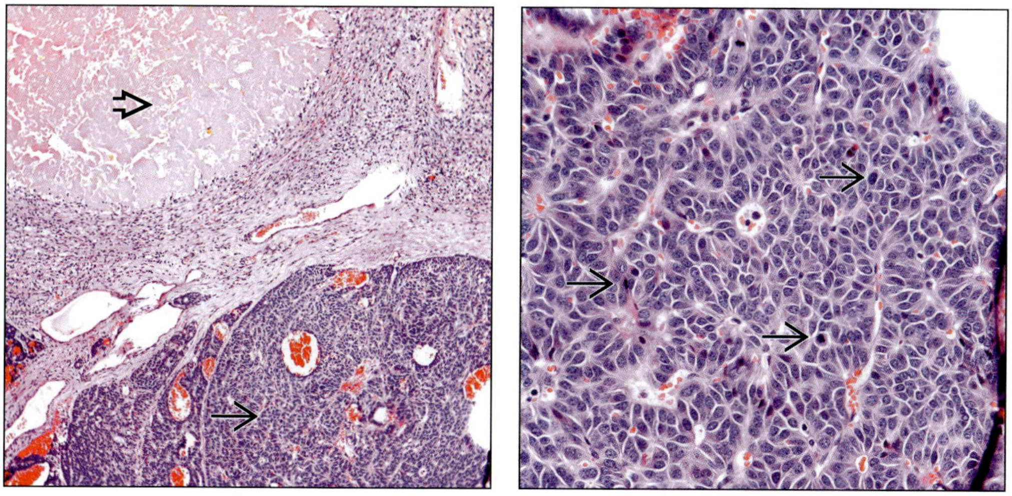

(Left) *Moderately differentiated neuroendocrine carcinoma shows extensive areas of necrosis* ⇨ *with areas of viable tumor* →. *It is very important to separate tumor necrosis from other possible causes of necrosis, such as necrosis secondary to needle biopsy.* ***(Right)*** *H&E shows well-organized pattern with rosettes and easily identifiable mitotic figures* →. *Although the pattern is fairly organized, the presence of mitotic figures is the most important criterion for grading these tumors.*

High-Grade NE Carcinoma, Small Cell Type

*(**Left**) H&E shows predominantly solid pattern of growth of neoplastic cells with high mitotic activity and prominent nuclear atypia. (**Right**) H&E shows solid pattern of neoplastic cells ➡ admixed with numerous inflammatory cells, predominantly lymphocytes ➩. In some cases, the inflammatory response may be very prominent. It is unusual to see this type of feature in small cell carcinomas.*

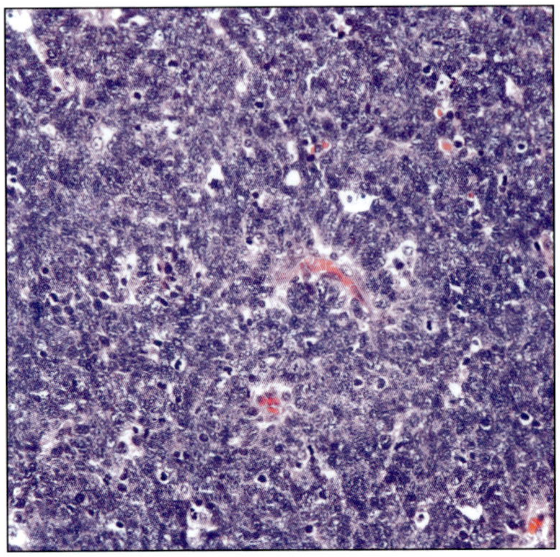

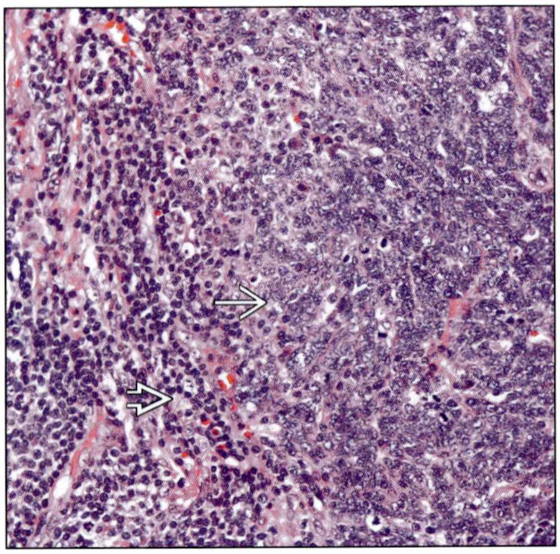

*(**Left**) H&E shows high-grade neuroendocrine carcinoma with extensive necrosis and sheets of neoplastic cells with a vague basaloid pattern. (**Right**) Closer view shows neoplastic cells in a high-grade neuroendocrine carcinoma. Note the absence of nucleoli, which is an important characteristic of these tumors. The features of small cell carcinomas in resected specimens may show better preservation than in biopsy specimens.*

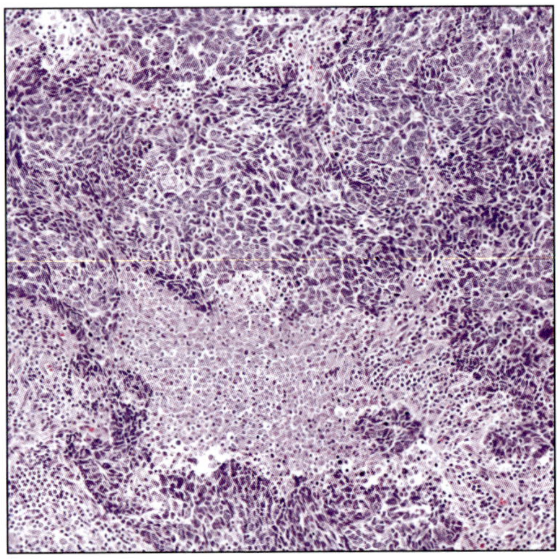

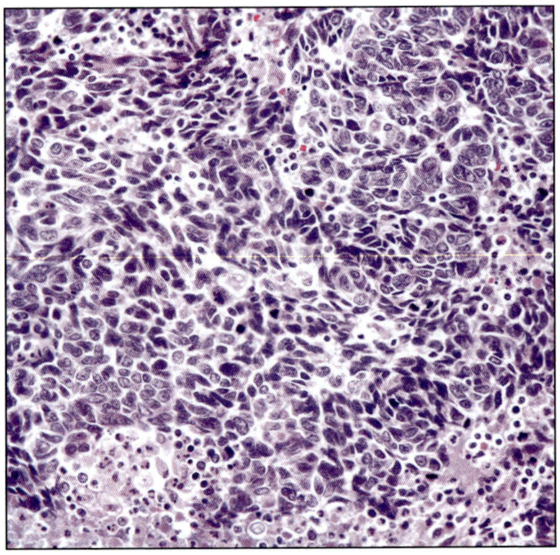

*(**Left**) H&E shows extensive necrosis and clusters of neoplastic cells. The tumor cytology is that of small cells with scant cytoplasm and inconspicuous nucleoli. Often the presence of extensive areas of necrosis is more commonly seen in high-grade tumors. (**Right**) H&E shows classic small cell morphology of small cells with nuclear molding and prominent atypia. However, in this example, the presence of mitoses is not marked.*

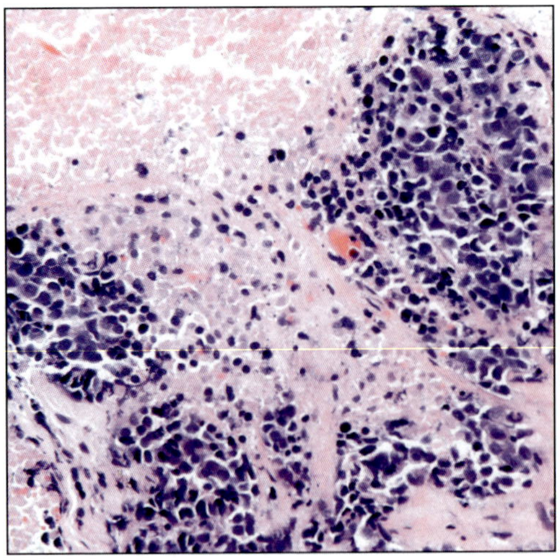

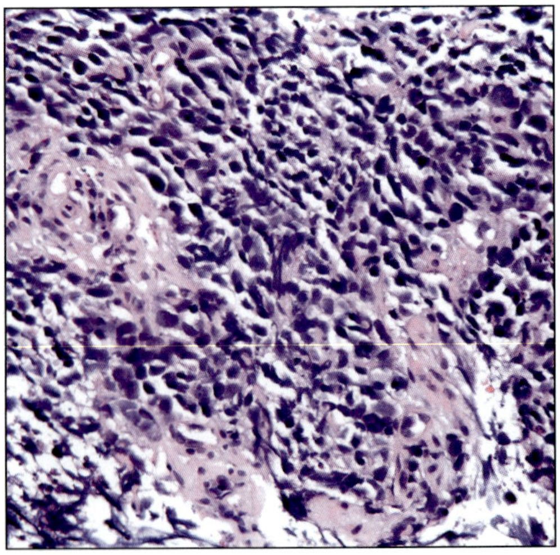

High-Grade NE Carcinoma, Large Cell Type

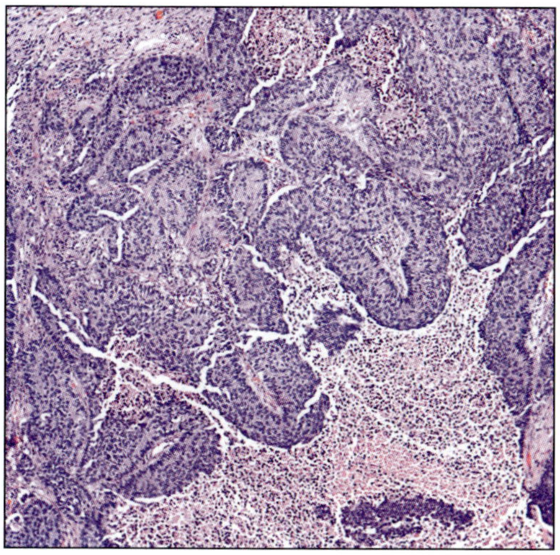

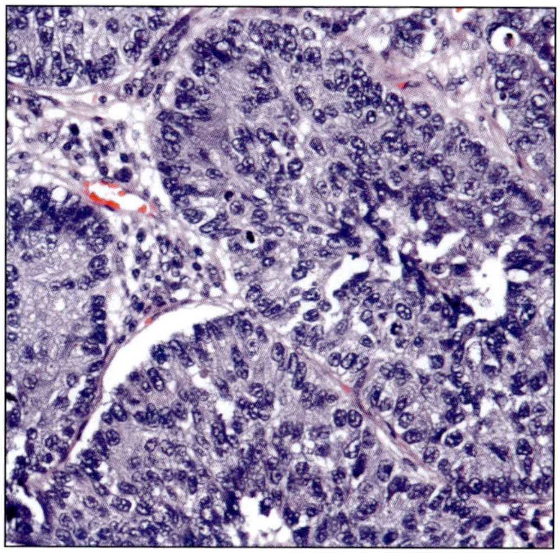

(Left) *H&E shows large cell neuroendocrine carcinoma with necrosis and organoid pattern of growth. This pattern, however, may be seen in tumors that do not show positive neuroendocrine markers.* ***(Right)*** *Closer view shows neoplastic cells displaying nuclear atypia and prominent nucleoli. However, it is the positive staining for neuroendocrine markers that confirms the diagnosis of large cell neuroendocrine carcinoma.*

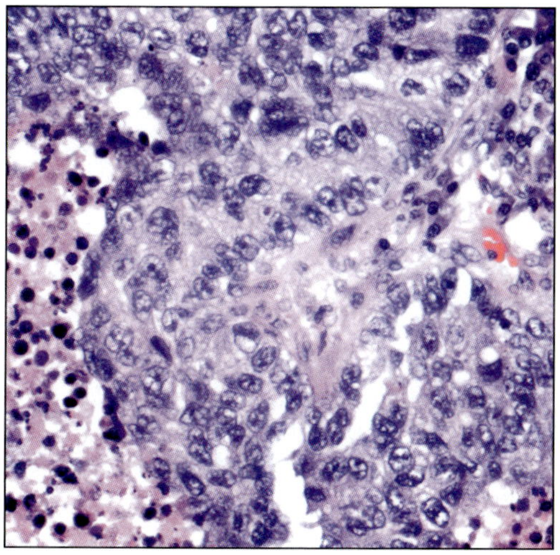

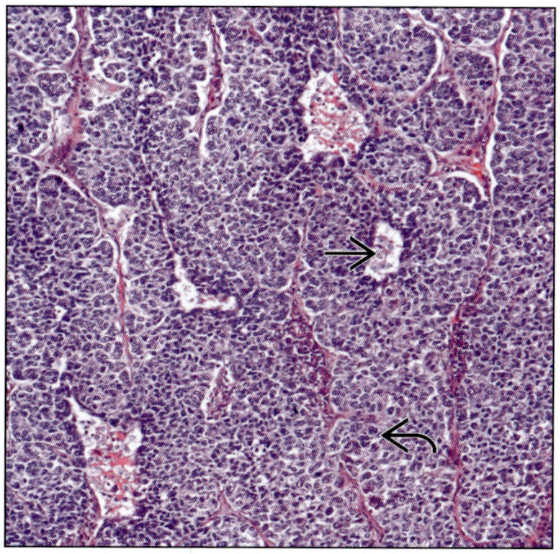

(Left) *High-power view shows larger cells with ample cytoplasm, round nuclei, and prominent nucleoli. These features are those of a non-small cell carcinoma.* ***(Right)*** *High-grade neuroendocrine carcinoma is shown with more conventional nesting pattern and absence of obvious necrosis. In some focal areas, there is a hint of comedo-like necrosis* → *and the presence of larger pleomorphic cells* ↶.

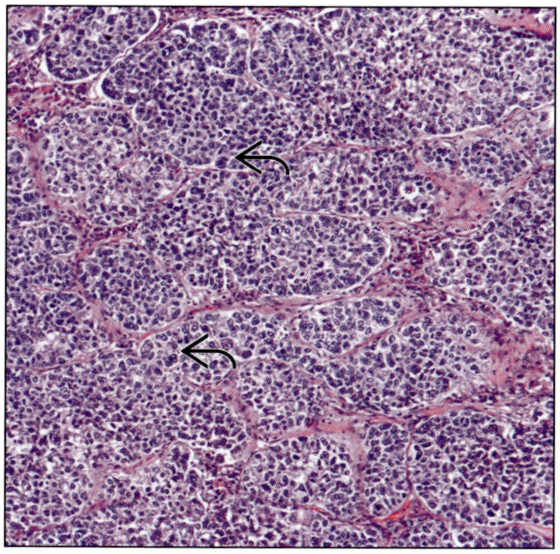

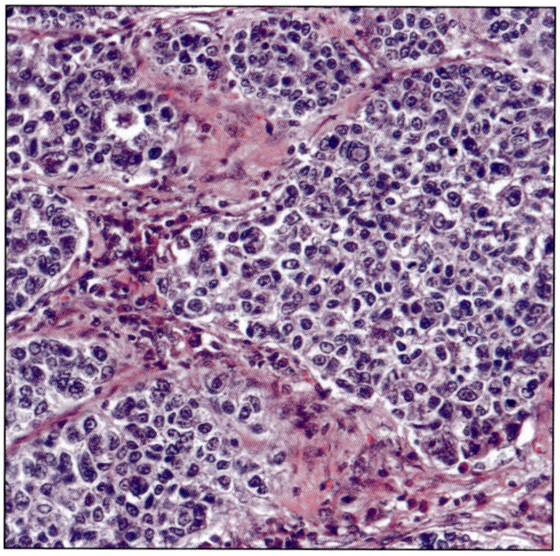

(Left) *High-grade neuroendocrine carcinoma is shown with a very organized pattern of growth. Necrosis is absent; however, note the presence of marked nuclear atypia* ↶*, which should raise the suspicion of a higher grade neoplasm.* ***(Right)*** *High-grade neuroendocrine carcinoma shows the classic characteristics of prominent nuclear atypia and increased mitotic activity; however, necrosis is absent.*

PLEUROPULMONARY BLASTOMA

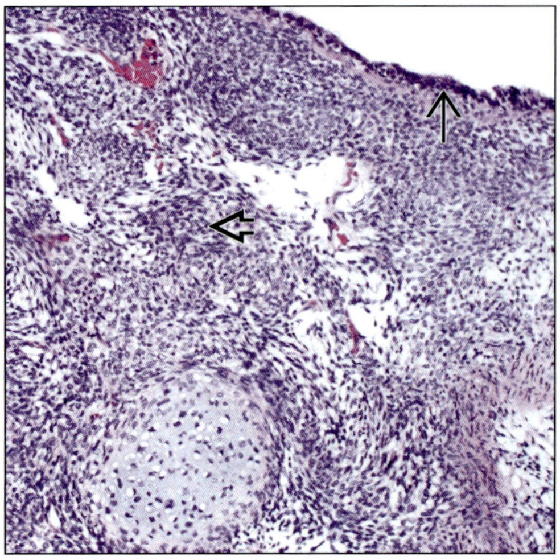

This low-power view of solid type III pleuropulmonary blastoma (PPB) shows benign epithelial component in the upper right ➔ overlying the malignant mesenchymal component ⇨.

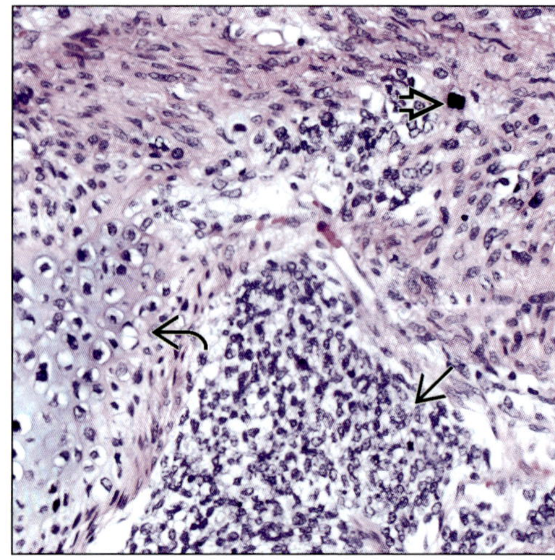

Solid component of PPB illustrated here consists of malignant cartilage ↩, blastema ➔, and spindle cell undifferentiated sarcoma with atypical mitotic figure ⇨.

TERMINOLOGY

Abbreviations

- Pleuropulmonary blastoma (PPB)

Synonyms

- Mesenchymal cystic hamartoma, malignant mesenchymoma, sarcoma arising in congenital cystic malformation

Definitions

- Embryonal tumor of lung and pleura with epithelial (benign) and mesenchymal (low- to high-grade malignant) components, presenting most often in early childhood
- A rare pediatric lung tumor that is often part of an inherited cancer syndrome
  - PBBs consist of mesenchymal cells that are susceptible to malignant transformation and cysts lined by epithelial cells
  - Sentinel disease in a familial tumor syndrome recently found to be associated with germline mutations in *DICER1*

ETIOLOGY/PATHOGENESIS

Genetic Abnormality

- 20% are familial and associated with other extrapulmonary lesions in same patient or family members
- Heterozygous germline mutations in *DICER1* have been identified in familial PPB
  - Loss of DICER1 protein expression specifically in lung epithelium overlying mesenchymal component
  - Loss of DICER1 in epithelium of developing lung alters regulation of diffusible factors that promote mesenchymal proliferation
- Extrapulmonary lesions include cystic nephroma (most common), thyroid hyperplasia, rhabdomyosarcoma, Sertoli-Leydig-type tumors, and other embryonal tumors
- Variety of karyotypic abnormalities have been described; gain of chromosome 8, usually as trisomy 8, is very common
  - Thus PPB may arise through a novel mechanism of non-cell-autonomous cancer initiation

CLINICAL ISSUES

Epidemiology

- Incidence
  - Extremely rare tumor, estimated incidence of 0.35-0.65 cases per 100,000 births
  - Most common malignancy of lung presenting in early childhood
- Age
  - Occurs almost exclusively in children, primarily in infants and toddlers
    - 94% present in children < 6 years old
    - Rare beyond 12 years of age

Presentation

- May be detected incidentally in utero or postnatally
- Most common presentation is respiratory distress ± pneumothorax
- May be solitary or multiple with additional lesions occurring synchronously or metachronously
- In a subset of patients, overgrowth of cysts by mesenchymal cells → sarcoma formation

Treatment

- Depends on type of PPB
  - PPB I (cystic): Complete surgical resection; adjuvant chemotherapy if resection is incomplete
  - PPB II (cystic and solid) and PPB III (solid): Complete surgical resection followed by adjuvant chemotherapy; radiation therapy for residual disease

PLEUROPULMONARY BLASTOMA

Key Facts

Terminology
- Embryonal tumor of lung and pleura with epithelial (benign) and mesenchymal (low- to high-grade malignant) components, presenting most often in early childhood

Etiology/Pathogenesis
- 20% are familial and associated with other extrapulmonary lesions in same patient or family members
- Heterozygous germline mutations in *DICER1* have been identified in familial pleuropulmonary blastoma (PPB)

Macroscopic Features
- Type I: Peripheral- and pleural-based cysts, sometimes protruding from pleural surface, no solid nodules
- Type II: Both solid and cystic areas in varying proportions
- Type III: All solid, although areas of necrosis and cystic degeneration may be present

Microscopic Pathology
- PPB type I: Large cysts lined by single layer of cuboidal to flattened benign epithelium; within wall, there are areas of hypercellularity composed of small blue to spindled cells, often forming cambium-like layer
- PPB types II and III have variable amount of solid areas composed of higher grade sarcomatous components (which may be undifferentiated), rhabdomyosarcomatous, or chondrosarcomatous

- Close clinical follow-up for recurrence, metastasis, multifocal lesions, extrapulmonary lesions

Prognosis
- 5-year survival is 83% for type I and 42% for types II and III PPB
- Type I may recur as higher grade (II or III) lesions
- Metastases occur in 30% of types II and III lesions and may occur late
- Sites of metastases include central nervous system and bone

Associated Tumors
- Cystic nephroma (CN)
  - Multilocular CN is a benign kidney tumor and is part of a family of kidney neoplasms including cystic partially differentiated nephroblastoma and Wilms tumor
  - CN is rarely familial or bilateral, but it occurs in ~ 10% of families in which PPB is present
- Medulloepithelioma
- Embryonal rhabdomyosarcoma is the most common childhood sarcoma and is a component of familial PPB predisposition syndrome
- Ovarian sex cord-stromal tumors (OSCST)
  - Primary ovarian neoplasms, particularly OSCST, are a manifestation of familial PPB syndrome and may be initial clinical presentation of *DICER1* mutations within a family
  - OSCST is also present in PPB kindred
- Multinodular hyperplasia
  - *DICER1* mutations are associated with both familial multinodular goiter (MNG) and MNG with Sertoli-Leydig cell tumor (SLCT), independent of PPB
- Nasal chondromesenchymal hamartoma (NCMH), an extremely rare benign tumor arising in sinonasal tract

IMAGE FINDINGS

General Features
- Best diagnostic clue
  - Radiographically seen as unilocular or multilocular cyst, mixed cystic or solid lesion, or large solid mass often distorting contour of lung, located in periphery or protruding from pleura

MACROSCOPIC FEATURES

Subclassification
- Based on gross morphology
- Type I: Purely cystic
- Type II: Solid and cystic
- Type III: Purely solid

Gross Features
- Type I: Peripheral- and pleural-based cysts, sometimes protruding from pleural surface, no solid nodules
- Type II: Both solid and cystic areas in varying proportions
- Type III: All solid, although areas of necrosis and cystic degeneration may be present

MICROSCOPIC PATHOLOGY

Histologic Features
- PPB type I: Large cysts lined by single layer of cuboidal to flattened benign epithelium; within wall, there are areas of hypercellularity composed of small blue to spindled cells, often forming cambium-like layer
- PPB types II and III have variable amount of solid areas composed of higher grade sarcomatous (which may be undifferentiated), rhabdomyosarcomatous, or chondrosarcomatous components
- Primitive/sarcomatous component is vimentin (+); may be focal myogenic differentiation on IHC staining

ANCILLARY TESTS

In Situ Hybridization
- Chromosome 8 copy number
  - Polysomy of chromosome 8 is a feature of PPB

PLEUROPULMONARY BLASTOMA

Immunohistochemistry

Antibody	Reactivity	Comment
TTF-1	Positive	In glandular component
EMA/MUC1	Positive	In glandular component
CEA-M	Positive	In glandular component
Chromogranin-A	Positive	In morules
p53	Positive	Scattered nuclei
Desmin	Positive	In muscle component
Myogenin	Positive	In muscle component
S100	Positive	In nerves and adipose tissue component

- Chromosome 8 gains are present in all mesenchymal elements, including undifferentiated blastematous, rhabdomyoblastic, fibroblastic, and chondroblastic areas
- Epithelial cells show no chromosome 8 gains

DIFFERENTIAL DIAGNOSIS

Congenital Pulmonary Airway Malformation Type 4 (CPAM 4)

- PPB type I has areas very similar to CPAM 4; however, latter has no immature/malignant component
- Cytogenetically, these are completely different lesions

Primary Sarcomas of Lung

- Synovial sarcoma can be distinguished by being focally keratin (+) and EMA(+), and by diagnostic t(X;18)
- Primary rhabdomyosarcoma of lung is very rare; many cases reported in older literature are probably PPB type III

DIAGNOSTIC CHECKLIST

Pathologic Interpretation Pearls

- Cystic lesions need to be sampled extensively to differentiate benign CPAM 4 from low-grade malignant PPB I
- PPB I may recur as PPB II or III
- Margins of resection must be assessed

SELECTED REFERENCES

1. Darrat I et al: Novel DICER1 mutation as cause of multinodular goiter in children. Head Neck. Epub ahead of print, 2013
2. de Kock L et al: Germ-line and somatic DICER1 mutations in a pleuropulmonary blastoma. Pediatr Blood Cancer. Epub ahead of print, 2013
3. Laird PW et al: Ciliary body medulloepithelioma associated with pleuropulmonary blastoma. Br J Ophthalmol. 97(8):1079, 2013
4. Lucia-Casadonte C et al: An unusual case of pleuropulmonary blastoma in a child with jejunal hamartomas. Case Rep Pediatr. 2013:140508, 2013
5. Schultze-Florey RE et al: DICER1 syndrome: a new cancer syndrome. Klin Padiatr. 225(3):177-8, 2013
6. Behery RE et al: Translocation t(12;17)(q24.1;q21) as the sole anomaly in a nasal chondromesenchymal hamartoma arising in a patient with pleuropulmonary blastoma. Pediatr Dev Pathol. 15(3):249-53, 2012
7. Doros L et al: DICER1 mutations in embryonal rhabdomyosarcomas from children with and without familial PPB-tumor predisposition syndrome. Pediatr Blood Cancer. 59(3):558-60, 2012
8. Heravi-Moussavi A et al: Recurrent somatic DICER1 mutations in nonepithelial ovarian cancers. N Engl J Med. 366(3):234-42, 2012
9. Shin SH et al: Follicular thyroid carcinoma arising after hematopoietic stem cell transplantation in a child with pleuropulmonary blastoma. Thyroid. 22(5):547-51, 2012
10. Venkatramani R et al: Pleuropulmonary blastoma: a single-institution experience. J Pediatr Hematol Oncol. 34(5):e182-5, 2012
11. Bhardwaj AK et al: Bilateral cystic nephroma with pleuropulmonary blastoma. BMJ Case Rep. 2011, 2011
12. Foulkes WD et al: Extending the phenotypes associated with DICER1 mutations. Hum Mutat. 32(12):1381-4, 2011
13. Rio Frio T et al: DICER1 mutations in familial multinodular goiter with and without ovarian Sertoli-Leydig cell tumors. JAMA. 305(1):68-77, 2011
14. Schultz KA et al: Ovarian sex cord-stromal tumors, pleuropulmonary blastoma and DICER1 mutations: a report from the International Pleuropulmonary Blastoma Registry. Gynecol Oncol. 122(2):246-50, 2011
15. Slade I et al: DICER1 syndrome: clarifying the diagnosis, clinical features and management implications of a pleiotropic tumour predisposition syndrome. J Med Genet. 48(4):273-8, 2011
16. Traubici J et al: Pleuropulmonary blastoma in a child with autosomal-recessive polycystic kidney disease. Pediatr Radiol. 41(11):1465-8, 2011
17. Bahubeshi A et al: Germline DICER1 mutations and familial cystic nephroma. J Med Genet. 47(12):863-6, 2010
18. Hill DA et al: DICER1 mutations in familial pleuropulmonary blastoma. Science. 325(5943):965, 2009
19. Gutweiler JR et al: A familial case of pleuropulmonary blastoma. Eur J Pediatr Surg. 18(3):192-4, 2008
20. Hill DA et al: Type I pleuropulmonary blastoma: pathology and biology study of 51 cases from the international pleuropulmonary blastoma registry. Am J Surg Pathol. 32(2):282-95, 2008
21. Taube JM et al: Pleuropulmonary blastoma: cytogenetic and spectral karyotype analysis. Pediatr Dev Pathol. 9(6):453-61, 2006
22. Vargas SO et al: Gains of chromosome 8 are confined to mesenchymal components in pleuropulmonary blastoma. Pediatr Dev Pathol. 4(5):434-45, 2001

Types of Pleuropulmonary Blastoma

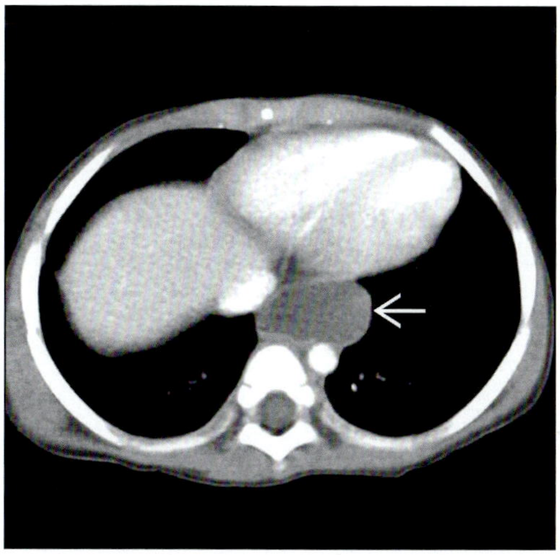

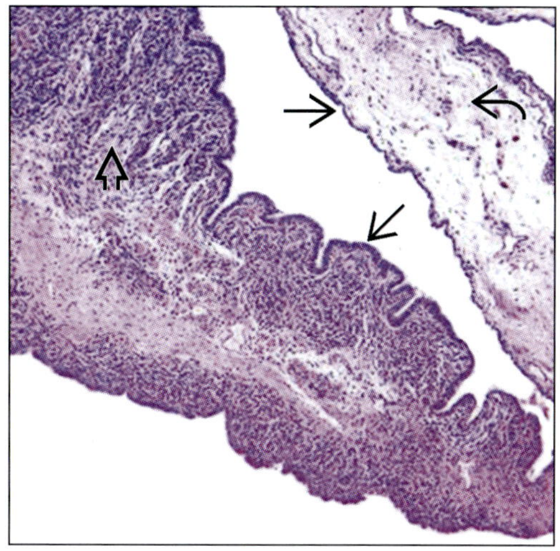

(Left) *CT scan of chest with type I PPB shows a pleural-based cystic lesion ➡ with no solid component. (Courtesy B. Shehata, MD.)* ***(Right)*** *This histologic section from a type I PPB shows the diagnostic cystic spaces lined by a single layer of epithelium →. The walls contain densely cellular (blastomatous) tumor ⇨ as well as loose hypocellular tissue ↪. (Courtesy B. Shehata, MD.)*

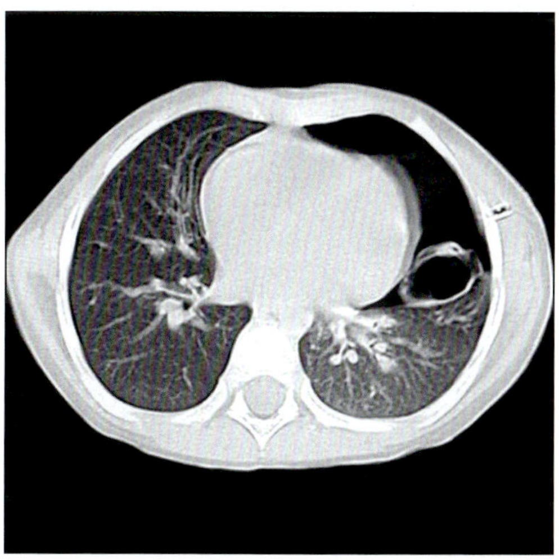

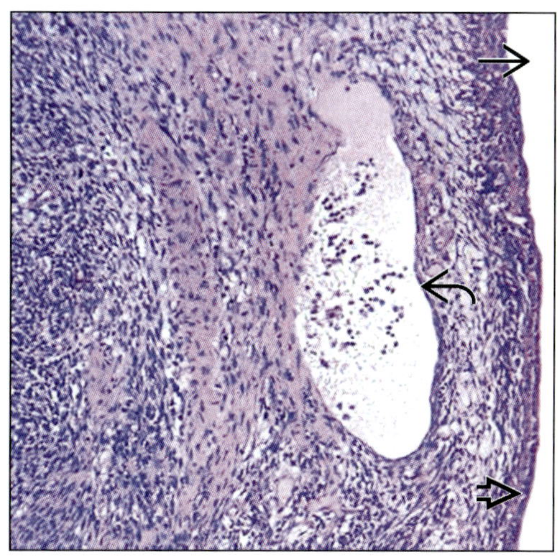

(Left) *CT scan of type II PPB shows a large cyst in the center of the left lung field, with some solid component in its wall. Part of the lung is collapsed. (Courtesy B. Shehata, MD.)* ***(Right)*** *This histologic section of a type II PPB has cystic space to the right →, which is lined by a single layer of cuboidal cells ⇨, beneath which is the solid cellular component of the tumor composed of primitive cells. In addition, there is a smaller cyst ↪. (Courtesy B. Shehata, MD.)*

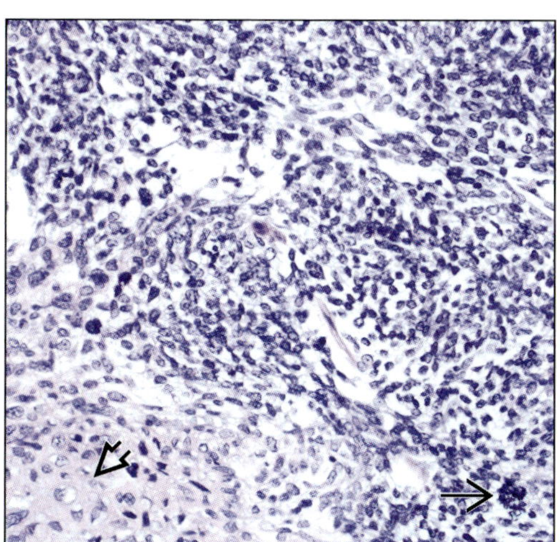

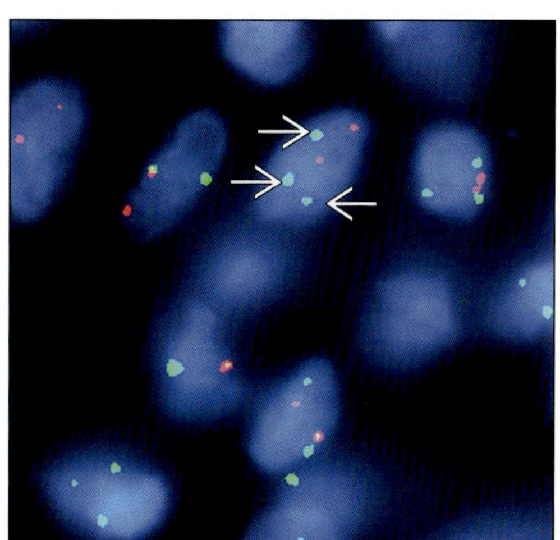

(Left) *High-power photomicrograph of a type III PPB shows a solid proliferation of malignant cells without any cyst formation. There is a blastomatous small cell component as well as focal cartilaginous differentiation ⇨. Note the atypical mitotic figure →.* ***(Right)*** *FISH shows trisomy 8 (green dots) ➡ in many of the tumor cells of this pleuropulmonary blastoma. There is no evidence of trisomy 18 (red dots). (Courtesy B. Shehata, MD.)*

Skin

BASAL CELL CARCINOMA

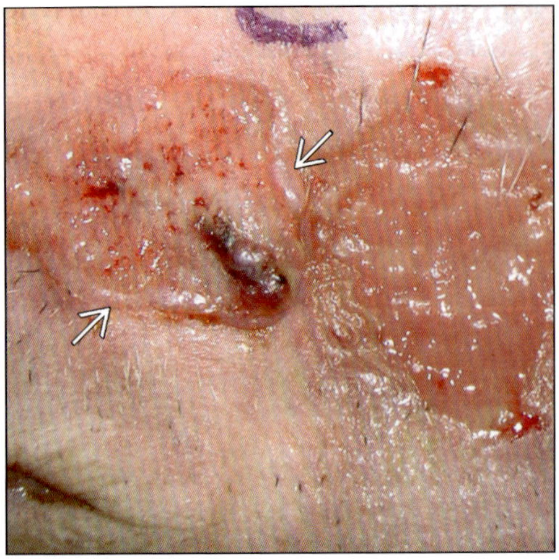

Clinical photograph of a large facial basal cell carcinoma (BCC) shows areas of ulceration and granulation-like tissue surrounded by a raised border ➡. (Courtesy S. Yashar, MD.)

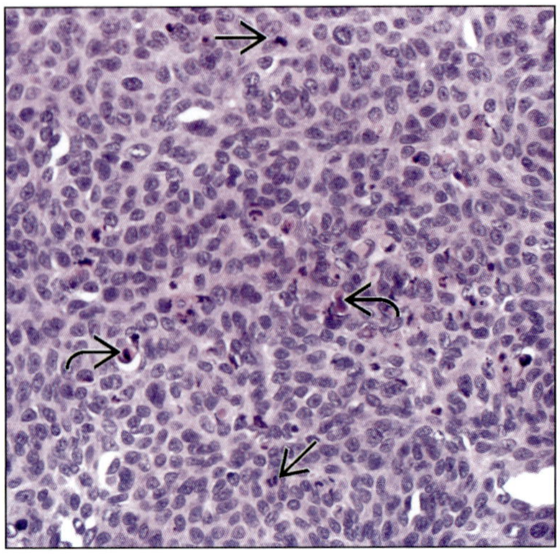

High magnification of a nodular BCC shows a sheet-like proliferation of atypical basaloid cells with high N:C ratios and numerous apoptotic ↪ and mitotic figures →.

TERMINOLOGY

Abbreviations

- Basal cell carcinoma (BCC)

Synonyms

- Basal cell epithelioma
- Trichoblastic carcinoma (not well accepted)

ETIOLOGY/PATHOGENESIS

Multifactorial

- Related to sun exposure (vast majority of cases)
  - Some cases may also be associated with radiation, immunosuppression (organ transplantation), burn scars
    - These cases tend to be more aggressive
- May actually be derived from follicular stem cells (hence, "trichoblastic carcinoma")

Genetics

- Rare cases are associated with genetic syndromes including
  - Nevoid basal cell nevus (Gorlin) syndrome
  - Xeroderma pigmentosum
  - Basex-Dupré-Christol syndrome
  - Rombo syndrome
- Genes implicated include *PTCH1* (Gorlin syndrome), *P53*, *SOX9*, *BMI1*, *BAX*, *RMRP*

CLINICAL ISSUES

Epidemiology

- Incidence
  - Extremely common: Most common cancer in humans when skin cancers are included
    - Accounts for 70% of primary cutaneous malignancies
- Age
  - Typically older adults
  - Sporadic BCC is presenting at younger ages (3rd and 4th decades)
    - Risk factors include red hair and tanning bed use
  - If patient age < 20 years, should consider a genetic syndrome
- Ethnicity
  - Light-skinned individuals; rare in darker skin types

Site

- Most common in head and neck region (up to 80% of cases)
  - ~ 15% occur on trunk and shoulders
  - Very rare cases involve lips, breast, axillae, groin, inguinal region, and genitalia
- If on palms or soles, a genetic syndrome should be considered

Presentation

- Typically pearly, papular, plaque-like, or nodular lesion with surface telangiectasias
  - Larger lesions often ulcerated with bleeding &/or overlying crusting
  - Minority of cases are pigmented, more often in patients with darker skin types

Treatment

- Surgical approaches
  - Complete excision or electrodessication and curettage (ED&C)
  - Mohs micrographic surgery often used in facial cases or other high-risk cases
- Radiation
  - Radiation therapy is an option, particularly if there are comorbidities

Prognosis

- Usually excellent, cured by local excision

BASAL CELL CARCINOMA

Key Facts

Terminology
- Low-grade malignancy of basal keratinocytes

Etiology/Pathogenesis
- Related to sun exposure, radiation, immunosuppression
- May have a genetically inherited component
- May be derived from follicular stem cells

Clinical Issues
- Very common: Most common cancer in humans
- Prognosis usually excellent, most cases cured by excision
- More aggressive subtypes: Infiltrative, micronodular, desmoplastic, and basosquamous
- Most commonly treated by complete excision or electrodessication and curettage

Microscopic Pathology
- Proliferation of nodules, nests, and cords of small basaloid cells with peripheral palisading, stromal retraction artifact, and mucinous material
- Numerous mitotic and apoptotic figures
- Cells show enlarged hyperchromatic nuclei with inconspicuous nucleoli and scant amounts of eosinophilic cytoplasm

Top Differential Diagnoses
- Squamous cell carcinoma
- Actinic keratosis (on superficial shave biopsy)
- Follicular neoplasms (trichoepithelioma and trichoblastoma)
- Merkel cell carcinoma

- More aggressive subtypes, including micronodular, infiltrative, desmoplastic, and basosquamous, have higher rate of recurrence and increased risk of metastasis
    - Overall risk of metastasis estimated at 0.05%

MACROSCOPIC FEATURES

Size
- Variable, small (few mm) to large (several cm)

MICROSCOPIC PATHOLOGY

Histologic Features
- Any microscopic variant of BCC can be seen in Gorlin syndrome
    - There are not microscopic clues, per se, as to presence of a genetic syndrome
- Proliferation of small basaloid cells with peripheral palisading in nodules, nests, &/or infiltrative cords
    - Overlying ulceration and serum crusting often present in large tumors
- Particularly in ulcerated or eroded lesions, there is squamatization, with increased eosinophilic cytoplasm and sometimes formation of keratin
- Stromal retraction artifact
    - Between tumor cells and stroma
- Mucinous material may be present
- Numerous mitotic and apoptotic figures present

Cytologic Features
- Oval nuclei with inconspicuous/small nucleoli and scant eosinophilic cytoplasm

Variants
- **Superficial-multicentric**: Superficial nests attached to epidermis separated by areas of uninvolved epidermis
- **Nodular**: Large, rounded, predominantly dermal-based nests with prominent peripheral palisading
- **Micronodular**: Predominantly dermal-based infiltrative proliferation of small nests
- **Infiltrative**: Small cords and nests, often deeply invasive
- **Desmoplastic/sclerosing/morpheaform**: Infiltrative strands and nests associated with dense sclerotic stroma
- **Infundibulocystic**: Cystic spaces containing keratinous material surrounded by ramifying cords of cells with pink cytoplasm
- **Basosquamous/metatypical**: Prominent areas of squamous differentiation (may mimic squamous cell carcinoma [SCC]), less peripheral palisading present
- **Fibroepithelioma of Pinkus**: Numerous small, anastomosing cords of basaloid cells attached to the epidermis
- Rare variants include adenoid, clear cell, signet ring cell, plasmacytoid/myoepithelial, and BCC with neuroendocrine differentiation or sebaceous differentiation

ANCILLARY TESTS

Immunohistochemistry
- Not necessary in most cases except when unusual features present
- Basal cell carcinoma vs. trichoepithelioma and trichoblastoma
    - BCC shows greater staining for Bcl-2, p53, and Ki-67
    - BCC lacks CK20(+) cells
    - CD10 tends to stain basaloid cells of BCC with only stromal staining in trichoepithelioma
    - BCC often stains for androgen receptor; desmoplastic trichoepithelioma is generally negative
- BCC vs. SCC
    - BCC is positive for BER-EP4; SCC generally negative
    - CK-PAN, HMWCKs, and p63 positive in both tumors

BASAL CELL CARCINOMA

DIFFERENTIAL DIAGNOSIS

Squamous Cell Carcinoma (SCC)

- Most cases are easily separated; however, basosquamous type of BCC shows prominent squamous differentiation
  - Usually, areas of more typical BCC are present, especially at periphery of tumor
  - Overlying actinic keratosis or Bowen disease often seen in association with SCC
  - BER-EP4 strongly positive in BCC, almost always negative in SCC
- Superficial shave biopsies of ulcerated/inflamed cases may be very difficult or impossible to accurately separate

Actinic Keratosis (AK)

- Can be difficult to distinguish from superficial type of BCC on very superficial shave biopsies
  - AK typically shows basilar budding of atypical squamous cells and overlying parakeratosis
  - No mucinous stroma, peripheral palisading, or tumor-stromal retraction artifact should be seen
  - Numerous apoptotic and mitotic figures favor BCC

Follicular Neoplasms (Trichoepithelioma and Trichoblastoma)

- Dermal-based basaloid adnexal neoplasms, may be large and nodular (trichoblastoma)
  - Usually symmetric and well circumscribed at scanning magnification
- Typically lack the degree of cytologic atypia, mitoses, and apoptotic figures of BCC
- May show peripheral palisading, but mucinous stroma and tumor-stromal retraction artifact typically lacking in benign follicular neoplasms
- Papillary mesenchymal bodies may be evident
- Immunohistochemistry may be helpful

Merkel Cell Carcinoma

- Nodular to sheet-like proliferation of highly atypical basaloid cells
  - Mucinous stroma and tumor-stromal retraction artifact only rarely identified
  - Peripheral palisading usually absent
- Nuclei typically show speckled (salt-and-pepper) chromatin pattern or nuclear clearing
- Perinuclear dot-like staining with CK20, pancytokeratin, and CAM5.2
- Positive immunoreactivity with neuroendocrine markers

Sebaceous Carcinoma

- Can show prominent areas of basaloid differentiation
- Focal atypical clear/multivacuolated cells with nuclear indentations should be present
- Lacks peripheral palisading, mucinous stroma, or stromal retraction artifact
- Immunohistochemistry may be useful
  - Androgen receptor is not necessarily helpful as it stains both sebaceous carcinoma and BCC
  - CAM5.2 and CK7 (+/-); typically negative in BCC
  - EMA often positive in clear cells, although it is often lost in poorly differentiated cases
  - Strong BER-EP4 and Bcl-2 favor BCC, but they are positive in some sebaceous carcinomas
  - Adipophilin is positive in sebaceous carcinoma and is negative in clear cell basal cell carcinoma

DIAGNOSTIC CHECKLIST

Clinically Relevant Pathologic Features

- Aggressive behavior associated with certain subtypes, deep dermal/subcutaneous invasion, and perineural invasion

SELECTED REFERENCES

1. Ferrucci LM et al: Host phenotype characteristics and MC1R in relation to early-onset basal cell carcinoma. J Invest Dermatol. 132(4):1272-9, 2012
2. Ferrucci LM et al: Indoor tanning and risk of early-onset basal cell carcinoma. J Am Acad Dermatol. 67(4):552-62, 2012
3. Heidarpour M et al: CD10 expression helps to differentiate basal cell carcinoma from trichoepithelioma. J Res Med Sci. 16(7):938-44, 2011
4. Ostler DA et al: Adipophilin expression in sebaceous tumors and other cutaneous lesions with clear cell histology: an immunohistochemical study of 117 cases. Mod Pathol. 23(4):567-73, 2010
5. Garcia C et al: Basosquamous carcinoma. J Am Acad Dermatol. 60(1):137-43, 2009
6. Krokowski M et al: Basal cell carcinoma with neuroendocrine differentiation arising in a scar: A case report. Dermatol Online J. 15(10):4, 2009
7. Cohen PR et al: Basal cell carcinoma with mixed histology: a possible pathogenesis for recurrent skin cancer. Dermatol Surg. 32(4):542-51, 2006
8. Farley RL et al: Aggressive basal cell carcinoma with invasion of the parotid gland, facial nerve, and temporal bone. Dermatol Surg. 32(2):307-15; discussion 315, 2006
9. Tschen JP et al: Pleomorphic basal cell carcinoma: case reports and review. South Med J. 99(3):296-302, 2006
10. Wadhera A et al: Metastatic basal cell carcinoma: a case report and literature review. How accurate is our incidence data? Dermatol Online J. 12(5):7, 2006
11. Ackerman AB et al: Fibroepithelial tumor of pinkus is trichoblastic (Basal-cell) carcinoma. Am J Dermatopathol. 27(2):155-9, 2005
12. Ting PT et al: Metastatic basal cell carcinoma: report of two cases and literature review. J Cutan Med Surg. 9(1):10-5, 2005
13. Bogdanov-Berezovsky A et al: Risk factors for incomplete excision of basal cell carcinomas. Acta Derm Venereol. 84(1):44-7, 2004
14. Saldanha G et al: Basal cell carcinoma: a dermatopathological and molecular biological update. Br J Dermatol. 148(2):195-202, 2003
15. Kim YC et al: Signet ring cell basal cell carcinoma: a basal cell carcinoma with myoepithelial differentiation. Am J Dermatopathol. 23(6):525-9, 2001
16. Meehan SA et al: Basal cell carcinoma with tumor epithelial and stromal giant cells: a variant of pleomorphic basal cell carcinoma. Am J Dermatopathol. 21(5):473-8, 1999

Microscopic Features

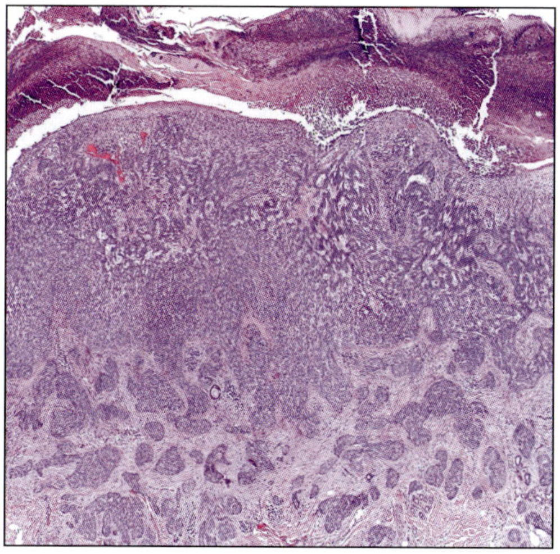

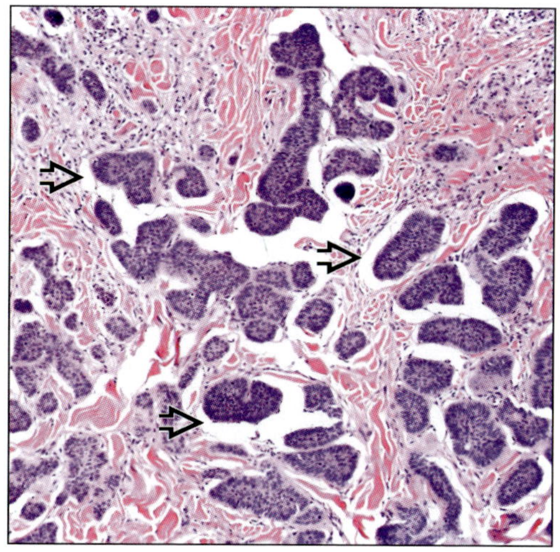

(Left) *Low magnification shows a large nodular- and micronodular-type BCC with diffuse overlying ulceration and dense serum crusting.* ***(Right)*** *Histologic section of a micronodular-type BCC shows a proliferation of small nests of basaloid cells with a prominent retraction artifact ⇨ in a somewhat sclerotic-appearing stroma.*

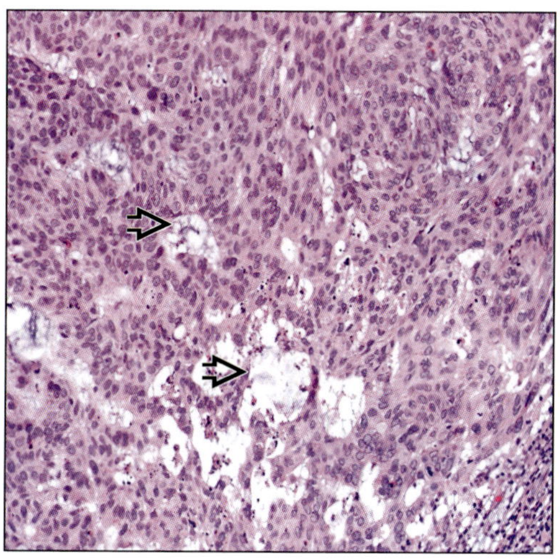

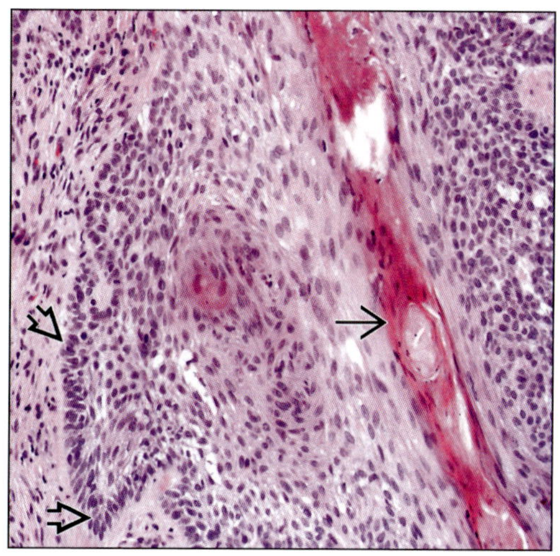

(Left) *Basosquamous-type BCC shows a proliferation of large, squamoid-appearing cells with abundant eosinophilic cytoplasm and focal mucin collections ⇨.* ***(Right)*** *Another example of basosquamous-type BCC shows traditional areas of BCC with peripheral palisading ⇨ surrounding collections of larger, squamoid-appearing cells associated with follicular differentiation and focal keratinization →.*

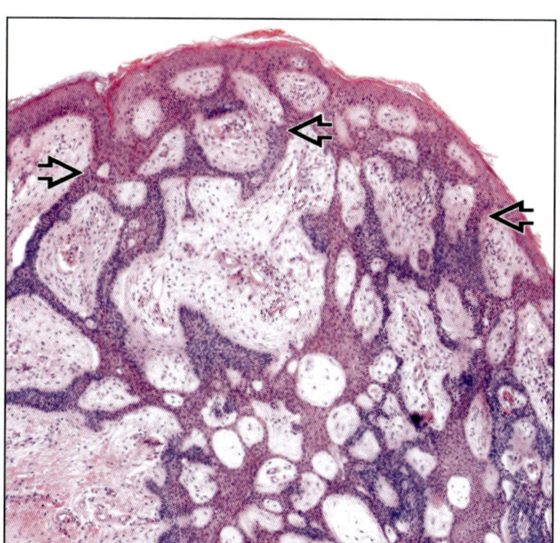

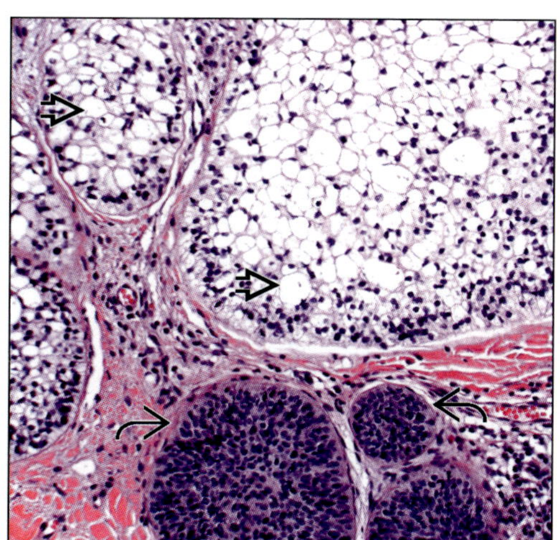

(Left) *Scanning magnification of a fibroepithelioma of Pinkus-type BCC is characterized by numerous small anastomosing cords of basaloid cells with multiple epidermal connections ⇨.* ***(Right)*** *Clear cell BCC is composed of large cells with abundant clear cytoplasm ⇨, and can mimic clear cell squamous cell carcinoma or sebaceous carcinoma in some cases. However, areas of more conventional-appearing BCC ↷ are often present, as are seen in the lower portion of this photomicrograph.*

BASAL CELL CARCINOMA

Microscopic and Immunohistochemical Features

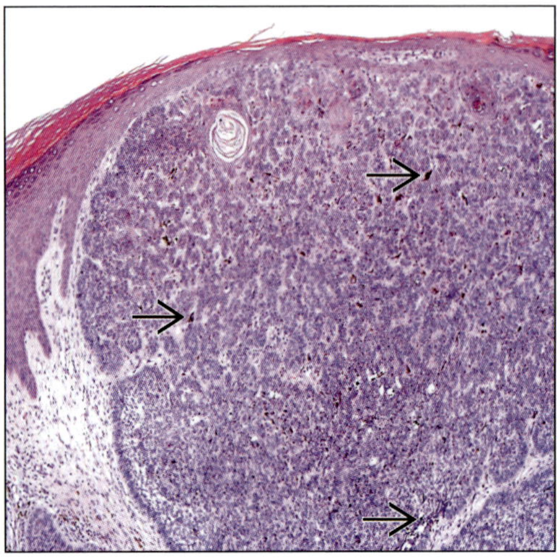
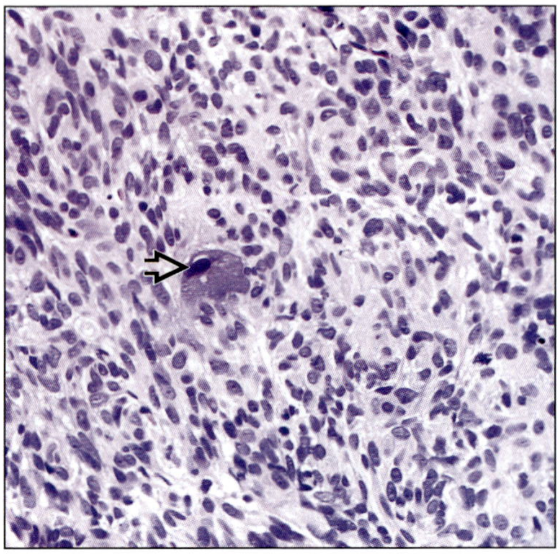

(Left) *Low-power view of a large pigmented nodular BCC shows prominent pigmentation → throughout the nodule.* ***(Right)*** *High magnification of a nodular BCC shows a rare markedly enlarged, pleomorphic tumor cell with a macronucleolus ⇨.*

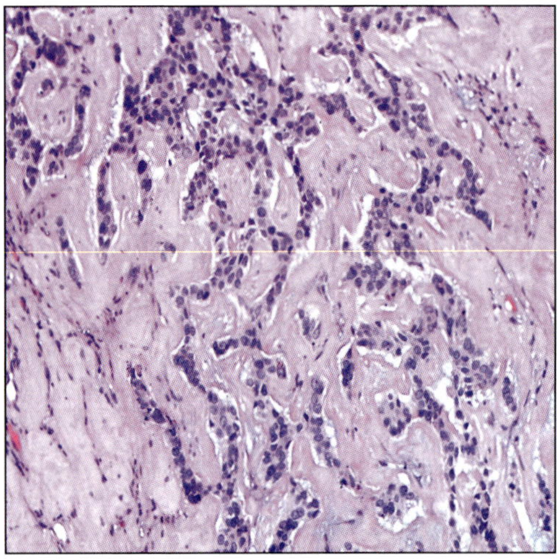
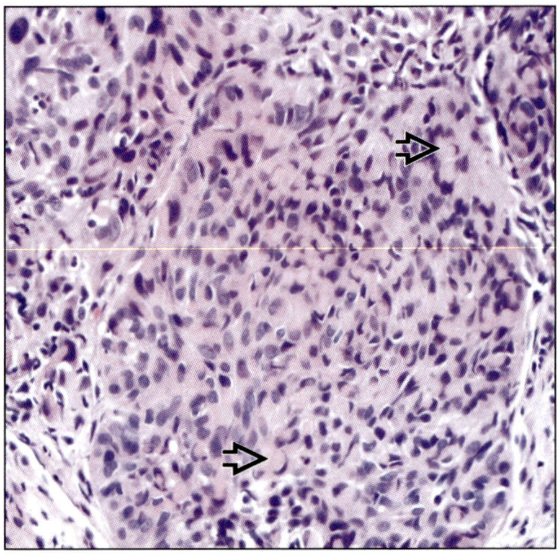

(Left) *Morpheaform (desmoplastic/sclerosing) BCC shows cords of atypical basaloid cells infiltrating a dense, desmoplastic stroma.* ***(Right)*** *High-power magnification of a plasmacytoid BCC shows dense eosinophilic cytoplasmic inclusions ⇨ and displaced nuclei. These cases have been shown to exhibit myoepithelial differentiation.*

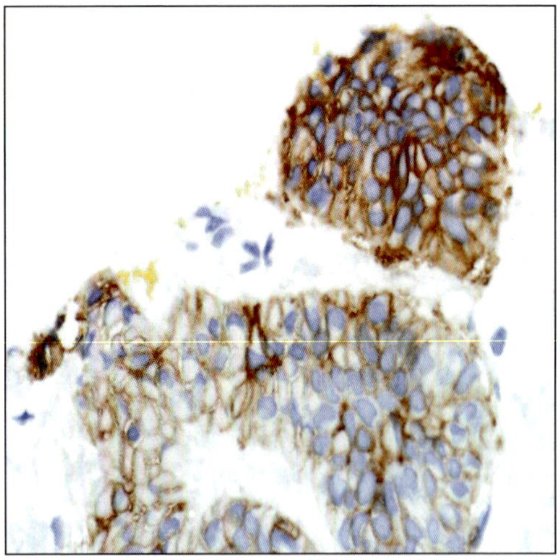
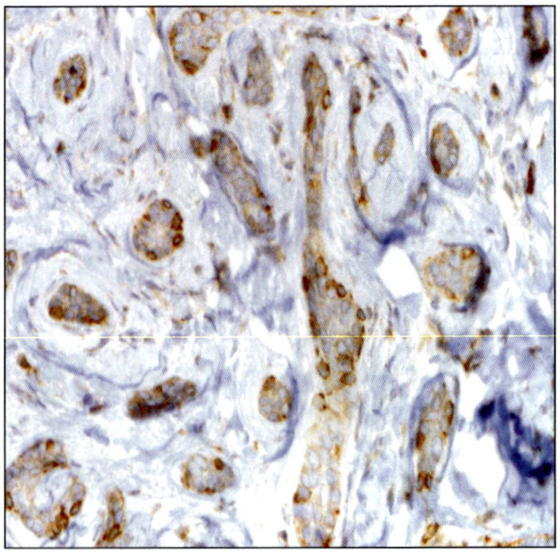

(Left) *BER-EP4/CD326 immunohistochemistry of a plasmacytoid BCC shows moderate to strong membranous staining of many of the tumor cells.* ***(Right)*** *Bcl-2 immunohistochemistry in a micronodular BCC shows moderate to strong cytoplasmic staining of the tumor cells.*

Differential Diagnosis

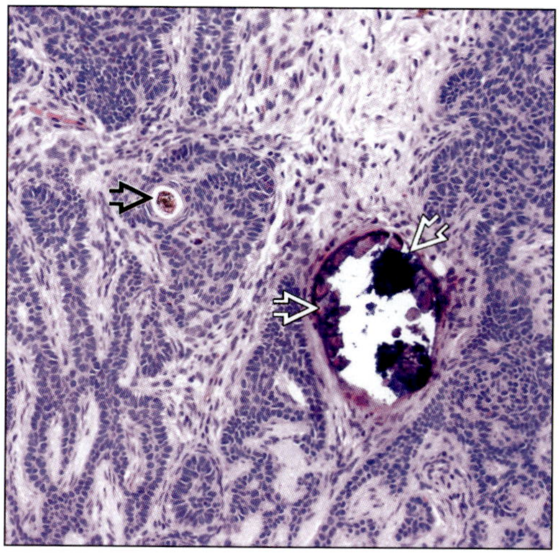

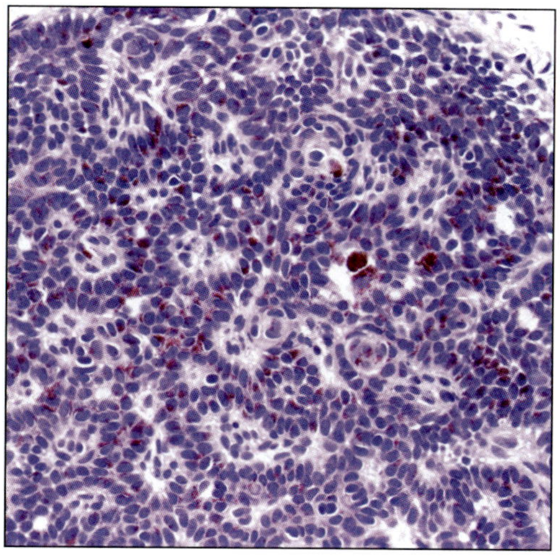

***(Left)** Histologic section of a trichoblastoma shows a bland-appearing basaloid tumor in a fibromyxoid stroma lacking tumor-stromal retraction artifact (as in BCC). There is focal pigmentation ➩ and an area of calcification ➩, findings typical of this neoplasm. **(Right)** High magnification shows a trichoblastoma with diffuse pigmentation. The lesion is composed of bland-appearing basaloid cells in anastomosing ribbons. Note the bland cytology and lack of mitotic or apoptotic figures.*

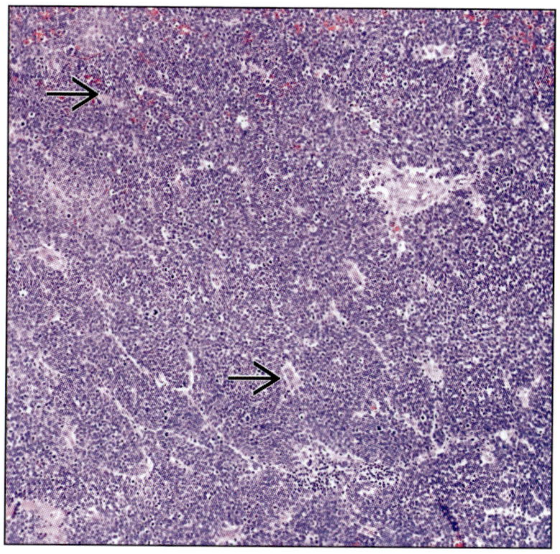

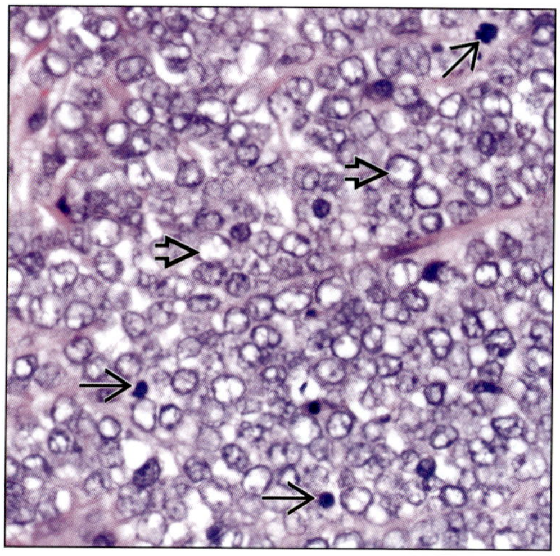

***(Left)** Merkel cell carcinoma is typically composed of broad cords and sheet-like collections of highly atypical basaloid cells. There is scant stroma → intervening between the neoplastic cells, and no tumor-stromal retraction, peripheral palisading, or mucinous material present. **(Right)** Nuclear clearing ➩ is often seen in Merkel cell carcinoma, a feature not seen in basal cell carcinoma. Note the numerous apoptotic and mitotic figures →.*

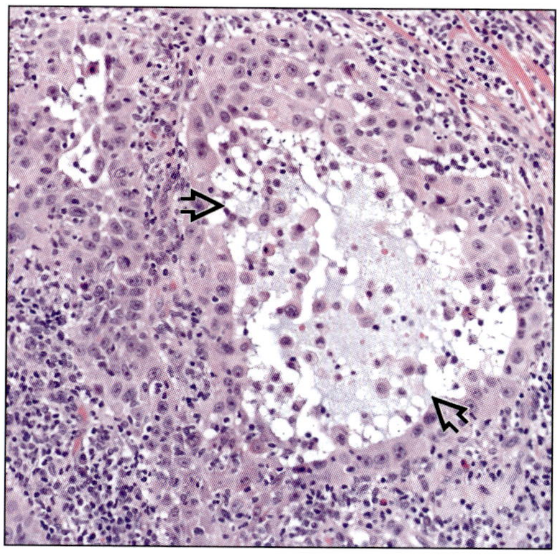

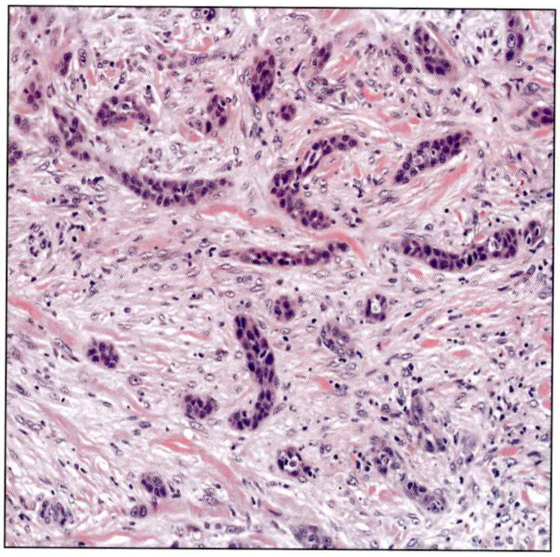

***(Left)** Squamous cell carcinoma can rarely show mucin production ➩, as in this example of acantholytic SCC, but it is typically found within the center of a tumor island, not in the stroma (as in BCC). **(Right)** Infiltrative SCC with cord-like structures associated with a desmoplastic stroma can mimic desmoplastic/morpheaform BCC or, less likely, microcystic adnexal carcinoma.*

CUTANEOUS MELANOMA

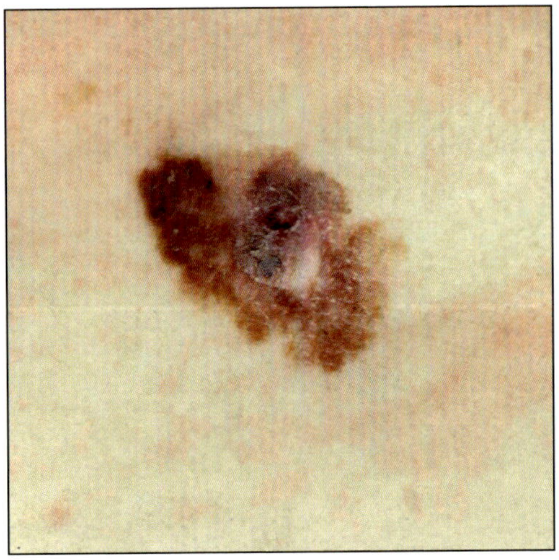

Clinical photograph shows a large melanoma with variegated color, jagged border, and irregular surface, all of which are concerning clinical signs. (Courtesy J. Hall, MD.)

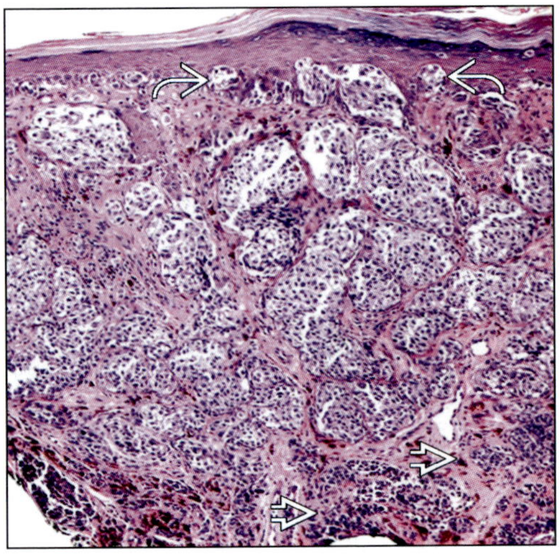

Melanoma is seen with pagetoid spread ➔ overlying the invasive melanoma. This case was complicated by a preexisting intradermal melanocytic nevus ➔. (Courtesy S. Dadras, MD.)

TERMINOLOGY

Synonyms

- Malignant melanoma

Definitions

- Malignant tumor of melanocytes

ETIOLOGY/PATHOGENESIS

Pathogenesis

- Environmental
  - > 85% of melanomas related to ultraviolet light-induced sporadic, activating mutations in *BRAF* and *NRAS*
- Genetics
  - Some melanomas have a genetic component with underlying germline mutations
  - Most common mutations are found in *CDKN2A*, a tumor suppressor gene
  - Other genetic disorders with DNA repair defects, such as xeroderma pigmentosum, can lead to accumulation of ultraviolet light-induced mutations at a young age, with development of melanoma at a young age

CLINICAL ISSUES

Epidemiology

- Age
  - Generally adults
    - Hereditary melanoma presents at a mean age of 34
  - Prepubertal melanoma is exceedingly rare
  - Presentation of melanoma in a young child, especially if not occurring within a large congenital nevus, should prompt consideration of a genetic syndrome (e.g., xeroderma pigmentosum)
- Gender
  - Males and females have different site predilections
- Ethnicity
  - Typically affects ethnicities with fairer skin (especially red hair and skin types I/II)
    - Linked to genetic risk; for example, red hair correlates with underlying *MC1R* mutations
- Geographic distribution
  - Highest incidence in Australia

Site

- Varies according to gender, on back (in men) and on legs (in women)
- Different types of melanoma associated with varying degrees of chronic sun exposure
  - Lentigo maligna type of melanoma in situ: Chronic sun exposure (e.g., face)
  - Acral melanoma: Generally non-sun-exposed sites (e.g., sole)
  - Superficial spreading melanoma: Often intermittently exposed areas (e.g., back)

Presentation

- Patient
  - Consider hereditary melanoma in a patient with
    - Multiple primary melanomas
    - Multiple clinically atypical nevi (often > 50)
    - > 2 or 3 first-degree relatives with cutaneous melanoma
    - Melanoma and a history of pancreatic cancer
  - Risk factors for melanoma
    - Endogenous factors: Number of melanocytic nevi, skin/eye color, family/personal history of melanoma and other skin cancer, degree of sun damage of skin
    - Environmental factors (e.g., tropical area)
- Tumor
  - Traditionally > 6 mm, but can be < 6 mm in diameter

CUTANEOUS MELANOMA

Key Facts

Terminology
- Malignant tumor of melanocytes

Etiology/Pathogenesis
- Majority of melanomas are sporadic
- Inherited predisposition to melanoma seen in minority of cases; may be associated with
  - Multiple, clinically atypical melanocytic nevi (often > 50)
  - Pancreatic cancer
  - Germline mutations in *CDKN2A* and other genes, *MC1R*, *BAP1*
  - Other syndromes, such as xeroderma pigmentosum

Clinical Issues
- Broad pigmented lesion, variegated colors, irregular borders
- Sites vary: Often back in men, legs in women
- Prognosis mainly dependent on depth of invasion in nonmetastatic lesions

Microscopic Pathology
- Microscopic features are not different in hereditary vs. sporadic melanomas
- Spread of atypical single cells and nests in epidermis
- Often abundant pagetoid scatter of atypical melanocytes into spinous layer
- Atypical melanocytes in dermis

Top Differential Diagnoses
- Severely atypical (dysplastic) melanocytic nevus
- Traumatized or special site melanocytic nevus
- Reed (pigmented spindle cell) nevus
- Spitz nevus

- Variegated color with shades of tan, brown, black, blue-black, red (due to inflammation or vascular ectasia), gray and white (zones of regression)
- Irregular borders

Treatment
- Surgical approaches
  - Complete excision with margins dependent on depth of invasion

Prognosis
- Dependent on variables such as depth of invasion, ulceration

MICROSCOPIC PATHOLOGY

Histologic Features
- Features of melanoma, whether sporadic or in inherited familial cancer setting, are the same; any microscopic variant of melanoma can be seen in inherited melanoma syndromes
  - Exception is cutaneous melanomas associated with *BAP1* mutations; these kindreds have risk of ocular melanoma
    - Melanoma composed of large, pleomorphic melanocytes; often with adjacent epithelioid nevus
- Melanoma variants/subtypes
  - Melanoma in situ (lentigo maligna is another term for melanoma in situ)
    - Limited to epidermis
  - Lentigo maligna melanoma
    - Predominantly single-cell melanocytic proliferation in epidermis with dermal invasion
  - Superficial spreading melanoma
    - Melanoma with large epidermal and dermal nests of atypical melanocytes
  - Nodular melanoma
    - Melanoma with at least 1 dermal mitosis **or**
    - Melanoma with a junctional component that does not extend beyond 3 rete ridges of invasive portion
  - Desmoplastic melanoma
    - Melanoma with a dermal component that has stromal desmoplasia and predominance of atypical spindled melanocytes, often with neurotropism
  - Acral lentiginous melanoma
    - Melanoma occurring on hands or feet with single melanocytes predominating
  - Nevoid melanoma
    - Melanoma that has histopathologic features mimicking melanocytic nevus
- Asymmetric, poorly circumscribed lesion with lateral expansion of large nests of atypical melanocytes
  - Irregular distribution of nests, which can be confluent
- Increased numbers of single atypical melanocytes involving both rete ridges and suprapapillary plates
- May have abundant pagetoid spread of atypical melanocytes located in spinous layer
  - Pagetoid spread at periphery of lesion (as opposed to only central focal spread in atypical and irritated nevi)
  - Pagetoid spread may be so extensive as to cause so-called consumption of epidermis
- Clefts between nests and epidermis above
- Absence of maturation with depth
- Generally at least 1 dermal mitosis
- Necrosis
- Dermal melanocytes often display large, purplish nucleoli
- Sometimes dense but irregularly distributed inflammatory dermal infiltrate
- Melanin pigment may be located deep in dermal nests and be distributed asymmetrically within the entire lesion
- Perineural or vascular invasion may be present
- Up to 1/3 of melanomas may be associated with a melanocytic nevus

- Regression
  - Absence of melanoma in epidermis or dermis with alteration of dermis (lymphocytic inflammation, melanophages, vascular alteration, fibroplasia)

Cytologic Features

- Cytoplasm
  - Pink and granular **or** with dusty melanin
  - Sometimes scant
- Nuclear hyperchromasia and pleomorphism
  - Large eosinophilic or purple nucleoli
  - Thick, irregular nuclear membranes
- Mitotic figures often present
- Occasional cytologic features include
  - Balloon cell (sebocyte-like) cells
  - Small cell size
  - Signet ring shapes
  - Rhabdoid
  - Myxoid
  - Clear cell

ANCILLARY TESTS

Immunohistochemistry

- Ki-67 often shows elevated nuclear proliferative rate (> 10-15%)
- HMB-45 may stain the base of tumor

DIFFERENTIAL DIAGNOSIS

Atypical (Dysplastic) Melanocytic (Clark) Nevus

- Should show symmetry and circumscription
  - Can be difficult to assess on partial biopsy
- Bridging of nests across rete ridges
- Lamellar fibroplasia of papillary dermis
- Pagetoid upward scatter of melanocytes is not prominent
  - If present, should be in center of lesion
- Dermal component typically small, nonatypical melanocytes in nests with maturation with depth; often located in center of junctional component
- Mitoses should be rare or absent

Melanocytic Nevi Subjected to External Forces (Irritated/Traumatized)

- May show parakeratosis &/or serum
- Ki-67 low

Spitz Nevus

- Hyperplastic (not atrophic) epidermis, lateral margins are sharply defined (no trailing off of single cells)
- Composed of epithelioid and spindle-shaped cells, which may be atypical but are often monomorphous
- Symmetric with circumscription
  - Can be difficult to assess on partial biopsy
- Kamino bodies (amorphous pink globs) often present in the epidermis
- Nests in epidermis may show clefting
- Maturation with depth
- If mitoses present, typically located in superficial portion of dermal component
- May have gain of chromosome 11p

Acral Nevus

- May have upward melanocytic scatter
- Generally small (< 6 mm diameter) with lateral circumscription
- Minimal melanocytic cytologic atypia
- Maturation of dermal component, if present

Genital Nevus

- May have similar histopathologic appearance to atypical (dysplastic) melanocytic nevus
- Generally symmetric, laterally circumscribed

Recurrent Nevus

- Usually any irregular junctional component delimited to epidermis above a scar
- Ideally, review of the preceding biopsy will show a banal melanocytic nevus

Nonmelanocytic Lesions

- Pagetoid scatter of nonmelanocytic cells can sometimes mimic melanoma
  - Paget disease of breast
  - Merkel cell carcinoma
  - Sebaceous carcinoma
  - Bowen disease
  - Pagetoid reticulosis
  - Clear cell papulosis
  - Pagetoid dyskeratosis

DIAGNOSTIC CHECKLIST

Pathologic Interpretation Pearls

- Anatomic (Clark) levels of invasion
  - I: Entirely intraepidermal
  - II: Invasive into papillary dermis
  - III: Expansion of papillary dermis (but confined to papillary dermis)
  - IV: Invasion of reticular dermis
  - V: Invasion of subcutaneous fat
- Case summaries should include, at the least, tumor thickness, anatomic level, ulceration, margin assessment, mitotic index, invasion (perineural, vascular), tumor-infiltrating lymphocytes, regression

SELECTED REFERENCES

1. Wiesner T et al: Toward an improved definition of the tumor spectrum associated with BAP1 germline mutations. J Clin Oncol. 30(32):e337-40, 2012
2. Frishberg DP et al: Protocol for the examination of specimens from patients with melanoma of the skin. Arch Pathol Lab Med. 133(10):1560-7, 2009
3. Barnhill RL et al: Pathology of melanocytic nevi and malignant melanoma. 2nd ed. New York: Springer-Verlag, 2004

Microscopic Features

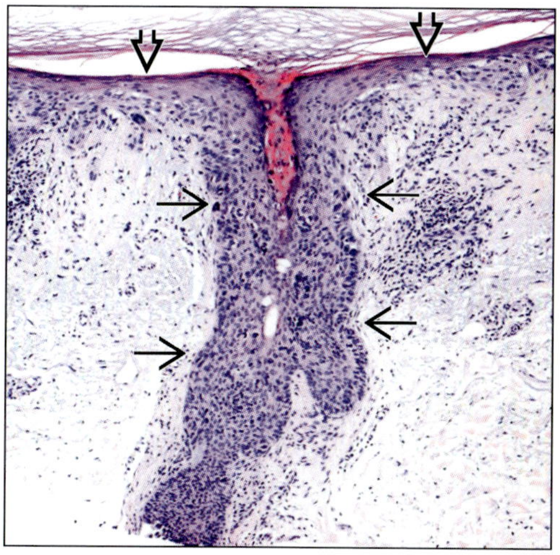

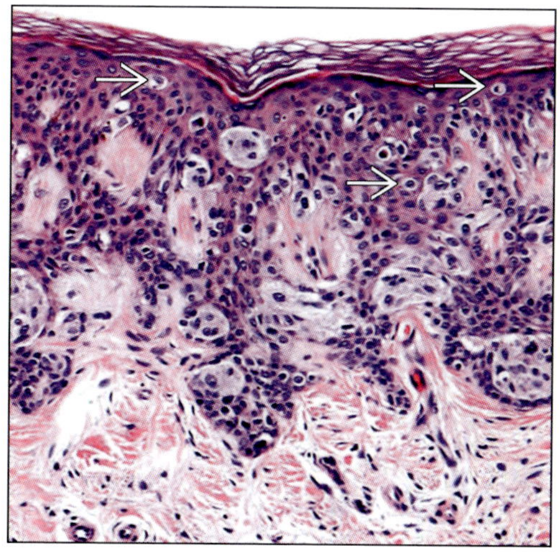

(Left) *Lentigo maligna (melanoma in situ) shows atypical melanocytes replacing the basilar layer in an atrophic epidermis [open arrow], extending down the follicular epithelium [arrow]. (Courtesy S. Dadras, MD.)* ***(Right)*** *Multifocal pagetoid scatter of atypical, epithelioid-shaped melanocytes is seen throughout all layers of the epidermis in a melanoma in situ [solid arrow].*

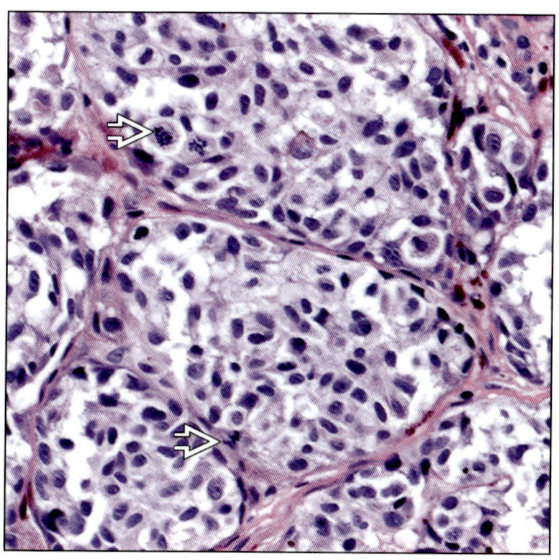

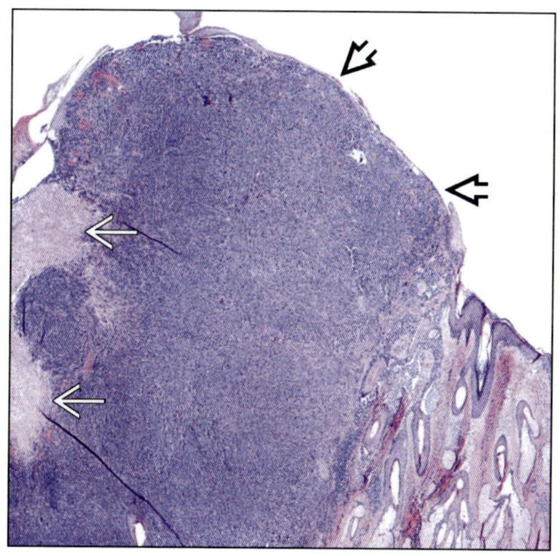

(Left) *The dermal component of this invasive melanoma fails to mature from the superficial to deeper dermis. Multiple mitoses [solid arrow] are easily found. (Courtesy S. Dadras, MD.)* ***(Right)*** *Scanning magnification of a nodular melanoma shows a large nodule with broad areas of overlying ulceration [open arrow] and large areas of necrosis [solid arrow]. (Courtesy S. Dadras, MD.)*

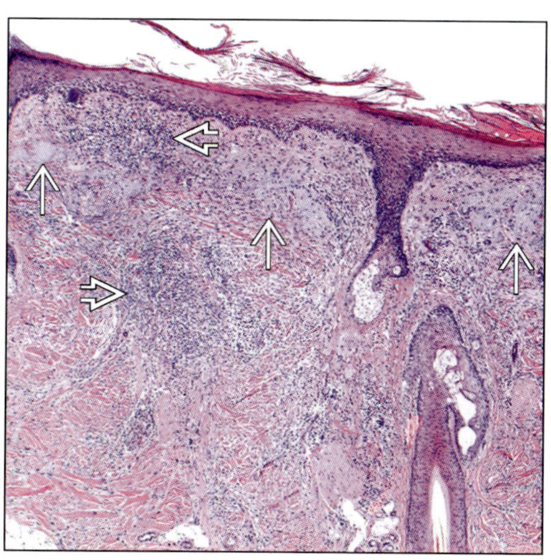

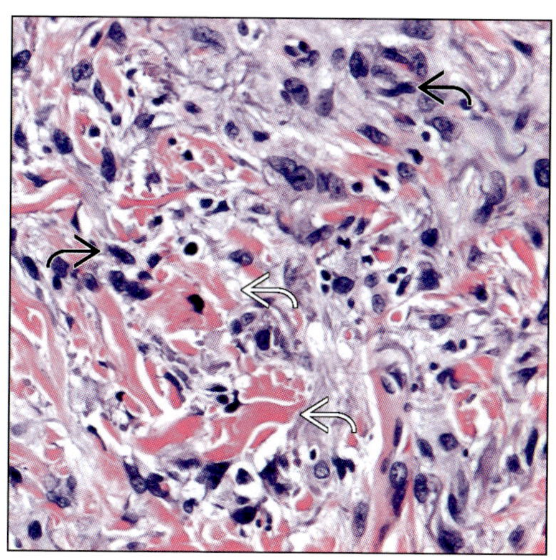

(Left) *Desmoplastic melanoma may resemble an inflamed scar on low-power examination. However, aggregates of lymphoid cells [solid arrow] and prominent solar elastosis [solid arrow] are usually identified and are helpful findings. (Courtesy S. Dadras, MD.)* ***(Right)*** *High-magnification examination of desmoplastic melanoma shows hyperchromatic, atypical spindle cells [curved arrow] surrounded by abundant collagen [solid curved arrow] bundles. (Courtesy S. Dadras, MD.)*

CUTANEOUS SQUAMOUS CELL CARCINOMA

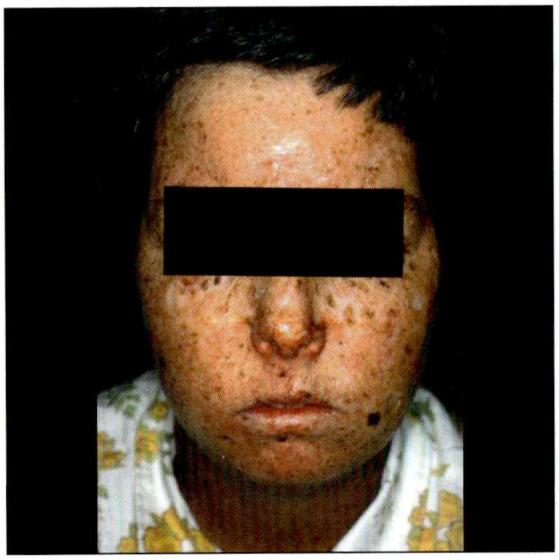

This child with xeroderma pigmentosum is predisposed to multiple skin cancers, including squamous cell carcinoma (SCC) at a young age. Many lentigines cover the face. (Courtesy, K. Kraemer, MD.)

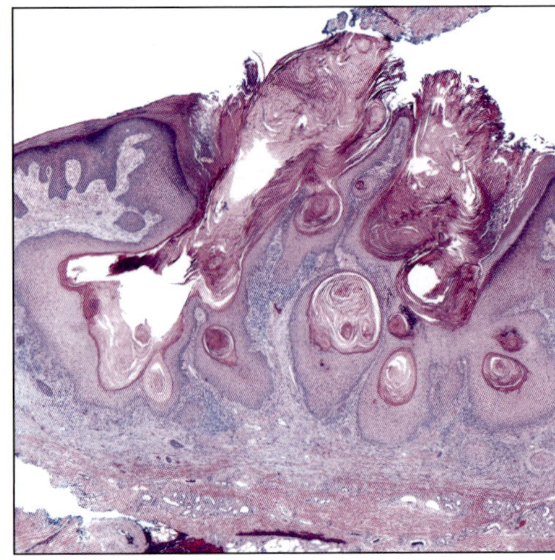

Keratoacanthoma (KA), a crateriform tumor considered by most to be a self-regressing subtype of squamous cell carcinoma, is sometimes associated with Muir-Torre syndrome. (Courtesy D. Cassarino, MD.)

TERMINOLOGY

Abbreviations

- Squamous cell carcinoma (SCC)

Synonyms

- Epidermoid carcinoma
- Sarcomatoid carcinoma, spindle cell carcinoma, carcinosarcoma, metaplastic carcinoma
- Acantholytic/adenoid/pseudoglandular SCC
- Verrucous carcinoma (well-differentiated variant)
- Keratoacanthoma (KA) (considered by some to be a well-differentiated, spontaneously regressing variant of cutaneous SCC)

Definitions

- Malignant tumor of squamous keratinocytes

ETIOLOGY/PATHOGENESIS

Environmental Exposure

- Most cases are related to ultraviolet (UV) radiation
- Some cases are likely related to chronic inflammation (e.g., SCC arising in burns, lupus, lichen planus)
- Other causes include previous radiation therapy and chronic wounds/scars, sometimes associated with more aggressive SCC
- HPV is associated with some cases
  - Especially verrucous carcinoma (low grade) and SCC in immunosuppressed patients (high grade)

Genetics

- Some cases with an underlying genetic predisposition
  - DNA repair defects in xeroderma pigmentosum lead to inability to repair mutations induced by UV radiation at an early age
  - Consider a genetic component in patients with SCC presenting in first 2 decades
  - Consider Muir-Torre syndrome or Ferguson-Smith disorder if multiple KAs, especially if age < 50 years

CLINICAL ISSUES

Epidemiology

- Age
  - Usually in elderly, especially solar-related lesions; however, can present in a wide age range (34-95 years)
  - Rare in children/young adults
    - Consider a genetic syndrome (e.g., xeroderma pigmentosum; Ferguson-Smith disorder or Muir-Torre syndrome if multiple KA)
- Gender
  - Slightly more common in males, overall

Presentation

- Slow-growing papular, nodular, or plaque lesion
- Often arises in sun-damaged skin (head and neck tumors)
  - Vast majority of cases associated with preexisting actinic keratosis (AK)
- May be ulcerated or bleeding
- Ear canal and middle ear tumors may present with pain, hearing loss, and discharge

Treatment

- Surgical approaches
  - Complete surgical excision (especially with Mohs surgery) is optimal and definitive therapy
- Drugs
  - Topical chemotherapeutics or immunomodulators may be used in patients who are not surgical candidates
- Radiation
  - May be used for very advanced cases in which surgical therapy is not curative

CUTANEOUS SQUAMOUS CELL CARCINOMA

Key Facts

Etiology/Pathogenesis
- Most cases are related to ultraviolet (UV) radiation
- Previous radiation therapy implicated in some cases, usually associated with more aggressive SCC
- Genetic component may be present, especially in SCC presenting in 1st or 2nd decades
  - Often the genetic defect is related to defective DNA repair (e.g., xeroderma pigmentosum, Muir-Torre syndrome)

Clinical Issues
- Genetic syndrome should be considered in very young patients
- Often arises in sun-damaged skin of elderly patients (usually head and neck) with preexisting actinic keratosis
- Complete surgical excision is optimal and definitive therapy
- Prognosis usually good in superficial and well-differentiated cases
- Worse prognosis with poorly differentiated, deeply invasive, or aggressive subtypes

Microscopic Pathology
- Proliferation of invasive atypical keratinocytes, often with areas of keratinization (keratin pearls) and squamous eddies
- Degree of differentiation is variable, ranging from well to moderately to poorly differentiated
- Multiple variants of differing malignant potential described
- KA associated with certain genetic syndromes, e.g., Muir-Torre syndrome

Prognosis
- Usually excellent in most cases
- Worse prognosis with poorly differentiated, deeply invasive, or rare aggressive subtypes
- Site of tumor important for prognosis
  - Lip and ear tumors more aggressive, regardless of degree of differentiation

MACROSCOPIC FEATURES

General Features
- Papular to nodular or plaque-like lesion; can be exophytic, ulcerated, or hemorrhagic

Size
- Variable; can be small or large

MICROSCOPIC PATHOLOGY

Histologic Features
- Microscopic features, per se, do not point to a genetic syndrome
  - Exception would be the well-differentiated, crateriform, KA type composed of glassy keratinocytes
    - Associated with Ferguson-Smith disorder, Muir-Torre syndrome (especially if mature sebocytes are intermixed in the KA); if subungual, incontinentia pigmenti
- Proliferation of invasive atypical keratinocytes
  - Cells are present in nests, sheets, and infiltrative cords
  - Often show areas of keratinization (keratin pearls) and squamous eddies
  - Attachments to overlying epidermis in most cases
  - Associated AK is very common; less likely, may be associated with SCC in situ (Bowen disease)
  - Cytologically, cells show abundant eosinophilic cytoplasm and large nucleus with vesicular chromatin and prominent nucleoli
  - Intercellular bridges (desmosomes) should be present on high-power examination
  - Presence of dyskeratotic cells (apoptotic keratinocytes) is reliable sign of squamous differentiation
  - If no definite squamous differentiation is present, immunohistochemistry should be used to confirm diagnosis
- Degree of differentiation is variable, ranging from well- to moderately to poorly differentiated
  - Amount of keratinization typically decreases and cytologic atypia increases with higher grades
  - Mitotic figures are usually numerous, and atypical forms are found especially in moderately to poorly differentiated cases
- Multiple variants of differing malignant potential described
  - Low-risk variants include well-differentiated SCC arising in AK, KA, verrucous carcinoma, and trichilemmal (variant of clear cell) carcinoma
  - Intermediate-risk variants include acantholytic (adenoid/pseudoglandular) and lymphoepithelioma-like carcinoma of skin (LELCS)
  - High-risk variants include spindle cell/sarcomatoid, basaloid, adenosquamous, and desmoplastic
    - Also radiation, burn scar, and immunosuppression-related SCCs
  - Rare variants of uncertain malignant potential include clear cell SCC, signet ring cell SCC, follicular SCC, papillary SCC, pigmented SCC, and SCC arising from adnexal ducts or cysts

Predominant Pattern/Injury Type
- Epithelioid/squamoid

ANCILLARY TESTS

Immunohistochemistry
- Not necessary in well-/moderately differentiated cases but may be needed in poorly differentiated and spindle cell cases

CUTANEOUS SQUAMOUS CELL CARCINOMA

- Cytokeratins are most important markers, especially high molecular weight cytokeratins (HMWCKs)
  - HMWCKs are most sensitive markers for poorly differentiated and spindle cell/sarcomatoid SCC
    - Pan keratin can be lost in poorly differentiated and spindle cell cases
  - p63 is also a very sensitive marker and can be used in addition to HMWCK to confirm diagnosis
- Vimentin may be positive in spindle cell/sarcomatoid cases
- Negative staining for other markers, including
  - S100, MART-1/Melan-A, and HMB-45 (melanoma)
  - CD10, CD68, and CD99 (AFX)
  - Actin-sm and desmin (leiomyosarcoma)
  - BER-EP4, androgen receptor (AR), and D2-40 (BCC and sebaceous carcinoma)

DIFFERENTIAL DIAGNOSIS

Basal Cell Carcinoma (BCC)

- Cells typically smaller, more hyperchromatic, and show peripheral palisading, mucinous stroma, and retraction artifact
- BER-EP4 and AR are almost always positive in BCC, negative in SCC

Atypical Fibroxanthoma (AFX)

- Usually a large nodular lesion in heavily sun-damaged skin (typically head and neck)
- SCC is typically positive for HMWCKs and p63; AFX is negative for these markers and often CD10(+) and CD99(+)

Poorly Differentiated Carcinoma (Including Metastatic)

- Clinical history and imaging studies are paramount, as immunohistochemistry may not be able to distinguish some cases from primary SCC
- Adenocarcinomas may show varying degree of ductal/glandular differentiation (highlighted with markers such as EMA and CEA)

Pseudoepitheliomatous Hyperplasia

- Can mimic SCC but does not show infiltrative features or high-grade cytologic atypia

Keratoacanthoma (KA)

- Considered by many to be a well-differentiated variant of SCC that spontaneously regresses in most cases
- Typically a large, crateriform (cup-like) lesion filled with abundant keratin
- Cells are enlarged, with abundant glassy-appearing/hyalinized cytoplasm
- Most cases regress, but giant KA and subungual KA can be aggressive

DIAGNOSTIC CHECKLIST

Clinically Relevant Pathologic Features

- Degree of differentiation
- Depth of invasion
  - Deeply invasive tumors have much higher rates of recurrence and metastasis
- Perineural invasion
  - Tumors with perineural invasion have high rates of local recurrence and increased risk of metastasis
  - More concerning if diameter of nerve is > 0.1 mm
- Location of tumor important (i.e., lip, mucosal lesions more aggressive)

SELECTED REFERENCES

1. Yang A et al: Primary cutaneous myxoid spindle cell squamous cell carcinoma: a clinicopathologic study and review of the literature. J Cutan Pathol. 37(4):465-74, 2010
2. Bridges MN et al: Cutaneous squamous cell carcinoma of the external auditory canal. Dermatol Online J. 15(2):13, 2009
3. McGuire JF et al: Nonmelanoma skin cancer of the head and neck I: histopathology and clinical behavior. Am J Otolaryngol. 30(2):121-33, 2009
4. Ross AS et al: Diameter of involved nerves predicts outcomes in cutaneous squamous cell carcinoma with perineural invasion: an investigator-blinded retrospective cohort study. Dermatol Surg. 35(12):1859-66, 2009
5. Garcia-Zuazaga J et al: Cutaneous squamous cell carcinoma. Adv Dermatol. 24:33-57, 2008
6. Ulrich C et al: Skin cancer in organ transplant recipients--where do we stand today? Am J Transplant. 8(11):2192-8, 2008
7. Yang HM et al: Immunohistochemical expression of D2-40 in benign and malignant sebaceous tumors and comparison to basal and squamous cell carcinomas. Am J Dermatopathol. 30(6):549-54, 2008
8. Renzi C et al: Sentinel lymph node biopsy for high risk cutaneous squamous cell carcinoma: case series and review of the literature. Eur J Surg Oncol. 33(3):364-9, 2007
9. Weinberg AS et al: Metastatic cutaneous squamous cell carcinoma: an update. Dermatol Surg. 33(8):885-99, 2007
10. Cassarino DS et al: Cutaneous squamous cell carcinoma: a comprehensive clinicopathologic classification--part one. J Cutan Pathol. 33(3):191-206, 2006
11. Cassarino DS et al: Cutaneous squamous cell carcinoma: a comprehensive clinicopathologic classification--part two. J Cutan Pathol. 33(4):261-79, 2006
12. Veness MJ et al: High-risk cutaneous squamous cell carcinoma of the head and neck: results from 266 treated patients with metastatic lymph node disease. Cancer. 106(11):2389-96, 2006
13. Leibovitch I et al: Cutaneous squamous cell carcinoma treated with Mohs micrographic surgery in Australia I. Experience over 10 years. J Am Acad Dermatol. 53(2):253-60, 2005
14. Lindelöf B et al: Cutaneous squamous cell carcinoma in organ transplant recipients: a study of the Swedish cohort with regard to tumor site. Arch Dermatol. 141(4):447-51, 2005
15. Baker NJ et al: Surgical management of cutaneous squamous cell carcinoma of the head and neck. Br J Oral Maxillofac Surg. 39(2):87-90, 2001
16. Weinstock MA: Epidemiologic investigation of nonmelanoma skin cancer mortality: the Rhode Island Follow-Back Study. J Invest Dermatol. 102(6):6S-9S, 1994
17. Rowe DE et al: Prognostic factors for local recurrence, metastasis, and survival rates in squamous cell carcinoma of the skin, ear, and lip. Implications for treatment modality selection. J Am Acad Dermatol. 26(6):976-90, 1992

Microscopic Features

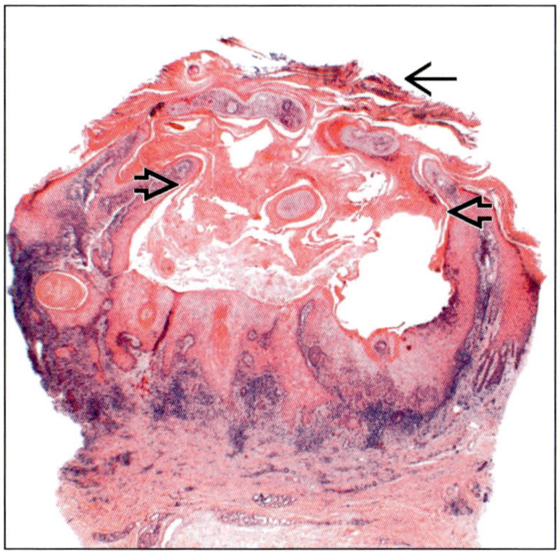

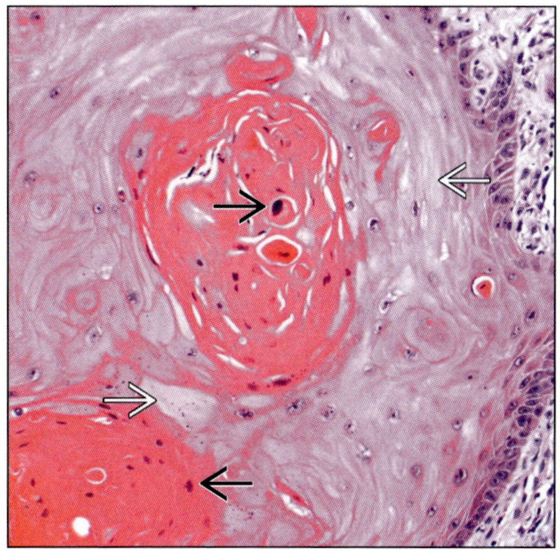

(Left) *Scanning power examination of a relatively small KA shows a symmetric-appearing atypical squamous proliferation with a dilated, central keratin-filled crater ⇨ and dense overlying parakeratosis →. (Courtesy D. Cassarino, MD.)* ***(Right)*** *High magnification shows enlarged keratinocytes with abundant, glassy amphophilic- ➡ to eosinophilic-staining cytoplasm. Note the numerous dyskeratotic cells → in the foci of keratinization. (Courtesy D. Cassarino, MD.)*

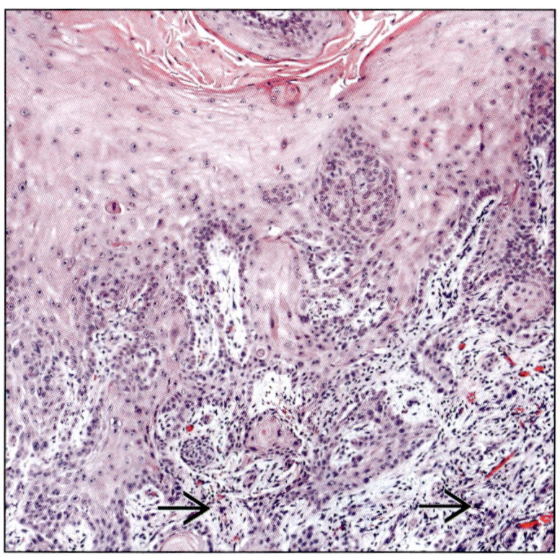

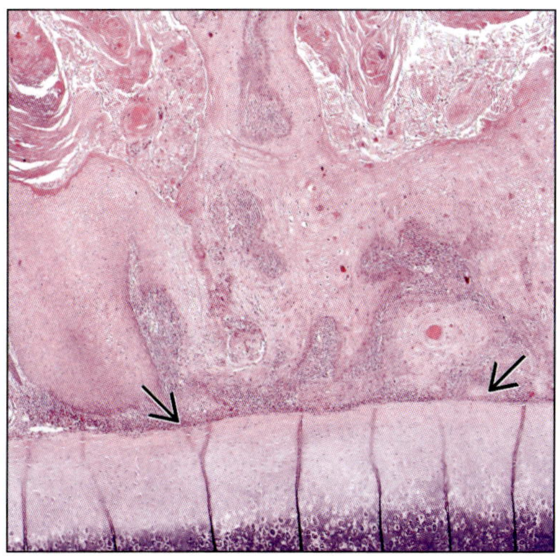

(Left) *This well-differentiated SCC has some features mimicking a KA, including enlarged squamous cells with abundant glassy-appearing eosinophilic cytoplasm. However, this tumor lacks a central keratin-filled crater and shows infiltrating single atypical cells in the dermis →. (Courtesy D. Cassarino, MD.)* ***(Right)*** *This well-differentiated SCC mimics a KA. This case arose on the ear and invaded deeply to abut the cartilage →. (Courtesy D. Cassarino, MD.)*

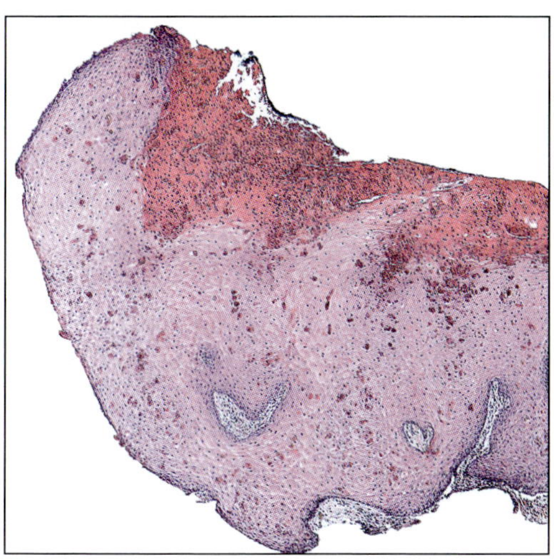

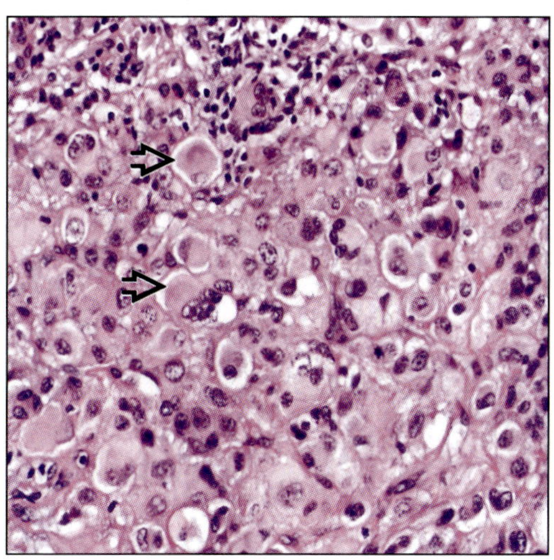

(Left) *This is a subungual keratoacanthoma. Although such tumors can present in patients without a genetic syndrome, multiple such tumors should cause consideration of incontinentia pigmenti.* ***(Right)*** *High-grade invasive SCC shows a sheet-like proliferation of atypical and pleomorphic epithelioid and multinucleated cells with hyperchromatic nuclei, prominent nucleoli, and abundant glassy-appearing eosinophilic cytoplasm ⇨.*

CUTANEOUS SQUAMOUS CELL CARCINOMA

Variant Microscopic Features

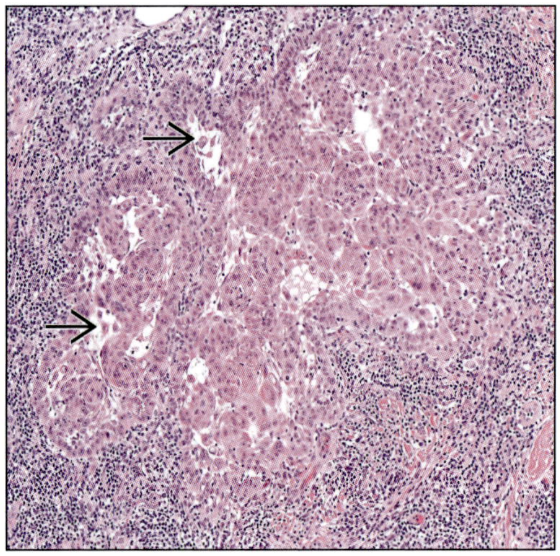

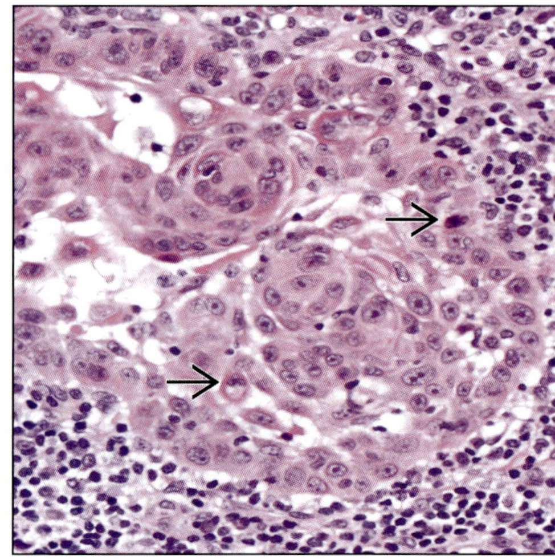

(Left) *Acantholytic (adenoid) type of invasive squamous cell carcinoma shows scattered cystic spaces containing dyscohesive squamous cells →. This variant of SCC may mimic adenocarcinoma (pseudoglandular SCC) or even angiosarcoma (pseudovascular SCC).* ***(Right)*** *High-power view of acantholytic SCC shows large epithelioid cells with dense eosinophilic cytoplasm and scattered dyskeratotic (apoptotic) cells →. There is an associated heavy inflammatory cell infiltrate.*

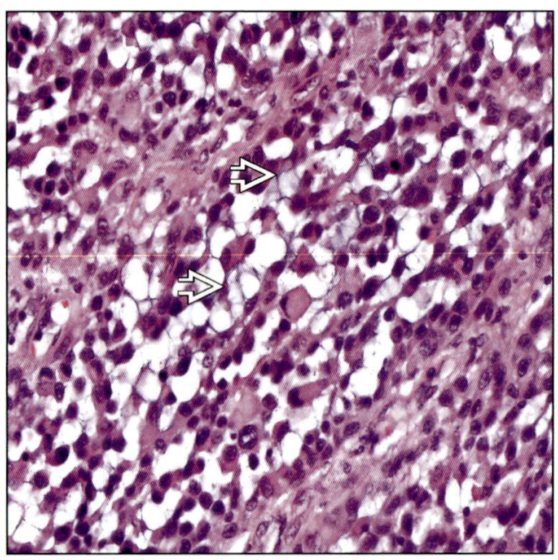

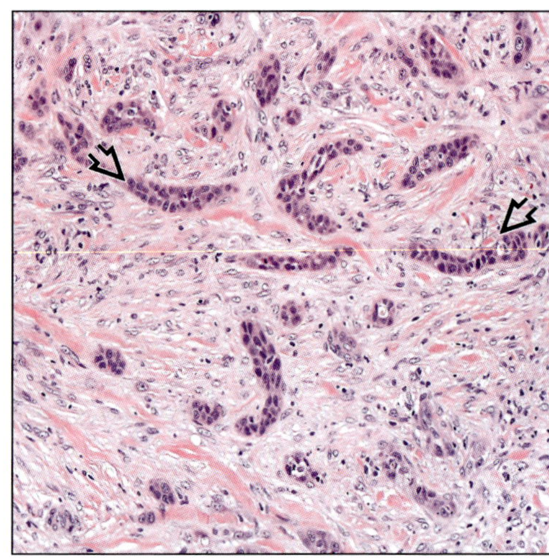

(Left) *Higher power view of poorly differentiated myxoid SCC shows epithelioid to signet ring-like eosinophilic-staining cells with focal extracellular mucin ⇨.* ***(Right)*** *H&E section shows poorly differentiated infiltrating squamous cell carcinoma forming cords, mimicking ductal structures ⇨. There is an associated dense desmoplastic stroma.*

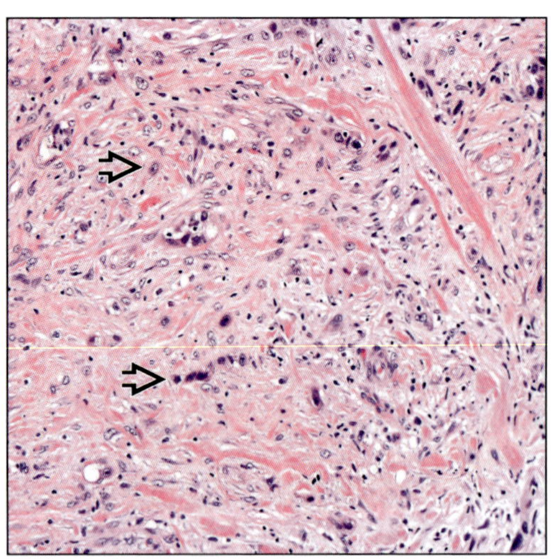

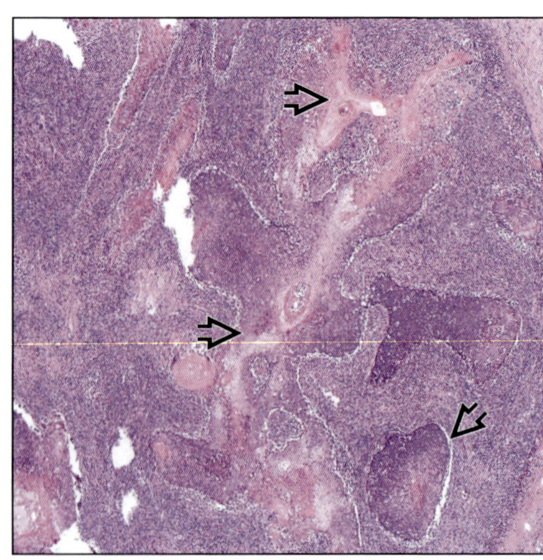

(Left) *Poorly differentiated infiltrating SCC ⇨ associated with a sclerotic (desmoplastic) stroma is shown. This is a high malignant potential variant of SCC.* ***(Right)*** *Heavily inflamed invasive SCC with moderately differentiated tumor islands ⇨ composed of basaloid to squamoid cells is surrounded by a sea of inflammatory cells, features suggestive of the lymphoepithelioma-like carcinoma of the skin (LELCS) variant.*

Immunohistochemical Features

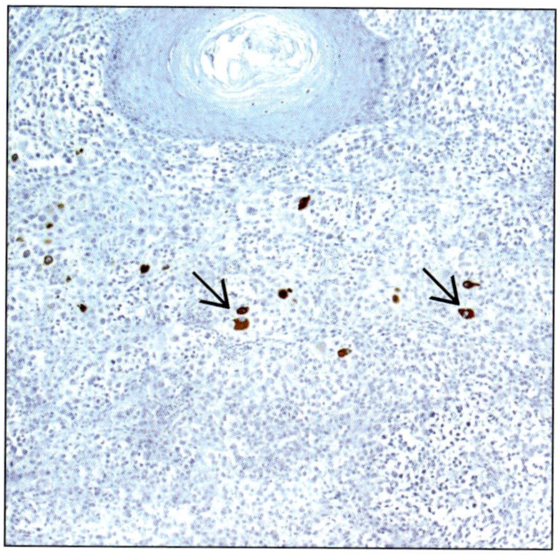

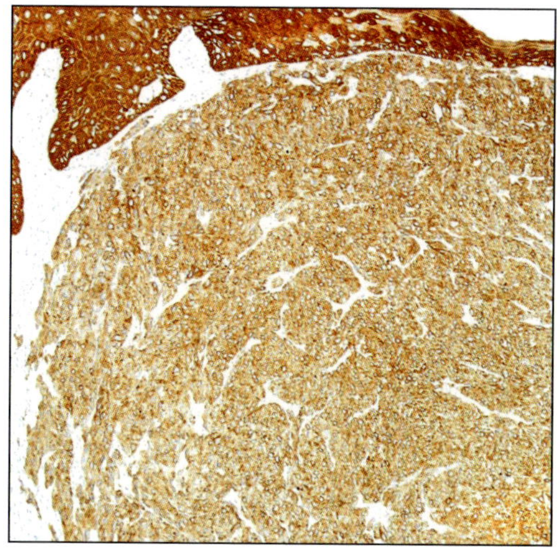

(Left) *CK-PAN immunohistochemistry (IHC) shows only focal staining of a few scattered single cells → in a case of poorly differentiated SCC. CK-PAN is much less sensitive than HMWCKs and p63 in identifying poorly differentiated and sarcomatoid SCC cases.* ***(Right)*** *CK903 (HMWCK) immunohistochemistry shows strong staining of an invasive, poorly differentiated SCC (with strong internal control staining of the overlying epidermis).*

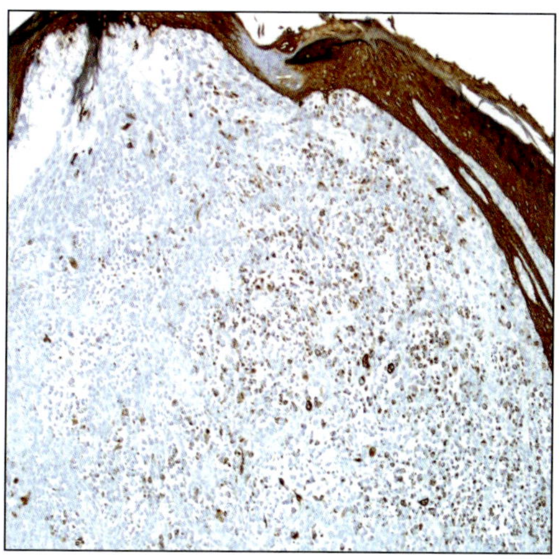

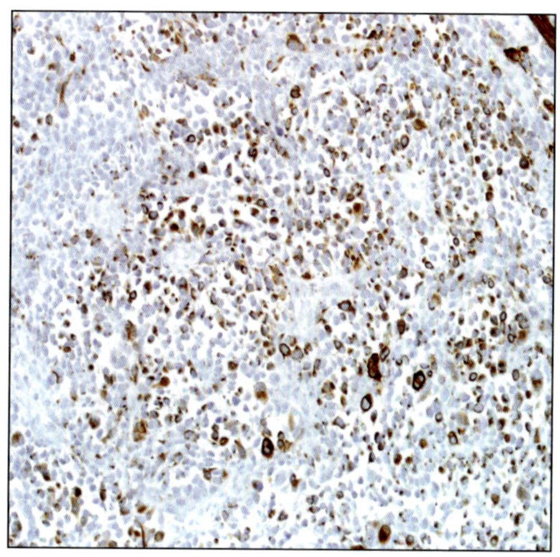

(Left) *CK5/6 (HMWCK) IHC shows strong staining of the epidermis and scattered single cells in a poorly differentiated SCC.* ***(Right)*** *Higher power view of CK5/6 shows moderate to strong cytoplasmic staining of many of the tumor cells.*

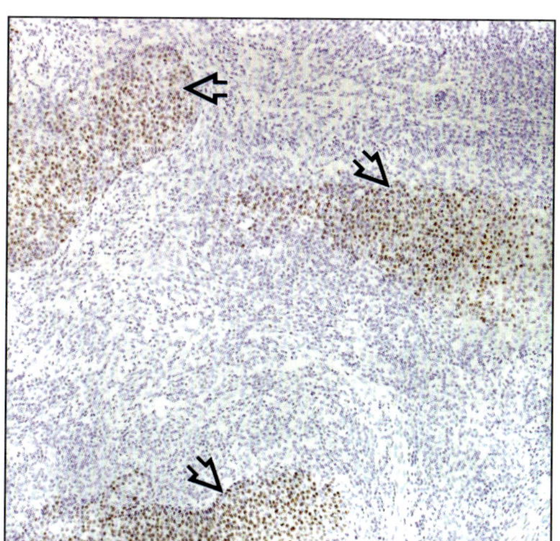

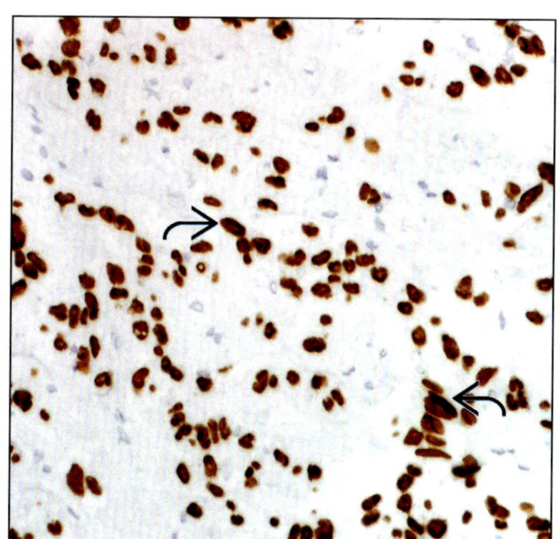

(Left) *IHC stain for p63 in an lymphoepithelioma-like carcinoma of the skin (LELCS) shows strong and diffuse nuclear staining in islands of epithelial tumor cells ⇒.* ***(Right)*** *High-power view of p63 immunohistochemistry shows strong and diffuse nuclear staining of large, irregularly shaped nuclei ↪ in a poorly differentiated infiltrating SCC.*

SEBACEOUS CARCINOMA

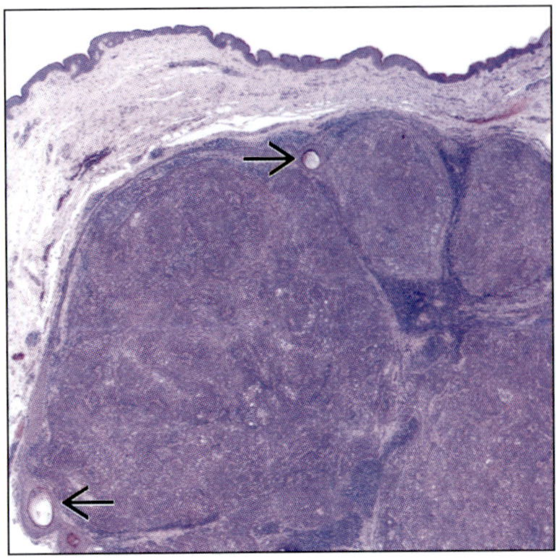

Scanning magnification of a sebaceous carcinoma shows a very large nodular tumor in the dermis. Note the lack of epidermal attachments; however, there are focal entrapped follicular structures ⇒.

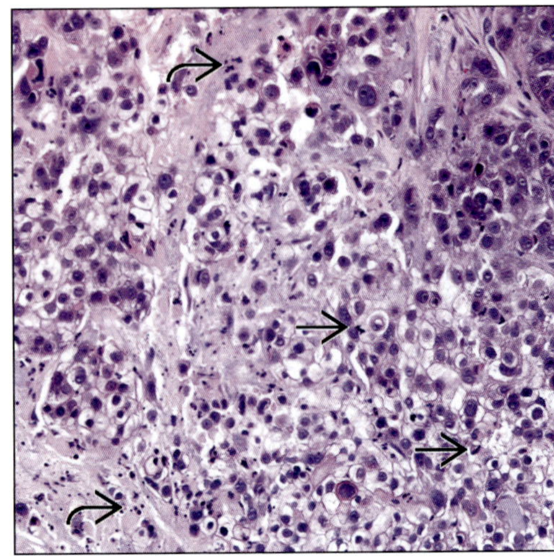

Higher power examination of sebaceous carcinoma shows a proliferation of markedly atypical clear cells with numerous mitotic figures ⇒ and abundant apoptotic cellular debris ↗.

TERMINOLOGY

Synonyms

- Sebaceous adenocarcinoma

Definitions

- Malignant adnexal tumor of sebaceous cells
- Often lacks clear cell features in poorly differentiated cases and may show basaloid or squamoid features, leading to high incidence of misdiagnosis

ETIOLOGY/PATHOGENESIS

Unknown in Most Cases

- Some cases likely due to solar (UV) damage, as most occur on sun-damaged skin of elderly
- Sporadic tumors may have loss of mismatch repair proteins, suggesting a defect in DNA mismatch repair

Genetic

- May be a marker of Muir-Torre syndrome (MTS)
  - Genes implicated include *MSH2* (majority of cases), *MLH1*, *MSH6*
    - Encode mismatch repair proteins
    - Mutations lead to microsatellite instability (MSI)
    - MSI assays and immunohistochemistry can be used to screen for MTS

CLINICAL ISSUES

Epidemiology

- Incidence
  - Uncommon tumors, but 1 of the more common types of adnexal carcinoma
- Age
  - Most occur in elderly patients
- Gender
  - Females have slightly higher incidence

Site

- Eyelids are by far the most common site (~ 75% of cases)
- Remainder of cases occur in other head and neck sites, followed by trunk, extremities
- Nonperiocular sebaceous carcinoma may be more likely than periocular carcinomas to be associated with MTS

Presentation

- Nodular, firm, yellow-tan lesions
- Often ulcerated

Treatment

- Surgical approaches
  - Complete excision is necessary to ensure local removal
  - Mohs excision is reported to be effective in most cases
  - Sentinel lymph node biopsy may be useful for staging purposes

Prognosis

- Aggressive tumors with high incidence of metastasis (> 30% of cases) and generally poor prognosis unless discovered early

MACROSCOPIC FEATURES

General Features

- Dermal-based firm, nodular lesion

Size

- Usually 1-4 cm

MICROSCOPIC PATHOLOGY

Histologic Features

- Dermal-based infiltrative, nodular to sheet-like tumor

SEBACEOUS CARCINOMA

Key Facts

Terminology
- Adnexal carcinoma that often lacks clear cell features in poorly differentiated cases

Etiology/Pathogenesis
- Strong association with MTS if patients have multiple sebaceous tumors

Clinical Issues
- Eyelids are most common site (~ 75% of cases)
- Mohs excision is effective in most cases
- Aggressive tumors with high incidence of metastasis (> 30%) and generally poor prognosis unless discovered early

Microscopic Pathology
- Dermal-based infiltrative, nodular to sheet-like tumor
- Often focal follicular &/or epidermal connections
- Well-differentiated tumors show clear cell changes
- Moderately and poorly differentiated tumors show few to rare clear cells
- Often show basaloid or squamoid features
- Mitotic figures are usually abundant
- Areas of comedonecrosis are common

Ancillary Tests
- EMA(+) in well-differentiated cases, but often lost in poorly differentiated tumors
- AR(+) in most cases, including poorly differentiated

Top Differential Diagnoses
- Clear cell squamous cell carcinoma (SCC)
- Clear cell basal cell carcinoma (BCC)
- Other primary cutaneous adnexal carcinomas
- Metastatic carcinoma to the skin

- Often with focal follicular &/or epidermal connections
  - Pagetoid involvement of epidermis may be seen in up to 30% of cases
- Tumor consists of variably differentiated epithelioid cells
  - Clear cells often present but vary greatly in number
  - Well-differentiated tumors show prominent clear cell changes
    - Cells contain abundant cytoplasmic lipid, often producing multiple vacuoles and nuclear indentation
    - Nuclei are enlarged and vesicular or hyperchromatic staining, with prominent nucleoli
  - Moderately and poorly differentiated tumors show few to rare clear cells
    - May be composed predominantly of basaloid or squamoid cells
    - Show prominent cytologic atypia and pleomorphism
    - Mitotic figures, including atypical forms, are usually abundant
  - Areas of necrosis, with comedonecrosis pattern, are common
  - Lymphovascular invasion present in significant percentage of cases
- Tumor-infiltrating lymphocytes may be a marker of defective mismatch repair

Cytologic Features
- Enlarged, epithelioid cells with abundant cytoplasm and hyperchromatic or vesicular nuclei with enlarged nucleoli
  - Clear cells usually show cytoplasmic vacuoles and nuclear indentation
  - Cells can also be basaloid (common) or squamoid (rare)

ANCILLARY TESTS

Histochemistry
- Sudan black B and oil red O (need frozen tissue)
  - Reactivity: Positive
  - Staining pattern
    - Cytoplasmic staining
- Periodic acid-Schiff
  - Reactivity: Usually negative (indicating lack of glycogen)

Immunohistochemistry
- EMA: Positive in most well-differentiated cases, but is often negative in poorly differentiated tumors
  - Negative in BCC, but often shows at least focal staining in SCC
  - Often highlights ductal structures in other adnexal carcinomas (i.e., porocarcinoma and hidradenocarcinoma), but not in sebaceous carcinoma
- Androgen receptor (AR) is positive (nuclear staining) in most cases, including poorly differentiated carcinomas
  - SCC and most other primary cutaneous carcinomas are negative for AR
  - AR is often positive in BCC (> 60% of cases) and some metastatic carcinomas to the skin
- Adipophilin often positive in most cases
- HMWCK (i.e., CK5/6 and CK903/34bE12) and p63 are typically strongly and diffusely positive
  - Help to exclude metastatic tumors (most of which are negative for both of these markers) but do not distinguish from other primary cutaneous tumors
- D2-40 (podoplanin) is positive in a subset of cases, especially in more basaloid sebaceous carcinomas
  - Can also highlight areas of lymphovascular invasion
- Other markers that may be positive include CAM5.2, BER-EP4, CK7 (~ 50% of cases), and CD10 (~ 50%)
- Negative for CEA-M, CK20, GCDFP-15, renal cell carcinoma antigen (RCA), TTF-1, S100
- Loss of staining for MLH1, MSH2, &/or MSH6 may be seen, regardless of whether patient has MTS

Molecular Genetics
- MTS defined as 1 sebaceous tumor and 1 internal organ malignancy

- Genes include *MSH2* (90% of cases), *MLH1*, *MSH6*
- Mutations lead to loss of mismatch repair capabilities
- Can be identified directly through PCR for specific mutations or indirectly through MSI studies
  - MSI studies are less sensitive than PCR

DIFFERENTIAL DIAGNOSIS

Squamous Cell Carcinoma (SCC)

- SCC with clear cell features can be difficult to distinguish from sebaceous carcinoma in some cases
- Often associated with overlying actinic keratosis or SCC in situ (Bowen disease)
- Clear cells in SCC are due to either degenerative changes or glycogen accumulation
  - Lack cytoplasmic lipid and nuclear indentations
  - PAS (without diastase) is positive in cases with cytoplasmic glycogen (negative in sebaceous carcinoma)
- Areas of squamous eddies and keratinization typically present (only rarely seen in sebaceous carcinoma)
- Sebaceous carcinoma is usually diffusely positive for EMA (weak/focal in SCC) and AR (negative in SCC)

Basal Cell Carcinoma (BCC)

- Most cases are not difficult to distinguish from sebaceous carcinoma
- Some cases of BCC are predominantly clear cell, **but** typically show at least focal areas of more conventional BCC with peripheral palisading and mucinous stroma
- BCC is usually negative with EMA and only focally positive with AR

Other Primary Cutaneous Adnexal Carcinomas

- Porocarcinoma and hidradenocarcinoma with clear cell features
- Porocarcinoma shows multiple epidermal attachments, whereas hidradenocarcinoma is a dermal-based tumor typically lacking epidermal connections
- Both tumors show at least focal ductal differentiation
  - May be highlighted by EMA and CEA
- Sebaceous carcinoma is usually diffusely positive for EMA and AR

Metastatic Carcinomas to Skin

- Metastatic carcinomas with clear cell features should be considered in the differential, especially if no epidermal or follicular connections are identified
- Metastatic clear cell renal cell carcinoma (RCC) is the most likely consideration
  - Prominent capillary-type vasculature present
  - Cells are typically relatively low-grade appearing
  - Show uniform cytoplasmic clearing
  - IHC: Positive for RCC antigen, pax-8, CD10 (positive in ~ 50% of sebaceous carcinomas); EMA is positive in both RCC and sebaceous carcinoma

DIAGNOSTIC CHECKLIST

Pathologic Interpretation Pearls

- Well-differentiated cells with cytoplasmic lipid, often producing multiple vacuoles and nuclear indentation
- Poorly differentiated cells often basaloid

SELECTED REFERENCES

1. Plocharczyk EF et al: Mismatch repair protein deficiency is common in sebaceous neoplasms and suggests the importance of screening for Lynch syndrome. Am J Dermatopathol. 35(2):191-5, 2013
2. Roberts ME et al: Screening for muir-torre syndrome using mismatch repair protein immunohistochemistry of sebaceous neoplasms. J Genet Couns. 22(3):393-405, 2013
3. Dasgupta T et al: A retrospective review of 1349 cases of sebaceous carcinoma. Cancer. 115(1):158-65, 2009
4. Buitrago W et al: Sebaceous carcinoma: the great masquerader: emgerging concepts in diagnosis and treatment. Dermatol Ther. 21(6):459-66, 2008
5. Singh RS et al: Site and tumor type predicts DNA mismatch repair status in cutaneous sebaceous neoplasia. Am J Surg Pathol. 32(6):936-42, 2008
6. Yang HM et al: Immunohistochemical expression of D2-40 in benign and malignant sebaceous tumors and comparison to basal and squamous cell carcinomas. Am J Dermatopathol. 30(6):549-54, 2008
7. Cabral ES et al: Desmoplastic tricholemmoma of the eyelid misdiagnosed as sebaceous carcinoma: a potential diagnostic pitfall. J Cutan Pathol. 34 Suppl 1:22-5, 2007
8. Ho VH et al: Sentinel lymph node biopsy for sebaceous cell carcinoma and melanoma of the ocular adnexa. Arch Otolaryngol Head Neck Surg. 133(8):820-6, 2007
9. Cabral ES et al: Distinction of benign sebaceous proliferations from sebaceous carcinomas by immunohistochemistry. Am J Dermatopathol. 28(6):465-71, 2006
10. Curry ML et al: Muir-Torre syndrome: role of the dermatopathologist in diagnosis. Am J Dermatopathol. 26(3):217-21, 2004
11. Nelson BR et al: Sebaceous carcinoma. J Am Acad Dermatol. 33(1):1-15; quiz 16-8, 1995
12. Cohen PR et al: Association of sebaceous gland tumors and internal malignancy: the Muir-Torre syndrome. Am J Med. 90(5):606-13, 1991
13. Nakamura S et al: Sebaceous carcinoma--with special reference to histopathologic differential diagnosis. J Dermatol. 15(1):55-9, 1988
14. Burgdorf WH et al: Muir-Torre syndrome. Histologic spectrum of sebaceous proliferations. Am J Dermatopathol. 8(3):202-8, 1986
15. Ratz JL et al: Sebaceous carcinoma of the eyelid treated with Mohs' surgery. J Am Acad Dermatol. 14(4):668-73, 1986
16. Wolfe JT 3rd et al: Sebaceous carcinoma of the eyelid. Errors in clinical and pathologic diagnosis. Am J Surg Pathol. 8(8):597-606, 1984
17. Russell WG et al: Sebaceous carcinoma of meibomian gland origin. The diagnostic importance of pagetoid spread of neoplastic cells. Am J Clin Pathol. 73(4):504-11, 1980

Microscopic Features

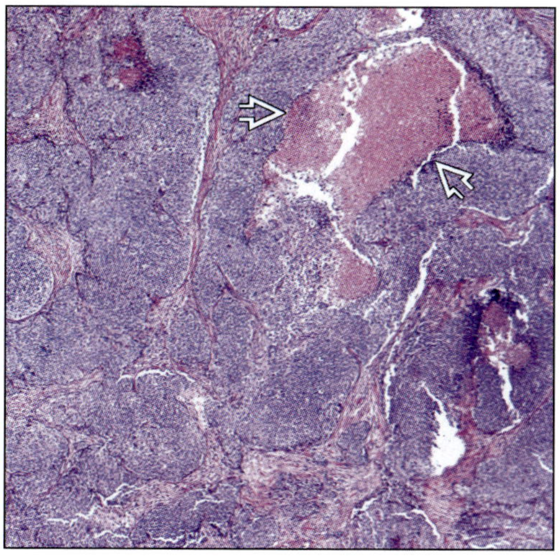
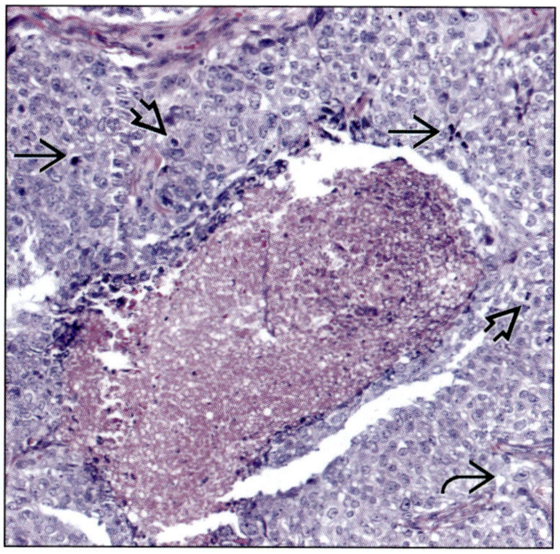

(Left) *Scanning magnification view shows an atypical cellular, nodular, basaloid-appearing proliferation with large areas of comedonecrosis.* ***(Right)*** *High magnification of an area of comedonecrosis is surrounded by atypical clear to basaloid cells with apoptotic bodies and mitoses. Some of the cells show clear cytoplasmic vacuoles.*

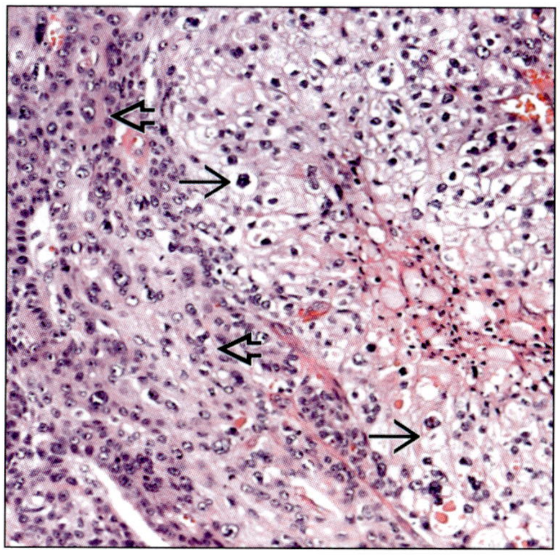
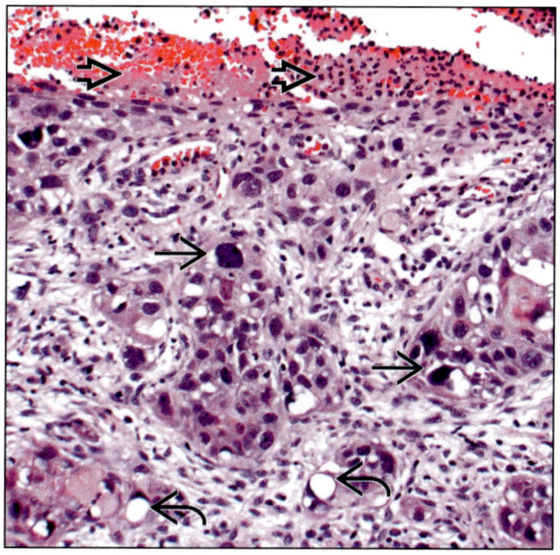

(Left) *Sebaceous carcinoma shows areas of squamous differentiation adjacent to more typical areas with clear cell differentiation.* ***(Right)*** *Invasive poorly differentiated sebaceous carcinoma with squamoid features shows markedly enlarged, atypical, and pleomorphic-appearing cells. Note the overlying epidermal ulceration with serum crusting and neutrophils. Scattered cells show nuclear indentations by cytoplasmic vacuoles.*

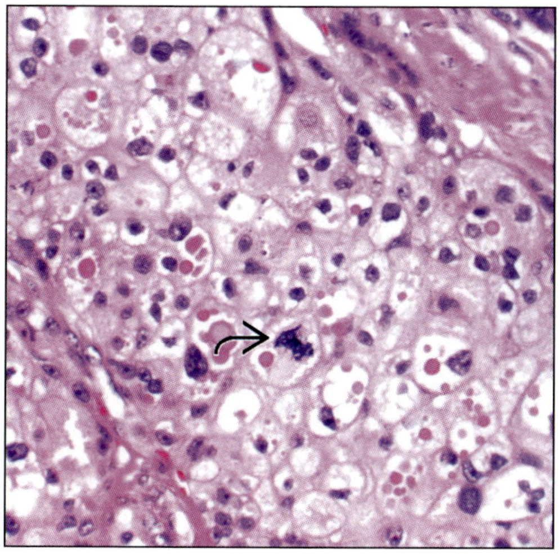
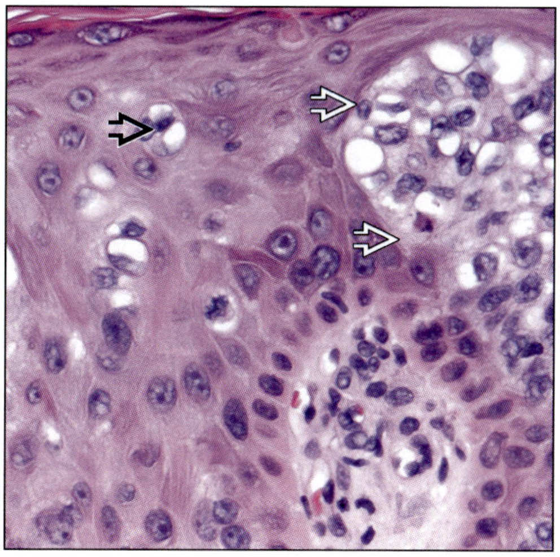

(Left) *High magnification shows a sebaceous carcinoma with abundant red blood cells, some of which appear to be within the cytoplasm of the atypical clear cells. However, the abundant vascularity of renal cell carcinoma is lacking. Note the central atypical mitotic figure.* ***(Right)*** *High magnification shows nests and atypical single pagetoid clear cells in the epidermis. Pagetoid involvement may be present in a minority of cases, and it may rarely be entirely in situ.*

SEBACEOUS CARCINOMA

Ancillary Techniques

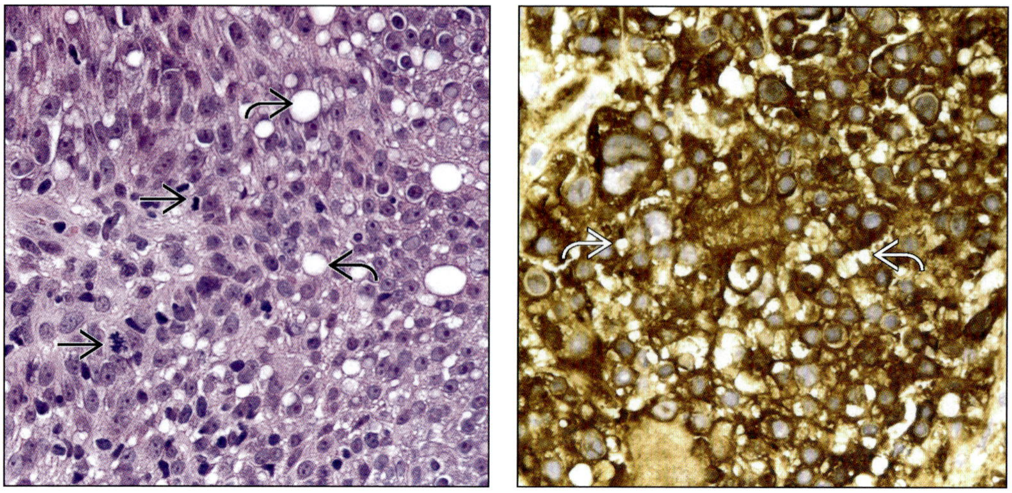

(Left) *High magnification shows a sebaceous carcinoma composed of atypical clear to basaloid cells with mitoses →. Many of the cells show multiple small to large clear cytoplasmic vacuoles ↷.* ***(Right)*** *Strong immunohistochemical staining for EMA, often positive in well- and moderately differentiated tumors, highlights the cytoplasmic membrane and intracytoplasmic vacuoles ↷.*

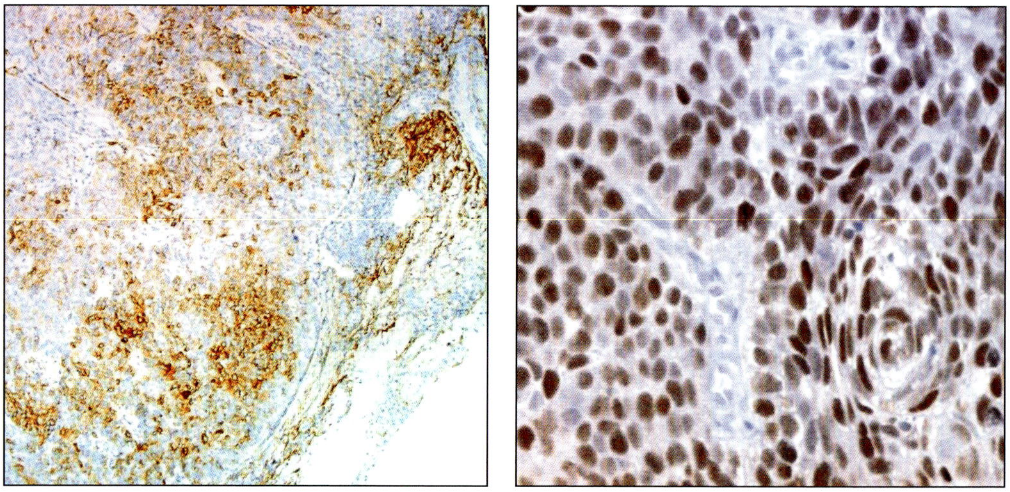

(Left) *CK7 may be positive, but only in approximately 50% of cases. It often shows patchy, moderate to strong cytoplasmic staining, as in this case.* ***(Right)*** *Androgen receptor (AR) immunohistochemistry is positive in most cases and shows moderate, diffuse nuclear staining in the majority of the tumor cells.*

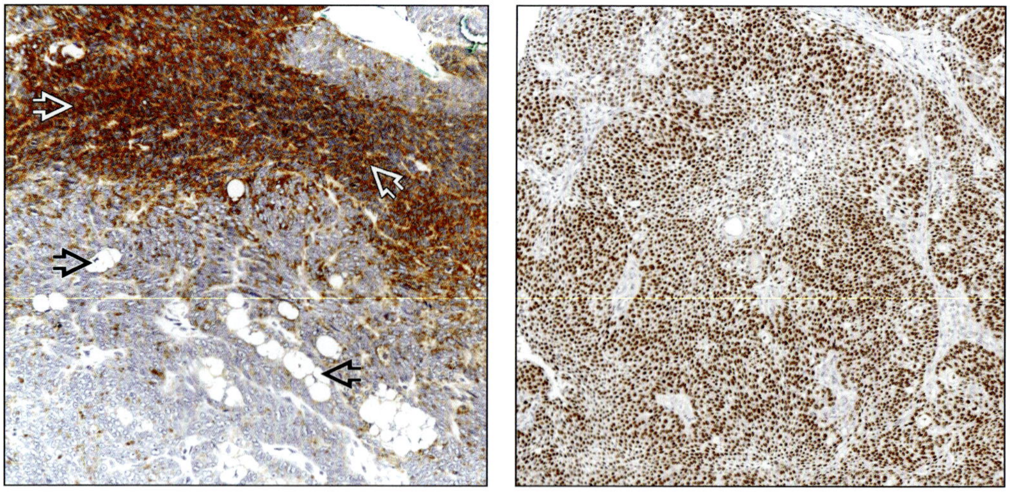

(Left) *D2-40 (podoplanin) is positive in some cases of sebaceous carcinoma, especially basaloid variants. This case shows strong cytoplasmic staining of many of the basaloid and spindled cells ➡ without significant staining of the well-differentiated clear cells ⇨.* ***(Right)*** *Diffuse nuclear staining for p53 is seen in this example of sebaceous carcinoma. p53 and Ki-67 are usually elevated in sebaceous carcinomas, and Bcl-2 is lost, compared with sebaceous adenomas and sebaceomas.*

Differential Diagnosis

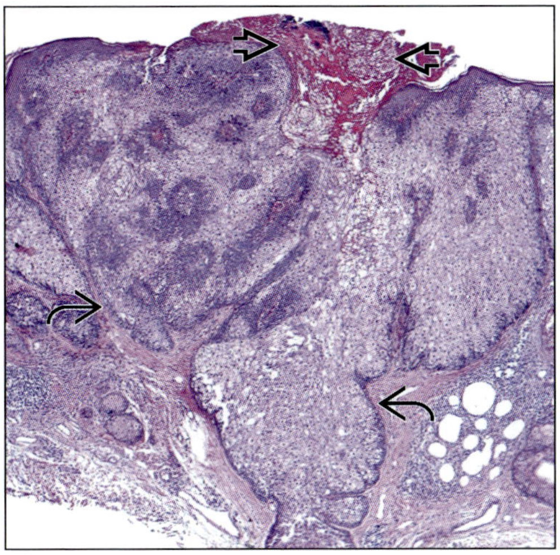

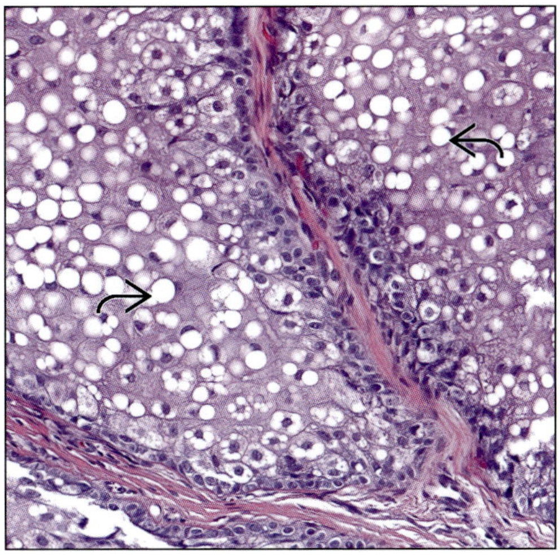

(Left) *Low magnification shows a large sebaceous adenoma. The tumor is a well-circumscribed, fusing lobular proliferation with superficial holocrine necrosis ➯ (recapitulating normal sebaceous glands), composed of bland clear cells surrounded by a thin layer of basaloid cells ↷.* ***(Right)*** *High magnification of a sebaceous adenoma shows the bland cytologic appearance of the mature sebocytes and surrounding basaloid cells. Note the prominent intracytoplasmic lipid vacuoles ↷.*

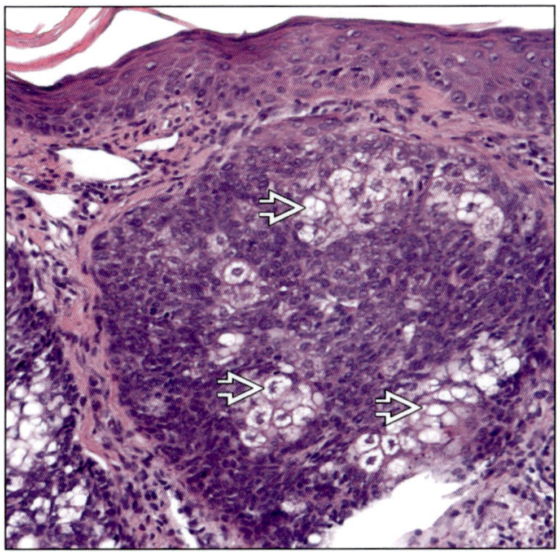

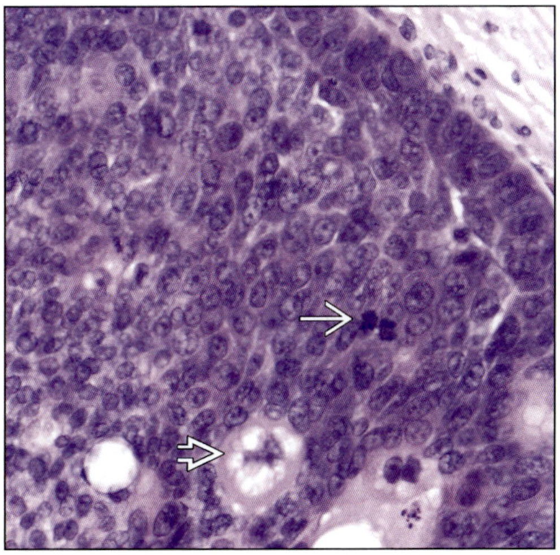

(Left) *Sebaceoma shows well-circumscribed lobules of predominantly basaloid cells with a smaller population of bland-appearing mature sebaceous cells ➯.* ***(Right)*** *High magnification of an atypical sebaceoma shows a predominantly basaloid population of enlarged, moderately atypical cells with nuclear hyperchromasia surrounding several large clear cells ➯ with abundant, multivacuolated cytoplasm. Several mitotic figures are seen →, but these can be quite numerous in some sebaceomas.*

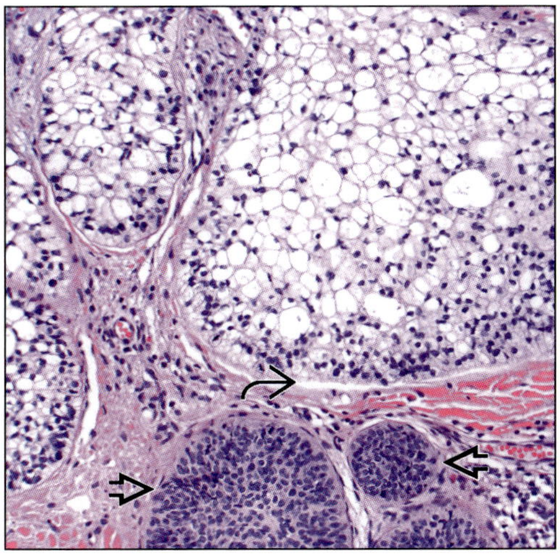

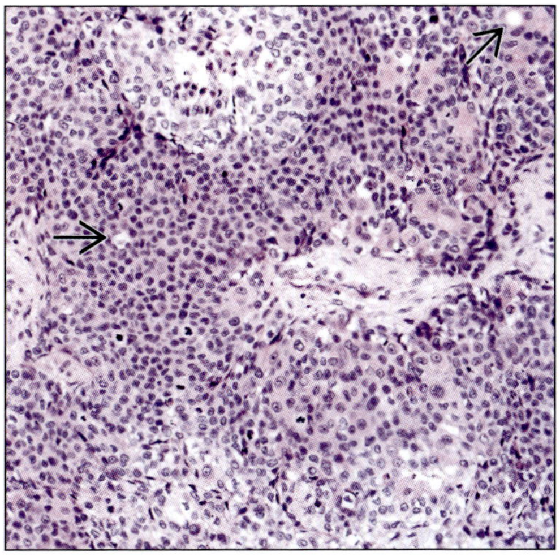

(Left) *Clear cell BCC shows uniform cytoplasmic clearing without the vacuoles and nuclear indentations seen in sebaceous carcinoma. Note the focal retraction artifact ↷ and adjacent areas of conventional-type BCC ➯.* ***(Right)*** *Hidradenocarcinoma is another malignant adnexal tumor that often shows clear cell features. However, the cells lack cytoplasmic vacuoles and nuclear indentations. In addition, a few ductal structures are often seen →, which are rare in sebaceous carcinoma.*

Breast

BREAST

Germline Mutations Associated With Increased Risk of Breast Cancer

Gene	Population Frequency	% of Hereditary Cancers	Risk by Age 70 (Penetrance)	Type of Breast Cancer	Other Cancers	Involvement in Sporadic Cancers	Comments
BRCA1 (17q21) Hereditary breast &/or ovarian cancer syndrome	0.1-0.3%	~ 50% (~ 2% of all cancers)	40-90%	Majority negative for ER, PR, and HER2; basal-like, early onset	Male breast (1-5% risk), ovary, fallopian tube, peritoneal, pancreas, cervix, uterus	Mutations rare, may be inactivated by methylation in medullary and metaplastic	Somatic *TP53* mutations common
BRCA2 (13q12.3) Hereditary breast &/or ovarian cancer syndrome	0.1-0.7%	~ 50% (~ 2% of all cancers)	~ 45-85%	Majority positive for ER, negative for PR and HER2, "luminal B," early or late onset	Male breast (7% risk), ovarian, fallopian tube, peritoneal, pancreas, prostate	Mutations and loss of expression rare	Homozygous germline mutations cause rare form of Fanconi anemia
TP53 (17p13.1) Li-Fraumeni syndrome	0.0025%	3% (< 1% of all cancers)	> 90%	ER positive, majority HER2 positive, "luminal B" or "HER2 enriched," early onset	Sarcomas, adrenal cortex, brain, leukemia, lepidic pattern lung cancer, colon	*TP53* is the most commonly mutated gene in sporadic cancers	
CDH1 (16q22.1) Familial gastric cancer and lobular breast cancer syndrome	0.005%	~ 0.2-1%	~ 40-50%	Lobular, ER positive, HER2 negative	Signet ring cell gastric cancer, signet ring cell colon cancer	Sporadic lobular carcinomas have somatic *CDH1* mutations	Very few women with lobular carcinoma have germline mutations
PTEN (10q23.3) Cowden syndrome	0.0005%	~ 0.3%	50-85%	No special features reported	Male breast, thyroid, uterus		10-50% of individuals may have de novo mutations
ATM (11q22-q23) ataxia-telangiectasia heterozygotes	0.5%	< 1%	~ 30%	No special features reported			Homozygosity results in ataxia-telangiectasia
CHEK2 (22q12.1)	0.5%	< 1-5% (~ 1 % of all cancers)	10-20%	No special features reported; late onset	Prostate, thyroid, kidney	Mutations rare; loss of expression by unknown mechanisms	May increase risk of breast cancer after radiation exposure
STK11/LKB1 (19p13.3) Peutz-Jeghers syndrome	0.001%	~ 0.6%	~ 40%	No special features reported; early onset	Colon, stomach, pancreas, small intestine, thyroid, lung, uterus, ovary, cervix		50% of individuals may have de novo mutations
BRIP1 (*FANCJ* or *BACH1*) (17q22.2)	0.1%	< 1%	~ 20%	No special features reported			Homozygosity results in Fanconi anemia
PALB2/FANCN (16p12.1)	0.1%	< 1%	~ 20% (limited information available)		Ovary, pancreas		Homozygosity results in Fanconi anemia
RAD51C (17q25.1)	~ 0.3%		~ 10% (limited information available)		Ovary		Homozygosity results in Fanconi anemia
BARD1 (2q34-q35)	~ 0.5%		~ 20% (limited information available)		Ovary		
RAD50 (5q31)	~ 0.3%		~ 20% (limited information available)		Ovary		Homozygosity results in Nijmegen breakage syndrome-like disorder
NBN (8q21)	~ 0.2%		~ 20% (limited information available)		Ovary		Homozygosity results in Nijmegen breakage syndrome
MRE11A (11q21)	~ 0.1%		~ 30% (limited information available)		Ovary		Homozygosity results in Ataxia telangiectasia-like disorder
MUTYH (1p34.1)	~ 0.1%		~ 10% (limited information available)		Colon, small intestine		Homozygosity results in MUTYH-associated polyposis

BRCA1 and BRCA2

Feature	BRCA1	BRCA2
Chromosome	17q21	13q12.3
Gene size	81 kb	84 kb
Protein size	1,863 amino acids	3,418 amino acids
Function	Tumor suppressor: Role in double-stranded DNA repair, transcriptional regulation	Tumor suppressor: Role in double-stranded DNA repair, transcriptional regulation
Mutations	> 1,000	> 1,000
Incidence of mutations in population	~ 0.1-0.3%	~ 0.1-0.7%
Groups with increased incidence	Ashkenazi Jews (2 mutations), Finns, French Canadians, others	Ashkenazi Jews (1 mutation), Icelandic, others
Risk of breast cancer by age 70	40-90%	45-85%
Risk of ovarian cancer	40-50%	10-20%
Risk of male breast cancer	1.8%	7%
Age of onset of female breast cancer	44 years	47 years
Age of onset of ovarian cancer	49-53 years	55-58 years
Proportion of families with breast cancer due to a single gene	~ 50%	~ 50%
Proportion of families with breast and ovarian cancer	80%	15%
Proportion of families with female and male breast cancer	< 4%	75%
Other associated cancers	Prostate, pancreas, cervix, uterus	Prostate, pancreas, stomach, bile duct, gallbladder, melanoma
Alterations in sporadic breast cancer	Mutations very rare (< 5%) inactivation may occur by methylation	Mutations very rare (< 5%)
Pathologic Features of Breast Cancers		
Histologic type	Many medullary or "medullary-like" (high nuclear grade, syncytial growth pattern, pushing borders, lymphocytic infiltrate)	Many lobular or with lobular features
DCIS	Absent or scant	Common
Grade	> 95% poorly differentiated	Majority moderately to poorly differentiated
Hormone receptors	70-80% negative	> 80% positive (but may be at low levels)
HER2	> 95% negative	> 95% negative
TP53 mutations	> 90% of cancers	30-65% of cancers
Molecular type	Majority basal-like	Majority "luminal B," HER2 negative

Blood and Bone Marrow

BLOOD AND BONE MARROW

Hereditary Syndromes With Blood and Bone Marrow Abnormalities and Predisposition to Myeloid Neoplasms

Syndrome	Affected Gene(s)	Clinical Features	Peripheral Blood Manifestations	Bone Marrow Manifestations	Incidence of MDS/AML	Inheritance Pattern
Bone Marrow Failure						
Congenital amegakaryocytic thrombocytopenia	Loss of function mutations in *MPL* (encodes thrombopoietin receptor)	No syndromic malformations/ dysmorphism, evolution to bone marrow failure	Severe thrombocytopenia, progression to pancytopenia	Absent or markedly reduced megakaryocytes (may be relatively normal in number at early age/initial presentation), progression to marrow aplasia	Lower than other bone marrow failure syndromes	AR
Diamond-Blackfan anemia	Mutations in genes encoding several ribosomal subunit proteins (25% of cases: *RPS19*)	40% with congenital manifestations such as cardiac and renal defects, hypertelorism, short stature, radial ray abnormalities	Isolated severe macrocytic anemia and reticulocytopenia	Erythroid maturation arrest (only rare erythroblasts), increased hematogones, other lineages preserved, normal marrow cellularity	Poorly defined (some report ≤ 1%)	AD (highly variable penetrance); also sporadic
Dyskeratosis congenita	Mutations in telomere maintenance genes: *TERT, TERC, DKC1, TINF2*	Variable findings, classically oral leukoplakia, abnormal nails, reticulate hyperpigmentation in 1st decade, and progression to bone marrow failure in 2nd decade, carcinoma risk: 40-50% by age 50	Gradual development of pancytopenia, reticulocytopenia	Aplastic anemia (in up to 85% of patients)	3-5%	AD, AR, and X-linked recessive
Severe congenital neutropenia	Mutations in *ELANE*, causing misfolding of the encoded protein (neutrophil elastase) and granulocyte apoptosis; *HAX1*, causing uncontrolled mitochondrion-dependent apoptosis; and *WAS*, causing increased activity (gain of function)	Usually no syndromic malformations/ dysmorphism, highly susceptible to infection	Isolated, profound neutropenia presenting at birth/ infancy	Sustained myeloid aplasia with maturation arrest (few myeloblasts and promyelocytes)	21% (cumulative incidence)	AD, AR, and X-linked recessive
Shwachman-Diamond syndrome	Mutations in *SBDS* (ribosomal biogenesis; mitotic spindle stabilization)	Exocrine pancreatic insufficiency (failure to thrive, malabsorption, steatorrhea, deficiency of fat-soluble vitamins), skeletal abnormalities including short stature	Initial neutropenia (may be intermittent), 25% progress to pancytopenia	Initially only granulocytic abnormalities (variable myeloid left-shift/ hypoplasia), 25% develop eventual marrow aplasia	10%	AR
DNA Damage Repair Deficiency						
Fanconi anemia	Mutations in genes encoding the Fanconi anemia pathway; proteins encoded by these genes sense DNA damage and initiate DNA repair (most frequently mutated: *FANCA*)	Up to 75% demonstrate low birth weight/short stature, hypoplastic or absent thumbs &/or radii, pigmentation, or ear, cardiac, renal, neurologic, endocrine, and gastrointestinal abnormalities	Thrombocytopenia progressing to pancytopenia in 1st decade of life, reticulocytopenia	Initially normocellular or hypercellular; eventual marrow aplasia	25% cumulative incidence of hematologic malignancy (compared to normal population, 600x increased risk of AML and 5,000x increased risk of MDS)	AR and X-linked recessive

AD: Autosomal dominant; AML: Acute myeloid leukemia; AR: Autosomal recessive; MDS: Myelodysplastic syndromes.

Microscopic Features

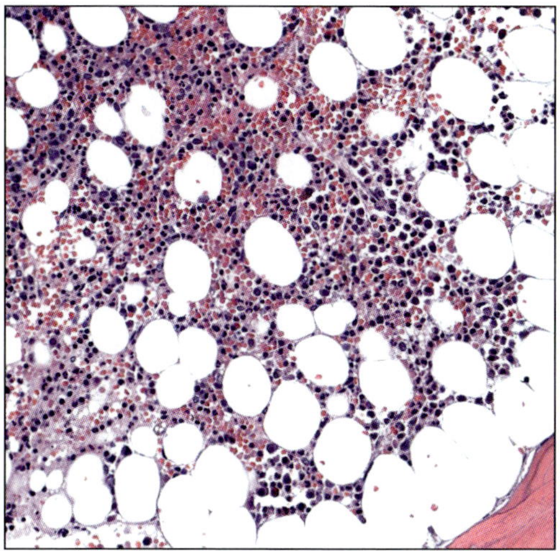
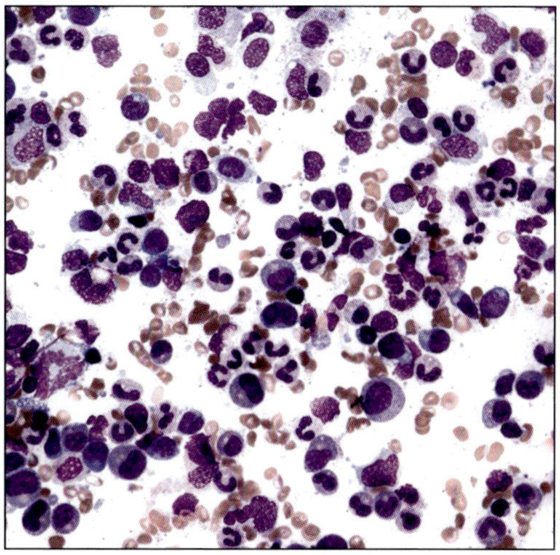

*(**Left**) Congenital amegakaryocytic thrombocytopenia is characterized by absent or markedly reduced megakaryocytes. Other lineages are unaffected, and early in the disease course, bone marrow cellularity is normal. (Courtesy D. Czuchlewski, MD.) (**Right**) Bone marrow aspirate smear from a patient with Diamond-Blackfan anemia shows only scattered erythroid elements within a background of adequate granulopoiesis. (Courtesy D. Czuchlewski, MD.)*

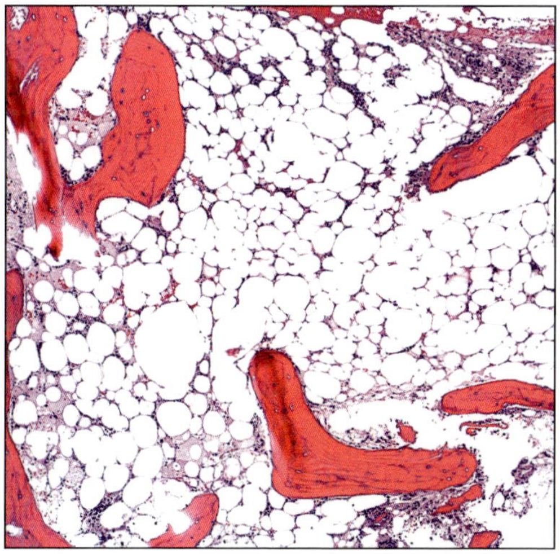
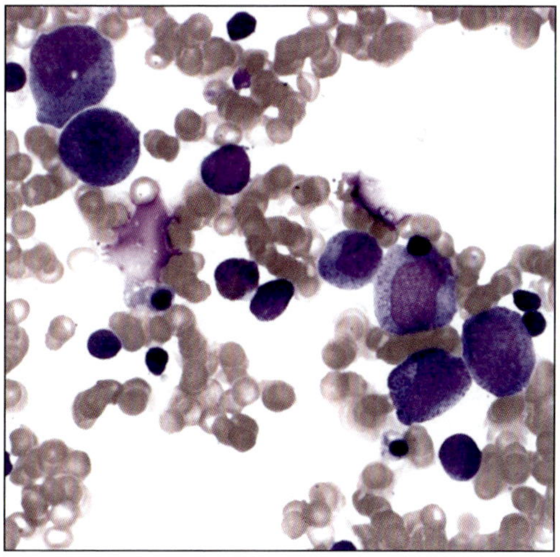

*(**Left**) The majority of patients with dyskeratosis congenita develop aplastic anemia. Bone marrow core biopsy will reveal marked hypocellularity as shown here. (Courtesy D. Czuchlewski, MD.) (**Right**) Bone marrow aspirate from a 2 year old with severe congenital neutropenia shows a so-called maturation arrest picture with a paucity of late-stage granulocytes. (Courtesy D. Czuchlewski, MD.)*

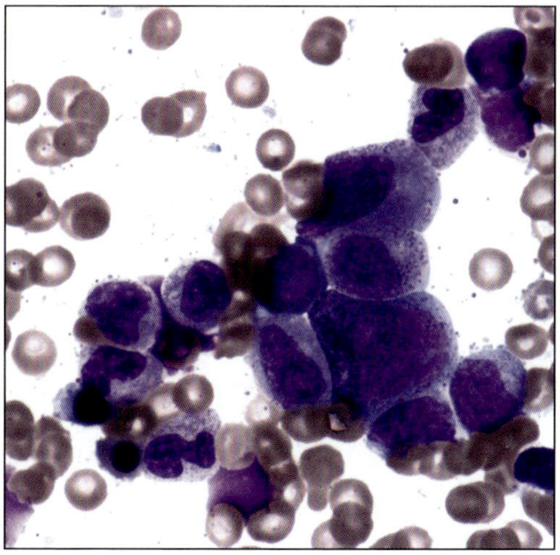
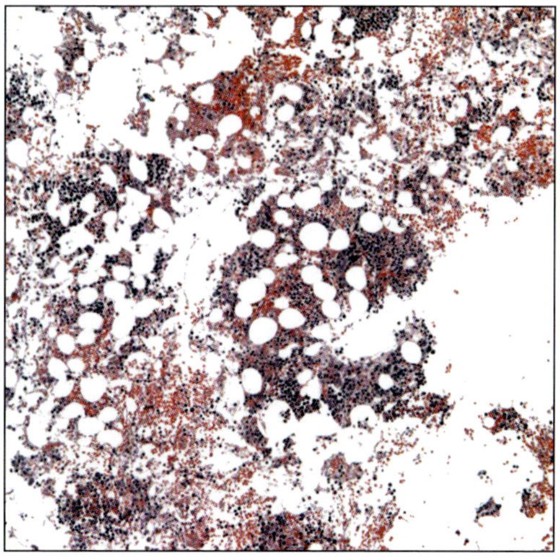

*(**Left**) The bone marrow appearance of Shwachman-Diamond syndrome can be variable, but cases may show hypoplastic &/or left-shifted myelopoiesis, as in this 1-year-old girl. (Courtesy D. Czuchlewski, MD.) (**Right**) A bone marrow clot section from a 6-year-old girl with new onset pancytopenia shows moderate hypocellularity. The patient progressed to fulminant bone marrow failure and aplasia in the setting of Fanconi anemia. (Courtesy D. Czuchlewski, MD.)*

Bone and Soft Tissue

Bone and Soft Tissue III-3-2

BONE AND SOFT TISSUE

Molecular and Cytogenetic Findings in Bone and Soft Tissue Tumors

Histologic Type	Translocation or Rearrangement	Fusion Gene or Other Feature	Frequency
Aggressive angiomyxoma	t(12q15)	*HMGA2*	> 20%
Alveolar soft part sarcoma	t(X;17)(p11;q25)	*ASPL-TFE3* fusion	> 90%
Aneurysmal bone cyst	t(16;17)(q22;p13)	*CDH11-USP6* fusion	20%
	t(17p13.2)	*USP6*	> 50%
Angiomatoid fibrous histiocytoma	t(12;22)(q13;q12)	*EWSR1-ATF1* fusion	Unknown
	t(12;16)(q13;p11)	*FUS-ATF1* fusion	Unknown
	t (2;22)(q33;q12)	*EWSR1-CREB1* fusion	Unknown
Bizarre parosteal osteochondromatous proliferation	t(1;17)(q32;q21)	Unknown	Breakpoint in 1q23 present in 100% of lesions
	t(1;17)(q42;q23)	Unknown	Unknown
Clear cell sarcoma of soft parts	t(12;22)(q13;q12)	*EWSR1-ATF1* fusion	> 75%
Clear cell sarcoma (gastrointestinal)	t(2;22)(q33;q12)	*EWSR1-CREB1* fusion	Unknown
Chondromyxoid fibroma	Deletion 6q	Unknown	> 75%
Dermatofibrosarcoma protuberans and variants	t(17;22)(q21;q13)	*COL1A1-PDGFB* fusion	> 75%
	Ring form of chromosomes 17 and 22	*COL1A1-PDGFB* fusion	> 75%
Desmoplastic fibroblastoma	t(2;11)(q31;q12)	Unknown	Unknown
Desmoplastic small round cell tumor	t(11;22)(p13;q12)	*EWSR1-WT1* fusion	> 95%
	t(21;22)(q22;q12)	*EWSR1-ERG* fusion	
Endometrial stroma sarcoma	t(7;17)(p15:q21)	*JAZF1-JJAZ1* fusion	30%
	t(6;7)(p21;p22)	*JAZF1-PHF1* fusion	10%
	t(10:17)(q22;p13)	Unknown	Unknown
Epithelioid hemangioendothelioma	t(1;3)(p36.3;q25)	Unknown	Unknown
	t(10;14)(p13;q24)	Gene for VEGF-related protein at 14q24	
Epithelioid sarcoma	Abnormalities of 22q: t/del(22q11.2)	*INI1* inactivation	Unknown
Ewing sarcoma/primitive neuroectodermal tumor	t(11;22)(q24;q12)	*EWSR1-FLI1* fusion	> 80%
	t(21;22)(q12;q12)	*EWSR1-ERG* fusion	5-10%
	t(7;22)(p22;q12)	*EWSR1-ETV1* fusion	< 5%
	t(2;22)(q33;q12)	*EWSR1-FEV* fusion	< 5%
	t(17;22)(q12;q12)	*EWSR1-E1AF* fusion	< 5%
	t(16;21)(p11;q22)	*FUS-ERG* fusion	Rare
	inv(22)(q12;q12)	*EWSR1-ZSG* fusion	< 5%
Extraskeletal myxoid chondrosarcoma	t(9;22)(q22;q12)	*EWSR1-NR4A3* fusion	> 75%
	t(9;17)(q22;q11)	*TAFII68-NR4A3* fusion	< 10%
	t(9;15)(q22;q21)	*TCF12-NR4A3* fusion	< 10%
Fibromatosis	Trisomies of 8 and 20		30%
	Deletion 5q21	*APC* mutation or inactivation and β-catenin mutation	10-20% and 50%, respectively
Fibromyxoid sarcoma, low grade	t(7;16)(q32-34;p11.2)	*FUS-CREB3L2* fusion	96%
	t(11;16)(p11;p11)	*FUS-CREB3L1* fusion	Rare
Fibrosarcoma, infantile	t(12;15)(p13;q26)	*ETV6-NTRK3* fusion	> 75%
	Trisomies 8, 11, 17, and 20		> 75%
Gastrointestinal stromal tumor		*KIT, PDGFRA, SDHB* mutations	> 90%
Giant cell tumor, diffuse type (PVNS)	t(1;2)(p13;q37)/t(1p13)	*COL6A3-CSF1* fusion	> 25%
Inflammatory myofibroblastic tumor	2p23 rearrangement, numerous	*ALK* fusions with various genes	Unknown
	t(1;2)(q22;p23)	*TPM3-ALK* fusion	Unknown
	t(2;19)(p23;p13)	*TPM4-ALK* fusion	Unknown
	t(2;17)(p23;q13)	*CLTC-ALK* fusion	Unknown
Leiomyosarcoma	Deletion of 1p		
Lipoblastoma	8q12 rearrangement	*PLAG1* oncogene	> 80%

BONE AND SOFT TISSUE

Lipoma			
Typical lipoma	t(12q15) or t(6p21)	*HMGA2* rearrangement	40% and 10%
Spindle cell or pleomorphic lipoma	Deletion 13q12 &/or 16q13, polysomy 12	*RB*/13q14 allelic loss	> 75%
Liposarcoma			
Well differentiated	Ring/giant markers chromosome 12 (12q13-q15)	*MDM2, HMGA2*	> 75%
Dedifferentiated	Ring forms and complex changes	12q14 amplicon including *MDM2, CDK4, HMGA2, ASK1,* and *JUN* amplification	Unknown
Spindle cell		*RB1* deletion	
Myxoid/round cell	t(12;16)(q13;p11), t(12;22)(q13;q12)	*FUS-DDIT3* fusion, *EWS-CHOP* fusion	> 75% and < 5%
	t(12;22)(q13;q12)	*EWSR1-DDIT3*	
Pleomorphic	Complex changes, multiple karyotypes		> 90%
		FUS-CREB3L1 (in a small number of cases)	
Malignant rhabdoid tumor	del/t(22)(q11.2)	*hSNF5/INI1* deletion and mutation with inactivation	> 90%
Malignant peripheral nerve sheath tumor	Complex changes	*NF1* inactivation, *INK4A* deletion	
Myxofibrosarcoma	Ring form of chromosome 12, complex changes		
Myxoinflammatory fibroblastic sarcoma	t(1;10)(p22;q24)	*TGFBR3-MGEA5* fusion	Unknown
Osteochondroma	Deletion 8q	*EXT1* inactivation	> 25%
Osteosarcoma	Ring chromosomes (low grade) and complex	*RB* and *TP53* inactivation	> 80%
Rhabdomyosarcoma			
Alveolar	t(2;13)(q35;q14)	*PAX3-FKHR*	> 75%
	t(1;13)(p36;q14)	*PAX7-FKHR*	10-20%
	t(2)(q35)	*PAX3*	
Embryonal	Trisomies 2q, 8, and 20	Loss of heterozygosity at 11p15.5	> 75%
Schwannoma and perineurioma	Deletion 22q	*NF2* inactivation	> 80%
Subungual exostosis	t(X;6)(q13-14;q22)	*COL4A5* and *COL12A1*	Unknown
Synovial sarcoma	t(X;18)(p11;q11)	*SYT* with *SSX1, SSX2,* or *SSX4* fusion	> 90%
	t(X;20)(p11;q13)	*SS18L1-SSX1* fusion	

Genetic Findings in Benign and Intermediate Soft Tissue Tumors

Histologic Type	Translocation or Rearrangement	Fusion Gene or Other Feature
Adipose tumors		
Lipoma	t(3;12)(q27-28;q15), *HMGA2* rearrangements at 12q15	*HMGA2-LPP* fusion
Spindle cell and pleomorphic lipoma	Loss of 13q12, 16q13, polysomy of 12	*RB*/13q14 allelic loss
Hibernoma	11q13 rearrangements	
Lipoblastoma	8q11-13 rearrangements	*PLAG1-HAS2* fusion
Chondroid lipoma	t(11;16)(q13;p12-13)	
Cellular angiofibroma	Loss at 13q	*RB*/13q14 allelic loss
Chondroma of soft tissue	*HMGA2* rearrangements	Unknown
Desmoplastic fibroblastoma	t(2;11)(q31;q12)	
Fibroma of tendon sheath	t(2;11)(q31-32;q12)	
Fibromatosis	Trisomies of 8 and 20 and deletion 5q21	
Sporadic deep		*CTNNB1* (β-catenin gene) mutations
In familial adenomatous polyposis		Germline *APC* inactivating mutations
Leiomyoma		
Cutaneous hereditary	1q42.3-q43 rearrangements	*MCUL1* mutations (fumarate hydratase)
Uterine	*HMGA2* rearrangements	
Nerve sheath tumors		
Neurofibroma	9p21-22 rearrangements	*NF1* deletion (17q11) in neurofibromatosis type 1

BONE AND SOFT TISSUE

Perineurioma	22q11.2-12 rearrangements	*NF2* loss
Sclerosing perineurioma	t(2;10)(p23;q24), monosomy 10	
Schwannoma	Changes in 22, 7, X, Y	*NF2* mutations in neurofibromatosis type 2
Mammary-type myofibroblastoma	Partial monosomy of 13q and 16q	Allelic loss at *RB*/13q14 and *FKHR*/13q14
Myoepithelioma	t(1;22)(q23;q12)	*EWSR1-PBX1* fusion
	t(19;22)(q13;q12)	*EWSR1-ZNF444* fusion
Plexiform fibrohistiocytic tumor	t(4;15)(q21;q15)	
Solitary fibrous tumor	12q15 rearrangements	
	t(8;12)(p11.2;q24.3)	
	t(12;17)(q15;q23)	
Tenosynovial giant cell tumor	t(1;2)(p13;q37) /t(1p13)	*CSF1-COL6A3* fusion

Familial Cancer Syndromes With Bone and Soft Tissue Tumors

Bone and Soft Tissue Tumor	Familial Cancer Syndromes
Chondrosarcoma	Hereditary multiple exostosis
	Li-Fraumeni syndrome
	Hereditary retinoblastoma
Chordoma	Familial chordoma
	Tuberous sclerosis
Soft tissue tumor and sarcoma	Basal cell nevus syndrome
	Li-Fraumeni syndrome
	Hereditary retinoblastoma
	Multiple hereditary exostosis
	Familial adenomatous polyposis
	Renal carcinoma with leiomyomas
	von Hippel-Lindau syndrome
	Werner syndrome
	Familial melanoma
Osteosarcoma	Li-Fraumeni syndrome
	Hereditary retinoblastoma
Rhabdomyosarcoma	Li-Fraumeni syndrome
	Beckwith-Wiedemann syndrome
	Neurofibromatosis type 1
	Hereditary retinoblastoma
	Costello syndrome
	Werner syndrome
Malignant peripheral nerve sheath tumor	Li-Fraumeni syndrome
	Familial melanoma
	Neurofibromatosis type 1
	Neurofibromatosis type 2
	Carney complex
	Multiple endocrine neoplasia 1
	Werner syndrome
Ossifying fibroma	Hyperparathyroidism-jaw tumor syndrome

Diagrammatic Features

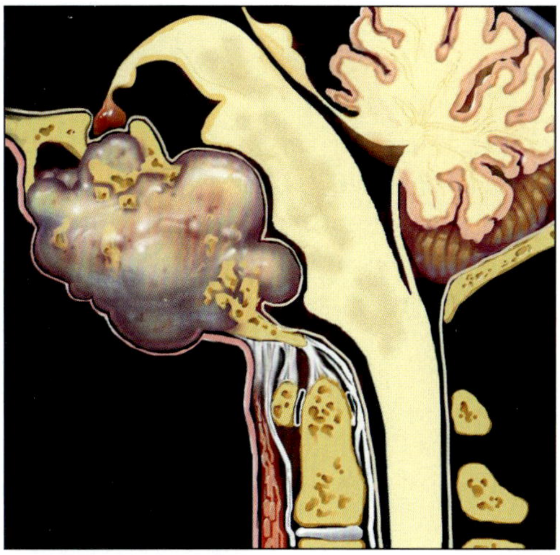

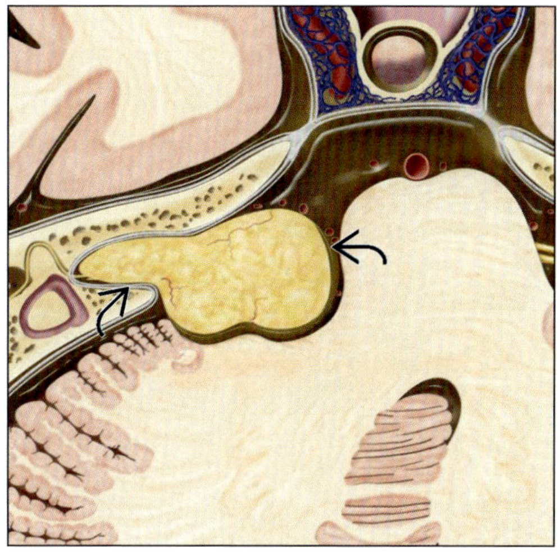

(Left) *Graphic shows a chordoma of the clivus extending into the sphenoid sinus. The tumor has a gray translucent appearance and expands and erodes the bone, causing focal destruction of the bony cortex. These tumors may be associated with familial chordoma or with tuberous sclerosis.* ***(Right)*** *Bilateral schwannomas involving the vestibular branch of cranial nerve 8 are a hallmark of neurofibromatosis type 2, present as a cerebropontine angle mass →, and may be multiple.*

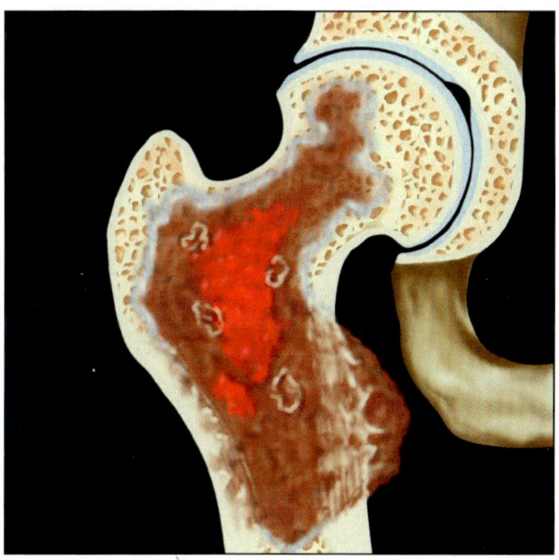

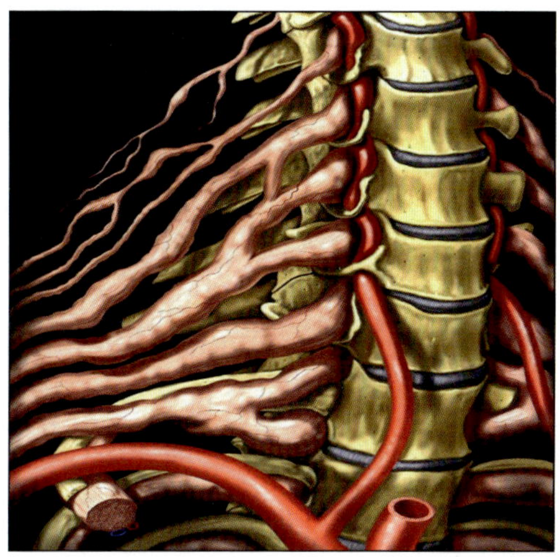

(Left) *Chondrosarcoma with a tan-gray glistening appearance fills the medullary cavity of the proximal diaphysis, greater trochanter, and base of the femoral neck. It can be present in hereditary multiple exostosis, Li-Fraumeni syndrome, and hereditary retinoblastoma.* ***(Right)*** *Graphic shows bilateral spinal nerve root and branchial plexus neurofibromas in NF1. There is lobulated tortuous expansion of the cervical nerve roots with widening of the neural foramina.*

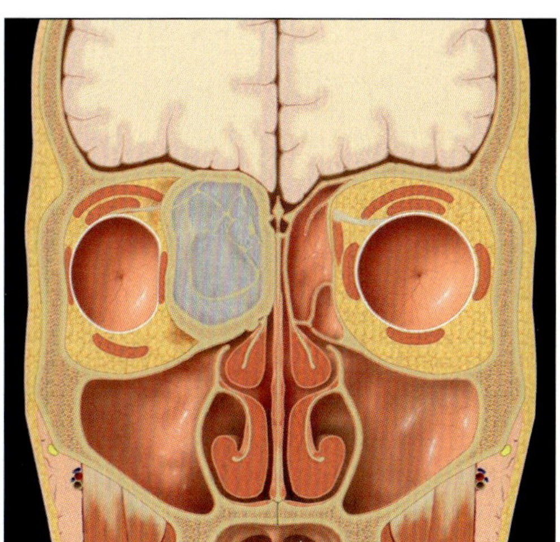

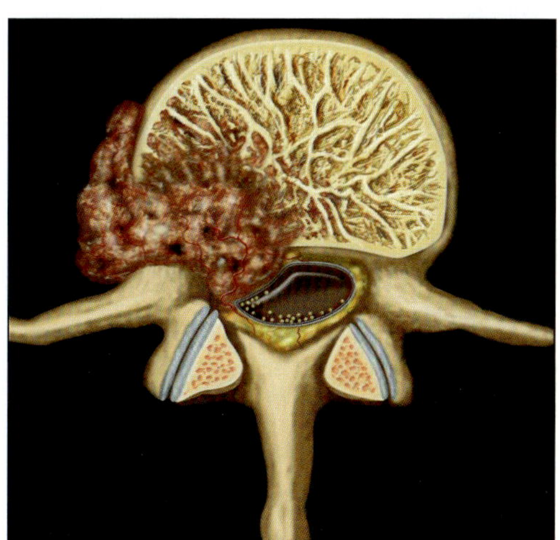

(Left) *Graphic depicts a nonossifying fibroma in a patient with hyperparathyroidism-jaw tumor syndrome, presenting as a large maxillary mass. Note that the mass obstructs one side of the nose and compresses the eye.* ***(Right)*** *Graphic depicts osteosarcoma arising from the lateral area of C5. The firm, pink, solid mass has transgressed the cortex and extended into the soft tissues. These tumors may be present in Li-Fraumeni syndrome, Werner syndrome, and hereditary retinoblastoma.*

Head and Neck

HEAD AND NECK

Familial Cancer Syndromes With Head and Neck Neoplasms

Syndrome	Gene	Head and Neck Tumor	Other Manifestations
Dyskeratosis congenita	*TERT, TERC, DKC1, TINF2*; other genes involved in telomere maintenance	SCCa of head and neck, SCCa of tongue	Skin cancer, anorectal carcinoma, gastric carcinoma, lung carcinoma, colon carcinoma, esophageal carcinoma, Hodgkin lymphoma, retinoblastoma, and others
Fanconi anemia	13 separate genes comprising the "Fanconi anemia pathway": *FANCx*	SCCa of head and neck	Short stature, eye abnormalities, Wilms tumor and other solid tumors, SCCa of cervix; hematologic neoplasms (by age 45, cumulative incidence of hematologic malignancy is 25%; median diagnosis age: 11-14 years); predominantly myeloid malignancies, acute myeloid leukemia, and other hematopoietic abnormalities, (600x increased risk of AML; 5,000x increased risk of MDS); solid tumors such as SCCa (esophageal, anogenital), hepatocellular carcinoma, brain tumors; breast cancer susceptibility
XP	Genes involved in nucleotide excision repair of ultraviolet light-induced damage (*XPA-XPG*)	SCCa of tongue (increase 100,000x in XP patients < 20 years compared to general population)	Carcinomas and sarcomas of skin, melanomas, ocular cancer, and other internal malignancies, such as brain tumors (medulloblastomas and glioblastomas); spinal cord astrocytomas; carcinomas of lung, uterus, breast, stomach, kidney, and testicles; leukemias; and multiple benign tumors
Bloom syndrome	*BLM* (a tumor-suppressor gene belonging to the family of RecQ DNA helicase)	SCCa of head and neck	Up to 50% of patients will develop a malignancy; ~ 10% of patients have ≥ 2 primary cancers, with fewer patients reported to have 3, 4, or even 5 primary neoplasms; hematolymphoid malignancies predominant in the first 2 decades of life; carcinomas predominant after the first 2 decades of life and arise in varied sites, e.g., skin, head and neck, gastrointestinal tract (including esophagus [both squamous cell carcinoma and adenocarcinoma], stomach, and colon), lung, uterus, and breast; medulloblastoma, Wilms tumor, osteogenic sarcoma
Retinoblastoma	*RB*	Carcinoma of nasal cavity	Retinoblastoma; 2nd cancers common in patients with *RB* mutations (i.e., osteosarcoma, leiomyosarcoma, fibrosarcoma, chondrosarcoma, rhabdomyosarcoma, Ewing sarcoma, melanoma, pinealoblastoma, Hodgkin lymphoma, breast carcinoma)
NF2	*NF2*	Vestibular schwannoma: Bilateral vestibular schwannomas a hallmark of NF2 (90-95% of patients)	Plexiform schwannoma (features occurring more frequently in NF2-associated schwannomas include whorl formation, multiple tumors involving a single nerve, and juxtaposition to meningioma), neurofibroma, meningoma, ependymoma, conventional MPNST and MPNST ex-schwannomas reported in NF2 but very rare
Basal cell nevus syndrome (Gorlin syndrome)	*PTCH1*	Odontogenic cysts, dentigerous cysts	Triggers that should prompt evaluation for Gorlin syndrome: Odontogenic keratocysts if age < 20 years old, basal cell carcinoma if age < 20 years old, palmar or plantar pits, lamellar calcification of falx cerebri, medulloblastoma, desmoplastic, characteristic facies with broad nasal root (and hypertelorism), numerous tumors, including basal cell carcinoma, medulloblastoma, meningoma, ovarian fibroma, cardiac fibroma
HPTH-jaw tumor syndrome	*HRPT2*	Fibroma of the jaw, ossifying fibroma of the jaw	Hyperparathyroidism develops late in adolescence in > 80% of patients: Parathyroid hyperplasia, adenoma, and carcinoma; renal cysts, hamartomas, and cortical adenomas; Wilms tumor; testicular germ cell tumor; papillary thyroid carcinoma, and other neoplasms
FAP	*APC*	Juvenile nasopharyngeal angiofibroma	≥ 100 colorectal adenomas (classical FAP), fundic gland polyps, antral adenomas, gastric cancer (rare), hepatoblastomas in male infants, hepatic adenomas and hepatocellular carcinomas, pancreatic adenocarcinoma and intraductal mucinous neoplasms of pancreas, adenocarcinoma of gallbladder, fibromatosis, multiple osteomas, congenital hypertrophy of the retinal pigmented epithelium, cribriform-morular variant of papillary thyroid carcinoma

AML: Acute myeloid leukemia; FAP: Familial adenomatous polyposis; HPTH: Hyperparathyroidism; MDS: Myelodysplastic syndrome; MPNST: Malignant peripheral nerve sheath tumor; NF2: Neurofibromatosis type 2; SCCa: Squamous cell carcinoma; XP: Xeroderma pigmentosum.

Diagrammatic, Clinical, and Gross Features

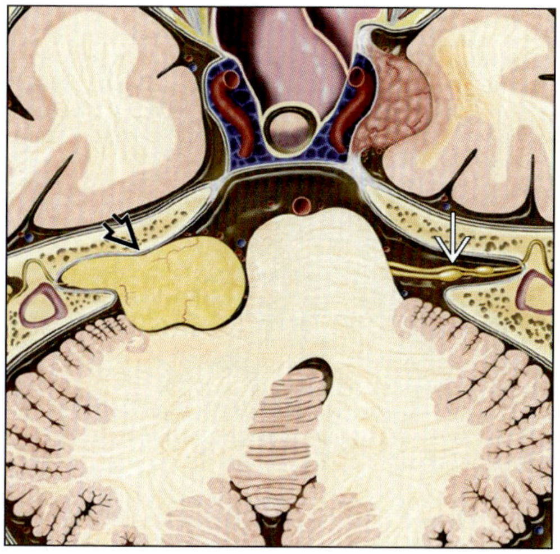

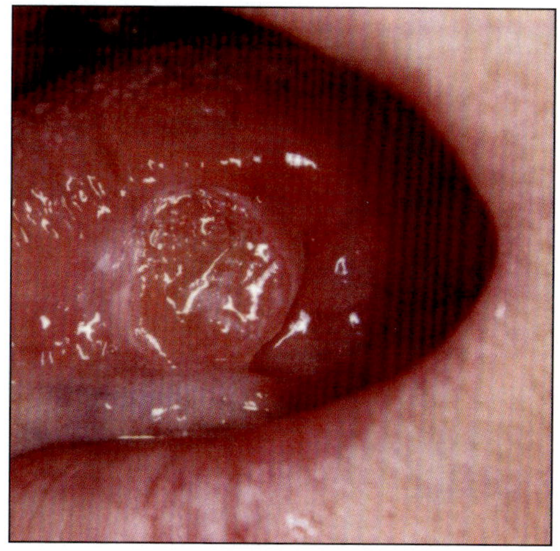

(Left) *Bilateral schwannomas involving the vestibular branch of cranial nerve 8 are a hallmark of neurofibromatosis type 2, present as a cerebellopontine angle mass →. These may be multiple →.* ***(Right)*** *Squamous cell carcinoma on the posterior lateral border of the tongue in a patient with dyskeratosis congenita presents as an exophytic, firm, indurated mass with rolled borders. (Courtesy S. Muller, DMD.)*

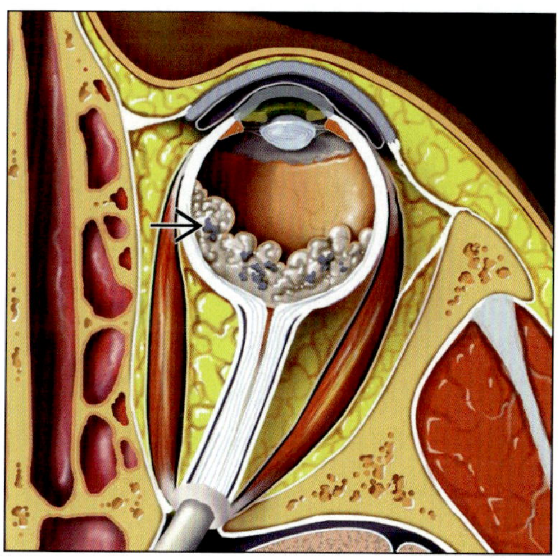

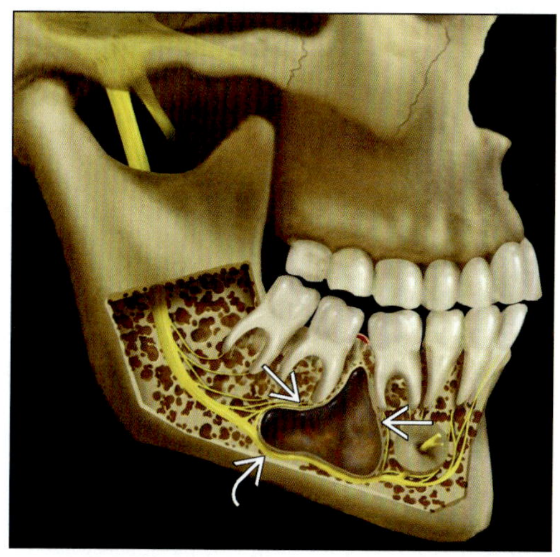

(Left) *Axial graphic shows retinoblastoma with lobulated tumor extending through the limiting membrane into the vitreous. Punctate calcifications → are characteristic. Hereditary retinoblastoma patients may develop carcinoma of the nasal cavity.* ***(Right)*** *Lateral graphic of the mandible (buccal cortex removed) illustrates features of a classic keratocytic odontogenic tumor →, splaying roots of the 1st and 2nd molar teeth, displacing the inferior alveolar nerve →.*

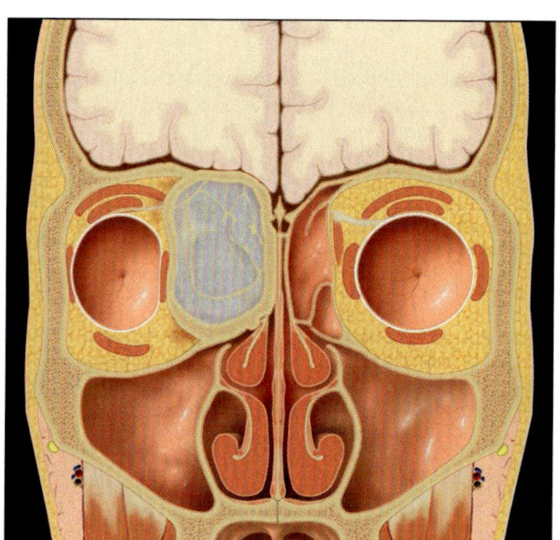

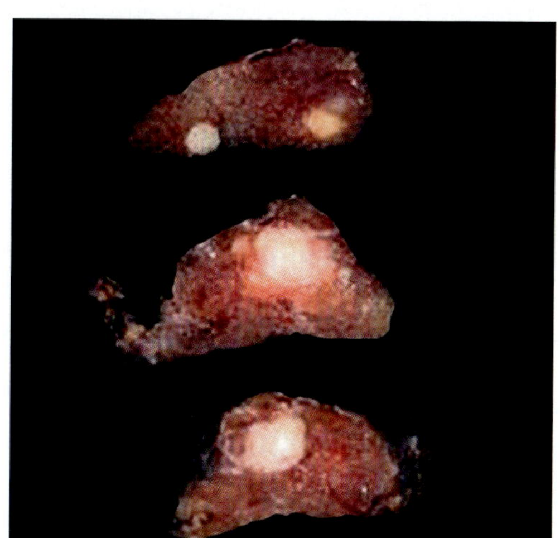

(Left) *Nonossifying fibroma shows a large, well-demarcated maxillary mass with mixed calcification and fibrosis. Note that the mass obstructs 1 side of the nose and compresses the eye in a patient with hyperparathyroidism-jaw tumor syndrome.* ***(Right)*** *Multiple thyroid tumors in a patient with familial adenomatous polyposis show white firm nodules in both thyroid lobes. The patient also had a juvenile nasopharyngeal angiofibroma.*

SALIVARY GLANDS

Familial Cancer Syndromes With Salivary Gland Neoplasms

Syndrome	Gene (Locus)	Inheritance	Salivary Gland Tumor	Other Manifestations
BSS and FC	*CYLD* (16q12-q13)	AD	Basal cell adenoma, membranous type[1]	Dermal cylindroma, trichoepithelioma, and eccrine spiradenoma
VHL	*VHL* (3p25-p26)	AD	Mucoepidermoid carcinoma[2]	Retinal and central nervous system hemangioblastoma; pheochromocytoma; renal cysts and renal cell carcinoma; pancreatic cysts, cystadenoma, carcinoma, and islet cell tumor; hepatic cysts; papillary cystadenoma of epididymis (men) and broad ligament (women); FATWO; endolymphatic sac tumor
AT	*ATM* (11q22.3)	AR	Mucoepidermoid carcinoma and acinic cell carcinoma[3]	Cerebellar ataxia-telangiectasia; hematolymphoid malignancies (B-cell lymphoma, ALL, chronic lymphocytic leukemia); gastric cancer (associated with IgA-deficient men); medulloblastoma; basal cell carcinoma; glioma; uterine cancer; ovarian dysgerminoma; heterozygotes show increased risk for breast cancer in younger women, colorectal cancer, gastric cancer, and T-cell ALL
RB	*RB1* (13q14)	AD	Mucoepidermoid carcinoma[4]	Osteosarcoma; pinealoblastoma; melanoma, nasal cavity cancers; leiomyosarcoma; fibrosarcoma; chondrosarcoma; rhabdomyosarcoma; Ewing sarcoma; leukemia and lymphoma; malignant phyllodes tumor; some tumors may be due in part to radiation therapy for retinoblastoma

AD: Autosomal dominant; ALL: Acute lymphocytic leukemia; AR: Autosomal recessive; AT: Ataxia-telangiectasia; BSS: Brooke-Spiegler syndrome; FATWO: Female adnexal tumor of probable Wolffian origin; FC: Familial cylindromatosis; RB: Retinoblastoma; VHL: von Hippel-Lindau syndrome. [1]Strong etiologic association of membranous type of basal cell adenoma with BSS and FC based on multiple reports. [2]Etiologic association with VHL disease is unclear; single case from authors' institution. [3]Etiologic association with AT is unclear; 2 case reports in literature. [4]Etiologic association with RB is unclear; 1 case report in literature.

Case Reports of Salivary Gland Neoplasms With Familial Clustering

Reference	Affected Family Members (Age in Years at Diagnosis)	Comment
Pleomorphic Adenoma		
Ahn MS et al (1999)	Sister (51), sister (age N/A)	Sister (51) with bilateral tumors; t(3;12)(p21;q15) identified in 1 of these tumors, presumably involving *HMGA2* gene on 12q15
Klausner RD and Handler SD (1993)	Brother (11), sister (15)	
Hayter JP and Robertson JM (1990)	Brother (27), brother (29)	
Cameron JM (1959)	Father (51), son (21), daughter (21)	
Warthin Tumor		
Gallego et al (2010)	Twin brothers (45, 47)	
Russo et al (1999)	Mother (73), son (51)	
Talmi et al (1994)	3 brothers (ages N/A)	
Noyek et al (1980)	Mother (76), son (57)	
Skerlavay et al (1976)	Brother (69), brother (65)	
Acinic Cell Carcinoma		
Delides et al (2005)	Father (89), son (64), daughter (27)	Son (64) with bilateral acinic cell carcinoma; other conditions in family include pituitary adenoma, oncocytic adenoma of parotid, Warthin tumor
Depowski et al (1999)	Father (35), daughter (16)	
Mucoepidermoid Carcinoma		
Newman et al (1981)	Brother (33), sister (32)	Brother (33) with moderately differentiated adenocarcinoma of submandibular gland; sister (32) with mucoepidermoid carcinoma
Low-Grade Neuroendocrine Carcinoma		
Michaels et al (1999)	Mother (67), sister (46), brother (34), sister (43), brother (33)	Tumors in siblings were composed primarily of cells with neuroendocrine differentiation, admixed with ductal and myoepithelial cells; histology of mother's tumor not reported; other conditions in family include vestibular schwannoma, sensorineural hearing loss, amelogenesis imperfecta
Lymphoepithelial Carcinoma		
Autio-Harmainen et al (1988)	Mother (64), daughter (43)	Other conditions in family include trichoepitheliomas, eccrine spiradenomas, cylindromas
Merrick et al (1986)	**Family 1:** Sister (31), sister (34), sister (50); **family 2:** Sister (37), sister (44)	Likely EBV related, but suspect additional genetic predisposition; other conditions in family include uterine cervical cancer, nasopharyngeal carcinoma, malignant neck mass (NOS) in maternal grandfather

EBV: Epstein-Barr virus; N/A: Not available. Case reports of salivary gland neoplasms showing familial clustering (without a known germline mutation) are summarized in this table.

SALIVARY GLANDS

Molecular Changes Described in Salivary Gland Tumors

Tumor	Locus	Implicated Gene(s)
Pleomorphic adenoma	8q12 translocations [t(3;8)p21;q12 is most common]	Fusion transcripts involving *PLAG1*
Carcinoma ex pleomorphic adenoma	12q14-15 translocations [t(9;12)(p12-22;q13-15) is most common]	Fusion transcripts involving *HMGA2* (also known as *HMGIC*)
Mammary analogue secretory carcinoma	t(12;15)(p13;q25)	*ETV6-NTRK3* fusion
Mucoepidermoid carcinoma	t(11;19)(q21;p13) and losses of 2q, 5p, 12p, 16p	*MECT1-MAML2* fusion (*MECT1* is also known as *CRTC1*, *TORC1*, and *WAMTP1*)
Warthin tumor	Rare cases with t(11;19) reported, but larger series have not reproduced this finding	
Adenoid cystic carcinoma	t(6;9)(q22-23;p23-24); LOH at 6q23-q25; and loss of 12q12-q13	*MYB-NFIB* fusion
Acinic cell carcinoma	Deletions of 6q; loss of Y; trisomy 8; and LOH at 4p, 5q, 6p, 17p	
Polymorphous low-grade adenocarcinoma	12q12-q13, 12q22, or 12p12.3 translocations	
Salivary duct carcinoma	LOH at 9p21, 6q, 17p, 17q	

LOH: Loss of heterozygosity. This table summarizes cytogenetic changes that have been observed in salivary gland neoplasms. Most of these cases represent somatic mutations in sporadic salivary gland tumors and are included here for reference.

Microscopic Features

(Left) *This basal cell adenoma, membranous type, was resected from the parotid gland of a patient with multiple dermal cylindromas. The tumor has multinodular architecture and is encased by dense fibrous stroma.* ***(Right)*** *Another area of the basal cell adenoma shows dense collagen bands and multiple tumor nodules. Within the nodules are nests of basaloid cells that are surrounded by eosinophilic hyaline material and arranged in a jigsaw puzzle-like pattern.*

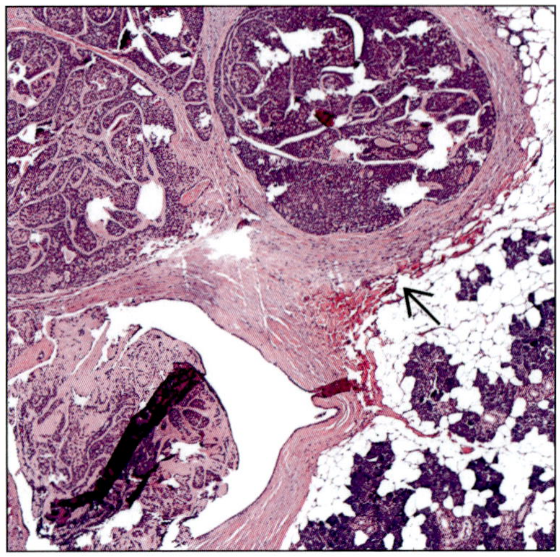

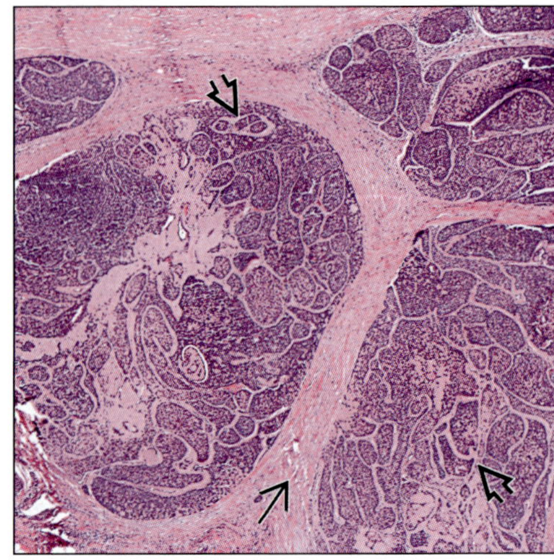

(Left) *On higher magnification, this membranous-type basal cell adenoma shows drop-like eosinophilic hyaline material of variable sizes and shapes in addition to the rim of basement membrane-like material separating the nests of basaloid cells.* ***(Right)*** *The basaloid cells in the centers of the nests are larger with fine chromatin; those at the periphery appear smaller with hyperchromatic nuclei. Peripheral palisading of the tumor cells is seen.*

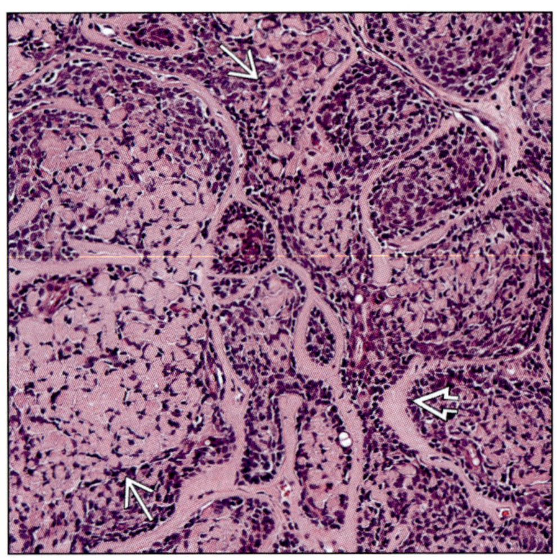

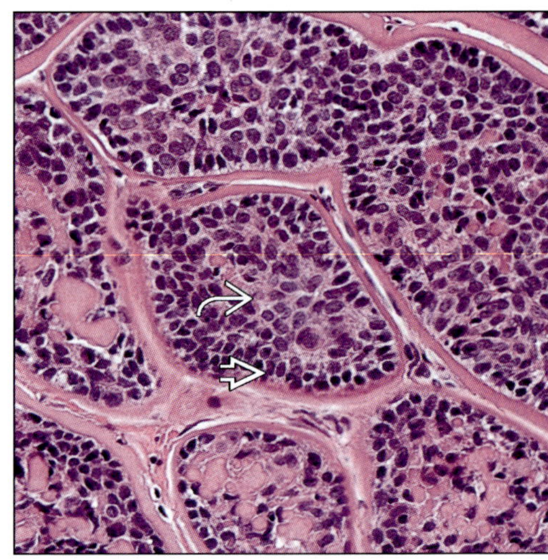

(Left) *This Romanowsky-stained, air-dried smear from a fine-needle aspiration of basal cell adenoma shows a sheet of medium-sized basaloid cells with a peripheral rim of hyaline material.* ***(Right)*** *Other areas of the smear showed multiple droplets of magenta-colored extracellular matrix material surrounded by basaloid tumor cells.*

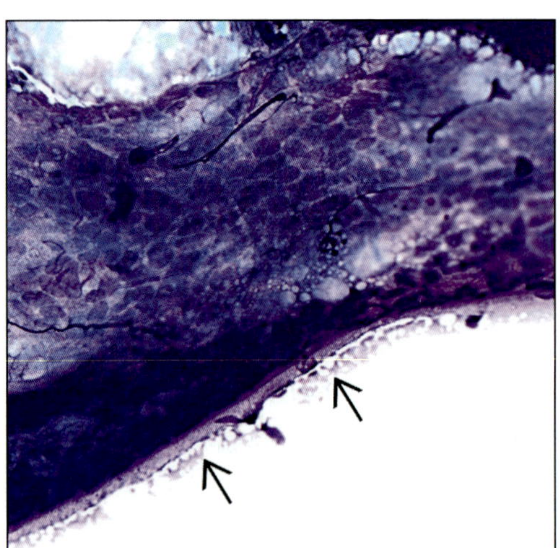

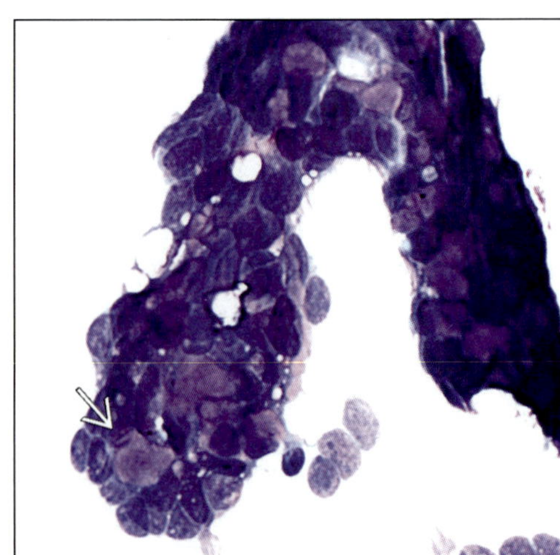

Microscopic Features

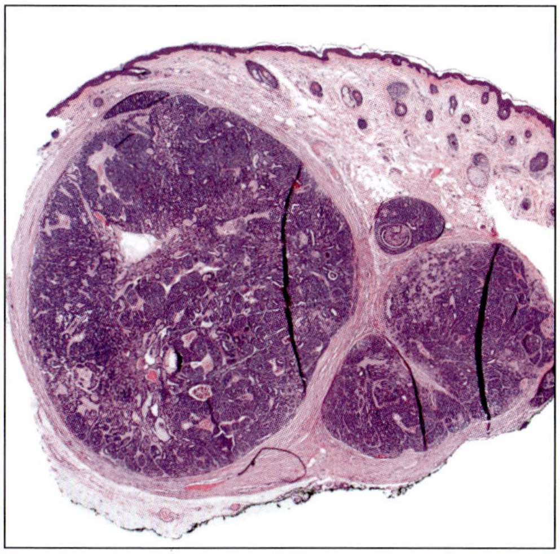

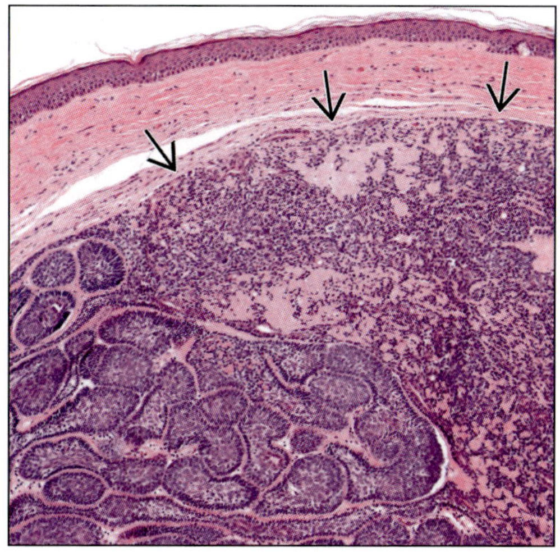

(Left) *In addition to basal cell adenoma in the parotid gland, this patient had multiple cutaneous cylindromas. This low-power view shows multiple nodules of basaloid cells in the dermis.* ***(Right)*** *This cylindroma from the same patient shows a typical jigsaw puzzle-like pattern (lower left) in addition to a more diffuse pattern → that overlaps with eccrine spiradenoma.*

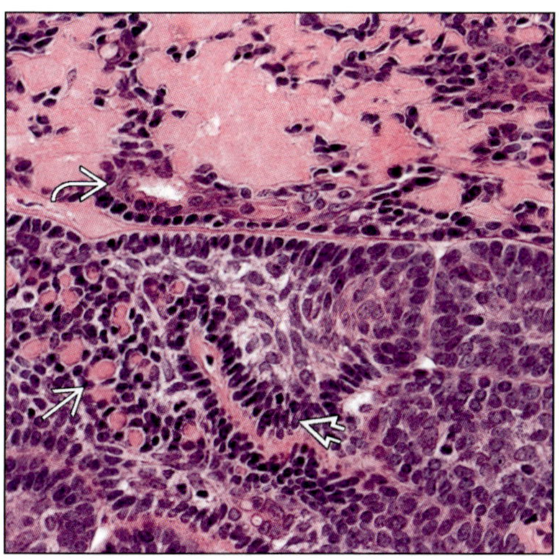

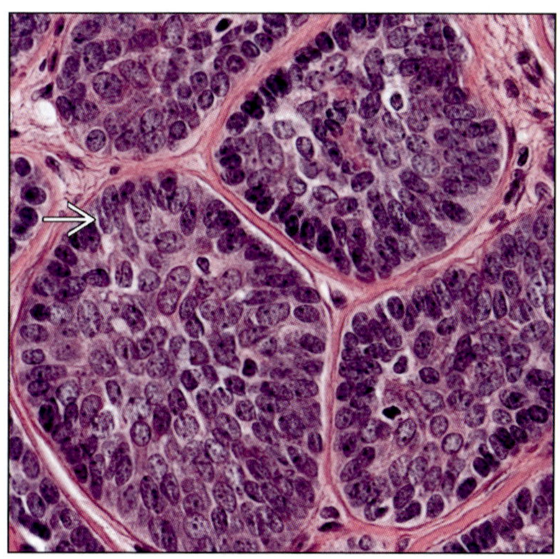

(Left) *Higher magnification highlights the hyaline droplets → and peripheral palisading of the basaloid cells →. The upper portion of the tumor shows cords of basaloid cells and increased stromal hyalinization. A sweat duct lumen is present →.* ***(Right)*** *The basaloid cytology and peripheral palisading → of the tumor cells are highlighted. The tumor nests are separated by hyaline material and appear identical to the membranous-type basal cell adenoma in the patient's parotid.*

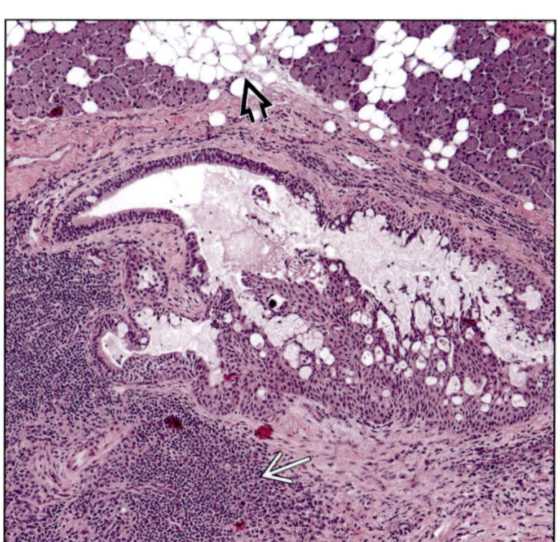

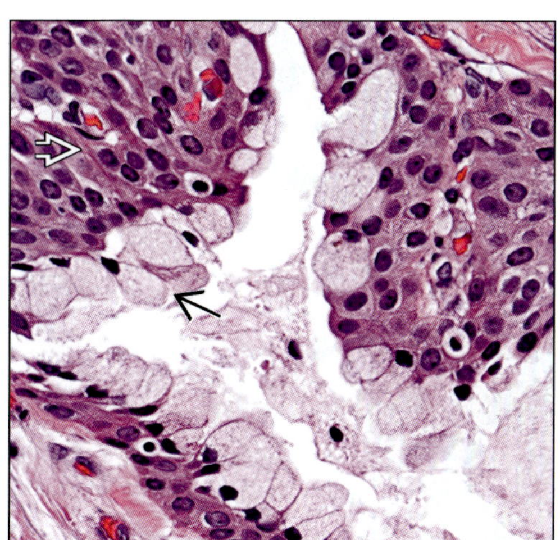

(Left) *This low-grade mucoepidermoid carcinoma was resected from the parotid gland of a patient with von Hippel-Lindau disease. On low magnification, a cystic space lined by epidermoid and mucous cells is present. A prominent lymphoid infiltrate is present →. Parotid parenchyma is present at the top of the image →.* ***(Right)*** *Multiple mucocytes → are supported by sheets of epidermoid/intermediate cells → with a transitional or squamous metaplastic appearance.*

Endocrine

ADRENAL CORTEX

Clinical Settings Associated With Cytomegalic Cells

Focal Cytomegalic Cells (Variably Present)	Diffusely Scattered Cytomegalic Cells
Extensive hemolysis	Beckwith-Wiedemann syndrome
Rhesus isoimmunization	X-linked congenital adrenal hypoplasia
Congenital lupus erythematosus	
Erythropoietic purpura	
Nonimmune hydrops	
Trisomy 13 and 18	
Diaphragmatic hernia	
Ectopic adrenal tissue	
Intrauterine viral infections	

Differential Diagnosis of Adrenal Cortical Adenoma

Neoplasm	Inhibin	Melan-A	Chromogranin	Synaptophysin	Hep-Par1	CD10
Adrenal cortical adenoma	Positive	Positive	Negative	Positive (57%)	Negative	Negative
Pheochromocytoma	Negative	Negative	Positive	Positive	Negative	Negative
Hepatocellular carcinoma	Negative	Negative	Negative	Negative	Positive	Positive (61%)
Renal cell carcinoma	Negative	Negative	Negative	Negative	Negative	Positive

Immunohistochemistry of Adrenal Cortical Adenomas

Antibody	Reactivity	Staining Pattern	Comment
Inhibin	Positive	Cell membrane and cytoplasm	
Mart-1	Positive	Cytoplasmic	
Melan-A103	Positive	Cytoplasmic	
Chromogranin-A	Negative		Helps to differentiate from pheochromocytoma
CK7	Negative		Helps to differentiate from other epithelial tumors
CK20	Negative		Helps to differentiate from other epithelial tumors
AE1/AE3	Negative		Helps to differentiate from other epithelial tumors
EMA	Negative		Helps to differentiate from other epithelial tumors
CD10	Negative		Helps to differentiate from renal cell carcinoma
Hep-Par1	Negative		Helps to differentiate from hepatocellular carcinoma
HMFG	Negative		
RCC	Negative		Helps to differentiate from renal cell carcinoma
HMB-45	Negative		

Clinical Features Suggesting Familial Adrenal Cortical Carcinoma

Personal History	Family History
Metachronous ACC	Family history of ACC
Bilateral ACC	Family history of known hereditary cancer susceptibility syndromes
Multiple primary tumors in other organs	Unusually high number of family members affected with cancer
Other rare cancers	Family history of other rare cancers
ACC diagnosed in childhood	
Development of ACC from precursor lesion	
Other endocrine diseases	
Cutaneous lesions associated with hereditary cancer susceptibility	
Other congenital defects	

ACC: Adrenal cortical carcinoma.

ADRENAL CORTEX

Criteria for Differentiation Between Adenoma and Carcinoma

Criteria	Adenoma	Carcinoma
Hormone production	Often functional	Usually nonfunctional
Gross	Weight < 50 g	Weight > 100 g
Tumor gross color	Variable	Variable; does not differentiate
Circumscription	Well circumscribed	Invasive
Hemorrhage	Absent	Frequent
Necrosis	Absent	Frequent
Capsular invasion	Absent	Usually present
Invasion into adjacent tissues	Absent	Usually present
Intratumoral fibrosis	May be present	May be present
Myxomatous degeneration	May be present	May be present
Cytology	May have cytologic atypia	Cytologic atypia present
Histology	Atypia may be present	Atypia present
Necrosis	Necrosis absent	Present; confluent necrosis
Mitosis	Rare	> 5/50 HPF
Venous invasion	Absent	Present

Adrenal Cortical Tumor as Part of Inherited Tumor Syndromes

Syndrome	Gene	Chromosomal Location	Adrenal Pathology	% Adrenal Involvement
Li-Fraumeni	*TP53*	17p13	ACC	6.5-9.9%
Beckwith-Wiedemann	*CDKN1C/NSD1*	11p15.5	ACA, ACC, NH	1.0%
MEN1	*MEN1*	11q13	ACA, ACC	45-55%
Carney complex	*PRKAR1A*	2p16	PPNAD, ACA	~ 100%
McCune-Albright	*GNAS1*	20q13.2	NH, ACA	
Congenital adrenal hyperplasia	*CYP21*	6p21.3	NH, ACA, ACC	
NF1	*NF1*	17	ACC	
FAP	*APC*	5q21-22	ACA, functional or nonfunctional; ACC	7.4-13%
HNPCC	*MLH1, MSH2, MSH6, PMS2*	Multiple	ACC	

ACA: Adrenal cortical adenoma; ACC: Adrenal cortical carcinoma; FAP: Familial adenomatous polyposis; HNPCC: Hereditary nonpolyposis colon cancer; MEN1: Multiple endocrine neoplasia type 1; NF1: Neurofibromatosis type 1; NH: Nodular hyperplasia; PPNAD: Primary pigmented nodular adrenal disease.

Pathology Findings and Syndromes Involving Adrenal Cortex

Adrenal Pathology	Syndrome Associated With Pathology
Adrenal cortical adenoma	MEN1, McCune-Albright Syndrome, Beckwith-Wiedemann syndrome, congenital adrenal hyperplasia, Carney complex
Adrenal cortical carcinoma	MEN1, Beckwith-Wiedemann syndrome, Li-Fraumeni syndrome
Primary pigmented adrenal cortical disease	Carney complex
Macronodular hyperplasia	MEN1, McCune-Albright syndrome, Beckwith-Wiedemann syndrome, congenital adrenal hyperplasia

MEN1: Multiple endocrine neoplasia 1.

Gross Features of Adrenal Cortical Lesions

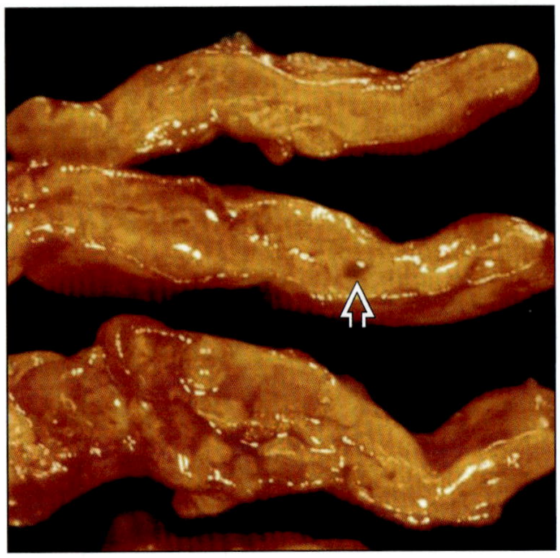

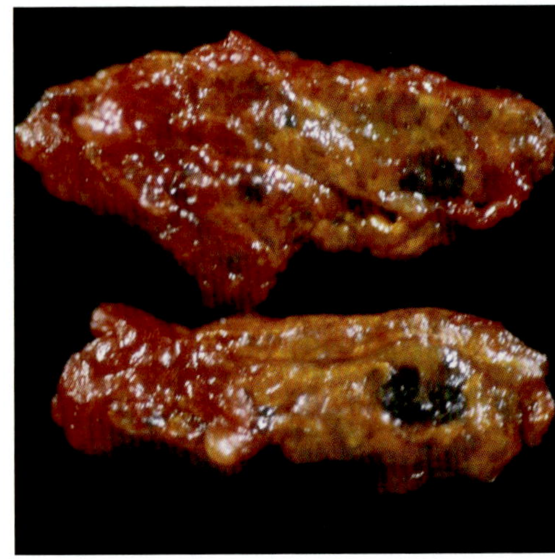

(Left) *Sections of the adrenal gland with primary pigmented adrenal nodular disease in a patient with Carney complex may appear almost unremarkable, with the exception of rare pigmented micronodules ⇨. The outer surface may have a micronodular contour.* ***(Right)*** *Sections of the adrenal gland are studded with pigmented micronodules and occasional macronodules that are due to confluence of smaller nodules. The outer surface has an irregular micronodular contour.*

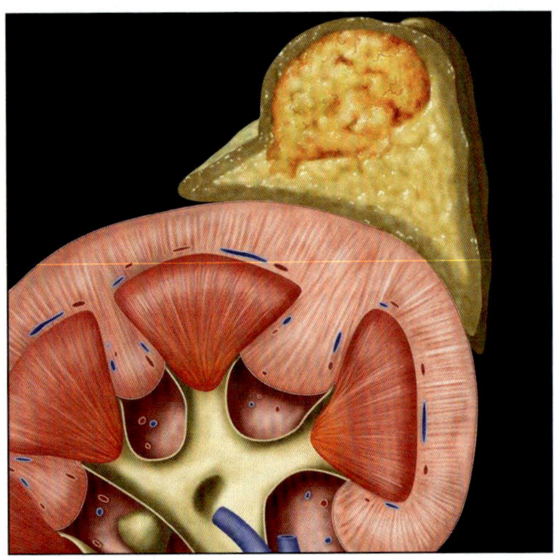

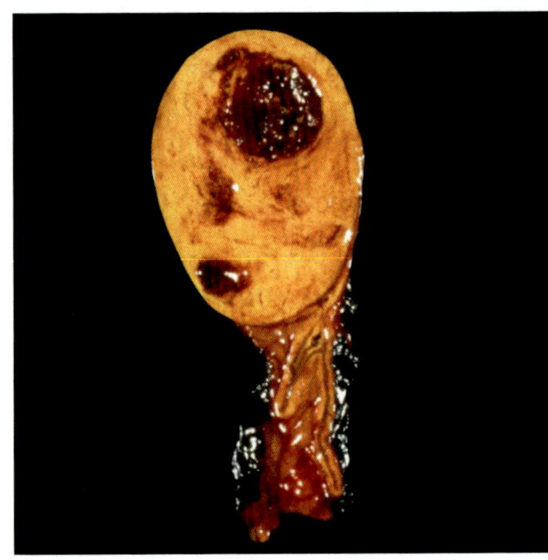

(Left) *This coronal graphic demonstrates an adrenal cortical adenoma. The tumor is < 5 cm in greatest dimension, without invasion of kidney or other adjacent organs.* ***(Right)*** *Cross section of a cortisol-secreting adrenal cortical adenoma shows the typical round, well-circumscribed golden-yellow appearance. This tumor also has an area of dark discoloration that can be attributed to an old hemorrhage.*

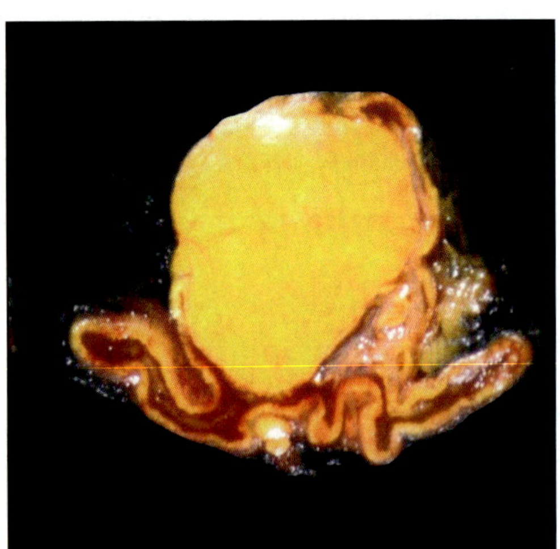

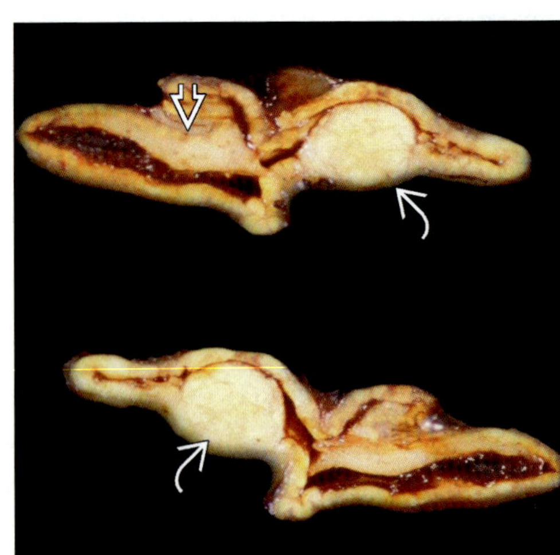

(Left) *A cross section through an adrenal mass shows the classic "canary yellow" color of an aldosterone-producing adenoma. Another characteristic of these tumors is the pushing borders.* ***(Right)*** *This cross section shows classical findings in aldosterone-producing tumors. A round, small, and well-circumscribed mass ➩ has pushing borders. Also seen is hyperplasia of the zona glomerulosa ⇨ located at the nontumoral adrenal gland, frequently present in aldosterone-secreting adenomas.*

Gross Features of Adrenal Tumors

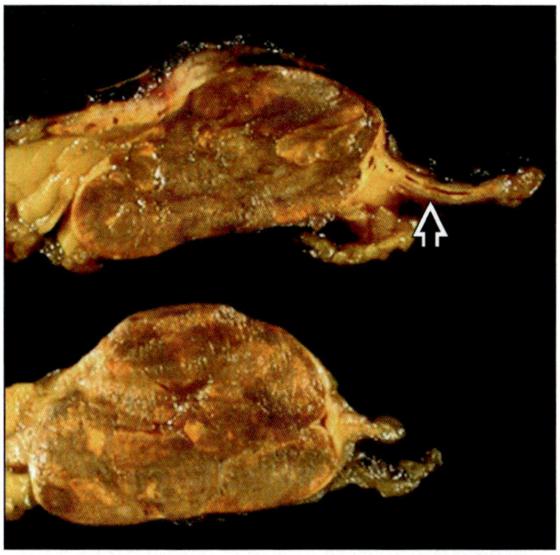

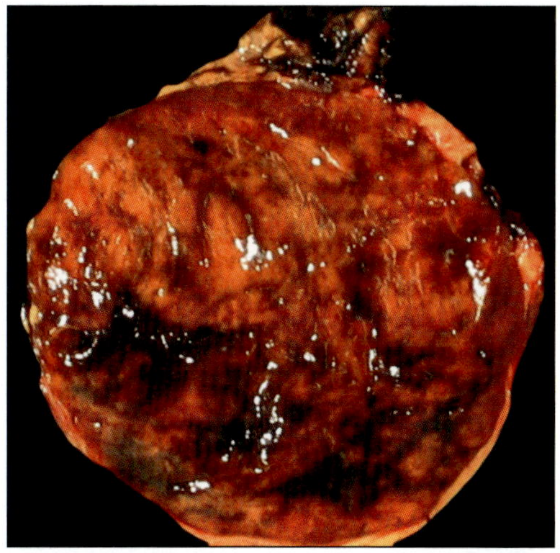

(Left) *This well-circumscribed adrenal cortical adenoma demonstrates a mottled appearance with areas of dark discoloration due to the compact eosinophilic cytoplasm of the tumor cells by lipid depletion and increased lipofuscin pigment. Note the marked atrophy of the adjacent adrenal cortex.* ***(Right)*** *Adrenal cortical adenoma in Cushing syndrome has a yellow-orange cut surface and mottled zones of dark pigmentation due to lipofuscin accumulation and depletion of lipid.*

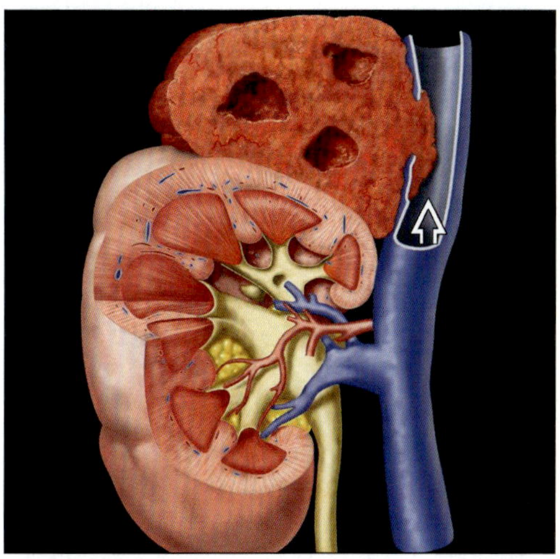

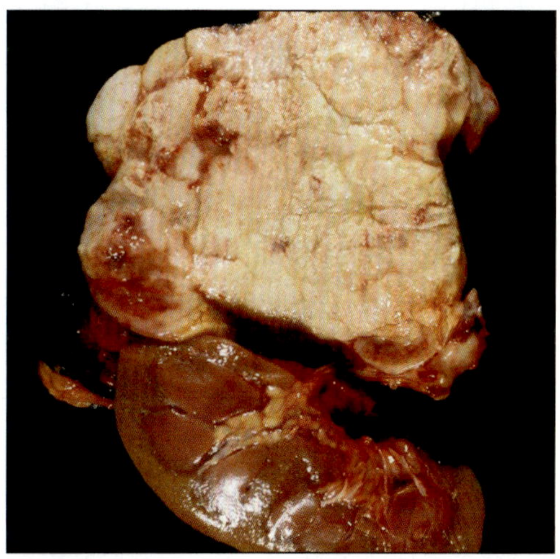

(Left) *Adrenal cortical carcinomas tend to be large, usually > 5 cm with irregular and invasive borders, and are usually unilateral. This graphic shows direct extension into the vena cava.* ***(Right)*** *Adrenal cortical carcinoma tends to appear grossly as a large solid mass in the suprarenal region. Focal areas of necrosis and hemorrhage are present.*

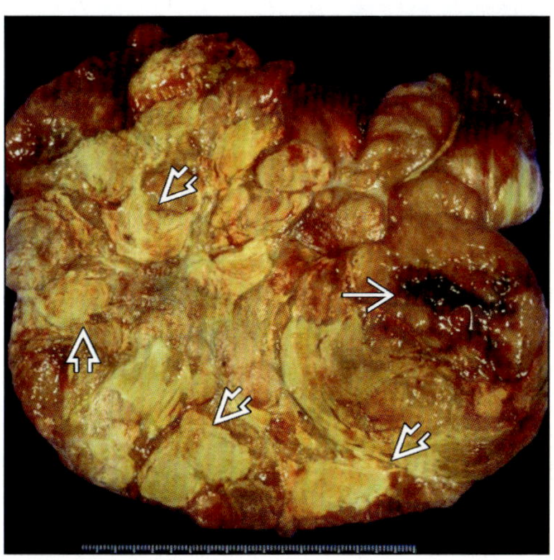

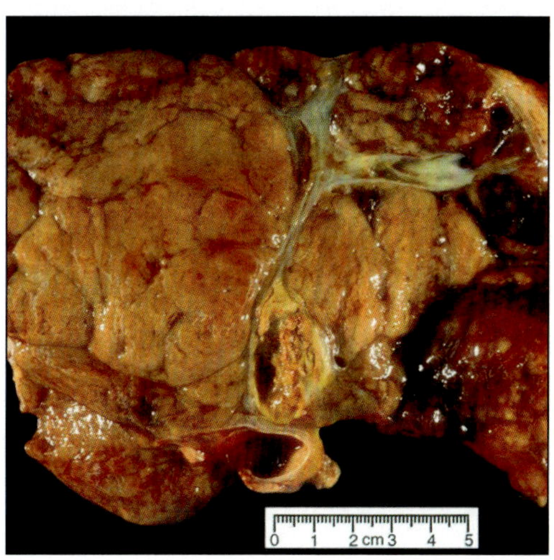

(Left) *This pediatric adrenal cortical carcinoma has a yellow, pink to light-brown variegated cut surface with extensive areas of necrosis, degenerative changes, and hemorrhagic areas.* ***(Right)*** *This adrenal cortical carcinoma presented as an irregular shaped, bulky, unilateral mass and has a light-brown variegated cut surface. Note also extensive necrosis, degenerative changes, hemorrhage, and calcification.*

ADRENAL MEDULLA

Clinical and Genetic Features of Familial Pheochromocytoma and Paraganglioma

Syndrome	Gene	Tumors in Paraganglia	Associated Neoplasms	Relative Frequency of PCC/PGL (%)
Familial PGL 1	*SDHD*	Multiple H&N PGL	Thyroid	5-6
Familial PGL 2	*SDHAF2*	Multiple H&N PGL	Unknown	< 1
Familial PGL 3	*SDHC*	Multiple PGL	Unknown	1
Familial PGL 4	*SDHB*	Single PGL	Renal cell carcinoma	6-8
Familial *SDHA*-related	*SDHA*	Predominant extraadrenal PGL	GIST	Rare
Carney-Stratakis syndrome	*SDHB, SDHC, SDHD*	PGL	GIST	Rare
MEN2	*RET*	Predominant adrenal Pheo	Medullary thyroid carcinoma, parathyroid adenoma or hyperplasia	5-6
von Hippel-Lindau	*VHL*	Predominant adrenal Pheo	Renal cell carcinoma, hemangioblastomas	9-12
Neurofibromatosis type 1	*NF1*	Predominant adrenal Pheo	Neurofibroma, glioma, other tumors	1-2
Familial Pheo 2q	*TMEM127*	Predominant adrenal Pheo	Unknown	1.7-2
Familial *MAX*-related	*MAX*	Predominant adrenal Pheo	Unknown	1.2
Familial *KIF1B*-related	*KIF1B*	Predominant adrenal Pheo	Neuroblastoma, medulloblastoma	Rare
Familial *PHD2*-related	*PHD2*	Unknown	Erythrocytosis	Rare

GIST: Gastrointestinal stromal tumor; H&N: Head and neck; PGL: Paraganglioma; Pheo: Pheochromocytoma.

Adrenal Medullary Hyperplasia and Pheochromocytoma

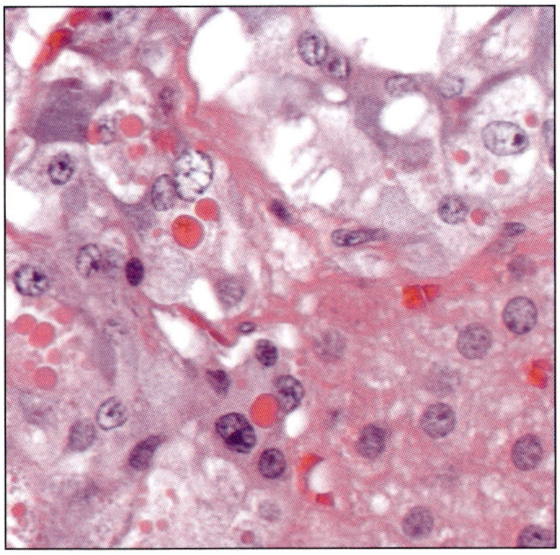

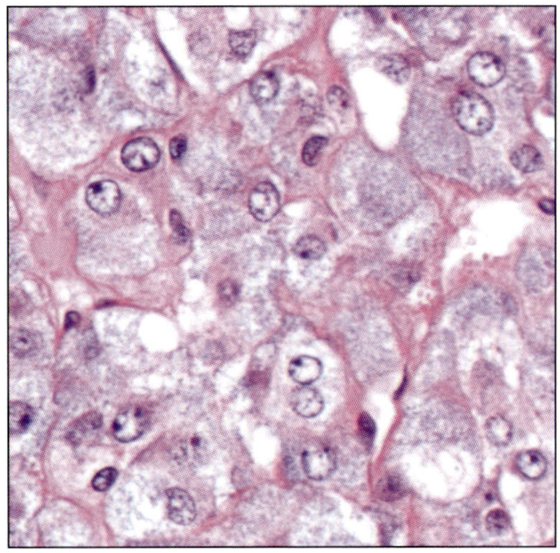

(Left) *Adrenal medullary hyperplasia in a patient with MEN2 syndrome shows medullary cells within the adrenal cortex. The presence of hyaline granules is usually present in MEN2.* ***(Right)*** *Bilateral adrenal medullary hyperplasia is a precursor of pheochromocytomas and was initially described in patients with MEN2A and MEN2B syndromes. This figure shows medullary adrenal hyperplasia composed of large cells with basophilic granular cytoplasm.*

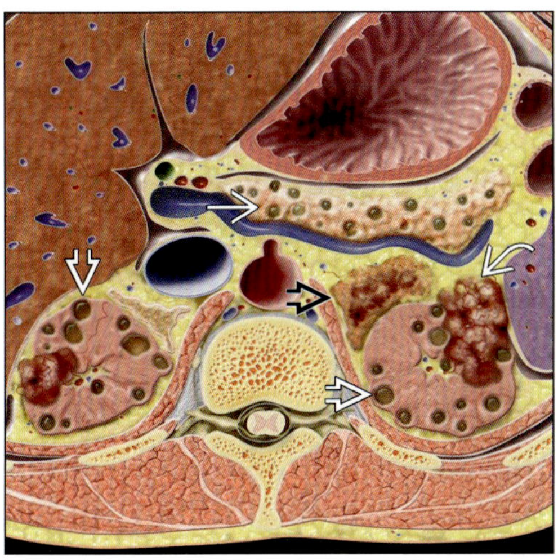

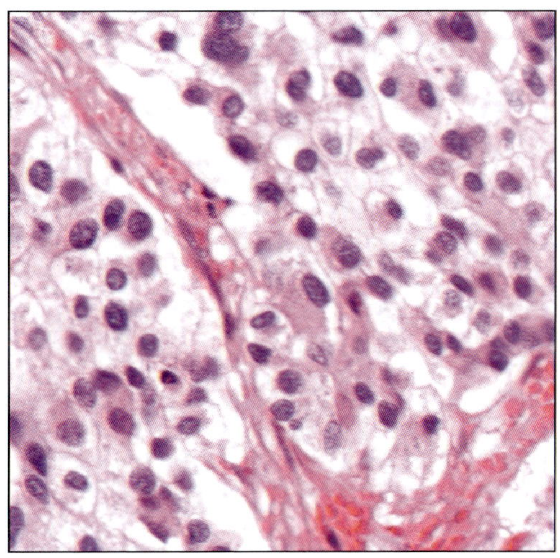

(Left) *Abdominal lesions in von Hippel-Lindau are varied and include bilateral renal cysts ➔, renal tumors, particularly renal cell carcinoma ➔, pancreatic cysts ➔, and pheochromocytoma ➔.* ***(Right)*** *This pheochromocytoma has the characteristic alveolar pattern (zellballen) with variably sized nests of tumor cells surrounded by thin-walled vessels and thin bands of fibrous tissue.*

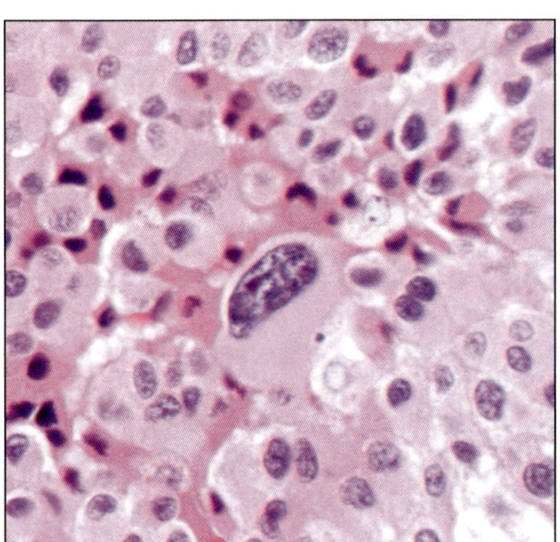

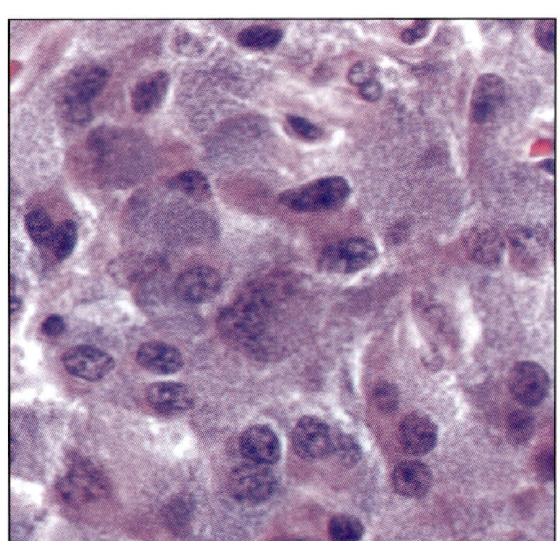

(Left) *Some pheochromocytomas lack the organoid pattern and instead may show a diffuse growth pattern composed of small cells with ample eosinophilic cytoplasm with occasional bizarre cells.* ***(Right)*** *Some pheochromocytomas show a mosaic-like pattern of often large cells with granular basophilic cytoplasm admixed with cells that have amphophilic to slightly eosinophilic cytoplasm.*

PANCREAS

Immunohistochemistry

Antibody	Reactivity	Staining Pattern	Comments
Synaptophysin	Positive	Cell membrane & cytoplasm	Nearly every tumor cell is positive; SPT and ACC may be focally positive
PGP9.5	Positive	Cytoplasmic	Nearly every tumor cell is positive
NSE	Positive	Cytoplasmic	Very low specificity
CD56	Positive	Cell membrane & cytoplasm	Usually accentuated on cell membrane
Chromogranin-A	Positive	Cytoplasmic	Granular reactivity, a reflection of neurosecretory granules; less staining in less granulated tumors; SPT negative; ACC may be focally positive
E-cadherin	Positive	Cell membrane	SPT negative; ACC positive
CK-PAN	Positive	Cytoplasmic	Nearly all tumors
CK8/18/CAM5.2	Positive	Cytoplasmic	Most tumor cells
CK19	Positive	Cytoplasmic	Expression correlated with outcome
PRP	Positive	Nuclear	If progesterone receptor positivity is lost, associated with worse prognosis
NFP	Positive	Cytoplasmic	Present in a few tumor cells
Trypsin	Negative		SPT negative; ACC positive
β-catenin	Negative		SPT positive; ACC negative

ACC: Acinar cell carcinoma; SPT: Solid pseudopapillary tumor.

Criteria for the Clinicopathological Classification of Tumors of the Endocrine Pancreas

WHO Tumor Type	Criteria for Clinicopathological Classification
Well-differentiated endocrine tumor: Benign behavior	Confined to pancreas; < 2.0 cm in diameter; < 2 mitoses/10 HPF, < 2% Ki-67 proliferative index; no lymphovascular invasion; no perineural invasion
Well-differentiated endocrine tumor: Uncertain behavior	Confined to pancreas and 1 or more of the following features: > 2.0 cm in diameter; 2-10 mitoses/10 HPF, > 2% Ki-67 proliferative index; lymphovascular invasion, perineural invasion
Well-differentiated endocrine carcinoma	Gross local invasion &/or metastases; low-grade malignant
Poorly differentiated endocrine carcinoma (small cell carcinoma)	High-grade malignant; > 10 mitoses/10 HPF
Mixed endocrine-exocrine carcinoma	Malignant mixed neoplasm in which endocrine and exocrine cells are intimally admixed (each component comprises at least 1/3 of tumor)

Adapted from Heitz PU et al: Pancreatic endocrine tumours. In DeLellis RA et al: World Health Organization Classification of Tumors. Pathology and Genetics of Tumors of Endocrine Organs. Lyon: IARC Press. 177-82, 2004.

Comparison of Different Features of Endocrine Pancreatic Tumors and Their Differential Diagnoses

Clinical Features	Solid Pseudopapillary Neoplasm	Pancreatic Endocrine Neoplasm	Acinar Cell Carcinoma	Pancreatoblastoma
Age	Young adults	50-70 years; younger in MEN1	50-60 years	Children < 10 years
Gender	Female	Equal gender distribution	Slight male predominance	Slight male predominance
Gross	Circumscribed; variegated, hemorrhagic, solid, and cystic	Circumscribed, usually solid	Circumscribed, soft with abundant hemorrhage	Circumscribed and lobulated, soft and fleshy
Microscopic	Pseudopapillae, necrosis, polygonal epithelial cells with eosinophilic to clear cytoplasm, uniform, round to oval nuclei with grooves, intracytoplasmic and extracytoplasmic hyaline globules	Trabecular, nested pattern; densely hyalinized stroma; cells are polygonal with amphophilic cytoplasm; round to oval, uniform in size and shape of nuclei; classic coarsely stippled salt-and-pepper chromatin; inconspicuous nucleoli	Tumor is arranged in cellular lobules separated by bands of collagenized stroma; acinar formation; granular eosinophilic cytoplasm; uniform and well-polarized nuclei with basal palisading at interface with stroma	Lighter- and darker-staining cells, reflecting different cell types of pancreatoblastoma; acinar formation and squamoid corpuscles; hypercellular stromal cells
Cytology	Papillary fragments; cytoplasmic vacuoles, nuclear grooves	Cellular, monotonous, small or medium-sized cells; granular chromatin and plasmacytoid morphology	Prominent acinar formation, cells with granular cytoplasm	Primitive stromal elements, squamoid corpuscles
Positive IHC markers	β-catenin, progesterone receptor, CD10, cyclin-D1	Chromogranin, synaptophysin, CD56	Trypsin, chymotrypsin	Markers of acinar, endocrine, and ductal differentiation

Pancreatic Tumor as Part of Inherited Tumor Syndrome

Syndrome	Gene	Pancreatic Pathology
Multiple endocrine neoplasia 1	*MEN1*	Islet cell hyperplasia, nesidioblastosis, and dysplasia; pancreatic endocrine tumors (e.g., Zollinger-Ellison syndrome, insulinoma, glucagonoma, VIPoma); usually associated with nesidioblastosis and microadenomas
von Hippel-Lindau syndrome	*VHL*	Pancreatic cysts and endocrine pancreatic tumors; usually functionally inactive with 30-40% with immunoexpression of somatostatin, glucagon, or insulin; usually not associated with nesidioblastosis or microadenomas; presence of foamy and clear cell changes is characteristic of VHL-associated PET
Neurofibromatosis type 1	*NF1*	Somatostatinoma (in pancreas, duodenum, and periampullary region)
Tuberous sclerosis	*TSC1* and *TSC2*	Benign and malignant pancreatic endocrine tumors, insulinoma

MEN1: Multiple endocrine neoplasia 1; PET: Pancreatic endocrine tumor; VHL: von Hippel-Lindau syndrome.

Genes Involved in Pancreatic Tumorigenesis

Gene	% Sporadic Pancreatic Endocrine Tumor With Mutation
MEN1	30% of sporadic PETs have *MEN1* mutation; found in 55% of gastrin-producing tumors, 50% of VIP-producing tumors, and 7% of insulin-producing tumors
VHL	Not found to be involved in the development of sporadic tumors
NF1	Not found to be involved in the development of sporadic tumors
TSC1 and *TSC2*	Not found to be involved in the development of sporadic tumors

PET: Pancreatic endocrine tumor.

Diagrammatic and Microscopic Features

__(Left)__ This graphic shows the anatomic relationship of the pancreas to the surrounding organs and vessels. A pancreatic endocrine tumor (PET) is shown in relationship to the lymph nodes seen along the upper border of the pancreas. ***(Right)*** *Islet dysplasia refers to slightly enlarged islets that contain neuroendocrine cells arranged in trabeculae that display mild atypia and show loss of the normal spatial cellular distribution and numbers of the 4 cell types. This is usually present in patients with MEN1 and VHL.*

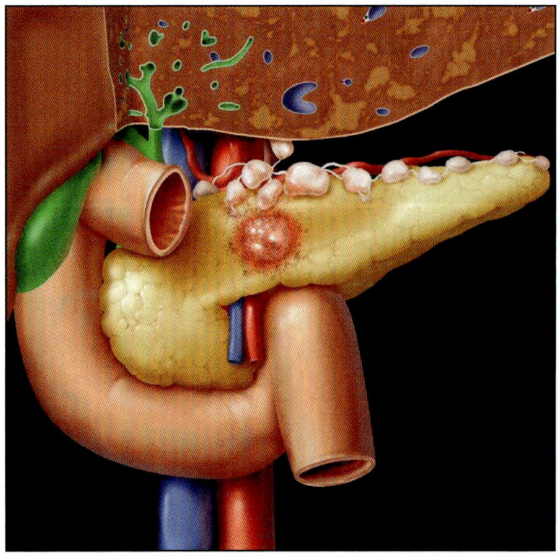

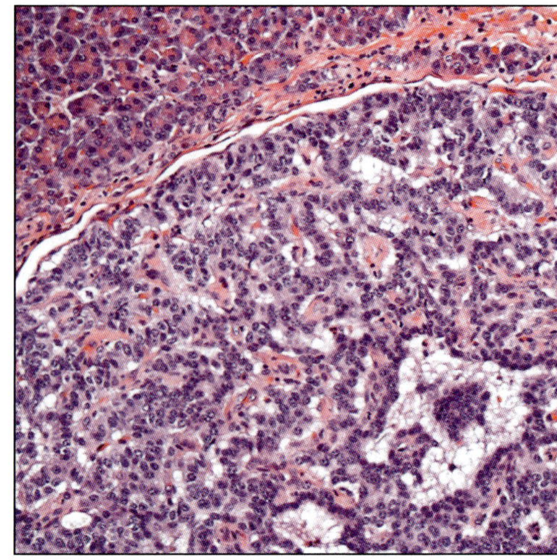

__(Left)__ Two distinct pancreatic endocrine cell proliferations are shown in a case of MEN1. The lesion on the left side of this figure has irregular borders, and the lesion on the right side is well demarcated and larger. ***(Right)*** *The smaller pancreatic endocrine lesion is uniformly positive for glucagon (microadenoma) whereas the larger lesion shows a pattern of distribution of glucagon similar to a normal island, indicating hyperplasia.*

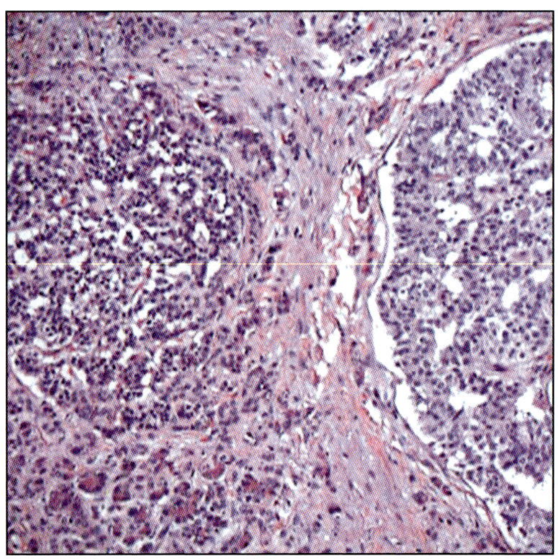

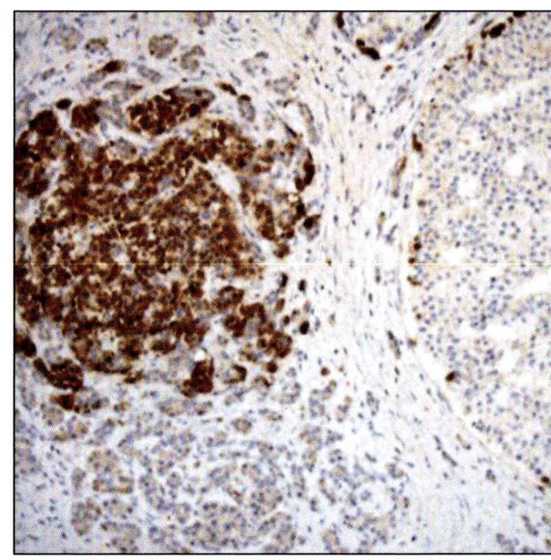

__(Left)__ In the pancreata of patients with MEN1, there are typically multiple small (< 5 mm) neuroendocrine tumors, a finding that has been referred to as microadenomatosis. Note the presence of a proliferation of endocrine cells within the acinar component. ***(Right)*** *Touch imprint from a pancreatic neuroendocrine tumor shows a monotonous population of round cells with eosinophilic cytoplasm and a coarse, "salt and pepper" chromatin.*

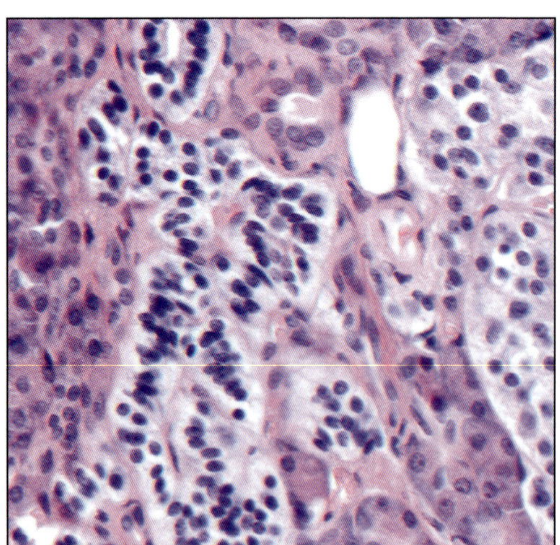

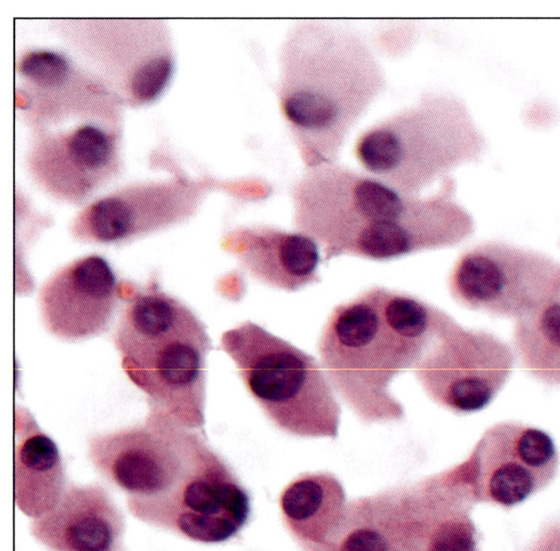

Microscopic Features

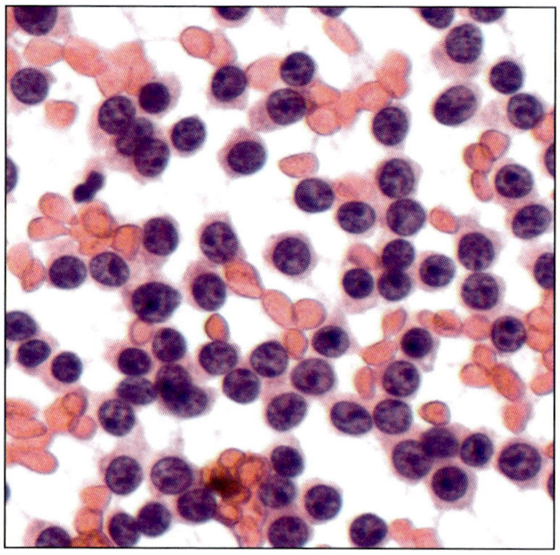

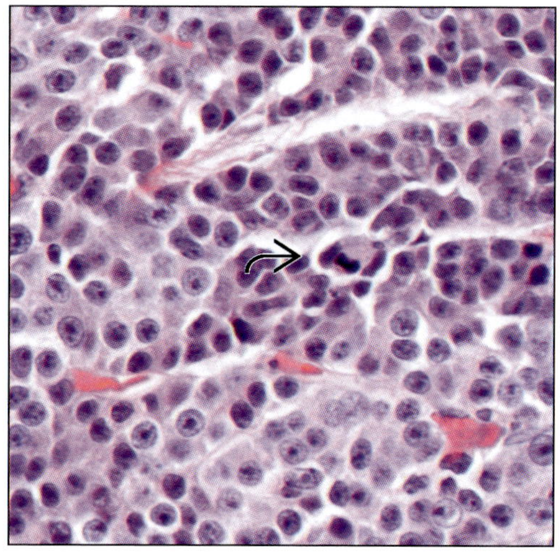

(Left) *The round monotonous nuclei with a coarse chromatin support the diagnosis of a pancreatic endocrine neoplasm. Note the presence of small amounts of cytoplasm.* ***(Right)*** *This pancreatic endocrine tumor in a 17-year-old young man with MEN1 syndrome is a large tumor associated with islet cell hyperplasia and microadenomas. Note the prominent nucleoli and mitosis →.*

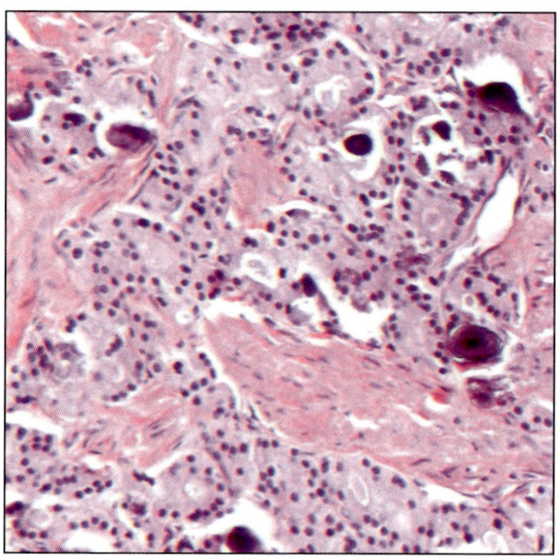

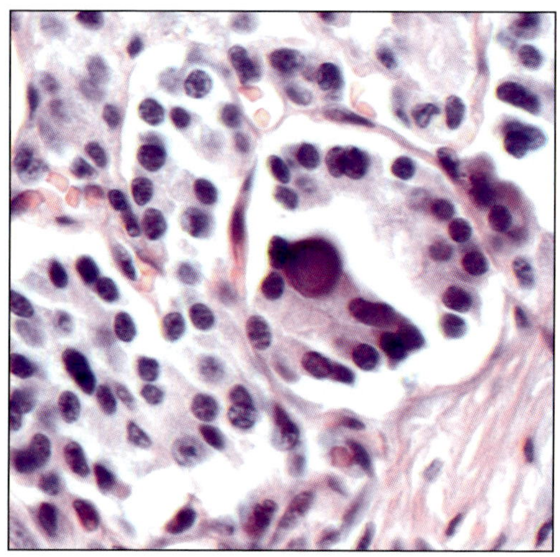

(Left) *This well-differentiated PET with a prominent acinar pattern with multifocal intraluminal calcifications is associated with pancreatic cysts in a patient with von Hippel-Lindau (VHL). These tumors are usually inactive, 30-40% with immunoexpression of somatostatin, glucagon, or insulin.* ***(Right)*** *High-power view shows the characteristic small to medium-sized cells with an eosinophilic, slightly granular cytoplasm. There is focal fibrosis and a psammoma body.*

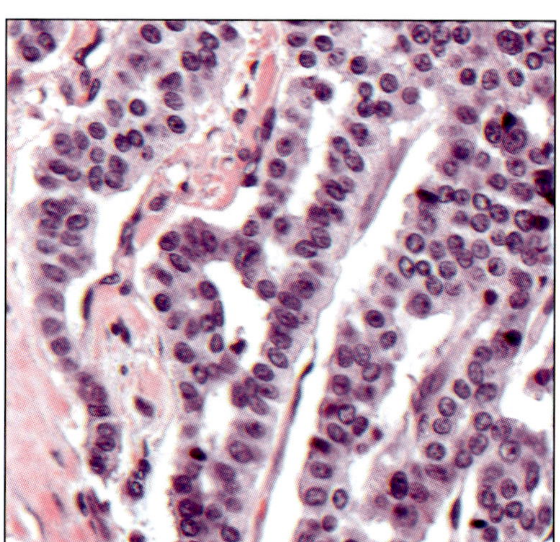

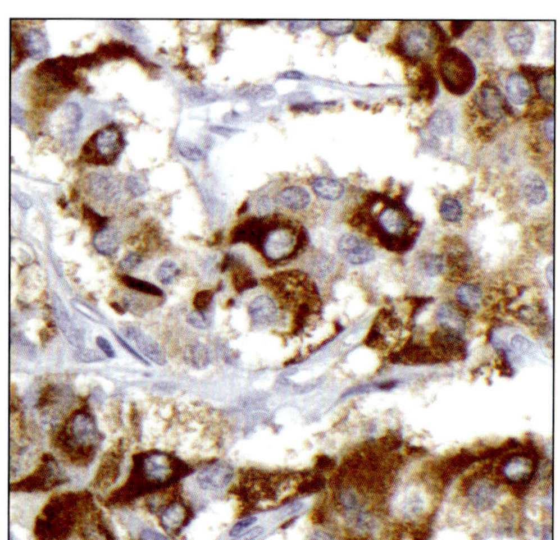

(Left) *A pancreatic endocrine neoplasm shows a prominent trabecular architecture. The monotony of the cells suggests neuroendocrine cell differentiation. The presence of foamy and clear cell changes is characteristic of VHL-associated PET.* ***(Right)*** *Multiple pancreatic microadenomas (< 0.5 cm) seen in patients with MEN1 and neurofibromatosis are often accompanied by 1 or more macroadenomas (diameter > 5 mm), some of which may become insulinomas, as seen in this picture.*

Differential Diagnosis Between Parathyroid Adenoma and Parathyroid Carcinoma

Feature	Parathyroid Adenoma	Parathyroid Carcinoma
Symptoms	Usually asymptomatic or vague symptoms	Often symptomatic
Serum calcium	Elevated	Markedly elevated (> 13 mg/dL)
Palpable mass	Unusual	Yes
Tumor size	Enlarged	Larger, but may overlap
Invasion into adjacent structures	No (but can have irregular growth and cells in capsule due to degenerative features)	Yes
Fibrous bands	Can be present due to degenerative features	Yes
Perineural invasion	No	Yes
Vascular invasion	No	Yes
Growth pattern	Patterns of growth (follicular, acinar, etc.)	Monotonous, sheet-like growth
Cellular features	Often mixed cell types, can show "endocrine atypia"	Often monotonous cytomorphology, prominent nucleoli
Mitoses	Few, scattered	Yes, more mitoses than adenomas
Proliferation markers (Ki-67, MIB1)	Low	Moderate to high

Differential Diagnosis: Parathyroid and Thyroid Immunohistochemistry

Tissue	Keratin	TTF-1	PTH	Chromogranin	Synaptophysin	Calcitonin
Parathyroid cells and tumors	Positive (particularly low molecular weight keratins, e.g., CAM5.2)	Negative	Positive but often not an overly robust stain	Positive	Positive	Negative
Thyroid follicular cells and neoplasms	Positive	Positive (strong nuclear staining)	Negative	Negative	Negative	Negative
Medullary thyroid carcinoma	Positive (particularly low molecular weight keratins, e.g., CAM5.2)	Positive (nuclear staining; may not be as strong as in follicular cells and neoplasms)	Negative	Positive	Positive	Positive

Differential Diagnosis of Parathyroid Carcinoma

Tumor	Chromogranin	Synaptophysin	Parathyroid Hormone	Thyroglobulin	TTF-1	Calcitonin
Parathyroid carcinoma	Positive	Positive	Positive	Negative	Negative	Negative
Medullary thyroid carcinoma	Positive	Positive	Negative	Negative	Positive	Positive
Follicular, Hürthle, or papillary thyroid carcinoma	Negative	Negative	Negative	Positive	Positive	Negative
Metastatic carcinoma	Usually negative	Usually negative	Negative	Negative	Positive/negative	Negative

Differential Diagnosis of Tumors Secondarily Involving Parathyroid

Tumor/Tissue	Chromogranin	Synaptophysin	Cytokeratin	TTF-1	Calcitonin	Other
Parathyroid	Positive	Positive	Positive (CAM5.2)	Negative	Negative but variable	Parathyroid hormone
Breast carcinoma	Negative	Negative	Variable	Negative	Negative	Mammoglobulin, GCDFP-15, estrogen
Follicular/papillary thyroid	Negative	Positive	Positive	Positive	Negative	Thyroglobulin
Medullary thyroid	Positive	Positive	Positive (CAM5.2)	Positive	Positive	CEA
Hepatocellular carcinoma	Negative	Negative	Positive	Negative	Negative	Hep-Par1, albumin
Prostatic adenocarcinoma	Negative	Negative	Positive	Negative	Negative	PSA, PAP
Malignant melanoma	Negative	Negative	Negative	Negative	Negative	S100, Melan-A, HMB-45
Hematolymphoid	Negative	Negative	Negative	Negative	Negative	CD45 (LCA)

Heritable Hyperparathyroidism

Syndrome	Gene	Locus	Parathyroid Pathology	Associated Tumors
Multiple endocrine neoplasia 1	*MEN1*	11q13	Parathyroid hyperplasia (80%)	Pituitary adenoma, pancreatic endocrine tumors, carcinoid tumors, adrenal cortical tumors
Multiple endocrine neoplasia 2	*RET*	10q11.2	Parathyroid hyperplasia (30%)	Medullary thyroid carcinoma, pheochromocytoma
Hyperparathyroidism-jaw tumor syndrome	*HRPT2*	1q25-q32	Cystic parathyroid adenoma; parathyroid carcinoma (15%)	Ossifying fibromas of the jaw, renal cysts and renal carcinomas, Wilms tumor
Familial hypocalciuric hypercalcemia	*CASR*/heterozygous	3q13.3-q21	Parathyroid hyperplasia, mild	
Neonatal severe primary hyperparathyroidism	*CASR*/homozygous	3q13.3-q21	Parathyroid hyperplasia	
Familial isolated hyperparathyroidism	*CASR*; *HRPT2*	3q13.3-q21; 1q25-q32	Parathyroid hyperplasia; parathyroid carcinoma	
Familial hypercalcemic hypercalciuria	*CASR*	3q13.3-q21	Parathyroid hyperplasia; parathyroid adenoma	

Parathyroid Gland: Anatomy and Pathology

*(**Left**) This axial graphic at the thyroid level depicts the thyroid lobes and the isthmus in the anterior visceral space. The figure also shows 2 normal parathyroid glands ➚ in the area of the tracheoesophageal groove. (**Right**) Cut surface of a parathyroid adenoma shows a homogeneous yellow-orange surface, with focal areas of hemorrhage. A small rim of normal parathyroid is appreciated ➡.*

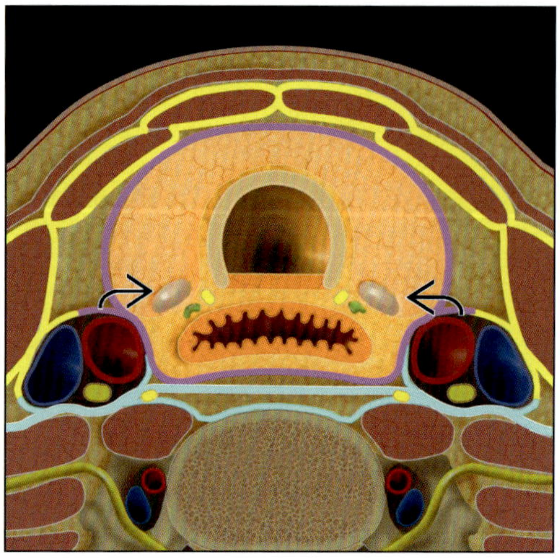

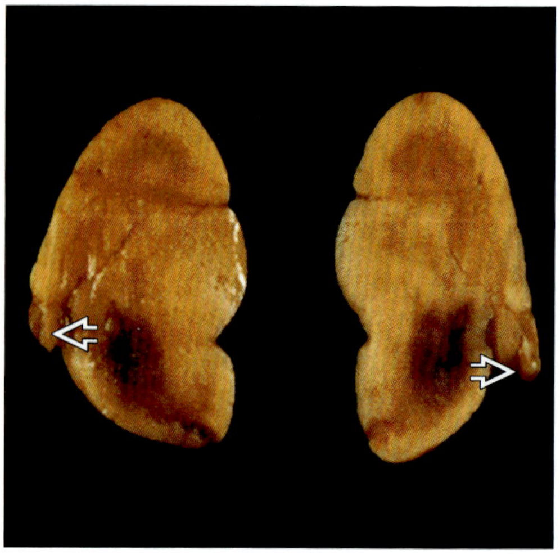

*(**Left**) This graphic shows a parathyroid adenoma ➡ and a normal parathyroid gland ➡. Parathyroid adenoma is a benign neoplasm and usually affects a single parathyroid gland. (**Right**) This smear of a parathyroid adenoma composed by oxyphil cells shows a monomorphic population of cells with abundant eosinophilic cytoplasm and a round nuclei.*

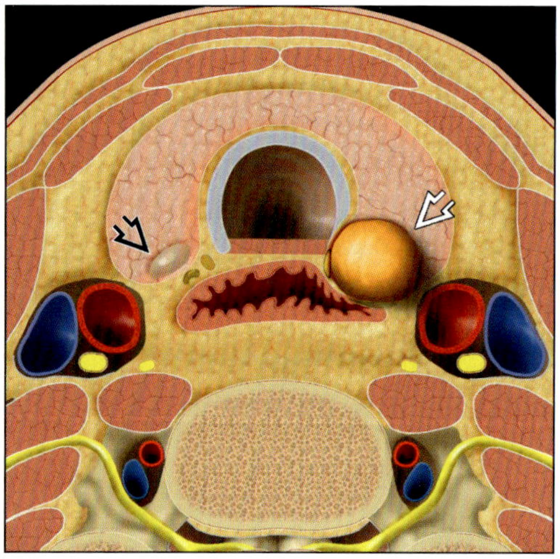

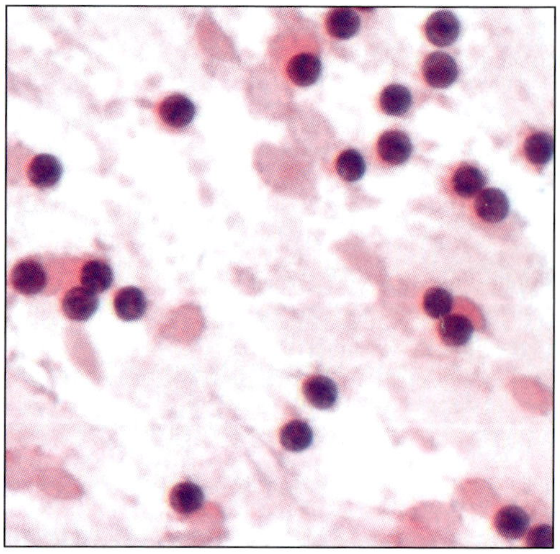

*(**Left**) Chief cell parathyroid adenoma shows a rim of normocellular parathyroid tissue. Parathyroid adenomas are usually composed of chief cells. Cells in the rim are usually smaller than those within the adenoma. (**Right**) Chief cell adenoma with a nested growth pattern shows prominent vascularity ➚. The nuclei are small, round, and dense. The cells show no nuclear pleomorphism or mitosis.*

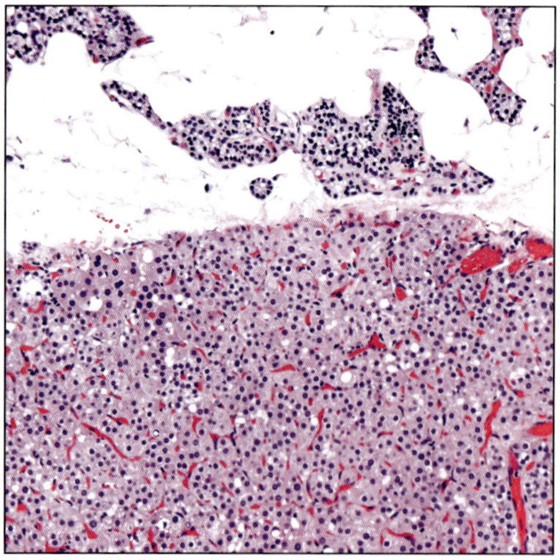

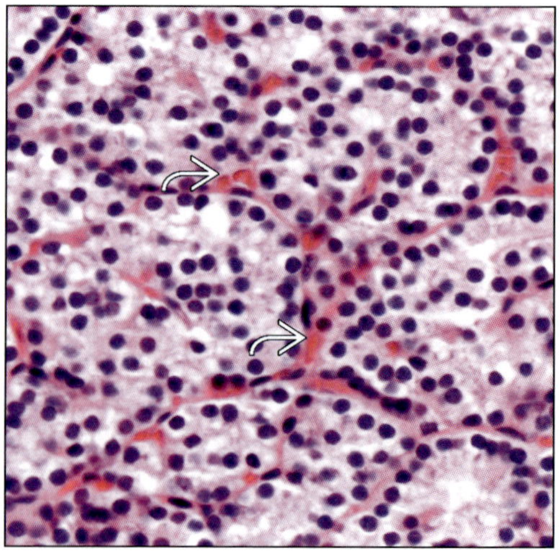

Gross and Microscopic Features of Parathyroid Lesions

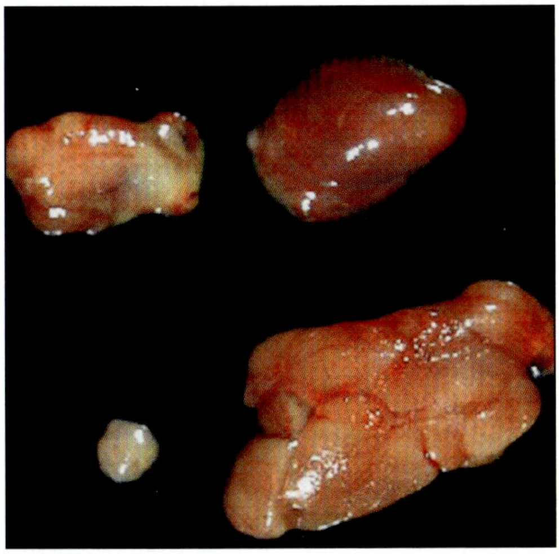

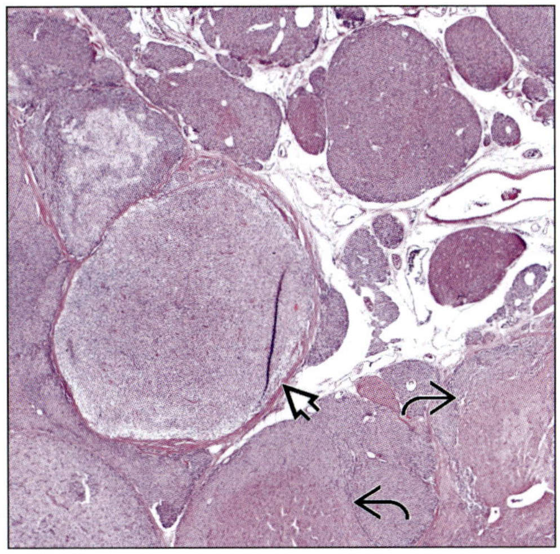

(Left) *Parathyroid hyperplasia is characterized by asymmetric hyperplasia with marked variation in extension of glandular involvement (pseudoadenomatous variant). The asymmetric hyperplasia is easily confused with adenoma or multiple adenomas.* ***(Right)*** *Parathyroid hyperplasia in MEN1 usually shows nodular growth pattern. The nodules are composed of populations of chief cells ⇨, which predominate, as well as nodules of oxyphil cells ⇨.*

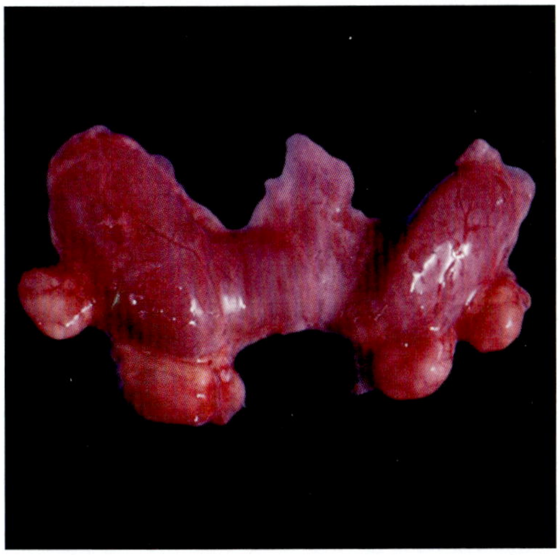

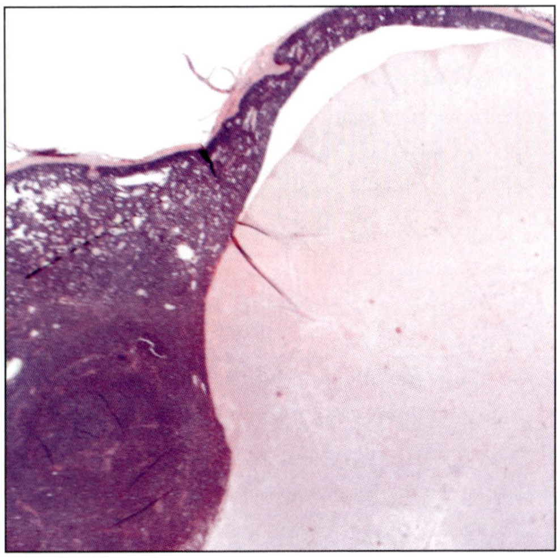

(Left) *In primary parathyroid hyperplasia, ~ 50% of patients present with symmetric enlargement of all 4 parathyroid glands, as seen in this gross picture, which differs from asymmetric hyperplasia.* ***(Right)*** *Cystic change is particularly common in larger parathyroid adenomas and those associated with hyperparathyroidism-jaw tumor syndrome (HPT-JT). This picture illustrates a chief cell adenoma with cystic changes in a patient with HPT-JT.*

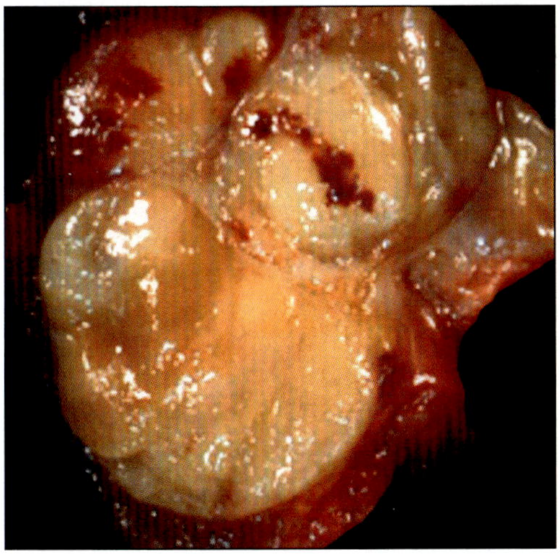

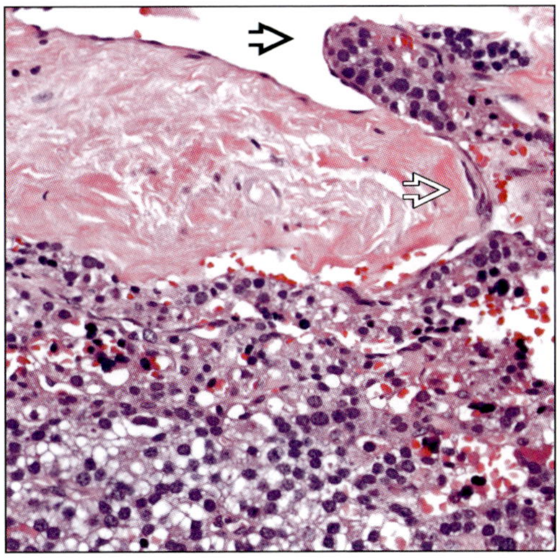

(Left) *Cut surface of a parathyroid carcinoma shows a firm yellow nodular surface. Parathyroid carcinomas are usually larger than parathyroid adenoma and show unequivocal capsular invasion, vascular invasion, perineural invasion, or invasion into adjacent structures. (Courtesy L. Erickson, MD.)* ***(Right)*** *Parathyroid carcinoma is characterized by capsular and vascular invasion. This picture illustrates a parathyroid carcinoma tumor invading through the tumor capsule ⇨ into the vascular space ⇨.*

PITUITARY

Pituitary Adenoma as Part of Inherited Tumor Syndromes

Syndrome	Gene	Pituitary Pathology	Notes
MEN1	*MEN1*	Prolactin-producing adenoma (66%); GH-producing adenoma; nonfunctional adenoma	40% of patients with MEN1 develop PA; *MEN1* mutation uncommon in sporadic cases
McCune-Albright syndrome	*GNAS1*	GH-producing adenoma; somatomammotrope hyperplasia	*GNAS1* mutation present in 40% of sporadic; high GH and IGF1 levels
Carney complex	*PRKAR1A*	GH-producing adenoma; characterized by multiple microadenomas and somatomammotrope hyperplasia	Acromegaly occurs in 10% of patients with Carney complex; pituitary hyperplasia is characteristic
FIPA	*AIP*	GH-producing adenoma; prolactin-producing adenoma; other subtypes of PA	*AIP* mutation is present in 15-20% of FIPAs, in 50% of familial acromegaly, and in a small proportion of sporadic PAs; almost 90% are GH-producing PAs; most patients with *AIP* mutation are men (70%), have macroadenomas (97%), and are younger at time of diagnosis than patients with other PAs
IFS	*AIP*	GH-producing adenoma	
MEN4	*CDKN1B*	GH-producing PA	Associated with hyperparathyroidism; few reported cases and families

FIPA: Familial isolated pituitary adenoma; GH: Growth hormone; IFS: Isolated familial somatotropinoma syndrome; MEN1: Multiple endocrine neoplasia 1; MEN4: Multiple endocrine neoplasia 4; PA: Pituitary adenoma.

Genetic Abnormalities in Pituitary Adenomas

Gene	Molecular Defect
RB1	Loss of 13q14; promoter methylation
CCND1	Allelic imbalance; overexpression
PTTG	Overexpression
FGFR2	Promoter methylation
EGFR	Overexpression
PTAG	Underexpression; promoter methylation
GNAS	Inactivating mutations
MEN1	Inactivating mutations
CDKN1B	Underexpression; germline nonsense mutation
PRKAR1A	Germline mutations
AIP	Germline mutations and LOH
PKC	Point mutation; overexpression
RAS	Point mutation; gene amplification
PIK3CA	Somatic mutation; gene amplification
CCNA1	Overexpression

Pituitary Adenomas

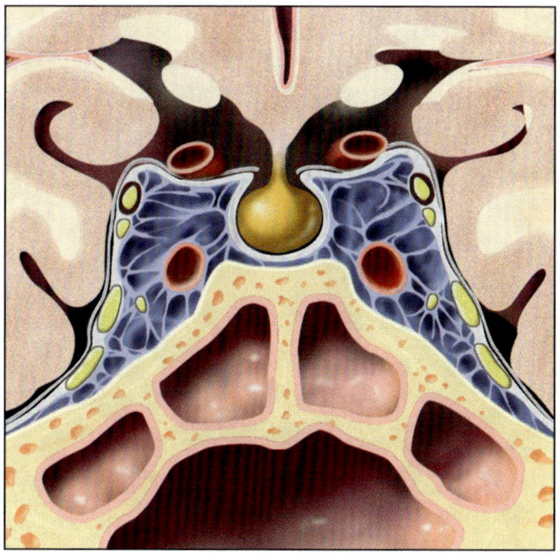

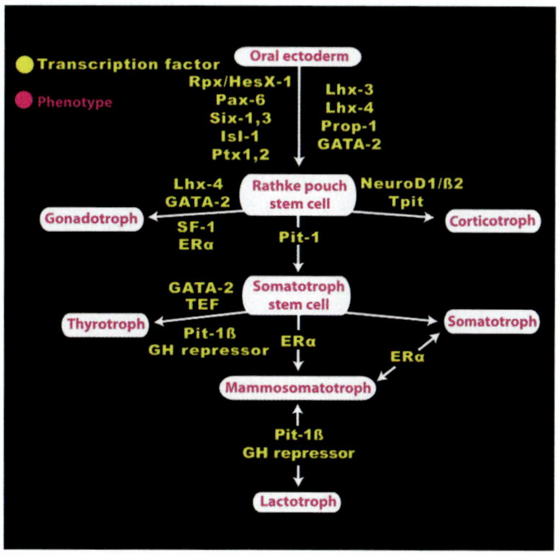

(Left) *The following cranial nerves traverse the cavernous sinus within the lateral wall of the cavernous sinus: Oculomotor nerve, trochlear nerve, and 1st and 2nd divisions of trigeminal nerve.* ***(Right)*** *Pituitary adenoma arising from PIT-1 lineage adenohypophyseal cells expresses mainly GH, PRL, and TSH and exhibit PRL-, GH-, and TSH-containing secretory granules. The familial pituitary adenomas are more frequently from the somatotrophic lineage.*

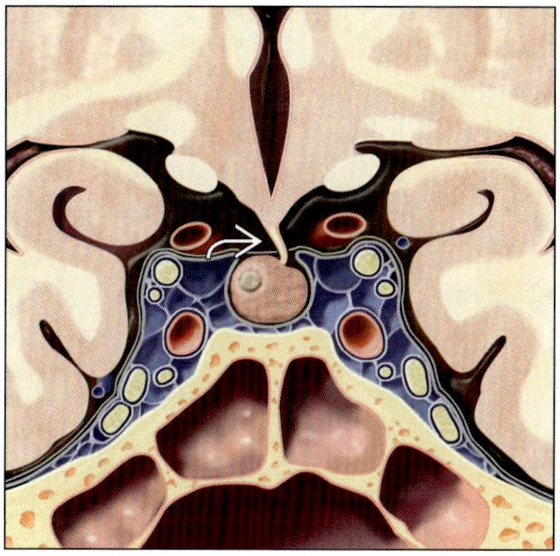

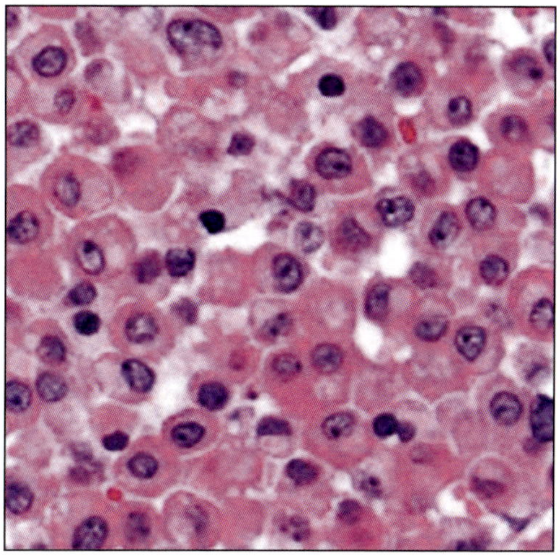

(Left) *Coronal graphic shows a small microadenoma that slightly enlarges the right side of the pituitary gland and deviates the infundibulum toward the left.* ***(Right)*** *Most of the familial-associated pituitary adenomas are GH-producing pituitary adenomas. Tumor cells of the densely granulated somatotroph adenomas have an eosinophilic cytoplasm and are positive for PIT-1 and α-subunit.*

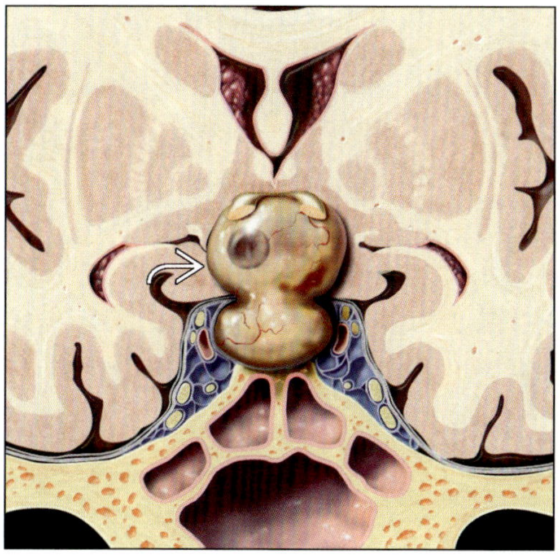

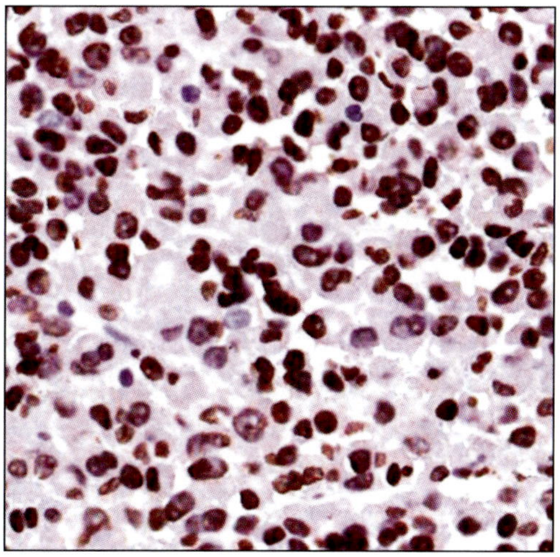

(Left) *Coronal graphic shows a snowman-shaped or "figure of eight" sellar/suprasellar mass with hemorrhage and cystic change. Familial somatotrophic adenomas may be a component of MEN1, Carney complex, McCune-Albright, MEN4, familial isolated pituitary adenoma, and somatotropinoma syndromes.* ***(Right)*** *Regardless of the subtype, all PRL-producing adenomas, GH-producing adenomas, and TSH-producing pituitary adenomas are positive for PIT-1.*

Microscopic Features

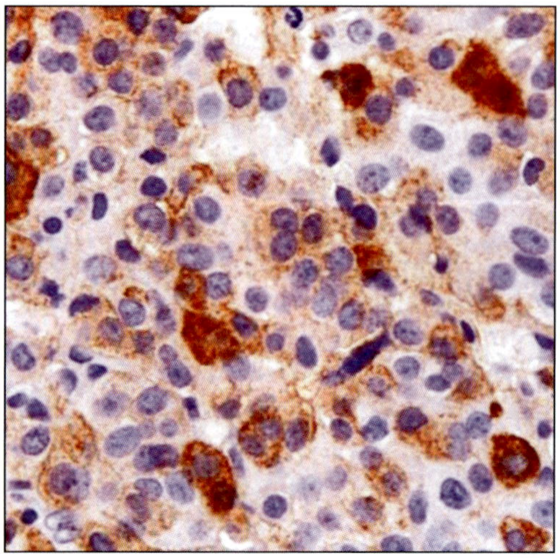

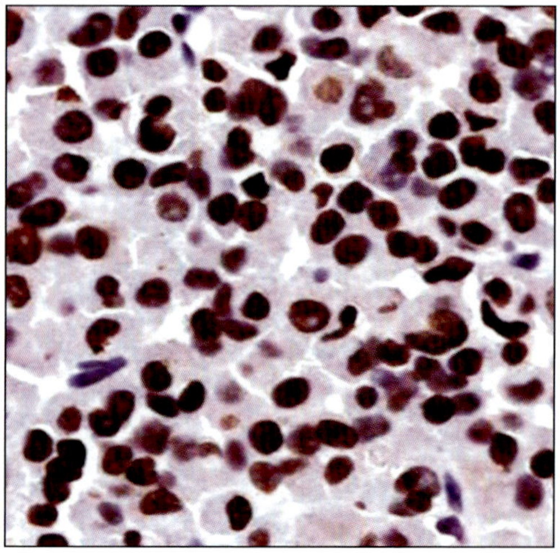

(Left) Familial densely granulated somatotroph adenomas harbor numerous GH-containing secretory granules that correlate with their eosinophilic, densely granulate cytoplasm on conventional histology. *(Right)* Regardless of the subtype, all GH-producing pituitary adenomas are strongly positive for PIT-1. PIT-1 is also expressed in PRL- and TSH-producing pituitary adenomas and in silent subtype III adenomas (aggressive monomorphous PIT-1 lineage plurihormonal adenomas).

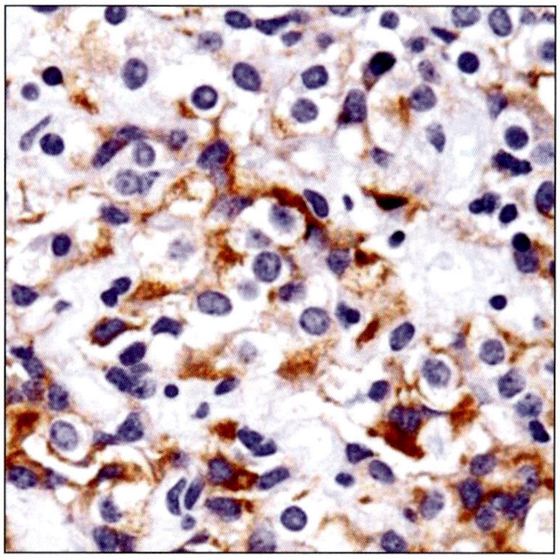

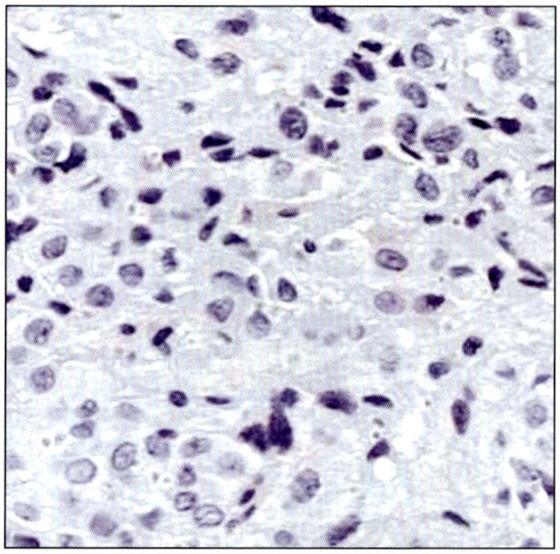

(Left) Familial densely granulated somatotroph adenomas are positive for α-subunit; however, sparsely granulated somatotroph adenomas are usually negative for α-subunit. *(Right)* α-subunit is usually negative in PRL-producing adenomas, as well as sparsely granulated GH-producing adenomas. Among the PIT-1 lineage pituitary adenoma members, α-subunit is usually expressed in densely granulated GH- and TSH-producing adenomas.

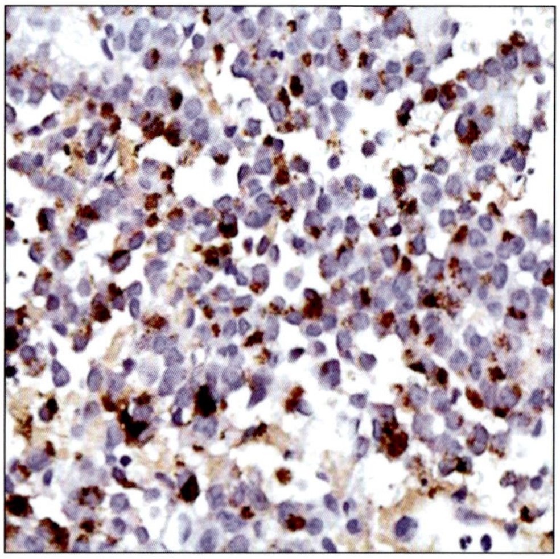

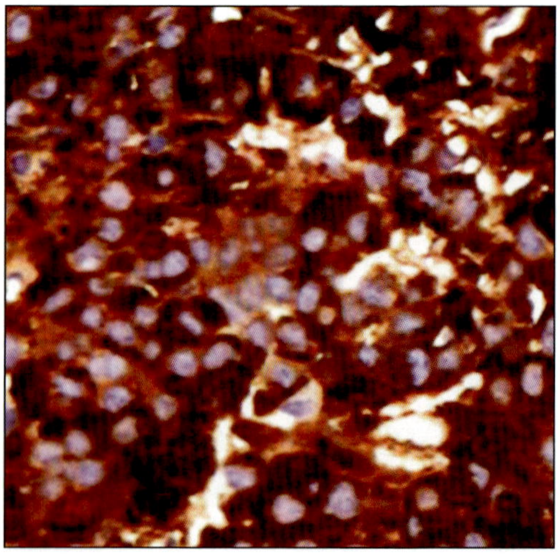

(Left) Familial sparsely granulated lactotroph adenomas are composed of chromophobic cells that reveal typical Golgi-type staining for PRL. *(Right)* Unlike sparsely granulated lactotroph adenomas, aggressive variants of PRL-producing adenomas (such as densely granulated lactotroph adenomas and acidophil stem cell adenomas) have diffuse cytoplasmic positivity for PRL and usually lack the characteristic Golgi pattern.

Diagrammatic and Microscopic Features

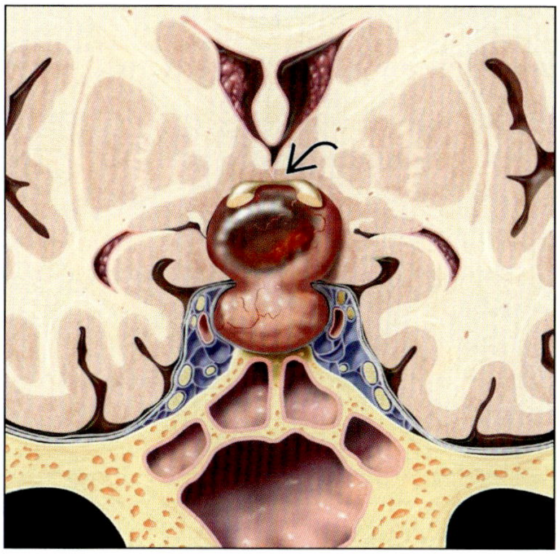

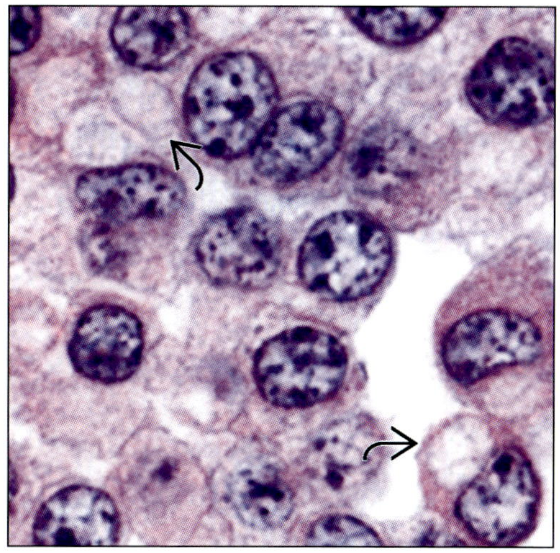

(Left) *Coronal graphic illustrates a large pituitary macroadenoma extending superiorly to compress the body of the chiasm, thus compressing the bulk of the crossing nasal retinal fibers →.* ***(Right)*** *This acidophil stem cell adenoma is composed of eosinophilic cells that exhibit cytoplasmic vacuolization → due to mitochondrial dilatation. These tumors also originate from the PIT-1 line of differentiation.*

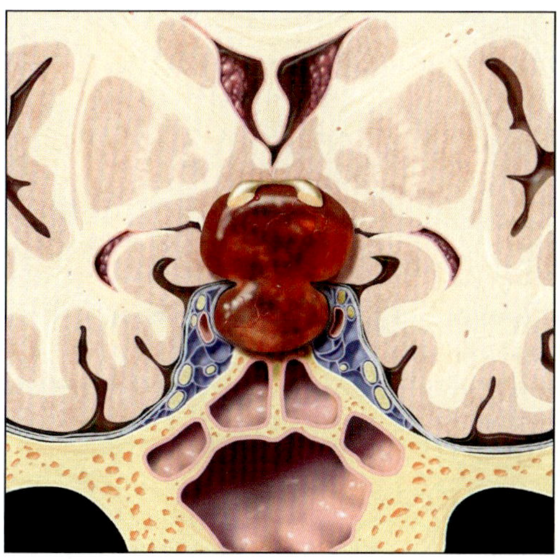

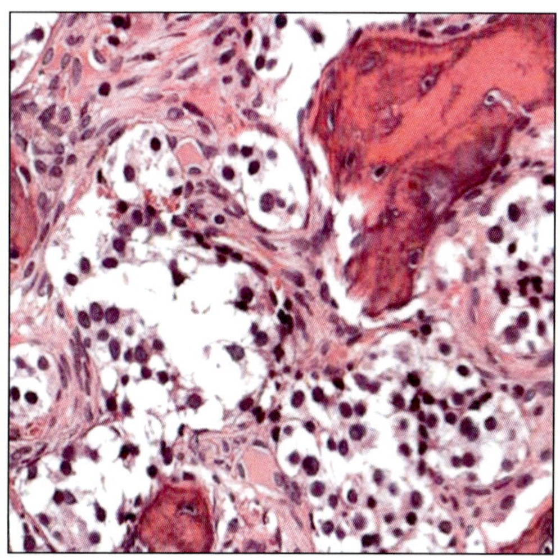

(Left) *Coronal graphic shows a large "figure of eight" sellar/suprasellar pituitary macroadenoma with acute hemorrhage causing pituitary apoplexy.* ***(Right)*** *Thyrotroph adenomas are usually large and invasive adenomas, which may invade bone, as demonstrated in this figure. These tumors are composed of polygonal, angulated, or spindle-shaped cells that exhibit indistinct cell borders.*

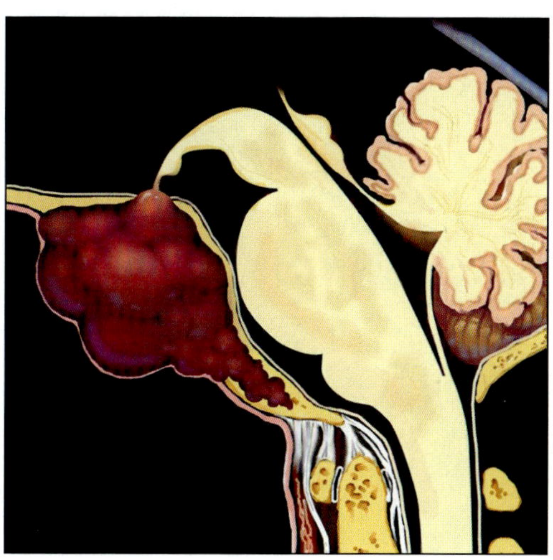

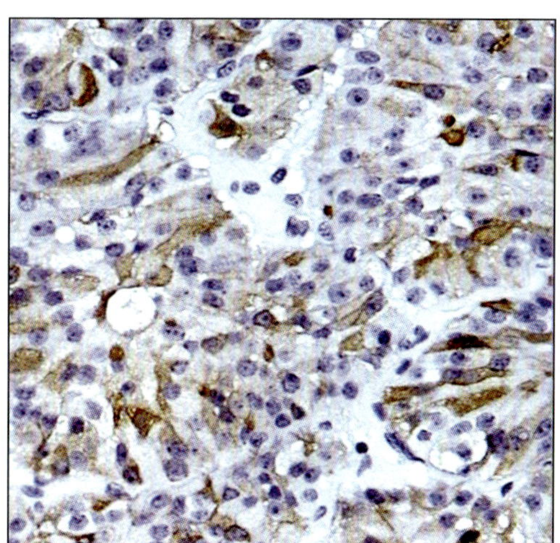

(Left) *Sagittal graphic depicts a giant pituitary macroadenoma. Notice that the normal pituitary gland is not seen. The lesion extends anteroinferiorly into the basisphenoid and posteroinferiorly into the basiocciput.* ***(Right)*** *The immunoreactivity for β-TSH varies from cell to cell in thyrotroph adenomas. The staining pattern allows recognition of the angular cell morphology of the tumor cells. Only rare inherited familial tumors are TSH-producing adenomas.*

THYROID, MEDULLARY

Differential Diagnosis Between Reactive/ Physiologic and Neoplastic C-Cell Hyperplasia

Features	Reactive C-Cell Hyperplasia	Neoplastic C-Cell Hyperplasia
Detectable on H&E stains	No	Yes
Cytologic atypia	No	Yes
Seen adjacent to MTC	No	Yes, usually found adjacent to MTC
Associated with MTC	No	Precursor lesion of MTC
Bilaterality	No	Yes
Calcitonin reactivity	Yes	Yes
RET mutation	No	These lesions harbor germline *RET* mutations
CEA reactivity	No	Yes/no
Chromogranin reactivity	Yes	Yes
Synaptophysin reactivity	Yes	Yes
Staining with NCAM	No	Yes

CEA: Carcinoembryonic antigen; MTC: Medullary thyroid carcinoma; NCAM: Neural cellular adhesion molecule.

Differential Diagnosis of Medullary Thyroid Carcinoma by Immunohistochemistry

Antibody	MTC	PTC	PDC	ATC	PA/C	Para	Met C
Cytokeratin	Positive	Positive	Positive	Positive/negative	Positive	Negative	Positive
Calcitonin	Positive	Negative	Negative	Negative	Negative	Negative	Negative
TTF-1	Positive	Positive	Positive	Negative	Negative	Negative	Negative
Thyroglobulin	Negative	Positive	Positive	Negative	Negative	Negative	Negative
Chromogranin	Positive	Negative	Negative	Negative	Positive	Positive	Positive/negative
Synaptophysin	Positive	Negative	Negative	Negative	Positive	Positive	Positive/negative
PTH	Negative	Negative	Negative	Negative	Positive	Negative	Negative
S100	Negative	Negative	Negative	Negative	Negative	Positive	Negative

ATC: Anaplastic thyroid carcinoma; Met C: Metastatic carcinoma; MTC: Medullary thyroid carcinoma; PA/C: Parathyroid adenoma/carcinoma; Para: Paraganglioma; PDC: Poorly differentiated carcinoma; PTC: Papillary thyroid carcinoma.

Incidence of Medullary Thyroid Carcinoma and Associated Diseases in Multiple Endocrine Neoplasia Syndrome Type 2

Findings	FMTC (% Association)	MEN2A (% Association)	MEN2B (% Association)
Medullary thyroid carcinoma	100	100	100
C-cell hyperplasia	100	100	100
Pheochromocytoma	0	10-60	100
Hyperparathyroidism	0	10-30	0
Lichen amyloidosis	0	0	< 10
Marfanoid habitus	0	0	100
Mucosal neuromas	0	0	70-100
Intestinal ganglioneuromatosis	0	0	60-90
Thick corneal nerves	0	Rare	60-90

FMTC: Familial medullary thyroid carcinoma; MEN2A: Multiple endocrine neoplasia type 2A; MEN2B: Multiple endocrine neoplasia type 2B.

ATA Age Recommendations for Prophylactic Thyroidectomy Depending on RET Mutation

RET Mutation	Recommended Age for Prophylactic Thyroidectomy
Codons 838, 918, 922	Within 1st year of life
Codons 768, 790, 791, 804, 891	Consider surgery < 5 years; may delay surgery up to 10 years if normal serum calcitonin, normal neck ultrasound, family history of less aggressive tumor
Codons 609, 611, 618, 620, 630	Consider surgery < 5 years; may delay surgery up to 10 years if normal serum calcitonin, normal neck ultrasound, family history of less aggressive tumor
Codon 634	< 5 years

ATA: American Thyroid Association. Table based on American Thyroid Association Guidelines Task Force et al: Medullary thyroid cancer: management guidelines of the American Thyroid Association. Thyroid. 19(6):565-612, 2009 and Grubbs EG et al: Do the recent American Thyroid Association (ATA) Guidelines accurately guide the timing of prophylactic thyroidectomy in MEN2A? Surgery. 148(6):1302-9; discussion 1309-10, 2010.

Familial Medullary Thyroid Carcinoma Characteristics

Characteristics	MEN2B	MEN2A	FMTC
Incidence of MEN2 syndromes	Comprises ~ 5% of cases with MEN2	Makes up the majority of MEN2 cases (70-80%)	Comprises ~ 10-20% of cases of MEN2
Age at diagnosis of MTC	Early development of MTC; usually < 5 years	Usually < 35 years	Age of onset of MTC is later than the other familial cases; usually 50 years
Presentation	Aggressive form of MTC; average age of death before early prophylactic thyroidectomy was 21 years	MTC is usually the initial presentation; up to 70% have LN metastases at time of presentation	MTC is the only clinical manifestation of FMTC
MTC incidence by syndrome	Most individuals with MEN2B develop MTC	70-95% of individuals with MEN2A develop MTC	MTC is characteristically present
RET mutation	~ 95% of individuals with MEN2B have single point mutation at codon 918		

FMTC: Familial medullary thyroid carcinoma-only syndrome; LN: Lymph node; MEN2A: Multiple endocrine neoplasia type 2A; MEN2B: Multiple endocrine neoplasia type 2B; MTC: Medullary thyroid carcinoma.

Pathological Features Distinguishing Familial From Sporadic Medullary Thyroid Carcinoma

Pathological Features	Familial	Sporadic
Gross features	Multicentric	Solitary mass
Laterality	Bilateral	Unilateral
Presence of C-cell hyperplasia	Associated with C-cell hyperplasia	Association with C-cell hyperplasia unknown
Neoplastic C-cell hyperplasia	Frequent (~ 90%)	Rare (< 15%)
Microscopic features	No distinct MTC histopathological features or MTC variants can distinguish from sporadic tumors	No distinct MTC features or MTC variants can distinguish sporadic from inherited forms
Lymph node metastasis	May be present at time of diagnosis	Usually present at time of diagnosis
RET mutation	Present in majority of hereditary forms	May be present in 6-9.5% of sporadic cases
RET mutation MEN2A	98% of families have *RET* mutation	
RET mutation MEN2B	~ 100% of families have *RET* mutation	
RET mutation FMTC	~ 95% of families have *RET* mutation	

FMTC: Familial medullary thyroid carcinoma-only syndrome; MTC: Medullary thyroid carcinoma.

THYROID, NONMEDULLARY

Familial Nonmedullary Thyroid Carcinoma Classification

Disease	Histological Subtype
Syndromic or Familial Tumor Syndrome with Preponderance of Nonthyroidal Tumors	
PTEN hamartoma tumor syndrome (Cowden disease)	FTC associated with follicular adenomas, multiple adenomatous nodules, and C-cell hyperplasia
FAP hamartoma tumor syndrome	PTC with cribriform and morular pattern with sclerosis
Carney complex	FTC associated with follicular adenomas, multiple adenomatous nodules, and PTC
Werner syndrome	FTC, PTC, and ATC
Pendred syndrome	FTC
Nonsyndromic or Familial Tumor Syndrome with Preponderance of Nonmedullary Thyroid Carcinoma	
Familial PTC	PTC, usual variant
Familial PTC with papillary renal cell neoplasia	PTC, usual papillary variant architecture
Familial nonmedullary thyroid carcinoma type 1	PTC, usual variant
Familial PTC and multinodular goiter	PTC and nodular hyperplasia

ATC: Anaplastic thyroid carcinoma; FAP: Familial adenomatous polyposis; FTC: Follicular thyroid carcinoma; PTC: Papillary thyroid carcinoma.

Familial Nonmedullary Thyroid Carcinoma in Familial Cancer Syndromes

Syndrome	Inheritance	Gene	Gene Location	Thyroid Involvement (%)
PTEN hamartoma tumor syndrome	Autosomal dominant	*PTEN*	10q23.2	50
Familial adenomatous polyposis	Autosomal dominant	*APC*	5q21	2-12
Carney complex	Autosomal dominant	*PRKAR1A*	2p12-17q22-24	60; 4
Pendred syndrome	Autosomal recessive	*SLC26A4* (pendrin)	7q21-24	1
Werner syndrome	Autosomal recessive	*WRN*	8p11-p12	18

Distinct Characteristics of Familial Thyroid Carcinoma and Sporadic Carcinoma

	Familial	Sporadic
Gross Characteristics		
	Usually multiple tumors	Usually single
	Usually bilateral	Unilateral
Microscopic Characteristics		
	Usually associated with a background of lymphocytic thyroiditis &/or multinodular hyperplasia	Background thyroid usually uninvolved
	Unique morphology in some familial cases: Cribriform morular thyroid carcinoma in familial adenomatous polyposis	All described variants occur
Lymph Node Metastases		
	Usually more frequent than sporadic cases	

FAP and PTEN Hamartoma Tumor Syndrome

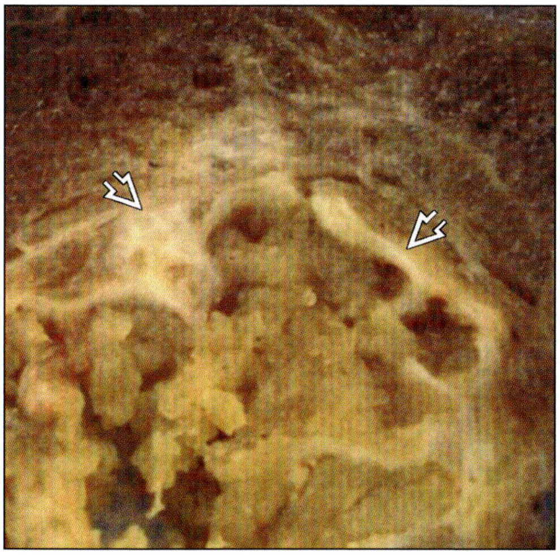

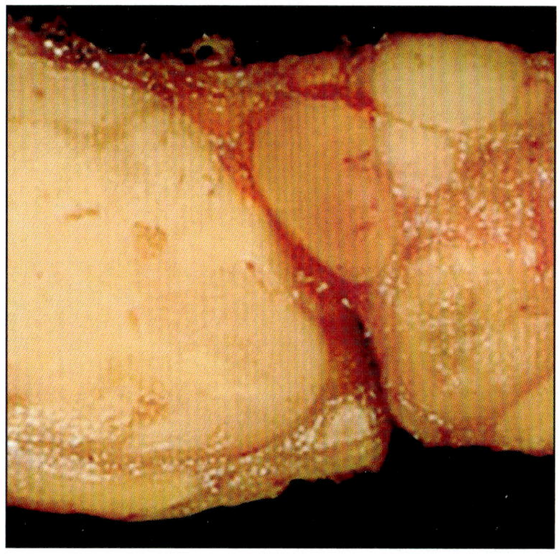

(Left) *Gross cut surface of a cribriform morular variant of papillary thyroid carcinoma (CMV-PTC) in a patient with FAP shows irregular areas of fibrosis* ➔ *and a pale, soft, and friable tumor mass. These tumors are usually multiple and bilateral in a familial setting.* ***(Right)*** *Gross cut surface of a thyroid from an 18-year-old woman with PHTS/Cowden disease shows multiple well-circumscribed nodules almost entirely replacing the thyroid parenchyma with a small amount of residual noninvolved thyroid.*

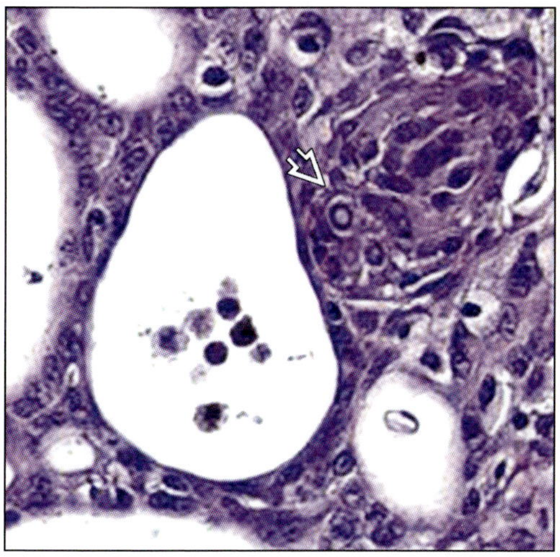

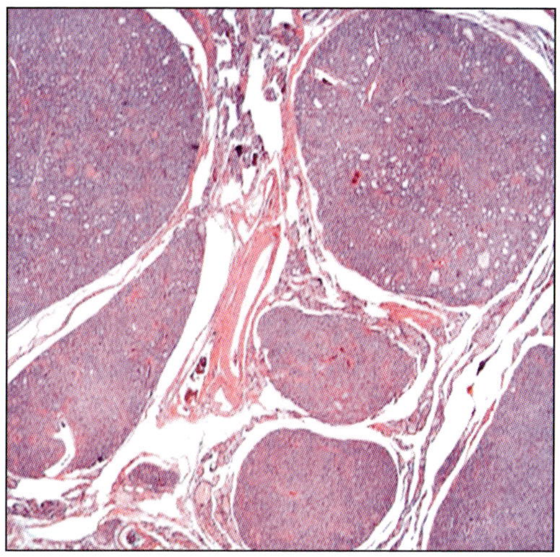

(Left) *High-power H&E demonstrates the characteristic peculiar nuclear clearing (PNC)* ➔ *seen within some of the nuclei in CMV-PTC. These PNCs are characteristically found within squamous morules.* ***(Right)*** *This photomicrograph of a thyroid from an 18-year-old woman with PTEN hamartoma tumor syndrome (PHTS) shows multiple well-circumscribed, nonencapsulated, adenomatous nodules with a small amount of compressed residual thyroid parenchyma.*

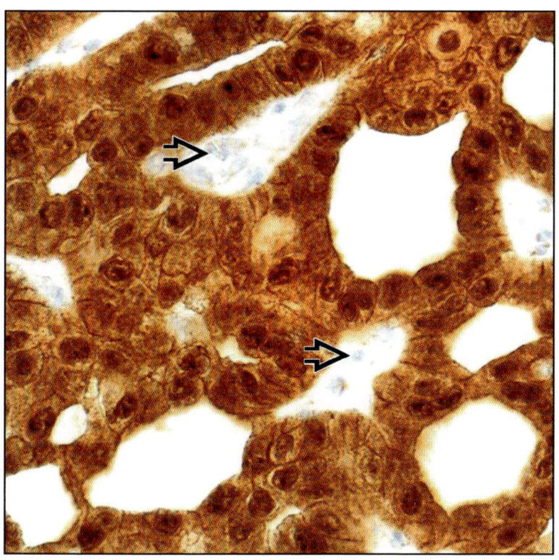

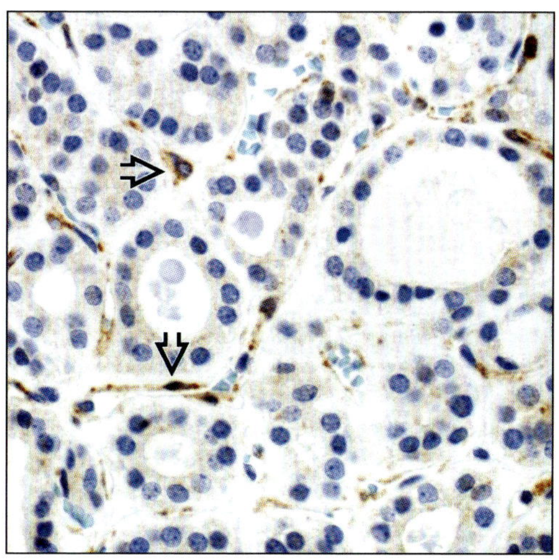

(Left) *High power of β-catenin immunostain in CMV-PTC demonstrates characteristic nuclear and cytoplasmic staining resulting from aberrant accumulation within the nucleus. Note the negativity of endothelial cells for β-catenin* ➔*.* ***(Right)*** *Immunohistochemistry for PTEN in a thyroidectomy specimen from an 18-year-old woman with PHTS/Cowden disease shows loss of staining of the follicular cells with preservation of staining of the endothelial cells* ➔*.*

Gastrointestinal

BILIARY TRACT/LIVER/PANCREAS

Familial Neoplasia of Biliary Tract, Liver, and Pancreas

Type of Tumor	Possible Syndromes	Gene
Ampullary adenoma/ carcinoma	FAP, MYH, Lynch, Peutz-Jeghers	*APC, MYH, MSH1, MSH2, MLH1, PMS2, LKB1*
Pancreaticobiliary adenocarcinoma	FAP, Lynch, Peutz-Jeghers, juvenile polyposis, hereditary breast and ovarian cancer syndrome, familial atypical multiple mole melanoma syndrome, hereditary pancreatitis, Li-Fraumeni	*APC, MSH1, MSH2, MLH1, PMS2, LKB1, SMAD4, BMPR1A, ENG, BRCA2, PALB2, BRCA1, P16/CDKN2A, PRSS1, PRSS2, SPINK1, CFTR, TP53, CHEK2*
Pancreatic endocrine tumor	Multiple endocrine neoplasia 1, von Hippel-Lindau disease, tuberous sclerosis	*MEN1, VHL, TSC1, TSC2*
Hepatocellular adenoma/ carcinoma	FAP, hemochromatosis, tyrosinemia, citrullinemia, α-1-antitrypsin deficiency, glycogen storage disease, Alagille, progressive familial intrahepatic cholestasis	*APC, HFE, FAH, HPD, TAT, SLC25A13, ASS1, SERPINA1, G6PC, AGL, PYGL, JAG1, NOTCH2, ATP8B1, ABCB11, MDR3*
Hepatoblastoma	FAP, Li-Fraumeni	*APC, TP53, CHEK2*

FAP: Familial adenomatous polyposis.

Familial Biliary Tract, Liver, and Pancreas Neoplasms by Syndromes

Syndrome	Gene(s)	Inheritance Pattern	Tumor	Other Manifestations
FAP	*APC*	Autosomal dominant	Ampullary adenomas and adenocarcinomas, hepatoblastoma, hepatic adenoma, hepatocellular carcinoma, pancreatic and biliary tract adenocarcinomas	Multiple colonic adenomas and carcinomas, gliomas, desmoids, CHRPE, osteomas and jaw cysts, adrenal cortical neoplasms, papillary thyroid carcinoma, cribriform-morular variant, parathyroid and pituitary adenomas
Peutz-Jeghers syndrome	*LKB1*	Autosomal dominant	Ampullary, biliary, and pancreatic adenocarcinomas	Hamartomatous polyps of the GI tract, adenocarcinoma of the colon, ovarian sex cord tumor with annular tubules, adenoma malignum of cervix, mucinous tumors of ovaries and fallopian tubes, breast carcinoma, bronchioalveolar carcinomas of the lung, testicular sex cord and Sertoli cell tumors, papillary thyroid carcinoma
Juvenile polyposis	*SMAD4, BMPR1A, ENG*	Autosomal dominant	Pancreatic adenocarcinoma	Hamartomatous polyps of the GI tract and adenocarcinoma of the stomach, small intestine, and colon
Multiple endocrine neoplasia 1	*MEN1*	Autosomal dominant	Pancreatic endocrine neoplasms	Endocrine neoplasms of the parathyroid and pituitary glands, adrenal cortical neoplasms, thymic and bronchial carcinoids, esophageal leiomyomas, renal angiomyolipomas, GISTs, spinal ependymomas, meningioma, astrocytoma, lipomas, collagenomas, and angiofibromas
von Hippel-Lindau disease	*VHL*	Autosomal dominant	Pancreatic serous cystadenomas, pancreatic endocrine neoplasms	CNS hemangioblastomas, renal cell carcinomas, pheochromocytomas, café au lait spots
Tuberous sclerosis	*TSC1, TSC2*	Autosomal dominant	Pancreatic endocrine neoplasms (*TSC2* mutations)	Angiomyolipomas, angiofibromas, astrocytomas, lymphangioleiomyomatosis, renal cysts, retinal hamartomas, cardiac rhabdomyoma, hypomelanotic skin macules, periungual fibromas, cortical tubers
Hereditary breast and ovarian cancer syndrome	*BRCA2, PALB2, BRCA1*	Autosomal dominant	Pancreatic and biliary tract adenocarcinomas	Breast, ovarian, fallopian tube, peritoneal, prostate, stomach, cervical, and endometrial carcinomas
Familial atypical multiple mole melanoma syndrome	*P16/CDKN2A*	Autosomal dominant	Pancreatic adenocarcinoma	Melanomas and dysplastic nevi
Lynch syndrome	*MLH1, PMS2, MSH2, MSH6*	Autosomal dominant	Ampullary, biliary, and pancreatic adenocarcinomas	Colonic adenomas and adenocarcinomas; carcinomas of the endometrium, ovaries, adrenal cortex, prostate, bladder, renal pelvis, and ureter; glioblastomas; and sebaceous neoplasms
Hereditary pancreatitis	*PRSS1, PRSS2, SPINK1, CFTR*	Autosomal dominant	Pancreatic adenocarcinoma	Pancreatitis
Hemochromatosis	*HFE*	Autosomal recessive	Hepatocellular carcinoma	Iron overload can lead to endocrine dysfunction, heart failure, arthritis, and cirrhosis of the liver
Tyrosinemia	*FAH, HPD, TAT*	Autosomal recessive	Hepatocellular adenoma and carcinoma	Failure to thrive, liver and renal failure, skin and ocular lesions
Citrullinemia	*SLC25A13, ASS1*	Autosomal recessive	Hepatocellular carcinoma	Liver dysfunction, hyperammonemia
α-1-antitrypsin deficiency	*SERPINA1*	Autosomal codominant	Hepatocellular carcinoma	Pulmonary disease
Glycogen storage disease	*G6PC, AGL, PYGL*	Autosomal recessive	Hepatocellular adenoma and carcinoma	Hypoglycemia, muscle disease, liver disease
Li-Fraumeni syndrome	*TP53, CHEK2*	Autosomal dominant	Hepatoblastoma, pancreatic and biliary adenocarcinoma	Breast carcinoma, osteosarcoma, and other soft tissue sarcomas; leukemias; adrenal cortical carcinoma; brain tumors
Alagille syndrome	*JAG1, NOTCH2*	Autosomal dominant	Hepatocellular carcinoma	Bile duct paucity, pulmonic stenosis, butterfly vertebrae, abnormal facial features
Progressive familial intrahepatic cholestasis (Byler disease)	*ATP8B1, ABCB11, MDR3*	Autosomal recessive	Hepatocellular carcinoma	Cholestatic liver disease

CHRPE: Congenital hypertrophy of retinal pigment epithelium; FAP: Familial adenomatous polyposis; GIST: Gastrointestinal stromal tumor.

COLON/RECTUM

Familial Neoplasia of the Colon and Rectum

Type of Tumor	Possible Syndromes	Gene
Adenoma	FAP, MYH-associated polyposis, Lynch syndrome, juvenile polyposis, hereditary mixed polyposis, Cowden/PTEN hamartoma syndrome (possible association), serrated polyposis (previously known as giant hyperplastic polyposis)	*APC, MYH, MLH1, PMS2, MSH2, MSH6, SMAD4, ENG, CRAC1, BMPR1A, PTEN*
Serrated polyp	Serrated polyposis (previously known as giant hyperplastic polyposis), hereditary mixed polyposis, MYH-associated polyposis	Unknown, possibly *CRAC1* for hereditary mixed polyposis, *MYH*
Adenomas, hamartomatous polyps, and serrated polyps	Hereditary mixed polyposis	*CRAC1* possible gene involved
Adenomas and hamartomatous polyps	Juvenile polyposis, Cowden/PTEN hamartoma syndrome	*SMAD4, BMPR1A, ENG, PTEN*
Adenocarcinoma	FAP, MYH-associated polyposis, Lynch syndrome, juvenile polyposis, hereditary mixed polyposis, Cowden/PTEN hamartoma syndrome (possible association), serrated polyposis, Peutz-Jeghers syndrome, Li-Fraumeni syndrome	*APC, MYH, MLH1, PMS2, MSH2, MSH6, SMAD4, ENG, CRAC1, BMPR1A, PTEN, LKB1, TP53*

FAP: Familial adenomatous polyposis.

Familial Colon and Rectum Tumors by Syndrome

Syndrome	Gene	Inheritance Pattern	Tumor	Other Manifestations
FAP	*APC*	Autosomal dominant	Adenomas and adenocarcinomas of the GI tract	Gastric fundic gland polyps with and without dysplasia, pancreaticobiliary tract adenocarcinomas, fibromatosis (Gardner syndrome), hepatoblastomas, hepatic adenomas, hepatocellular carcinomas, osteomas (Gardner syndrome), supernumerary teeth, congenital hypertrophy of retinal pigment epithelium, epidermal inclusion cysts of face and scalp, papillary thyroid carcinoma (cribriform morular variant), adrenal cortical neoplasms, pancreatic islet cell neoplasms, parathyroid and pituitary adenomas, medulloblastomas (Turcot syndrome), nasopharyngeal angiofibromas
MYH-associated polyposis	*MYH*	Autosomal recessive	Adenomas and adenocarcinomas of the GI tract	Gastric fundic gland polyps with and without dysplasia, fibromatosis, osteomas, supernumerary teeth, congenital hypertrophy of retinal pigment epithelium, epidermal inclusion cysts of face and scalp; ovarian, bladder, and skin cancers that may mimic Lynch syndrome have been reported; given the rarity of the MYH, it is unknown whether all of the lesions associated with FAP can be seen
Lynch syndrome (HNPCC)	*MLH1, PMS2, MSH2, MSH6*	Autosomal dominant	Adenomas and adenocarcinomas of the GI tract	Ampullary, biliary, and pancreatic adenocarcinomas; carcinomas of the endometrium, ovaries, adrenal cortex, prostate, bladder, renal pelvis, and ureter; glioblastomas; and sebaceous neoplasms
Peutz-Jeghers syndrome	*LKB1*	Autosomal dominant	Hamartomatous polyps and adenocarcinomas of the GI tract	Adenocarcinoma of the stomach, small bowel, and pancreas; ovarian sex cord tumor with annular tubules; adenoma malignum of cervix; mucinous tumors of ovaries and fallopian tubes; breast carcinoma; bronchioalveolar carcinomas of the lung; testicular sex cord and Sertoli cell tumors; papillary thyroid cancer
Juvenile polyposis	*SMAD4, BMPR1A, ENG*	Autosomal dominant	Hamartomatous polyps and adenocarcinomas of the GI tract	Adenocarcinomas of the stomach, small intestine, and pancreas
Cowden/PTEN hamartoma syndrome	*PTEN*	Autosomal dominant	Hamartomatous polyps, adenomas, and adenocarcinomas of the GI tract	Thyroid, breast, endometrial and renal carcinomas; mucocutaneous lesions; fibrocystic breast disease; leiomyomas of the uterus; macrocephaly
Serrated polyposis (giant hyperplastic polyposis)	Unknown	Both autosomal dominant and recessive patterns reported	Serrated polyps, adenomas, adenocarcinomas of the colon and rectum	Risk of extracolonic tumors appears to be no greater than in normal population
Hereditary mixed polyposis	*CRAC1?*	Autosomal dominant?	Adenomas, serrated polyps, and juvenile polyps as well as adenocarcinomas of the GI tract	Unknown
Li-Fraumeni syndrome	*TP53*	Autosomal dominant	Adenocarcinomas of the colon and rectum	Breast carcinoma, osteosarcoma, and other soft tissue sarcomas; leukemias; adrenal cortical carcinoma; brain tumors
Bloom syndrome	*BLM*	Autosomal recessive	Adenocarcinomas of the GI tract and squamous cell carcinoma of the esophagus	Lymphoma and leukemia, short stature, immunodeficiency, medulloblastoma, Wilms tumor, osteogenic sarcoma, and skin, head and neck, lung, and uterine cancers
Hereditary diffuse gastric cancer	*CDH1*	Autosomal dominant	Signet ring cell carcinoma of the colon and rectum	Diffuse gastric cancer, lobular carcinoma of the breast, prostate cancer

FAP: Familial adenomatous polyposis; HNPCC = familial nonpolyposis colorectal cancer.

ESOPHAGUS/STOMACH/SMALL BOWEL

Familial Esophageal, Gastric, and Small Intestinal Tumors by Syndromes

Syndrome	Gene	Inheritance Pattern	Tumor	Other Manifestations
Tylosis (type A nonepidermolytic palmoplantar keratoderma)	*RHBDF2*	Autosomal dominant	Squamous cell carcinoma of the esophagus	Hyperkeratosis of the palms and soles, leukoplakia
Familial Barrett esophagus	Unknown gene or genes	Thought to be autosomal dominant with incomplete penetrance	Dysplasia and adenocarcinoma of the esophagus and the gastroesophageal junction	Unknown
Familial adenomatous polyposis	*APC*	Autosomal dominant	Fundic gland polyps ± dysplasia, adenomas, adenocarcinomas	Multiple colonic adenomas and carcinomas, ampullary neoplasms, gliomas, desmoids, CHRPE, osteomas and jaw cysts, hepatoblastoma, hepatic adenoma, hepatocellular carcinoma, adrenal cortical neoplasms, papillary thyroid cancer, parathyroid and pituitary adenomas, pancreatic and biliary tract adenocarcinomas
MYH polyposis	*MYH*	Autosomal recessive	Fundic gland polyps ± dysplasia, adenomas, adenocarcinomas	Similar to FAP but with a more attenuated phenotype
Hereditary diffuse gastric cancer	*CDH1*	Autosomal dominant	Diffuse gastric adenocarcinoma, signet ring cell carcinoma in situ	Lobular carcinoma of the breast in women, prostate cancer in men, signet ring cell colon cancer
Germline *KIT* mutation	*KIT*	Autosomal dominant	GISTs	Multiple GISTs at younger age than sporadic, hyperpigmentation, urticaria pigmentosa
Carney-Stratakis syndrome	*SDH* subunits B, C, D	Autosomal dominant	Epithelioid GISTs	Epithelioid gastric GISTs and paragangliomas in children and young adults
Germline platelet-derived growth factor-α mutation	*PDGFRA*	Autosomal dominant	Epithelioid GISTs	Multiple GISTs at a younger age, lipomas, large hands, intestinal neurofibromatosis
Neurofibromatosis type 1	*NF1*	Autosomal dominant	Small intestinal GISTs and adenocarcinomas	Neurofibromas, plexiform neurofibromas, malignant peripheral nerve sheath tumors, CNS gliomas, café au lait spots, Lisch nodules in iris, tibial dysplasia, pheochromocytomas, glomus tumors, carcinoid tumors, gastrointestinal schwannomas, juvenile myelomonocytic leukemia, breast cancer, rhabdomyosarcoma
Lynch syndrome	*MLH1, MSH2, MSH6, PMS2*	Autosomal dominant	Gastric, small intestinal, and periampullary adenocarcinomas	Colonic adenomas and adenocarcinomas; carcinomas of the endometrium, ovaries, adrenal cortex, prostate, bladder, renal pelvis, ureter, and biliary tract; glioblastomas, and sebaceous neoplasms
Peutz-Jeghers syndrome	*LKB1*	Autosomal dominant	Hamartomatous polyps of the gut, adenocarcinoma of the stomach and small intestine	Adenocarcinoma of the colon and pancreas, ovarian sex cord tumor with annular tubules, adenoma malignum of cervix, mucinous tumors of ovaries and fallopian tubes, breast carcinoma, bronchioalveolar carcinomas of the lung, testicular sex cord and Sertoli cell tumors, papillary thyroid cancer
Juvenile polyposis	*SMAD4, BMPR1A, ENG*	Autosomal dominant	Hamartomatous polyps of the gut, adenocarcinoma of the stomach and small intestine	Adenocarcinoma of the colon and pancreas
GAPPS	Unknown	Autosomal dominant	Fundic gland polyps and adenocarcinoma of the stomach	None known

CHRPE: Congenital hypertrophy of retinal pigment epithelium; FAP: Familial adenomatous polyposis; GAPPS: Gastric adenocarcinoma and proximal polyposis of the stomach; GIST: Gastrointestinal stromal tumor.

Familial Neoplasia of Esophagus, Stomach, and Small Intestine

Type of Tumor	Possible Syndromes	Gene	Tests Available
Adenocarcinoma of the esophagus (arising in Barrett mucosa)	Familial Barrett esophagus	Unknown	None
Squamous cell carcinoma of the esophagus	Tylosis	*RHBDF2*	Sequencing of *RHBDF2*
Fundic gland polyps ± dysplasia	FAP, MYH polyposis, gastric adenocarcinoma and GAPPS (most fundic gland polyps are sporadic and associated with gastric acid suppression therapy); multiple polyps with dysplasia should raise issue of polyposis	*APC* or *MYH*	Sequence *FAP* gene first; if normal, look for 2 common mutations in *MYH* gene; gene for GAPPS is unknown
Gastric adenoma	FAP or MYH polyposis (most are sporadic)	*APC* or *MYH*	Sequence *FAP* gene first; if normal, look for 2 common mutations in *MYH* gene
Diffuse gastric cancer	HDGC or Lynch syndrome	*CDH1* (E-cadherin) for HDGC, *MLH1*, *MSH2*, *MSH6*, or *PMS2* for Lynch syndrome	*CDH1* gene mutation in 30-40% of HDGC, presence of signet ring cell carcinoma in situ diagnostic of HDGC; loss of E-cadherin immunostaining in up to 77% of tumors in HDGC; loss of mismatch repair proteins in Lynch syndrome
Intestinal-type gastric cancer	FAP, MYH polyposis, Peutz-Jeghers syndrome, juvenile polyposis, GAPPS	*APC*, *MYH*, *LKB1*, *SMAD4*, *BMPR1A*, *ENG*	Sequencing of genes
GIST	Familial GIST, Carney-Stratakis syndrome (epithelioid GIST with paragangliomas), NF1	*KIT*, *PDGFRA*, *NF1*, and succinate dehydrogenase gene complex	Germline mutational analysis of *KIT* (usually exon 11), *PDGFRA*, *NF1*, or succinate dehydrogenase; loss of immunostaining for succinate dehydrogenase in Carney-Stratakis but not specific for the syndrome
Small intestinal adenoma (usually periampullary duodenum)	FAP or MYH polyposis	*APC* or *MYH*	Sequence *FAP* gene first; if normal, look for 2 common mutations in *MYH* gene
Small intestinal adenocarcinoma	FAP, MYH polyposis, Lynch syndrome, Peutz-Jeghers syndrome, juvenile polyposis, NF1	*APC*, *MYH*, *MLH1*, *MSH2*, *MSH6*, *PMS2*, *LKB1*, *SMAD4*, *BMPR1A*, *ENG*, *NF1*	Sequencing of all genes, immunostaining for MLH1, MSH2, MSH6, and PMS2 as well as microsatellite instability testing (Lynch)

FAP: Familial adenomatous polyposis; GAPPS: Gastric adenocarcinoma and proximal polyposis of the stomach; GIST: Gastrointestinal stromal tumor; HDGC: Hereditary diffuse gastric cancer; NF1: Neurofibromatosis type 1.

Genitourinary

BLADDER

High-Grade Poorly Differentiated Carcinoma

Antibody	Prostate Carcinoma	Urothelial Carcinoma
PSMA	> 95% (best)	0%
PSA	68-94%	0%
PAP	78-95%	0%
p63	0-18%	70-75%
HMWCK (34bE12)	6-10%	65-100%
GATA3	0-3%	67%
S100	0-1%	78-86%
Uroplakin-3	0%	57-60%
Thrombomodulin	0%	49-69%

Flat Urothelial Lesions With Atypia

Antibody	Normal Urothelium	Reactive Urothelium	Carcinoma In Situ
CK20	Umbrella layer only	Umbrella layer only	Full-thickness urothelium
CD44	Basal layer only	Intermediate cells to full thickness	Basal layer only or loss of expression
p53 (nuclear)	Rare cells; weak reactivity	Rare cells; weak reactivity	Diffuse, strong reactivity

Urothelial Carcinoma-Associated Markers in Metastatic Setting

Antibody	Sensitivity for Urothelial Carcinoma
p63	60-90%
S100p	78-86%
GATA3	67%
CK7/CK20	65%
Thrombomodulin	49-69%
Uroplakin-3	57-60%

2010 AJCC Staging for Bladder Cancer

Stage	Definition
Primary Tumor (pT)	
pT0	No evidence of primary tumor
pTa	Noninvasive papillary carcinoma
pTis	Carcinoma in situ: "Flat tumor"
pT1	Tumor involves subepithelial connective tissue
pT2	Tumor invades muscularis propria
pT2a	Tumor invades superficial muscularis propria (inner half)
pT2b	Tumor invades deep muscularis propria (outer half)
pT3	Tumor invades perivesical tissue
pT3a	Microscopically
pT3b	Macroscopically (extravesical mass)
pT4	Tumor invades any of the following: Prostatic stroma, seminal vesicles, uterus, vagina, pelvic wall, abdominal wall
pT4a	Tumor invades prostatic stroma, uterus, vagina
pT4b	Tumor invades pelvic wall, abdominal wall
Regional Lymph Nodes (pN)	
N0	No lymph node metastasis
N1	Single regional lymph node metastasis in the true pelvis (hypogastric, obturator, external iliac, or presacral lymph node)
N2	Multiple regional lymph node metastasis in the true pelvis (hypogastric, obturator, external iliac, or presacral lymph node)
N3	Lymph node metastasis to the common iliac lymph nodes
Distant Metastasis (M)	
M0	No distant metastasis
M1	Distant metastasis

Bladder Cancer Staging

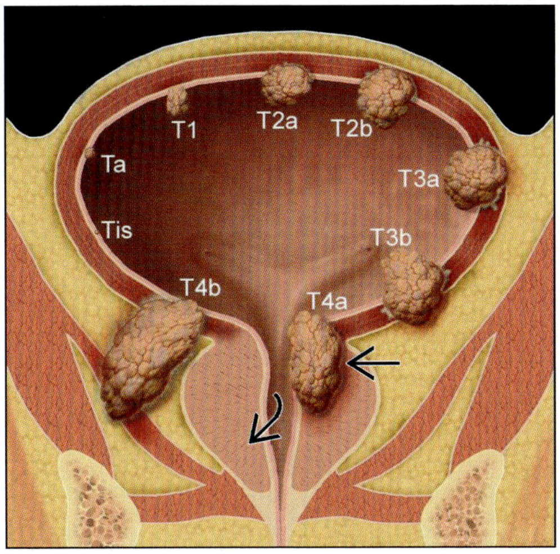

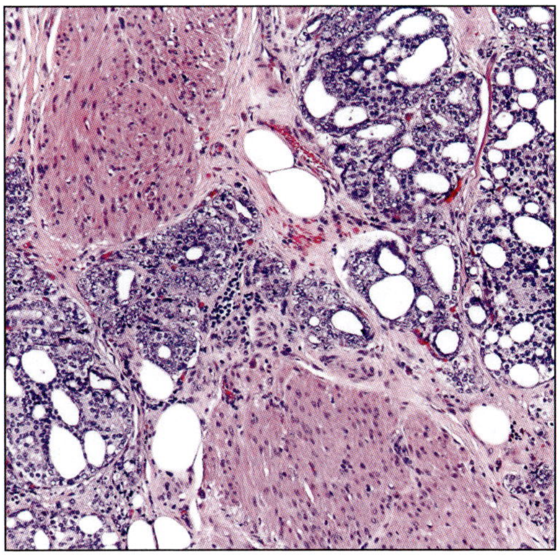

(Left) *Graphic image shows different pT stages of bladder cancer. Bladder cancer pT staging is defined by the level of invasion of bladder wall and adjacent structures. In the 2010 AJCC system, intraurethral extension into prostate ↷ was excluded from pT4a tumors, which now includes only transmural invasion into prostate →.* **(Right)** *H&E shows urothelial carcinoma invading into the muscularis propria (MP) (pT2). MP is composed of large compact muscle bundles. Note presence of intra-MP fat.*

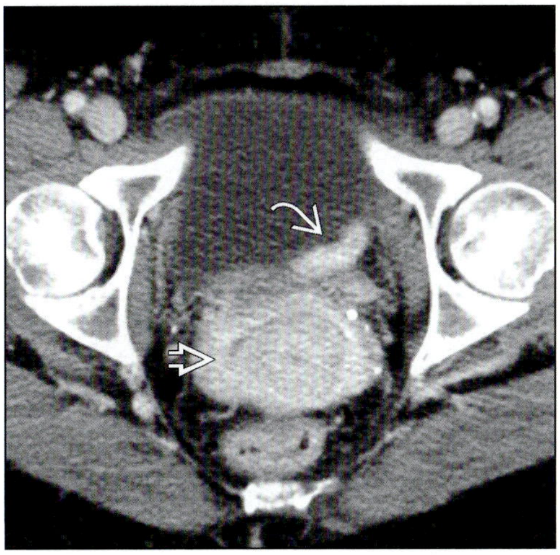

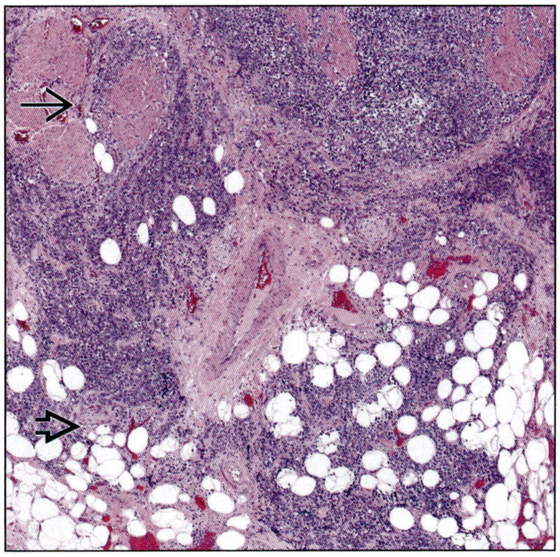

(Left) *Axial CECT shows a sessile mass in the bladder ↷ with enhancement greater than that of the bladder wall. The mass straddles the ureterovesical junction. The cervix is noted ➔ for orientation.* **(Right)** *Low-power view shows urothelial carcinoma infiltrating through the MP → and extending into perivesical fat (pT3) ⇨. The MP-perivesical fat boundary is usually irregular because of fat extension into MP, complicating assessment of microscopic perivesical tissue invasion.*

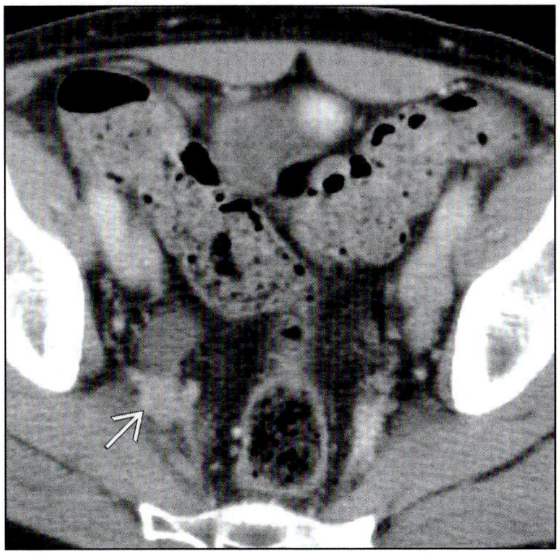

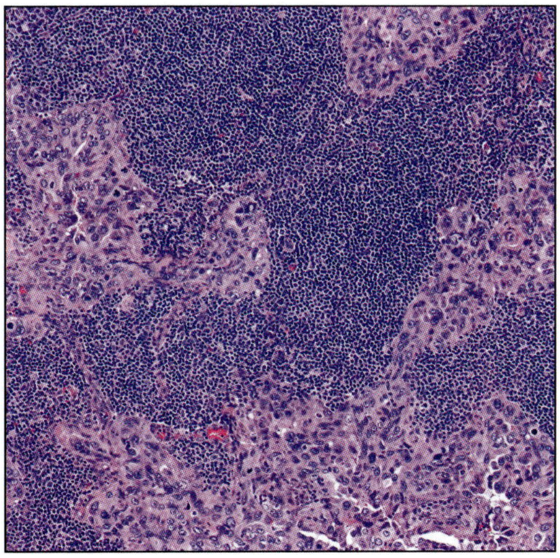

(Left) *Axial CECT shows a pelvic lymphadenopathy ➔ due to bladder cancer.* **(Right)** *H&E shows a pelvic lymph node involved by metastatic urothelial carcinoma. Metastatic foci can be discrete in a post-neoadjuvant setting in which there is shrinkage of tumor. It is important to document the number and location of positive nodes for pN substaging. Involvement of common iliac lymph node is staged as pN3. Size of lymph node metastasis is suggested to have prognostic significance.*

Immunohistochemical Features

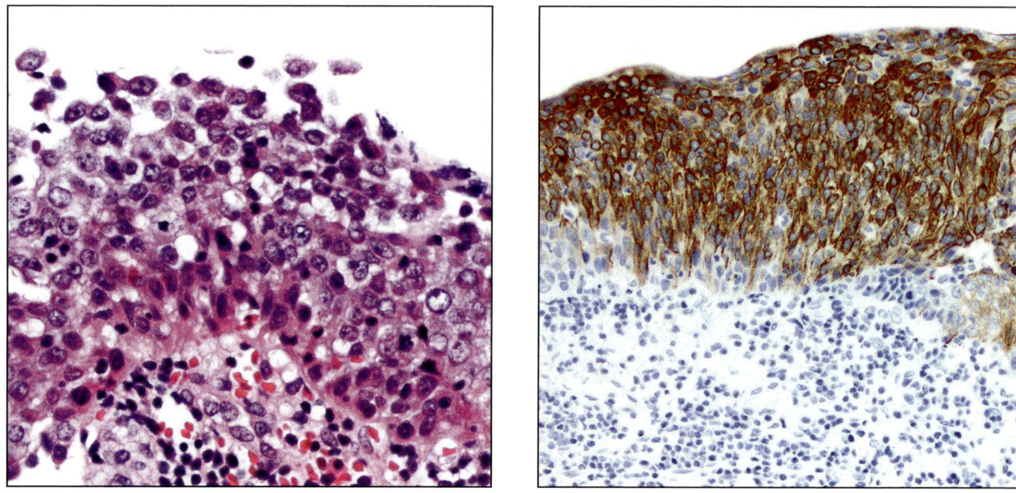

(Left) *H&E shows CIS with nuclear pleomorphism and prominent nucleoli. In some instances, distinction between CIS and reactive atypia can be difficult, necessitating use of ancillary immunostains (CK20, CD44, and p53).* ***(Right)*** *CK20 shows full-thickness staining of urothelium in CIS. In normal and reactive urothelium, CK20 is expressed only in the surface umbrella cell layer. When interpreting immunoreactivity in CIS, it is crucial to match the exact focus to the corresponding H&E stain.*

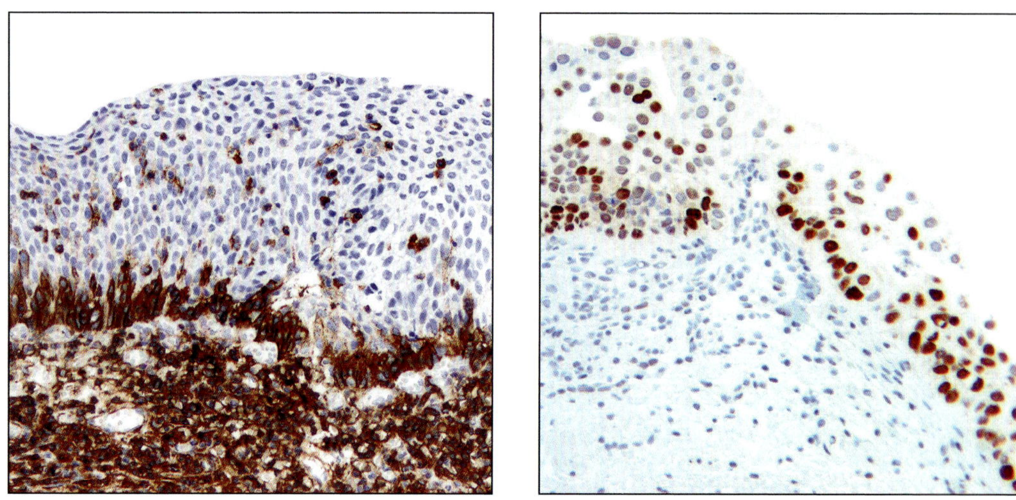

(Left) *CD44 in CIS shows staining in basal and few parabasal cells and with no staining in most cells. In reactive urothelium, CD44 staining extends to intermediate cells or is full thickness (not shown). Note the positive staining in lymphocytes, which serves as internal positive control.* ***(Right)*** *p53 shows diffuse (> 50%) nuclear staining in CIS. Full-thickness nuclear p53 staining is diagnostic of CIS. It is recommended that CK20, CD44, and p53 should be performed together as a panel.*

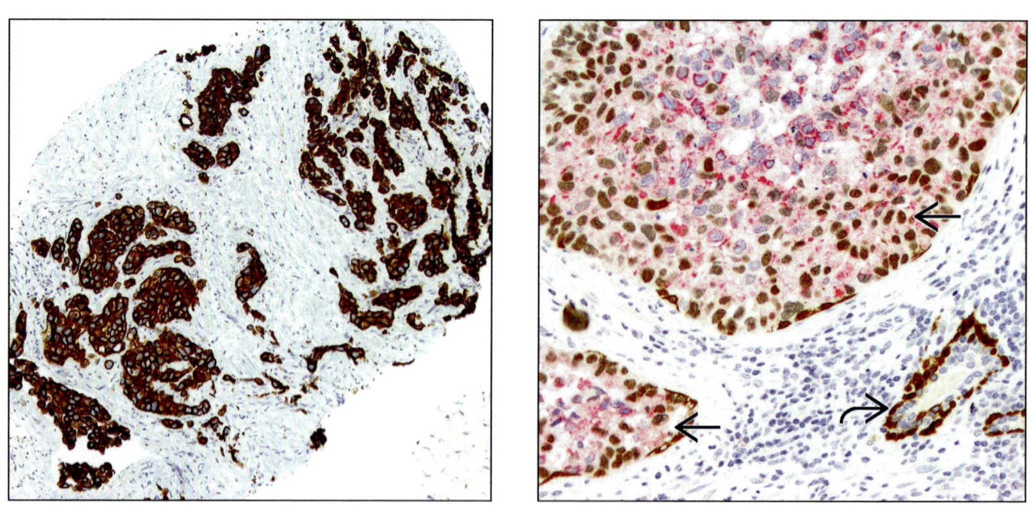

(Left) *Needle biopsy shows urothelial carcinoma involving prostate parenchyma highlighted by diffuse HMWCK staining. Prostate carcinoma is typically negative for HMWCK.* ***(Right)*** *Dual chromogen stain of AMACR (red) and prostatic basal cell markers (HMWCK and p63) (brown) shows nuclear p63 staining and some cytoplasmic AMACR staining in this urothelial carcinoma → involving the prostate. Note the adjacent benign prostatic glands positive for basal cell markers and no AMACR staining ↪.*

Immunohistochemical Features

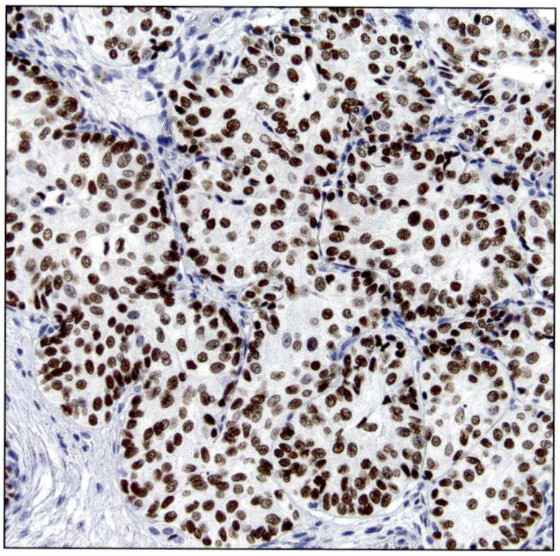

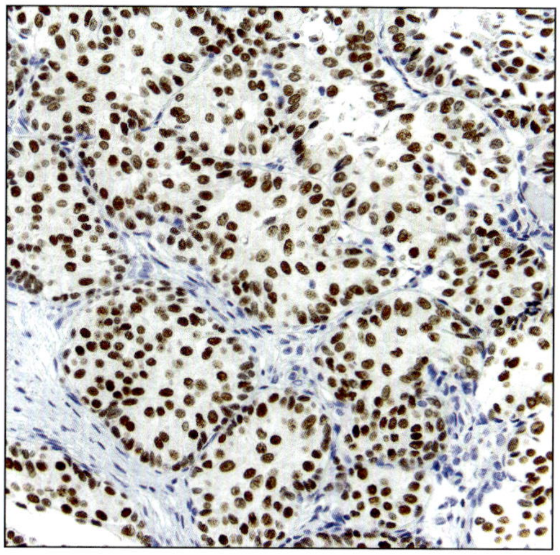

(Left) p63 shows diffuse nuclear staining in urothelial carcinoma. In the GU tract, p63 is helpful when distinguishing urothelial carcinoma from prostate or renal cell carcinomas, which are both p63 negative. *(Right)* GATA3 shows diffuse nuclear staining in urothelial carcinoma. Compared to p63, GATA3 is more urothelial lineage specific and is helpful in the metastatic setting. Other GATA3-positive tumors include ductal breast carcinoma and some uterine cervical carcinomas.

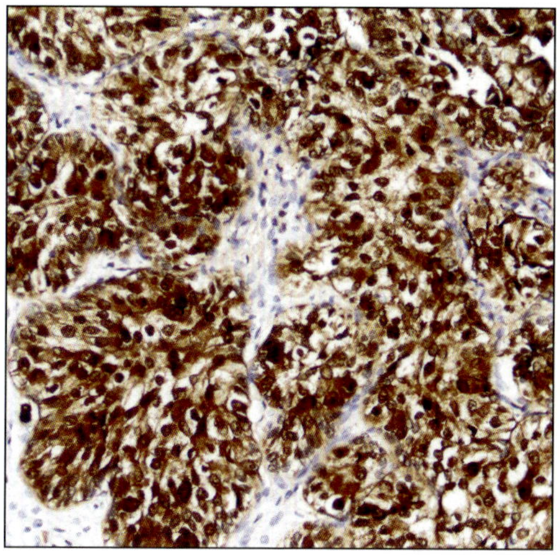

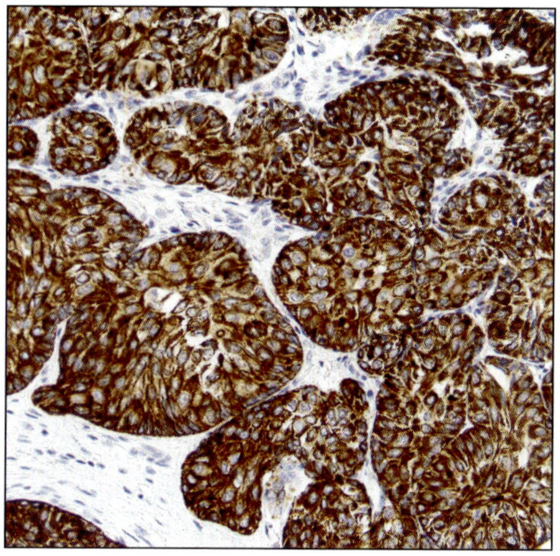

(Left) S100-pla shows nuclear and cytoplasmic positivity in urothelial carcinoma. S100-pla is generally not expressed in squamous cell carcinoma and like GATA3 is helpful when making a distinction from urothelial carcinoma. *(Right)* HMWCK shows strong diffuse cytoplasmic staining in urothelial carcinoma. HMWCK is helpful when distinguishing urothelial carcinoma from prostatic carcinoma. In the prostate, HMWCK is typically expressed only by prostatic basal cells, which are lost in prostate carcinoma.

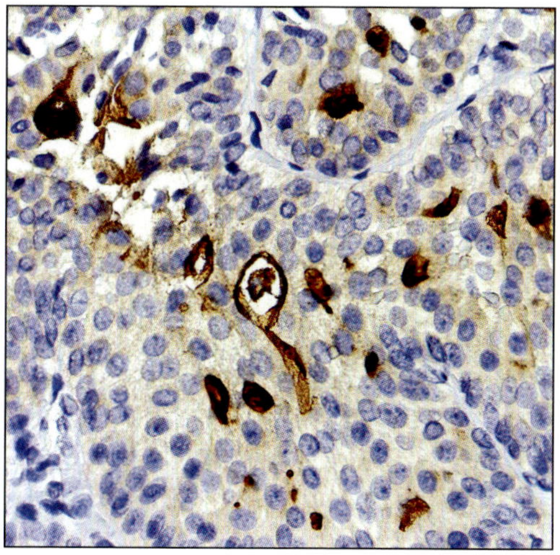

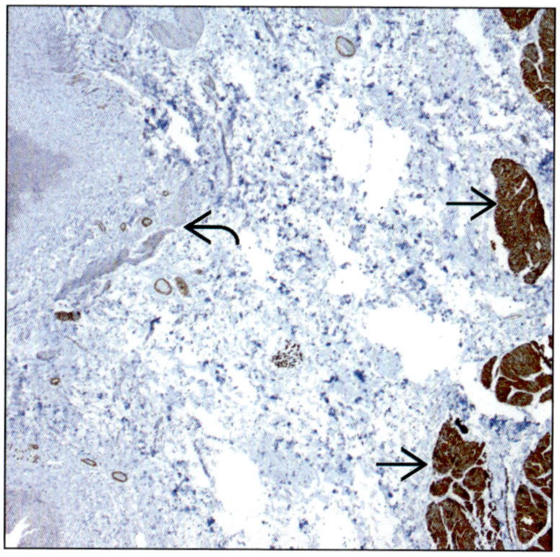

(Left) Uroplakin-3 shows some plaque-like positivity in urothelial carcinoma. Uroplakin-3 is the most specific marker for urothelial lineage. However, sensitivity is not high and reactivity is often focal with this stain. *(Right)* Smoothelin shows differential staining between MP (strong and diffuse staining) → and hyperplastic muscularis mucosae (MM) (weak to absent staining) ↶. Smoothelin can be helpful when distinguishing MP from hyperplastic MM in staging muscle-invasive urothelial carcinoma.

Familial Renal Tumors

Conditions	Gene	Renal Tumors
Tuberous sclerosis	*TSC1* and *TSC2*	Angiomyolipoma, clear cell RCC, benign epithelial cyst, and renal oncocytoma
von Hippel-Lindau	*VHL*	Clear cell RCC and "clear cell tumorlets"
Constitutional chromosome 3 translocation	Unknown; candidate genes: *FHIT*, *TRC8*, *DIRC1*, *DIRC2*, *DIRC3*, *HSPBAP1*, *LSAMP*, *NORE1*, *KCNIP4* and *FBXW7*	Clear cell RCC
Familial clear cell RCC	Unknown	Clear cell RCC
Familial oncocytoma	Unknown	Renal oncocytoma (association with renal oncocytosis or hybrid oncocytic tumors unknown)
Birt-Hogg-Dubé	*FLCN* or *BHD*	Hybrid oncocytic tumors, renal oncocytoma, renal oncocytosis, chromophobe RCC, and clear cell RCC
Hereditary papillary RCC	*MET*	Papillary RCC type 1
Papillary thyroid carcinoma with associated neoplasia	Unknown; candidate genes: *NRAS* and *NTRK1*	Papillary RCC and papillary adenoma; possibly renal oncocytoma
Hereditary hyperparathyroidism-jaw tumor syndrome	*CDC73* or *HRPT2*	Papillary RCC, Wilms tumor, cortical adenoma, and benign epithelial cyst
Hereditary leiomyomatosis and renal cancer	*FH*	Papillary RCC, NOS (mostly classified as papillary RCC type 2 previously)
Succinate dehydrogenase B-associated hereditary paraganglioma/ pheochromocytoma	*SDHB*	RCC, NOS (mostly classified as renal oncocytoma previously)
Familial Wilms tumor	*FWT1*, *FWT2*, and at least 1 unknown gene	Wilms tumor
WT1-associated Wilms tumor (WAGR, DDS, and FS)	*WT1*	Wilms tumor
Overgrowth syndromes (BWS, SGBS, IHH, and PS)	BWS: Most caused by altered expression of *KCNQ1OT1*, *CDKN1C*, *LIT1* or *H19*, and *IGF2* and *CDKN1C* mutation; SGBS: *GPC3*; IHH: Subset with Chr 11p15 abnormality; PS: Unknown, but GPC3 suggested	Wilms tumor

BWS: Beckwith-Wiedemann syndrome; DDS: Denys-Drash syndrome; FS: Frasier syndrome; IHH: Isolated hemihypertrophy; PS: Perlman syndrome; RCC: Renal cell carcinoma; SGBS: Simpson-Golabi-Behmel syndrome; WAGR: Wilms tumor, aniridia, genitourinary malformations, and mental retardation syndrome.

Renal Tumors With Clear/Light-Staining Cytoplasm

Antibody	Clear Cell RCC	Chromophobe RCC	MiTF/TFE Family Translocation-Associated Carcinoma	Clear Cell Papillary RCC	Epithelioid Angiomyolipoma
pax-2	+	+	+	+	-
pax-8	+	+	+	+	-
CAIX	+ (diffuse)	-	- (some focal +)	+ (diffuse)	-
CK7	-	+ (diffuse, occasionally patchy)	-	+ (diffuse, almost 100% tumor cells)	-
CD10	+ (membranous)	- (rarely +)	+ (but often - in TFEB carcinoma)	-	-
Vimentin	+	- (rarely +)	-/+	+	-
Ksp-cadherin	-	+	- (usually)	ND	-
CD117	-	+ (diffuse, often peripheral membranous accentuation	-	ND	-
AMACR	- (rarely focal +)	-	+ (usually)	-	-
EMA/MUC1	+	+	- (rarely focal +)	+	-
PAN-CK (AE1/AE3)	+	+	- (rarely focal +)	+	-
TFE3/TFEB	-	-	+	-	-
Parvalbumin	-	+	-	-	-
Melan-A (MART-1)	-	-	+ in TFEB carcinoma, rarely + in TFE3	-	+
HMB-45	-	-	+ in TFEB carcinoma, rarely + in TFE3	-	+
MITF	-	-	+ in TFEB carcinoma, rarely + in TFE3	-	+
Actin-sm	-	-	-	-	+/-

ND: No data; RCC: Renal cell carcinoma.

Renal Tumors With Papillary or Tubulopapillary Architecture

Antibody	Papillary RCC	Collecting Duct Carcinoma	Metanephric Adenoma	Mucinous Tubular and Spindle Cell Carcinoma	Clear Cell Papillary RCC
CK7	+	+	- (may be + in branching tubules or papillary structures)	+	+
CD10	+ (often luminal pattern)	-	-	-/+ (focal)	-
RCC	+	-	-	V	-/+
AMACR	+	-	-/+	+	-
EMA/MUC1	+	+	- (may be + in branching tubules or papillary structures)	+	+
WT1	-	-	+	-	-
HMWCK (34bE12)	-	+/-	-	-/+	-
CD57	-	ND	+	-	ND
INI1	+	+ (lost in renal medullary carcinoma)	+	+	+
CAIX	- (+ perinecrotic areas and papillary tips)	-/+ (perinecrotic area)	ND	ND	+

ND: No data; RCC: Renal cell carcinoma; V: Variable.

Renal Tumors With Granular/Eosinophilic Cytoplasm

Antibody	Clear Cell RCC, Eosinophilic	Chromophobe RCC, Eosinophilic	Oncocytoma	MiTF/TFE Family Translocation-Associated Carcinoma	Epithelioid Angiomyolipoma
CAIX	+	-	-	- (+ in some cases)	-
Vimentin	+/-	- (rarely +)	-	-/+	+
CD117	-	+	+	-	-
pax-2	+	+/-	+	+/-	-
RCC	+	-/+	-/+	+	-
CK7	-	+/- (scattered to diffuse +)	- (occasionally scattered +)	-	-
CD10	+	-/+	+	+ in TFE3 carcinoma, often - in TFEB	-
Ksp-cadherin	-	+	+	- (usually)	-
Parvalbumin	-	+	+	ND	-
TFE3/TFEB	-	-	-	+	-
Melan-A (MART-1)	-	-	-	+ in TFEB carcinoma, rarely + in TFE3	+
HMB-45	-	-	-	+ in TFEB carcinoma, rarely + in TFE3	+
MiTF	-	-	-	+ in TFEB carcinoma, rarely + in TFE3	+
Actin-sm	-	-	-	-	+/-
EMA/MUC1	+	+ (occasionally only focal +)	- (occasionally only focal +)	- (occasionally only focal +)	-

RCC: Renal cell carcinoma.

KIDNEY

Small Blue Round Cell Tumors of Kidney

Antibody	Wilms Tumor	Ewing Sarcoma/ PNET	Small Cell Carcinoma	Lymphoma	Desmoplastic Small Round Cell Tumor	Synovial Sarcoma, Poorly Differentiated
Vimentin	+	+	-	-	+	+
WT1	+	-	-	-	+	-
S100	-	-	-	-	V	-/+
FLI-1	-	+	-	-	-	-
CD99	+/-	+	-	+/-	-/+	-/+
NSE	-	-	-/+	-	+	ND
HMWCK (34bE12)	-	-/+	+ (often dot-like)	-	-	-/+
EMA/MUC1	-/+	-	-/+	-	-	-/+
CD45 (LCA)	-	-	-	+	-	-
Chromogranin	-	-	+	-	-	-
Desmin	-	-	-	-	+	-
pax-2	+	ND	ND	ND	ND	ND
PAN-CK (AE1/ AE3)	+ (in tubules)	+/- (focal)	+ (often dot-like)	-	+	-/+

ND: No data; PNET: Primitive neuroectodermal tumor; V: Variable.

2010 AJCC Staging System for Kidney Cancer

Stage	Definition
Primary Tumor (T)	
TX	Primary tumor cannot be assessed
T0	No evidence of primary tumor
T1	Tumor ≤ 7 cm in greatest dimension, limited to kidney
T1a	Tumor ≤ 4 cm in greatest dimension, limited to kidney
T1b	Tumor > 4 cm but ≤ 7 cm in greatest dimension, limited to kidney
T2	Tumor > 7 cm in greatest dimension, limited to kidney
T2a	Tumor > 7 cm but ≤ 10 cm in greatest dimension, limited to kidney
T2b	Tumor > 10 cm, limited to kidney
T3	Tumor extends into major veins or perinephric tissues but not into ipsilateral adrenal gland and not beyond Gerota fascia
T3a	Tumor grossly extends into renal vein or its segmental (muscle-containing) branches, or tumor invades perirenal &/or renal sinus fat but not beyond Gerota fascia
T3b	Tumor grossly extends into vena cava below diaphragm
T3c	Tumor grossly extends into vena cava above diaphragm or invades wall of vena cava
T4	Tumor invades beyond Gerota fascia (including contiguous extension into ipsilateral adrenal gland)
Regional Lymph Nodes (N)	
NX	Regional lymph nodes cannot be assessed
N0	No regional lymph node metastasis
N1	Metastasis in regional lymph node(s)
Distant Metastasis (M)	
M0	No distant metastasis
M1	Distant metastasis

Adapted from 7th edition AJCC Staging Forms (2010).

Kidney Cancer Staging

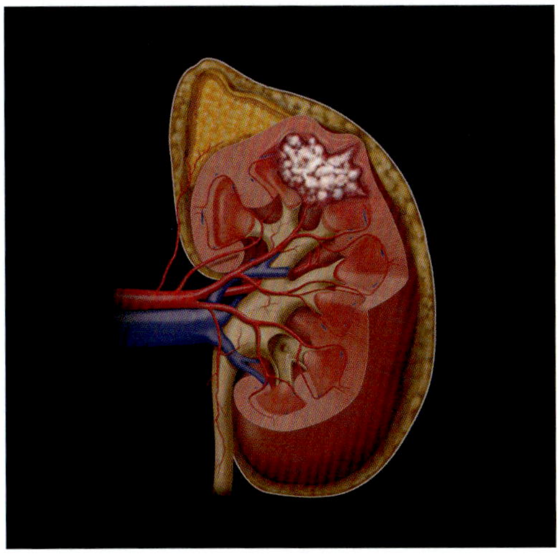

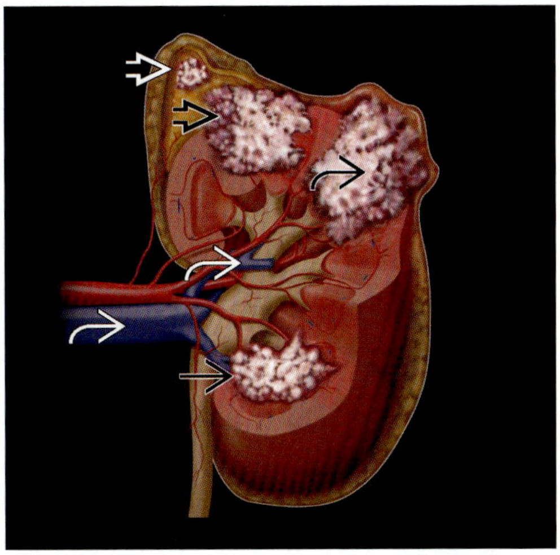

(Left) *Renal cell tumors confined to the kidney and ≤ 7 cm in diameter are assigned stage pT1 (up to 4 cm, pT1a; 4-7 cm, pT1b). Tumors > 7 cm and confined to the kidney are regarded as pT2.* ***(Right)*** *The size criterion does not apply to tumors with extrarenal extension. Tumors with renal sinus ➔ or perirenal fat ➔ or renal vascular ➔ invasion are all assigned stage pT3a. Tumors directly invading the adrenal ➔ are considered pT4, and those with discontinuous adrenal invasion ➔ as pM1.*

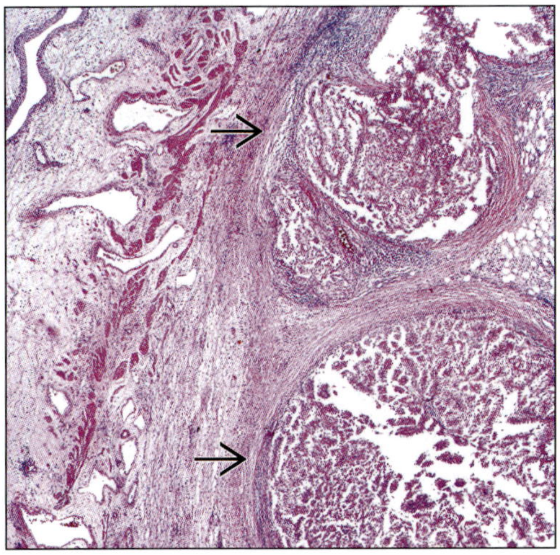

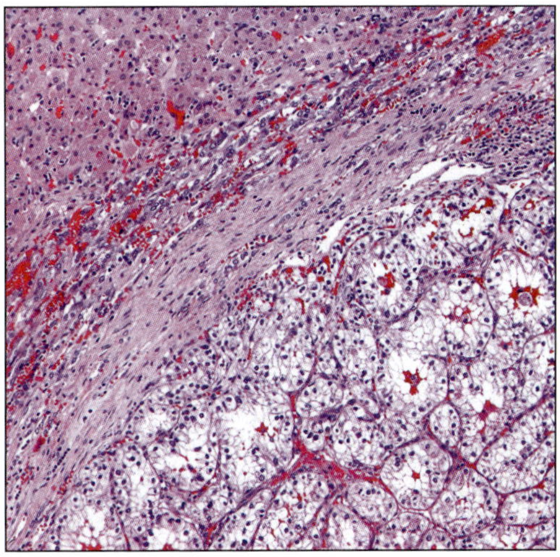

(Left) *Low-power view shows RCC invading the renal sinus ➔ (pT3a). Renal sinus invasion occurs more often via the sinus vessels or by direct infiltration of adipose tissue. Renal sinus should be routinely sampled in nephrectomy specimens to assess for invasion, which significantly upstages small tumors.* ***(Right)*** *This clear cell RCC involves the adrenal gland. Direct contiguous extension into the adrenal is considered pT4 whereas discontinuous involvement is regarded as metastasis (pM1).*

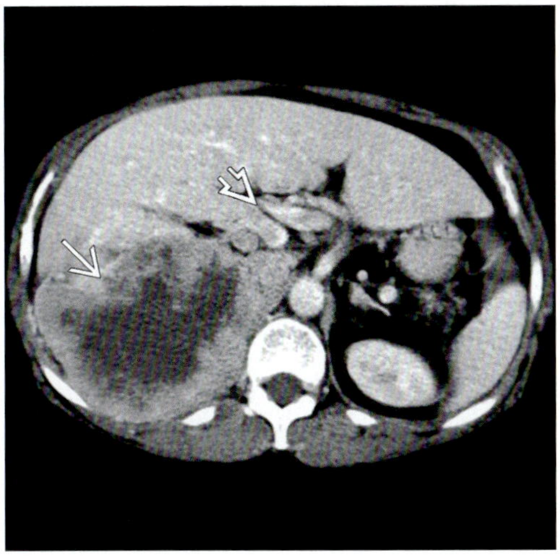

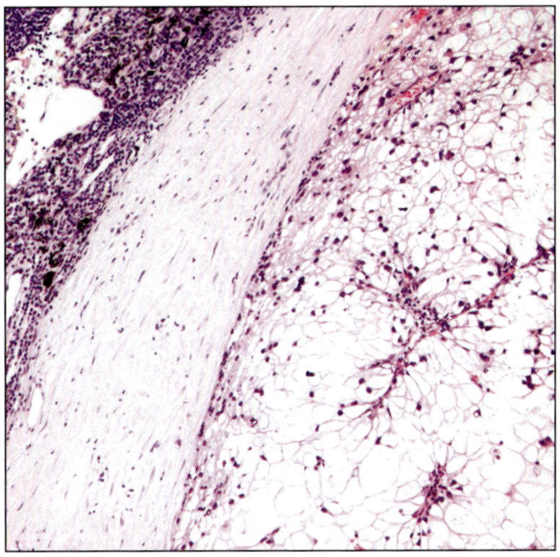

(Left) *Axial CECT shows a large, centrally necrotic mass ➔ invading the posterior margin of the liver (T4). The mass completely engulfs the adrenal gland and has invaded the entire perirenal and pararenal spaces. The IVC ➔ is not invaded but is displaced anteriorly.* ***(Right)*** *This clear cell RCC has metastasized into a pulmonary hilar lymph node. Involvement of distant nonregional lymph nodes is regarded as M1. Diagnosis of metastatic clear cell RCC can often be made by morphology alone.*

Immunohistochemical Features

*(**Left**) pax-2 shows nuclear immunoreactivity in this collecting duct carcinoma. pax-2 is expressed by most RCC subtypes and is helpful in the metastatic setting. (**Right**) Needle core biopsy shows diffuse CAIX immunoreactivity in this clear cell RCC. Diffuse CAIX immunoreactivity is helpful in distinguishing clear cell RCC from its mimics such as eosinophilic chromophobe RCC and renal oncocytoma, which are usually negative. Clear cell papillary RCC also exhibits diffuse CAIX positivity.*

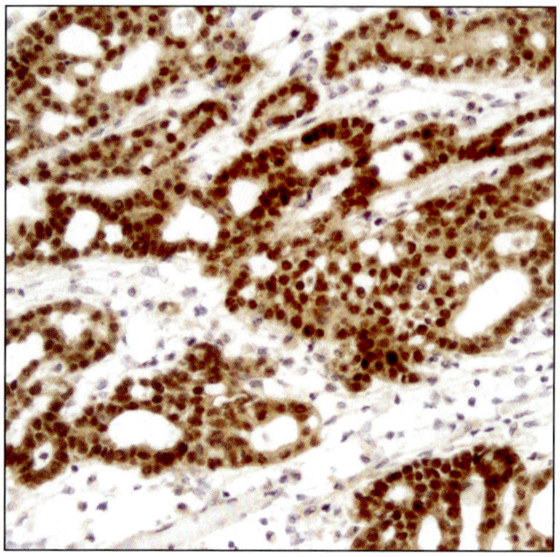

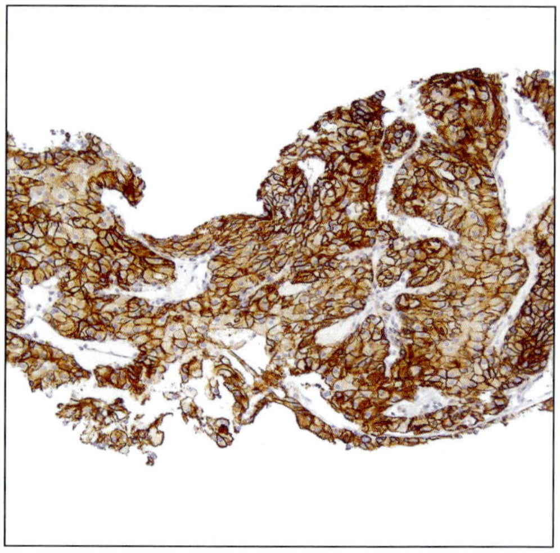

*(**Left**) AMACR shows strong diffuse cytoplasmic immunoreactivity in this papillary RCC. Mucinous tubular and spindle cell carcinoma is diffusely AMACR positive. Other renal tumors with papillae, such as clear cell papillary RCC and collecting duct carcinoma, show absent AMACR staining. Some metanephric adenoma, however, may express AMACR. (**Right**) This clear cell papillary RCC shows diffuse CK7 reactivity. This tumor is also positive for CAIX and negative for AMACR, in contrast to papillary RCC.*

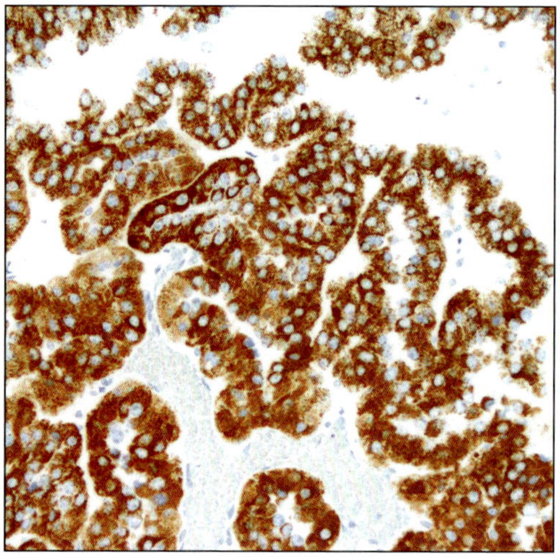

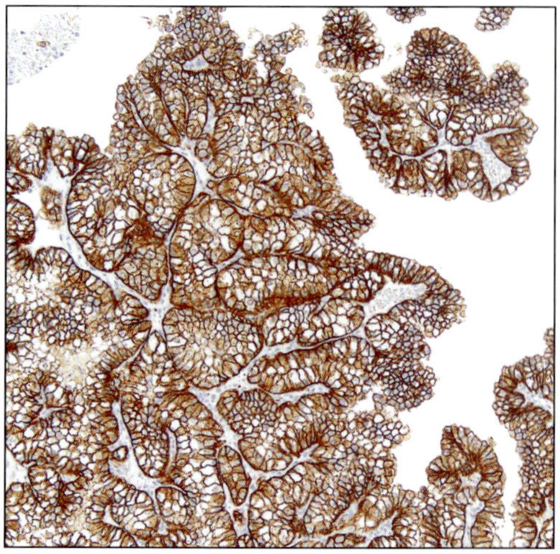

*(**Left**) C-Kit (CD117) is diffusely immunoreactive in this chromophobe RCC. Renal oncocytoma is also diffusely positive with C-Kit and is not helpful to distinguish this tumor. Clear cell RCC with eosinophilic cytoplasm, however, is typically negative with this marker. (**Right**) CK7 shows cytoplasmic positivity in some chromophobe RCC cells. CK7 staining in chromophobe RCC can be diffuse or focal; diffuse staining may help distinguish from oncocytoma, which usually shows scattered or absent staining.*

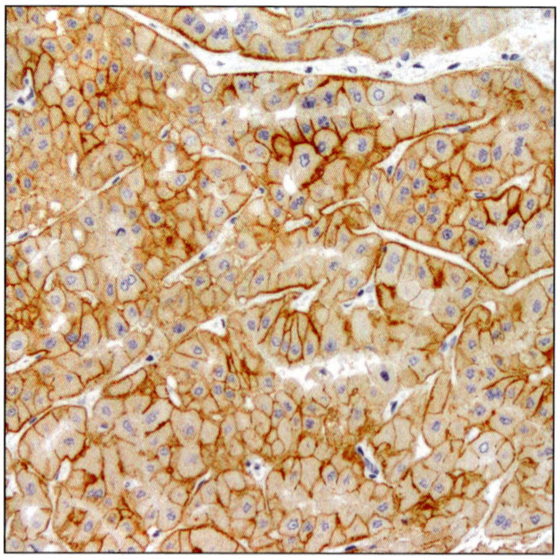

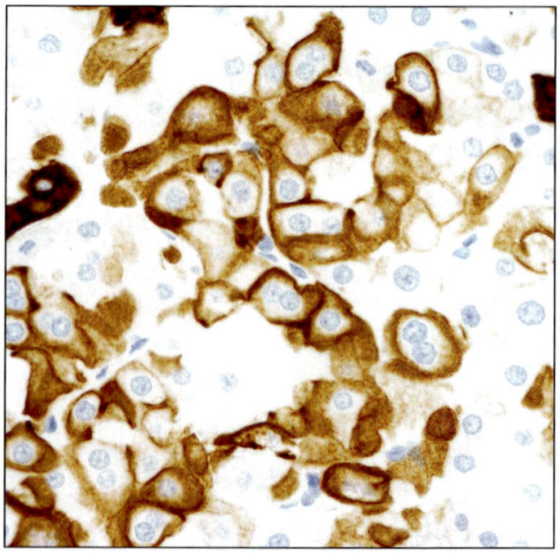

Immunohistochemical Features

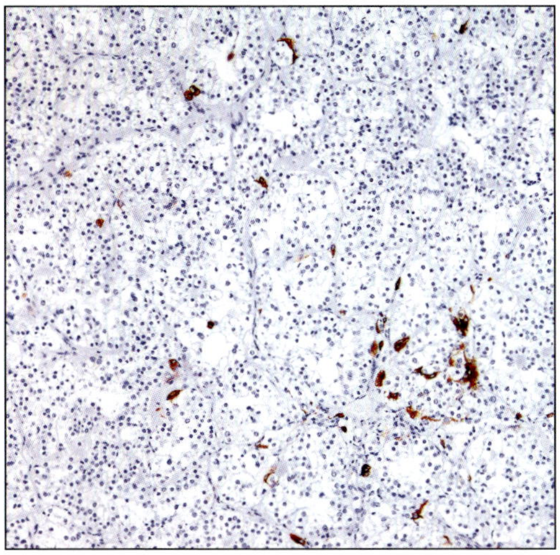
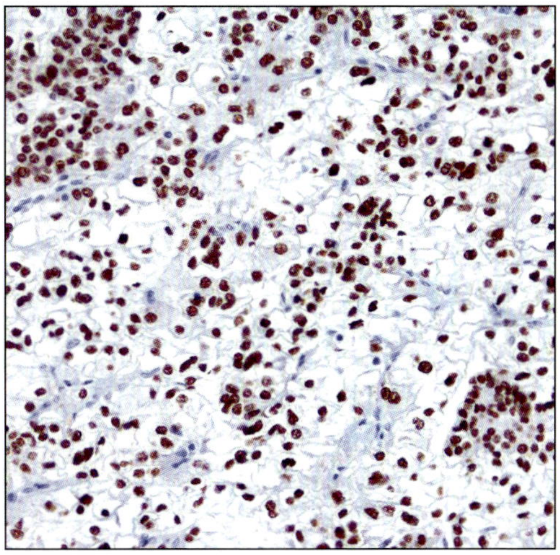

(Left) *CK-PAN shows scattered immunoreactivity in this translocation-associated RCC, where staining is often focal or absent. Lack of CK-PAN is a helpful when translocation-associated RCC is suspected. Clear cell RCC often shows diffuse staining with CK-PAN.* ***(Right)*** *This antibody to TFE3 shows diffuse nuclear positivity in this translocation-associated carcinoma. Specificity of this antibody is still not proven and FISH confirmation may be necessary for cases with atypical morphology.*

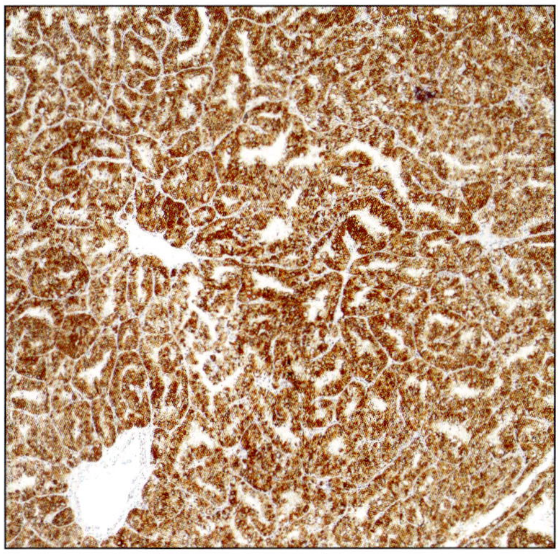
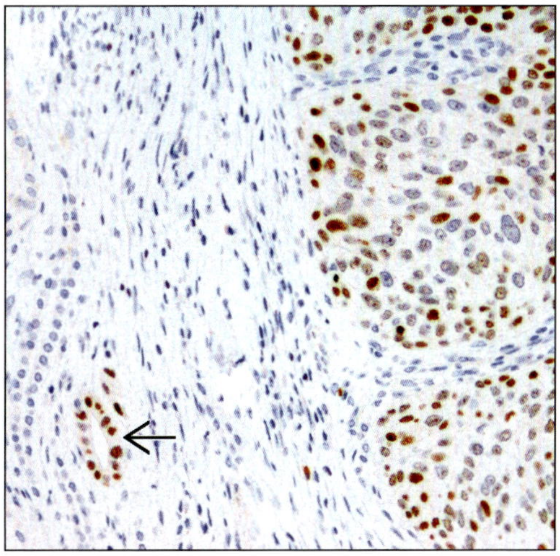

(Left) *This TFEB carcinoma shows diffuse MART-1 staining. Other melanocytic markers such HMB-45 and MITF are often positive in this tumor and are helpful when distinguishing from clear cell RCC, where these are generally negative.* ***(Right)*** *GATA3 shows nuclear positivity in this renal urothelial carcinoma. In contrast, renal carcinomas are often GATA3 negative. Note GATA3 positivity in some collecting tubules. GATA3 is a good compliment for pax-2/ pax-8, which are positive in renal carcinoma.*

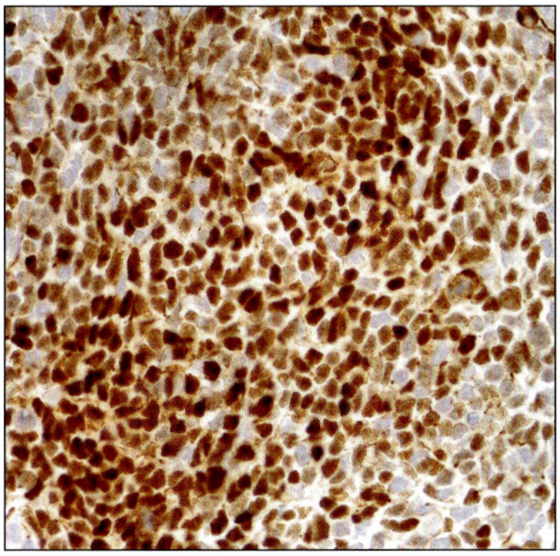
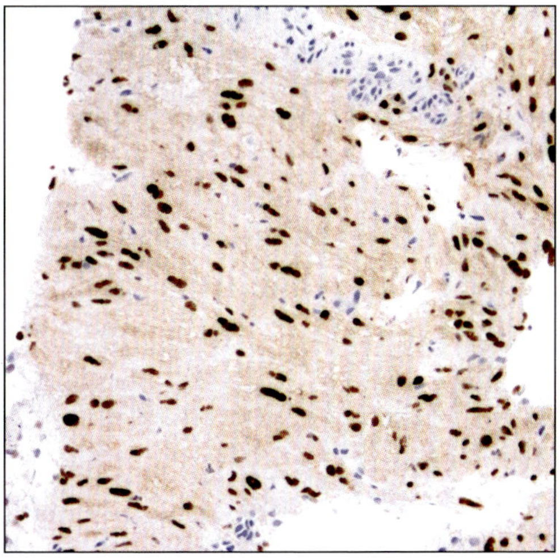

(Left) *WT1 shows diffuse nuclear reactivity in this Wilms tumor. WT1 immunoreactivity is usually seen in blastemal and epithelial components. Metanephric adenoma also exhibits nuclear WT1 positivity.* ***(Right)*** *This fat-poor angiomyolipoma shows diffuse nuclear positivity for MITF. Other melanocytic markers such as MART-1 and HMB-45 are also expressed by this tumor, which helps confirm the diagnosis. Immunoreactivity is usually present in the spindle cell component.*

PROSTATE

Significance of Normal Histoanatomic Structures in Prostate Pathology

Structures	Remarks
Peripheral zone (PZ)	Most common origin for prostate carcinoma (70-75%)
	Most susceptible to inflammation and most common to undergo atrophy
	Uncommon site for benign prostatic hyperplasia (BPH)
Transition zone (TZ)	Most common site for BPH and its myriad morphologic patterns
	Common site for atypical adenomatous hyperplasia (AAH)
	Less commonly, site of origin of prostate carcinoma (15-20%), which tends to be lower grade
Central zone (CZ)	Relatively resistant to prostate carcinoma and inflammation
	CZ glands mimic glands of BPH and prostatic intraepithelial neoplasia (PIN)
Periurethral gland region	Possible origin of uncommon pure primary urothelial carcinoma of prostate
Corpora amylacea	Common in benign prostate glands and rarely seen in carcinoma
Intraluminal crystalloids	Common in prostate carcinoma but may also be seen in benign glands
	Presence in benign glands not a risk factor for subsequent diagnosis of prostate carcinoma
Lipofuscin pigment	Not exclusive for seminal vesicle and ejaculatory duct epithelium and may also be seen uncommonly in benign and malignant prostate glands
Striated muscles in anterior fibromuscular stroma (AFS) and apical region	Benign glands may be seen admixed with striated muscles and thus are not necessarily an invasive or malignant feature
	Adenocarcinoma involving striated muscles at these sites does not constitute extraprostatic extension (EPE)
Prostate capsule	Although not a true capsule, serves as histoanatomic boundary for organ-confined prostate cancer
	Absent in base and not clearly defined in apex, complicating interpretation of EPE at these sites
Nerve	Perineural glands not exclusively associated with carcinoma, unless glands completely circle or are present within a nerve
	1 of the pathways for EPE by carcinoma
Prostatic urethra (PU)	May give rise to urothelial carcinoma (common), squamous carcinoma, adenocarcinoma of prostate, and primary carcinoma of urethra
	Florid nephrogenic adenoma from this site may extend to prostate and mimic prostate carcinoma
	Urothelial carcinoma of PU invading prostate may occur in patients with bladder urothelial carcinoma and should not be staged as pT4 bladder cancer
Verumontanum	May undergo florid glandular hyperplasia, which may be confused with prostate carcinoma
Seminal vesicle (SV)	Rare site for primary malignancy
	Secondary involvement by prostate carcinoma relatively more common and denotes higher tumor stage (pT3b)
	Pseudomalignant features of epithelium may be confused with malignancy in limited sample
Ejaculatory duct (ED)	Involvement by cancer in needle biopsy should not be confused as SV involvement, which denotes higher tumor stage
	Pseudomalignant features of epithelium may be confused with malignancy in limited sample
	Distinction from SV is based on absence of distinct smooth muscle wall
Cowper gland	Resembles minor salivary gland tissue; may mimic low-grade prostate carcinoma
Periprostatic adipose tissue	Involvement by prostate carcinoma constitutes EPE, including needle biopsy specimens
	May be absent over large areas of prostatic surface in prostatectomy specimen, making evaluation of EPE difficult
Paraganglia	May mimic prostate carcinoma with hypernephroid features
	Involvement by carcinoma not always equivalent to EPE, since it may be present rarely within prostate

Important Immunohistochemical Stains in Diagnosis of Prostate Carcinoma

Immunostain	Rationale
Basal cell-associated markers HMWCK (34bE12), CK5/6, p63, basal cell cocktail	Benign vs. malignant proliferation; complete absence of basal cell layer is defining criterion for invasive prostate carcinoma
Prostate carcinoma-associated marker AMACR (p504S)	Benign vs. malignant proliferation; absence of basal cell-associated markers favors invasive prostate carcinoma
Epithelial lineage PAN-CK(AE1/AE3)	Identification of subtle infiltrating cells in post-treatment setting; in differential diagnosis of carcinoma vs. nonepithelial process or malignancy
Prostate lineage-specific marker PSA, PAP, PSMA	Prostatic vs. nonprostatic origin, e.g., Cowper gland, mesonephric remnant, nephrogenic adenoma, seminal vesicle vs. prostate cancer

Benign Mimics of Prostate Carcinoma

Antibody	Seminal Vesicle Ejaculatory Duct	Cowper Gland	Mesonephric Remnants	Verumontanum Hyperplasia	Nephrogenic Adenoma
PSA/PAP	-/+	-/+	-	+/-	-/+
Basal cell marker	+ (basal cell)	+	-/+	+ (basal cell)	-/+
AMACR	-/NS	-	-	-	+/-

NS: Nonspecific, frequently marks pigment. Mesonephric remnants are also positive for CD10, calretinin, and vimentin.

Atypical Small Glandular Proliferations

Antibody	Benign Glands	Postatrophic Hyperplasia and Atrophy	Prostatic Adenocarcinoma	Basal Cell Hyperplasia	Outpouching of High-Grade PIN	AAH (Adenosis)
Basal cell-associated markers	+	+ (patchy)	-	+	+	+/- (patchy)
AMACR	-/+ (rare)	-/+	+ (strong circumferential)	-	+	-/+

AAH: Atypical adenomatous hyperplasia; PIN: Prostatic intraepithelial neoplasia.

Single/Individual Cell Patterns

Antibody	Gleason Pattern 5 Prostate Carcinoma	Post-Treatment Carcinoma	Marked Inflammation	Granulomatous Prostatitis
PAN-CK (AE1/AE3)	+	+	-	-
Basal cell marker	-	-	-	-
AMACR	+	+/-	-	-

2010 AJCC Pathologic Staging of Prostate Cancer

Stage	Definition
*Primary Tumor (pT)**	
pT2	Organ confined
pT2a	Unilateral, 1/2 of 1 side or less
pT2b	Unilateral, involving > 1/2 of side but not both sides
pT2c	Bilateral disease
pT3	Extraprostatic extension
pT3a	Extraprostatic extension or microscopic invasion of bladder neck
pT3b	Seminal vesicle invasion
pT4	Invasion of rectum, levator muscles, &/or pelvic wall
Regional Lymph Nodes (pN)	
pNX	Regional lymph nodes not sampled
pN0	No positive regional lymph nodes
pN1	Metastasis in regional lymph node(s)
Distant Metastasis (M)	
M0	No distant metastasis
M1	Distant metastasis
M1a	Nonregional lymph nodes(s)
M1b	Bone(s)
M1c	Other site(s) with or without bone disease

*Adapted from 7th edition AJCC Staging Forms (2010). *There is no pathologic pT1 classification.*

PROSTATE

Normal Anatomy and Histology

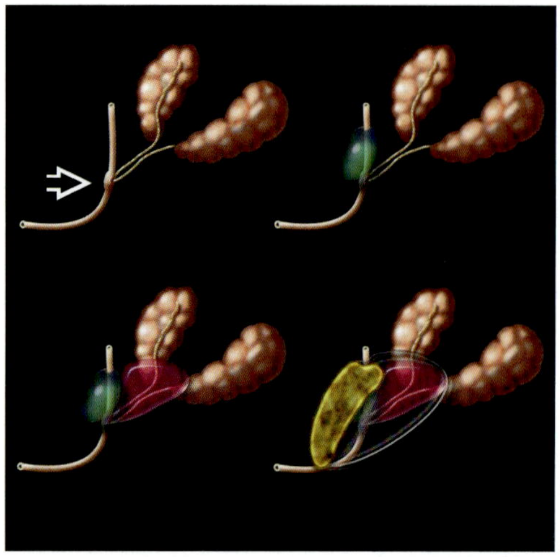
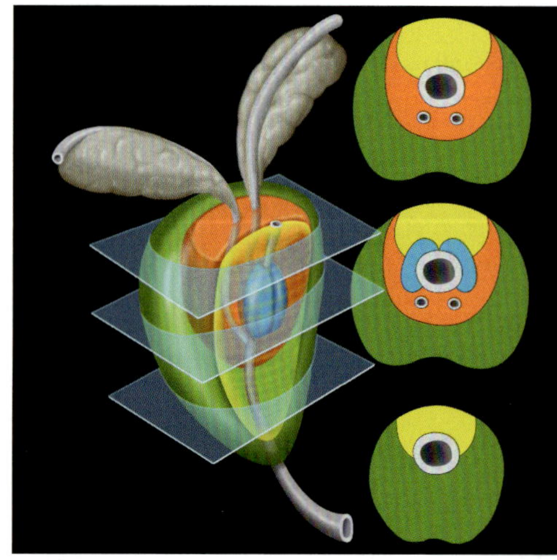

(Left) *PU is divided into proximal PU and distal PU by a mid angulation at the verumontanum where the ED exits ➡. TZ (blue) and CZ (magenta) encase proximal PU and ED, respectively. PZ (transparent) surrounds CZ and distal PU posteriorly. Nonglandular AFS (yellow) is situated anteriorly.* ***(Right)*** *McNeal model uses PU as key anatomic landmark and divides the prostate glandular component into PZ (green), CZ (orange), TZ (blue), and PUGR (white). The AFS (yellow) comprises the midanterior portion.*

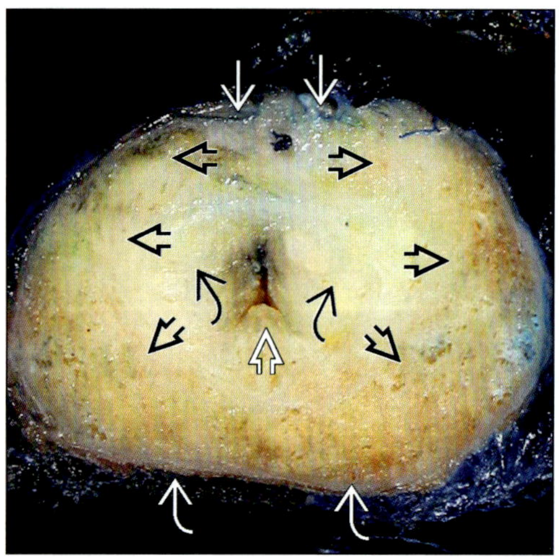
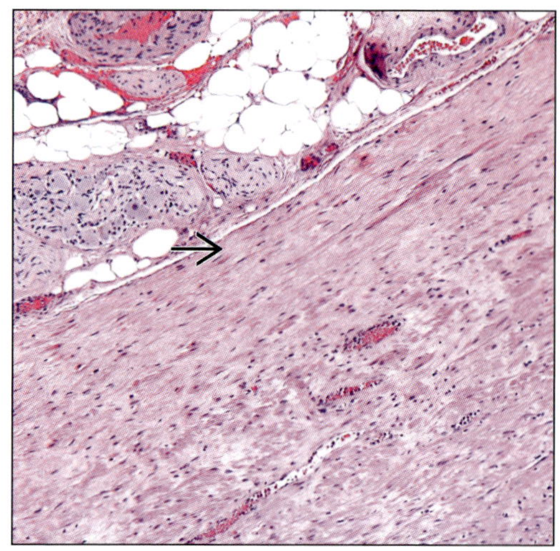

(Left) *Coronal section of the prostate at the verumontanum ➡ shows the peripheral zone ⇨ extending from posterior aspect ➦, surrounding part of transition zone ↷, and abutting the AFS ➡. The central urethra is enveloped by the transition zone.* ***(Right)*** *The prostate "capsule" → is not a true capsule but a condensation of fibromuscular tissue that is an inseparable component of the prostatic stroma. Periprostatic adipose tissues and nerves are present. Involvement of adipose tissue by prostatic carcinoma constitutes EPE.*

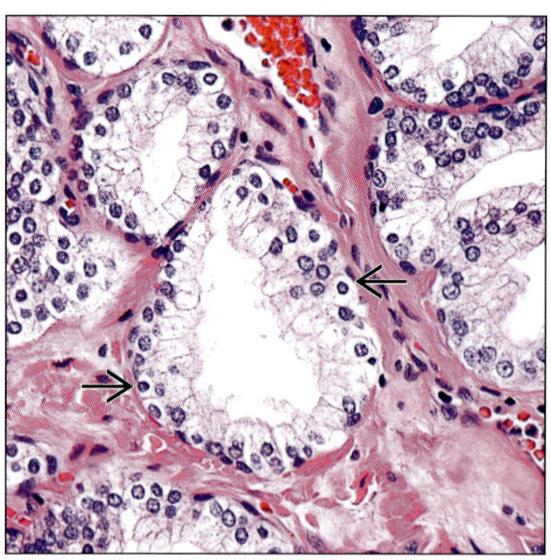
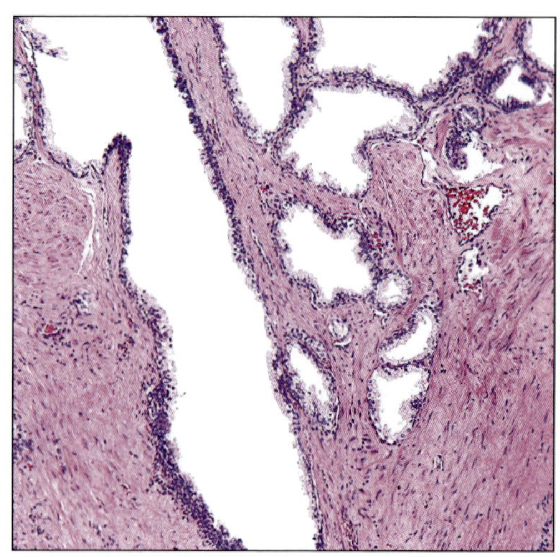

(Left) *Typical benign acini show columnar secretory cells with pale cytoplasm and round, regular, basally oriented nuclei, with indistinct nucleoli. Basal cells → are situated internal to glandular basement membrane outline and contain scant cytoplasm.* ***(Right)*** *The lining of the prostatic duct is similar to that of the adjacent acini. On cross section, ducts and acini are not reliably distinguished unless the longitudinal dimension of the duct is appreciated.*

Cancer Staging

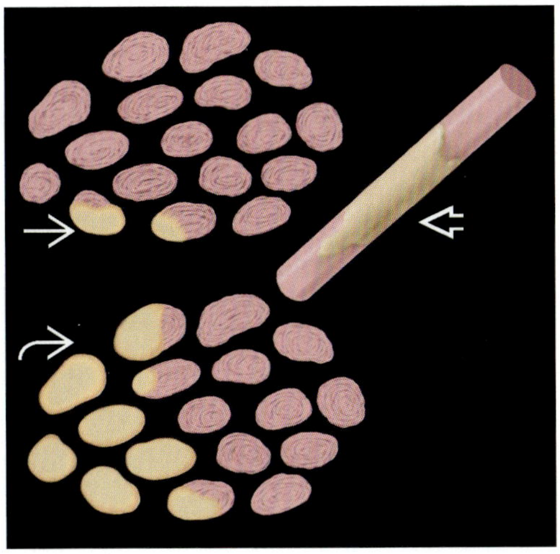

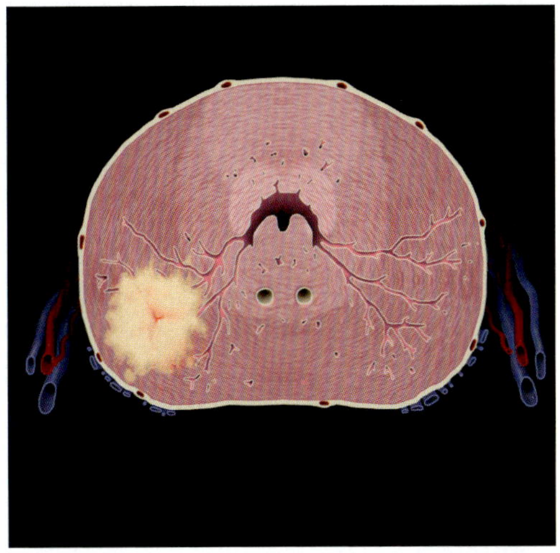

(Left) *Graphic shows examples of incidental T1 prostate carcinoma divided into T1a, < 5% tumor in tissue resected (TURP); T1b, > 5% tumor in tissue resected (TURP); and T1c, tumor identified by needle biopsy (e.g., because of elevated PSA). If unsuspected prostate carcinoma is identified in tissue submitted and is < 5%, then remainder of tissue should be submitted for histologic evaluation.* ***(Right)*** *pT2a shows tumor involving not more than 1/2 of 1 lobe of the prostate.*

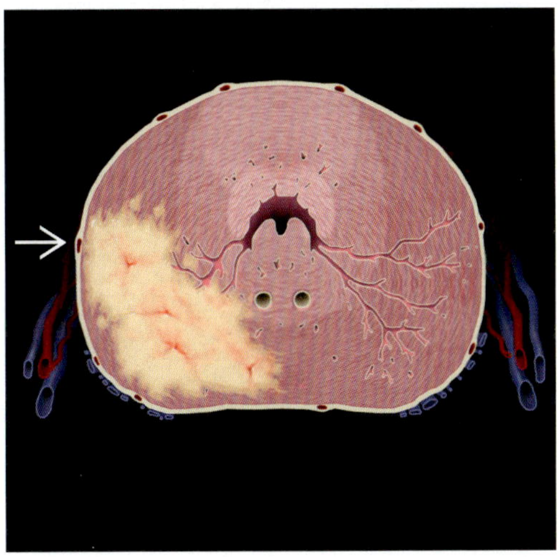

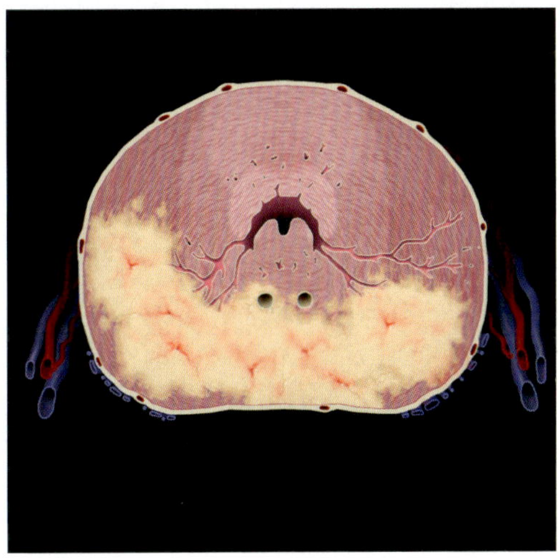

(Left) *pT2b shows tumor involving more than 1/2 of 1 lobe of prostate. This pattern of tumor involvement is uncommon, since prostate carcinoma is usually located at the posterior aspect, and larger tumors tend to involve bilateral posterior sides (pT2c), even without anterior involvement.* ***(Right)*** *pT2c shows organ-confined tumor involving both lobes of the prostate. pT2 subdivisions may act as surrogate for estimating prostate carcinoma volume, which correlates with disease relapse.*

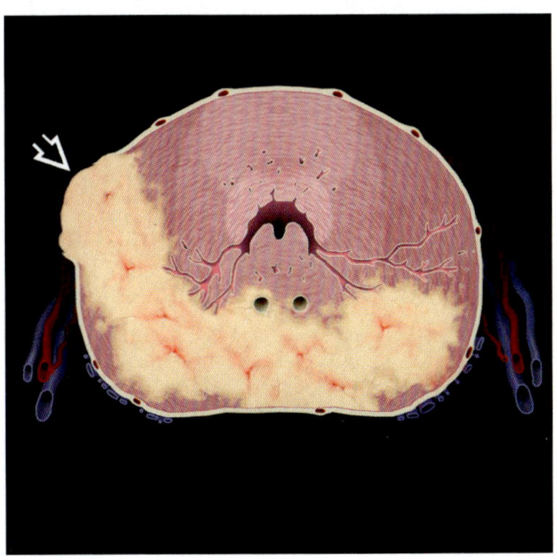

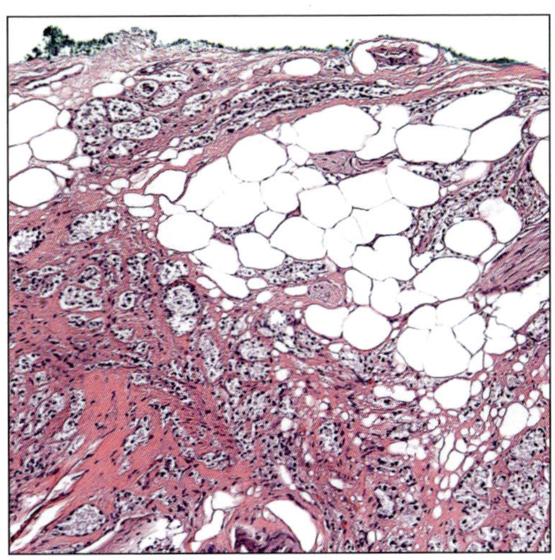

(Left) *EPE by prostate carcinoma indicates pT3 disease. Detection of EPE is most reliably made by histologic examination. DRE and radiographic studies are not sensitive in detecting EPE.* ***(Right)*** *EPE with tumor extension into periprostatic fat is shown, which is the most objective evidence for EPE. Intraprostatic fat is vanishingly rare; thus, fat involvement by prostate carcinoma is considered diagnostic for EPE. EPE most commonly occurs at the posterior and posterolateral aspects of prostate.*

PROSTATE

Cancer Staging

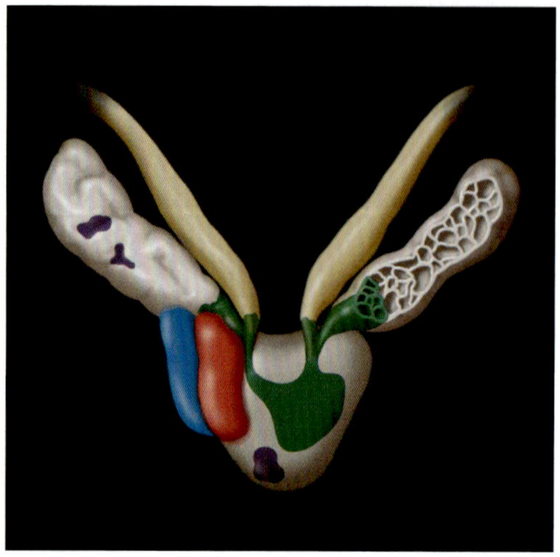

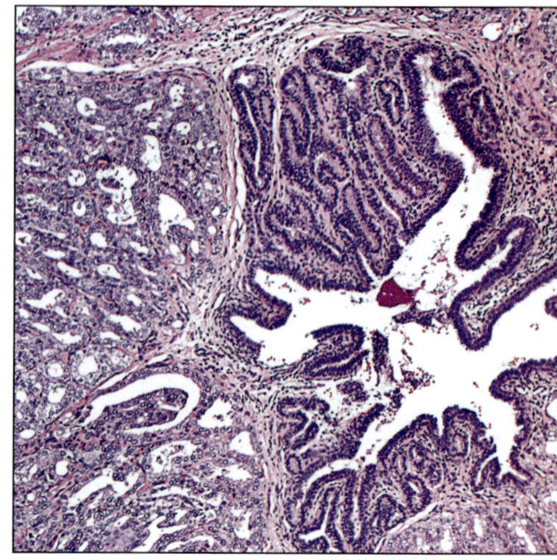

(Left) *Mechanisms of SV involvement by prostate cancer include spread via (a) ejaculatory duct tissue into SV (green), (b) direct extra- (blue) or intraprostatic (red) spread into SV, or (c) noncontiguous metastasis to SV (purple).* ***(Right)*** *Prostate cancer involving the ED shows a tumor adjacent to ED epithelium. Prostate cancer may extend to SV via invasion through the wall and not within the lumen of ED. SV invasion is considered only when there is involvement of SV muscular wall.*

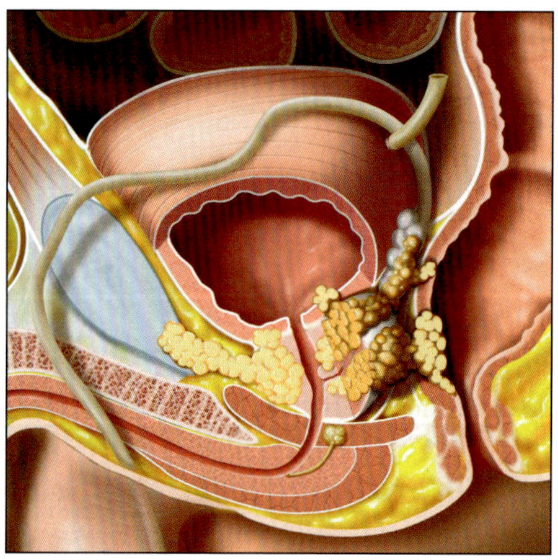

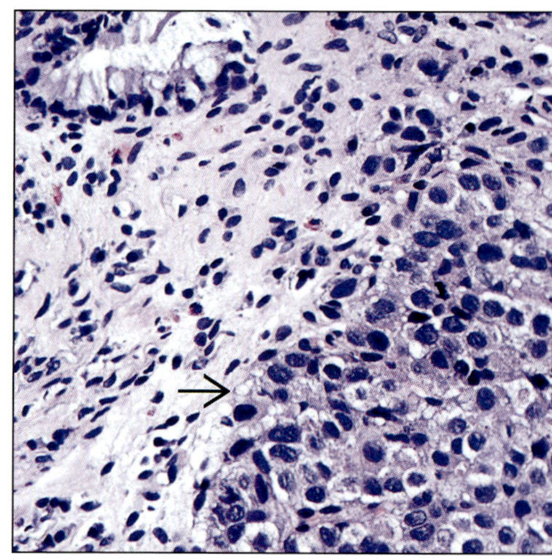

(Left) *pT4 prostate cancer shows tumor invading structures other than SV, such as the bladder, rectum, and anterior pelvic wall. This tumor extent is managed with radiotherapy or hormonal therapy. RP with lymph node dissection may be performed in selected patients (e.g., low volume, no fixation).* ***(Right)*** *Rectal biopsy shows poorly differentiated prostate carcinoma ➔ involving rectal mucosa. This, the highest pT stage, is confirmed histologically, and criteria for pT staging is fulfilled without removal of the tumor.*

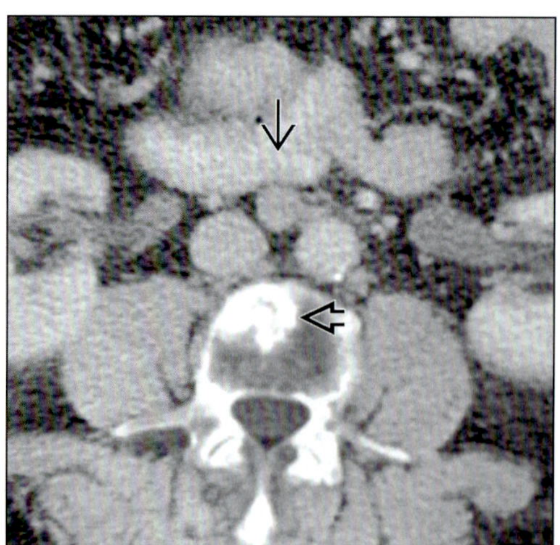

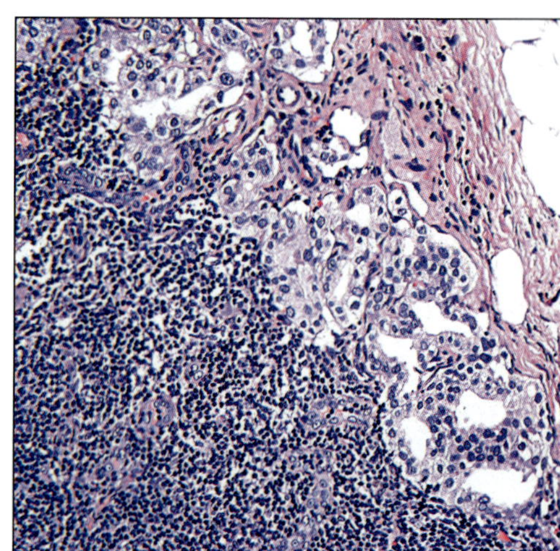

(Left) *Axial CT shows retroperitoneal lymphadenopathy ➔ and sclerotic vertebral metastasis by prostate cancer ➲. Staging pelvic CT or MR is performed for T3 or T4 or in localized prostate cancer with high nomogram probability for lymph node involvement. Due to false positivity, staging MR/CT is usually not performed if GS < 7 or PSA < 20 ng/mL.* ***(Right)*** *Lymph node shows subcapsular metastatic prostate carcinoma. It is important to specify the number of nodes involved.*

Immunohistochemical Features

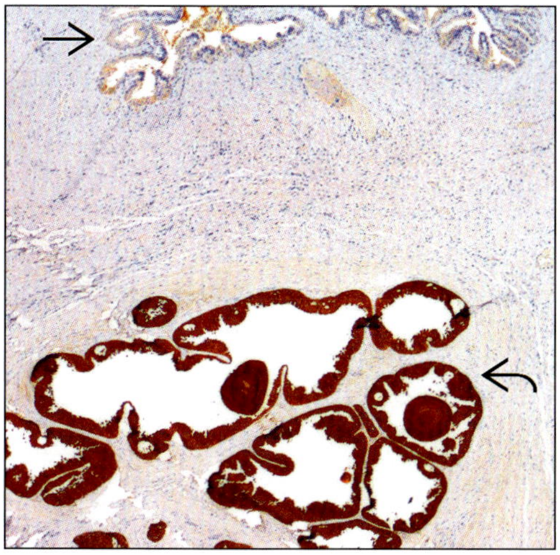
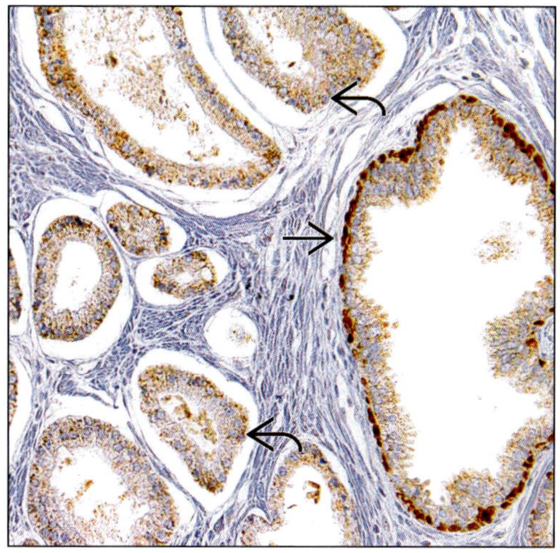

(Left) *PSA shows strong positive reaction in the prostatic acini ⮫ whereas staining is negative in the SV epithelium →.* ***(Right)*** *p63 shows nuclear positivity of basal cells in the benign gland →. Carcinoma glands show absence of p63 staining ⮫. Complete absence of basal cell layer is defining criterion for invasive prostate carcinoma. All glands in the same atypical focus should similarly show complete absence of basal cells as some benign cancer mimics may have patchy basal cell staining.*

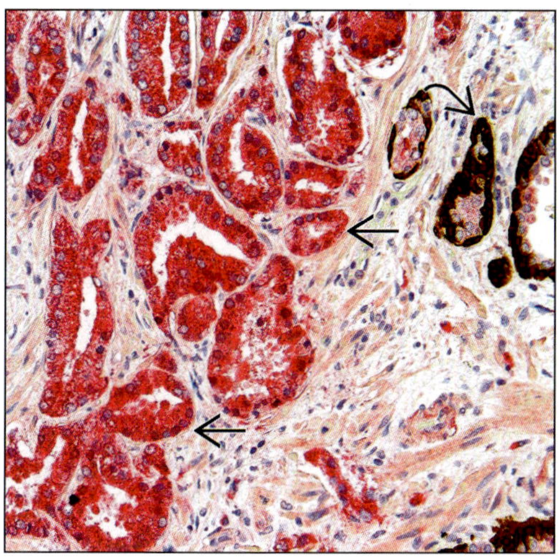
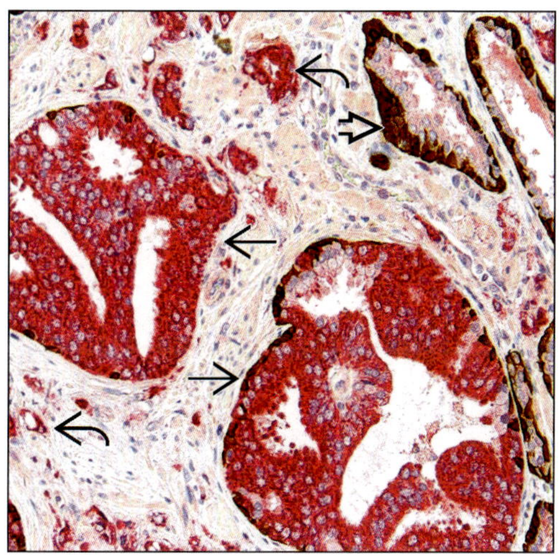

(Left) *Dual chromogen immunostain shows overexpression of AMACR (red) in carcinoma glands → and basal cell markers (HMWCK and p63) (brown) positivity only in benign glands ⮫. AMACR staining in carcinoma is typically granular and circumferential.* ***(Right)*** *Dual chromogen immunostain shows overexpression of AMACR (red) and basal cell markers (brown) positivity in HGPIN glands →. Carcinoma glands show AMACR overexpression ⮫. Benign glands show basal cell markers staining ⇨.*

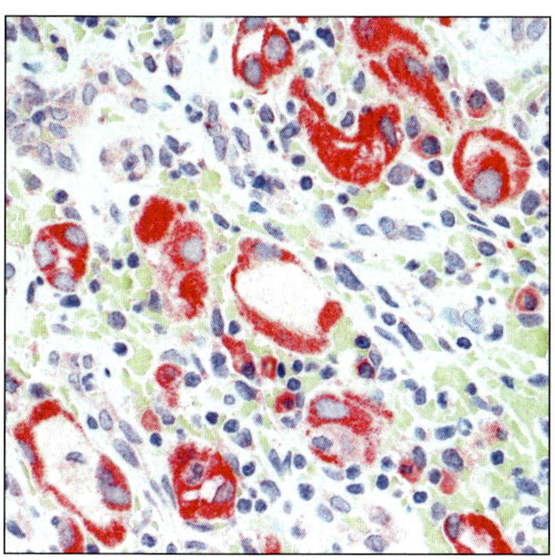
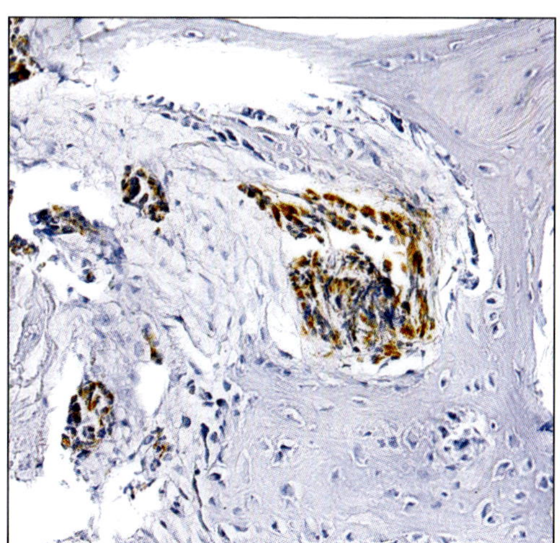

(Left) *AMACR immunostain shows cytoplasmic staining in tubules of nephrogenic adenoma. Prostatic urethral nephrogenic adenoma may proliferate inward into the prostate and mimic a Gleason grade 3 acinar carcinoma, confounded by the similar AMACR staining.* ***(Right)*** *Bone biopsy shows foci of metastatic prostate carcinoma highlighted by PSMA staining. Prostate-lineage markers PSMA, PSA, and PAP have good sensitivity in the metastatic setting. Among these, PSMA is considered the most sensitive.*

RENAL PELVIS AND URETER

Diagnosis of Lynch (HNPCC) Syndrome Upper Urinary Tract UCa

Examination	Findings
Clinical	Patient < 60 years old
	History of HNPCC-associated cancer (e.g., colon cancer, uterine cancer)
	First-degree relative < 50 years of age with HNPCC-associated cancer
	2 first-degree relatives with HNPCC-associated cancer
Pathologic	Upper tract UCa more often with inverted growth pattern (sensitivity and specificity of 0.82 for high frequency MSI [MSI-H])
Immunohistochemical screening with antibodies against MLH1, MSH2, PMS2, and MSH6	Loss of nuclear staining with normal nuclear staining in internal control cells (such as normal lymphocytes) indicates loss of that protein
MSI testing by PCR using NCI consensus panel of 2 mononucleotide (BAT25 and BAT26) and 3 dinucleotide (D2S123, D5S346, and D17S250) markers	MSI phenotypes: **MSI-H** if size alterations or shifts observed in ≥ 2 markers, low MSI (**MSI-L**) if only 1 marker shows instability, and microsatellite stable (**MSS**) if none of the markers show instability

HNPCC: Hereditary nonpolyposis rectal cancer; MSI: Microsatellite instability; NCI: National Cancer Institute; UCa: Urothelial carcinoma.

Carcinomas Involving Kidney &/or Renal Pelvis

Antibody	Urothelial Carcinoma	Collecting Duct Carcinoma	Renal Cell Carcinoma, NOS
p63	+	-	-
GATA3	+	- (data limited)	-
CK7	+	+	-/+
CK20	+/-	- (rarely focal +)	-
HMWCK (34bE12)	+	-/+	-
Thrombomodulin	+/-	-	-
Uroplakin-3	+/-	-	-
pax-8	- (rarely focal +)	+/-	+
pax-2	- (rarely focal +)	+/-	+
RCC	-	-	+/-
Vimentin	-/+	+	+/-
INI1	+	+ (loss in medullary)	+

2010 AJCC Staging System for Renal Pelvis and Ureter Cancer

Stage	Definition
Primary Tumor (pT)	
pTX	Primary tumor cannot be assessed
pT0	No evidence of primary tumor
pTa	Papillary noninvasive carcinoma
pTis	Carcinoma in situ
pT1	Tumor invades subepithelial connective tissue
pT2	Tumor invades the muscularis
pT3	For renal pelvis only: Tumor invades beyond muscularis into peripelvic fat or the renal parenchyma
	For ureter only: Tumor invades beyond muscularis into periureteric fat
pT4	Tumor invades adjacent organs or through the kidney into the perinephric fat
Regional Lymph Nodes (pN)	
pNX	Regional lymph nodes cannot be assessed
pN0	No regional lymph node metastasis
pN1	Metastasis in a single lymph node, ≤ 2 cm in greatest dimension
pN2	Metastasis in a single lymph node, > 2 cm but not > 5 cm in greatest dimension; or multiple lymph nodes, none > 5 cm in greatest dimension
pN3	Metastasis in a lymph node, > 5 cm in greatest dimension
Distant Metastasis (M)	
M0	No distant metastasis
M1	Distant metastasis

Adapted from 7th edition AJCC Staging Forms (2010).

Staging and Immunohistochemical Features

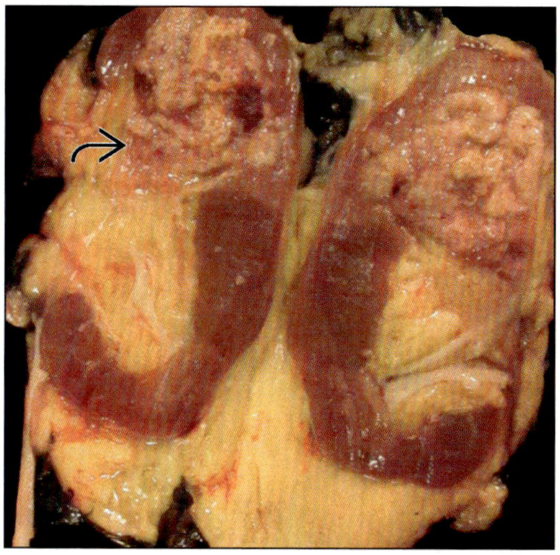

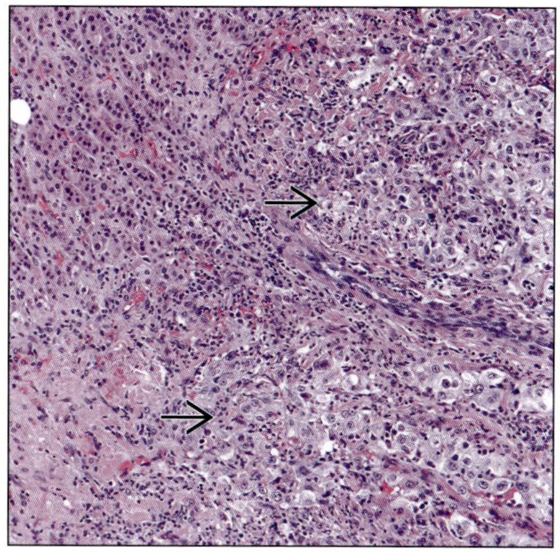

(Left) *Gross image shows urothelial carcinoma ↗ arising from upper renal pelvis and infiltrating into the renal parenchyma without involving the perinephric fat (pT3). Urothelial carcinoma shows an infiltrative border in contrast to most renal carcinomas.* ***(Right)*** *Low-power view shows adrenal cortex involved by urothelial carcinoma →. Extension by renal urothelial carcinoma into adrenal or perinephric fat is considered pT4. Five-year specific survival of pT4 renal urothelial carcinoma is < 10%.*

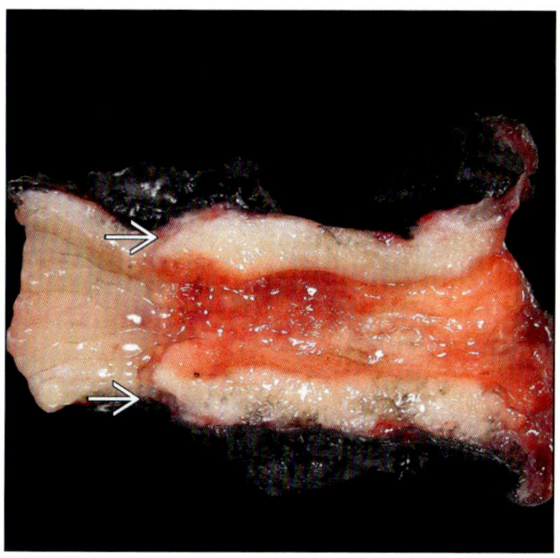

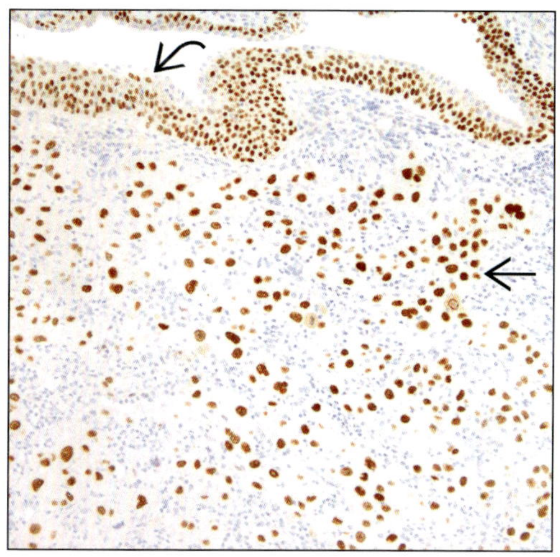

(Left) *Gross photograph shows a segment of ureter thickened by invasive urothelial carcinoma ➡. Ureteral urothelial carcinoma may present as obstruction that mimics a stricture. In this case, the tumor infiltrates full thickness of the wall and extends into the periureteric fat (pT3).* ***(Right)*** *p63 shows diffuse nuclear positivity in this infiltrating renal urothelial carcinoma →. A portion of overlying benign urothelium ↗ similarly shows diffuse nuclear positivity, which serves as an internal control.*

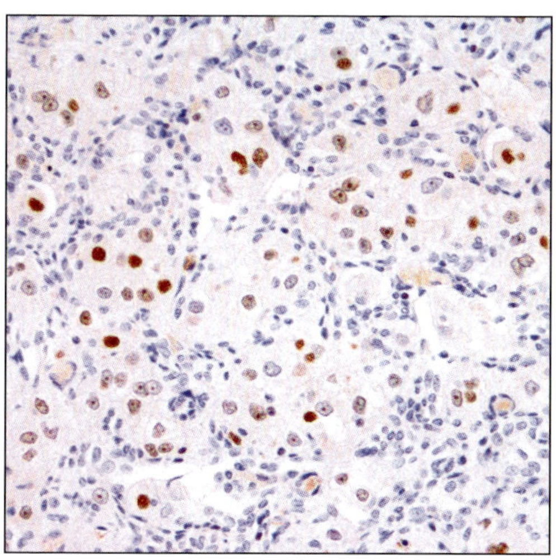

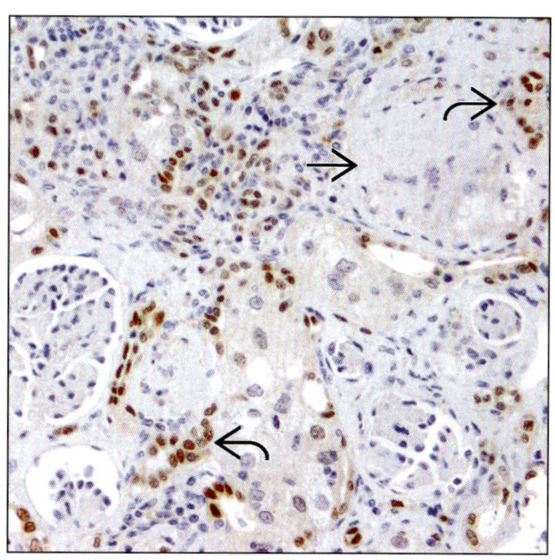

(Left) *GATA3 shows nuclear positivity in this renal pelvis invasive urothelial carcinoma. Note the variability of staining, weaker in areas where there are squamoid features.* ***(Right)*** *pax-8 shows negative staining in urothelial carcinoma → infiltrating the renal parenchyma. Renal tubules ↗ exhibit nuclear positivity and serve as internal control. Combination of p63 and pax-8/pax-2 is helpful to distinguish urothelial carcinoma (p63[+]/pax-8 or pax-2[-]) from renal carcinoma (p63[-]/pax-8 or pax-2[+]).*

TESTICLE

Familial Testicular Tumors

Conditions	Gene	Testicular Tumors
Familial testicular GCT (female relatives with familial ovarian GCT)	Several genes implicated; *KITLG*, *SPRY4*, and *BAK1* confirmed by genome-wide association studies	ITGCN and GCT (tumors reported are postpubertal types)
Peutz-Jeghers syndrome	*STK11/LKB1*	ILCHSCN, LCCSCT, and Sertoli cell tumor
Carney complex	*PRKAR1A* (mutations seen in 45-80%)	LCCSCT is a component of Carney complex

GCT: Germ cell tumor; ILCHSCN: Intratubular large cell hyalinizing Sertoli cell neoplasia; ITGCN: Intratubular germ cell neoplasia; LCCSCT: Large cell calcifying Sertoli cell tumor.

Tumors With Diffuse Arrangement and Pale and Clear Cytoplasm

Antibody	Classic Seminoma	Spermatocytic Seminoma	Embryonal Carcinoma	Yolk Sac Tumor	Sertoli Cell Tumor	Lymphoma	Renal Cell Carcinoma	Melanoma
CD117	+	+	-	-/+	-	-/+	V	V
OCT3/4	+	-	+	-	-	-	-	-
CD30 (BER-H2)	-/+ (rare focal cells)	-	+	-	-	V	ND	-
α-fetoprotein	-	-	-	+	-	ND	-	-
Glypican-3	-	-	-	+	-	-	-	-
PAN-CK (AE1/AE3)	-	-	+	+	+/-	-	+	-
CK7	V	ND	+	-/+	-	ND	V	-
EMA	-	-	-	-/+	-	-	+	-
Inhibin	- (+ STC)	ND	-	-	+	-	+	-
CD45 (LCA)	-	-	-	-	-	+	-	-
S100	-	-	-	-	V	-	-	+
RCC	-	ND	V	-	-	-	+	-

ND: No data; STC: Syncytiotrophoblast; V: Variable.

Tumors With Glandular/Tubular Pattern

Antibody	Embryonal Carcinoma	Seminoma	Yolk Sac Tumor	Sertoli Cell Tumor	Rete Testis Tumor	Metastatic Adenocarcinoma
OCT3/4	+	+	-	-	-	-
CD30 (BER-H2)	+	-/+ (rare focal cells)	Rarely +		-	V
CD117	-	+	-/+	-	-	V
Inhibin	-	-	-	+	-	-
EMA	-	-	-/+	-	V	+
SALL4	+	+	+	-	-	-
α-fetoprotein	-	-	+	-	-	-
Calretinin	-	-	-	+	+	-/+
Chromogranin	-	-	-	+	-	-
Glypican-3	-	-	+	-	-	- (+ in hepatocellular carcinoma)

Tumors With Oxyphilic Cytoplasm

Antibody	Leydig Cell Tumor	Large Cell Calcifying Sertoli Cell	Sertoli Cell Tumor, NOS	Carcinoid	Plasmacytoma
Inhibin	+	+	+	-	-
PLAP	-	-	-	-	-
PAN-CK (AE1/AE3)	-/+	-/+	+/-	+	-
Vimentin	+	+	V	V	V
S100	V	+	V	V	V
Synaptophysin	V	ND	V	+	-

ND: No data; V: Variable.

2010 AJCC Staging System for Testicular Cancer

Stage	Definition
Primary Tumor (pT)	
pTX	Primary tumor cannot be assessed
pT0	No evidence of primary tumor (e.g., histologic scar in testis)
pTis	Intratubular germ cell neoplasia (carcinoma in situ)
pT1	Tumor limited to the testis and epididymis without vascular/lymphatic invasion; tumor may invade into the tunica albuginea but not the tunica vaginalis
pT2	Tumor limited to the testis and epididymis with vascular/lymphatic invasion, or tumor extending through the tunica albuginea with involvement of the tunica vaginalis
pT3	Tumor invades the spermatic cord with or without vascular lymphatic invasion
pT4	Tumor invades the scrotum with or without vascular/lymphatic invasion
Regional Lymph Nodes (pN)	
pNX	Regional lymph nodes cannot be assessed
pN0	No regional lymph node metastasis
pN1	Metastasis with a lymph node mass ≤ 2 cm in greatest dimension and ≤ 5 nodes positive, none > 2 cm in greatest dimension
pN2	Metastasis with a lymph node mass > 2 cm but not > 5 cm in greatest dimension; or > 5 lymph nodes positive, none > 5 cm; or evidence of extranodal tumor extension
pN3	Metastasis with a lymph node mass > 5 cm in greatest dimension
Distant Metastasis (M)	
M0	No distant metastasis
M1	Distant metastasis
M1a	Nonregional nodal or pulmonary metastasis
M1b	Distant metastasis other than to nonregional lymph nodes or lung

Adapted from 7th edition AJCC Staging Forms (2010).

Normal Testicular Histoanatomy and Cancer Staging

(Left) Schematic diagram of testis and paratestis is shown. The testicular parenchyma is separated by fibrous septae. The tubules converge and exit to the rete testis, efferent ducts, epididymis, and vas deferens. *(Right)* Schematic diagram shows seminiferous tubule with spermatogenesis (spermatogonia, spermatocytes, spermatids, spermatozoa). Cellular maturation progresses from base to lumina. Sertoli cells and Leydig cells are also shown.

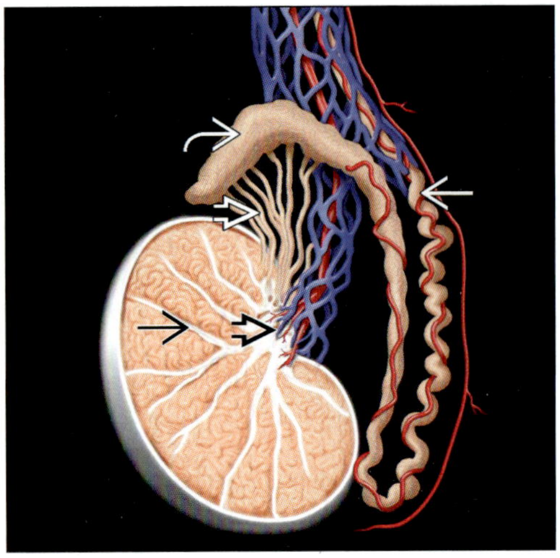

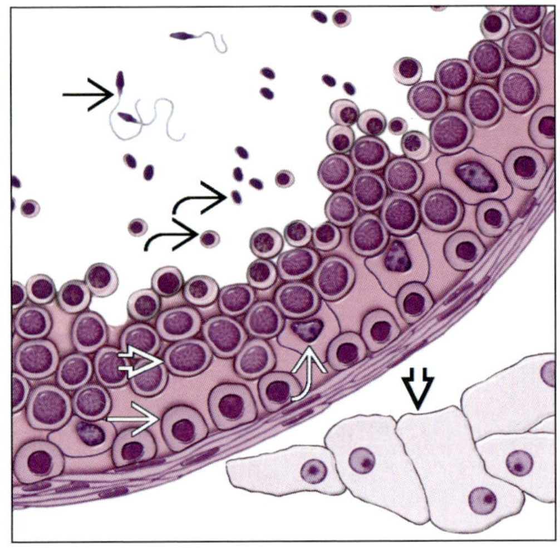

(Left) Seminiferous tubule (ST) shows spermatogenesis. The largest cell in a normal ST is the primary spermatocyte, usually situated about halfway toward the lumen. Primary spermatocytes have beaded (spireme) nuclear chromatin. In ITGCN, large atypical cells with nucleoli are seen usually adjacent to basement membrane. Note the Leydig and Sertoli cells. *(Right)* Axial CECT shows a complex enhancing mass in the left scrotum, compatible with testicular cancer.

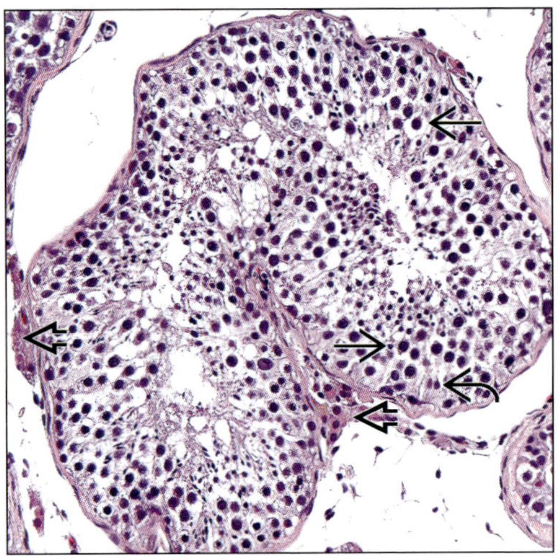

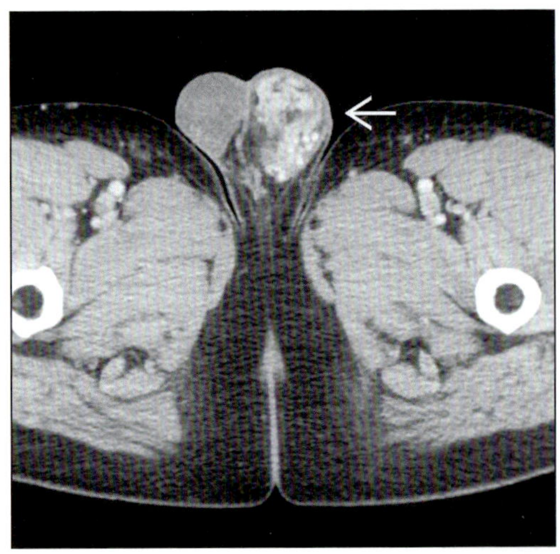

(Left) Longitudinal ultrasound shows a large seminoma, which has essentially replaced the testis. There is a thin crescent of normal remaining parenchyma. Despite its large size, it remains homogeneous without evidence of necrosis. *(Right)* Gross photograph of resected testis shows the seminoma to be uniform in texture without necrosis or hemorrhage, resulting in its homogeneous echogenicity on ultrasound. The testicular tunica is grossly uninvolved by tumor.

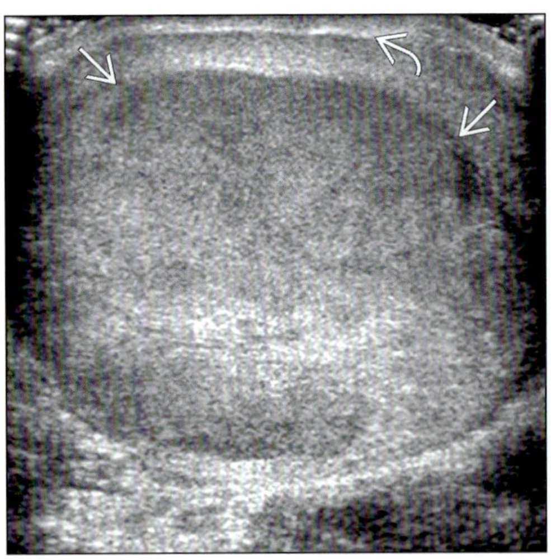

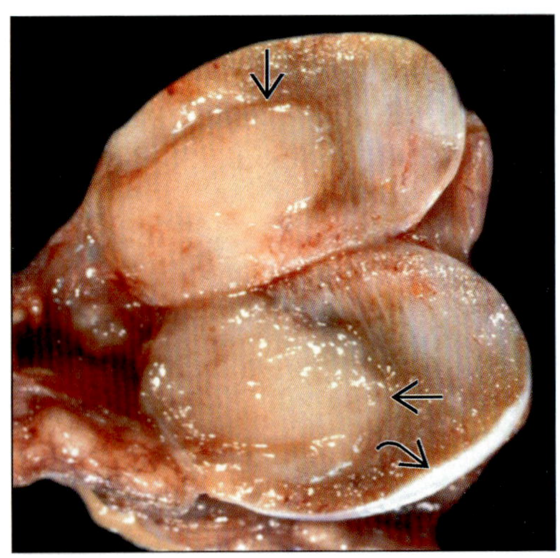

Testicular Cancer Staging

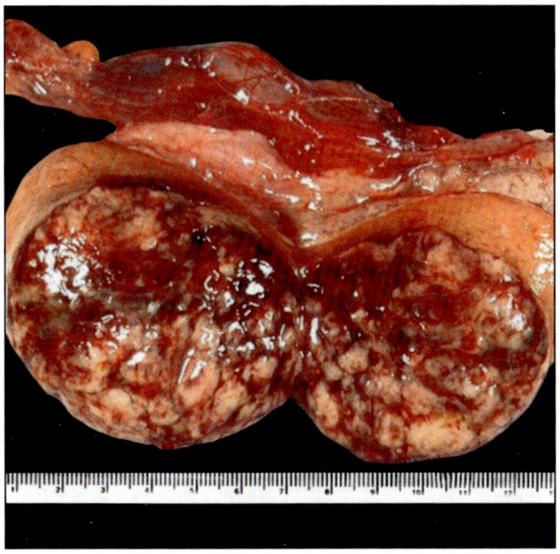

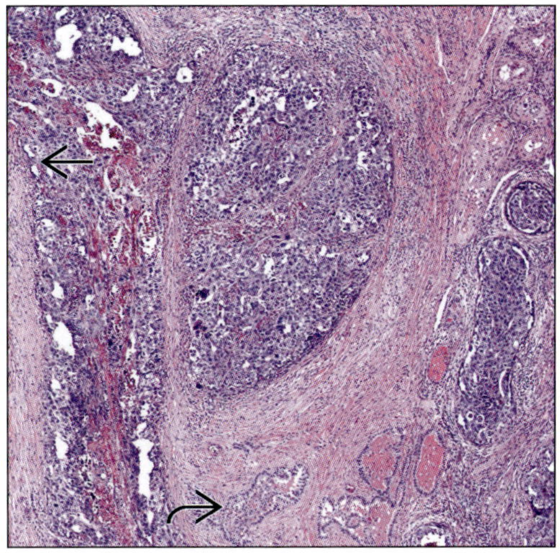

(Left) *Embryonal carcinoma shows circumscribed variegated hemorrhagic tumor surrounded by a rim of normal testicular parenchyma. Primary tumor size is not a variable when staging testicular cancer. Staging is based on extent of invasion to surrounding structures and by lymphovascular invasion.* ***(Right)*** *Low-power view shows embryonal carcinoma invading the rete testis ↪ and into the spermatic cord (pT3) →. Invasion of the rete testis is suggested to be an adverse prognostic indicator.*

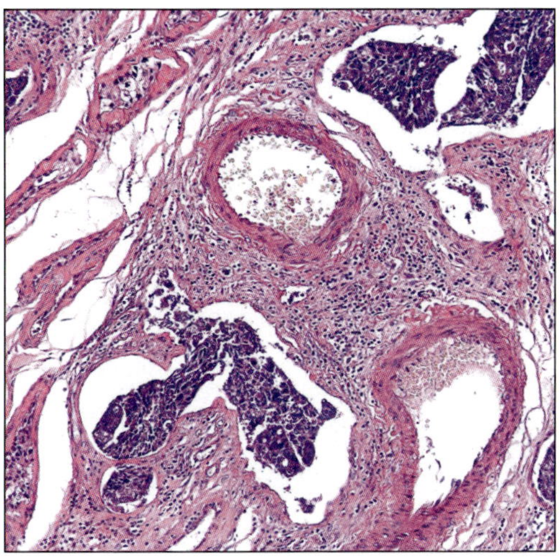

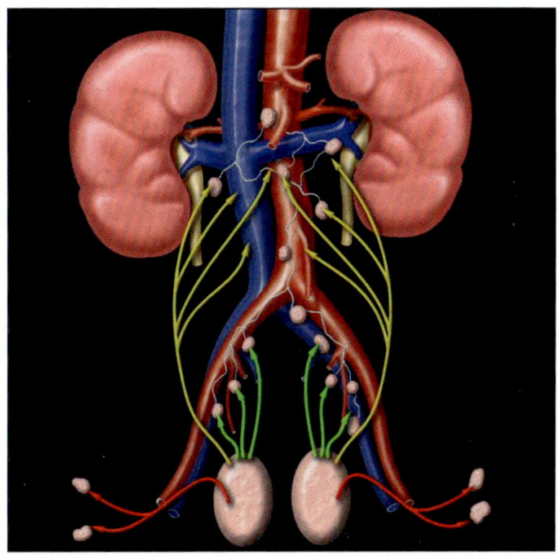

(Left) *Multiple tumor emboli are seen inside the vessel lumina. Note the tumor clusters follow the vessel contour. Presence of lymphovascular invasion upstages a testis-confined tumor from pT1 to pT2 and should be diligently searched in orchiectomy specimens.* ***(Right)*** *Schematic drawing shows testicular lymphatic drainage. The primary pathway (yellow) follows the testicular veins. If tumor has invaded through the tunica vaginalis into the scrotal skin, the inguinal nodes may be involved.*

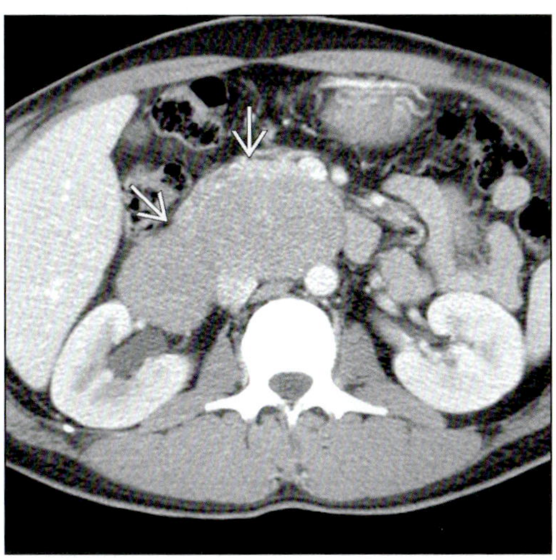

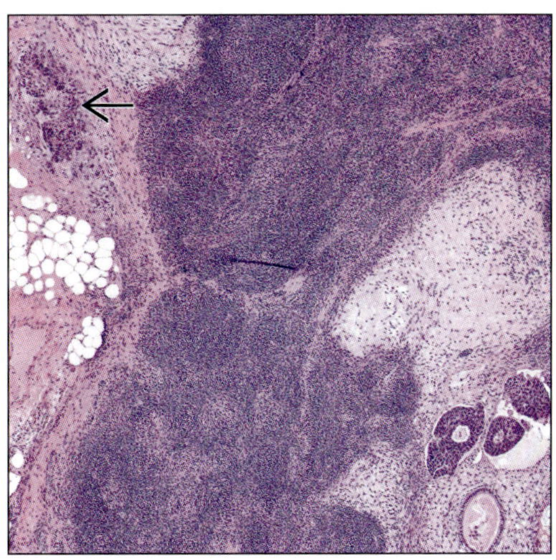

(Left) *Axial CECT in a patient with a right testicular carcinoma shows bulky retroperitoneal adenopathy ➔. The right testis lymphatics drain to the aorto-caval nodes just inferior to the right renal hilum.* ***(Right)*** *This mixed germ cell tumor has metastasized into a retroperitoneal lymph node. Note presence of extranodal tumor extension →. Size of nodal metastasis (pN1 ≤ 2 cm, pN2 = 2-5 cm, and pN3 > 5 cm) and presence of extranodal extension (pN2) are used in substaging pN status.*

TESTICLE

Immunohistochemical Features

(Left) *PLAP shows cytoplasmic and membranous immunoreactivity in intratubular germ cell neoplasia (ITGCN). PLAP is generally not expressed in normal spermatocytes and has high sensitivity in highlighting presence of ITGCN.* ***(Right)*** *PLAP shows strong and diffuse immunoreactivity in this embryonal carcinoma. PLAP is immunoreactive in all germ cell tumors (GCTs) and is only helpful in testis when distinguishing GCTs from non-GCT tumors, particularly sex cord-stromal tumors.*

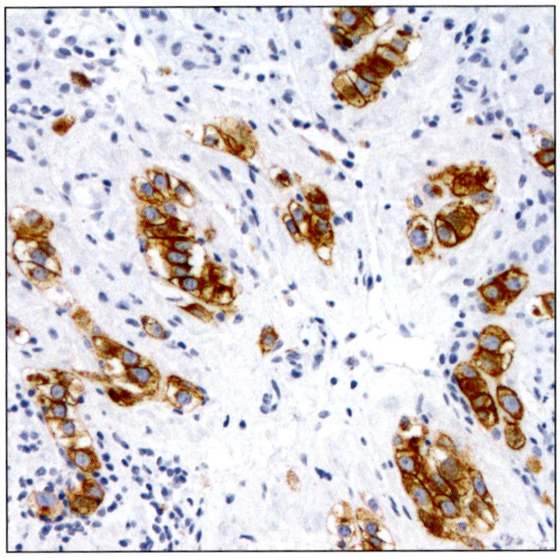

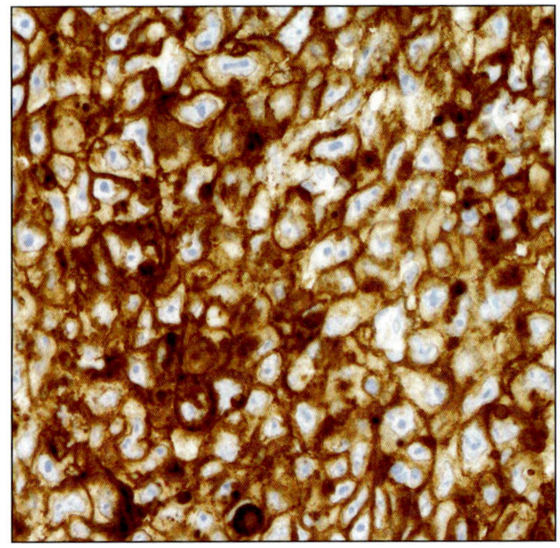

(Left) *OCT3/4 shows nuclear and some membranous positivity in this ITGCN. OCT3/4 is not expressed by normal spermatocytes.* ***(Right)*** *OCT3/4 shows diffuse immunoreactivity in this embryonal carcinoma. OCT3/4 can be positive in ITGCN, classic seminoma, and embryonal carcinoma. This marker is useful when distinguishing seminoma and embryonal carcinoma from other GCTs exhibiting solid growth, such as solid yolk sac tumor and spermatocytic seminoma.*

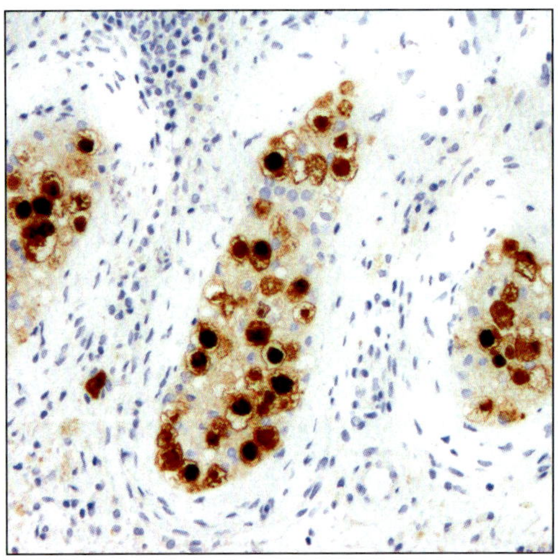

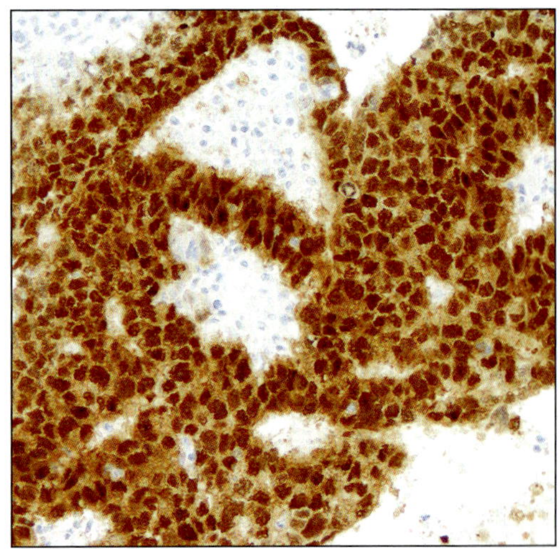

(Left) *CD117 is diffusely (+) in this classic seminoma. It is also immunoreactive in ITGCN and spermatocytic seminoma and is useful when distinguishing seminoma from embryonal carcinoma and solid yolk sac tumor, which are both negative for CD117.* ***(Right)*** *CD30 shows diffuse membranous immunoreactivity in this embryonal carcinoma (EC). CD30 is highly specific for EC and is often done to compliment CD117 when distinguishing EC from seminoma (CD30[-] and CD117[+]).*

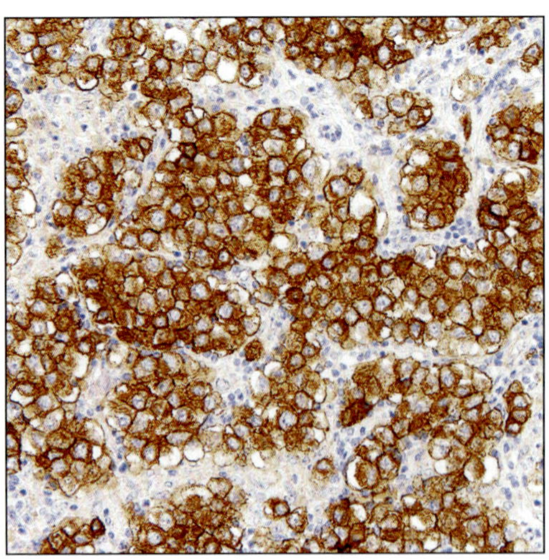

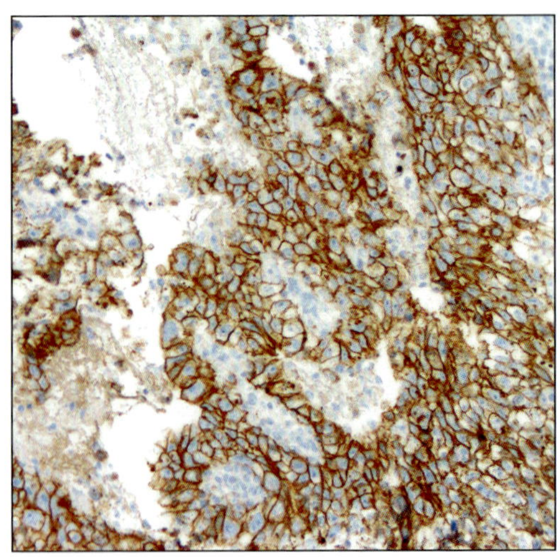

Immunohistochemical Features

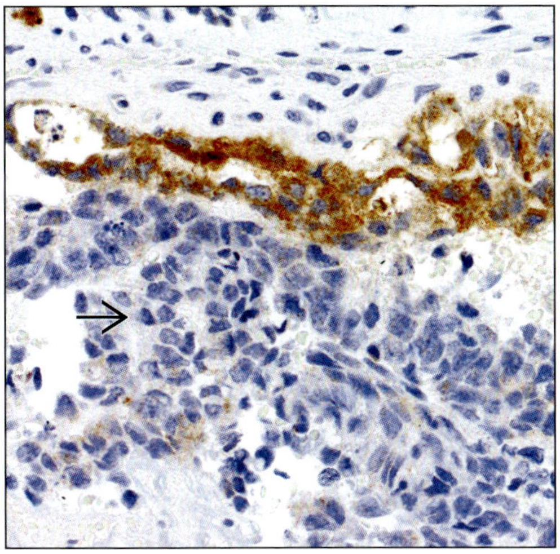

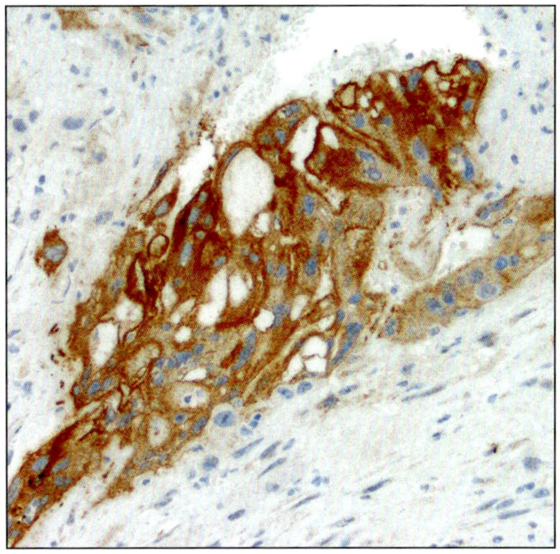

(Left) *Glypican-3 highlights yolk sac element in mixed germ cell tumor. Note the embryonal carcinoma component is completely negative →. Glypican-3 may also be positive in some teratomas.* ***(Right)*** *HCG-β highlights a multinucleated syncytiotrophoblasts. HCG-β can be used to confirm diagnosis of choriocarcinoma and detect presence of syncytiotrophoblasts admixed in GCTs such as seminoma or embryonal carcinoma. Use of HCG-β is sometimes limited by its nonspecific background staining.*

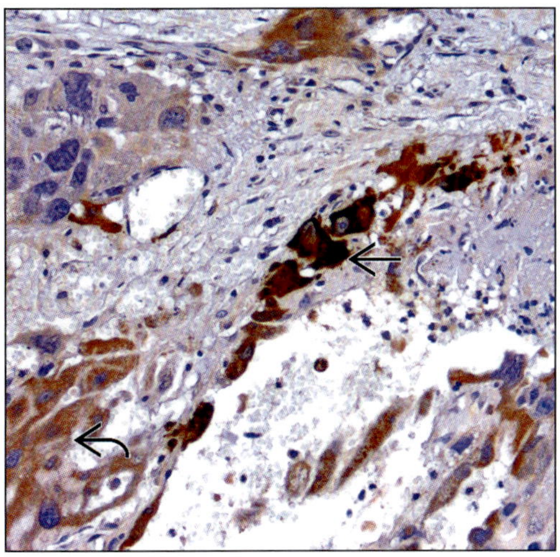

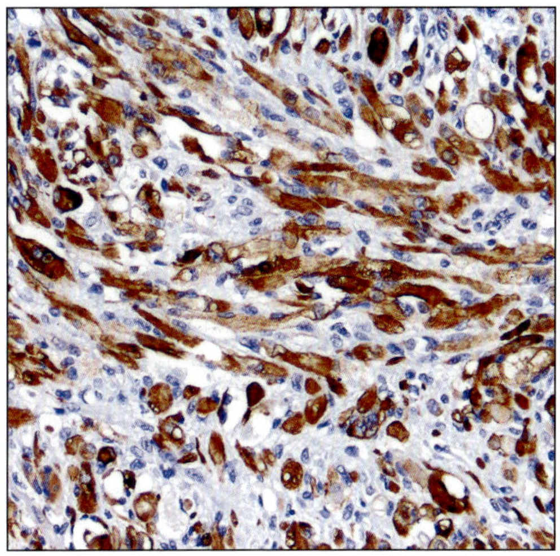

(Left) *HPL in choriocarcinoma shows intense cytoplasmic reactivity in syncytiotrophoblasts →. The large mononucleated (intermediate) trophoblasts usually show weaker cytoplasmic staining ↷. Cytotrophoblasts are typically negative for HPL (not shown).* ***(Right)*** *Desmin shows cytoplasmic positivity in this rhabdomyosarcoma (RMS) arising from teratoma. Nonsarcomatous myogenic differentiation may also occur in teratoma after therapy and should be distinguished morphologically from RMS.*

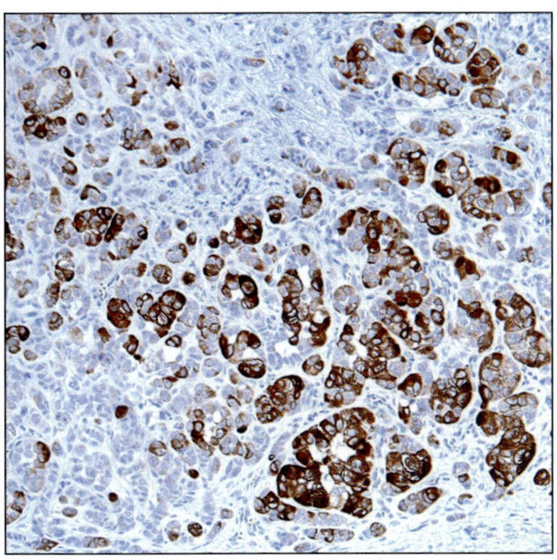

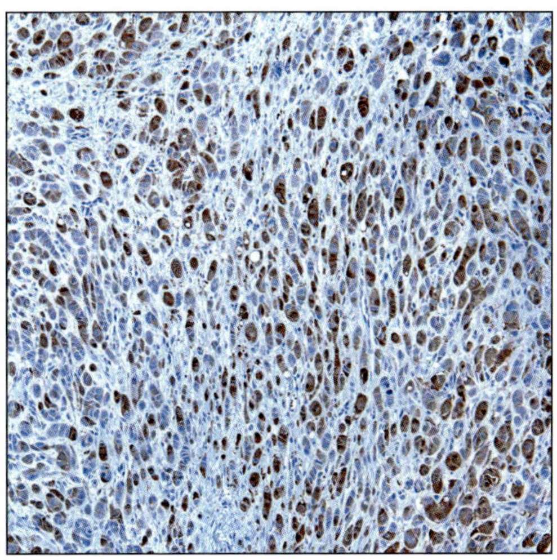

(Left) *Inhibin shows occasional positivity in this Sertoli cell tumor. Inhibin is expressed by all sex cord-stromal tumors (SCSTs) and is often used to complement PLAP when distinguishing SCSTs from GCTs (inhibin [-] and PLAP[+]).* ***(Right)*** *Calretinin shows positivity in this Sertoli cell tumor. GCTs that also exhibit tubular features such as seminoma, yolk sac tumor, and embryonal carcinoma are negative for calretinin. Beware that calretinin is also expressed by paratesticular adenomatoid tumor.*

Gynecology

GYNECOLOGIC NEOPLASMS

Familial Cancer Syndromes With Gynecologic Manifestations

Syndrome	Sites Affected	Genetics	Lifetime Risk	Histologic Types	Tumor Characteristics	Diagnostic Testing
Lynch syndrome	Endometrium, ovaries	*MLH1*, *MSH2*, *MSH6*, *PMS2*	60% for endometrial cancer; 11% for ovarian cancer	Endometrioid, serous, clear cell, carcinosarcoma	Tumor infiltrating lymphocytes; synchronous endometrial and ovarian endometrioid adenocarcinomas	Immunohistochemistry for MLH1, MSH2, MSH6, and PMS2; *MLH1* promoter hypermethylation; microsatellite instability testing; sequencing of *MLH1*, *MSH2*, *MSH6*, *PMS2*
Hereditary breast and ovarian cancer	Ovaries, peritoneum, fallopian tubes	*BRCA1*, *BRCA2*	Ovarian cancer: 35-60% for *BRCA1*, 12-25% for *BRCA2*	Ovaries: Most are high-grade invasive serous carcinomas; fallopian tubes: Most are serous intraepithelial carcinomas	Limited data	Sequencing of *BRCA1* and *BRCA2*; testing for gene rearrangements
PTEN hamartoma tumor syndrome (Cowden syndrome)	Uterus	*PTEN*	5-42% for endometrial cancer	Endometrial adenocarcinoma, uterine leiomyomas	Limited data	*PTEN* sequencing and large deletion analysis
Peutz-Jeghers syndrome	Ovaries, cervix, endometrium	*STK11* (*LKB1*)	9% for endometrial cancer; limited data for ovarian and cervical tumors	Ovarian SCTAT, cervical minimal deviation adenocarcinoma, endometrial adenocarcinoma	SCTATs are small, calcified, multifocal, bilateral	*STK11* sequencing and large deletion analysis
Germline mutations of Fanconi anemia-BRCA pathway and others	Ovaries, potentially fallopian tubes and peritoneum	*RAD51C*, *RAD51D*, *BRIP1*, *RAD50*, *NBN*, *MRE11A*	Limited data	Limited data	Limited data	Limited data
Hereditary leiomyomatosis and renal cell carcinoma	Uterus	Fumarate hydratase (*FH*)	77% for uterine leiomyoma	Leiomyomas	Multiple leiomyomas	*FH* sequencing
Hereditary esophageal-vulvar syndrome	Vulva	Some associated with Alport syndrome	Limited data	Leiomyomas	Multiple leiomyomas	Limited data
von Hippel-Lindau syndrome	Mesosalpinx and broad ligament	*VHL*	Limited data	Clear cell papillary cystadenoma	Limited data	*VHL* sequencing and deletion/duplication analysis

SCTAT: Sex cord-stromal tumors with annular tubules.

Microscopic Features

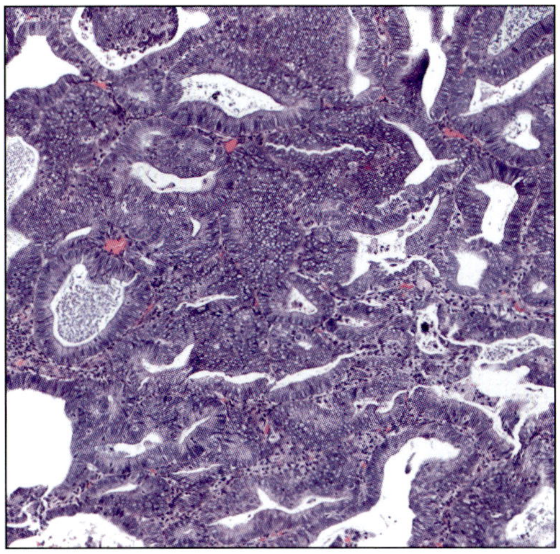

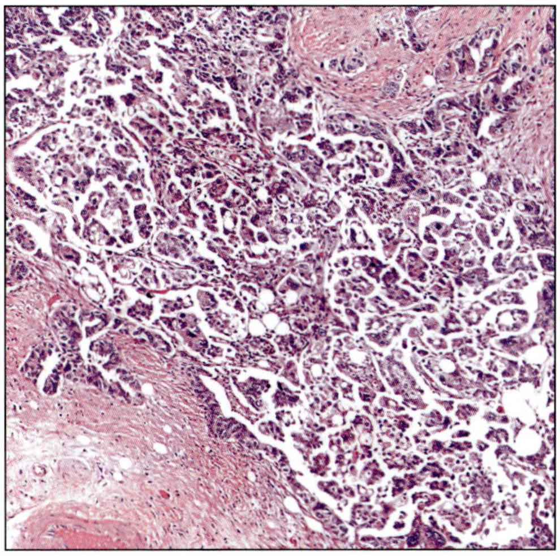

(Left) *Endometrioid adenocarcinoma shows confluent glands. Lynch syndrome, PTEN hamartoma tumor syndrome, and Peutz-Jeghers syndrome are associated with increased risk of endometrial adenocarcinoma.* ***(Right)*** *High-grade serous carcinoma diffusely infiltrates the peritoneum. Hereditary breast and ovarian cancers lead to the development of serous carcinomas, which can originate in the ovaries, fallopian tubes, or peritoneum.*

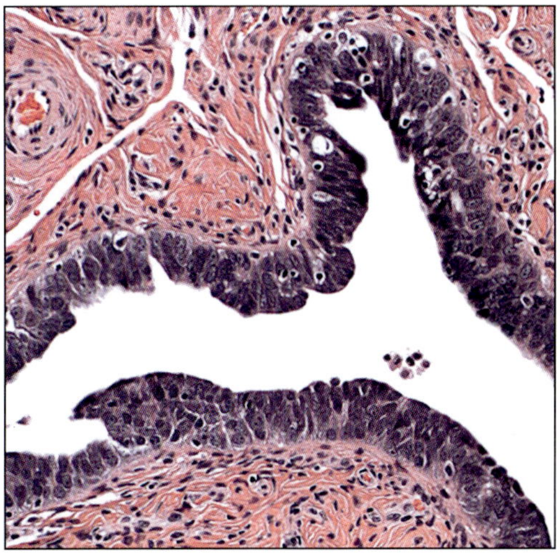

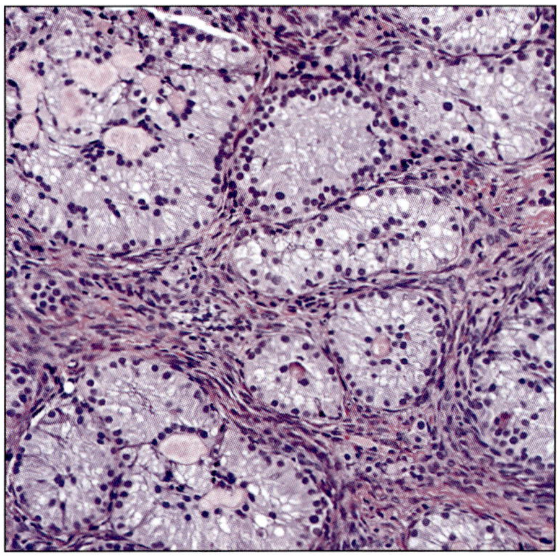

(Left) *In 5-7% of cases, risk-reducing salpingo-oophorectomies in patients with hereditary breast and ovarian cancer reveal high-grade serous carcinoma at the in situ stage, known as serous intraepithelial carcinomas.* ***(Right)*** *Sex cord-stromal tumor with annular tubules (SCTAT) is associated with Peutz-Jeghers syndrome.*

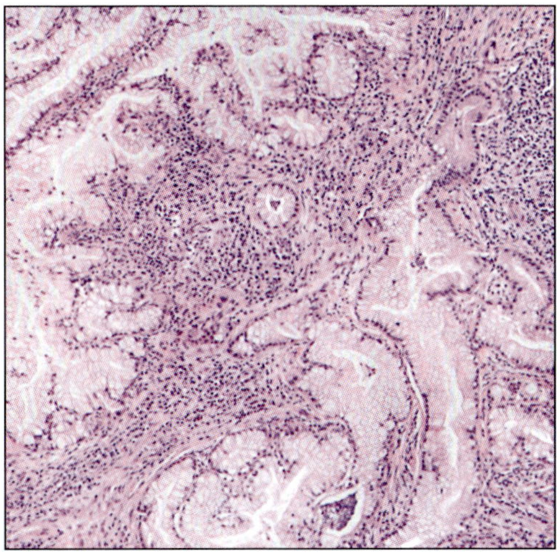

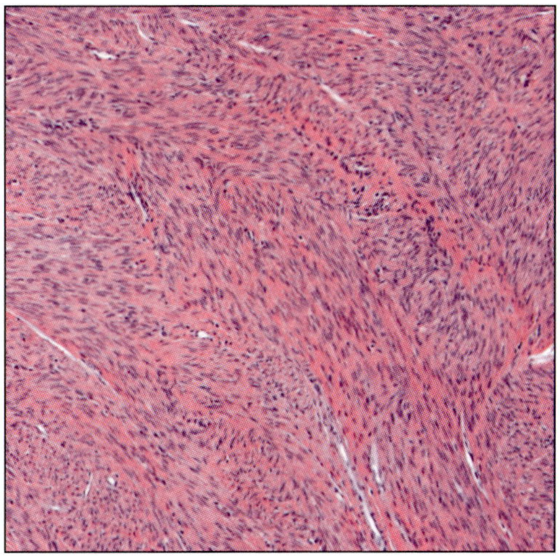

(Left) *Adenoma malignum is associated with Peutz-Jeghers syndrome. Well-differentiated mucinous glands with minimal atypia deeply infiltrate the cervical stroma.* ***(Right)*** *Benign leiomyomas are associated with multiple syndromes, including hereditary leiomyomatosis and renal cell carcinoma and hereditary esophageal-vulvar syndrome.*

Nervous System

CENTRAL NERVOUS SYSTEM

Genetic Syndromes Associated With CNS Neoplasms

Syndromes	Gene(s)	Gene Regions	Cell Pathways	CNS Tumors	Non-CNS Tumors	Nonneoplastic Manifestations
Neurofibromatosis type 1	*NF1*	17q11.2	RAS/MAPK/PI3K/mTOR/cAMP	Astrocytic tumors (grade I-IV), glioneuronal tumors	Neurofibromas, MPNST, pheochromocytoma, carcinoid tumors, juvenile myelomonocytic leukemia	Lisch nodules, café au lait spots, skeletal dysplasias, vasculopathy
Neurofibromatosis type 2	*NF2*	22q12.2	Integrin, RAC/PAK, WNT, YAP/Hippo, MAPK, PI3K, CRL4	Meningioma, ependymoma, glioma NOS	Schwannoma	Retinal hamartoma, skeletal abnormalities, café au lait spots (few), subcapsular cataract
von Hippel-Lindau syndrome	*VHL*	3p25.3	HIF (angiogenesis)	Hemangioblastoma	Renal cell carcinoma, pheochromocytoma, pancreatic endocrine tumors, endolymphatic sac tumor, papillary cystadenoma	Cysts of pancreas, kidney, adrenal gland, testis, and ovary
Gorlin syndrome	*PTCH1* > > *PTCH2*, *SUFU*	9q22.3, 1p34.1, 10q24.32	Sonic hedgehog	Medulloblastoma	Basal cell carcinoma	Odontogenic keratocysts, skeletal anomalies, calcification of falx cerebri, palmar/plantar pits
Turcot type 1 (Lynch)	*MLH1*, *MSH2*, *MSH6*, *PMS2*	3p, 2p, 2p, 7p	Mismatch repair	Astrocytic tumors (grade II-IV)	GI carcinomas, endometrium, adrenal carcinoma, osteomas, sebaceous neoplasms	
Turcot type 2 (familial adenomatous polyposis)	*APC*	5q21-q22	WNT	Medulloblastoma/PNET	FAP colorectal cancer, GI polyps, desmoid tumor (fibromatosis), papillary thyroid carcinoma (cribriform-morular variant)	Congenital hypertrophy of retinal pigment epithelium, osteomas, teeth impaction
Constitutional mismatch repair deficiency syndrome	*MLH1*, *MSH2*, *MSH6*, *PMS2*	3p, 2p, 2p, 7p	Mismatch repair	Astrocytic tumors (grade II-IV)	Lymphoma + cancers associated with Turcot type 1	Café au lait spots
Tuberous sclerosis complex	*TSC1*, *TSC2*	9q34, 16p13.3	mTOR	Subependymal giant cell astrocytoma (SEGA)	Angiomyolipoma, angioleiomyomatosis, rhabdomyoma, angiofibroma	Cortical tubers, subependymal nodules, ungual fibroma, macules, nevi
Li-Fraumeni syndrome	*TP53*	17p13.1	DNA damage response, apoptosis, cell cycle	Astrocytic tumors (grade II-IV) > > medulloblastoma, choroid plexus tumors	Sarcomas, osteosarcomas, breast carcinoma, adrenal cortical carcinoma, hematolymphoid	
Melanoma-astrocytoma syndrome	*CDKN2A*	9p21	Cell cycle (CDKs) (p16), DNA damage response (p14)	Astrocytic tumors	Melanoma, pancreatic adenocarcinoma, atypical nevi	
Familial uveal melanoma	*BAP1*	3p21	DNA repair (BRCA1 pathway)	Astrocytic tumors, meningioma	Uveal melanoma, renal cell carcinoma, mesothelioma, atypical melanocytic lesions	
Rhabdoid predisposition syndrome	*INI1* (*SMARCB1*)	22q11.23	Chromatin dynamics	Atypical teratoid-rhabdoid tumor	Renal and extrarenal rhabdoid tumors	
Hereditary retinoblastoma	*RB1*	13q14.2	Cell cycle (CDKs)	Pineoblastoma, PNET	Retinoblastoma, bone and soft tissue sarcomas	
Cowden/Lhermitte-Duclos syndrome	*PTEN*	10q23.3	mTOR	Dysplastic gangliocytoma of cerebellum	Breast/endometrial carcinoma, thyroid carcinoma and adenoma, trichilemmomas, renal cell carcinoma	Acral keratoses, multiple thyroid nodules, intestinal polyps, intellectual disabilities
Noonan syndrome	*PTPN11*, *NF1*, *KRAS*, *RAF1*, *SOS1*	12q24 (*PTPN11* most common)	RAS/MAPK	Pilocytic astrocytoma, glioneuronal tumors	None	Pulmonary valve stenosis, learning disabilities, pectus excavatum, characteristic facies
Aicardi syndrome	Unknown	X-linked dominant	Unknown	Choroid plexus papilloma	None	Agenesis of corpus callosum, chorioretinal lacunae, infantile spasms
Pleuropulmonary blastoma	*DICER1*	14q32.13	microRNA machinery	Pineoblastoma	Pleuropulmonary blastoma, medulloepithelioma (eye), Wilms tumor, sex cord-stromal tumors	Lung cysts
Multiple meningioma syndromes	*INI1*, *SUFU*, *SMARCE1*	22q, 10q, 17q	Chromatin dynamics, Shh	Meningiomas, clear cell subtype (*SMARCE1*)	Schwannomatosis (*INI1*)	

Imaging and Microscopic Features

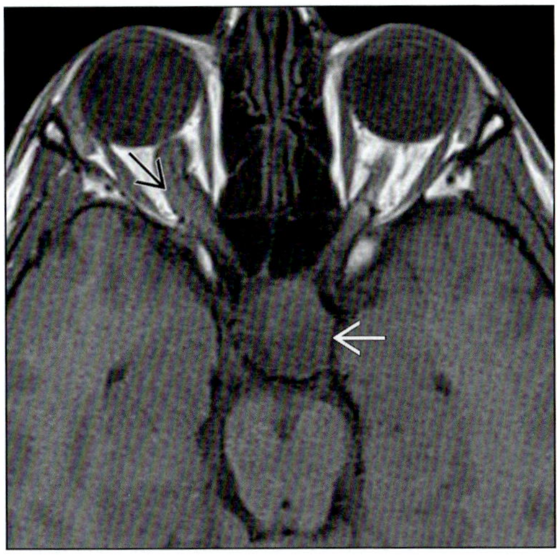

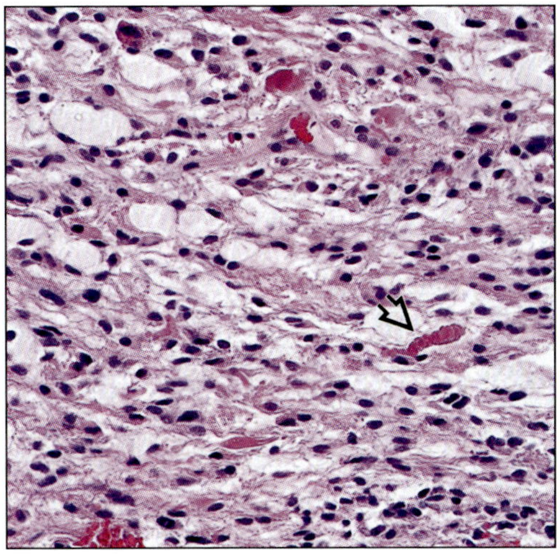

(Left) *The central nervous system hallmark of NF1 is multiple (bilateral) involvement of the optic pathways by low-grade gliomas. These may affect the optic nerve proper ⇨ as well as the chiasm ➡.* ***(Right)*** *The overwhelming majority of optic pathway gliomas are pilocytic astrocytomas. In this NF1-associated case, areas of tissue compaction, microcysts, and Rosenthal fibers ⇨ are evident. The tumors grow slowly and may even be followed without treatment in most cases.*

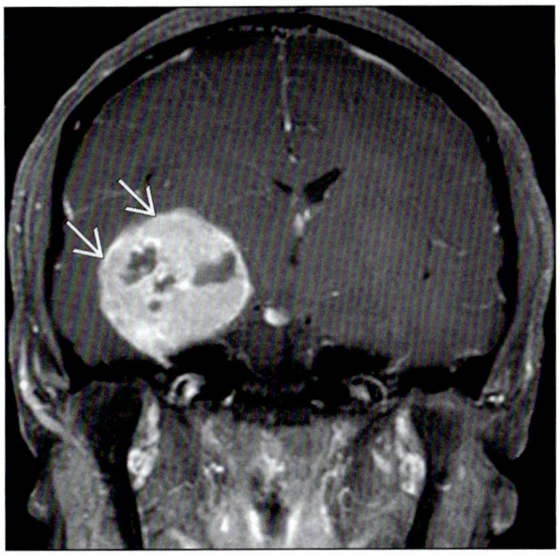

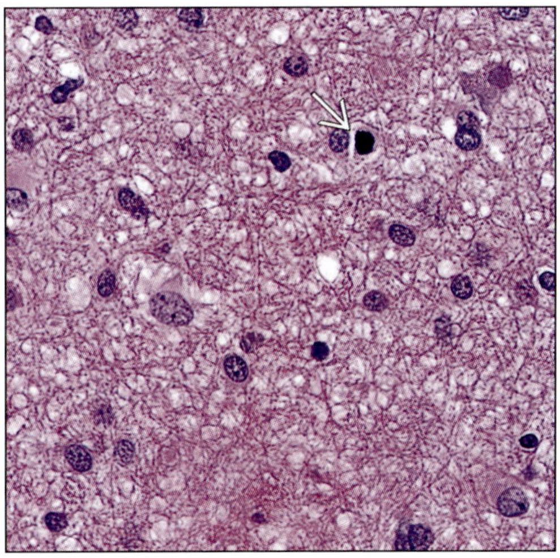

(Left) *Although pilocytic astrocytoma is the most frequent glioma in patients with NF1, all astrocytic subtypes develop including high-grade astrocytomas, as seen in this example. Heterogeneous contrast enhancement ➡ is evident in this tumor.* ***(Right)*** *High-grade astrocytomas in patients with NF1 are graded using similar criteria as in sporadic tumors. Parenchymal infiltration, atypia, and mitotic activity ➡ are present in this anaplastic (WHO grade III) astrocytoma.*

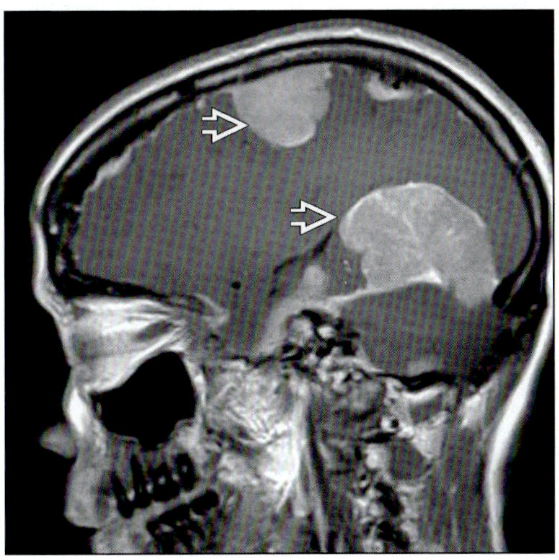

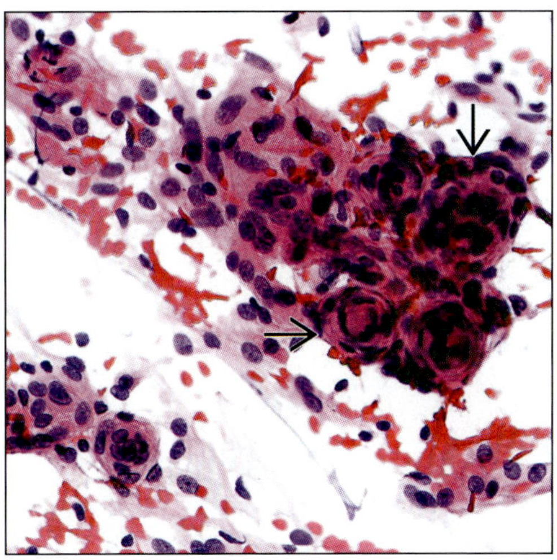

(Left) *Meningiomas are the 2nd most common neoplasms in patients with NF2. They are usually dura-based, multiple, and demonstrate strong, homogeneous contrast enhancement after administration of gadolinium in T1-weighted MR sequences ➡.* ***(Right)*** *The cytologic features of meningiomas are evident in intraoperative smears. Features include "flat" cells with ample eosinophilic cytoplasm containing bland oval nuclei as well as whorls ⇨.*

Imaging and Microscopic Features

(Left) Axial T1-weighted post-contrast MR shows 2 of several cerebellar hemangioblastomas ➔, a finding that is so characteristic as to be diagnostic of VHL syndrome by itself. The presence of multiple cysts and tumors in other organs is also characteristic of this disorder. (Right) The characteristic neoplasm involving the CNS and retina in patients with VHL syndrome is hemangioblastoma, a vascularized tumor containing vacuolated stromal cells ➔.

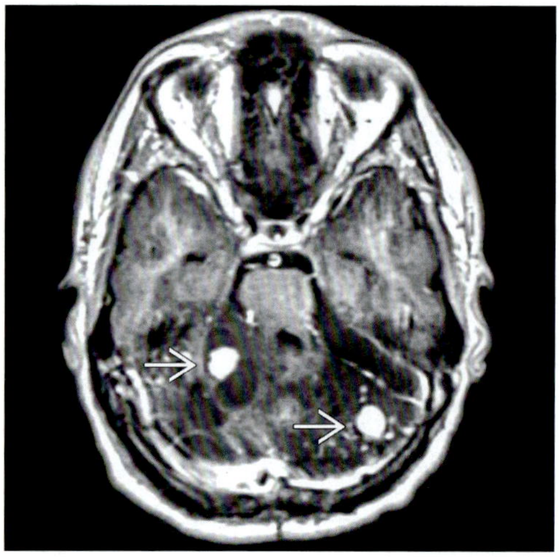

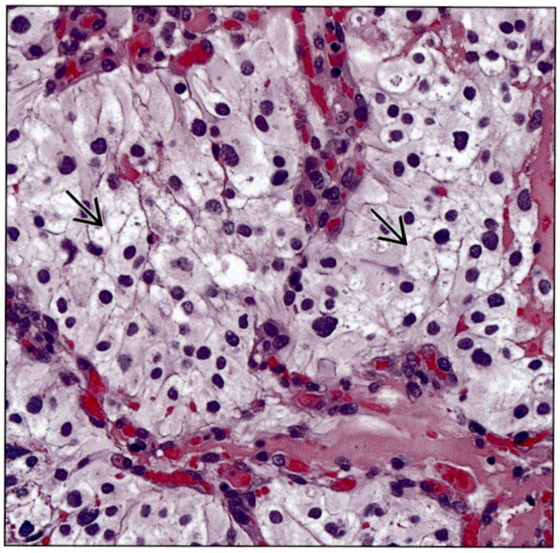

(Left) Subependymal giant cell astrocytomas (SEGAs)are typical of tuberous sclerosis complex, characterized by contrast-enhancing intraventricular masses near the foramen of Monro ➔. A subtle cortical tuber is also present ➔ in this patient with tuberous sclerosis complex. (Right) SEGAs are characterized by colorful, large cells with prominent nucleoli, features particularly recognizable in smear preparations. Variable cytoplasmic processes and pleomorphism may also be present.

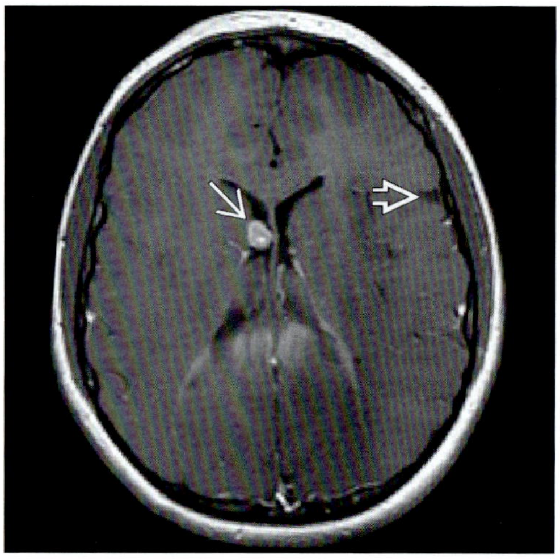

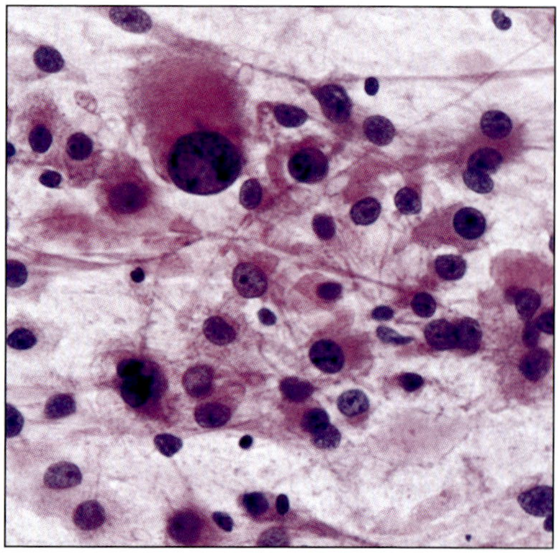

(Left) Choroid plexus carcinomas are malignant neoplasms that almost always develop in young children and demonstrate variable contrast enhancement ➔. (Courtesy T. Vanegas, MD.) (Right) Choroid plexus carcinomas usually have a papillary architecture, at least in part, and variable pleomorphism. This young patient developed a rhabdomyosarcoma subsequently, which strongly suggests Li-Fraumeni syndrome.

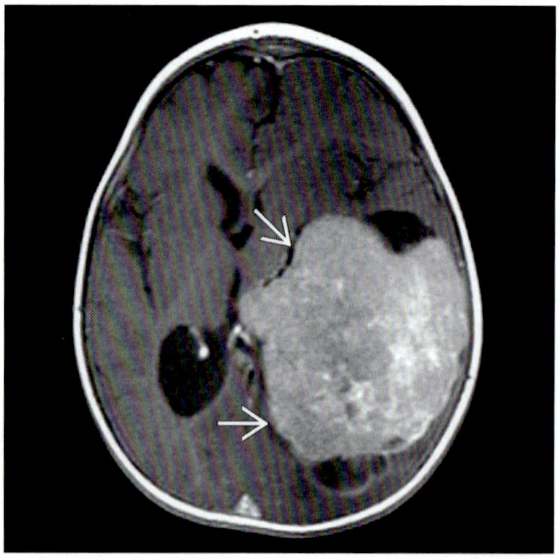

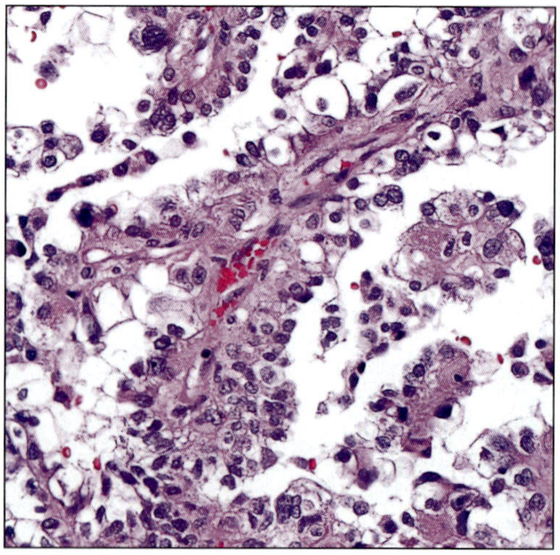

Imaging, Diagrammatic, and Microscopic Features

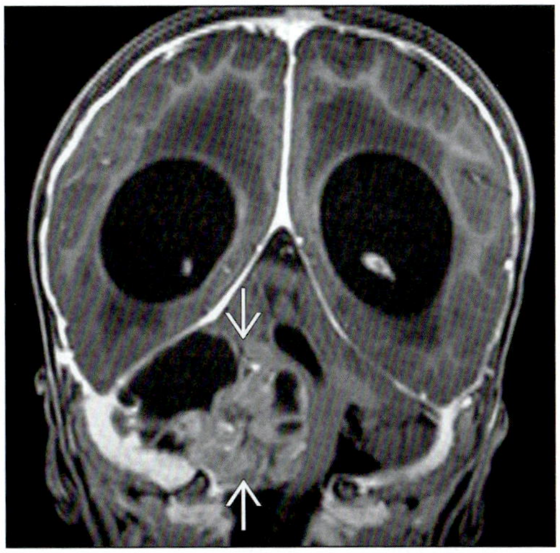

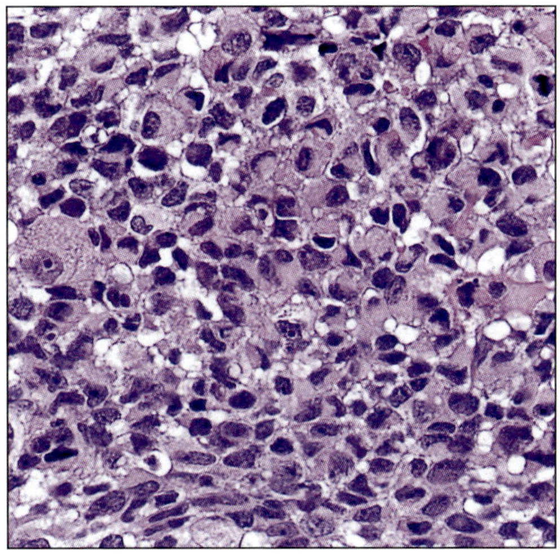

(Left) *The cerebellopontine angle is a classic location for AT/RT ➡. These tumors may form large heterogeneous masses involving the posterior fossa, but they may also affect other CNS sites. (Courtesy C. Specht, MD.)* ***(Right)*** *Atypical teratoid rhabdoid tumors contain variable proportions of rhabdoid cells, characterized by eccentric nuclei with nucleoli and eosinophilic cytoplasm. This patient had a constitutional chromosome 22 abnormality and multiple associated congenital anomalies.*

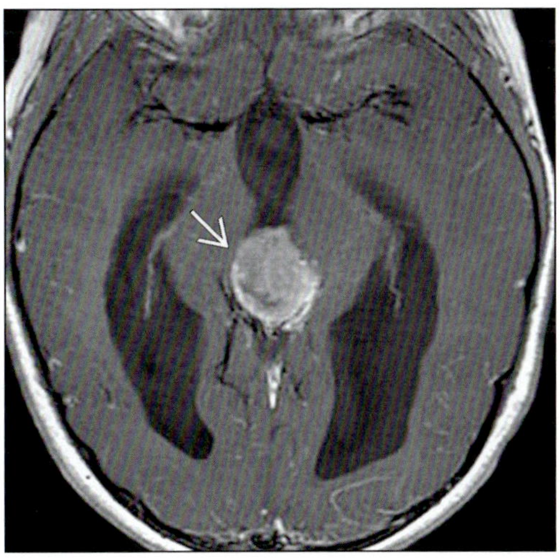

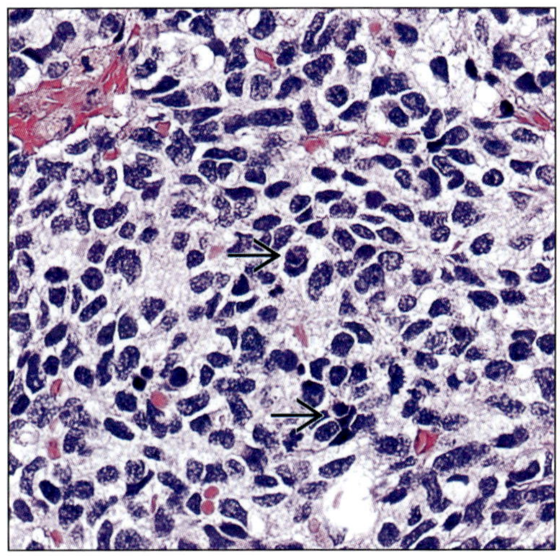

(Left) *Pineoblastomas are malignant neoplasms presenting as contrast-enhancing masses in the pineal region ➡. Associated hydrocephalus is a frequent finding. Pineoblastomas may occur sporadically or in association with tumor predisposition syndromes such as familial retinoblastoma.* ***(Right)*** *Pineoblastomas are high-grade neoplasms composed of cells with high nuclear to cytoplasmic ratios. Cell-cell wrapping may be present as in other embryonal neoplasms ➡.*

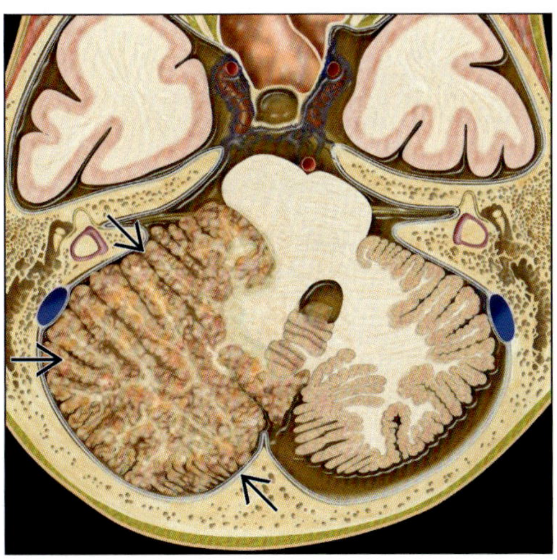

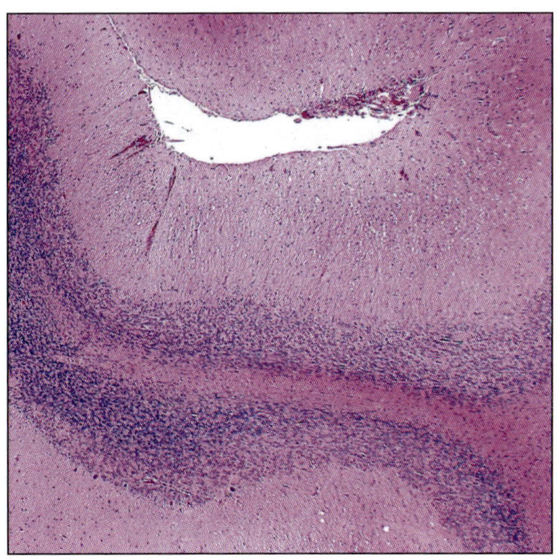

(Left) *The hallmark of CNS involvement by Cowden syndrome secondary to constitutional PTEN mutations is Lhermitte-Duclos disease, which has a characteristic gross/radiographic appearance (i.e., asymmetric expansion of cerebellar folia ➡).* ***(Right)*** *Lhermitte-Duclos (or dysplastic gangliocytoma of the cerebellum) is characterized by replacement of the internal granular layer of the cerebellum by large, dysplastic ganglion cells, with relative architectural preservation.*

EYE

Genetic Syndromes and Neoplasms Involving Eye and Ocular Adnexa

Syndromes	Gene(s)	Gene Region	Cell Pathways	Eye Tumors	Extraocular Tumors	Nonneoplastic Manifestations
Neurofibromatosis type 1	*NF1*	17q11.2	RAS/MAPK/PI3K/mTOR/cAMP	Optic nerve glioma (pilocytic astrocytoma), orbital and intraocular neurofibromas	Astrocytomas, glioneuronal tumors, neurofibromas, MPNST, pheochromocytoma, carcinoid tumors, juvenile myelomonocytic leukemia	Lisch nodules, café au lait spots, skeletal, vasculopathy
Neurofibromatosis type 2	*NF2*	22q12.2	Integrin, RAC/PAK, WNT, YAP/Hippo, MAPK, PI3K, CRL4	Orbital meningioma, orbital and intraocular schwannoma	Meningioma, schwannoma	Retinal hamartoma, skeletal abnormalities, café au lait spots (few), subcapsular cataract
von Hippel-Lindau syndrome	*VHL*	3p25.3	HIF (angiogenesis)	Hemangioblastoma	Renal cell carcinoma, pheochromocytoma, pancreatic endocrine tumors, endolymphatic sac tumor, papillary cystadenoma	Cysts of pancreas, kidney, adrenal gland, testis, and ovary
Muir-Torre (Lynch)	*MSH2* > *MLH1*	2p21, 3p21.3	Mismatch repair	Sebaceous neoplasms involving eyelid, conjunctiva	Astrocytomas, GI carcinomas, endometrial and adrenal carcinoma, osteomas, sebaceous neoplasms	
Tuberous sclerosis complex	*TSC1*, *TSC2*	9q34, 16p13.3	mTOR	Giant cell astrocytoma/ astrocytic hamartomas	Subependymal giant cell astrocytoma, angiomyolipoma, angioleiomyomatosis, rhabdomyoma, angiofibroma	Cortical tubers, subependymal nodules, ungual fibroma, macules, nevi
Familial uveal melanoma	*BAP1*	3p21.31-p21.2	DNA repair (BRCA1 pathway)	Uveal melanoma	Astrocytoma, meningioma, renal cell carcinoma, mesothelioma, atypical melanocytic lesions	
Hereditary retinoblastoma	*RB1*	13q14.2	Cell cycle (CDKs)	Retinoblastoma (often bilateral)	Pineoblastoma, CNS-PNET, retinoblastoma, bone and soft tissue sarcomas	
Pleuropulmonary blastoma	*DICER1*	14q32.13	microRNA machinery	Medulloepithelioma	Pineoblastoma, pleuropulmonary blastoma, Wilms tumor, sex cord-stromal tumors	Lung cysts
Xeroderma pigmentosum	Multiple (*XPA-G*, *POLH*)	Multiple	Nucleotide excision DNA repair	Ocular surface squamous cell carcinoma (SCCa); basal cell carcinoma and melanoma (eyelids/ conjunctiva)	SCCa of tongue, sarcomas	Telangiectasias, cataracts, keratitis, CNS dysfunction
Norrie disease	*NDP*	Xp11.4	WNT pathway	Pseudoglioma of retina		Cataracts, eye globe shrinkage; abnormalities of iris, CNS, and hearing

MPNST: Malignant peripheral nerve sheath tumor.

Genetic Tumor Syndromes and Nonneoplastic Ocular Manifestations

Syndromes	Gene(s)	Gene Region	Nonneoplastic Ocular Manifestations	Extraocular Neoplasms	Other Nonneoplastic Manifestations
Aicardi syndrome	Unknown	X-linked dominant	Chorioretinal lacunae	Choroid plexus papilloma	Agenesis of corpus callosum, infantile spasms
Ataxia-telangiectasia	*ATM*	11q22-23	Conjunctival telangiectasias	Hematolymphoid neoplasms, ovarian and breast carcinoma, smooth muscle tumors	Progressive ataxia, dermatitis, café au lait spots, hypogonadism, short stature, insulin resistance
WAGR	Multiple	11p	Aniridia	Wilms tumor, gonadoblastoma	Genitourinary anomalies, mental retardation
Gorlin syndrome	*PTCH1* >> *PTCH2*, *SUFU*	9q22.3, 1p34.1, 10q24.32	Microphthalmos, cataracts, glaucoma, coloboma	Basal cell carcinoma, medulloblastoma	Odontogenic keratocysts, skeletal anomalies, calcification of falx cerebri, palmar/plantar pits
Fanconi anemia	Genes coding for Fanconi anemia core complex	Multiple	Microphthalmia	Hematolymphoid, solid tumors (e.g., SCCa)	Multiple congenital anomalies, endocrine dysfunction
Werner syndrome/ progeria	*WRN* (*RECQL2*)	8p12	Cataracts	Epithelial and nonepithelial cancers	Premature aging, short stature, bird-like facies

Microscopic Features

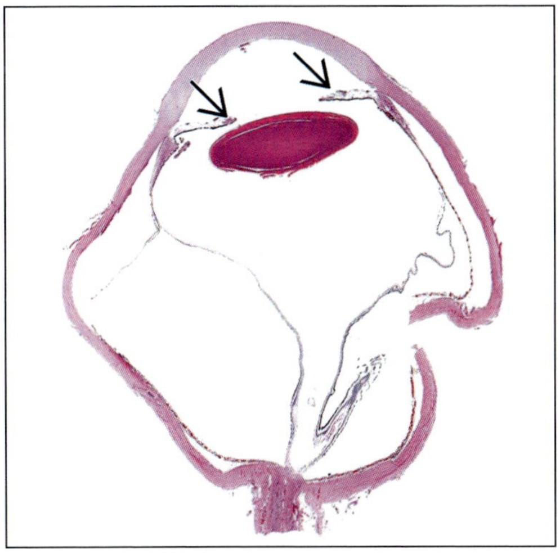

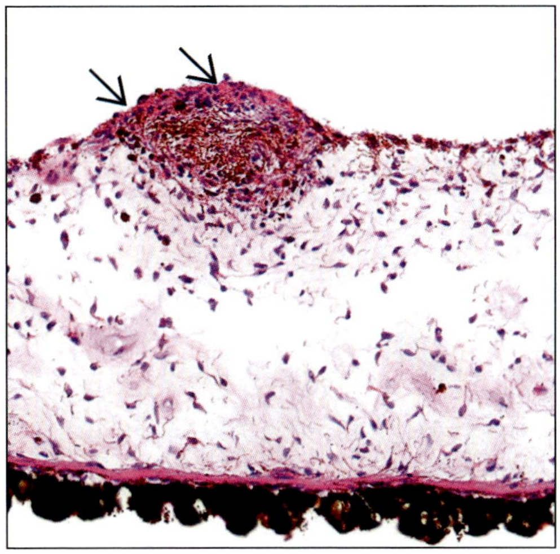

(Left) *A diagnostically important ocular manifestation of neurofibromatosis type 1 (NF1) is the Lisch nodule, an aggregate of pigmented cells in the anterior surface of the iris →.* ***(Right)*** *Lisch nodules are composed of melanin-containing cells that form superficial aggregates in the iris →. They usually do not affect vision and have no malignant potential.*

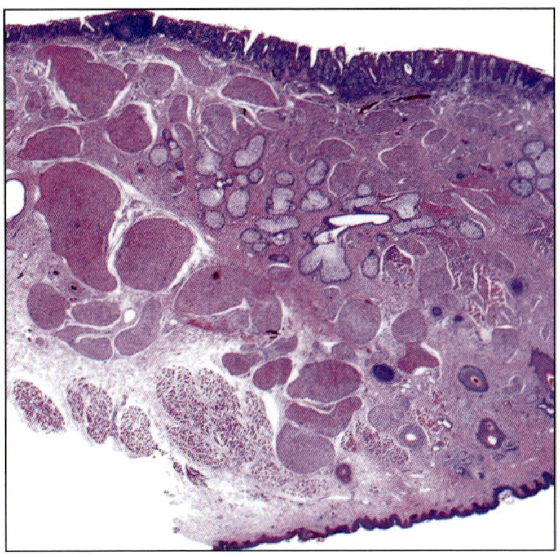

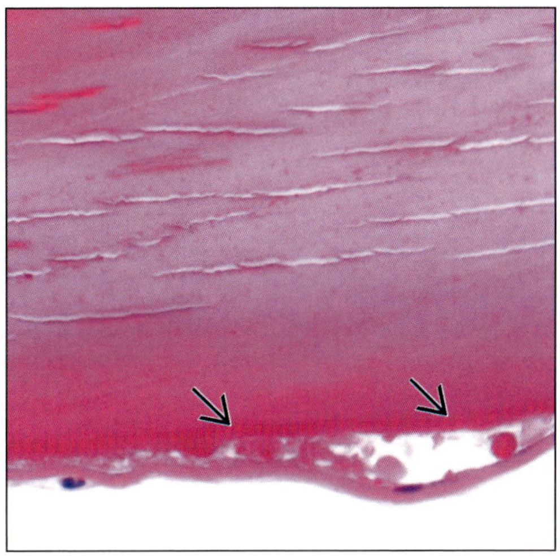

(Left) *Plexiform neurofibroma is a hallmark of NF1 and often affects the eyelid and orbital tissues. This eyelid example demonstrates the characteristic multinodular appearance resulting from multiple nerve fascicle involvement.* ***(Right)*** *Posterior subcapsular cataracts → represent a hallmark of neurofibromatosis type 2 (NF2) and are incorporated in the clinical diagnostic criteria for the syndrome.*

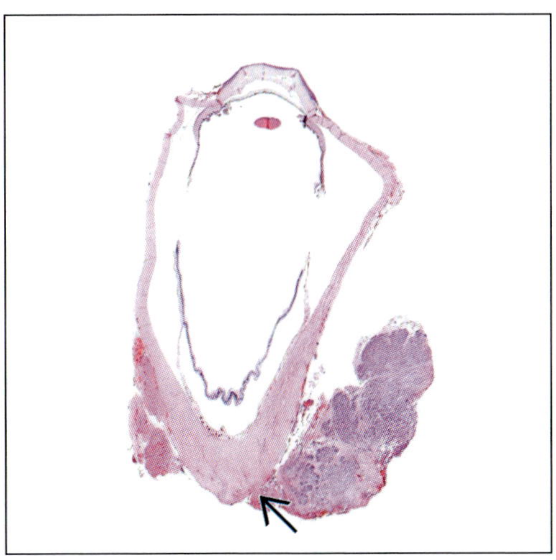

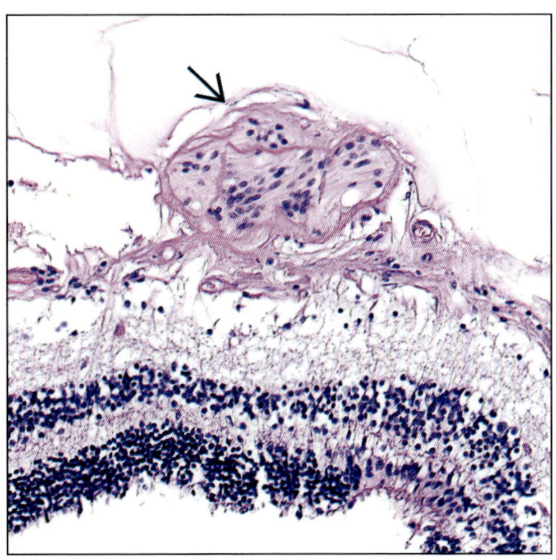

(Left) *Meningiomas in NF2 patients are usually multiple and may arise in any anatomic site, including the orbit. Many intraorbital meningiomas develop in close relation to the optic nerve sheath →.* ***(Right)*** *Glial hamartomas are characterized by benign glial proliferations → involving the retina superficially. They may occur in the setting of NF2 or tuberous sclerosis complex (TSC). This particular example developed in an NF2 patient.*

Microscopic Features

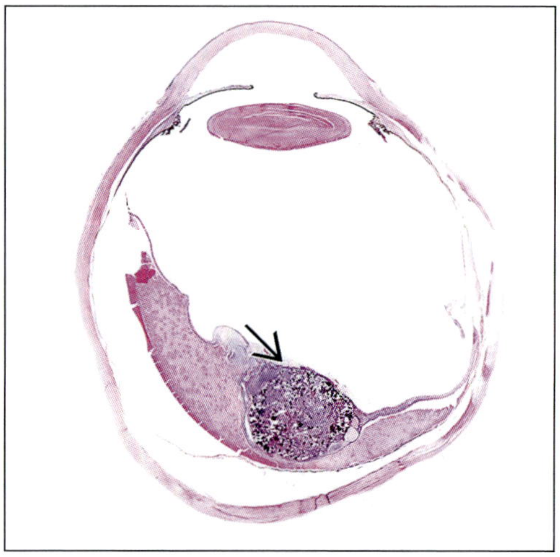
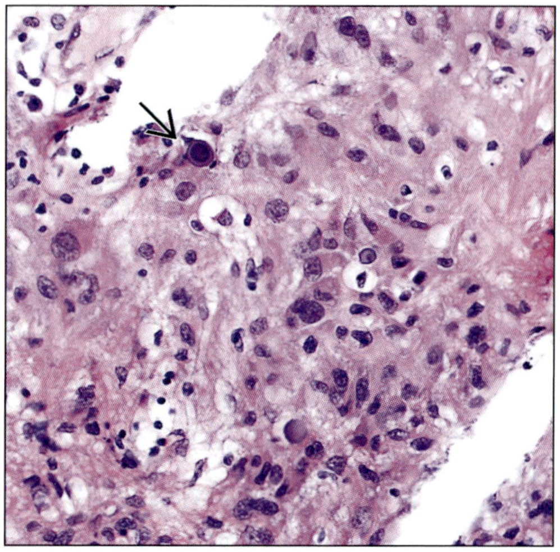

(Left) *The typical intraocular manifestation of TSC is the astrocytic hamartoma/ astrocytoma. This proliferation is characterized by slow growth and bland cytology, and it is frequently multiple in TSC but may form a dominant mass →.* ***(Right)*** *Retinal astrocytic lesions in tuberous sclerosis patients are histologically similar to subependymal nodules/subependymal giant cell astrocytoma. Scattered microcalcifications were present in this example →.*

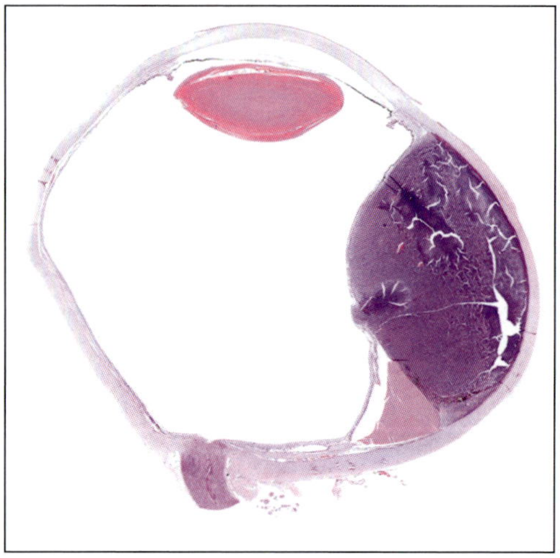
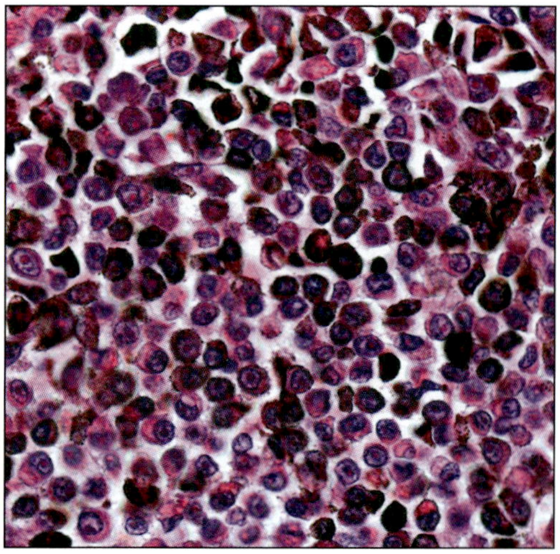

(Left) *Uveal melanomas arise predominantly in the choroid and form well-circumscribed masses. Most uveal melanomas arise sporadically, but they may also develop in the setting of a tumor predisposition syndrome characterized by BAP1 mutations.* ***(Right)*** *The presence of epithelioid cells in uveal melanoma is a negative prognostic factor and is associated with class 2 (high-risk) tumors and BAP1 mutations. These cells contain ample cytoplasm, round nuclei, and macronuclei.*

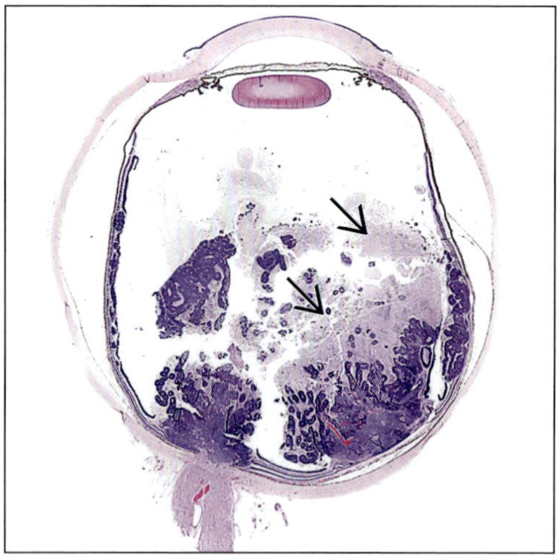
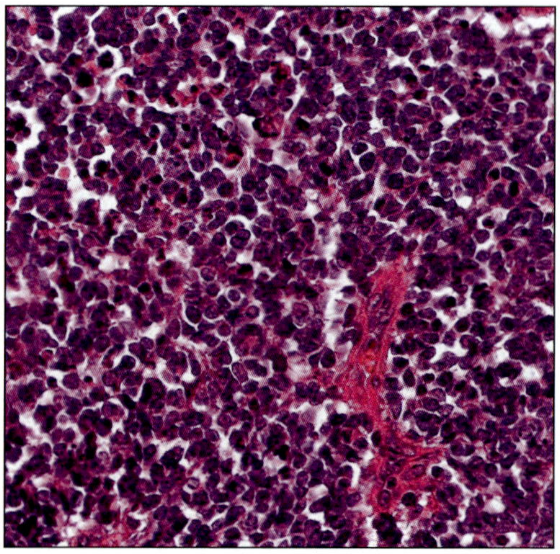

(Left) *Retinoblastoma is a proliferative tumor with frequent necrosis →, centered in the retina. It is the main tumor developing in patients with germline RB1 mutations and may be multiple &/or bilateral in these patients.* ***(Right)*** *Retinoblastoma is histologically a round blue cell tumor, highly cellular, and composed of sheets or nests of proliferative neoplastic cells.*

Microscopic Features

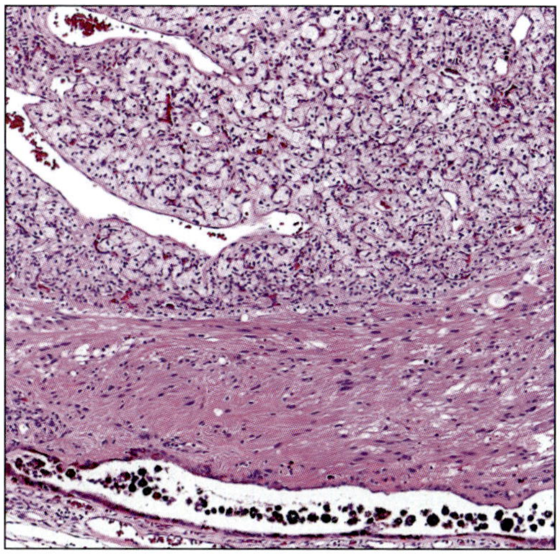

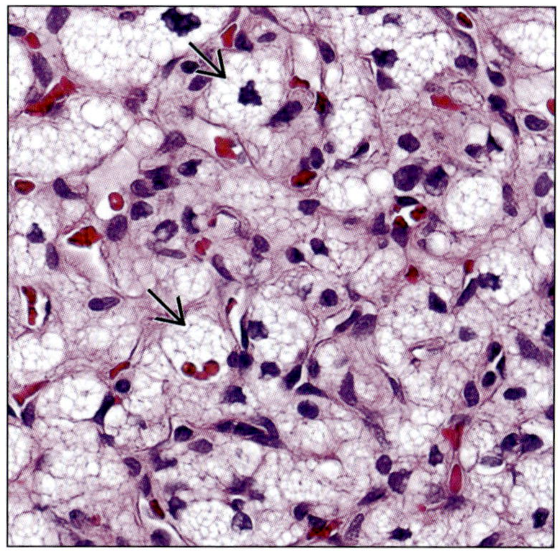

(Left) *Although named hemangiomas in the past, given their rich vascular supply, retinal tumors afflicting von Hippel-Lindau syndrome (VHL) patients are hemangioblastomas, histologically identical to tumors involving the CNS.* ***(Right)*** *The characteristic neoplasm involving the CNS and retina in patients with VHL syndrome is hemangioblastoma, a vascularized tumor containing vacuolated stromal cells →. This particular example is intraocular in a VHL patient.*

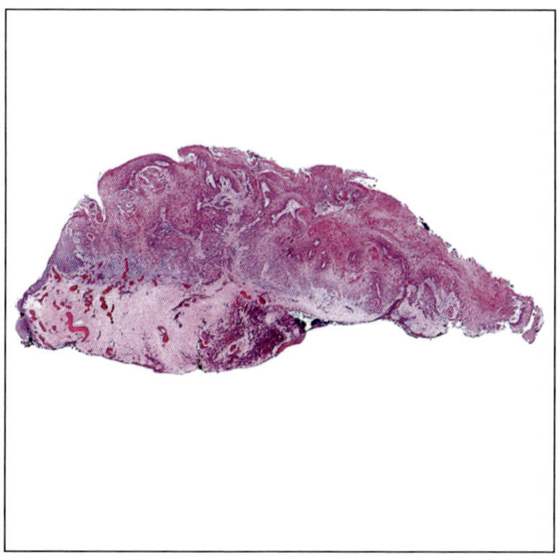

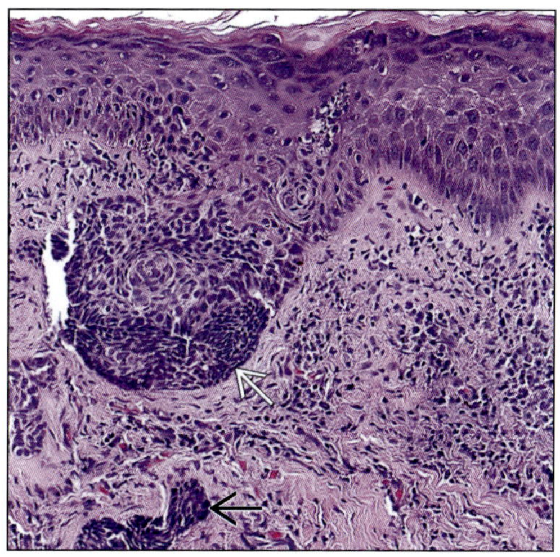

(Left) *Patients with xeroderma pigmentosum (XP) are predisposed to neoplasms developing in sun-exposed areas. This excision of a bulbar conjunctival lesion in a child with XP demonstrates a well-differentiated squamous cell carcinoma.* ***(Right)*** *XP patients also develop basal cell carcinomas in a variety of cutaneous sites, including the eyelids, as this example shows →.*

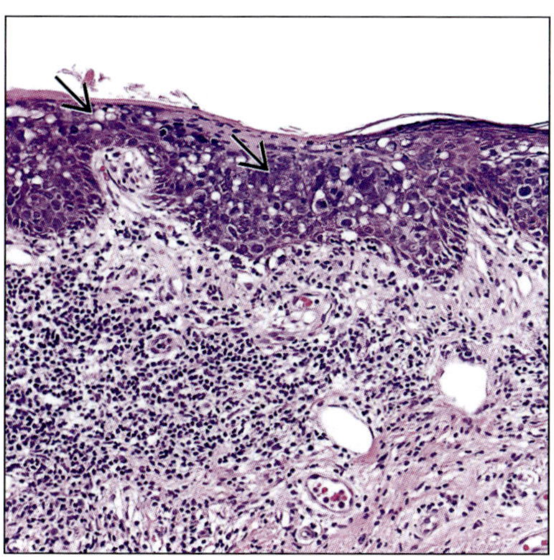

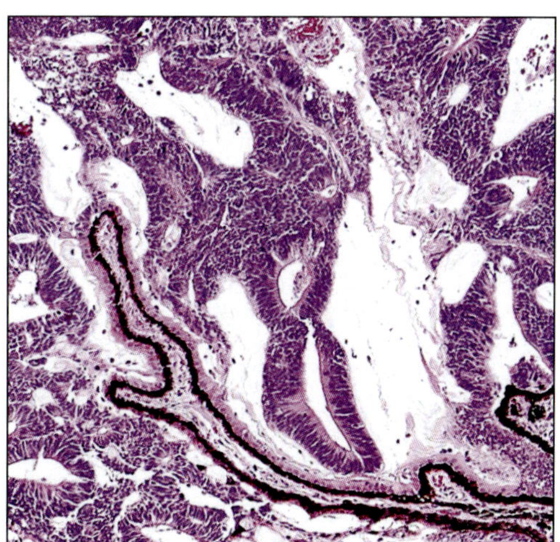

(Left) *Patients with alterations in genes encoding for mismatch repair enzymes are predisposed to a variety of superficial and visceral neoplasms. Sebaceous tumors characterize Muir-Torre syndrome. Sebaceous carcinomas frequently involve the eyelids →.* ***(Right)*** *Medulloepithelioma is a distinct ocular neoplasm arising in the ciliary body. It is a recently recognized component of a tumor predisposition syndrome characterized by DICER1 mutations.*

PERIPHERAL NERVOUS SYSTEM

Syndromes With Genetic Predisposition for Peripheral Nerve Neoplasia

Feature	NF1	NF2	Schwannomatosis	Carney Complex
Incidence	1 in 2,500-3,000 births	1 in 30,000-40,000 births	1 in 30,000-40,000 births	Very rare
Geography/ethnic predilection	None	None	None	None
Inheritance	Familial ~ sporadic (autosomal dominant)	Familial ~ sporadic (autosomal dominant)	Sporadic > familial (autosomal dominant)	Familial > sporadic (autosomal dominant)
Gene	*NF1*	*NF2*	*INI1 (SMARCB1, BAF47, hSNF5)*	*PRKAR1A*
Gene location	17q11.2	22q12.2	22q11.23	17p22-24, 2p16
Protein	Neurofibromin	Merlin	SMARCB1 (SWI/SNF complex)	Regulatory R1 α-subunit of protein kinase A (PKA)
Pathway/cellular function	RAS/MAPK/PI3K/mTOR/cAMP	Integrin, RAC/PAK, WNT, YAP/Hippo, MAPK, PI3K, CRL4	Chromatin remodeling	cAMP
Mosaicism	Yes ("segmental neurofibromatosis")	Yes	Yes (segmental in 1/3)	No
Peripheral nervous system neoplasms	Neurofibromas (localized, diffuse, plexiform, massive soft tissue), intestinal ganglioneuromatosis, gastrointestinal schwannoma, benign hybrid nerve sheath tumor, MPNST	Schwannomas > > neurofibromas (cutaneous), benign hybrid nerve sheath tumor, MPNST (very rare, probably post radiation)	Schwannomas, benign hybrid nerve sheath tumor, neurofibromas (very rare)	Melanotic schwannomas (psammomatous)
Central nervous system neoplasms	Astrocytomas (grade I-IV), indeterminate astrocytomas, glioneuronal tumors	Ependymomas > meningiomas > > nonependymal gliomas	Meningiomas (rare)	
Other neoplasms	Pheochromocytoma, sarcomas (rhabdomyosarcoma), gastrointestinal stromal tumor, carcinoids, glomus tumor, juvenile myelomonocytic leukemia, breast carcinoma			Myxomas (cutaneous, mucosal, cardiac), GH adenoma, blue nevi, breast duct adenoma, breast myxomatosis, osteochondromyxoma, thyroid carcinoma/nodules, large cell calcifying Sertoli cell tumor, fibromas
Nonneoplastic nervous system manifestations	Macrocephaly, cognitive disabilities, developmental delays, and behavioral disturbances	Meningioangiomatosis, glial microhamartoma, peripheral neuropathy	Neuropathic pain	
Eye manifestations	Lisch nodules	Posterior subcapsular cataract, retinal hamartoma, epiretinal membranes		
Cutaneous manifestations	Café au lait spots, intertriginous skin freckling	Hairy plaques, café au lait spots (rare)		Spotty skin pigmentation (lips, conjunctiva, inner or outer canthi, vagina, penis), freckling, café au lait spots, pilonidal sinus, skin tags
Skeletal manifestations	Sphenoid wing dysplasia/ hypoplasia, scoliosis, pseudoarthrosis, bowing of long bones	Scoliosis		
Endocrine manifestations	Increased catecholamines/ hypertension (secondary to pheochromocytoma)			Acromegaly, hyperprolactinemia, pigmented nodular adrenal cortical disease (Cushing disease)
Cardiovascular manifestations	Cerebral arteriopathy (moyamoya disease), pulmonary artery stenosis			Cardiomyopathy
Differential diagnosis	Noonan syndrome, Legius syndrome, constitutional mismatch repair syndrome, McCune-Albright syndrome, proteus syndrome, familial café au lait spots, MEN2B	Schwannomatosis, NF1	NF2	Peutz-Jeghers, McCune-Albright syndrome, LEOPARD, Cowden disease and Bannayan-Ruvalcaba-Riley syndrome (PTEN hamartoma tumor syndromes)

MEN2B: Multiple endocrine neoplasia 2B; NF1: Neurofibromatosis type 1; NF2: Neurofibromatosis type 2.

DIAGNOSTIC CRITERIA

Neurofibromatosis Type 1

- **NIH (1991)**
  - 2 or more of the following features
    - Café au lait macules (≥ 6), with a diameter of 0.5 cm in children or 1.5 cm after puberty
    - Cutaneous or subcutaneous neurofibromas (≥ 2) or plexiform neurofibroma
    - Freckling of the axillary or groin region
    - Glioma of the optic pathways
    - Lisch nodules identified by slit-lamp examination (≥ 2)
    - Dysplasias of skeletal system (sphenoid wing, long bone bowing, pseudoarthrosis)
    - Diagnosis of NF1 in a 1st-degree relative

Neurofibromatosis Type 2

- **Manchester criteria (1992)**
  - Any of the following
    - Bilateral vestibular schwannoma
    - NF2 in 1st-degree relative plus unilateral vestibular schwannoma or any 2 of the following
      - Neurofibroma
      - Meningioma
      - Glioma
      - Schwannoma
      - Posterior subcapsular lens opacity
    - Unilateral vestibular schwannoma plus any 2 of the following
      - Neurofibroma
      - Meningioma
      - Glioma
      - Schwannoma
      - Posterior subscapular lens opacity
    - ≥ 2 meningiomas plus unilateral vestibular schwannoma or any 2 of the following
      - Neurofibroma
      - Glioma
      - Schwannoma
      - Cataract
- **Baser Criteria-Additive scoring system**
  - Criteria
    - NF2 in 1st-degree relative → 2 points
    - Vestibular schwannoma (unilateral)
      - If present at age ≤ 30 years → 2 points
      - If present at age > 30 years → 1 point
    - Vestibular schwannoma (2nd)
      - If present at age ≤ 30 years → 4 points
      - If present at age > 30 years → 3 point
    - Meningioma(s)
      - If present at age ≤ 30 years → 2 points
      - If present at age > 30 years → 1 point
    - Cutaneous schwannoma(s)
      - If present at age ≤ 30 years → 2 points
      - If present at age > 30 years → 1 point
    - Neoplasm of cranial nerves
      - If present at age ≤ 30 years → 2 points
      - If present at age > 30 years → 1 point
    - Mononeuropathy
      - If present at age ≤ 30 years → 2 points
      - If present at age > 30 years → 1 point
    - Cataract(s)
      - If present at age ≤ 30 years → 2 points
      - If present at age > 30 years → 0 points
  - Points added
    - Points ≥ 6: Definite NF2
    - Points 4-5: *NF2* mutational analysis required
    - Points < 4: NF2 unlikely

Schwannomatosis

- **Baser et al (2006)**
  - Definite schwannomatosis
    - Age > 30 years **plus** 2 or more schwannomas (not dermal), at least 1 with histologic confirmation
    - Schwannoma (pathologically confirmed) **plus** 1st-degree relative who meets the above criteria
  - Possible schwannomatosis
    - Age < 30 years **plus** 2 or more schwannomas (not dermal), at least 1 with histologic confirmation
    - Age > 45 years **plus** 2 or more schwannomas (not dermal), at least 1 with histologic confirmation
    - Evidence of a schwannoma (by radiology) and 1st-degree relative meeting the criteria for definite schwannomatosis
  - Must **not** have
    - NF2 by criteria
    - Vestibular schwannoma (by high-resolution MRI)
    - NF2 in 1st-degree relative
    - Germline *NF2* mutation
- **International Schwannomatosis Workshop (2011)**
  - Molecular diagnosis
    - Both
      - Schwannomas or meningiomas (≥ 2 pathologically proven)
      - ≥ 2 tumors with chromosome 22 loss of heterozygosity + 2 different *NF2* mutations
    - Or schwannoma or meningioma + germline *SMARCB1* mutation
  - Clinical diagnosis
    - Both
      - ≥ 2 schwannomas (not intradermal), 1 pathologically confirmed
      - No vestibular schwannomas on high-quality MR study
    - Or either
      - Schwannoma, pathologically confirmed
      - Intracranial meningioma and 1st-degree relative with schwannomatosis
  - Possible schwannomatosis
    - ≥ 2 schwannomas (not intradermal) without pathologic confirmation
  - Any of the following excludes schwannomatosis
    - NF2 by criteria
    - Germline *NF2* mutation
    - 1st-degree relative with NF2
    - Multiple schwannomas in a prior irradiated field only

Diagrammatic, Imaging, and Microscopic Features

(Left) *Expansion of numerous nerve roots by neurofibromas is typical of neurofibromatosis type 1. Many of these neurofibromas may be classified as plexiform neurofibromas, defined by involvement of multiple nerve fascicles.* ***(Right)*** *Plexiform neurofibroma is a distinctive subtype defined by architectural features (i.e., involvement of multiple nerve fascicles) and demonstrates a multinodular pattern of growth. When large and deep, plexiform neurofibroma is almost pathognomonic of NF1.*

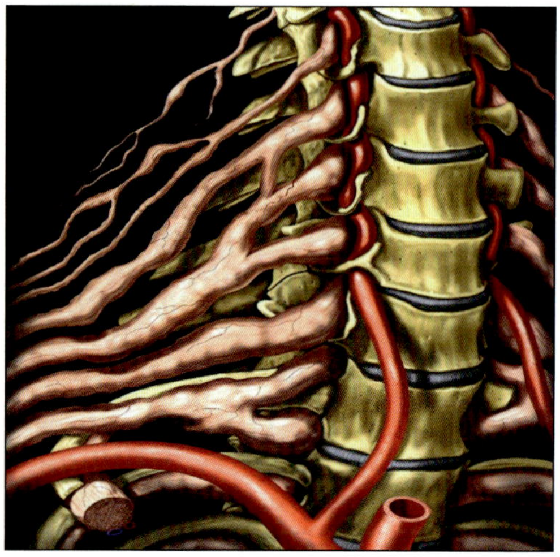

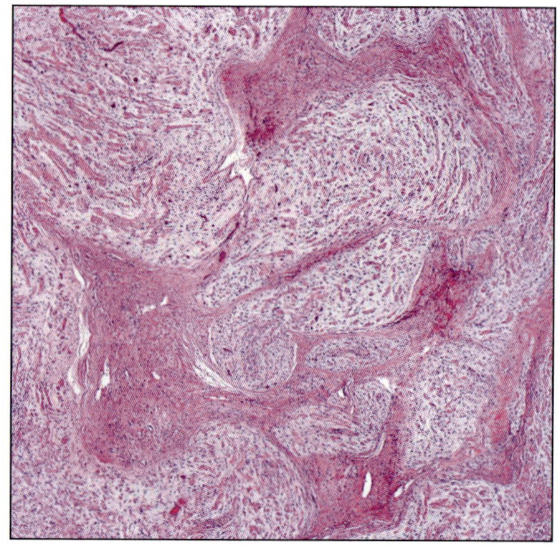

(Left) *Neurofibromas of all types may affect NF1 patients. The typical neurofibroma contains wavy neoplastic Schwann cells in a myxoid background and delicate collagen fibers. Mast cells are frequent →. In the context of NF1, mast cells facilitate tumor growth by providing trophic signals to the Schwann cell component.* ***(Right)*** *Spinal neurofibromas often involve sensory ganglia in NF1. These entrapped ganglion cells are distributed singly and contain numerous satellite cells →.*

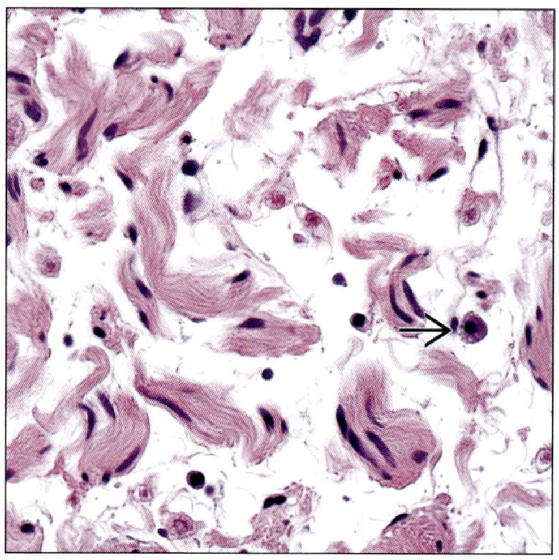

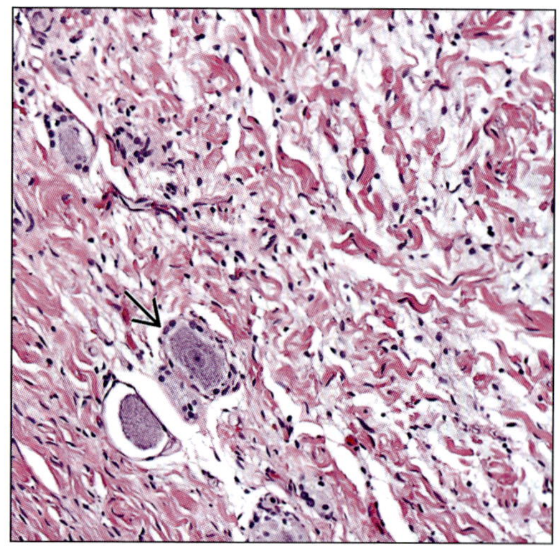

(Left) *Malignant peripheral nerve sheath tumors (MPNST) represent the main malignancies afflicting NF1 patients. This large contrast-enhancing mass → afflicting a patient with NF1 was characterized by sudden growth, which is a worrisome clinical feature. The histologic features were diagnostic of MPNST.* ***(Right)*** *MPNSTs are characterized by a cellular, fascicular pattern of growth. Mitotic activity is not subtle in this NF1-associated MPNST →.*

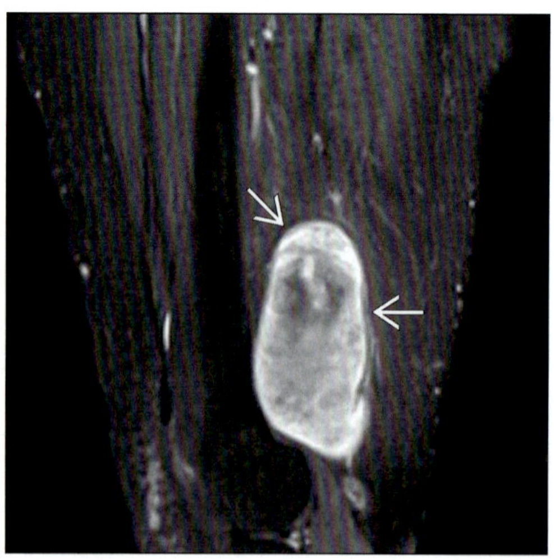

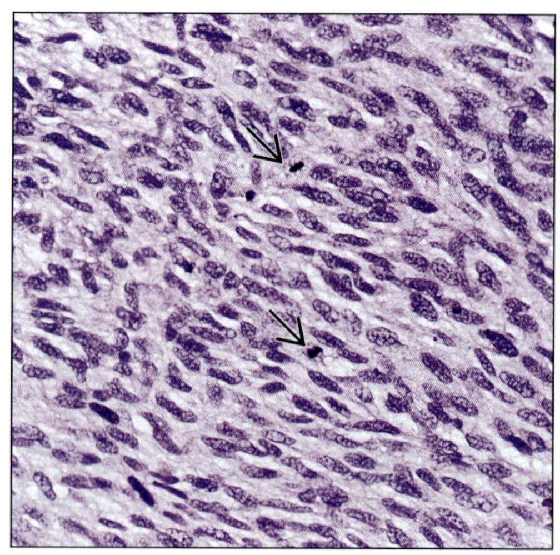

Microscopic Features

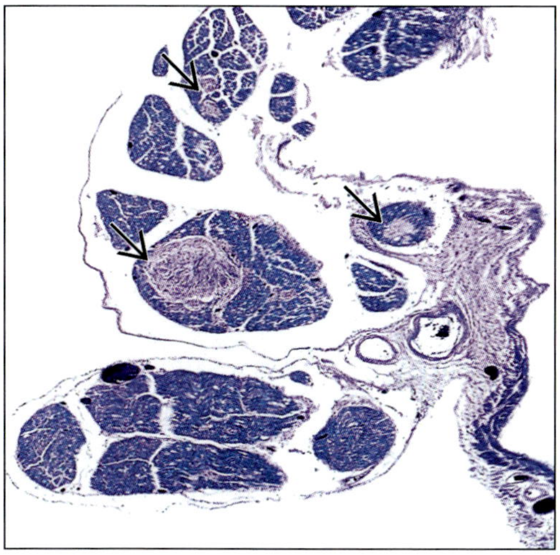
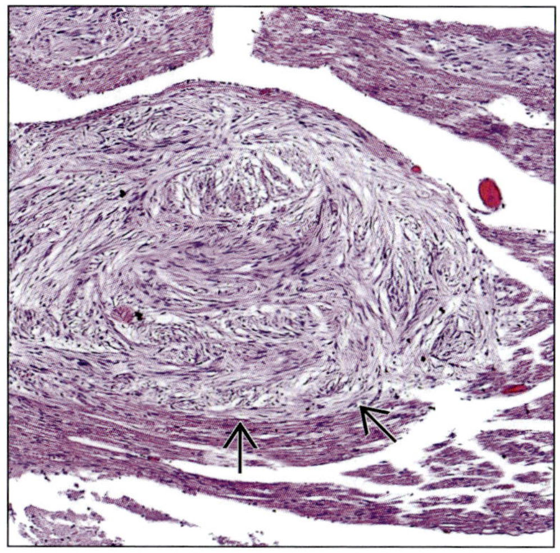

(Left) *Well-circumscribed schwannomas of various sizes are evident in nerve roots in this patient with NF2 at autopsy. These schwannomas stand out as areas of pallor* → *in a background of myelinated nerve fibers.* ***(Right)*** *In contrast to neurofibromas, schwannomas form well-circumscribed masses composed almost exclusively of neoplastic Schwann cells, as this NF2-associated example demonstrates. A sharp edge with associated nerve is typical* →*, which facilitates surgical excision.*

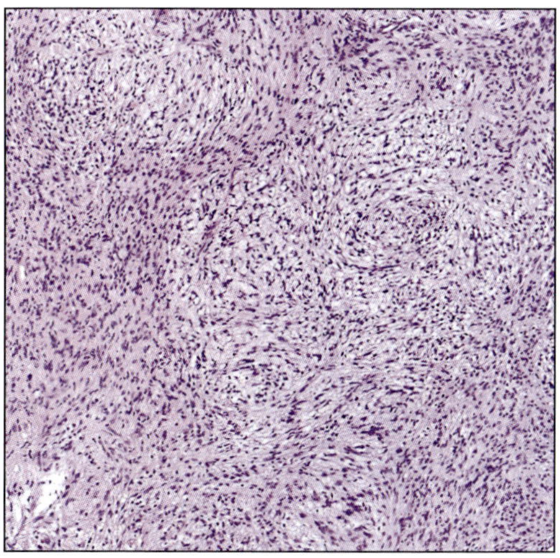
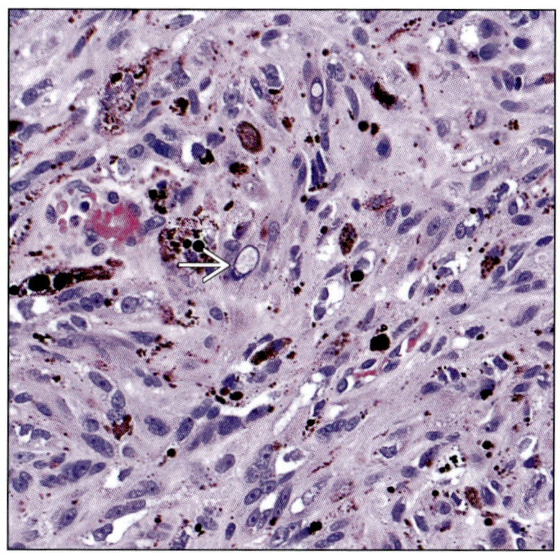

(Left) *Schwannomas characterized by a predominance of myxoid stroma ("myxoid schwannomas") are not infrequent in the setting of schwannomatosis, as this example shows.* ***(Right)*** *Melanotic schwannoma is a distinctive, rare subtype characterized by prominent melanotic content, pleomorphism, and nuclear pseudoinclusions* →*. On isolation, melanotic schwannomas raise an important differential diagnosis with melanocytic neoplasms of various grades.*

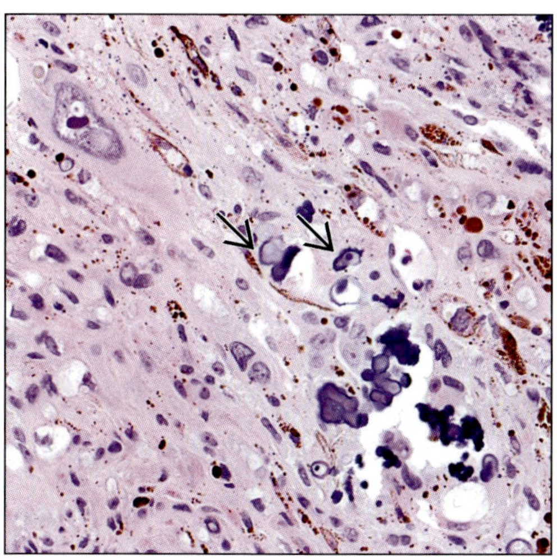
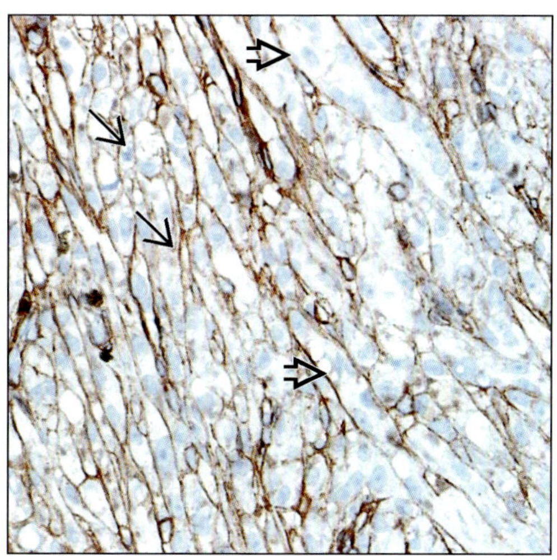

(Left) *Patients with melanotic schwannomas containing microcalcifications and psammoma bodies* → *(psammomatous melanotic schwannoma) should be clinically evaluated for the possibility of Carney complex. A significant proportion of such tumors develop in the setting of this rare syndrome.* ***(Right)*** *Pericellular* → *and perilobular* ⇨ *collagen IV staining, identifying basal lamina typical of Schwann cells, is typical of melanotic schwannomas. A perilobular pattern may predominate.*

Pulmonary

Lung III-10-2

Familial Cancer Syndromes With Lung Neoplasms

Syndrome	Type of Tumor	Associated Neoplasms
Tuberous sclerosis	LAM	Major features: Cortical tuber, subependymal nodule, SEGA, facial angiofibroma/forehead plaque, ungual/periungual fibroma, > 3 hypomelanotic macules, Shagreen patch, multiple retinal hamartomas, cardiac rhabdomyoma, renal angiomyolipoma/ lymphangioleiomyomatosis Minor features: White matter migration lines, transmantle cortical dysplasia, retinal patch, hamartomatous rectal polyps, gingival fibroma, dental pits, hypomelanotic clustered skin lesions, bone cysts, renal cysts, nonrenal hamartomas
Carney triad	Pulmonary chondroma	Gastric stromal sarcomas, extraadrenal paragangliomas, adrenal cortical neoplasms, esophageal tumors
Familial pleuropulmonary blastoma due to germline *DICER1* mutation	PPB	Manifestations of the syndrome have been identified including cystic nephroma, medulloepithelioma, Sertoli-Leydig cell tumor, embryonal rhabdomyosarcoma, and others *DICER1* mutations are associated with both familial multinodular thyroid hyperplasia and multinodular thyroid hyperplasia with Sertoli-Leydig cell tumor of the ovary, independent of PPB
Bloom syndrome	Lung adenocarcinoma	Leukemias, both acute myeloid leukemia and acute lymphoblastic leukemia; carcinomas arise in varied sites including skin, head and neck, gastrointestinal tract including esophagus (both squamous cell carcinoma and adenocarcinoma), stomach and colon, lung, uterus and breast; medulloblastoma, Wilms tumor, osteogenic sarcoma
Breast-ovarian *BRCA2*	Lung adenocarcinoma	Carcinoma of breast, ovary, fallopian tubes and peritoneal; carcinoma of prostate, pancreas, gall bladder, bile duct, and stomach
Li-Fraumeni	Lung adenocarcinoma, lepidic pattern	Any childhood cancer or sarcoma, brain tumor, or adrenal cortical carcinoma before age 45; soft tissue sarcoma, osteosarcoma, premenopausal breast cancer, brain tumor, adrenal cortical carcinoma, leukemia
Peutz-Jeghers	Lung adenocarcinoma, lepidic pattern	Pigmentation of lips and oral and genital mucosa; polyps arise in stomach, small bowel, and colon; adenocarcinoma of small bowel, colon, pancreas, stomach; carcinoma of breast; ovarian sex cord tumors with annular tubules, adenoma malignum of cervix, mucinous tumors of ovaries and fallopian tubes, testicular sex cord and Sertoli cell tumors, papillary thyroid carcinoma
Hereditary retinoblastoma	Early onset of small cell lung carcinoma; some non-small cell carcinoma	Retinoblastoma, pineoblastoma/CNS-PNET; soft tissue and bone sarcomas including leiomyosarcoma, fibrosarcoma, rhabdomyosarcoma, pleomorphic sarcoma, liposarcoma/lipomatous tumors; melanoma of skin; carcinomas of bladder, upper respiratory tract, and skin; tumors of the central nervous system/meningiomas
Xeroderma pigmentosum	Carcinoma, both adenocarcinoma and squamous cell carcinoma	Skin carcinomas and sarcoma, especially basal cell carcinoma and squamous cell carcinoma; cutaneous malignant melanoma, ocular cancer, tongue cancer, brain tumors, and carcinoma of uterus, breast, stomach, kidney, and testis

LAM: Lymphangioleiomyomatosis; PNET: Primitive neuroectodermal tumor; PPB: Pleuropulmonary blastoma; SEGA: Subependymal giant cell astrocytoma.

Gross and Microscopic Features

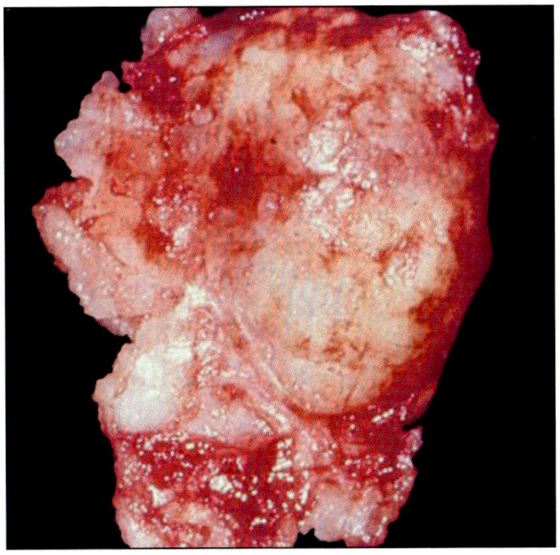

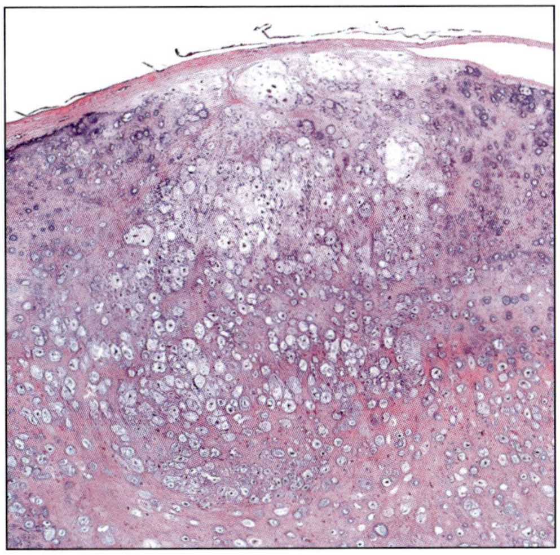

(Left) *One of the tumors associated with Carney triad is pulmonary chondroma. This gross picture of a pulmonary chondroma shows a cartilaginous cut surface appearance. (Courtesy J. A. Carney, MD.)* ***(Right)*** *Carney triad is a rare multitumoral syndrome composed by neoplasms of the stomach, lungs, paraganglionic system, adrenal cortex, and esophagus. The pulmonary chondroma is covered by a thin, fibrous pseudocapsule without entrapped epithelium and fat.*

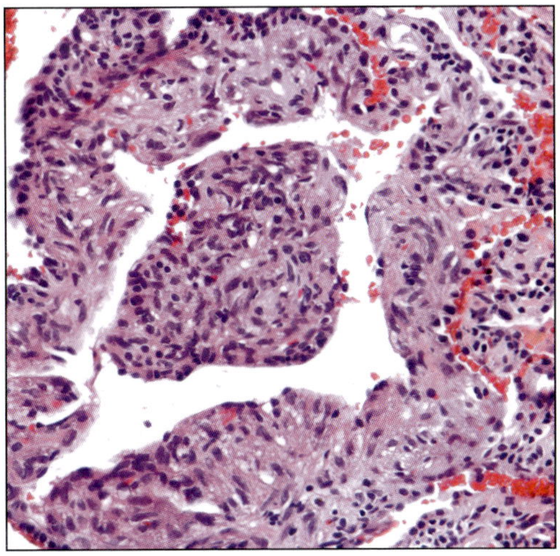

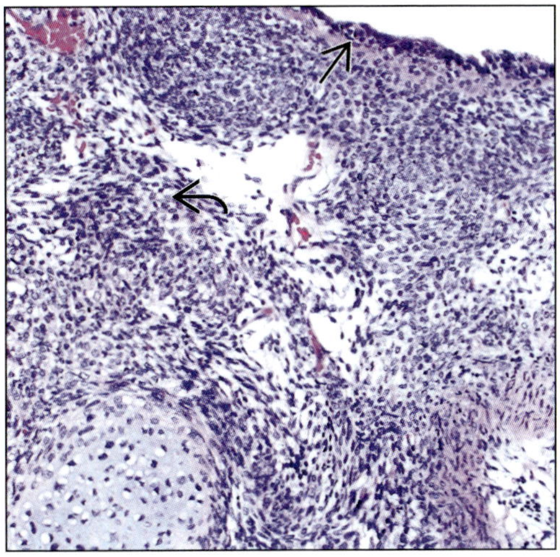

(Left) *High-power magnification of lymphangioleiomyomatosis in a patient with tuberous sclerosis shows the classical presence of smooth muscle proliferation within the alveolar wall that has obliterated the normal alveolar lining.* ***(Right)*** *Familial pleuropulmonary blastoma (PPB) is associated with DICER1 mutation. This low-power view of solid type III PPB shows benign epithelial component at upper right ⇒ overlying the malignant mesenchymal component ➡.*

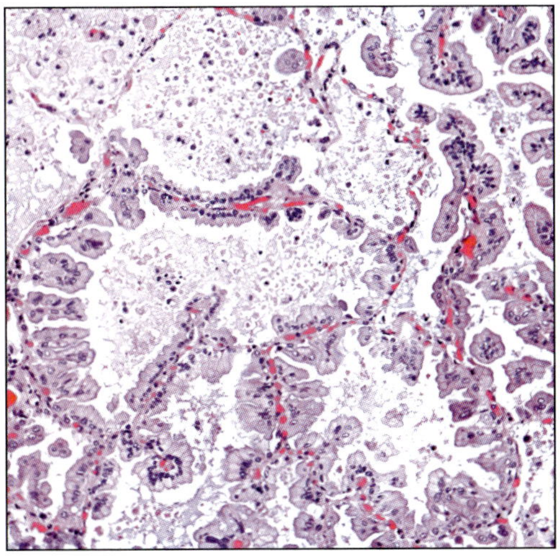

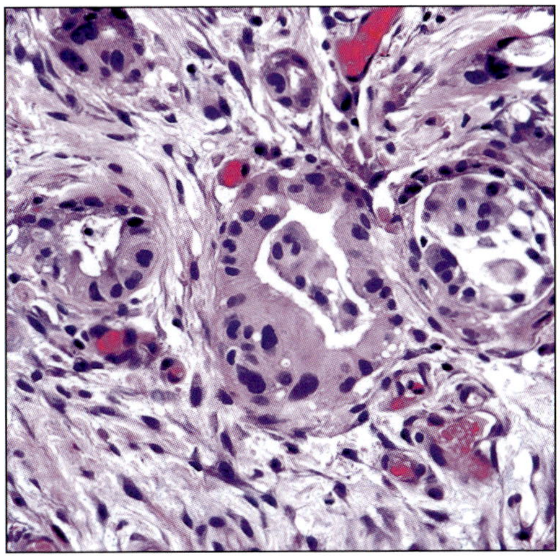

(Left) *Lung adenocarcinoma, lepidic pattern shows a classical pattern of lepidic growth, characteristically associated with Li-Fraumeni syndrome. Note the presence of neoplastic cells lining the alveolar wall.* ***(Right)*** *Well-differentiated adenocarcinomas seen in association with familial syndromes are similar to the sporadic tumors. The acinar growth pattern is composed of small glandular proliferation, arranged in a haphazard pattern with fibrotic and inflammatory stroma.*

Skin

Skin **III**-11-2

SKIN

Selected Cutaneous Neoplasms and Associated Hereditary Cancer Syndromes

Cutaneous Neoplasm	Hereditary Cancer Syndrome
Basal cell carcinoma	Gorlin syndrome (basal cell nevus syndrome), xeroderma pigmentosum, Bazex-Dupré-Christol syndrome, Rombo syndrome, hereditary infundibulocystic basal cell carcinoma
Squamous cell carcinoma	Xeroderma pigmentosum
Malignant melanoma	Hereditary multiple melanoma, melanoma/pancreatic carcinoma syndrome, xeroderma pigmentosum, Werner syndrome
Sebaceous adenoma	Muir-Torre syndrome, Lynch syndrome
Sebaceoma	Muir-Torre syndrome, Lynch syndrome
Sebaceous carcinoma	Muir-Torre syndrome, Lynch syndrome
Trichilemmoma	Cowden syndrome
Fibrofolliculoma/trichodiscoma	Birt-Hogg-Dubé syndrome
Fibrous papule (angiofibroma)	Tuberous sclerosis, multiple endocrine neoplasia type 1, Birt-Hogg-Dubé syndrome
Leiomyoma	Reed syndrome

Selected Hereditary Cancer Syndromes With Skin Manifestations

Syndrome	Common Skin Manifestations
Gorlin syndrome (basal cell nevus syndrome)	Basal cell carcinoma, palmoplantar pitting
Muir-Torre syndrome	Sebaceous neoplasms
Lynch syndrome	Sebaceous neoplasms
Hereditary multiple melanoma syndrome	Melanoma, atypical nevi
Melanoma/pancreatic carcinoma syndrome	Melanoma, atypical nevi
Birt-Hogg-Dubé syndrome	Fibrofolliculoma/trichodiscoma, perifollicular fibroma, skin tags
Cowden syndrome (*PTEN*-hamartoma syndrome)	Trichilemmoma, verrucous keratosis, acral keratosis, oral papilloma, sclerotic fibroma, lipoma
Reed syndrome	Leiomyoma
Tuberous sclerosis	Angiofibroma, hypopigmented macule, collagenoma
Multiple endocrine neoplasia type 1	Angiofibroma, collagenoma, lipoma, hypopigmented macule
Multiple endocrine neoplasia type 2B	Mucosal > cutaneous neuroma
Multiple endocrine neoplasia type 2A	Lichen amyloidosis
Gardner syndrome (familial polyposis of colon)	Epidermoid cyst, pilomatrical cyst, desmoid tumor, fibroma
Hereditary breast/ovarian carcinoma	Melanoma
Beckwith-Wiedemann syndrome	Hemihyperplasia, abdominal wall defects, anterior ear lobe creases, posterior helical pits, nevus flammeus
Xeroderma pigmentosum	Skin cancers, lentigines, poikiloderma
Werner syndrome	Melanoma, skin atrophy
Howel-Evans syndrome	Palmoplantar keratoderma
Costello syndrome	Papillomas, palmoplantar keratoderma
Dyskeratosis congenita	Palmoplantar keratoderma, reticulate hyperpigmentation

Microscopic Features

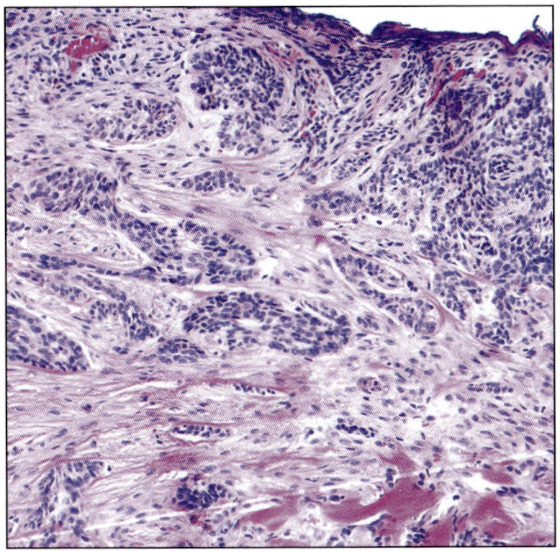

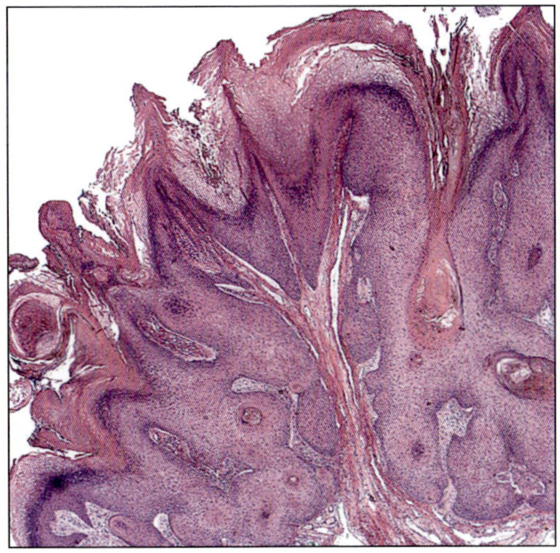

(Left) *This is a morpheaform basal cell carcinoma. Multiple basal cell carcinomas are seen in Gorlin syndrome.* ***(Right)*** *This verrucous keratosis has some features of trichilemmoma but does not have a truly lobular configuration with peripheral palisading and central clear/pale cells. This verrucous keratosis was removed from a patient with Cowden syndrome.*

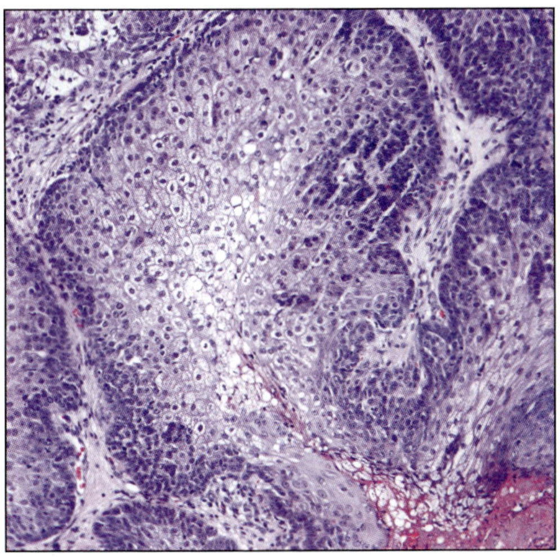

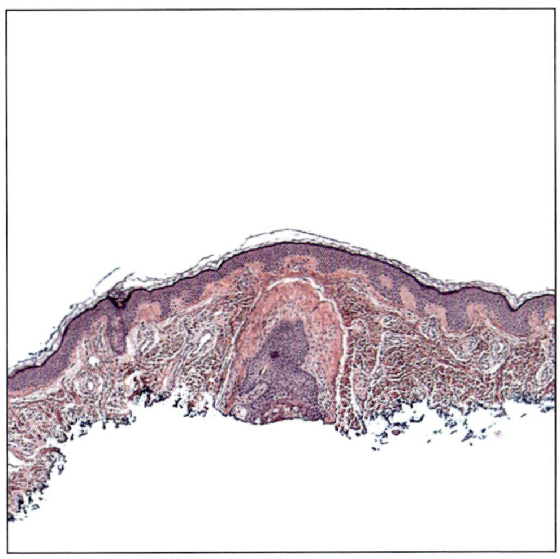

(Left) *This is a sebaceous adenoma, which may be seen in the setting of Muir-Torre syndrome. The tumor may display loss of staining with mismatch repair proteins.* ***(Right)*** *There is prominent perifollicular fibrosis around the central hair follicle, compatible with a perifollicular fibroma. This particular lesion was removed from a patient with Birt-Hogg-Dubé syndrome.*

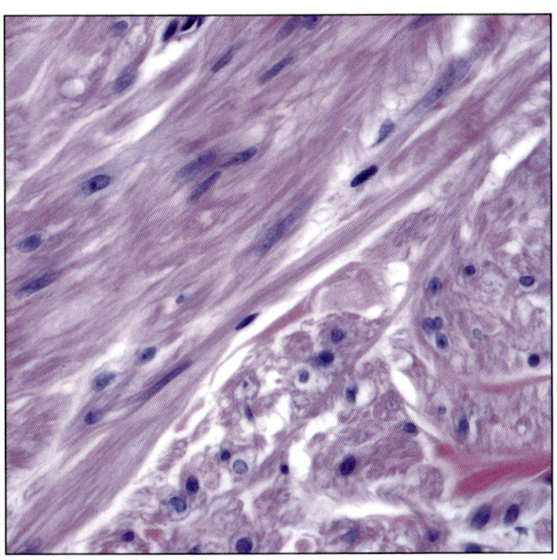

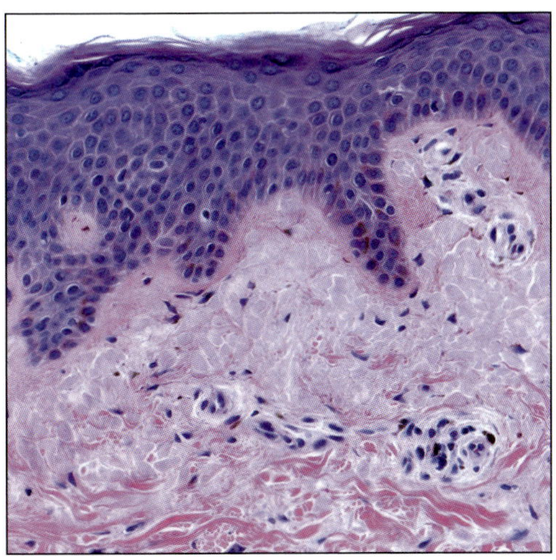

(Left) *This is a high-magnification view of a pilar leiomyoma. Such tumors can be seen in the setting of Reed syndrome.* ***(Right)*** *There are amorphous pink deposits and pigment incontinence in the papillary dermis below a hyperplastic epidermis, compatible with lichen amyloidosis. Lichen amyloidosis is sometimes seen in association with multiple endocrine neoplasia type 2A.*

Molecular Factors

MOLECULAR FACTORS INDEX

Molecular Factors Discussed

Gene	Gene Location	Official Gene Symbol and Name	Chapter Term Found
ABCB11	2q24	ABCB11; ATP-binding cassette, sub-family B (MDR/TAP), member 11	Biliary Tract/Liver/Pancreas
ABF1	8q21	MSC; musculin	Hodgkin Lymphoma
AGL	1p21	AGL; amylo-alpha-1, 6-glucosidase, 4-alpha-glucanotransferase	Biliary Tract/Liver/Pancreas
AIP	11q13.3	AIP; aryl hydrocarbon receptor interacting protein	Pituitary; Pituitary Adenoma
AKT1	14q32.32	AKT1; v-akt murine thymoma viral oncogene homolog 1	Meningioma; Neurofibromatosis Type 1; PTEN-Hamartoma Tumor Syndromes
ALDH2	12q24.2	ALDH2; aldehyde dehydrogenase 2 family (mitochondrial)	Esophageal Squamous Cell Carcinoma
ALK	2p23	ALK; anaplastic lymphoma receptor tyrosine kinase	Bone and Soft Tissue; Diffuse Large B-Cell Lymphoma; Hereditary Neuroblastoma; Neuroblastoma
ALX4	11p11.2	ALX4; ALX homeobox 4	Hereditary Multiple Exostosis
AML1	21q22.3	RUNX1; runt-related transcription factor 1	Familial Acute Myeloid Leukemia
APC	5q21	APC; adenomatosis polyposis coli	Adrenal Cortex; Adrenal Cortical Neoplasms in Children; Astrocytoma; Biliary Tract/Liver/Pancreas; Bone and Soft Tissue; Central Nervous System; Colon Adenoma; Colon/Rectum; Esophagus; Familial Adenomatous Polyposis; Familial Nonmedullary Thyroid Carcinoma; Familial Thyroid Carcinoma; Gastrointestinal Stromal Tumor; Head and Neck; Hereditary Pancreatic Cancer Syndrome; Medulloblastoma/CNS-PNET; MYH-associated Polyposis; Pineoblastoma; Small Bowel Adenocarcinoma; Thyroid, Nonmedullary
API2-MALT1	t(11;18)(q22;q21)	BIRC3-MALT1	Lymphoplasmacytic Lymphoma/ Waldenström Macroglobulinemia
ASIP	20q11.2-q12	ASIP; agouti signaling protein	Hereditary Multiple Melanoma
ASK1	6q22.33	ASK1; MAP3K5;mitogen-activated protein kinase kinase kinase 5	Bone and Soft Tissue
ASPL-TFE3	t(X;17)(p11.2;q25)	ASPSCR1-TFE3	Bone and Soft Tissue
ASS1	9q34.1	ASS1; argininosuccinate synthase 1	Biliary Tract/Liver/Pancreas
ATG13	11p11.2	ATG13; autophagy related 13	Familial Plasma Cell Myeloma
ATM	11q22.3	ATM; ataxia telangiectasia mutated	Ataxia-Telangiectasia; Breast; Breast Carcinoma, Female; Eye; Hereditary Pancreatic Cancer Syndrome; Melanoma; Melanoma/Pancreatic Carcinoma Syndrome; Salivary Glands
ATP8B1	18q21.31	ATP8B1; ATPase, aminophospholipid transporter, class I, type 8B, member 1	Biliary Tract/Liver/Pancreas
BACH1	21q22.11	BACH1; BTB and CNC homology 1, basic leucine zipper transcription factor 1	Breast; Breast Carcinoma, Female
BAK1	6p21.3	BAK1; BCL2-antagonist/killer 1	Familial Testicular Tumor; Testicle
BAP1	3p21.31-p21.2	BAP1; BRCA1 associated protein-1 (ubiquitin carboxy-terminal hydrolase)	Central Nervous System; Cutaneous Melanoma; Eye; Familial Uveal Melanoma; Hereditary Multiple Melanoma
BARD1	2q34-q35	BARD1; BRCA1 associated RING domain 1	Breast; Breast Carcinoma, Female
BAX	19q13.3-q13.4	BAX; BCL2-associated X protein	Basal Cell Carcinoma
BCL10-IGH	t(1;14)(p22;q32)		Lymphoplasmacytic Lymphoma/ Waldenström Macroglobulinemia
BCL2	18q21.3	BCL2; B-cell CLL/lymphoma 2	Colon Adenoma; Diffuse Large B-Cell Lymphoma; Familial Non-Hodgkin Lymphoma; Prostate Carcinoma
BCL6	3q27	BCL6; B-cell CLL/lymphoma 6	Diffuse Large B-Cell Lymphoma; Follicular Lymphoma; Hodgkin Lymphoma
BCR-ABL1	t(9;22)(q34;q11)		Myeloid Neoplasms
BHD	17p11.2	FLCN; folliculin	Hereditary Renal Epithelial Tumors, Others; Kidney

MOLECULAR FACTORS INDEX

BLM	15q26.1	RECQL3; Bloom syndrome, RecQ helicase-like	Bloom Syndrome; Colon/Rectum; Head and Neck; Myeloid Neoplasms; Squamous Cell Carcinoma, Head and Neck; Xeroderma Pigmentosum
BMI1	10p11.23	BMI1; BMI1 polycomb ring finger oncogene	Basal Cell Carcinoma
BMPR1A	10q22.3	BMPR1A; bone morphogenetic protein receptor, type IA	Biliary Tract/Liver/Pancreas; Colon/Rectum; Esophagus; Juvenile Polyposis
BOB1	3q11.2-q13.1	GPR15; G protein-coupled receptor 15	Hodgkin Lymphoma
BRAF	7q34	BRAF; v-raf murine sarcoma viral oncogene homolog B	Astrocytoma; Colon Adenoma; Costello Syndrome; Cutaneous Melanoma; Familial Nonmedullary Thyroid Carcinoma; Familial Uveal Melanoma; Hereditary Multiple Melanoma; Lynch Syndrome
BRCA1	17q21	BRCA1; breast cancer 1, early onset	Biliary Tract/Liver/Pancreas; Breast; Breast Carcinoma, Female; Breast Carcinoma, Male; Fallopian Tube Carcinoma; Familial Uveal Melanoma; Gynecologic Neoplasms; Hereditary Breast/Ovarian Cancer Syndrome: BRCA1; Hereditary Breast/Ovarian Cancer Syndrome: BRCA2; Hereditary Multiple Melanoma; Hereditary Pancreatic Cancer Syndrome; Ovarian Carcinoma; Pancreatic Ductal Adenocarcinoma; Pathology of Familial Tumor Syndromes
BRCA2	13q12.3	BRCA2; breast cancer 2, early onset	Adenocarcinoma, Lung; Biliary Tract/Liver/Pancreas; Breast; Breast Carcinoma, Female; Breast Carcinoma, Male; Fallopian Tube Carcinoma; Gynecologic Neoplasms; Hereditary Breast/Ovarian Cancer Syndrome: BRCA1; Hereditary Breast/Ovarian Cancer Syndrome: BRCA2; Hereditary Multiple Melanoma; Hereditary Pancreatic Cancer Syndrome; Hereditary Prostate Cancer; Li-Fraumeni Syndrome/Li-Fraumeni-Like Syndrome; Lung; Melanoma; Melanoma/Pancreatic Carcinoma Syndrome; Ovarian Carcinoma; Pancreatic Ductal Adenocarcinoma; Parathyroid Carcinoma; Pathology of Familial Tumor Syndromes; Prostate Carcinoma; Wilms Tumor-Associated Syndromes
BRIP1	17q22.2	BRIP1; BRCA1 interacting protein C-terminal helicase 1	Breast; Breast Carcinoma, Female; Gynecologic Neoplasms; Li-Fraumeni Syndrome/Li-Fraumeni-Like Syndrome; Ovarian Carcinoma
CASR	3q13.3-21	CASR; calcium-sensing receptor	Familial Isolated Hyperparathyroidism; Parathyroid; Parathyroid Hyperplasia
CBFA2	21q22.3	RUNX1; runt-related transcription factor 1	Familial Acute Myeloid Leukemia
CBL	11q23.3	CBL; Cas-Br-M (murine) ecotropic retroviral transforming sequence	Myeloid Neoplasms
CCNA1	13q12.3-q13	CCNA1; cyclin-A1	Pituitary
CCND1	11q13	CCND1; cyclin-D1	Parathyroid Adenoma; Parathyroid Carcinoma; Parathyroid Hyperplasia; Pituitary; Plasma Cell Myeloma; Squamous Cell Carcinoma, Head and Neck
CCND1-IGH	t(11;14)(q13;q32)	CCND1-IGH	Mantle Cell Lymphoma
CCND3	6p21	CCND3; cyclin D3	Plasma Cell Myeloma
CD19	16p11.2	CD19; CD19 molecule	Hodgkin Lymphoma
CDC73/HRPT2	1q25	CDC73; cell division cycle 73	Familial Isolated Hyperparathyroidism; Hereditary Renal Epithelial Tumors, Others; Kidney
CDH1	16q22.1	CDH1; cadherin 1, type 1	Breast; Breast Carcinoma, Female; Colon/Rectum; Esophagus; Gastric Adenocarcinoma; Hereditary Diffuse Gastric Cancer
CDH11	16q21	CDH11; cadherin 11, type 2	Bone and Soft Tissue
CDK4	12q14	CDK4; cyclin-dependent kinase 4	Bone and Soft Tissue; Hereditary Multiple Melanoma

MOLECULAR FACTORS INDEX

CDKN1B	12p13.1-p12	CDKN1B; cyclin-dependent kinase inhibitor 1B	Pituitary; Pituitary Adenoma; Prostate Carcinoma
CDKN1C	11p15.5	CDKN1C; cyclin-dependent kinase inhibitor 1C	Adrenal Cortex; Adrenal Cortical Neoplasms in Children; Beckwith-Wiedemann Syndrome; Kidney; Rhabdomyosarcoma; Wilms Tumor; Wilms Tumor-Associated Syndromes
CDKN2A/P16	9p21	CDKN2A; cyclin-dependent kinase inhibitor 2A	Astrocytoma; Biliary Tract/Liver/Pancreas; Central Nervous System; Cutaneous Melanoma; Cutaneous Melanoma; Familial Plasma Cell Myeloma; Familial Uveal Melanoma; Follicular Lymphoma; Hereditary Multiple Melanoma; Hereditary Pancreatic Cancer Syndrome; Melanoma/Pancreatic Carcinoma Syndrome; Neurofibromatosis Type 1; Pancreatic Endocrine Tumor; Squamous Cell Carcinoma, Head and Neck
CEBPA	19q13.1	CEBPA; CCAAT/enhancer binding protein (C/EBP), alpha	Familial Acute Myeloid Leukemia; Myeloid Neoplasms
CFTR	7q31.2	CFTR; cystic fibrosis transmembrane conductance regulator (ATP-binding cassette sub-family C, member 7)	Biliary Tract/Liver/Pancreas; Hereditary Pancreatic Cancer Syndrome
CHEK1	11q24.2	CHEK1; checkpoint kinase 1	Breast Carcinoma, Female
CHEK2	22q12.1	CHEK2; checkpoint kinase 2	Biliary Tract/Liver/Pancreas; Breast; Breast Carcinoma, Female; Breast Carcinoma, Male; Li-Fraumeni Syndrome/Li-Fraumeni-Like Syndrome; Prostate Carcinoma
CLTC-ALK	t(2;17)(p23;q23)	CLTC-ALK	Bone and Soft Tissue
COL12A1	6q12-q13	COL12A1; collagen, type XII, alpha 1	Bone and Soft Tissue
COL1A1-PDGFB	t(17;22)(q21;q13)	COL1A1-PDGFB	Bone and Soft Tissue
COL4A5	Xq22	COL4A5; collagen, type IV, alpha 5	Bone and Soft Tissue
COL6A3-CSF1	t(1;2)(p13;q37)	COL6A3-CSF1	Bone and Soft Tissue
CRAC1	15q13-q21	CRAC1; colorectal adenoma and carcinoma 1	Colon/Rectum
CTC1	17p13	CTC1; CTS telomere maintenance complex component 1	Dyskeratosis Congenita
CTCL	Xp11.2	TSPYL2; TSPY-like 2	Diffuse Large B-Cell Lymphoma
CTNNB1	3p21	CTNNB1; catenin (cadherin-associated protein), beta 1	Bone and Soft Tissue; Wilms Tumor
CXORF5	Xp22	OFD1; oral-facial-digital syndrome 1	Beckwith-Wiedemann Syndrome
CYLD	16q12.1	CYLD; cylindromatosis (turban tumor syndrome)	Birt-Hogg-Dubé Syndrome; Salivary Glands
CYP21	6p21.3	CYP21A2; cytochrome P450, family 21, subfamily A, polypeptide 2	Adrenal Cortex; Adrenal Cortical Neoplasms in Children
DICER1	14q32.13	DICER1; dicer 1, ribonuclease type III	Central Nervous System; Clinical Diagnosis and Management of Familial; Eye; Lung; Pineoblastoma; Pleuropulmonary Blastoma
DIRC1	2q33	DIRC1; disrupted in renal carcinoma 1	Hereditary Renal Epithelial Tumors, Others; Kidney
DIRC2	2q33	DIRC2; disrupted in renal carcinoma 1	Hereditary Renal Epithelial Tumors, Others; Kidney;
DIRC3	2q35	DIRC3; disrupted in renal carcinoma 3	Hereditary Renal Epithelial Tumors, Others; Kidney
DIS3L2	2q37.1	DIS3L2; DIS3 mitotic control homolog (S. cerevisiae)-like 2	Beckwith-Wiedemann Syndrome
DKC1	Xq28	DKC1; dyskeratosis congenita 1, dyskerin	Blood and Bone Marrow; Dyskeratosis Congenita; Head and Neck; Howel-Evans Syndrome/Keratosis Palmares and Plantares With Esophageal Cancer; Squamous Cell Carcinoma, Head and Neck
DND1	5q31.3	DND1; DND microRNA-mediated repression inhibitor 1	Familial Testicular Tumor
DOG1	11q13.3	ANO1; anoctamin 1, calcium activated chloride channel	Gastrointestinal Stromal Tumor
EBF1	5q34	EBF1; early B-cell factor 1	Hodgkin Lymphoma
EGFR	7p12	EGFR; epidermal growth factor receptor	Adenocarcinoma, Lung; Neurofibromatosis Type 1; Pituitary; Squamous Cell Carcinoma, Head and Neck
EGLN1/PHD2	1q42.1	EGLN1; egl-9 family hypoxia-inducible factor 1	Adrenal Medulla; Hereditary Paraganglioma/Pheochromocytoma Syndromes; Paraganglioma

MOLECULAR FACTORS INDEX

ELAC2	17p11.2	ELAC2; elaC ribonuclease Z 2	Hereditary Prostate Cancer; Prostate Carcinoma
ELANE	19p13.3	ELANE; elastase, neutrophil expressed	Blood and Bone Marrow
ENG	9q34.11	ENG; endoglin	Biliary Tract/Liver/Pancreas; Colon/Rectum; Esophagus; Juvenile Polyposis;
EPCAM	2p21	EPCAM; epithelial cell adhesion molecule	Endometrial Carcinoma; Lynch Syndrome ;
ERCC6	10q11.23	ERCC6; excision repair cross-complementing rodent repair deficiency, complementation group 6	Werner Syndrome/Progeria; Xeroderma Pigmentosum
ERCC8	5q12.1	ERCC8; excision repair cross-complementing rodent repair deficiency, complementation group 8	Werner Syndrome/Progeria; Xeroderma Pigmentosum
ERG	21q22.3	ERG; v-ets erythroblastosis virus E26 oncogene homolog	Prostate Carcinoma
ETS	11q23.3	ETS; v-ets avian erythroblastosis virus E26 oncogene homolog 1	Prostate Carcinoma
ETV1	7p21.3	ETV1; ets variant 1	Prostate Carcinoma
ETV4	17q21	ETV4; ets variant 4	Prostate Carcinoma
ETV5	3q28	ETV5; ets variant 5	Prostate Carcinoma
ETV6-NTRK3	t(12;15)(p13;q25)	ETV6-NTRK3	Bone and Soft Tissue; Salivary Glands
EWSR1/EWS	22q12	EWSR1; EWS RNA-binding protein 1	Osteosarcoma
EWSR1-ATF1/EWS-ATF1	t(12;22)(q13;q12)	EWSR1-ATF1	Bone and Soft Tissue; Gastrointestinal Stromal Tumor; Malignant Peripheral Nerve Sheath Tumor
EWSR1-CREB1/EWS-CREB1	t(2;22)(q34;q12)	EWSR1-CREB1	Bone and Soft Tissue; Gastrointestinal Stromal Tumor; Malignant Peripheral Nerve Sheath Tumor
EWSR1-DDIT3/EWS-CHOP	t(12;22)(q13;q12)	EWSR1-DDIT3	Bone and Soft Tissue
EWSR1-E1AF	t(17;22)(q21;q12)	EWSR1-ETV4	Bone and Soft Tissue
EWSR1-ERG	t(21;22)(q22;q12)	EWSR1-ERG	Bone and Soft Tissue; Malignant Peripheral Nerve Sheath Tumor
EWSR1-ETV1	t(7;22)(p21.3;q12)	EWSR1-ETV1	Bone and Soft Tissue
EWSR1-FEV	t(2;22)(q36;q12)	EWSR1-FEV	Bone and Soft Tissue
EWSR1-FLI1	t(11;22)(q24;q12)	EWSR1-FLI1	Bone and Soft Tissue; Malignant Peripheral Nerve Sheath Tumor; Neuroblastoma; Rhabdomyosarcoma
EWSR1-NR4A3	t(9;22)(q22;q12)	EWSR1-NR4A3	Bone and Soft Tissue
EWSR1-PBX1	(1;22)(q23;q12)	EWSR1-PBX1	Bone and Soft Tissue
EWSR1-WT1	t(11;22)(p13;q12)	EWSR1-WT1	Bone and Soft Tissue
EWSR1-ZNF444	t(19;22)(q13;q12)	EWSR1-ZNF444	Bone and Soft Tissue
EWSR1-ZSG	t(22;22)(q12;q12)	EWSR1-PATZ1	Bone and Soft Tissue
EXT1	8q24.11	EXT1; exostosin 1	Bone and Soft Tissue; Hereditary Multiple Exostosis
EXT2	11p12-p11	EXT2; exostosin 2	Hereditary Multiple Exostosis
EXT3	19p	EXT3; exostoses (multiple) 3	Hereditary Multiple Exostosis;
FAH	15q25.1	FAH; fumarylacetoacetate hydrolase (fumarylacetoacetase)	Biliary Tract/Liver/Pancreas
FAM129A	1q25	FAM129A; family with sequence similarity 129, member A	Pineoblastoma
FANCA	16q24.3	FANCA; Fanconi anemia, complementation group A	Blood and Bone Marrow; Fanconi Anemia
FANCB	Xp22.2	FANCB; Fanconi anemia, complementation group B	Fanconi Anemia
FANCC	9q22.3	FANCC; Fanconi anemia, complementation group C	Fanconi Anemia
FANCD1	13q12.3	BRCA2; breast cancer 2, early onset	Fanconi Anemia
FANCD2	3p26	FANCD2; Fanconi anemia, complementation group D2	Fanconi Anemia
FANCE	6p22-p21	FANCE; Fanconi anemia, complementation group E	Fanconi Anemia
FANCF	11p15	FANCF; Fanconi anemia, complementation group F	Fanconi Anemia
FANCG	9p13	FANCG; Fanconi anemia, complementation group G	Fanconi Anemia
FANCI	15q26.1	FANCI; Fanconi anemia, complementation group I	Fanconi Anemia
FANCJ	17q22.2	BRIP1; BRCA1 interacting protein C-terminal helicase 1	Breast; Breast Carcinoma, Female; Fanconi Anemia
FANCL	2p16.1	FANCL; Fanconi anemia, complementation group L	Fanconi Anemia
FANCM	14q21.2	FANCM; Fanconi anemia, complementation group M	Fanconi Anemia

MOLECULAR FACTORS INDEX

FANCN	16p12.2	PALB2; partner and localizer of BRCA2	Breast; Fanconi Anemia
FANCx	multiple	Fanconi anemia, complementation groups	Head and Neck; Squamous Cell Carcinoma, Head and Neck
FAP	2q23	FAP; fibroblast activation protein, alpha	Esophagus
FBXW7	4q31.3	FBXW7; F-box and WD repeat domain containing 7, E3 ubiquitin protein ligase	Hereditary Renal Epithelial Tumors, Others; Kidney
FGFR2	10q26	FGFR2; fibroblast growth factor receptor 2	Pituitary
FGFR3	4p16.3	FGFR3; fibroblast growth factor receptor 3	Bladder Carcinoma; Plasma Cell Myeloma
FH	1q42.1	FH; fumarate hydratase	Gynecologic Neoplasms; Hereditary Leiomyomatosis and Renal Cell Carcinoma/ Reed Syndrome; Hereditary Renal Epithelial Tumors, Others; Kidney
FHIT	3p14.2	FHIT; fragile histidine triad	Hereditary Renal Epithelial Tumors, Others; Kidney; Squamous Cell Carcinoma, Head and Neck
FKHR	13q14.1	FOXO1; forkhead box O1	Bone and Soft Tissue
FLCN	17p11.2	FLCN; folliculin	Birt-Hogg-Dubé Syndrome; Hereditary Renal Epithelial Tumors, Others; Kidney; Renal Oncocytoma, Chromophobe, and Hybrid Oncocytic Tumors
FLT3	13q12	FLT3; fms-like tyrosine kinase 3	Myeloid Neoplasms
FNIP1	5q23.3	FNIP1; folliculin interacting protein 1	Birt-Hogg-Dubé Syndrome
FUS-ATF1	t(12;16)(q13;p11.2)	FUS-ATF1	Bone and Soft Tissue
FUS-CREB3L1	t(11;16)(p11.2;p11.2)	FUS-CREB3L1	Bone and Soft Tissue
FUS-CREB3L2	t(7;16)(q34;p11.2)	FUS-CREB3L2	Bone and Soft Tissue
FUS-DDIT3	t(12;16)(q13;p11.2)	FUS-DDIT3	Bone and Soft Tissue
FUS-ERG	t(16;21)(p11.2;q22.3)	FUS-ERG	Bone and Soft Tissue
FWT1	17q12-q21	WT4; Wilms tumor 4	Familial Wilms Tumor; Kidney; Wilms Tumor
G6PC	17q21	G6PC; glucose-6-phosphatase, catalytic subunit	Biliary Tract/Liver/Pancreas
GATA2	3q21.3	GATA2; GATA binding protein 2	Familial Acute Myeloid Leukemia
GATA3	10p15	GATA3; GATA binding protein 3	Familial Hodgkin Lymphoma
GJB6	13q12	GJB6; gap junction protein, beta 6, 30kDa	Howel-Evans Syndrome/Keratosis Palmares and Plantares With Esophageal Cancer
GLI2	2q14	GLI2; GLI family zinc finger 2	Medulloblastoma/CNS-PNET
GNA11	19p13.3	GNA11; guanine nucleotide binding protein (G protein), alpha 11 (Gq class)	Familial Uveal Melanoma
GNAQ	9q21	GNAQ; guanine nucleotide binding protein (G protein), q polypeptide	Familial Uveal Melanoma
GNAS/GNAS1	20q13.3	GNAS; GNAS complex locus	Adrenal Cortex; Adrenal Cortical Neoplasms in Children; Carney Complex Including LAMB Syndrome; Follicular Carcinoma; Neurofibromatosis Type 1; Pituitary; Pituitary Adenoma
GPC3	Xq26.1	GPC3; Glypican 3	Beckwith-Wiedemann Syndrome; Kidney; Wilms Tumor; Wilms Tumor-Associated Syndromes;
gr/gr	Yq11.2	genetic linkage region (no specific gene identified)	Familial Testicular Tumor
GSTM1	1p13.3	GSTM1; glutathione S-transferase mu 1	Hereditary Multiple Melanoma
GSTP1	11q13	GSTP1; glutathione S-transferase pi 1	Prostate Carcinoma
H19	11p15.5	H19; imprinted maternally expressed transcript (non-protein coding)	Adrenal Cortical Carcinoma; Adrenal Cortical Neoplasms in Children; Beckwith-Wiedemann Syndrome; Kidney; Wilms Tumor; Wilms Tumor-Associated Syndromes
HAX1	1q21.3	HAX1; HCLS1 associated protein X-1	Blood and Bone Marrow
HER2	17q12	ERBB2; v-erb-b2 avian erythroblastic leukemia viral oncogene homolog 2	Breast Carcinoma, Female
HFE	6p21.3	HFE; hemochromatosis	Biliary Tract/Liver/Pancreas
HLA-DRA	6p21.3	HLA-DRA; major histocompatibility complex, class II, DR alpha	Familial Hodgkin Lymphoma
HMGA2/HMGIC	12q15	HMGIC; high mobility group AT-hook 2	Bone and Soft Tissue; Salivary Glands

MOLECULAR FACTORS INDEX

HMGA2-LPP	t(3;12)(q28;q15)	HMGIC-LPP	Bone and Soft Tissue
HPD	12q24.31	HPD; 4-hydroxyphenylpyruvate dioxygenase	Biliary Tract/Liver/Pancreas
HRAS	11p15.5	HRAS; v-Ha-ras Harvey rat sarcoma viral oncogene homolog	Bladder Carcinoma; Costello Syndrome; Familial Nonmedullary Thyroid Carcinoma; Pituitary Carcinoma
HRPT2	1q25	CDC73; cell division cycle 73	Head and Neck; Hereditary Hyperparathyroidism-Jaw Tumor Syndrome; Hereditary Renal Epithelial Tumors, Others; Kidney; Parathyroid; Parathyroid Adenoma; Parathyroid Carcinoma; Parathyroid Hyperplasia
HSPBAP1	3q21.1	HSPBAP1; HSPB (heat shock 27kDa) associated protein 1	Hereditary Renal Epithelial Tumors, Others; Kidney;
ID2	2p25	ID2; inhibitor of DNA binding 2, dominant negative helix-loop-helix protein	Hodgkin Lymphoma
IDH1	2q33.3	IDH1; isocitrate dehydrogenase 1 (NADP+), soluble	Astrocytoma; Chondrosarcoma; Medulloblastoma/CNS-PNET; Osteosarcoma
IDH2	15q26.1	IDH2; isocitrate dehydrogenase 2 (NADP+), mitochondrial	Chondrosarcoma; Osteosarcoma
IGF2	11p15.5	IGF2; insulin-like growth factor 2	Adrenal Cortical Carcinoma; Adrenal Cortical Neoplasms in Children; Beckwith-Wiedemann Syndrome; Kidney; Rhabdomyosarcoma; Wilms Tumor; Wilms Tumor-Associated Syndromes
IGH	14q32.33	IGH; immunoglobulin heavy locus	Chronic Lymphocytic Leukemia; Plasma Cell Myeloma; Lymphoplasmacytic Lymphoma/Waldenström Macroglobulinemia
IGH-BCL2	t(14;18)(q32;q21)	IGH-BCL2	Follicular Lymphoma
IGH-BCL6	t(3;14)(q27;q32)	IGH-BCL6	Hodgkin Lymphoma
IGH-MALT1	t(14;18)(q32;q21)	IGH-MALT1	Lymphoplasmacytic Lymphoma/ Waldenström Macroglobulinemia
IL10	1q31-q32	IL10; interleukin 10	Familial Non-Hodgkin Lymphoma
INK4A	9p21	CDKN2A; cyclin-dependent kinase inhibitor 2A	Bone and Soft Tissue; Malignant Peripheral Nerve Sheath Tumor
JAG1	20p12.1-p11.23	JAG1; jagged 1	Biliary Tract/Liver/Pancreas
JAK2	9p24	JAK2; Janus kinase 2	Myeloid Neoplasms
JAZF1-JJAZ1	t(7;17)(p15;q11)	JAZF1-JJAZ1	Bone and Soft Tissue
JAZF1-PHF1	t(6;7)(p21;p15)	JAZF1-PHF1	Bone and Soft Tissue
JUN	1p32-p31	JUN; jun proto-oncogene	Bone and Soft Tissue
KCNIP4	4p15.32	KCNIP4; Kv channel interacting protein 4	Hereditary Renal Epithelial Tumors, Others; Kidney;
KCNQ1	11p15.5	KCNQ1; potassium voltage-gated channel, KQT-like subfamily, member 1	Adrenal Cortical Neoplasms in Children; Beckwith-Wiedemann Syndrome
KCNQ1OT1/LIT1	11p15	KCNQ1OT1; KCNQ1 opposite strand/antisense transcript 1 (non-protein coding)	Adrenal Cortical Neoplasms in Children; Beckwith-Wiedemann Syndrome; Kidney; Wilms Tumor; Wilms Tumor-Associated Syndromes;
KIF1B	1p36.2	kinesin family member 1B	Adrenal Medulla; Hereditary Paraganglioma/Pheochromocytoma Syndromes; Paraganglioma; Pheochromocytoma/Paraganglioma
KIT	4q11-q12	KIF1B; v-kit Hardy-Zuckerman 4 feline sarcoma viral oncogene homolog	Bone and Soft Tissue; Esophagus; Familial Gastrointestinal Stromal Tumor; Familial Testicular Tumor; Gastrointestinal Stromal Tumor; Myeloid Neoplasms; Neurofibromatosis Type 1; Prostate Carcinoma
KITLG	12q22	KITLG; KIT ligand	Familial Testicular Tumor; Testicle
KLF4	9q31	KLF4; Kruppel-like factor 4 (gut)	Meningioma
KLF6	10p15	KLF6; Kruppel-like factor 6	Prostate Carcinoma
KLHDC8B	3p21.31	KLHDC8B; kelch domain containing 8B	Familial Hodgkin Lymphoma
KLLN	10q23	KLLN; killin, p53-regulated DNA replication inhibitor	PTEN-Hamartoma Tumor Syndromes
KRAS	12p12.1	KRAS; v-Ki-ras2 Kirsten rat sarcoma viral oncogene homolog	Astrocytoma; Central Nervous System; Colon Adenoma; Costello Syndrome; Familial Nonmedullary Thyroid Carcinoma;

MOLECULAR FACTORS INDEX

			Myeloid Neoplasms; MYH-associated Polyposis; Neurofibromatosis Type 1; Pancreatic Endocrine Tumor; Plasma Cell Myeloma
KRT16	17q21.2	KRT16; keratin 16	Howel-Evans Syndrome/Keratosis Palmares and Plantares With Esophageal Cancer
KRT17	17q21.2	KRT17; keratin 17	Howel-Evans Syndrome/Keratosis Palmares and Plantares With Esophageal Cancer
KRT6	12q13.13	KRT72; keratin 72	Howel-Evans Syndrome/Keratosis Palmares and Plantares With Esophageal Cancer
LIN28	1p36.11	LIN28; lin-28 homolog A	Medulloblastoma/CNS-PNET
LMNA	1q22	LMNA; lamin A/C	Werner Syndrome/Progeria
LSAMP	3q13.2-q21	LSAMP; limbic system-associated membrane protein	Hereditary Renal Epithelial Tumors, Others; Kidney;
MAF	16q22-q23	MAF; v-maf musculoaponeurotic fibrosarcoma oncogene homolog	Plasma Cell Myeloma
MAFB	20q11.2-q13.1	MAFB; v-maf avian musculoaponeurotic fibrosarcoma oncogene homolog B	Plasma Cell Myeloma
MAX	14q23	MAX; MYC associated factor X	Adrenal Medulla; Hereditary Paraganglioma/Pheochromocytoma Syndromes; Paraganglioma; Pathology of Familial Tumor Syndromes; Pheochromocytoma/Paraganglioma
MC1R	16q24.3	MC1R; melanocortin 1 receptor (alpha melanocyte stimulating hormone receptor)	Cutaneous Melanoma; Hereditary Multiple Melanoma
MCUL1	1q42.1	FH; fumarate hydratase	Bone and Soft Tissue
MDM2	12q15	MDM2; MDM2 oncogene, p53 E3 ubiquitin protein ligase homolog	Bone and Soft Tissue; Hereditary Retinoblastoma
MDM4	1q32	MDM4; Mdm4 p53 binding protein homolog	Hereditary Retinoblastoma
MDR1	7q21.12	ABCB1; ATP-binding cassette, sub-family B (MDR/TAP), member 1	Adrenal Cortical Carcinoma
MDR3	7q21.1	ABCB4; ATP-binding cassette, sub-family B (MDR/TAP), member 4	Biliary Tract/Liver/Pancreas
MECT1	19p13	MECT1; mucoepidermoid carcinoma translocated 1	Salivary Glands
MECT1-MAML2	t(11;19)(q21-22;p13)		Salivary Glands
MEK1	15q22.1-q22.33	MAP2K1; mitogen-activated protein kinase kinase 1	Costello Syndrome; Familial Nonmedullary Thyroid Carcinoma
MEK2	19p13.3	MEK2; mitogen-activated protein kinase kinase 2	Costello Syndrome; Familial Nonmedullary Thyroid Carcinoma;
MEN1	11q13	MEN1; multiple endocrine neoplasia I	Adrenal Cortex; Adrenal Cortical Carcinoma; Adrenal Cortical Neoplasms in Children; Biliary Tract/Liver/Pancreas; Familial Isolated Hyperparathyroidism; Hereditary Pancreatic Cancer Syndrome; Hereditary Paraganglioma/Pheochromocytoma Syndromes; Hereditary Renal Epithelial Tumors, Others; Multiple Endocrine Neoplasia Type 1; Pancreas; Pancreatic Endocrine Tumor; Parathyroid; Parathyroid Adenoma; Parathyroid Carcinoma; Parathyroid Hyperplasia; Pituitary; Pituitary Adenoma
MET	7q31	MET; met proto-oncogene (hepatocyte growth factor receptor)	Familial Nonmedullary Thyroid Carcinoma; Hereditary Papillary Renal Cell Carcinoma; Hereditary Renal Epithelial Tumors, Others; Kidney; Papillary Renal Cell Carcinoma
MICB	6p21.3	MICB; MHC class I polypeptide-related sequence B	Familial Hodgkin Lymphoma
MLH1	3p21.3	MLH1; mutL homolog 1	Adrenal Cortex; Adrenal Cortical Neoplasms in Children; Astrocytoma; Biliary Tract/Liver/Pancreas; Central Nervous System; Colon/Rectum; Endometrial Carcinoma; Esophagus; Eye; Gynecologic Neoplasms; Hereditary Pancreatic Cancer Syndrome; Lynch Syndrome ; Ovarian Carcinoma; Renal Urothelial Carcinoma; Sebaceous Carcinoma
MMSET	4p16.3	WHSC1; Wolf-Hirschhorn syndrome candidate 1	Plasma Cell Myeloma

MPL	1p34	MPL; myeloproliferative leukemia virus oncogene	Blood and Bone Marrow
MRE11A	11q21	MRE11A; MRE11 meiotic recombination 11 homolog A	Ataxia-Telangiectasia; Breast; Breast Carcinoma, Female; Gynecologic Neoplasms
MSH2	2p21	MSH2; mutS homolog 2	Adrenal Cortex; Adrenal Cortical Neoplasms in Children; Astrocytoma; Biliary Tract/Liver/Pancreas; Central Nervous System; Colon/Rectum; Endometrial Carcinoma; Esophagus; Eye; Gynecologic Neoplasms; Hereditary Pancreatic Cancer Syndrome; Lynch Syndrome ; Ovarian Carcinoma; Renal Urothelial Carcinoma; Sebaceous Carcinoma; Ureter Urothelial Carcinoma
MSH6	2p16	MSH6; mutS homolog 6	Adrenal Cortex; Adrenal Cortical Neoplasms in Children; Astrocytoma; Biliary Tract/Liver/Pancreas; Central Nervous System; Colon/Rectum; Endometrial Carcinoma; Esophagus; Gynecologic Neoplasms; Hereditary Pancreatic Cancer Syndrome; Lynch Syndrome ; Ovarian Carcinoma; Renal Urothelial Carcinoma; Sebaceous Carcinoma
MSR1	8p22	MSR1; macrophage scavenger receptor 1	Prostate Carcinoma
MUTYH/MYH	1p34.1	MUTYH; mutY homolog	Breast; Breast Carcinoma, Female; Biliary Tract/Liver/Pancreas; Colon/Rectum; Esophagus; Familial Adenomatous Polyposis; Hereditary Pancreatic Cancer Syndrome; MYH-associated Polyposis; Pathology of Familial Tumor Syndromes
MYB-NFIB	t(6;9)(q22-23;p24)	MYB-NFIB	Salivary Glands
MYC	8q24	MYC; v-myc myelocytomatosis viral oncogene homolog	Adrenal Cortical Carcinoma; Diffuse Large B-Cell Lymphoma; Follicular Lymphoma; Hereditary Hyperparathyroidism-Jaw Tumor Syndrome; Hodgkin Lymphoma; Medulloblastoma/CNS-PNET; Prostate Carcinoma
MYCN	2p24.3	MYCN; v-myc myelocytomatosis viral related oncogene, neuroblastoma derived	Hereditary Neuroblastoma; Neuroblastoma; Wilms Tumor
MYD88	3p22	MYD88; myeloid differentiation primary response 88	Lymphoplasmacytic Lymphoma/ Waldenström Macroglobulinemia
NBN/NBS1	8q21	NBN; nibrin	Breast; Breast Carcinoma, Female; Gynecologic Neoplasms; Ataxia-Telangiectasia; Prostate Carcinoma
NDP	Xp11.4	NDP; Norrie disease (pseudoglioma)	Eye
NF1	17q11.2	NF1; neurofibromin 1	Adrenal Cortex; Adrenal Cortical Neoplasms in Children; Adrenal Medulla; Astrocytoma; Bone and Soft Tissue; Central Nervous System; Clinical Diagnosis and Management of Familial; Esophagus; Eye; Familial Gastrointestinal Stromal Tumor; Gastrointestinal Stromal Tumor; Hereditary Paraganglioma/ Pheochromocytoma Syndromes; Malignant Peripheral Nerve Sheath Tumor; Myeloid Neoplasms; Neurofibromatosis Type 1; Pancreas; Pancreatic Endocrine Tumor; Paraganglioma; Peripheral Nervous System; Pheochromocytoma/Paraganglioma; Schwannoma
NF2	22q12.2	NF2; neurofibromin 2	Astrocytoma; Bone and Soft Tissue; Central Nervous System; Clinical Diagnosis and Management of Familial; Ependymoma; Eye; Head and Neck; Meningioma; Neurofibromatosis Type 1; Neurofibromatosis Type 2; Peripheral Nervous System; Schwannoma; Schwannomatosis
NHP2	5q35.3	NHP2; NHP2 ribonucleoprotein	Dyskeratosis Congenita
NKX3-1	8p21.2	NKX3-1; NK3 homeobox 1	Prostate Carcinoma
NMTC1	2q21	NMTC1; Nonmedullary thyroid carcinoma 1	Familial Nonmedullary Thyroid Carcinoma

MOLECULAR FACTORS INDEX

PIK3CA	3q26.3	PIK3CA; phosphatidylinositol-4,5-bisphosphate 3-kinase, catalytic subunit alpha	Follicular Carcinoma; Pituitary; PTEN-Hamartoma Tumor Syndromes
PIM1	6p21.2	PIM1; pim-1 oncogene	Hodgkin Lymphoma
PKC	16p11.2	PKC; proline-rich transmembrane protein 2	Pituitary
PLAG1	8q12	PLAG1; pleiomorphic adenoma gene 1	Bone and Soft Tissue; Salivary Glands
PLAG1-HAS2	t(8;8)(q12;q24)	PLAG1-HAS2	Bone and Soft Tissue
PML-RARA	t(15;17)(q22;q21)	PML-RARA	Myeloid Neoplasms
PMS1	2q31.1	PMS1; PMS1 postmeiotic segregation increased 1	Astrocytoma
PMS2	7p22.2	PMS2; PMS2 postmeiotic segregation increased 2	Adrenal Cortex; Adrenal Cortical Neoplasms in Children; Astrocytoma; Biliary Tract/Liver/Pancreas; Breast Carcinoma, Female; Central Nervous System; Colon/Rectum; Endometrial Carcinoma; Esophagus; Gynecologic Neoplasms; Hereditary Pancreatic Cancer Syndrome; Lynch Syndrome ; Ovarian Carcinoma; Renal Urothelial Carcinoma
POLH	6p21.1	POLH; polymerase (DNA directed), eta	Eye; Hereditary Multiple Melanoma; Xeroderma Pigmentosum
POU5F1P1	8q24.21	POU5F1B; POU class 5 homeobox 1B	Hereditary Prostate Cancer
PRAD1	11q13	CCND1; cyclin-D1	Parathyroid Hyperplasia
PRKAR1A	17q23-q24	PRKAR1A; protein kinase, cAMP-dependent, regulatory, type I, alpha	Adrenal Cortex; Adrenal Cortical Carcinoma; Adrenal Cortical Neoplasms in Children; Carney Complex Including LAMB Syndrome; Clinical Diagnosis and Management of Familial; Familial Nonmedullary Thyroid Carcinoma; Familial Testicular Tumor; Familial Thyroid Carcinoma; Follicular Carcinoma; Peripheral Nervous System; Pituitary; Pituitary Adenoma; Primary Pigmented Nodular Adrenocortical Disease; Testicle; Testicular Sertoli Cell Neoplasms; Thyroid, Nonmedullary
PRSS1	7q34	PRSS1; protease, serine, 1 (trypsin 1)	Biliary Tract/Liver/Pancreas; Hereditary Pancreatic Cancer Syndrome
PRSS2	7q34	PRSS2; protease, serine, 2 (trypsin 2)	Biliary Tract/Liver/Pancreas; Hereditary Pancreatic Cancer Syndrome
PTAG	22q12.2	RHBDD3; rhomboid domain containing 3	Pituitary
PTCH1	9q22.3	PTCH1; patched 1	Basal Cell Carcinoma; Basal Cell Nevus Syndrome/Gorlin Syndrome; Central Nervous System; Eye; Head and Neck; Medulloblastoma/CNS-PNET
PTCH2	1p34.1	PTCH2; patched 2	Central Nervous System; Eye; Medulloblastoma/CNS-PNET
PTEN	10q23.31	PTEN; phosphotase and tensin homolog	Birt-Hogg-Dubé Syndrome; Breast; Breast Carcinoma, Female; Breast Carcinoma, Male; Carney Complex Including LAMB Syndrome; Central Nervous System; Colon/Rectum; Endometrial Carcinoma; Familial Nonmedullary Thyroid Carcinoma; Familial Thyroid Carcinoma; Follicular Carcinoma; Gynecologic Neoplasms; Hereditary Multiple Melanoma; Juvenile Polyposis; Neurofibromatosis Type 1; Pathology of Familial Tumor Syndromes; Prostate Carcinoma; PTEN-Hamartoma Tumor Syndromes; Skin; Thyroid, Nonmedullary
PTPN11	12q24	PTPN11; protein tyrosine phosphatase, non-receptor type 11	Astrocytoma; Central Nervous System; Costello Syndrome; Myeloid Neoplasms; Neurofibromatosis Type 1
PTTG	5q35.1	PTTG1; pituitary tumor-transforming 1	Pituitary
PU.1	11p11.2	SPI1; spleen focus forming virus (SFFV) proviral integration oncogene	Hodgkin Lymphoma
PVT1	8q24	PVT1; Pvt1 oncogene (non-protein coding)	Familial Hodgkin Lymphoma
PYGL	14q21-q22	PYGL; phosphorylase, glycogen, liver	Biliary Tract/Liver/Pancreas
RAD50	5q31	RAD50; RAD50 homolog	Breast; Breast Carcinoma, Female; Gynecologic Neoplasms

MOLECULAR FACTORS INDEX

RAD51B	14q23-q24.2	RAD51B; RAD51 paralog B	Breast Carcinoma, Female
RAD51C	17q22	RAD51C; RAD51 paralog C	Breast; Breast Carcinoma, Female; Gynecologic Neoplasms; Li-Fraumeni Syndrome/Li-Fraumeni-Like Syndrome; Ovarian Carcinoma
RAD51D	17q11	RAD51D; RAD51 paralog D	Breast Carcinoma, Female; Gynecologic Neoplasms; Ovarian Carcinoma
RAF1	3p25	RAF1; v-raf-1 murine leukemia viral oncogene homolog 1	Astrocytoma; Central Nervous System; Costello Syndrome; Neurofibromatosis Type 1
RAS	multiple	RAS; Rat sarcoma oncogene	Follicular Carcinoma; Myeloid Neoplasms; Pheochromocytoma/Paraganglioma; Pituitary
RB1/RB	13q14.2	RB1; retinoblastoma 1	Adrenal Cortical Carcinoma; Bladder Carcinoma; Bone and Soft Tissue; Bone and Soft Tissue; Central Nervous System; Eye; Head and Neck; Hereditary Multiple Melanoma; Hereditary Retinoblastoma; Neuroendocrine Carcinoma, Lung; Osteosarcoma; Parathyroid Carcinoma; Pineoblastoma; Pituitary; Plasma Cell Myeloma; Prostate Carcinoma; Retinoblastoma; Salivary Glands
RECQL4	8q24.3	RECQL4; RecQ protein-like 4	Bloom Syndrome; Werner Syndrome/ Progeria; Xeroderma Pigmentosum
REL	2p13-p12	REL; v-rel reticuloendotheliosis viral oncogene homolog; c-REL	Familial Hodgkin Lymphoma
RET	2p13-p12	RET; v-rel reticuloendotheliosis viral oncogene homolog; c-REL	Adrenal Medulla; Adrenal Medullary Hyperplasia; C-Cell Hyperplasia; Familial Isolated Hyperparathyroidism; Familial Nonmedullary Thyroid Carcinoma; Familial Thyroid Carcinoma; Hereditary Paraganglioma/Pheochromocytoma Syndromes; Medullary Thyroid Carcinoma; Multiple Endocrine Neoplasia Type 2/ Familial Medullary Thyroid Carcinoma; Neurofibromatosis Type 1; Paraganglioma; Parathyroid; Parathyroid Adenoma; Parathyroid Carcinoma; Parathyroid Hyperplasia; Pheochromocytoma/ Paraganglioma; Thyroid, Medullary
RHBDF2	17q25.1	RHBDF2; rhomboid 5 homolog 2	Esophageal Squamous Cell Carcinoma; Esophagus; Howel-Evans Syndrome/ Keratosis Palmares and Plantares With Esophageal Cancer
RHOH	4p13	RHOH; ras homolog family member H	Hodgkin Lymphoma
RMRP	9p21-p12	RMRP; RNA component of mitochondrial RNA processing endoribonuclease	Basal Cell Carcinoma
RNASEL	1q25	RNASEL; ribonuclease L (2',5'-oligoisoadenylate synthetase-dependent)	Hereditary Prostate Cancer; Prostate Carcinoma
RPS19	19q13.2	RPS19; ribosomal protein S19	Blood and Bone Marrow; Myeloid Neoplasms
RTEL1	20q13.3	RTEL1; regulator of telomere elongation helicase 1	Dyskeratosis Congenita
RUNX1	21q22.3	RUNX1; runt-related transcription factor 1	Familial Acute Myeloid Leukemia; Myeloid Neoplasms
RUNX1-RUNX1T1	t(8;21)(22;22.3)		Myeloid Neoplasms
SBDS	7q11.21	SBDS; Shwachman-Bodian-Diamond syndrome	Blood and Bone Marrow
SDH/SDHx	multiple	succinate dehydrogenase complex	Adrenal Medullary Hyperplasia; Familial Gastrointestinal Stromal Tumor; Paraganglioma; Pathology of Familial Tumor Syndromes; PTEN-Hamartoma Tumor Syndromes
SDHA	5p15	SDHA; succinate dehydrogenase complex, subunit A, flavoprotein	Adrenal Medulla; Hereditary Paraganglioma/Pheochromocytoma Syndromes; Paraganglioma; Pathology of Familial Tumor Syndromes; Pheochromocytoma/Paraganglioma
SDHAF2	11q12.2	SDHAF2; succinate dehydrogenase complex assembly factor 2	Adrenal Medulla; Hereditary Paraganglioma/Pheochromocytoma

			Syndromes; Paraganglioma; Pheochromocytoma/Paraganglioma
SDHB	1p36	SDHB; succinate dehydrogenase complex, subunit B, iron sulfur	Adrenal Medulla; Adrenal Medullary Hyperplasia; Esophagus; Hereditary Paraganglioma/Pheochromocytoma Syndromes; Hereditary Renal Epithelial Tumors, Others; Kidney; Paraganglioma; Pheochromocytoma/Paraganglioma
SDHC	1q21-23	SDHC; succinate dehydrogenase complex, subunit C, integral membrane protein	Adrenal Medulla; Esophagus; Hereditary Paraganglioma/Pheochromocytoma Syndromes; Paraganglioma; Pheochromocytoma/Paraganglioma
SDHD	11q23	SDHD; succinate dehydrogenase complex, subunit D, integral membrane protein	Adrenal Medulla; Esophagus; Hereditary Paraganglioma/Pheochromocytoma Syndromes; Paraganglioma; Pheochromocytoma/Paraganglioma
SEC31A-ALK	t(2;4)(p23;q21.22)		Diffuse Large B-Cell Lymphoma
SERPINA1	14q32.1	SERPINA1; serpin peptidase inhibitor, clade A (alpha-1 antiproteinase, antitrypsin), member 1;	Biliary Tract/Liver/Pancreas
SF3B1	2q33.1	SF3B1; splicing factor 3b, subunit 1, 155kDa	Chronic Lymphocytic Leukemia
SHH	7q36	SHH; sonic hedgehog	Medulloblastoma/CNS-PNET
SHOC2	10q25	SHOC2; soc-2 suppressor of clear homolog	Costello Syndrome
SLC25A13	7q21.3	SLC25A13; solute carrier family 25 (aspartate/glutamate carrier), member 13	Biliary Tract/Liver/Pancreas
SLC26A4	7q31	SLC26A4; solute carrier family 26, member 4	Familial Nonmedullary Thyroid Carcinoma; Familial Thyroid Carcinoma; Thyroid, Nonmedullary
SMAD4	18q21.1	SMAD4; SMAD family member 4	Biliary Tract/Liver/Pancreas; Colon/Rectum; Esophagus; Juvenile Polyposis; Pancreatic Endocrine Tumor; Small Bowel Adenocarcinoma
SMARCA4/BRG1	19p13.2	SMARCA4; SWI/SNF related, matrix associated, actin dependent regulator of chromatin, subfamily a, member 4	Rhabdoid Predisposition Syndrome
SMARCB1/INI1/BAF47/hSNF5	22q11	SMARCB1; SWI/SNF related, matrix associated, actin dependent regulator of chromatin, subfamily b, member 1	Bone and Soft Tissue; Central Nervous System; Meningioma; Peripheral Nervous System; Rhabdoid Predisposition Syndrome; Schwannomatosis
SMARCE1	17q21.2	SMARCE1; SWI/SNF related, matrix associated, actin dependent regulator of chromatin, subfamily e, member 1	Central Nervous System; Meningioma
SMO	7q32.3	SMO; smoothened, frizzled family receptor	Medulloblastoma/CNS-PNET; Meningioma
SOS1	2p21	SOS1; son of sevenless homolog 1	Astrocytoma; Central Nervous System; Costello Syndrome; Neurofibromatosis Type 1
SOX9	17q23	SOX9; SRY (sex determining region Y)-box 9	Basal Cell Carcinoma
SPINK1	5q32	SPINK1; serine peptidase inhibitor, Kazal type 1	Biliary Tract/Liver/Pancreas; Hereditary Pancreatic Cancer Syndrome
SPOP	17q21.33	SPOP; speckle-type POZ protein	Prostate Carcinoma
SPRED1	15q14	SPRED1; sprouty-related, EVH1 domain containing 1	Neurofibromatosis Type 1
SPRY4	5q31.3	SPRY4; sprouty homolog 4	Familial Testicular Tumor; Testicle
SRP72	4q11	SRP72; signal recognition particle 72kDa	Familial Acute Myeloid Leukemia
SS18/SYT	18q11.2	SS18; synovial sarcoma translocation, chromosome 18	Bone and Soft Tissue; Malignant Peripheral Nerve Sheath Tumor
SS18L1-SSX1	t(X;20)(p11.23;q13.3)	SS18L1-SSX1	Bone and Soft Tissue
SSX	multiple	synovial sarcoma, X	Malignant Peripheral Nerve Sheath Tumor
SSX1	Xp11.23	SSX1; synovial sarcoma, X breakpoint 1	Bone and Soft Tissue
SSX2	Xp11.22	SSX2; synovial sarcoma, X breakpoint 2	Bone and Soft Tissue
SSX4	Xp11.23	SSX4; synovial sarcoma, X breakpoint 4	Bone and Soft Tissue
STAT5B/STAT5	17q11.2	STAT5B; signal transducer and activator of transcription 5B	Prostate Carcinoma
STK11/LKB1	19p13.3	STK11; serine/threonine kinase 11	Biliary Tract/Liver/Pancreas; Breast; Breast Carcinoma, Female; Cervical Carcinoma; Colon/Rectum; Endometrial Carcinoma; Esophagus; Familial Testicular Tumor; Gynecologic Neoplasms; Hereditary

MOLECULAR FACTORS INDEX

			Pancreas; Pancreatic Endocrine Tumor; Tuberous Sclerosis Complex
TSC2/PKD1	16p13.3	TSC2; tuberous sclerosis 2	Angiomyolipoma; Astrocytoma; Biliary Tract/Liver/Pancreas; Birt-Hogg-Dubé Syndrome; Central Nervous System; Eye; Familial Chordoma; Hereditary Pancreatic Cancer Syndrome; Hereditary Renal Epithelial Tumors, Others; Kidney; Pancreas; Pancreatic Endocrine Tumor; Tuberous Sclerosis Complex
TSHR	14q31	TSHR; thyroid stimulating hormone receptor	Familial Nonmedullary Thyroid Carcinoma
TYR	11q14.3	TYR; tyrosinase	Hereditary Multiple Melanoma
TYRP1	9p23	TYRP1; tyrosinase-related protein 1	Hereditary Multiple Melanoma
ULK4	3p22.1	ULK4; unc-51 like kinase 4	Familial Plasma Cell Myeloma
USB1/C16orf57	16q21	USB1; U6 snRNA biogenesis 1	Dyskeratosis Congenita
USP6	17p13	USP6; ubiquitin specific peptidase 6 (Tre-2 oncogene)	Bone and Soft Tissue
VDR	12q13.11	VDR; vitamin D (1,25- dihydroxyvitamin D3) receptor	Hereditary Multiple Melanoma
VHL	3p25.3	VHL; von Hippel-Lindau tumor suppressor	Adrenal Medulla; Biliary Tract/Liver/Pancreas; Central Nervous System; Clear Cell Renal Cell Carcinoma; Clinical Diagnosis and Management of Familial; Endolymphatic Sac Tumor; Eye; Gynecologic Neoplasms; Hereditary Leiomyomatosis and Renal Cell Carcinoma/Reed Syndrome; Hereditary Pancreatic Cancer Syndrome; Hereditary Paraganglioma/Pheochromocytoma Syndromes; Hereditary Renal Epithelial Tumors, Others; Kidney; Pancreas; Pancreatic Endocrine Tumor; Paraganglioma; Pheochromocytoma/Paraganglioma; Salivary Glands; von Hippel-Lindau Syndrome
WAS	Xp11.4-p11.21	WAS; Wiskott-Aldrich syndrome	Blood and Bone Marrow
WNT	multiple	wingless-type family	Medulloblastoma/CNS-PNET
WRN/RECQL2	8p12	WRN; Werner syndrome, RecQ helicase-like	Bloom Syndrome; Eye; Familial Nonmedullary Thyroid Carcinoma; Familial Thyroid Carcinoma; Follicular Carcinoma; Hereditary Multiple Melanoma; Thyroid, Nonmedullary; Werner Syndrome/Progeria
WT1	11p13	WT1; Wilms tumor 1	Beckwith-Wiedemann Syndrome; Denys-Drash Syndrome; Familial Wilms Tumor; Kidney; Wilms Tumor; Wilms Tumor-Associated Syndromes
WT1-EWSR1	t(11;22)(p13;q12)	WT1-EWSR1	Rhabdomyosarcoma
WT2	19q13.4	genetic linkage region (no specific gene identified)	Familial Wilms Tumor; Kidney; Wilms Tumor
WTX/FAM123B	Xq11.2	AMER1; APC membrane recruitment protein 1	Wilms Tumor
XPA	9q22.3	XPA; xeroderma pigmentosum, complementation group A	Hereditary Multiple Melanoma; Xeroderma Pigmentosum
XPA-XPG	multiple	xeroderma pigmentosum, complementation group A through G	Eye; Head and Neck; Squamous Cell Carcinoma, Head and Neck
XPB	2q21	ERCC3; excision repair cross-complementing rodent repair deficiency, complementation group 3	Hereditary Multiple Melanoma; Xeroderma Pigmentosum
XPC	3p25	XPC; xeroderma pigmentosum, complementation group C	Hereditary Multiple Melanoma; Xeroderma Pigmentosum
XPD	19q13.3	ERCC2; excision repair cross-complementing rodent repair deficiency, complementation group 2	Hereditary Multiple Melanoma; Xeroderma Pigmentosum
XPE	11q12-q13	DDB1; damage-specific DNA binding protein 1	Hereditary Multiple Melanoma; Xeroderma Pigmentosum
XPF	16p13.12	ERCC4; excision repair cross-complementing rodent repair deficiency, complementation group 4	Hereditary Multiple Melanoma; Xeroderma Pigmentosum
XPG	13q33	ERCC5; excision repair cross-complementing rodent repair deficiency, complementation group 5	Hereditary Multiple Melanoma; Xeroderma Pigmentosum

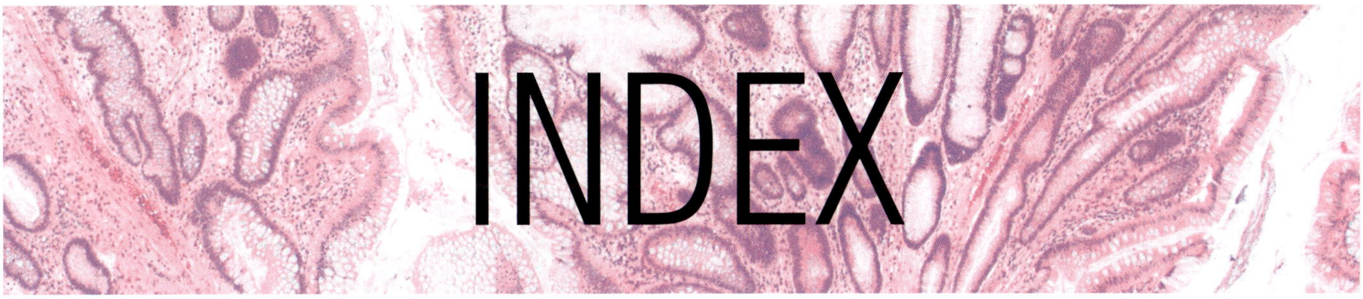

INDEX

A

INDEX

INDEX

INDEX

B

INDEX

INDEX

INDEX

C

INDEX

INDEX

INDEX

INDEX

INDEX

INDEX

INDEX

E

INDEX

F

INDEX

INDEX

INDEX

INDEX

INDEX

INDEX

INDEX

INDEX

INDEX

INDEX

INDEX

J

K

INDEX

INDEX

INDEX

INDEX

INDEX

INDEX

N

INDEX

INDEX

O

INDEX

P

INDEX

INDEX

INDEX

INDEX

INDEX

INDEX

INDEX

INDEX

S

INDEX

INDEX

T

U

INDEX

V

W